MRI of Short- and Ultrashort-T$_2$ Tissues

Jiang Du • Graeme M. Bydder

Editors

MRI of Short- and Ultrashort-T$_2$ Tissues

Making the Invisible Visible

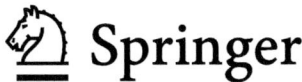 Springer

Editors
Jiang Du
Radiology
University of California, San Diego
La Jolla, CA, USA

Graeme M. Bydder
Radiology
University of California, San Diego
La Jolla, CA, USA

Mātai Medical Research Institute
Tairāwhiti Gisborne, New Zealand

ISBN 978-3-031-35196-9   ISBN 978-3-031-35197-6   (eBook)
https://doi.org/10.1007/978-3-031-35197-6

This Springer imprint is published by the registered company Springer Nature Switzerland AG
The registered company address is: Gewerbestrasse 11, 6330 Cham, Switzerland

Printed on acid-free paper

Foreword

MRI is a highly regarded imaging method for clinical diagnosis. It provides exceptional soft tissue contrast, is non invasive, and has a wide range of applications. It is particularly useful for the musculoskeletal system, especially for monitoring cartilage, tendons, ligaments, and other collagen-rich tissues. However, the use of MRI extends far beyond this and covers a wide range of fields.

The accurate morphological and quantitative imaging of short- and ultrashort-T_2 tissues requires the use of correspondingly short echo times. The development of short and ultrashort echo time (UTE) sequences has opened up the possibility of imaging a wide range of tissues, including tendons, calcified cartilage, cortical bone, lung, myelin, and others. There are now many intriguing UTE and zero echo time (ZTE) sequences with various acquisition schemes, including hybrid variants such as pointwise encoding time reduction with radial acquisition (PETRA), serving different purposes and each having its own advantages and disadvantages.

Over the years, advancements in technology such as higher field strengths, improved coil designs, and stronger gradients have led to significant increases in signal-to-noise ratio, higher spatial resolution, and shorter echo times. These improvements, in conjunction with the development of new and more refined MR sequences, have made morphological and quantitative imaging available in a wide range of tissues where this was not previously possible.

The book is organized into four sections, each focusing on a different aspect of short- and ultrashort-T_2 tissue imaging. The first section covers data acquisition, including the different sequences available for detecting signal from these types of tissues.

The second section delves into contrast mechanisms, highlighting some slightly less commonly used but equally exciting techniques such as spectroscopic and phase imaging.

The third section focuses on various quantification techniques such as T_1 and T_2* quantification, as well as perfusion and diffusion, and on novel applications of deep learning for automatic segmentation and quantitative imaging.

The last section provides a comprehensive overview of the wide range of applications of short and UTE sequences and highlights the many different types of tissues that the sequences can be used to study.

This book is a comprehensive work for anyone who wants to gain a deeper understanding of short- and ultrashort-T_2 tissues and their measurement. It is aimed both at newcomers to the field, such as Ph.D. students, as well as established scientists and clinicians who will find a wealth of excellent information within its pages.

The contributors to this book are an impressive group of experts in the field, and I am honored to have played a role in the creation of this book by contributing a chapter on the Cartesian variable echo time sequence, along with my research group and Xeni Deligianni from the University Hospital Basel. It is a privilege to be a part of such an impressive book!

Finally, I would like to express my sincere gratitude to Jiang Du, Ph.D., Professor of Radiology at the University of California, San Diego, and Graeme M. Bydder, MB ChB, Emeritus Professor of Radiology at the University of California, San Diego, for their dedication and efforts in making this book possible.

Department of Biomedical Imaging and Image-guided Therapy   Siegfried Trattnig
Medical University of Vienna
Wien, Austria

Preface

When clinical MRI began in the early 1980s, lung, cortical bone, and other musculoskeletal tissues appeared black on MR images, and the thinking was that these tissues produced no useful signals, were not suitable for clinical MRI and would probably remain so. Only large abnormalities could be seen in the lung and musculoskeletal tissues with MRI; more subtle changes could not be recognized and tissue properties could not be quantified. The lack of detectable signal from short- and ultrashort-T_2 tissues was regarded as a fundamental limitation of MRI and meant that the technique was not competitive in areas of considerable clinical importance.

The advent of UTE imaging which produced detectable signal in the lung [1], tendons and ligaments [2], and cortical bone [3] was therefore a most welcome development. It meant that these tissues could be regarded as part of mainstream MRI, and research on imaging techniques and visualization could progress in the way that it had for other tissues and organs.

Progress in the first decade of clinical imaging of short- and ultrashort-T_2 tissues was summarized in a book published in 2012 [4]. Since that time there has been increased interest and major progress in technical aspects of imaging short- and ultrashort-T_2 tissues. There has also been a notable expansion in clinical applications. These developments are the subject of this book.

We are very grateful to the authors who have, without exception, produced up-to-date, thoughtful and wide-ranging accounts of their work, and so have provided abundant raison d'être for the book.

Our thanks go to Patricia Hamilton for meticulous manuscript preparation and review, as well as to Duncan Stovell and Stuart Crozier from Magnetica who have provided generous financial support. Thanks also to Vinodh Thomas and Margaret Moore from Springer who have provided valuable advice and direction.

At a personal level, we are very grateful for the unstinting support from all of those involved in this project and have greatly appreciated the opportunity to get to know authors and their work in depth.

References

1. Bergin CJ, Pauly JM, Macovski A. Lung parenchyma: projection reconstruction MR imaging. Radiology. 1991;179(3):777–81.
2. Gold GE, Thedens DR, Pauly JM, Fechner KP, Bergman G, Beaulieu CF, Macovski A. MR imaging of articular cartilage of the knee: new methods using ultrashort TEs. AJR Am J Roentgenol. 1998;170(5):1223–6.
3. Robson MD, Gatehouse PD, Bydder M, Bydder GM. Magnetic resonance: an introduction to ultrashort TE (UTE) imaging. J Comput Assist Tomogr. 2003;27(6):825–46.
4. Bydder GM, Fullerton GD, Young IR, editors. MRI of tissues with short T_2s or $T_2{}^*$s. New York: Wiley; 2012.

La Jolla, CA   Jiang Du

La Jolla, CA   Graeme M. Bydder

16 February 2023

Contents

Contributors

Nivedita Agarwal Istituto di Ricovero e Cura a Carattere Scientifico (IRCCS), Eugenio Medea Bosisio Parini, Lecco, Italy

Aria Ashir Department of Radiology, University of California, San Diego, La Jolla, CA, USA

Research Service, VA San Diego Healthcare System, San Diego, CA, USA

Santa Barbara Cottage Hospital, Santa Barbara, USA

Jiyo Athertya Department of Radiology, University of California, San Diego, La Jolla, CA, USA

Emily Louise Baadsvik Institute for Biomedical Engineering, ETH Zurich and University of Zurich, Zurich, Switzerland

Layale Bazzi Department of Physics, University of Windsor, Windsor, ON, Canada

Fernando E. Boada Department of Radiology, Center for Biomedical Imaging, New York University Grossman School of Medicine, New York, NY, USA

Noah B. Bonnheim Department of Orthopaedic Surgery, University of California, San Diego, La Jolla, CA, USA

Philipp Braun Department of Diagnostic and Interventional Radiology, Klinikum rechts der Isar, TUM School of Medicine, Technical University of Munich, Munich, Germany

Stephan J. Breda, MD, PhD Department of Radiology and Nuclear Medicine, Erasmus MC University Medical Center, Rotterdam, The Netherlands

Ryan E. Breighner Department of Radiology and Imaging, Hospital for Special Surgery, New York, NY, USA

Susan V. Bukata Department of Orthopaedics, University of California, San Diego, La Jolla, CA, USA

Graeme M. Bydder Department of Radiology, University of California, San Diego, La Jolla, CA, USA

Mātai Medical Research Institute, Tairāwhiti Gisborne, New Zealand

Mark Bydder Department of Radiological Sciences, David Geffen School of Medicine, University of California Los Angeles, Los Angeles, CA, USA

Michael Carl GE Healthcare, San Diego, CA, USA

Eric Y. Chang Department of Radiology, University of California, San Diego, La Jolla, CA, USA

VA San Diego Healthcare System, San Diego, CA, USA

Research Service, Veterans Affairs San Diego Healthcare System, San Diego, CA, USA

Cynthia Chin Department of Radiology and Biomedical Imaging, University of California, San Diego, La Jolla, CA, USA

Christine B. Chung Department of Radiology, University of California, San Diego, La Jolla, CA, USA

VA San Diego Healthcare System, San Diego, CA, USA

Research Service, Veterans Affairs San Diego Healthcare System, San Diego, CA, USA

Paul Condron Mātai Medical Research Institute, Tairāwhiti Gisborne, New Zealand

Department of Anatomy and Medical Imaging and Centre for Brain Research, Faculty of Medical and Health Sciences, University of Auckland, Auckland, New Zealand

Daniel M. Cornfeld Mātai Medical Research Institute, Tairāwhiti Gisborne, New Zealand

Department of Anatomy and Medical Imaging and Centre for Brain Research, Faculty of Medical and Health Sciences, University of Auckland, Auckland, New Zealand

Xeni Deligianni Division of Radiological Physics, Department of Radiology, University of Basel Hospital, Basel, Switzerland

Research Coordination Team, Department of Radiology, University Hospital Basel, Basel, Switzerland

Basel Muscle MRI, Department of Biomedical Engineering, University of Basel, Allschwil, Switzerland

Mark D. Does Institute of Image Science, Vanderbilt University Medical Center, Nashville, TN, USA

Biomedical Engineering, Vanderbilt University, Nashville, TN, USA

Radiology and Radiological Sciences, Vanderbilt University Medical Center, Nashville, TN, USA

Electrical Engineering, Vanderbilt University Medical Center, Nashville, TN, USA

Annette von Drygalski Department of Medicine, University of California, San Diego, La Jolla, CA, USA

Jiang Du Department of Radiology, University of California, San Diego, La Jolla, CA, USA

Department of Bioengineering, University of California, San Diego, La Jolla, CA, USA

VA San Diego Healthcare System, San Diego, CA, USA

Georg Feuerriegel Department of Diagnostic and Interventional Radiology, Klinikum rechts der Isar, TUM School of Medicine, Technical University of Munich, Munich, Germany

Aaron J. Fields Department of Orthopaedic Surgery, University of California, San Diego, La Jolla, CA, USA

Maggie Fung GE Healthcare, New York, NY, USA

Alexandra Gersing Department of Diagnostic and Interventional Radiology, Klinikum rechts der Isar, TUM School of Medicine, Technical University of Munich, Munich, Germany

David Grodzki Siemens Healthcare GmbH, Magnetic Resonance, Erlangen, Germany

Department of Neuroradiology, Friedrich-Alexander-Universität Erlangen-Nürnberg, Erlangen, Germany

Benedikt Hager Department of Biomedical Imaging and Image-guided Therapy, High Field MR Centre, Medical University of Vienna, Vienna, Austria

CD Laboratory for MR Imaging Biomarkers (BIOMAK), Vienna, Austria

Austrian Cluster for Tissue Regeneration, Ludwig Boltzmann Institute for Experimental and Clinical Traumatology, Vienna, Austria

Misung Han Department of Radiology and Biomedical Imaging, University of California, San Diego, La Jolla, CA, USA

Claudia M. Hillenbrand Research Imaging NSW, Division of Research and Enterprise, University of New South Wales, Sydney, NSW, Australia

Samantha J. Holdsworth Mātai Medical Research Institute, Tairāwhiti Gisborne, New Zealand

Department of Anatomy and Medical Imaging and Centre for Brain Research, Faculty of Medical and Health Sciences, University of Auckland, Auckland, New Zealand

Hyungseok Jang Department of Radiology, University of California, San Diego, La Jolla, CA, USA

Saeed Jerban Department of Radiology, University of California, San Diego, La Jolla, CA, USA

Department of Orthopaedic Surgery, University of California, San Diego, La Jolla, CA, USA

Brandon C. Jones Department of Radiology, Perelman School of Medicine, University of Pennsylvania, Philadelphia, PA, USA

Department of Bioengineering, School of Engineering and Applied Sciences, University of Pennsylvania, Philadelphia, PA, USA

Vladimir Juras Department of Biomedical Imaging and Image-guided Therapy, High Field MR Centre, Medical University of Vienna, Vienna, Austria

CD Laboratory for MR Imaging Biomarkers (BIOMAK), Vienna, Austria

Austrian Cluster for Tissue Regeneration, Ludwig Boltzmann Institute for Experimental and Clinical Traumatology, Vienna, Austria

Dimitrios C. Karampinos Department of Diagnostic and Interventional Radiology, Klinikum rechts der Isar, TUM School of Medicine, Technical University of Munich, Munich, Germany

Axel J. Krafft Siemens Healthcare GmbH, Erlangen, Germany

Sophia Kronthaler Department of Diagnostic and Interventional Radiology, Klinikum rechts der Isar, TUM School of Medicine, Technical University of Munich, Munich, Germany

Roland Krug Department of Radiology and Biomedical Imaging, University of California, San Diego, La Jolla, CA, USA

Peder Larson Department of Radiology and Biomedical Imaging, University of California, San Francisco, CA, USA

James Lo Department of Bioengineering, University of California, San Diego, La Jolla, CA, USA

Ralf B. Loeffler Research Imaging NSW, Division of Research and Enterprise, University of New South Wales, Sydney, NSW, Australia

Letizia Losa Istituto di Ricovero e Cura a Carattere Scientifico (IRCCS), Eugenio Medea Bosisio Parini, Lecco, Italy

Aiming Lu Division of Medical Physics, Department of Radiology, Mayo Clinic, Rochester, MN, USA

Xing Lu Department of Radiology, University of California, San Diego, La Jolla, CA, USA

Yajun Ma Department of Radiology, University of California, San Diego, La Jolla, CA, USA

Dina Moazamian Department of Radiology, University of California, San Diego, La Jolla, CA, USA

Aurea Mohana-Borges Department of Radiology, University of California, San Diego, La Jolla, CA, USA

Jeffry S. Nyman Institute of Image Science, Vanderbilt University Medical Center, Nashville, TN, USA

Biomedical Engineering, Vanderbilt University, Nashville, TN, USA

Department of Veterans Affairs, Tennessee Valley Healthcare System, Nashville, TN, USA

Orthopaedic Surgery and Rehabilitation, Vanderbilt University Medical Center, Nashville, TN, USA

Center for Bone Biology, Vanderbilt University Medical Center, Nashville, TN, USA

Edwin H. G. Oei, MD, PhD Department of Radiology and Nuclear Medicine, Erasmus MC University Medical Center, Rotterdam, The Netherlands

Denis Peruzzo Istituto di Ricovero e Cura a Carattere Scientifico (IRCCS), Eugenio Medea Bosisio Parini, Lecco, Italy

John D. Port Department of Radiology, Mayo Clinic, Rochester, MN, USA

Hollis G. Potter Department of Radiology and Imaging, Hospital for Special Surgery, New York, NY, USA

Klaas P. Pruessmann Institute for Biomedical Engineering, ETH Zurich and University of Zurich, Zurich, Switzerland

Yongxian Qian Department of Radiology, Center for Biomedical Imaging, New York University Grossman School of Medicine, New York, NY, USA

Chamith S. Rajapakse Department of Radiology, Perelman School of Medicine, University of Pennsylvania, Philadelphia, PA, USA

Department of Orthopaedic Surgery, Perelman School of Medicine, University of Pennsylvania, Philadelphia, PA, USA

Jerban Saeed Department of Radiology, University of California, San Diego, La Jolla, CA, USA

Tobias Schaeffter Physikalisch-Technische Bundesanstalt (PTB), Braunschweig and Berlin, Germany

Medical Engineering, Technical University of Berlin and Einstein Centre Digital Future, Berlin, Germany

Division of Imaging Sciences and Biomedical Engineering, King's College London, London, UK

Fritz Schick Department of Diagnostic and Interventional Radiology, Section of Experimental Radiology, University of Tübingen, Tübingen, Germany

Volkmar Schulz Department of Physics of Molecular Imaging Systems, Institute for Experimental Molecular Imaging, RWTH Aachen University, Aachen, Germany

Institute of Physics IIIB, RWTH Aachen University, Aachen, Germany

Hyperion Hybrid Imaging Systems GmbH, Aachen, Germany

Fraunhofer Institute for Digital Medicine MEVIS, Aachen, Germany

Sam Sedaghat Department of Radiology, University of California, San Diego, La Jolla, CA, USA

Soo Hyun Shin Department of Radiology, University of California, San Diego, La Jolla, CA, USA

Department of Bioengineering, University of California, San Diego, La Jolla, CA, USA

Ana Beatriz Solana GE Healthcare, Munich, Germany

Center for Neuroimaging, Institute of Psychiatry, Psychology and Neuroscience (IoPPN), King's College London, London, UK

Arya Suprana Department of Bioengineering, University of California, San Diego, La Jolla, CA, USA

Pavol Szomolanyi Department of Biomedical Imaging and Image-guided Therapy, High Field MR Centre, Medical University of Vienna, Vienna, Austria

CD Laboratory for MR Imaging Biomarkers (BIOMAK), Vienna, Austria

Austrian Cluster for Tissue Regeneration, Ludwig Boltzmann Institute for Experimental and Clinical Traumatology, Vienna, Austria

Department of Imaging Methods, Institute of Measurement Science, Slovak Academy of Sciences, Bratislava, Slovakia

Siegfried Trattnig Department of Biomedical Imaging and Image-guided Therapy, High Field MR Centre, Medical University of Vienna, Vienna, Austria

CD Laboratory for MR Imaging Biomarkers (BIOMAK), Vienna, Austria

Austrian Cluster for Tissue Regeneration, Ludwig Boltzmann Institute for Experimental and Clinical Traumatology, Vienna, Austria

Institute for Clinical Molecular MRI in the Musculoskeletal System, Karl Landsteiner Society, St. Pölten, Austria

Markus Weiger Institute for Biomedical Engineering, ETH Zurich and University of Zurich, Zurich, Switzerland

Kilian Weiss Philips GmbH, Hamburg, Germany

Florian Wiesinger GE Healthcare, Munich, Germany

Center for Neuroimaging, Institute of Psychiatry, Psychology and Neuroscience (IoPPN), King's College London, London, UK

Mei Wu Department of Radiology, University of California, San Diego, La Jolla, CA, USA

Dan Xiao Department of Physics, University of Windsor, Windsor, ON, Canada

Olgica Zaric Department of Medicine, Faculty of Medicine and Dentistry, Danube Private University GmbH (DPU), Krems an der Donau, Austria

Institute for Clinical Molecular MRI in the Musculoskeletal System, Karl Landsteiner Society, St. Pölten, Austria

Chun Zeng Department of Radiology, University of California, San Diego, La Jolla, CA, USA

Department of Radiology, the First Affiliated Hospital of Chongqing Medical University, Chongqing, China

Abbreviations

1D	One-dimensional
2D	Two-dimensional
3D	Three-dimensional
4D	Four-dimensional
α	Alpha, flip angle
A^1IR	Added inversion recovery
AB	Anterior band
aBMD	Areal bone mineral density
ABS	Acrylonitrile butadiene styrene
AC	Attenuation correction
ACL	Anterior cruciate ligament
ACLR	Anterior cruciate ligament reconstruction
ACLT	Anterior cruciate ligament transection
ACR	American College of Radiology
ADC (i)	Analog digital conversion
ADC (ii)	Apparent diffusion coefficient
ADEM	Acute disseminated encephalomyelitis
$AdiabT_{1\rho}$	Adiabatic $T_{1\rho}$
AF	Annulus fibrosis
AFI	Actual flip angle imaging
AFP	Adiabatic full passage
AGE	Advanced glycation end product
AHP	Adiabatic half passage
AI	Artificial intelligence
AIR (i)	Added inversion recovery
AIR (ii)	Adiabatic inversion recovery
AIR-UTE	Adiabatic inversion recovery ultrashort echo time
AL	Attention layer
ANR	Acoustic noise reduction
ANT	Advanced normalization tool
App	Application
AQ	Acquired, Acquisition
AR	Algebraic reconstruction
ASL	Arterial spin labeling
ATT	Anterior tibialis tendon
AUTOMAP	Automated transform by manifold approximation
AWSOS	Acquisition-weighted stack of spirals
b	Diffusion sensitivity parameter
B_0	Static magnetic field
B_1	Radiofrequency magnetic field
BAT	Brown adipose tissue
BH	Breath hold

BMD	Bone mineral density
BME	Bone marrow edema
BOLD	Blood oxygenation level-dependent
BSI	Bone stress injury
bSSFP	Balanced steady-state free precession
BW (i)	Bandwidth
BW (ii)	Bound water
BWPD	Bound water proton density
C_{ab}, C_{fr}	C_{ab} = absolute contrast, C_{fr} = fractional contrast
C_{bw}	Bound water concentration
C_{pw}	Pore water concentration
CCT	Central contrast theorem
CEP	Cartilage endplate
CEST	Chemical exchange saturation transfer
CF	Cystic fibrosis
CHESS	Chemical shift selective
CKD	Chronic Kidney disease
CNFS	Cervical neural foraminal stenosis
CNN	Convolutional neural network
CNR	Contrast-to-noise ratio
COSMOS	Calculation of susceptibility through multiple orientation sampling
CPMG	Carr-Purcell-Meiboom-Gill
cr	Cardiorespiratory
CS	Compressed sensing
CSE	Chemical shift encoding
CSF	Cerebrospinal fluid
CSI	Chemical shift imaging
CSPI	Continuous single-point imaging
CT	Computed tomography
CTAC	Computed tomography-based attenuation correction
CTI	Constant time imaging
CV	Coefficient of variation
CW	Continuous wave
CWPE	Continuous wave power equivalent
D	Delta, difference
d	Divided
D*	Apparent diffusion coefficient
DAFP	Double adiabatic full passage
DAFP-UTE	Double adiabatic full-passage ultrashort echo time
DAQ	Data acquisition window
DB-UTE	Dual-band saturation-prepared ultrashort echo time
DC	Data collection
DC/TMD	Diagnostic criteria for temporomandibular disorder
DCE-MRI	Dynamic contrast-enhanced magnetic resonance imaging
DCNN	Deep convolutional neural network
DDH	Developmental dysplasia of the hip
DESIRE	Double echo sliding inversion recovery
DESIRE-UTE	Double echo sliding inversion recovery ultrashort echo time
DESS	Double echo steady state
DEXA	Dual-Energy X-ray absorptiometry
dIR	Divided inversion recovery
DIR	Double inversion recovery
Double-IR-UTE	Double adiabatic inversion recovery ultrashort echo time

dRHE-MRAC	Dual-echo ramped hybrid encoding-based magnetic resonance-based attenuation correction
DRONE	Deep RecOnstruction NEtwork
drSIR	Divided reverse subtraction inversion recovery
drSIREDS	Divided reverse subtraction inversion recovery echo and diffusion subtraction
drSIRES	Divided reverse subtraction inversion recovery echo subtraction
DS	Diffusion subtraction
dSIR	Divided subtracted inversion recovery
DTI	Diffusion tensor imaging
Dual-IR-UTE	Dual adiabatic inversion recovery ultrashort echo time
DW	Diffusion-weighted
DWI	Diffusion-weighted imaging
DW-SE-EPI	Diffusion-weighted spin echo-based echo planar imaging
DXA	Dual X-ray absorptiometry
ECM	Extracellular matrix
ECV	Extracellular volume
EDSS	Expanded disability status scale
EPI	Echo planar imaging
EPR	Electron paramagnetic resonance
ES	Echo subtraction
F	Fibula
FA	Flip angle
FAI	Femoroacetabular impingement
FAPI	Fibroblast activation protein inhibitors
FAT-SAT	Fat saturation
FB	Free breathing
FCD	Fixed charge density
FEA	Finite element analysis
FE-UTE	Frequency encoding-based ultrashort echo time
FFT	Fast Fourier transform
FID	Free induction decay
FIR	Fitted inversion recovery
FLAWS	Fluid and white matter suppression
fMRI	Functional magnetic resonance imaging
FOV	Field of view
F_{racl}	Short-T_2 fraction
FS	Fat saturated
FSE	Fast spin echo
FT	Fourier transformation
FW	Free (pore) water
FWHM	Full width at half maximum
G	Gradient
GAG	Glycosaminoglycan
GAN	Generative adversarial network
GBCA	Gadolinium-based contrast agent
GE	Gradient echo
GIRF	Gradient impulse response function
GM (i)	Gradient modulated
GM (ii)	Gradient moment
GM (iii)	Gray matter
GM_L	Long-T_2 gray matter
GM_{myelin}	Myelin in gray matter

GRE	Gradient recalled echo
G_{read}	Readout gradient
GRE-$T_{1\rho}$	Gradient recalled echo-based $T_{1\rho}$
G_{RF}	Gradient during RF excitation
GT	Ground truth
HA	Hemophilic arthropathy
HIC	Hepatic iron content
HJHS	Hemophilia Joint Health Score
HPF	High-pass filtering
HU	Hounsfield units
HYFI	Hybrid filling
HYFI-ZTE	Hybrid filling zero echo time
ICC	Intraclass correlation coefficient
IDEAL	Iterative decomposition of water and fat with echo asymmetry and least square estimation
IFFT	Inverse fast Fourier transformaction
IFT	Inverse Fourier transformaction
IHE	Interleaved hybrid encoding
ihMT	Inhomogeneous magnetization transfer
iLSQR	Improved sparse linear equation and least square
iMoCo	Iterative motion compensation
IONP	Iron oxide nanoparticle
IP	In-phase
IPSG	International Prophylaxis Study Group
IR	Inversion recovery
IRB	Institutional Review Board
IRES	Inversion recovery echo subtraction
IR-FS-UTE	Inversion recovery and fat saturation ultrashort echo time
IR-HE	Inversion recovery-based hybrid encoding
IR-IHE	Inversion recovery-based interleaved hybrid encoding
IR-PRUTE	Inversion recovery-based projection radial ultrashort echo time
IR-RHE	Inversion recovery prepared ramped hybrid encoding
IR-SE	Inversion recovery spin echo
IR-UTE	Inversion recovery ultrashort echo time
IR-UTE-ES	Single adiabatic inversion recovery ultrashort echo time with echo subtraction
IVD	Intervertebral disc
iW^r	Image weighting ratio
IZ	Intermediate zone
KL	Kellgren–Lawrence
L	Lorentzian
LAC	Linear attenuation coefficient
LAM	Lymphangioleiomyomatosis
LBP	Low back pain
LCN	Lacunar-canalicular network
LFB	Luxol fast blue
LOR	Line of response
$Loss_{map}$	l1 loss
$Loss_{MSQ}$	Total loss
$Loss_{pcMSQ}$	pcMSQ-net loss
$Loss_{phy}$	Physical-constraint loss
$Losss_{eg}$	Segmentation loss
LTI	Linear time-invariant

M (i)	Magnetization
M (ii)	Menisci
m	Magnitude
MANTIS	Model-augmented neural network with incoherent *k*-space sampling
MAPSS	Magnetization-prepared angle-modulated partitioned *k*-space spoiled gradient echo snapshots
MAS	Magic angle spinning
MASDIR	Multiplied, added, subtracted, and/or divided inversion recovery
MBP	Myelin basic protein
MCIR	Motion-compensated image reconstruction
mD	Middle domain
MEDI	Morphology-enabled dipole inversion
MF	Motion fields
MIOP	Magnetic iron oxide particles
MIP	Maximum intensity projection
MIR	Multiplied inversion recovery
ML	Machine learning
MMF	Macromolecular fraction
MMPD	Macromolecular proton density
MOLLI	Modified look-locker inversion recovery
MP2RAGE	Magnetization-prepared 2 rapid acquisition gradient echo
MPF	Macromolecular proton fraction
MPnRAGE	Magnetization-prepared n rapid acquisition gradient echo
MPR	Multiplanar reformatting
MP-RAGE	Magnetization-prepared rapid acquisition gradient echo
MRA	MR angiography
MRAC	Magnetic resonance-based attenuation correction
MRF	Magnetic resonance fingerprinting
MRF-EPI	Magnetic resonance fingerprinting echo planar imaging
MRI	Magnetic resonance imaging
MRS	Magnetic resonance spectroscopy
MRSI	Magnetic resonance spectroscopic imaging
MS	Multiple sclerosis
MSFC	Multiple sclerosis functional composite
MSK	Musculoskeletal
MSMQ-Net	Multi-tissue segmentation multi-parameter quantification net
MSQ-Net	Multi-tissue segmentation and quantification net
MT	Magnetization transfer
MTF	Modulation transfer function
MTJ	Muscle–tendon junction
MTR	Magnetization transfer ratio
NAGM	Normal-appearing gray matter
NASH	Nonalcoholic steatohepatitis
NAWM	Normal-appearing white matter
NEX	Number of excitations
NGM	Normal gray matter
NIRSI	Near-infrared spectral imaging
NMO	Neuromyelitis optica
NMSI	Normalized mean signal intensity
NP	Nucleus pulposus
N_{sp}	Number of spokes
NWM	Normal white matter
OA	Osteoarthritis

OCJ	Osteochondral junction
OP (i)	Osteoporosis
OP (ii)	Out-of-phase
OPe	Osteopenia
OPo	Osteoporosis
OVS	Outer volume suppression
PB	Posterior band
PBS	Phosphate-buffered saline
PC	Phase contrast
PCL	Posterior cruciate ligament
pcMSQ-Net	Physical constraint multi-tissue segmentation and quantification net
PD	Proton density
PDF	Projection onto a dipole field
PDFF	Proton density fat fraction
PD-FSE	Proton density-weighted fast spin echos
PET	Positron emission tomography
PETRA	Pointwise encoding time reduction with radial acquisition
PG	Proteoglycan
PGSE	Pulsed gradient spin echo
PH	Phase
PI	Porosity index
PLM	Polarized light microscopy
PNS	Peripheral nervous system
Po	Porosity
POCS	Projection onto convex set
PR (i)	Projection radial
PR (ii)	Projection reconstruction
PREFUL	Phase-resolved functional lung
PRFS	Proton resonance frequency shift
PS	Phase sensitive
PSF	Point spread function
PSMA	Prostate-specific membrane antigen
PSR	Picrosirius red
PT	Patellar tendinopathy
PTT	Posterior tibialis tendon
PW	Pore water
PWPD	Pore water proton density
QALAS	Quantification using an interleaved look-locker acquisition sequence
QCT	Quantitative computed tomography
QMRI	Quantitative magnetic resonance imaging
QSM	Quantitative susceptibility mapping
QT	Quadriceps tendon
qUTE-DESS	Quantitative ultrashort echo time-based double echo steady-state
r	Reversed
R1w	Spin-lattice relaxation rate
RAD	Radiologist
rBW	Readout bandwidth
RDC/TMD	Research diagnostic criteria for temporomandibular disorder
ReLu	Rectifier linear unit
RF	Radiofrequency
RFPA	Radiofrequency power amplifier
RHE	Ramped hybrid encoding
RM_{0m}	Exchange rate

RNN	Recurrent neural network
RO	Readout direction
ROD	Renal osteodystrophy
ROI	Region of interest
RP	Rectangular pulse
rSIR	Reversed subtraction inversion recovery
rSIREDS	Reverse subtracted inversion recovery echo and diffusion subtraction
rSIRES	Reverse subtracted inversion recovery echo subtraction
RUFIS	Rotating ultrafast imaging sequence
RX	Receive mode
S	Signal
SAR	Specific absorption rate
scMRI	Synergistic contrast magnetic resonance imaging
SD	Standard deviation
SE	Spin echo
SGE	Spoiled gradient echo
shMOLLI	Shortened modified look-locker imaging
SIJs	Sacroiliac joints
SIR (i)	Subtracted inversion recovery
SIR (ii)	Signal intensity ratio
SIREDS	Subtracted inversion recovery echo and diffusion subtracted
SIRES	Subtracted inversion recovery echo subtracted
SIRF	Synergistic reconstruction for biomedical imaging
SL (i)	Slice
SL (ii)	Spin lock
SL (iii)	Super-Lorentzian
SLR	Shinnar-Le Roux
SNR	Signal-to-noise ratio
SPAIR	Spectral adiabatic inversion recovery
SPGR	Spoiled gradient recalled echo
SPI	Single-point imaging
SPIR (i)	Spectral inversion recovery
SPIR (ii)	Spectral presaturation with inversion recovery
SPRITE	Single-point ramped imaging with T_1 enhancement
SR (i)	Saturation recovery
SR (ii)	Slew rate
SR (iii)	Suppression ratio
SR-SWIFT	Saturation recovery sweep imaging with Fourier transformation
SR-UTE	Saturation recovery prepared ultrashort echo time
SSFP	Steady-state free precession
SSIM	Structural similarity
STAIRES	Short repetition time adiabatic inversion recovery echo subtraction
STAIR-UTE	Short repetition time adiabatic inversion recovery prepared ultrashort echo time
STAR-QSM	Streaking artifact reduction for quantitative susceptibility mapping
STEAM	Stimulated echo acquisition mode
STEAM-UTE-DWI	Stimulated echo acquisition mode ultrashort echo time diffusion-weighted imaging
STE-MTR	Short echo time-based magnetization transfer ratio
STIR	Short tau inversion recovery
SWI	Susceptibility-weighted imaging
SWIFT	Sweep imaging with Fourier transform
sW^r	Sequence weighting ratio

T	Tibia
T/R	Transmit and receive
T_1	Longitudinal relaxation time
T_{1-BW}	Bound water T_1
T_1-FSE	T_1-weighted fast spin echo
T_2	Transverse relaxation time
T_2-FLAIR	T_2-weighted fluid attenuated inversion recovery
T_{2l}	Long transverse relaxation time
T_{2m}	Macromolecular proton transverse relaxation time
T_{2s}	Short transverse relaxation time
TA	Total acquisition
TBI	Total body iron
TE	Echo time
TE_1	First echo time
TE_{enc}	Encoding echo time
TE_{min}	Minimum echo time
TI	Inversion time
TKA	Total knee arthroplasty
TKR	Total knee replacement
TMD	Temporomandibular disorder
TMJ	Temporomandibular joint
TOF	Time-of-flight
TP	Tissue property
TP-filters	Tissue property filters
TPI	Twisted projection imaging
TR	Repetition time
TSL	Spin-locking time
TSR	Saturation recovery time
Tsvd	Truncated singular value decomposition
TW	Total water
TWPD	Total water proton density
US	Ultrasound
USPF	Ultrashort-T_2 proton fraction
UTE	Ultrashort echo time
UTE-AdiabT$_{1\rho}$	Ultrashort echo time-based adiabatic $T_{1\rho}$
UTE-AFI	Ultrashort echo time actual flip angle imaging
UTE-AFI-VFA	Ultrashort echo time actual flip angle imaging and variable flip angle
UTE-Cones-DESS	Ultrashort echo time cones-based double echo steady state
UTE-CSI	Ultrashort echo time chemical shift imaging
UTE-DESS	Ultrashort echo time double echo steady state
UTE-DWI	Ultrashort echo time diffusion-weighted imaging
UTE-IDEAL	Ultrashort echo time iterative decomposition of water and fat with echo asymmetry and least square estimation
UTE-MMF	Ultrashort echo time magnetization transfer modeling of macromolecular fraction
UTE-MT	Ultrashort echo time magnetization transfer
UTE-MTR	Ultrashort echo time magnetization transfer ratio
UTE-PD	Ultrashort echo time proton density
UTE-QSM	Ultrashort echo time quantitative susceptibility mapping
UTE-SE	Ultrashort echo time spin echo
UTESI	Ultrashort echo time spectroscopic imaging
UTE-STR	Ultrashort echo time with a short repetition time
UTE-$T_{1\rho}$	Ultrashort echo time-based $T_{1\rho}$

UTE-T$_2$*	Ultrashort echo time-based T$_2$*
UTE-VFA	Ultrashort echo time variable flip angle
UTE-VTR	Ultrashort echo time with variable repetition time
VARPRO	Variable projection
VERSE	Variable-rate selective excitation
VFA	Variable flip angle
VOE	Volumetric overlap error
vTE	Variable echo time
VTR	Variable repetition time
w	Weighting
W/V	Weight/volume
WASPI	Water- and fat-suppressed proton projection MRI
WAT	White adipose tissue
WHO	World Health Organization
WM	White matter
WM$_L$	Long-T$_2$ white matter
WM$_{myelin}$	Myelin in white matter
WORMS	Whole-organ magnetic resonance imaging score
zGRF-RHE	Zero gradient radiofrequency-ramped hybrid encoding
ZIP	Zero interpolation filling
ZTE	Zero echo time

Part I

Data Acquisition

Introduction to MRI of Short- and Ultrashort-T_2 Tissues

Jiang Du and Graeme M. Bydder

History

In the earliest days of human MRI from 1976 to 1985, very low or zero signals were observed in normal human cortical bone, tendons, ligaments, and menisci with a variety of pulse sequences, and this was generally attributed to the low tissue mobile proton density (ρ_m) and/or the short-T_2 of these tissues. The very low or zero signal from these normal tissues was a useful source of background contrast for identifying lesions in the tissues when the lesions had sufficiently higher ρ_ms and/or longer T_2s to make signal from them detectable and appear visible with the pulse sequences in use at that time. However, the lack of signal predicated against detailed study of these tissues. Whatever sequence preparation was used, there was no signal detectable from the normal tissues with conventional clinical pulse sequences so there was no opportunity to manipulate the contrast of the tissues. Likewise, the lack of signal meant that the normal tissues could not be characterized by measurement of their ρ_m, T_1, T_2, and/or T_2^* or other tissue properties (TPs) [1]. In addition, more subtle diseases might change TPs, but if these changes were of the wrong type, or insufficient to reach the thresholds for increase in ρ_m and T_2 to enable signal to be detected, the abnormalities were not usually observable, and the changes in TPs could not be quantified [1–3]. It rendered MRI insensitive to disease in short- and ultrashort-T_2 tissues and tissue components.

With increasing static field strength and gradient performance, it became possible to shorten echo times (TEs) and use conventional gradient echo (GE) sequences to detect some signals from tendons, ligaments, and menisci, but not from normal lung parenchyma, cortical bone, or myelin. Detection of signal from these tissues was dependent on the use of ultrashort TE (UTE) and/or zero TE (ZTE) type sequences with TEs less than 1 ms. These were first used clinically in 1992 [4].

Using small-bore MR systems with much superior gradient and radiofrequency (RF) performance, it was possible to achieve TEs much shorter than those attainable with clinical MR systems and images at high static field strengths with improved signal-to-noise ratios (SNRs). This merged into solid-state MRI where quite specific techniques such as magic angle spinning are used for detecting signals and creating lesion contrast. It is usually not possible to implement these techniques on lower-performance clinical MR systems, but studies of small animals and tissues using these systems may be very useful for morphological observations and characterizing tissues to provide guidance for clinical studies.

The book essentially describes the last 20 years of development in imaging of short- and ultrashort-T_2 tissues, often by the people who originated the techniques and/or did the first studies with them. Tissues that were previously "invisible", and frequently ignored in the past, are now the focus of morphological and quantitative imaging.

This introduction aims to describe some general concepts and principles as background to the detailed description of various UTE- and ZTE-type data acquisition strategies, contrast mechanisms, quantification techniques, and clinical applications that follow and begins with an outline of relevant TPs.

J. Du
Department of Radiology, University of California, San Diego, La Jolla, CA, USA

Department of Bioengineering, University of California, San Diego, La Jolla, CA, USA

VA San Diego Healthcare System, San Diego, CA, USA
e-mail: jiangdu@health.ucsd.edu

G. M. Bydder (✉)
Department of Radiology, University of California, San Diego, La Jolla, CA, USA

Mātai Medical Research Institute, Tairāwhiti Gisborne, New Zealand
e-mail: gbydder@health.ucsd.edu

Tissue Properties (TPs): Normal Values, Changes in Disease, and Changes with Contrast Agents

Normal Values of T_1, T_2, and Mobile Proton Density (ρ_m)

There are over 20 tissue properties (TPs) that contribute to the signals detected in clinical MRI. Some of these TPs such as ρ_m, diffusion, and flow are quite general and are applicable very widely, whereas others such as the longitudinal and transverse relaxation times T_1 and T_2 are specific for magnetic resonance [1–3]. In this section, and subsequently, the term TPs is used to include fluid properties as well, unless otherwise specified.

Mobile proton density (ρ_m) brings in the concept of nuclear or molecular mobility since immobile protons, as in crystalline solids, have extremely short T_2s (e.g., a few μs) making them impossible to detect directly with conventional approaches [5, 6]. This is incorporated into the concept of ρ_m, which is the MR detectable proton density. It implies that the protons are not held so rigidly that their T_2s are extremely short and that their mobility is associated with a longer T_2 so that signal is detectable with clinically relevant data acquisitions. ρ_m is less precisely defined than chemical proton density but represents the density of protons that can be detected and used in clinical MRI. It is also affected by shortening effects due to susceptibility, chemical shift, and other factors where signals can shorten the observed T_2 decay designated as T_2^*. These effects may be quite profound and drastically shorten the observed value of T_2^* to the level that signal becomes undetectable.

The range of normal T_1s of tissues encountered in clinical practice covers over three orders of magnitude from about 150 ms in cortical bone to fluids of about 4000 ms. The T_1s for tissues increase with field strength though those of fluids change very little. The relevant range of T_2s in tissues is even greater from <0.01 ms for protons in proteins to 4000 ms for fluids. It is useful to divide these T_2s into five broad groups: <0.01 ms (supershort), 0.01–1 ms (ultrashort), 1–10 ms (short), 10–100 ms (intermediate), and 100–4000 ms (long).

In clinical systems, this generally corresponds to the detectability of the tissues. Supershort-T_2s are usually only indirectly detectable through magnetization transfer (MT) [7]. Ultrashort-T_2s are only detectable with UTE or ZTE-type sequences, including 2D and 3D UTE [4–6], single-point imaging (SPI) [8], single-point ramped imaging with T_1 enhancement (SPRITE) [9], Cartesian variable TE (vTE) [10], water- and fat-suppressed proton projection MRI (WASPI) [11], sweep imaging with Fourier transformation (SWIFT) [12], hybrid acquisition-weighted stack of spirals (AWSOS) [13], pointwise encoding time reduction with radial acquisition (PETRA) [14], ramped hybrid encoding (RHE) [15], ZTE [16], and Looping Star [17]. Short-T_2s are detectable with GE sequences (shorter T_2 in the short-T_2 range) and spin echo (SE) sequences (longer T_2 in the short-T_2 range). Intermediate and long-T_2s are detectable with SE sequences. Sequences that can detect shorter T_2 signals can also detect longer T_2 signals.

Another important concept is to divide tissues into those with a majority of short- and/or ultrashort-T_2 components such as parenchymal lung, cortical bone, tendons, and ligaments, and those with a minority of short- and ultrashort-T_2 components such as brain, muscle, and most other tissues. With tissues with a majority of short- and ultrashort-T_2 components, direct imaging may be all that is necessary, but with tissues in which the short- and ultrashort-T_2 tissues are in a minority, it is usually necessary to suppress signals from more abundant intermediate- or long-T_2 tissue components, both to develop useful contrast and to provide accurate quantitation of the TPs of the short- and ultrashort-T_2 components [6].

Collagen-containing tissues vary in the ρ_m and T_2 with highly organized collagen as in tendons and ligaments having a moderate ρ_m and a short-T_2. These tissues are subject to the magic angle effect whereby the T_2 of the tissue varies widely with the orientation of fibers to B_0 [18]. Values, when the fibers are parallel to B_0, may be short (e.g., <5 ms), but when fibers are at, or near, the magic angle (about 55°) to B_0, T_2s are longer (e.g., 15–30 ms) [19]. This normal increase in T_2 may be much greater than the increases in T_2 produced by disease.

While backbone protons in collagen and other macromolecules (T_2s about 10 μs or less) are not directly detectable with conventional MRI and UTE sequences [20], water bound to collagen has a longer T_2 and this may be detectable as collagen-bound water and act as a surrogate for tissues of interest such as the matrix itself [21–23].

Myelin is an example of a tissue component that has a specific ultrashort-T_2 of about 0.2 ms [24–26], allowing it to be detected with UTE sequences even though it is present in much lower concentration than water in both white and gray matter of the brain.

Change in TPs in Disease

ρ_m changes are generally much less than those in T_1 and T_2 although in some situations they can be the dominant effect [1]. The most common TP change in disease in clinical practice is an increase in T_1 and T_2. This occurs in infarction, inflammation, infection, edema, and tumors. The reverse change of a decrease in T_1 and T_2 occurs in stages of hemorrhage, as well as with iron and other paramagnetic accumulation.

Diffusion is increased in many diseases but in some acute diseases, including infarction and infection, diffusion is decreased. It is also decreased in many tumors.

Changes in TPs with Contrast Agents

Clinical Gadolinium-based contrast agents (GBCAs) are paramagnetic and decrease T$_1$, T$_2$, and T$_2$* [27]. This effect increases with concentration. The effect is opposite to the increase in T$_1$ and T$_2$ produced by many diseases, and the two effects may cancel out, particularly at low concentrations of GBCAs.

Approaches to Imaging and Quantitation of Short-, Ultrashort- and Supershort-T$_2$ Tissues

The clinical approach to studying short-, ultrashort-, and supershort-T$_2$ tissues follows from a knowledge of their TPs [1–3].

The first part of the book describes various data acquisition strategies that can detect signal from short- and ultrashort-T$_2$ tissues of interest. The working rule is that the effective TE of the sequence should be of the same order as that of the T$_2$ of the tissue of interest. Data acquisition strategies, including SPRITE [9], 2D UTE [5], 3D UTE [28], ZTE [16], PETRA [14], RHE [15], AWSOS [13], vTE [10], and Looping Star [17], are described in detail.

The second part of the book deals with tissue contrast and, in particular, techniques to render abnormalities visible on images. This work is concerned with detecting wanted signals and suppressing unwanted signals from intermediate and long-T$_2$ water and fat tissues or tissue components. The contrast mechanisms include UTE with subtraction [29], long-T$_2$ saturation [30], adiabatic inversion recovery (IR) based techniques [5, 6], water excitation [31], water/fat separation [32, 33], UTE spectroscopic imaging (UTESI) [34], phase imaging [35], chemical shift artifacts [36], TP-filters [1], and multiplied, added, subtracted, and/or divided inversion recovery (MASDIR) [3]. Techniques may be used both for sensitivity to detect abnormalities, in general, and for specificity to show a particular tissue component (e.g., bound water in bone and myelin in white matter).

The third part of the book is on quantitation. This involves the two previous sections of signal acquisition and suppression of unwanted signals and adds to them modeling for different TPs and techniques to measure them accurately and consistently. This section covers quantitative MRI techniques, including UTE-based T$_1$ [37, 38], T$_2$* [39], T$_{1\rho}$ [40–42], mobile proton density [43–46], MT [47], susceptibility [48–50], perfusion [51–53], diffusion [54, 55], and deep learning methods [56].

The fourth part of the book is on clinical applications, which include the use of data acquisitions, contrast mechanisms for visualization of abnormalities, and quantitation for determining their extent as well as showing and characterizing disease, particularly where it is not recognizable using qualitative image assessment. Changes in short- and ultrashort-T$_2$ tissues can be evaluated with UTE-type sequences, which may have critical applications in the musculoskeletal (e.g., osteoarthritis (OA) [57], osteoporosis (OP) [43], tendinopathy [58], hemophilia arthropathy (HA) [59], rotator cuff injury [60], TMD [61], and spine degeneration [62]), as well as in the nervous (e.g., multiple sclerosis (MS) [63]), respiratory (e.g., lung diseases [64]), and gastrointestinal systems (e.g., liver iron overload [65]). MR-based attenuation correction and the silent feature of ZTE-type sequences are also discussed in this section.

Data Acquisitions

These are directly related to MR machine performance. Major considerations are static field strength (B_0), gradient strength, and slew rate, as well as RF strength (B_1 field strength). Clinical systems are generally at a major disadvantage compared with high field-small-bore systems used for small animal studies and microscopy. There are also safety constraints applicable to in vivo studies.

From a clinical point of view, the common conventional acquisitions, such as GE, SE, fast spin echo (FSE), and Dixon, are widely available and have been in clinical use for over 30 years. With improved gradient performance, the minimum TE available with these sequences in clinical applications has become shorter. The specific sequences used for short- and ultrashort-T$_2$ studies are broadly divided into four main groups: SPI where a single k-space point is acquired after each short RF excitation [8], UTE where the RF pulse is applied initially, and gradients are enabled after this [5], ZTE where gradients are initially enabled and the RF pulse is applied after this [16], and vTE where shorter TEs are used at the center of k-space with small phase encoding gradients [10]. With the ZTE approach, there is a period after the center of the RF pulse and before the receiver is enabled where data is not detectable, and this leaves a central area of k-space that must be filled by some other means. The vTE sequence uses a conventional acquisition but variable phase encoding durations. Other data acquisition strategies, including SPRITE [9], Cones [66], PETRA [14], RHE [15], AWSOS [13], and Looping Star [17], are similar to or hybrid combinations of the above four groups.

Once data acquisition is enabled, acquisition then proceeds with radial mapping of k-space, or a variant of this, from the center (or close to it with ZTE) outwards to allow acquisition of central or mainly central data in k-space before the received signal decays to very low levels. Variants of these approaches and combinations of them are used to address specific issues.

Contrast Mechanisms

The acquisitions can be classified and related to the types of tissue from which they can detect signal. Important to this is: (1) developing contrast between normal and abnormal tissues in the short- and ultrashort-T_2 domains, and (2) suppressing unwanted signals from intermediate and long-T_2 water and fat. This involves consideration of pulse sequence preparations, acquisitions, and basic image processing techniques such as addition, subtraction, and division of acquired images [1–3].

Inversion pulses fully invert intermediate and long-T_2 tissues where T_2s are much longer than the duration of the pulse (i.e., much longer than about 8 ms). However, this is not the case for short- or ultrashort-T_2 tissues where transverse magnetization decays during the inversion pulse, so that their longitudinal magnetizations are only partially inverted or are saturated during the inversion pulse. As a result, the inversion pulse can be a source of T_2 contrast, particularly when it is coupled with an inversion time (TI) chosen to null the signal from intermediate or long-T_2 components [6]. When linked with UTE or ZTE acquisition, this then provides images in which short-T_2 tissues show high signal, and long-T_2 tissues show low or zero signal. This is the reverse of the pattern seen with conventional T_2-weighted SE sequences.

Subtraction of a longer TE image from a shorter one is another method of suppressing or reducing unwanted signals from intermediate or long-T_2 components [29]. Long-T_2 saturation [30], off-resonance saturation [67], water excitation [31], fat/water separation [32, 33], spectroscopic imaging [34], and phase imaging [35] can also be used to create short-T_2 contrast.

Adiabatic IR-based sequences can be combined in the form of MASDIR sequences, and these provide additional options for developing and increasing contrast [3]. It is possible to develop synergistic contrast where a single TP such as T_1 and T_2 is used twice or more in one sequence to increase contrast, and/or two or more TPs are used in the same sequence for the same purpose [1–3]. These techniques can also be used with high signal suppression (e.g., for intermediate or long-T_2 water and fat-containing tissues) and are able to substantially increase contrast.

Quantitation

Many of the requirements for quantitation follow from consideration of the TPs of the tissues of interest. If there are a majority of short-T_2 components, a single exponential T_2 decay may be an adequate model, but if short- or ultrashort-T_2 tissues are in a minority, long-T_2 signal suppression or biexponential modeling may be required [6].

Fat may be a significant source of signal contamination and particular techniques suited to the tissue of interest (e.g., with susceptibility differences in trabecular bone) are needed to achieve effective fat suppression and accurate quantitation [36].

A combination of signal suppression techniques may be more effective than one alone, and MT modeling may be necessary with acquisitions specifically designed to acquire data for the model [47].

Quantitation techniques can be broadly divided into two categories: relaxometry including UTE-based T_1 [37, 38], T_2^* [39], $T_{1\rho}$ [40–42], and T_2 mapping; and other tissue properties including mobile proton density [43–46], MT ratio (MTR) [68], MT modeling of macromolecular proton fraction (MMF) [47], susceptibility [48–50], perfusion [51–53], and diffusion mapping [54, 55].

Quantitation usually requires specific techniques in order to achieve accuracy and consistency rather than just performing quantitation as a spin-off from sequences used for morphological purposes. This may require additional time, but in some circumstances (e.g., bone densitometry) it may be the only type of acquisition needed.

Clinical Applications

These often follow from general considerations about what is needed clinically, what is available with other MR techniques, other imaging modalities, and other investigative techniques.

Clinical work on short- and ultrashort-T_2 tissues began with the lung [4], but motion and the effectiveness of high-resolution breath-hold CT have meant that lung imaging has been a relatively small application for UTE- and ZTE-based techniques.

The short- and ultrashort-T_2 tissues in the musculoskeletal (MSK) system followed, and this has been a productive area with studies on all the major MSK tissues [5, 69]. UTE-type imaging of both long- and short-T_2 tissues makes it possible for a "whole-organ" disease approach, thereby improving the diagnosis of various MSK diseases such as OA [57], OP [43], tendinopathy [58], HA [59], rotator cuff injury [60], temporomandibular disease (TMD) [61], and spine degeneration [62].

The specific MR properties of myelin (T$_2 \approx 0.2$ ms) and its clinical significance have meant that the brain has been an important target, too [63]. Given the essential role of myelin in developing and maintaining elaborate cognitive functions, direct imaging of myelin may help understand the pathogenesis of many neurological diseases, such as MS, Alzheimer's disease (AD), Parkinson's disease (PD), traumatic brain injury (TBI), and epilepsy.

Accumulation of T$_2$-shortening iron has led to specific disease-related applications in hemophilia [59], thalassemia [70], and liver iron overload [65]. There are short- and ultrashort-T$_2$ components in many other tissues and organs that have yet to be studied in detail.

Other applications such as iron-labeled stem cell tracking [71], temperature mapping [72], and treatment monitoring remain to be systematically investigated.

Key Concepts

Listed below are some key concepts which help in understanding MRI of short- and ultrashort-T$_2$ tissues:

1. The name TE is often a misnomer since frequently no echo is acquired since the acquisition is a free induction decay (FID), but the concept of TE is used descriptively because it does provide a guide to contrast.
2. The definition of TE, including the timing from when it starts and when it finishes, has been the subject of debate. With UTE sequences, the effective starting point for measuring TE varies with T$_2$. The end of TE is usually taken as the time when acquisition starts, usually at the center of k-space.
3. Short-T$_2$ tissues can be divided into two major categories: (a) those with a majority of short- and/or ultrashort-T$_2$ tissues (e.g., bone, menisci, ligaments, and tendons), and (b) those with a minority of short- and/or ultrashort-T$_2$ tissues (e.g., trabecular bone and myelin). Generally, the latter group is much more challenging for selective imaging. Special considerations are needed to minimize signal contamination from long-T$_2$ water and fat when imaging these tissues.
4. Collagen is ubiquitous and in highly ordered form may produce magic angle effects. Water bound to collagen may be imaged rather than collagen itself as collagen backbone protons have T$_2$s that are too short for direct UTE or ZTE imaging [20].
5. Magic angle effects are major confounding factors in both morphological imaging and quantitative assessment of short-T$_2$ relaxation times and tissue properties [6, 18, 73].

6. The concept of ρ_m incorporates the idea of short-, ultrashort-, and supershort-T$_2$s ("invisible") which are not detectable with the acquisition in use.
7. Short-T$_2$ components typically have short T$_1$s, facilitating direct UTE imaging which otherwise may be challenging due to their usually lower ρ_ms than surrounding or associated long-T$_2$ tissues.
8. Phase imaging is an important source of contrast and typically requires relatively long TEs for appreciable phase evolution. Phase contrast can be generated for collagen-rich short-T$_2$ tissues associated with orientation-dependent frequency and phase shifts. Phase differences accrue in short- and ultrashort-T$_2$ tissues during the RF excitation and data acquisition portion of UTE imaging.
9. Data acquisition can be basically subdivided into SPI, UTE, ZTE, and vTE groups or a hybrid combination depending on the order of the RF pulse and gradient activation k-space mapping for the center of k-space.
10. The ZTE sequence applies RF excitation and data acquisition after setting the radial encoding gradients [16]. It effectively copes with rapidly decaying signals because it encodes fresh transverse magnetization immediately at full k-space speed and with zero signal delay (see Chap. 5, "Zero Echo Time (ZTE) MRI").
11. Inversion pulses can be used to create T$_2$ and T$_1$ contrast. The inversion and nulling of long-T$_2$ magnetization highly depend on T$_1$ relaxation as well as the choice of TR and TI, creating T$_1$-dependent contrast. Meanwhile, fast transverse relaxation during an adiabatic hyperbolic secant pulse can forestall complete inversion of the longitudinal magnetization but partial inversion or saturation of short-T$_2$ tissues, creating T$_2$-dependent contrast.
12. Echo subtraction suppresses long T$_2$ components and reverses T$_2$ contrast. Short-T$_2$ contrast is acquired by subtracting a second echo image from a first echo image which is equivalent to T$_2$ bandpass filtering.
13. Multiple IR sequences can be combined for improved long-T$_2$ signal suppression. The dual or double adiabatic inversion pulses allow more accurate nulling of long-T$_2$ water and fat signals by considering their significant differences in T$_1$s, thereby creating much improved short-T$_2$ contrast.
14. Synergistic contrast is valuable for short-T$_2$ tissues by combining a single and/or two or more different TPs to suppress unwanted high signals from long-T$_2$ components. It can be used to increase sensitivity and/or specificity in short- and ultrashort-T$_2$ tissues.
15. High T$_2$ contrast is possible with UTE and ZTE acquisitions in spite of their ultrashort TEs. Echo subtraction (i.e., shorter TE filter minus longer TE filter) leads to reversal of the sign of short-T$_2$ tissues, producing overall synergistic positive T$_2$ contrast.

16. UTE-type sequences can directly image nonaqueous myelin protons with ultrashort-T_2^*s of ~0.2 ms. Adiabatic IR-based techniques, especially the STAIR-UTE approach, allow efficient suppression of various water components and thereby facilitate robust mapping of myelin density and relaxation times (e.g., T_1 and T_2^*).

17. Short-T_2 imaging is subject to various artifacts related to chemical shift, susceptibility, long-T_2 signal contamination, and motion. Center-out radial or spiral mapping of k-space leads to off-resonance artifacts manifested as spatial blurring due to the ring-shaped point spread function. Partial volume and long-T_2 signal contamination may significantly affect short-T_2 quantification. UTE imaging is generally less sensitive to motion artifacts due to averaging of central k-space data.

18. Fat signal suppression and separation are critically important. Short-T_2 signal is typically much lower than fat signal if unsuppressed. Fat contamination and related off-resonance artifacts are potential sources of error with UTE imaging and can significantly affect the quantification of MR relaxation times and tissue properties.

19. Short-T_2 imaging is typically associated with spatial blurring and low signal because of the fast signal decay during data sampling and the relatively low ρ_ms of many tissues of interest. A short sampling window helps to minimize spatial blurring.

20. ZTE images are generally less blurry than UTE images. Stronger RF and gradient systems are expected to benefit all UTE-type sequences.

21. Quantitation of short- and ultrashort-T_2 tissues requires consideration of fast relaxation during RF excitation, spatial encoding, magnetization preparation, B_1 and B_0 inhomogeneities, chemical shift artifacts, and long-T_2 signal contamination.

22. Higher RF power and stronger gradient systems allow more accurate quantification of short- and ultrashort-T_2 tissues. Often effective long-T_2 signal suppression is necessary to avoid signal contamination and obtain accurate measurements for short-T_2 components such as the osteochondral junction, the cartilaginous endplate, trabecular bone, and myelin.

23. UTE type sequences allow mapping of T_1, T_2, $T_{1\rho}$, and T_2^* for bone, deep cartilage, menisci, ligaments, tendons, lung, iron overload, and myelin, making it possible to evaluate these TPs in clinically "invisible" short- and ultrashort-T_2 tissues.

24. Macromolecular fraction and exchange information in bone and other short-T_2 tissues can be derived through UTE-based MT modeling.

25. Relatively fiber orientation-independent biomarkers including UTE-MT modeling of MMF [74] and UTE-AdiabT$_{1\rho}$ [75] are likely more effective than traditional T_2, $T_{1\rho}$, and T_2^* mapping in evaluating degeneration of collagenous short-T_2 tissues.

26. The range of clinical applications of short- and ultrashort-T_2 imaging includes musculoskeletal (OA, OP, HA, TMD, tendinopathy, spine degeneration, etc.), nervous (MS, AD, PD, TBI, epilepsy, etc.), respiratory (lung fibrosis, etc.), and gastrointestinal diseases (liver iron overload, etc.). Other applications include PET-MRI attenuation correction, iron-labeled stem cell tracking, temperature mapping, and treatment monitoring.

Conclusion

This introductory chapter has provided background and a structure for understanding the imaging of short- and ultrashort-T_2 tissues. The book is designed to provide: (1) an overview of techniques and applications for those new to the field, (2) an introduction to the achievements of those active in the field, (3) an update on current concepts, and (4) an outline of current clinical work. It also provides a summary of over 20 years' work, often written by those who originated the advances they describe and those who performed the initial clinical studies.

References

1. Young IR, Szeverenyi NM, Du J, Bydder GM. Pulse sequences as tissue property filters (TP-filters): a way of understanding the signal, contrast and weighting of magnetic resonance images. Quant Imaging Med Surg. 2020;10(5):1080–120.
2. Ma YJ, Shao H, Fan S, Lu X, Du J, Young IR, et al. New options for increasing the sensitivity, specificity and scope of synergistic contrast magnetic resonance imaging (scMRI) using Multiplied, Added, Subtracted and/or FiTted (MASTIR) pulse sequences. Quant Imaging Med Surg. 2020;10(10):2030–65.
3. Ma YJ, Moazamian D, Cornfeld DM, Condron P, Holdsworth SJ, Bydder M, et al. Improving the understanding and performance of clinical MRI using tissue property filters and the central contrast theorem, MASDIR pulse sequences and synergistic contrast MRI. Quant Imaging Med Surg. 2022;12(9):4658–90.
4. Bergin CJ, Pauly JM, Macovski A. Lung parenchyma: projection reconstruction MR imaging. Radiology. 1991;179(3):777–81.
5. Robson MD, Gatehouse PD, Bydder M, Bydder GM. Magnetic resonance: an introduction to ultrashort TE (UTE) imaging. J Comput Assist Tomogr. 2003;27(6):825–46.
6. Ma Y, Jang H, Jerban S, Chang EY, Chung CB, Bydder GM, et al. Making the invisible visible-ultrashort echo time magnetic resonance imaging: technical developments and applications. Appl Phys Rev. 2022;9(4):041303.
7. Henkelman RM, Huang X, Xiang QS, Stanisz GJ, Swanson SD, Bronskill MJ. Quantitative interpretation of magnetization transfer. Magn Reson Med. 1993;29(6):759–66.
8. Beyea SD, Balcom BJ, Prado PJ, Cross AR, Kennedy CB, Armstrong RL, et al. Relaxation time mapping of short T*₂ nuclei with single-point imaging (SPI) methods. J Magn Reson. 1998;135(1):156–64.

9. Balcom BJ, Macgregor RP, Beyea SD, Green DP, Armstrong RL, Bremner TW. Single-point ramped imaging with T$_1$ enhancement (SPRITE). J Magn Reson A. 1996;123(1):131–4.

10. Deligianni X, Bar P, Scheffler K, Trattnig S, Bieri O. High-resolution Fourier-encoded sub-millisecond echo time musculoskeletal imaging at 3 Tesla and 7 Tesla. Magn Reson Med. 2013;70(5):1434–9.

11. Wu Y, Chesler DA, Glimcher MJ, Garrido L, Wang J, Jiang HJ, et al. Multinuclear solid-state three-dimensional MRI of bone and synthetic calcium phosphates. Proc Natl Acad Sci U S A. 1999;96(4):1574–8.

12. Idiyatullin D, Corum C, Park JY, Garwood M. Fast and quiet MRI using a swept radiofrequency. J Magn Reson. 2006;181(2):342–9.

13. Qian Y, Williams AA, Chu CR, Boada FE. High-resolution ultrashort echo time (UTE) imaging on human knee with AWSOS sequence at 3.0 T. J Magn Reson Imaging. 2012;35(1):204–10.

14. Grodzki DM, Jakob PM, Heismann B. Ultrashort echo time imaging using pointwise encoding time reduction with radial acquisition (PETRA). Magn Reson Med. 2012;67(2):510–8.

15. Jang H, Wiens CN, McMillan AB. Ramped hybrid encoding for improved ultrashort echo time imaging. Magn Reson Med. 2016;76(3):814–25.

16. Weiger M, Pruessmann KP, Hennel F. MRI with zero echo time: hard versus sweep pulse excitation. Magn Reson Med. 2011;66(2):379–89.

17. Wiesinger F, Menini A, Solana AB. Looping star. Magn Reson Med. 2019;81(1):57–68.

18. Bydder M, Rahal A, Fullerton GD, Bydder GM. The magic angle effect: a source of artifact, determinant of image contrast, and technique for imaging. J Magn Reson Imaging. 2007;25(2):290–300.

19. Du J, Pak BC, Znamirowski R, Statum S, Takahashi A, Chung CB, et al. Magic angle effect in magnetic resonance imaging of the Achilles tendon and enthesis. Magn Reson Imaging. 2009;27(4):557–64.

20. Ma YJ, Chang EY, Bydder GM, Du J. Can ultrashort-TE (UTE) MRI sequences on a 3-T clinical scanner detect signal directly from collagen protons: freeze-dry and D$_2$O exchange studies of cortical bone and Achilles tendon specimens. NMR Biomed. 2016;29(7):912–7.

21. Horch RA, Gochberg DF, Nyman JS, Does MD. Clinically compatible MRI strategies for discriminating bound and pore water in cortical bone. Magn Reson Med. 2012;68(6):1774–84.

22. Biswas R, Bae W, Diaz E, Masuda K, Chung CB, Bydder GM, et al. Ultrashort echo time (UTE) imaging with bi-component analysis: bound and free water evaluation of bovine cortical bone subject to sequential drying. Bone. 2012;50(3):749–55.

23. Du J, Bydder GM. Qualitative and quantitative ultrashort-TE MRI of cortical bone. NMR Biomed. 2013;26(5):489–506.

24. Sheth V, Shao H, Chen J, Vandenberg S, Corey-Bloom J, Bydder GM, et al. Magnetic resonance imaging of myelin using ultrashort Echo time (UTE) pulse sequences: phantom, specimen, volunteer and multiple sclerosis patient studies. NeuroImage. 2016;136:37–44.

25. Fan SJ, Ma Y, Zhu Y, Searleman A, Szeverenyi NM, Bydder GM, et al. Yet more evidence that myelin protons can be directly imaged with UTE sequences on a clinical 3T scanner: bicomponent T$_2$* analysis of native and deuterated ovine brain specimens. Magn Reson Med. 2018;80(2):538–47.

26. Ma YJ, Jang H, Wei Z, Cai Z, Xue Y, Lee RR, et al. Myelin imaging in human brain using a short repetition time adiabatic inversion recovery prepared ultrashort echo time (STAIR-UTE) MRI sequence in multiple sclerosis. Radiology. 2020;297(2):392–404.

27. Carr DH, Brown J, Bydder GM, Steiner RE, Weinmann HJ, Speck U, et al. Gadolinium-DTPA as a contrast agent in MRI: initial clinical experience in 20 patients. AJR Am J Roentgenol. 1984;143(2):215–24.

28. Rahmer J, Bornert P, Groen J, Bos C. Three-dimensional radial ultrashort echo-time imaging with T$_2$ adapted sampling. Magn Reson Med. 2006;55(5):1075–82.

29. Du J, Bydder M, Takahashi AM, Carl M, Chung CB, Bydder GM. Short T$_2$ contrast with three-dimensional ultrashort echo time imaging. Magn Reson Imaging. 2011;29(4):470–82.

30. Larson PE, Gurney PT, Nayak K, Gold GE, Pauly JM, Nishimura DG. Designing long-T$_2$ suppression pulses for ultrashort echo time imaging. Magn Reson Med. 2006;56(1):94–103.

31. Ma YJ, Jerban S, Jang H, Chang EY, Du J. Fat suppression for ultrashort echo time imaging using a novel soft-hard composite radiofrequency pulse. Magn Reson Med. 2019;82(6):2178–87.

32. Kronthaler S, Boehm C, Feuerriegel G, Bornert P, Katscher U, Weiss K, et al. Assessment of vertebral fractures and edema of the thoracolumbar spine based on water-fat and susceptibility-weighted images derived from a single ultra-short echo time scan. Magn Reson Med. 2022;87(4):1771–83.

33. Jang H, Carl M, Ma Y, Jerban S, Guo T, Zhao W, et al. Fat suppression for ultrashort echo time imaging using a single-point Dixon method. NMR Biomed. 2019;32(5):e4069.

34. Du J, Hamilton G, Takahashi A, Bydder M, Chung CB. Ultrashort echo time spectroscopic imaging (UTESI) of cortical bone. Magn Reson Med. 2007;58(5):1001–9.

35. Carl M, Chiang JT. Investigations of the origin of phase differences seen with ultrashort TE imaging of short T$_2$ meniscal tissue. Magn Reson Med. 2012;67(4):991–1003.

36. Bydder M, Carl M, Bydder GM, Du J. MRI chemical shift artifact produced by center-out radial sampling of k-space: a potential pitfall in clinical diagnosis. Quant Imaging Med Surg. 2021;11(8):3677–83.

37. Ma YJ, Lu X, Carl M, Zhu Y, Szeverenyi NM, Bydder GM, et al. Accurate T(1) mapping of short T(2) tissues using a three-dimensional ultrashort echo time cones actual flip angle imaging-variable repetition time (3D UTE-Cones AFI-VTR) method. Magn Reson Med. 2018;80(2):598–608.

38. Ma YJ, Zhao W, Wan L, Guo T, Searleman A, Jang H, et al. Whole knee joint T(1) values measured in vivo at 3T by combined 3D ultrashort echo time cones actual flip angle and variable flip angle methods. Magn Reson Med. 2019;81(3):1634–44.

39. Williams A, Qian Y, Golla S, Chu CR. UTE-T$_2$* mapping detects sub-clinical meniscus injury after anterior cruciate ligament tear. Osteoarthr Cartil. 2012;20(6):486–94.

40. Du J, Carl M, Diaz E, Takahashi A, Han E, Szeverenyi NM, et al. Ultrashort TE T$_1$rho (UTE T$_1$rho) imaging of the Achilles tendon and meniscus. Magn Reson Med. 2010;64(3):834–42.

41. Ma YJ, Carl M, Shao H, Tadros AS, Chang EY, Du J. Three-dimensional ultrashort echo time cones T($_1$rho) (3D UTE-cones-T($_1$rho)) imaging. NMR Biomed. 2017;30(6):3709.

42. Ma YJ, Carl M, Searleman A, Lu X, Chang EY, Du J. 3D adiabatic T($_1$rho) prepared ultrashort echo time cones sequence for whole knee imaging. Magn Reson Med. 2018;80(4):1429–39.

43. Li C, Seifert AC, Rad HS, Bhagat YA, Rajapakse CS, Sun W, et al. Cortical bone water concentration: dependence of MR imaging measures on age and pore volume fraction. Radiology. 2014;272(3):796–806.

44. Manhard MK, Horch RA, Gochberg DF, Nyman JS, Does MD. In vivo quantitative MR imaging of bound and pore water in cortical bone. Radiology. 2015;277(3):221–9.

45. Jerban S, Ma Y, Li L, Jang H, Wan L, Guo T, et al. Volumetric mapping of bound and pore water as well as collagen protons in cortical bone using 3D ultrashort echo time cones MR imaging techniques. Bone. 2019;127:120–8.

46. Ma YJ, Jang H, Wei Z, Wu M, Chang EY, Corey-Bloom J, et al. Brain ultrashort T(2) component imaging using a short TR adiabatic inversion recovery prepared dual-echo ultrashort TE sequence

with complex echo subtraction (STAIR-dUTE-ES). J Magn Reson. 2021;323:106898.

47. Ma YJ, Chang EY, Carl M, Du J. Quantitative magnetization transfer ultrashort echo time imaging using a time-efficient 3D multi-spoke Cones sequence. Magn Reson Med. 2018;79(2):692–700.

48. Dimov AV, Liu Z, Spincemaille P, Prince MR, Du J, Wang Y. Bone quantitative susceptibility mapping using a chemical species-specific R_2* signal model with ultrashort and conventional echo data. Magn Reson Med. 2018;79(1):121–8.

49. Jang H, Lu X, Carl M, Searleman AC, Jerban S, Ma Y, et al. True phase quantitative susceptibility mapping using continuous single-point imaging: a feasibility study. Magn Reson Med. 2019;81(3):1907–14.

50. Jerban S, Lu X, Jang H, Ma Y, Namiranian B, Le N, et al. Significant correlations between human cortical bone mineral density and quantitative susceptibility mapping (QSM) obtained with 3D Cones ultrashort echo time magnetic resonance imaging (UTE-MRI). Magn Reson Imaging. 2019;62:104–10.

51. Robson MD, Gatehouse PD, So PW, Bell JD, Bydder GM. Contrast enhancement of short T_2 tissues using ultrashort TE (UTE) pulse sequences. Clin Radiol. 2004;59(8):720–6.

52. Gatehouse PD, He T, Puri BK, Thomas RD, Resnick D, Bydder GM. Contrast-enhanced MRI of the menisci of the knee using ultrashort echo time (UTE) pulse sequences: imaging of the red and white zones. Br J Radiol. 2004;77(920):641–7.

53. Wan L, Wu M, Sheth V, Shao H, Jang H, Bydder G, et al. Evaluation of cortical bone perfusion using dynamic contrast enhanced ultrashort echo time imaging: a feasibility study. Quant Imaging Med Surg. 2019;9(8):1383–93.

54. Chaudhari AS, Sveinsson B, Moran CJ, McWalter EJ, Johnson EM, Zhang T, et al. Imaging and T(2) relaxometry of short-T(2) connective tissues in the knee using ultrashort echo-time double-echo steady-state (UTEDESS). Magn Reson Med. 2017;78(6):2136–48.

55. Jang H, Ma Y, Carl M, Jerban S, Chang EY, Du J. Ultrashort echo time Cones double echo steady state (UTE-Cones-DESS) for rapid morphological imaging of short T(2) tissues. Magn Reson Med. 2021;86(2):881–92.

56. Xue YP, Jang H, Byra M, Cai ZY, Wu M, Chang EY, et al. Automated cartilage segmentation and quantification using 3D ultrashort echo time (UTE) cones MR imaging with deep convolutional neural networks. Eur Radiol. 2021;31(10):7653–63.

57. Chu CR, Williams AA, West RV, Qian Y, Fu FH, Do BH, et al. Quantitative magnetic resonance imaging UTE-T_2* mapping of cartilage and meniscus healing after anatomic anterior cruciate ligament reconstruction. Am J Sports Med. 2014;42(8):1847–56.

58. Breda SJ, Oei EHG, Zwerver J, Visser E, Waarsing E, Krestin GP, et al. Effectiveness of progressive tendon-loading exercise therapy in patients with patellar tendinopathy: a randomised clinical trial. Br J Sports Med. 2021;55(9):501–9.

59. Jang H, von Drygalski A, Wong J, Zhou JY, Aguero P, Lu X, et al. Ultrashort echo time quantitative susceptibility mapping (UTE-QSM) for detection of hemosiderin deposition in hemophilic arthropathy: a feasibility study. Magn Reson Med. 2020;84(6):3246–55.

60. Ashir A, Ma Y, Jerban S, Jang H, Wei Z, Le N, et al. Rotator cuff tendon assessment in symptomatic and control groups using quantitative MRI. J Magn Reson Imaging. 2020;52(3):864–72.

61. Sanal HT, Bae WC, Pauli C, Du J, Statum S, Znamirowski R, et al. Magnetic resonance imaging of the temporomandibular joint disc: feasibility of novel quantitative magnetic resonance evaluation using histologic and biomechanical reference standards. J Orofac Pain. 2011;25(4):345–53.

62. Fields AJ, Han M, Krug R, Lotz JC. Cartilaginous end plates: quantitative MR imaging with very short echo times-orientation dependence and correlation with biochemical composition. Radiology. 2015;274(2):482–9.

63. Waldman A, Rees JH, Brock CS, Robson MD, Gatehouse PD, Bydder GM. MRI of the brain with ultra-short echo-time pulse sequences. Neuroradiology. 2003;45(12):887–92.

64. Burris NS, Johnson KM, Larson PE, Hope MD, Nagle SK, Behr SC, et al. Detection of small pulmonary nodules with ultrashort echo time sequences in oncology patients by using a PET/MR system. Radiology. 2016;278(1):239–46.

65. Krafft AJ, Loeffler RB, Song R, Tipirneni-Sajja A, McCarville MB, Robson MD, et al. Quantitative ultrashort echo time imaging for assessment of massive iron overload at 1.5 and 3 Tesla. Magn Reson Med. 2017;78(5):1839–51.

66. Gurney PT, Hargreaves BA, Nishimura DG. Design and analysis of a practical 3D cones trajectory. Magn Reson Med. 2006;55(3):575–82.

67. Du J, Takahashi AM, Bydder M, Chung CB, Bydder GM. Ultrashort TE imaging with off-resonance saturation contrast (UTE-OSC). Magn Reson Med. 2009;62(2):527–31.

68. Springer F, Martirosian P, Machann J, Schwenzer NF, Claussen CD, Schick F. Magnetization transfer contrast imaging in bovine and human cortical bone applying an ultrashort echo time sequence at 3 Tesla. Magn Reson Med. 2009;61(5):1040–8.

69. Afsahi AM, Ma Y, Jang H, Jerban S, Chung CB, Chang EY, et al. Ultrashort echo time magnetic resonance imaging techniques: met and unmet needs in musculoskeletal imaging. J Magn Reson Imaging. 2022;55(6):1597–612.

70. Hall-Craggs MA, Porter J, Gatehouse PD, Bydder GM. Ultrashort echo time (UTE) MRI of the spine in thalassaemia. Br J Radiol. 2004;77(914):104–10.

71. Kaggie JD, Markides H, Graves MJ, MacKay J, Houston G, El Haj A, et al. Ultra short echo time MRI of iron-labelled mesenchymal stem cells in an ovine osteochondral defect model. Sci Rep. 2020;10(1):8451.

72. Butts K, Sinclair J, Daniel BL, Wansapura J, Pauly JM. Temperature quantitation and mapping of frozen tissue. J Magn Reson Imaging. 2001;13(1):99–104.

73. Du J, Statum S, Znamirowski R, Bydder GM, Chung CB. Ultrashort TE T1rho magic angle imaging. Magn Reson Med. 2013;69(3):682–7.

74. Ma YJ, Shao H, Du J, Chang EY. Ultrashort echo time magnetization transfer (UTE-MT) imaging and modeling: magic angle independent biomarkers of tissue properties. NMR Biomed. 2016;29(11):1546–52.

75. Wu M, Ma YJ, Kasibhatla A, Chen M, Jang H, Jerban S, et al. Convincing evidence for magic angle less-sensitive quantitative T(1rho) imaging of articular cartilage using the 3D ultrashort echo time cones adiabatic T(1rho) (3D UTE cones-AdiabT(1rho)) sequence. Magn Reson Med. 2020;84(5):2551–60.

Single-Point Ramped Imaging with T$_1$ Enhancement (SPRITE)

Dan Xiao and Layale Bazzi

Introduction

Single-point ramped imaging with T$_1$ enhancement (SPRITE) [1] is best known in the magnetic resonance material science community where it is used for the study of porous media [2]. These show large susceptibility differences between solid matrix and the fluids in pore space which lead to very short signal lifetimes. SPRITE has been employed in the study of biomaterials [3], mummified human organs [4], in vivo animal imaging [5], myelin mapping [6], and in vivo sodium brain imaging [7, 8], as well as in electron paramagnetic resonance (EPR) imaging [9, 10].

SPRITE is a single-point imaging (SPI) technique that has a faster data acquisition than more traditional forms of SPI [11, 12]. The gradient switching and associated acoustic noise are much reduced with SPRITE. As a pure phase encoding method, SPRITE is largely immune to static magnetic field inhomogeneity since the signal evolution time is constant for all k-space points, and a very short encoding time is used.

Pulse Sequence

The SPRITE pulse sequence is shown in Fig. 2.1. The magnetic field gradient is switched on and stabilized before the radiofrequency (RF) pulse is applied. A single point in k-space is acquired after the short signal encoding time (T$_p$). The gradient is not turned off after data acquisition. This minimizes switching, which also passively spoils the transverse magnetization. At the end of TR, the gradient is ramped up or down to its next value. Additional spoiling gradients may be required around the k-space center. Any residual magnetization can also be removed by phase cycling [13]. SPRITE is a 3D imaging sequence.

D. Xiao (✉) · L. Bazzi
Department of Physics, University of Windsor,
Windsor, ON, Canada
e-mail: Dan.Xiao@uwindsor.ca

In frequency encoding schemes, k-space data is acquired at different signal evolution times, leading to a change in the amplitude and/or phase of the modulation transfer function (MTF). This may result in resolution loss and spatial misregistration, depending on the k-space trajectory, signal lifetime, and magnetic field offset. On the contrary, with pure phase encoding methods, all the k-space data points have the same signal evolution time T$_p$. The signal equation is then:

$$S(\vec{k}) = \int \rho(\vec{r}) e^{-i2\pi\vec{r}\cdot\vec{k}} e^{-\frac{T_p}{T_2^*(\vec{r})}} e^{-i\gamma\Delta B(\vec{r})T_p} d(\vec{r}), \qquad (2.1)$$

where $\rho(\vec{r})$ may include a T$_1$ relaxation term, which will be discussed below. $\Delta B(\vec{r})$ refers to the macroscopic magnetic field inhomogeneity that has a spatial variation on the scale of an image voxel. When microscopic magnetic field variation is significant, intravoxel dephasing leads to rapid signal decay, and the effect is expressed in T$_2^*$ attenuation. Because the T$_2^*$ and ΔB terms are not $\vec{k}$ dependent, this signal equation can be written as:

$$S(\vec{k}) = \int \hat{\rho}(\vec{r}) e^{-i2\pi\vec{r}\cdot\vec{k}} d(\vec{r}) \qquad (2.2)$$

where

$$\hat{\rho}(\vec{r}) = \rho(\vec{r}) e^{-\frac{T_p}{T_2^*(\vec{r})}} e^{-i\gamma\Delta B(\vec{r})T_p} \qquad (2.3)$$

T$_2^*$ is a contrast factor in the image, instead of a point spread function (PSF). Similarly, local phase evolution due to B_0 offset is consistent in all the k-space data points, leading to simple phase variation in the image. The true image resolution is not limited by the signal T$_2^*$, and static magnetic field inhomogeneity does not distort the image.

SPRITE is a powerful method when sources of severe magnetic field inhomogeneity are present, such as around metal [14, 15]. An example from Ref. [16] is shown in Fig. 2.2, where the SPRITE image (Fig. 2.2a) of a suspended titanium nut in a gel phantom is compared to a gradient recalled echo (GRE) image of the same nut (Fig. 2.2b). A 200 µs T$_p$ was used with SPRITE for an isotropic voxel of 1 mm^3. The minimum achievable GRE echo time (TE) for the given voxel size was 1.8 ms and this was

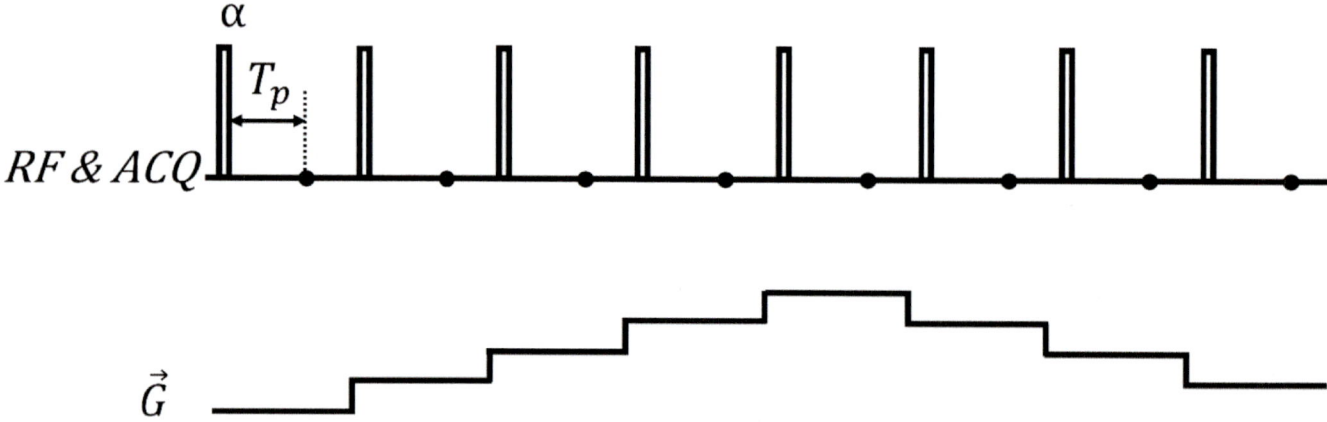

Fig. 2.1 SPRITE pulse sequence. A single point in *k*-space is acquired at the signal encoding time T_p after the RF pulse. At the end of TR, the gradient is ramped up or down to the next value

Fig. 2.2 A gel phantom with a suspended titanium nut imaged at 1 T with an isotropic voxel of 1 mm³. The distortion-free SPRITE ($T_p = 200 \mu s$) image (**a**) is compared with a GRE (TE = 1.8 ms) image (**b**) in which artifacts are obvious (arrows). Some signal enhancement was observed close to the metal in (**a**), but there is no geometric distortion. The magnetic field around the metal was mapped with multipoint SPRITE (**c**). Excellent agreement with the theoretical calculation in terms of the shape and magnitude of the distortion (**d**) was achieved. (Reproduced with permission from Ref. [16])

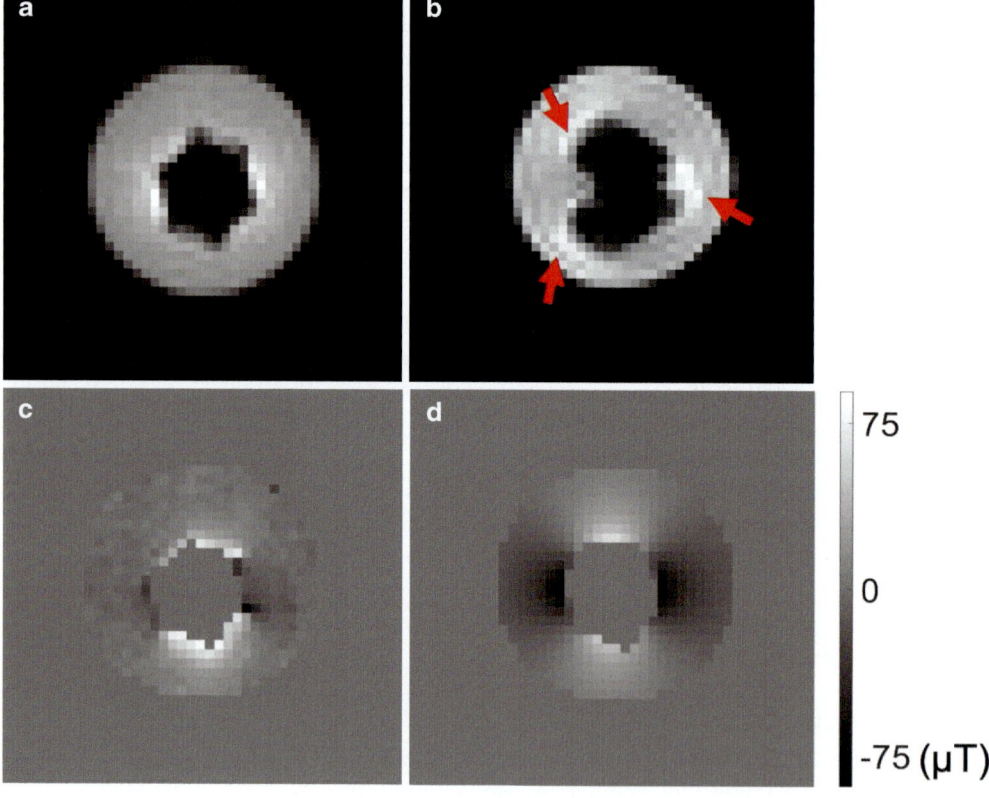

employed in Fig. 2.2b. Severe geometric distortion is observed in the GRE image where the hexagonal shape of the nut is not discernible. Intravoxel dephasing resulted in signal cancellation in regions close to the metal. Spatial misregistration also occurred in the frequency encoding direction as the magnetic field offset led to extra phase accrual during the data acquisition window. The SPRITE image (Fig. 2.2a) captured signals next to the metal. The image was free from geometric distortion due to the short and constant T_p. The image actually had an elevated intensity in regions close to the metal due to RF enhancement [17]. The robustness of SPRITE imaging has also been exploited to map B_1 fields near metal [18].

K-Space Trajectory

As a single-point imaging technique, the Cartesian *k*-space is traversed point by point, and the coverage is very flexible. The gradient can be stabilized for a relatively long period, of the order of milliseconds, before applying RF pulses, so there is virtually no constraint on the gradient slew rate and gradient waveform fidelity. SPRITE is very easy to implement in this respect. For a chosen T_p, the maximum *k* value is determined by the available gradient amplitude, which may be a limiting factor with some scanners.

The SPRITE k-space trajectory is defined in a nonconventional manner, where an interleaf or sector corresponds to a group of RF excitations. The interleaf can have a regular or irregular pattern. It is usually preferable to acquire a new data point in close proximity to the preceding k-space point within an interleaf, so that gradient switching is minimized. In principle, all the 3D k-space data can be acquired with a single interleaf.

The TR is usually much shorter than T_1. Without dummy cycles, saturation toward longitudinal steady state leads to an MTF that is determined by the k-space trajectory. Quantitative proton density-weighted imaging starts with an interleaf at the k-space center [19, 20], resulting in low-pass filtering of the k-space data. Signal-to-noise-ratio (SNR) is generally higher compared to other trajectories as the magnetization amplitude is highest at the k-space origin. The compromise is some loss of resolution. The width of the low-pass filter can be reduced by increasing TR, within the limit of acceptable gradient duty cycles. Reducing the excitation flip angle also leads to a narrower filter but with a decrease in the image SNR. A more practical approach is to use multiple shorter interleaves. A delay at the end of each interleaf for T_1 recovery also lowers the gradient duty cycle. Multiple-centric-interleaf acquisition is typical when magnetization preparation precedes the spatial encoding module as discussed below.

Alternatively, the trajectory can start at the periphery of k-space to maintain the image resolution, which is similar to applying dummy cycles. This leads to T_1 contrast and a reduced SNR.

Pure phase encoding is very compatible with k-space undersampling for accelerated data acquisition. It is trivial to execute an undersampling pattern that is incoherent in all dimensions [21, 22]. However, compressed sensing is not very commonly employed, as the SNR is usually not sufficient to support nonlinear image reconstruction. Signal averaging is often required in the most common SPRITE applications. Keyhole sampling [23, 24] has been applied to mitigate long scan times.

Multipoint Acquisition

In SPRITE, although only one point in k-space is acquired after the RF excitation, multiple time-domain points with increasing T_ps can be collected at virtually no additional cost. These points can be utilized to increase image resolution [25]. More often, multiple pure phase encoding images are reconstructed. The image FOV decreases with T_p after a simple inverse fast Fourier Transform (IFFT) and can be corrected by interpolation [26, 27]. These images can be summed to increase SNR. Alternatively, the image series can be analyzed to map the T_2^* [28, 29] and/or ΔB [16], based on Eq. (2.3).

Since the T_p can be very short and of the order of microseconds, severe magnetic field distortion $\Delta B(\vec{r})$ can be measured using the available gradient amplitude as long as the intravoxel dephasing does not lead to signal cancellation. Phase wrapping can be controlled by properly choosing the dwell time ΔT_p. An example of magnetic field mapping around metal is shown in Fig. 2.2c [16]. It was acquired with a range of T_ps between 200 and 300 μs. Excellent agreement is seen with the theoretical calculation shown in Fig. 2.2d, in terms of the shape and magnitude of the magnetic field distortion. Good quality field maps are only possible if images of all T_p values are distortion free. A similar principle has been applied to measure time-varying magnetic fields [30] and vocal fold oscillation [31] using pure phase encoded MRI.

Flip Angle and RF Power

The RF flip angle may affect resolution, contrast, and SNR, depending on the k-space trajectory. The use of the Ernst angle is generally preferred. SPRITE differs from frequency encoding methods in that the sample bandwidth varies with k-space values. To achieve a short T_p and/or high spatial resolution, very high-amplitude gradients may be required for k-space points in the periphery. The excitation bandwidth and receiver bandwidth in the multipoint acquisition scheme may only be sufficient for the central region of k-space, leading to additional filter and degradation in image resolution. A short duration, high-power rectangular RF pulse may exceed the MR system hardware or specific absorption rate (SAR) limits. The compromises may be the use of a lower excitation flip angle, longer encoding time, or lower spatial resolution. Corrections for excitation bandwidth can be applied at the image reconstruction stage [32]. Variable flip angle and/or bandwidth excitations have been proposed [33]. By including a variable TR, a reduced SAR was achieved with an increased SNR and/or reduced data acquisition time [33]. Variable acquisition filter bandwidth has been used to increase SNR [34].

Higher-order effects, such as phase accumulation during RF excitation, have been investigated [35]. More complex RF pulses with frequency and amplitude modulation, as employed in zero echo time (ZTE) [36, 37], can be considered in SPRITE. Applying a low-amplitude gradient during the RF excitation, followed by a ramping gradient, has been proposed to enable pure phase encoding around metal implants [38]. The hybrid-SPRITE method [39] was developed to address gradient and RF limitations.

Hybrid-SPRITE

Hybrid-SPRITE [39] employs some time-domain points for data from the periphery of k-space. The data acquisition is similar to multipoint SPRITE but with many fewer phase encoding steps. A single image is reconstructed instead of multiple frames. Because the center of k-space is more important in determining image quality, hybrid phase-frequency encoding largely retains the benefit of pure phase encoding and reduces gradient amplitude and RF power requirements. The proportion of phase versus frequency encoding points can be chosen based on the hardware constraints, the desired data acquisition time, and image quality. Compared to zero-filling of high k value SPRITE [40], hybrid-SPRITE improves image quality by incorporating experimentally acquired high-frequency information, though the data are not as ideal as those obtained with a pure phase encoded acquisition.

The method is similar to pointwise encoding time reduction with radial acquisition (PETRA) [41] and hybrid filling (HYFI) [42] but was motivated by reducing the gradient and RF duty cycles of SPRITE. A variable phase encoding interval technique essentially achieves the same purpose but acquires each time-domain point with a separate RF pulse [43]. In hybrid-SPRITE, a pseudo-polar grid was proposed for efficient k-space coverage and image reconstruction, as shown in Fig. 2.3. The black dots are phase encoding points that determine the image acquisition time and maximum sample bandwidth. The blue dots are frequency encoding points acquired immediately after the connected black dots. The pseudo-polar scheme enables simple image reconstruction without regridding.

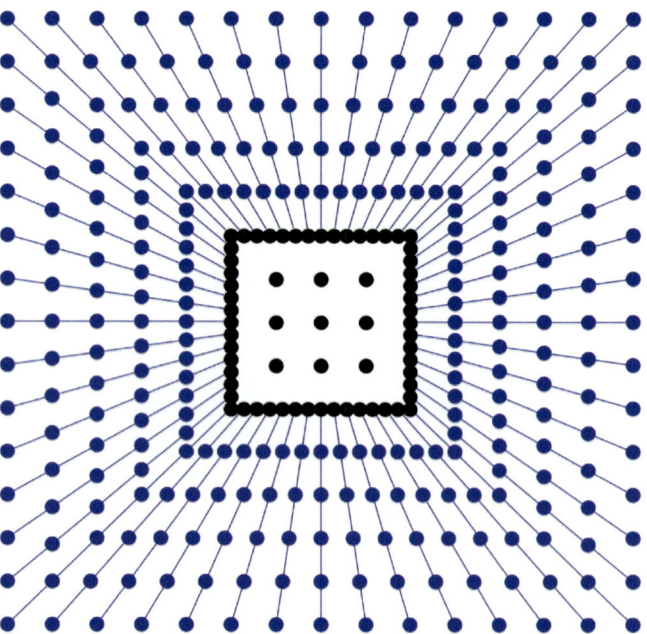

Fig. 2.3 Hybrid-SPRITE k-space trajectory on a pseudo-polar grid. The black dots are pure phase encoding points, with the central portion plotted on a Cartesian grid. The blue dots are frequency encoding points acquired after the connected black dots. The pseudo-polar scheme enables simple image reconstruction without regridding

Time-domain points can be acquired at no cost following the other phase encoding points in the central region of k-space, such as the three-by-three black dots in Fig. 2.3. These were not incorporated into the hybrid-SPRITE method. Recent work has been performed to utilize all the time-domain points in a regularized reconstruction. The goal is to acquire the T_2^* map as in the multipoint SPRITE scheme but with much reduced data sampling and hardware constraints [16].

Magnetization Preparation and Motion Encoding

SPRITE can be combined with magnetization preparation modules such as spin lock and inversion recovery [44], spin echo [45], as well as diffusion and flow [46–48] to study systems that are challenging for other MRI techniques. Centric scanning is usually used with a SPRITE spatial encoding module so that the k-space center is first acquired after the preparation. An extended k-space interleaf may lead to inaccurate results, as some data can be dominated by the freshly recovered magnetization after numerous RF excitations. This additional factor must be considered in designing the pulse sequence.

Alternatively, the magnetization preparation can be repeated for each k-space point. Motion-sensitized SPRITE is a very powerful technique for studying turbulent flow [49]. Very fast flow of up to 10 m/s can be quantified thanks to the use of a very short T_p. The pulse sequence is shown in Fig. 2.4. The dashed line is the spatial encoding gradient which is the same as in Fig. 2.1. A symmetrical excursion on either side of the spatial encoding gradient is applied. The gradient switching occurred at $T_p/2$ so that the integrated area of gradient waveform from the RF pulse to the data acquisition is the same as shown by the dashed line in Fig. 2.4. The gradient is not switched back to the spatial encoding value after data acquisition. Instead, it is ramped to the next step at the end of TR, where the motion-sensitizing gradient is again included. Accurate motion encoding is achieved for each point in k-space. Since SPRITE is immune to large susceptibility differences, turbulent flow through a dysfunctional bi-leaflet mechanical heart valve was successfully measured [50]. Diffusion tensor imaging of anisotropic turbulent flow with Reynolds numbers as high as 60,000 has been reported [51]. These motion encoding schemes have also been applied to study other challenging systems, such as the X-nuclei gas (sulfur hexafluoride) [52] and water spray [53].

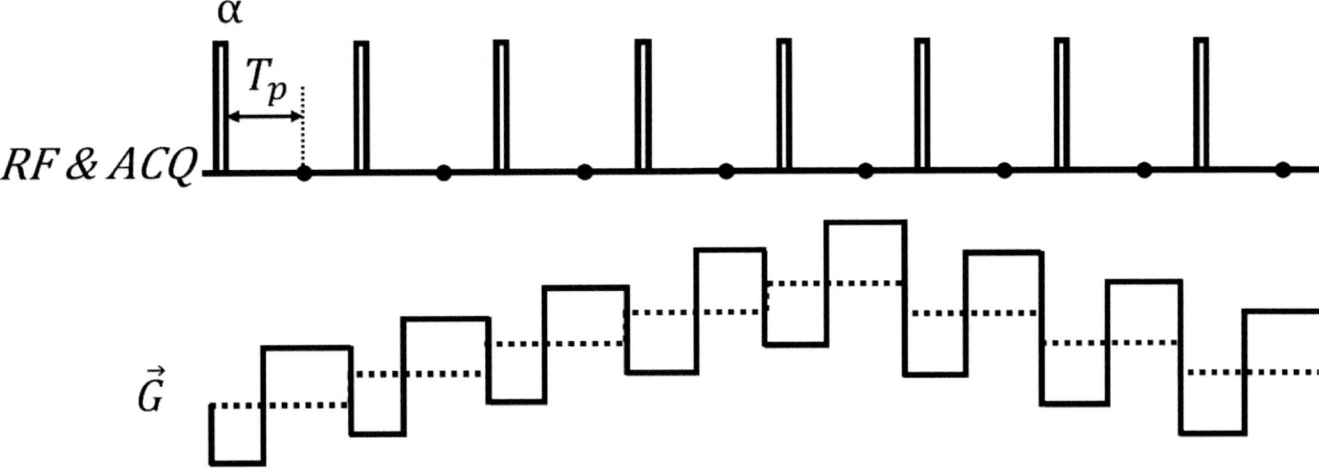

Fig. 2.4 Motion-sensitized SPRITE sequence. The gradient has a symmetrical excursion on either side of the spatial encoding gradient (dashed line)

Conclusion

SPRITE is a robust MRI technique used for the capture of short lifetime signals. The pure phase encoding method is immune to magnetic field distortion. It is a powerful method to map the magnetic field around metal. SPRITE acquisitions can also be combined with magnetization preparations to study situations that are not accessible with other MRI methods, such as the fast turbulent flow.

The biomedical applications have been limited by the long data acquisition time as well as by high gradient and RF duty cycles. These can be mitigated by the use of a hybrid scheme incorporating some frequency encoding points. The recent development of advanced constrained data processing may provide similar information to that obtained with fully sampled multipoint SPRITE, using only a fraction of the phase encoding steps. This could enable more biomedical applications.

References

1. Balcom BJ, Macgregor RP, Beyea SD, Green DP, Armstrong RL, Bremner TW. Single-point ramped imaging with T_1 enhancement (SPRITE). J Magn Reson A. 1996;123(1):131–4.
2. Muir CE, Balcom BJ. Pure phase encode magnetic resonance imaging of fluids in porous media. Annu Rep NMR Spectrosc. 2012;77:81–113.
3. Mastikhin IV, Balcom BJ. Chapter 5: Centric SPRITE MRI of biomaterials with short T_2^*s. In: Bydder GM, Fullerton GD, Young IR, editors. MRI of tissues with short T_2s or T_2^*s; 2012. p. 61–7.
4. Özen AC, Ludwig U, Öhrström LM, Rühli FJ, Bock M. Comparison of ultrashort echo time sequences for MRI of an ancient mummified human hand. Magn Reson Med. 2016;75(2):701–8.
5. Protti A, Herlihy A, Tessier J, Bell J. In-vivo diagonal-SPRITE imaging at 9.4T. Proc Intl Soc Mag Reson Med. 2006:3027.
6. Baadsvik EL, Weiger M, Froidevaux R, Faigle W, Ineichen BV, Pruessmann KP. Mapping the myelin bilayer with short-T_2 MRI: methods validation and reference data for healthy human brain. Magn Reson Med. 2023;89(2):665–77.
7. Romanzetti S, Halse M, Kaffanke J, Zilles K, Balcom BJ, Shah NJ. A comparison of three SPRITE techniques for the quantitative 3D imaging of the ^{23}Na spin density on a 4T whole-body machine. J Magn Reson. 2006;179(1):64–72.
8. Reetz K, Romanzetti S, Dogan I, Saß C, Werner CJ, Schiefer J, et al. Increased brain tissue sodium concentration in Huntington's disease - a sodium imaging study at 4T. NeuroImage. 2012;63(1):517–24.
9. Subramanian S, Devasahayam N, Murugesan R, Yamada K, Cook J, Taube A, et al. Single-point (constant-time) imaging in radiofrequency Fourier transform electron paramagnetic resonance. Magn Reson Med. 2002;48(2):370–9.
10. Matsumoto K, Kishimoto S, Devasahayam N, Chandramouli GVR, Ogawa Y, Matsumoto S, et al. EPR-based oximetric imaging: a combination of single point-based spatial encoding and T_1 weighting. Magn Reson Med. 2018;80(5):2275–87.
11. Jezzard P, Attard JJ, Carpenter TA, Hall LD. Nuclear magnetic resonance imaging in the solid state. Prog Nucl Magn Reson Spectrosc. 1991;23(1):1–41.
12. Emid S, Creyghton JHN. High resolution NMR imaging in solids. Phys Sect B+C. 1985;128(1):81–3.
13. Kaffanke JB, Stöcker T, Romanzetti S, Dierkes T, Leach MO, Shah NJ. Phase-cycled averaging for the suppression of residual magnetisation in SPI sequences. J Magn Reson. 2009;199(2):117–25.
14. Marble AE, Mastikhin IV, MacGregor RP, Akl M, LaPlante G, Colpitts BG, et al. Distortion-free single point imaging of multi-layered composite sandwich panel structures. J Magn Reson. 2004;168(1):164–74.
15. Ramos-Cabrer P, Van Duynhoven JPM, Van Der Toorn A, Nicolay K. MRI of hip prostheses using single-point methods: in vitro studies towards the artifact-free imaging of individuals with metal implants. Magn Reson Imaging. 2004;22(8):1097–103.
16. Bazzi L. Quantitative magnetic resonance imaging methodology development. University of Windsor; 2022.
17. Graf H, Steidle G, Lauer UA, Schick F. rf enhancement and shielding in MRI caused by conductive implants: dependence on electrical parameters for a tube model. Med Phys. 2005;32(2):337–42.

18. Vashaee S, Goora F, Britton MM, Newling B, Balcom BJ. Mapping B_1-induced eddy current effects near metallic structures in MR images: a comparison of simulation and experiment. J Magn Reson. 2015;250:17–24.

19. Halse M, Rioux J, Romanzetti S, Kaffanke J, MacMillan B, Mastikhin I, et al. Centric scan SPRITE magnetic resonance imaging: optimization of SNR, resolution, and relaxation time mapping. J Magn Reson. 2004;169(1):102–17.

20. Khrapitchev AA, Newling B, Balcom BJ. Sectoral sampling in centric-scan SPRITE magnetic resonance imaging. J Magn Reson. 2006;178(2):288–96.

21. Speidel T, Paul J, Wundrak S, Rasche V. Quasi-random single-point imaging using low-discrepancy k-space sampling. IEEE Trans Med Imaging. 2018;37(2):473–9.

22. Parasoglou P, Malioutov D, Sederman AJ, Rasburn J, Powell H, Gladden LF, et al. Quantitative single point imaging with compressed sensing. J Magn Reson. 2009;201(1):72–80.

23. Parasoglou P, Sederman AJ, Rasburn J, Powell H, Johns ML. Optimal k-space sampling for single point imaging of transient systems. J Magn Reson. 2008;194(1):99–107.

24. Xiao D, Balcom BJ. Restricted k-space sampling in pure phase encode MRI of rock core plugs. J Magn Reson. 2013;231:126–32.

25. Kaffanke JB, Romanzetti S, Dierkes T, Leach MO, Balcom BJ, Shah NJ. Multi-frame SPRITE: a method for resolution enhancement of multiple-point SPRITE data. J Magn Reson. 2013;230:111–6.

26. Rioux J, Halse M, Aubanel E, Balcom BJ, Kaffanke J, Romanzetti S, et al. An accurate nonuniform Fourier transform for SPRITE magnetic resonance imaging data. ACM Trans Math Softw. 2007;33(3):16-es.

27. Kaffanke J, Dierkes T, Romanzetti S, Halse M, Rioux J, Leach MO, et al. Application of the chirp z-transform to MRI data. J Magn Reson. 2006;178(1):121–8.

28. Beyea SD, Balcom BJ, Prado PJ, Cross AR, Kennedy CB, Armstrong RL, et al. Relaxation time mapping of short T_2^* nuclei with single-point imaging (SPI) methods. J Magn Reson. 1998;135(1):156–64.

29. Marica F, Chen Q, Hamilton A, Hall C, Al T, Balcom BJ. Spatially resolved measurement of rock core porosity. J Magn Reson. 2006;178(1):136–41.

30. Zhong Z, Sun K, Karaman MM, Zhou XJ. Magnetic resonance imaging with submillisecond temporal resolution. Magn Reson Med. 2021;85(5):2434–44.

31. Fischer J, Özen AC, Ilbey S, Traser L, Echternach M, Richter B, et al. Sub-millisecond 2D MRI of the vocal fold oscillation using single-point imaging with rapid encoding. MAGMA. 2022;35(2):301–10.

32. Grodzki DM, Jakob PM, Heismann B. Correcting slice selectivity in hard pulse sequences. J Magn Reson. 2012;214(1):61–7.

33. Shah NJ, Kaffanke JB, Romanzetti S. Repetition time and flip angle variation in SPRITE imaging for acquisition time and SAR reduction. J Magn Reson. 2009;199(2):136–45.

34. García-Naranjo JC, Glover PM, Marica F, Balcom BJ. Variable bandwidth filtering for magnetic resonance imaging with pure phase encoding. J Magn Reson. 2010;202(2):234–8.

35. McDonald T, MacMillan B, Newling B, Balcom BJ. Systematic image alteration due to phase accumulation during RF pulse excitation in pure phase encode magnetic resonance imaging. Concepts Magn Reson A. 2016;45A(6):e21425.

36. Li C, Magland JF, Seifert AC, Wehrli FW. Correction of excitation profile in zero echo time (ZTE) imaging using quadratic phase-modulated RF pulse excitation and iterative reconstruction. IEEE Trans Med Imaging. 2014;33(4):961–9.

37. Schieban K, Weiger M, Hennel F, Boss A, Pruessmann KP. ZTE imaging with enhanced flip angle using modulated excitation. Magn Reson Med. 2015;74(3):684–93.

38. Wiens CN, Artz NS, Jang H, McMillan AB, Koch KM, Reeder SB. Fully phase-encoded MRI near metallic implants using ultra-short echo times and broadband excitation. Magn Reson Med. 2018;79(4):2156–63.

39. Xiao D, Balcom BJ. Hybrid-SPRITE MRI. J Magn Reson. 2013;235:6–14.

40. Mastikhin IV, Mullally H, MacMillan B, Balcom BJ. Water content profiles with a 1D centric SPRITE acquisition. J Magn Reson. 2002;156(1):122–30.

41. Grodzki DM, Jakob PM, Heismann B. Ultrashort echo time imaging using pointwise encoding time reduction with radial acquisition (PETRA). Magn Reson Med. 2012;67(2):510–8.

42. Froidevaux R, Weiger M, Rösler MB, Brunner DO, Pruessmann KP. HYFI: hybrid filling of the dead-time gap for faster zero echo time imaging. NMR Biomed. 2021;34(6):e4493.

43. Latta P, Gruwel MLH, Volotovskyy V, Weber MH, Tomanek B. Single-point imaging with a variable phase encoding interval. Magn Reson Imaging. 2008;26(1):109–16.

44. Mastikhin IV, Balcom BJ, Prado PJ, Kennedy CB. SPRITE MRI with prepared magnetization and centrick-space sampling. J Magn Reson. 1999;136(2):159–68.

45. Khrapitchev AA, Newling B, Balcom BJ. Centric-scan SPRITE magnetic resonance imaging with prepared magnetisation. J Magn Reson. 2006;181(2):271–9.

46. Li L, Chen Q, Marble AE, Romero-Zerón L, Newling B, Balcom BJ. Flow imaging of fluids in porous media by magnetization prepared centric-scan SPRITE. J Magn Reson. 2009;197(1):1–8.

47. Romanenko K, Xiao D, Balcom BJ. Velocity field measurements in sedimentary rock cores by magnetization prepared 3D SPRITE. J Magn Reson. 2012;223:120–8.

48. Mastikhin IV, Hetherington NL, Emms R. Oscillating gradient measurements of fast oscillatory and rotational motion in the fluids. J Magn Reson. 2012;214(1):189–99.

49. Newling B, Poirier CC, Zhi Y, Rioux JA, Coristine AJ, Roach D, et al. Velocity imaging of highly turbulent gas flow. Phys Rev Lett. 2004;93(15):154503.

50. Adegbite O, Kadem L, Newling B. Purely phase-encoded MRI of turbulent flow through a dysfunctional bileaflet mechanical heart valve. MAGMA. 2014;27(3):227–35.

51. Gauthier ARP, Stocek N, Newling B. Diffusion tensor imaging of anisotropic inhomogeneous turbulent flow. Phys Rev E. 2022;106(1–2):015108.

52. Gauthier ARP, Newling B. Gas flow mapping in a recorder: an application of SPRITE MRI. Appl Magn Reson. 2018;49(10):1151–62.

53. Mastikhin I, Arbabi A, Bade KM. Magnetic resonance imaging measurements of a water spray upstream and downstream of a spray nozzle exit orifice. J Magn Reson. 2016;266:8–15.

Two-Dimensional Ultrashort Echo Time (2D UTE) Imaging

Aiming Lu

Introduction

There is increased interest in direct imaging of tissues with short transverse relaxation times (T_2s). When imaged with conventional clinical MRI sequences, the so-called short-T_2 tissues show little or no signal. They require more advanced techniques, such as single-point imaging (SPI) and ultrashort echo time (UTE) sequences [1–7]. Single-point imaging (SPI) sequences often require relatively long acquisition times which limit their clinical applications [1–3]. Two-dimensional (2D) and three-dimensional (3D) UTE imaging techniques have therefore been more frequently used for morphological and quantitative imaging of short-T_2 tissues [4–7].

UTE sequences acquire the free induction decay (FID) signal immediately following the radiofrequency (RF) excitation with center-out k-space sampling trajectories (e.g., radial or spiral trajectories). The simplest UTE sequence uses a short RF pulse for excitation followed by 3D radial readout trajectories. In this case, the minimal echo time (TE) achievable is only limited by the hardware switch time from transmit to receive, which ranges from a few microseconds to a couple of 100 μs. The sequence allows vast undersampling in the angular direction, so fast volumetric imaging can be achieved although with the penalty of diffused background noise. Advanced strategies such as parallel imaging, compressed sensing, and more efficient sampling trajectories such as 3D Cones and twisted projection imaging can be used to further improve 3D UTE image quality and shorten the acquisition time [8–11]. Despite these techniques, the acquisition times of 3D UTE sequences can still be long for applications where high spatial and temporal resolution is needed. For example, an important potential application of UTE MRI is to monitor the progress of the freeze-thaw cycle in tissues during cryoablation, where the tissue temperature,

as well as the cooling and warming rates, may vary significantly across relatively small regions of interest with short T_2/T_2* times. For this application, a faster 2D UTE sequence is preferred instead of 3D UTE imaging in order to achieve near real-time imaging with high spatial resolution, so dynamic tissue signal changes with temperature can be captured.

The 2D UTE Sequence

In 2D imaging, slice-selective excitation is usually achieved by playing out a shaped RF pulse (e.g., truncated SINC pulse) in the presence of the slice-select gradient. A typical conventional 2D imaging sequence is shown in Fig. 3.1a, where G_z, G_x, and G_y are the slice-select, frequency encoding, and phase encoding axes, respectively. The G_z gradient applied during the RF pulse is the slice-select gradient, and slice-rephasing gradient is the trapezoidal gradient applied following the RF pulse with opposite gradient polarity. The purpose of the slice-rephasing gradient is to unwind the phase dispersion of the transverse magnetization after its generation due to the remainder of the slice-select gradient. The required area under the rephasing gradient waveform depends on the isodelay of the RF pulse, which is the effective precession or dephasing time that results in the phase dispersion of the spins during the RF pulse. For symmetric/linear phase RF pulses, the isodelay is typically half the RF duration. By applying a negative gradient waveform with the same area as that under the slice-select gradient waveform after the isodelay, the phase accumulation due to the gradients cancels, and the k-space trajectory in the slice-select direction (usually denoted as the logical Z-axis) is returned to the origin. The minimal TE available with conventional 2D sequences is often of the order of milliseconds, as determined by the sum of the RF isodelay, the ramp-down duration of the slice-select gradient, and the maximal duration among the slice-rephasing gradient, the phase encoding gra-

A. Lu (✉)

Division of Medical Physics, Department of Radiology, Mayo Clinic, Rochester, MN, USA

e-mail: lu.aiming@mayo.edu

© The Author(s), under exclusive license to Springer Nature Switzerland AG 2023

J. Du, G. M. Bydder (eds.), *MRI of Short- and Ultrashort-T₂ Tissues*, https://doi.org/10.1007/978-3-031-35197-6_3

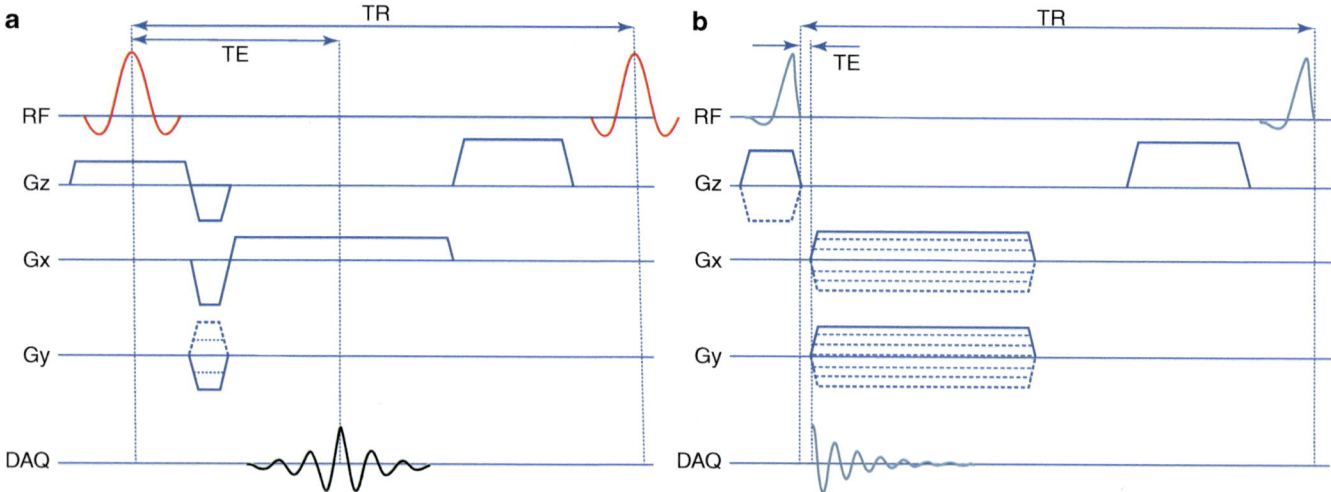

Fig. 3.1 (**a**) Pulse sequence diagram for a typical 2D sequence using a conventional full-pulse RF pulse for slice-selective excitation. The sequence acquires *k*-space data on regular Cartesian grids. (**b**) Pulse sequence diagram for a 2D UTE sequence with half-pulse excitation, where data are sampled along radial lines in *k*-space

dient, and the pre-phasing lobe of the frequency encoding gradient.

To achieve an ultrashort TE for imaging species with short T_2/T_2^* values, 2D UTE sequences employ a self-refocused half-pulse RF pulse for excitation with a center-out radial or spiral readout trajectory [12]. The half-pulse RF pulse is generated by taking the first half of a conventional symmetric full pulse. A typical 2D UTE sequence with a radial readout is shown in Fig. 3.1b. With zero isodelay, the half-pulse RF excitation does not require a refocusing gradient and the k_z trajectory ends at $k_z = 0$. The use of a radial acquisition samples the central *k*-space data first, eliminating the need for the phase encoding gradient and the pre-phasing gradient for the readout. The TE in this sequence is defined as the time from the end of the RF pulse to the beginning of data acquisition and is only limited by the hardware transit time. For rapid imaging, UTE sequences are usually implemented in the spoiled gradient echo mode (e.g., SPGR, or spoiled gradient recalled acquisition in steady state) to achieve short repetition times (TRs).

The phantom and in vivo canine prostate images shown in Fig. 3.2 were acquired using a conventional 2D sequence with a TE of 2.5 ms (Fig. 3.2a, c) and a 2D UTE sequence (Fig. 3.2b, d) with a TE of 0.1 ms. The phantom contains six vials with different T_2 values (five with T_2 values of 1–3 ms and one with a longer T_2 of about 12 ms). The vials with short T_2 components appear as signal voids in the conventional 2D image (Fig. 3.2a), while the vials demonstrate appreciable signals in the UTE image (Fig. 3.2b). Figure 3.2c, d were acquired during in vivo canine prostate cryoablation experiments. The frozen tissue in the prostate appears as a localized signal void in the image acquired using a conven-

tional 2D sequence. However, the image acquired using a 2D UTE sequence clearly demonstrates a temperature dependent signal intensity gradient in the two frozen regions. This could potentially allow UTE MRI to be used for monitoring cryoablation.

Half-Pulse Excitation

Playing out the RF pulse in the presence of the slice-select gradient(s) applies weighting along the *k*-space path determined by [13]:

$$k_z(t) = -\gamma \int_t^{t_1} G_z(\tau)\,d\tau \tag{3.1}$$

where γ is the gyromagnetic ratio, $G_z(t)$ includes the slice-select gradient, and in the case of conventional full RF pulse, the slice-refocusing gradient as well. t_1 is the end time of the slice rephasing gradient lobe with a conventional full RF pulse and the end time of the slice-select gradient in the case of half-pulse excitation. The RF energy deposition/*k*-space weighting along the *k*-space path for a symmetric full-pulse RF excitation is illustrated in Fig. 3.3a. The k_z trajectory starts from one end in *k*-space, passes the center, and moves to the other end. It returns to the *k*-space center again at the end of the slice-refocusing gradient lobe, so the dephasing effect due to the slice-select gradient is unwound. The highest weighting is applied at the *k*-space center when it is traversed the first time during the RF pulse.

In the half-pulse excitation case shown in Fig. 3.3b, only the first half of the conventional RF pulse is played out. By eliminating the second half of the conventional slice-select

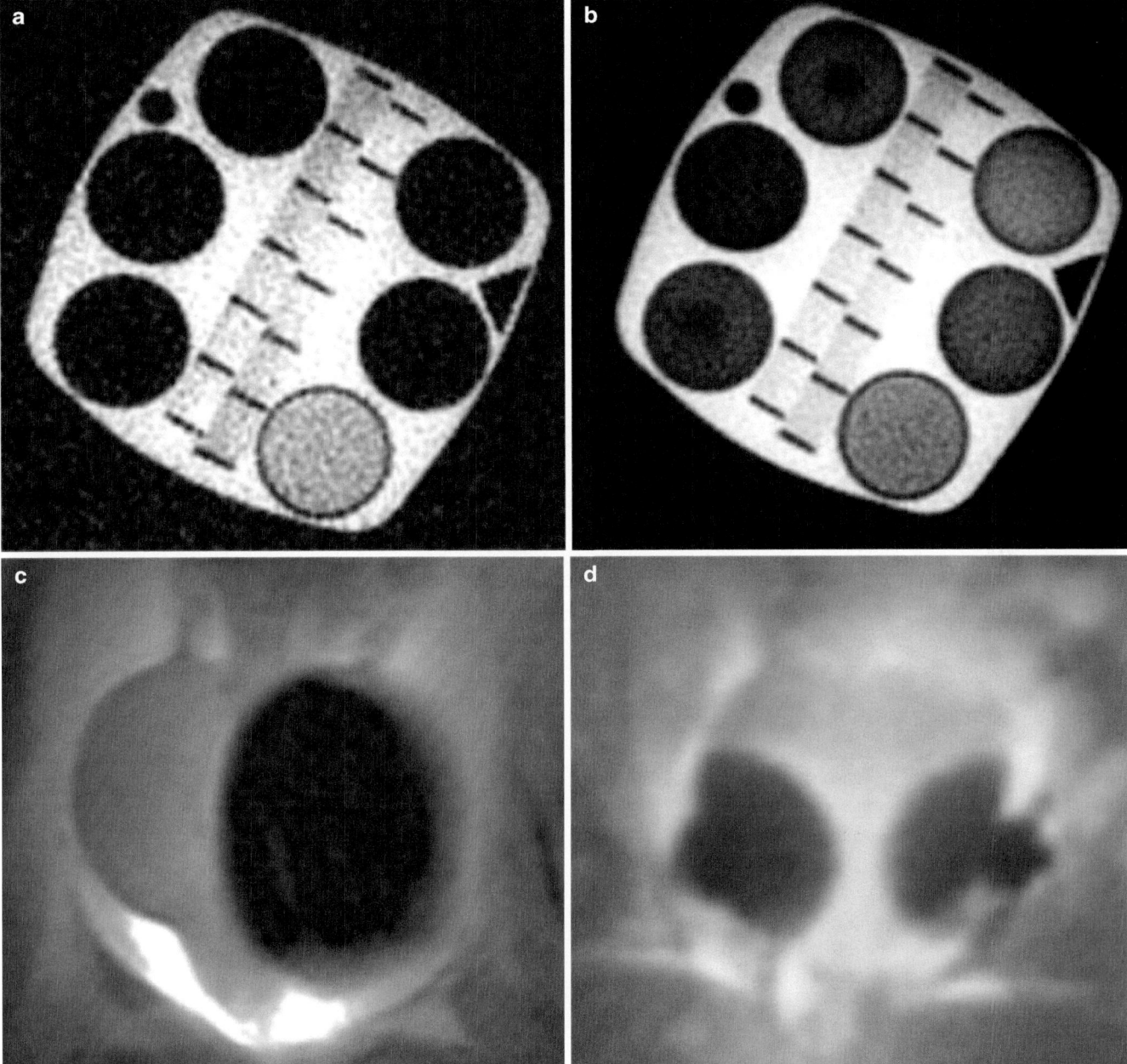

Fig. 3.2 Images acquired with a conventional sequence and a UTE sequence showing the capability of UTE MRI for imaging short-T_2 species. (**a**) Phantom image demonstrates that the vials with short T_2s values appear as signal voids using a conventional sequence. (**b**) Imaged using the UTE sequence, appreciable signals are visualized within the vials. (**c**) Using a conventional 2D sequence during an in vivo canine prostate cryoablation experiment, the frozen tissue in the prostate appears as a localized signal void. A single cryoprobe was used in this case. (**d**) Image acquired using a 2D UTE sequence clearly demonstrates a temperature-dependent signal intensity gradient in the two frozen regions in the prostate created using two cryoprobes

gradient and consequently the need for the slice-refocusing gradient, shorter TEs can be achieved with center-out read-out trajectories. 2D UTE sequences with half-pulse excitations require sampling k-space twice with longitudinal magnetizations excited using opposite slice-select gradient polarities. During each acquisition, the half-pulse excitation applies weighting along one-half of the full k_z trajectory. The traversed half k_z trajectories in the two acquisitions start from opposite edges in k-space and both end at the k-space center. The combination of the two acquisitions results in the same k-space weighting along the k-space path as a conventional full pulse and consequently the same excitation profile.

Fig. 3.3 (**a**) A typical slice-selective excitation sequence with conventional full-pulse RF pulse and its corresponding *k*-space trajectory. The RF pulse is applied during the constant portion of the slice-select gradient, which traverses the full extent of slice-selection *k*-space. The slice-refocusing gradient is used to align the RF energy deposition with the *k*-space trajectory centered at $k_z(t) = 0$. (**b**) The half-pulse excitation approach uses two excitations to achieve the same RF energy deposition along the same *k*-space trajectory. Each excitation covers one-half of the *k*-space. No refocusing is needed since the half-pulses end at the *k*-space center

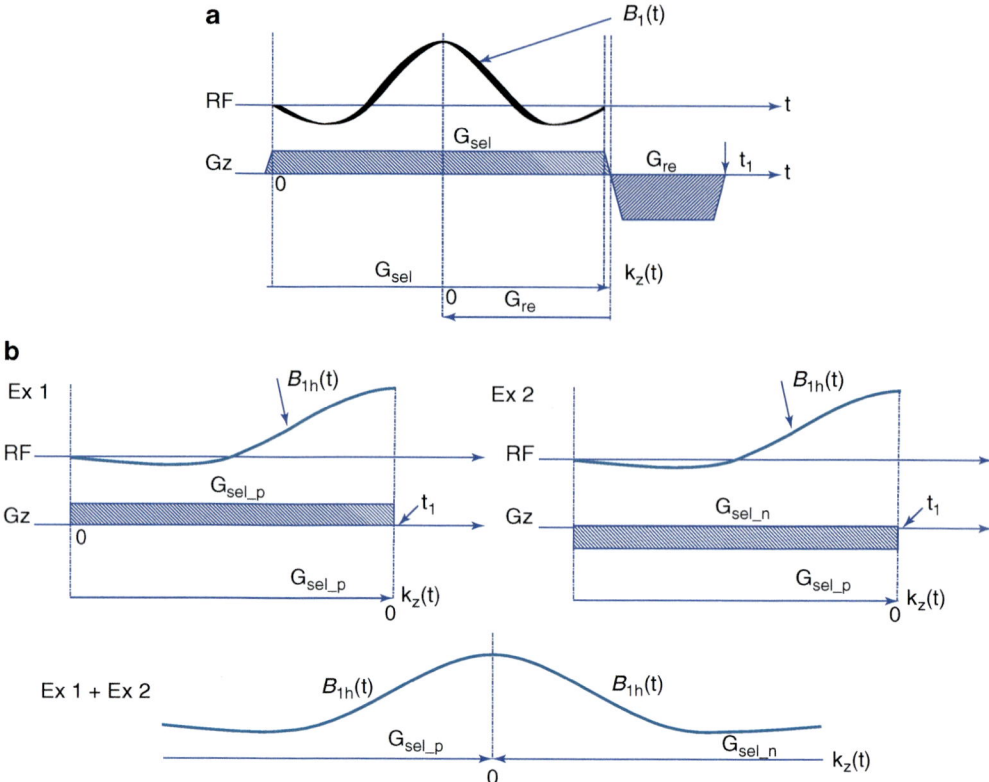

Half-Pulse Excitation with Varying Slice-Select Gradient

The plots in Fig. 3.3b assume that the slice-select gradient can be turned off instantaneously so the half pulse and the gradient end simultaneously. However, the gradient system usually has a limited slew rate, and it takes time to ramp up or ramp down the gradient. Ramping down the gradient after the excitation pulse would introduce magnetization dephasing and necessitate the addition of a refocusing gradient lobe to cancel the effect. Both the gradient ramping down and refocusing gradient would increase the TE. To avoid this, the variable-rate selective excitation (VERSE) technique can be used [14]. Instead of applying the RF pulse during a constant slice-select gradient, VERSE allows a time-varying gradient to be used during RF excitation without changing the spatial excitation profile for on-resonance spins by appropriately modifying the RF pulse shape. In Fig. 3.4, the half pulse is modified using VERSE to account for the ramp-down gradient (and although not critical, the ramp-up gradient as well if so desired), so the RF pulse and the ramp-down gradient end at the same time.

An example of excitation with a VERSE half pulse and the corresponding excited slice profiles is shown in Fig. 3.5. The excited slice profiles from the two excitations with dif-

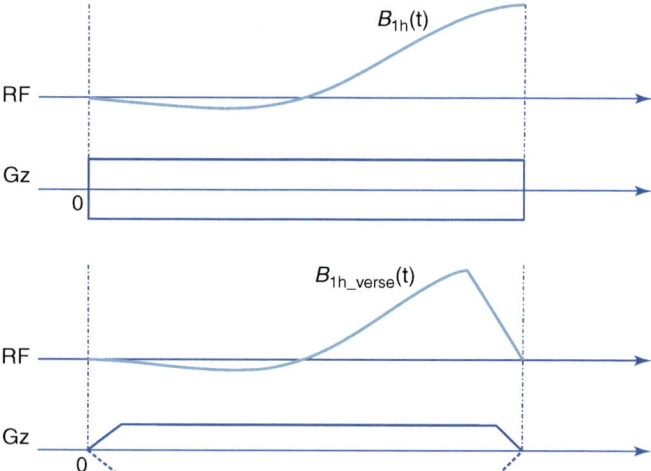

Fig. 3.4 Due to the limited slew rate of the gradient system, the VERSE technique is used to allow RF pulses to be applied in the presence of a time-varying gradient without compromising the slice profile

ferent slice-select gradient polarities show undesirable, broad magnitude profiles and variable phases in the slice direction. After combining the two excitations, a much better slice profile is achieved (sharper and flatter magnitude profile and constant phase in the selected slice).

Fig. 3.5 Plots showing a typical half pulse and the corresponding slice-select gradient used to select a 2 mm thick slice with a 30° flip angle, as well as the corresponding slice profiles from each of the two excitations and the combined slice profile. A much sharper slice profile is achieved after the combination of the two excitations. This is seen as a flat phase response in the excited slice

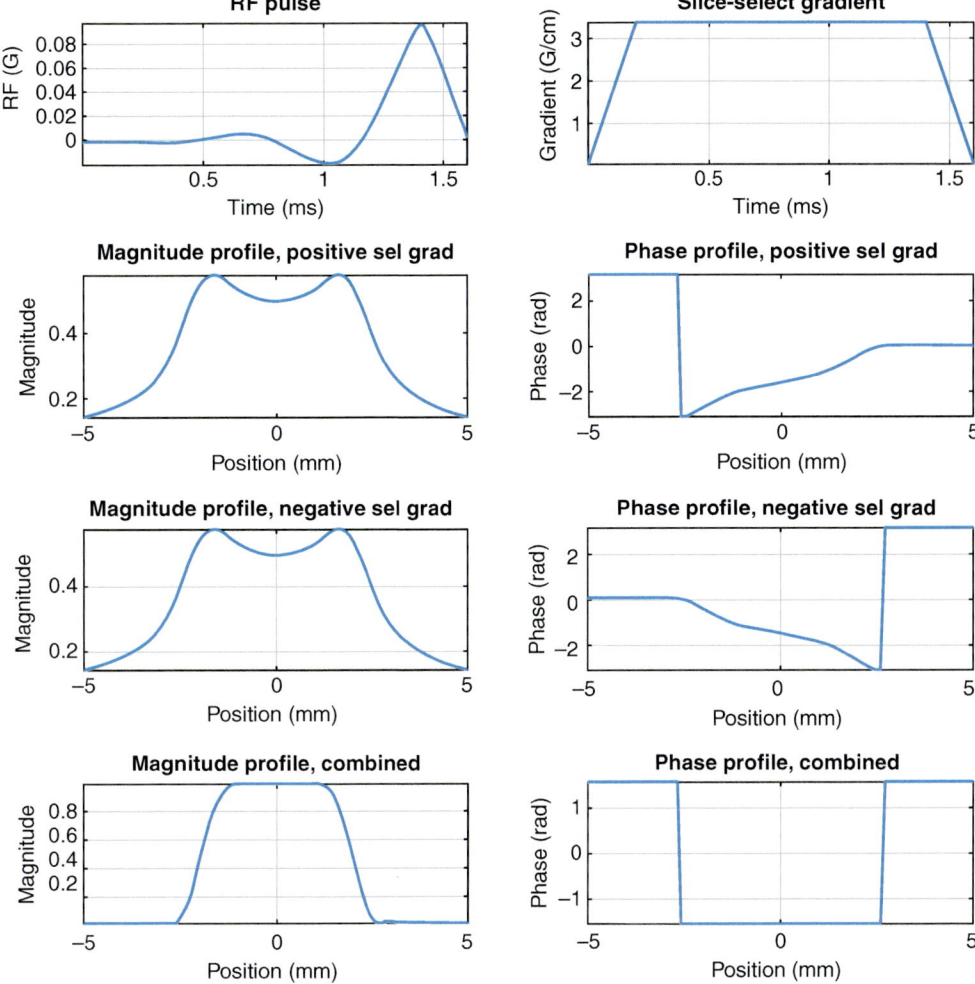

Half-Pulse Design

The half pulse is obtained by taking the first half of a conventional full pulse. Care must be taken to design the conventional full pulse with a flip angle twice that of the desired half pulse to achieve the desired slice profile. For half pulses with small flip angles (<45°), the full pulse can be designed using the small flip angle approximation approach. The full large flip angle pulse can be designed using methods such as the Shinnar–Le Roux (SLR) algorithm for larger flip angles. For example, a 90° excitation half pulse can be obtained by taking the first half of a full 180° refocusing pulse.

Exciting an Off-Isocenter Slice

With conventional full-pulse excitation applied in the presence of a constant slice-select gradient, exciting a slice at any off-isocenter location can be achieved by simply adjusting the transmitter frequency. As time-varying gradients are used in half-pulse excitation, imaging at any locations other than

the isocenter is more complicated. To excite a slice at positions z, in general, the RF waveform needed is:

$$B_{1z}(t) = B_1(t)e^{ik_z(t)z} \tag{3.2}$$

where $k_z(t)$ is the integral of the remaining slice-select gradient as defined in Eq. (3.1), and $B_1(t)$ is the envelope of the RF pulse. Note that there is no RF phase accumulation at the isocenter with $z = 0$. The phase term shifts the excited slice to position z and ensures the signal phase at the end of the RF pulse is consistent for both excitations, which is critical to make certain that the two signals add coherently. As can be seen from Eq. (3.2), the phase of the RF pulse is different for the excitations with positive and negative gradient polarities and needs to be calculated for each slice location. MRI systems provide a phase channel and/or a frequency channel for phase modulation. To modulate the phase using the frequency channel, a scaled version of the slice-select gradient waveform (in case of constant slice-select gradient, the modulation frequency offset is also constant) is loaded into the frequency channel. The slice location can be shifted by scaling the frequency channel accordingly. With this approach, a bipolar gradient waveform with zero net gradient area can be used with the RF pulse applied during the second half of the waveform to ensure the phase of the RF pulse ends at zero.

K-Space Sampling and Imaging Reconstruction

With the half-pulse UTE MRI approach, *k*-space data are sampled using the same readout trajectories after both excitations. The most straightforward approach to reconstruct the images is to first resample the *k*-space data onto Cartesian grids, and then use fast Fourier transformation to obtain the images. Advanced imaging methods such as parallel imaging and compressed sensing can be exploited to improve the acquisition speed and/or the quality of images.

Practical Considerations

Other factors that affect the MR signal during both excitation and acquisition need to be considered to achieve optimal image quality with 2D UTE sequences, and these are dealt with below.

Excitation

Compared to the conventional full-pulse excitation, the half-pulse excitation approach is more susceptible to practical challenges, including the impact of timing errors between the RF pulse and the slice-select gradient, gradient waveform infidelity due to eddy currents, off-resonance effects, the impact of T_2 decay during excitation on the slice profile, and so on.

The Impact of Gradient Timing Error

To achieve the desired slice profile, applying the appropriate weighting at the correct *k*-space location is critical. Since the half-pulse excitation approach relies on the combination of two excitations that each covers a half trajectory in *k*-space, the timing error between the RF pulse and slice-select gradient pulse causes misalignment of the desired *k*-space weighting and the *k*-space trajectory. The impact of this timing error on the slice profile can be appreciated in the simulation in Fig. 3.6, where the RF pulse was applied 8 μs ahead of the intended start time, on time, and 8 μs after the intended gradient start time. A better slice profile with less out-of-slice signal is achieved when there is no timing error.

The timing error occurs mainly because the gradient pulse cannot be generated instantaneously by the gradient system. It can be either measured using special sequences or empirically estimated based on the excited slice profile or image quality [15–17]. The timing error between the RF pulse and

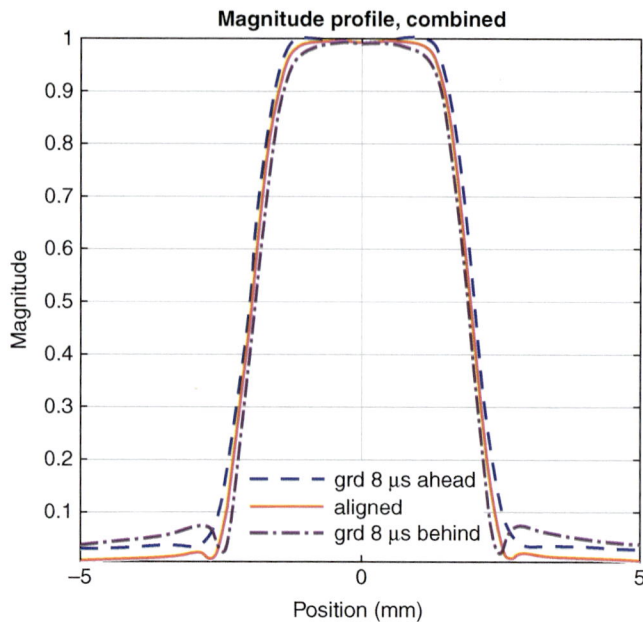

Fig. 3.6 Timing errors between the slice-select gradient and the RF pulse lead to degradation in the excited slice profile. The profile is more tolerant of timing errors when the slice-select gradient precedes the RF pulse

the slice-select gradient in the pulse sequence can be corrected based on the value obtained.

The Impact of Eddy Currents

The excitation profile achieved using half-pulse excitation is sensitive to eddy currents induced by the slice-select gradient. Eddy currents can be represented by a series of polynomial components as functions of the spatial coordinates. Among these components, the lower order polynomial terms, namely, the spatially invariant term (B_0 eddy currents) and the linearly spatially dependent term (linear eddy currents), are often of the most interest. B_0 eddy currents result in an unwanted constant phase offset between the two acquisitions with positive and negative slice-select gradient polarities, while linear eddy currents are effectively superimposed on the applied gradients and cause *k*-space trajectory distortions and consequent mismatch between the *k*-space weighting (RF pulse) and the *k*-space trajectory. Both eddy current terms cause distortions in the excited slice profile.

Pre-compensating Slice-Select Gradient

To correct for the linear eddy currents, the slice-select gradient can be pre-compensated using an empirical system impulse response function [18]. The B_0 eddy currents can be measured by acquiring one-dimensional (1D) slice profiles with both positive and negative slice-select gradient polarities. The slice profiles of the two excitations can be obtained by Fourier transformation of the data acquired with a readout gradient in the slice-select direction. The phase difference at the center of the slice profiles is then the phase offset due to B_0 eddy currents. The main issue with this approach is that the system impulse response function needed for correcting the linear eddy currents is difficult to obtain accurately.

Instead of using an explicit system impulse function, the pre-compensated slice-select gradient can also be derived from the measured slice-select gradient [6]. A drawback of this approach is that the calculated pre-compensated slice-select gradient waveform is sensitive to noise in the measured gradient waveform.

Pre-compensating Both the RF Pulse and the Slice-Select Gradient

Eddy current correction can also be achieved by pre-compensating both the RF pulse and the selective gradient simultaneously based on the measured eddy currents. Both B_0 and linear eddy currents can be characterized using a generalized approach [19–21]. Figure 3.7a, b shows examples of the measured gradient waveform and phase accumulation by B_0 eddy currents induced by the slice-select gradient. Both eddy current terms have relatively long time constant components as evidenced by the long tails after the nominal slice-select gradient.

Linear eddy currents during RF pulses can be compensated for by redesigning the RF pulse based on the measured gradient using VERSE. To correct for linear eddy currents extended beyond the RF pulse, the tail of the linear eddy current profile is inverted and appended to the end of the ideal trapezoidal gradient to form a new slice-select gradient. As shown in the measured gradient for the new slice-select gradient in Fig. 3.7c, the tail of linear eddy currents is greatly

suppressed after pre-compensation. B_0 eddy current effects during excitation can be compensated for by dynamically varying the RF phase, as is done to excite an off-isocenter slice. The B_0 eddy current correction can be combined with the phase modulation required for shifting the slice location. Long time constant components of B_0 eddy currents extended into the data acquisition can be corrected by dynamically adjusting the receiver phase, or by correcting the phase of the acquired signal on a per data point basis during image reconstruction. Example 2D slice profiles obtained on a spherical phantom using half-pulse RF excitation with and without eddy current compensation are shown in Fig. 3.8. As can be seen, a sharp slice is achieved using the half pulse after compensating for both B_0 and linear eddy currents. Example 2D UTE images acquired during an in vivo canine prostate cryo-ablation experiment with and without application of the eddy current correction strategy described above are shown in Fig. 3.9. The images with and without eddy current correction were acquired in an interleaved fashion with a cryoprobe inserted on each side of the prostate. Two "iceballs" can be visualized in the images as regions with lower but still appreciable signals in the magnitude images and elevated R_2^* in the R_2^* maps. After eddy current correction, both the magnitude image and the R_2^* map show improved image quality with much reduced streaking artifacts.

Since both B_0 and linear eddy currents are characteristics of the gradient system and scale with the gradient amplitude, they only need to be measured once on each of the three physical axes for the slice-select gradient for a given RF pulse, unless there are changes made to the gradient system. The correction can be scaled on the physical axes to excite a

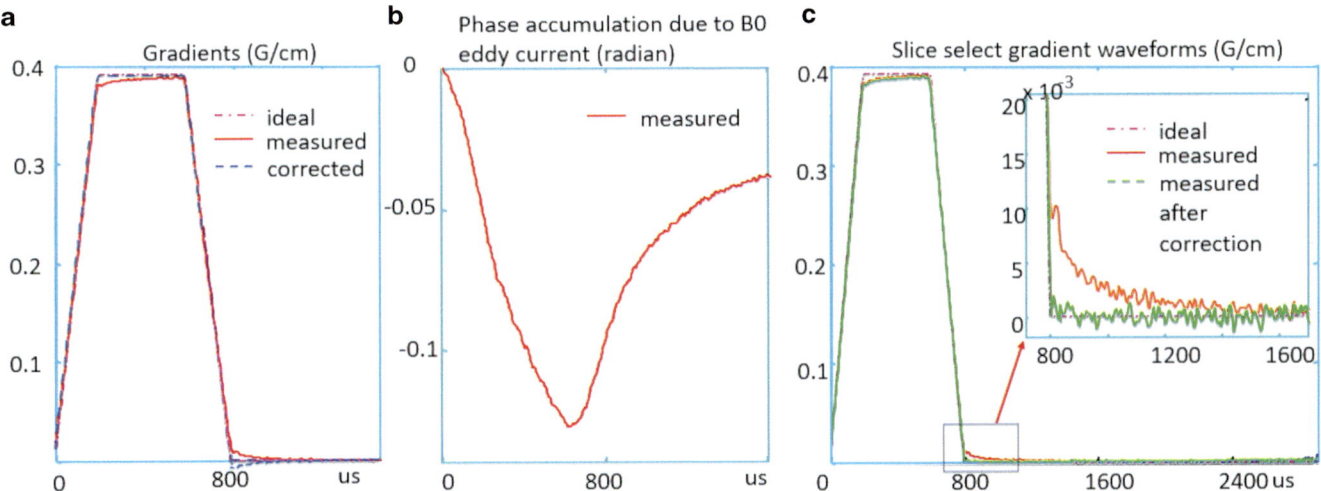

Fig. 3.7 (**a**) Ideal (dot-dashed), measured (solid) and corrected (dashed) waveforms for the slice-select gradient. The corrected gradient waveform is obtained by attaching the inverted tail of the measured gradient waveform to the ideal gradient waveform. The RF pulse is redesigned using VERSE based on the measured gradient waveform. (**b**) Measured B_0 eddy current introduced phase accumulation which is corrected by modulating the phase of the RF pulse. (**c**) Measured gradient waveform after linear eddy current correction. After correction, the tail of the linear eddy currents is reduced

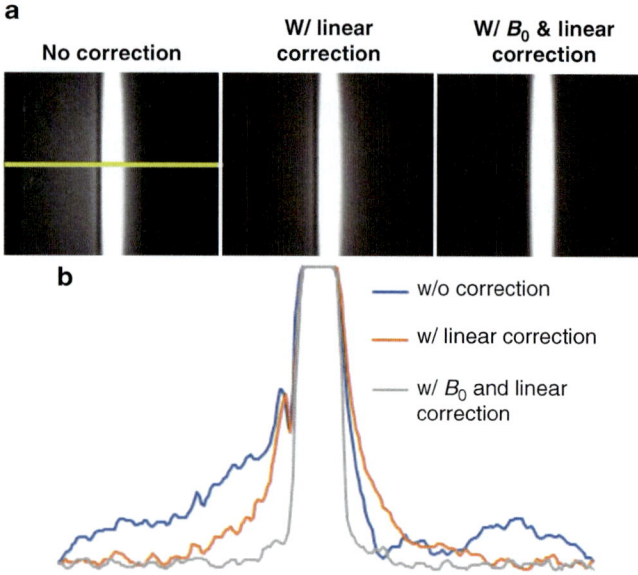

Fig. 3.8 (**a**) Images of the acquired slice profiles in the middle of a uniform spherical phantom, from left to right, without eddy current correction, with only linear eddy current correction, and with both B_0 and linear eddy current correction. (**b**) Slice profiles obtained from a row indicated by the horizontal line in (**a**) in the corresponding images. The slice profile images were obtained by imaging a slice playing out the readout gradient in the slice-selection direction. Without eddy current correction, there is a signal from outside the slice. This out-of-slice signal is decreased with linear eddy current correction and is essentially eliminated with both B_0 and linear eddy current corrections

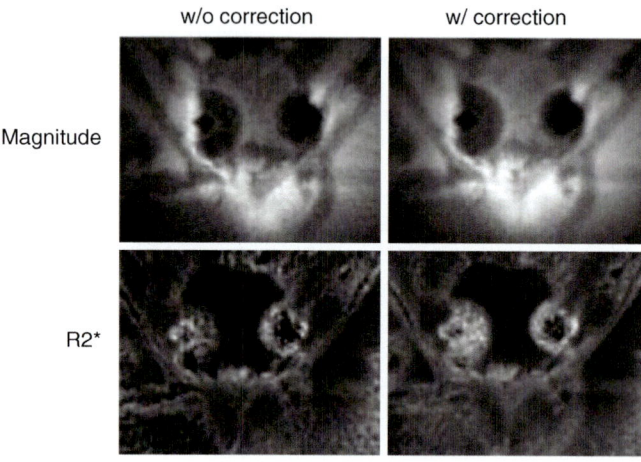

Fig. 3.9 2D UTE images acquired during an in vivo canine prostate cryoablation experiment using two cryoprobes demonstrate improved image quality with eddy current correction. The uncorrected magnitude image and R_2^* map show lower signal-to-noise ratio and more severe streaking artifacts than the magnitude image and R_2^* map acquired with both B_0 and linear eddy current correction

slice of any desired thickness. Excitation of an oblique slice is possible but requires redesigning the RF pulse based on the combination of the linear eddy currents from all three physical axes for each oblique angle.

Other Strategies to Mitigate the Impact of Eddy Currents

A few other techniques have also been proposed to achieve ultrashort TEs for 2D imaging while reducing the sensitivity of the excited slice profile to eddy currents induced by the slice-select gradient. The double half-pulse approach uses time-reversed half-pulse pairs for this purpose [22]. Ideally, the long-T_2 spins experience both half RF pulses and thus effectively experience either a conventional RF pulse or zero net excitation. It is assumed that the received signal from the short-T_2 component comes from the second half pulse, as that generated by the first half pulse has already vanished before the second RF pulse. As a result, the performance of this technique relies on the difference between the long and short T_2 values in the tissues and the interval between the two half pulses. Eddy currents can still produce signal contamination from out-of-slice short-T_2 tissue components. Moreover, the impact of the first half pulse on the longitudinal magnetization needs to be considered when designing the sequence.

To minimize the sensitivity to eddy currents with the half-pulse excitation, outer volume suppression (OVS) techniques have also been proposed to improve the slice profile by suppressing the signal from out-of-slice tissues [23]. However, spatial saturation on both sides of the imaging slice with long saturation RF pulses can significantly increase the data acquisition time.

The Impact of Off-Resonance

Factors such as main magnetic field inhomogeneity, magnetic susceptibility, chemical shift, and metal implants can lead to B_0 inhomogeneity and consequently a nonuniform precession frequency of the spins. With conventional full-pulse excitation, a constant resonance frequency offset over the slice results in a shift of the excited slice position, while spatially varying frequency offsets result in a "potato chip" shaped slice. The impact of off-resonance on the excited slice profile is more complicated in the case of the half-pulse excitation. As illustrated in Fig. 3.10, a constant resonance frequency offset causes the excited slice profiles to shift in opposite directions with different slice-select gradient polarities. Consequently, the combined slice profile is less selective as compared to that in the on-resonance scenario. Therefore, care must be taken to ensure excellent shimming is achieved to minimize the off-resonance effect.

The Impact of T_2 Decay

Signal decay during the excitation for the short T_2 species is a known concern with conventional full-pulse RF excitation. It remains a concern even when the peak RF energy is deposited toward the end of the excitation using the half-pulse excitation sequence. The effect of T_2 delay during half-pulse

Fig. 3.10 Compared to on-resonance spins, the slice profiles of the 200 Hz off-resonance spins are shifted in opposite directions with opposite slice-select gradient polarities in the two excitations. As a result, the combined slice profile has more contamination from out-of-slice signal

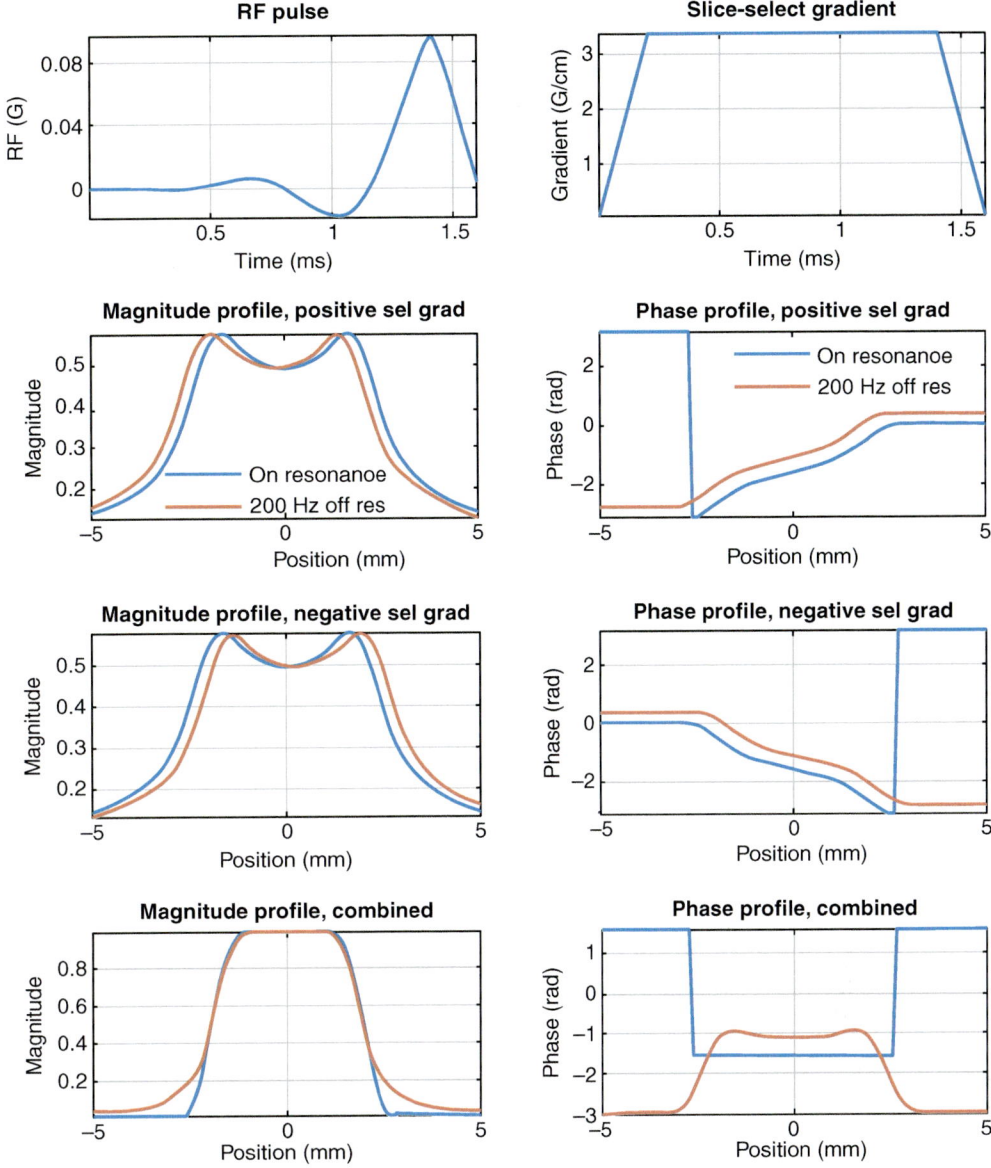

excitation is shown in Fig. 3.11, where the slice profiles from the two excitations with opposite slice-select gradient polarities and the combined signal are simulated for two species with long (100 ms) and short (1 ms) T_2s, respectively. The half pulse is 1.6 ms in duration. As can be seen, faster T_2 decay during the RF pulse results in a lower effective flip angle/signal and blurrier slice profile. In some cases, the impact of T_2 decay can be reduced by using shorter RF pulses.

Data Acquisition and Reconstruction

2D UTE MRI uses radial acquisition-based trajectories such as radial lines and spirals to sample k-space. These k-space sampling strategies are also sensitive to gradient timing errors, eddy currents induced by the readout gradients, off-resonance effects, and fast T_2 decay. These effects can be corrected/mitigated during either data acquisition or image reconstruction.

Gradient Timing Errors and Eddy Currents

Like gradient timing errors between the slice-select gradient and the RF excitation, gradient timing errors during data acquisition can come from timing differences between the gradient coils on different axes, as well as timing errors between the readout gradients and data sampling. Eddy currents during data acquisition can be introduced by readout gradient amplitude changes or the long time constant eddy current components from the slice-select gradient. Both gradient timing errors and eddy currents cause deviation of k-space trajectories from the nominal ones and mismatch

Fig. 3.11 Simulation of the effect of T_2 decay during half-pulse excitations. The slice profiles from the two excitations with opposite slice-select gradient polarities (to achieve a nominal flip angle of 30°) are shown in the second and third rows, and the combined signal from them is shown in the fourth row. This is for two species with a long T_2 (100 ms) (blue curves) and a short T_2 (1 ms) (red curves). Faster T_2 decay (red curves) results in a lower effective flip angle and a less sharp slice profile

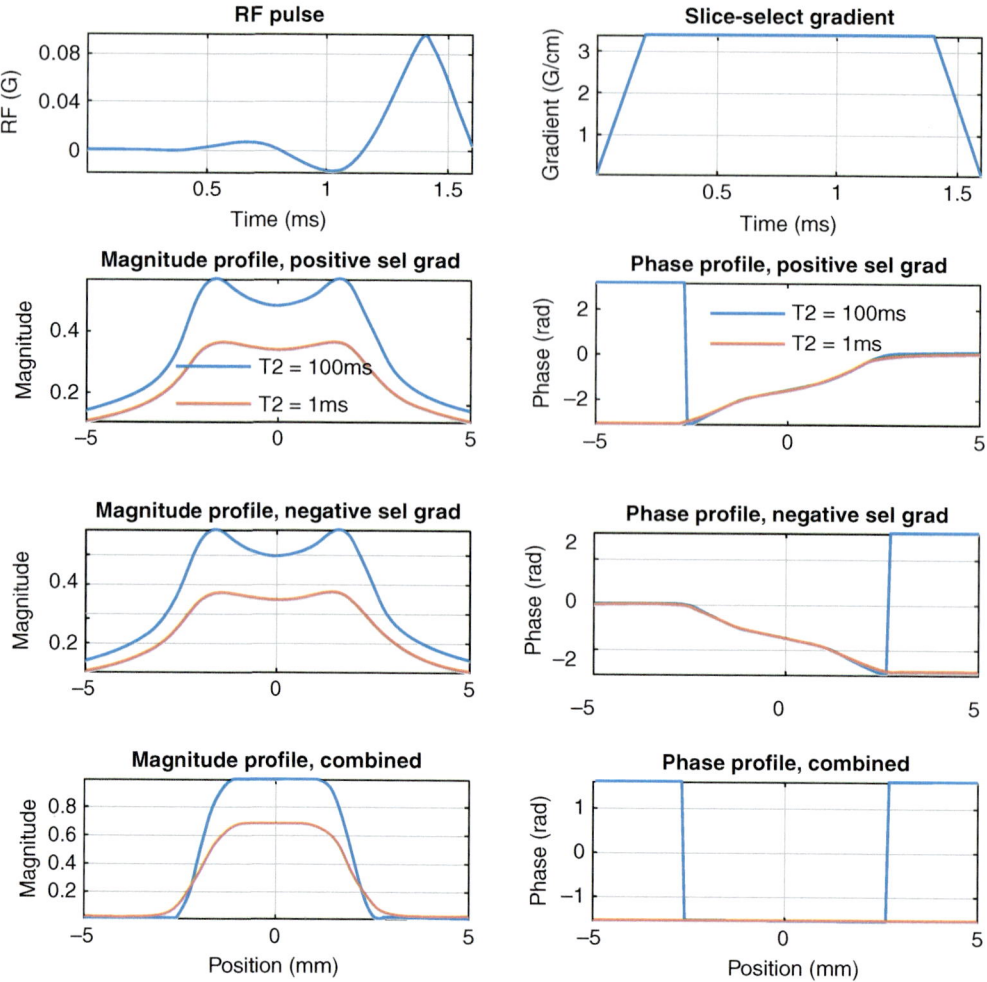

between the sampled data and their k-space locations if left uncorrected. As described earlier, gradient timing errors and B_0 and linear eddy current terms can be measured. The measured gradient timing errors can be used to align the readout gradient on each axis with the data acquisition. B_0 eddy currents can be corrected by removing the corresponding phases from the acquired data on a per-point basis along the trajectory. In contrast, linear eddy currents can be corrected by matching the acquired data with the measured k-space trajectories during image reconstruction. If the readout trajectories are rotation invariant (e.g., radial trajectories), linear combinations of the measured B_0 and linear eddy current terms on the orthogonal axes can be used to calculate the corrections needed for trajectories at arbitrary angles.

Off-Resonance Effects

Off-resonance effects can lead to signal loss, geometric distortions, and blurring in MRI images during data acquisition. UTE MRI is more resilient to signal loss due to off-resonance than conventional sequences as the use of

ultrashort TEs results in reduced intravoxel dephasing. Since radial and spiral trajectories rotate in different directions in k-space, the point spread function (PSF) or impulse response of off-resonance during readout is a ring-like function with a radius proportional to the off-resonance frequency. As a result, off-resonance causes blurring in the images. In contrast, in Cartesian acquisitions, it results in a linear shift in the readout/frequency encoding direction. Several methods have been proposed to correct for off-resonance effects during readout for non-Cartesian acquisitions [24–26].

T_2 Decay

In UTE MRI, T_2 decay during data acquisition effectively applies a low-pass filter to the acquired data. For imaging short-T_2 species, the fast T_2 delay limits the spatial resolution that can be achieved. To minimize the impact of T_2 decay during readout, shorter readout durations can be used, for example, by increasing the acquisition bandwidth.

Imaging Multiple Slices

Similar strategies, as used for acquiring multiple slices in conventional 2D imaging using full pulses for excitation, can be adopted to image multiple slices with 2D UTE MRI. However, care needs to be taken to minimize the impact of the relatively broad profiles of the excited slices with half pulses.

Conclusion

2D UTE imaging allows visualization of tissues with short T_2/T_2^* values using relatively short acquisition times. This chapter describes basic strategies needed to achieve 2D UTE images. Practical issues, such as imaging off-isocenter slices, the impact of gradient timing errors and eddy currents, off-resonance effects, and their impacts on image quality during both excitation and data acquisition, are described. Strategies to address or mitigate these effects are presented.

References

1. Balcom BJ, Macgregor RP, Beyea SD, Green DP, Armstrong RL, Bremner TW. Single-point ramped imaging with T_1 enhancement (SPRITE). J Magn Reson A. 1996;123(1):131–4.
2. Emid S, Creyghton JHN. High resolution NMR imaging in solids. Phys B+C. 1985;128(1):81–3.
3. Axelson DE, Kantzas A, Eads T. Single point H-1 magnetic-resonance-imaging of rigid solids. Canad J Appl Spectrosc. 1995;40(1):16–26.
4. Bergin CJ, Pauly JM, Macovski A. Lung parenchyma: projection reconstruction MR imaging. Radiology. 1991;179(3):777–81.
5. Gold GE, Pauly JM, Glover GH, Moretto JC, Macovski A, Herfkens RJ. Characterization of atherosclerosis with a 1.5-T imaging system. J Magn Reson Imaging. 1993;3(2):399–407.
6. Butts K, Sinclair J, Daniel BL, Wansapura J, Pauly JM. Temperature quantitation and mapping of frozen tissue. J Magn Reson Imaging. 2001;13(1):99–104.
7. Gatehouse PD, Bydder GM. Magnetic resonance imaging of short T_2 components in tissue. Clin Radiol. 2003;58(1):1–19.
8. Deshmane A, Gulani V, Griswold MA, Seiberlich N. Parallel MR imaging. J Magn Reson Imaging. 2012;36(1):55–72.
9. Lustig M, Donoho DL, Santos JM, Pauly JM. Compressed sensing MRI. IEEE Signal Process Mag. 2008;25(2):72–82.
10. Gurney PT, Hargreaves BA, Nishimura DG. Design and analysis of a practical 3D cones trajectory. Magn Reson Med. 2006;55(3):575–82.
11. Boada FE, Gillen JS, Shen GX, Chang SY, Thulborn KR. Fast three dimensional sodium imaging. Magn Reson Med. 1997;37(5):706–15.
12. Pauly JM, Conolly S, Nishimura D, Macovski A. Slice-selective excitation for very short T_2 species. Proc Soc Mag Reson Med. 1989:28.
13. Pauly J, Nishimura D, Macovski A. A k-space analysis of small-tip-angle excitation. 1989. J Magn Reson. 2011;213(2):544–57.
14. Conolly S, Nishimura DG, Macovski A, Glover G. Variable-rate selective excitation. J Magn Reson. 1988;78(3):440–58.
15. Robison RK, Devaraj A, Pipe JG. Fast, simple gradient delay estimation for spiral MRI. Magn Reson Med. 2010;63(6):1683–90.
16. Lu A, Atkinson IC, Vaughn JT, Thulborn KR. Impact of gradient timing error on the tissue sodium concentration bioscale measured using flexible twisted projection imaging. J Magn Reson. 2011;213(1):176–81.
17. Moussavi A, Untenberger M, Uecker M, Frahm J. Correction of gradient-induced phase errors in radial MRI. Magn Reson Med. 2014;71(1):308–12.
18. Schroeder C, Boernert P, Rahmer J. Slice excitation for ultrashort TE imaging. Proc Int Soc Mag Reson Med. 2004:628.
19. Lu A, Daniel BL, Pauly JM, Pauly KB. Improved slice selection for R_2^* mapping during cryoablation with eddy current compensation. J Magn Reson Imaging. 2008;28(1):190–8.
20. Duyn JH, Yang Y, Frank JA, Veen JW. Simple correction method for k-space trajectory deviations in MRI. J Magn Reson. 1998;132(1):150–3.
21. Gurney P, Pauly JM, Nishimura DG. A simple method for measuring B_0 eddy currents. Proc Int Soc Mag Reson Med. 2005:866.
22. Josan S, Pauly JM, Daniel BL, Pauly KB. Double half RF pulses for reduced sensitivity to eddy currents in UTE imaging. Magn Reson Med. 2009;61(5):1083–9.
23. Josan S, Kaye E, Pauly JM, Daniel BL, Pauly KB. Improved half RF slice selectivity in the presence of eddy currents with out-of-slice saturation. Magn Reson Med. 2009;61(5):1090–5.
24. Noll DC, Pauly JM, Meyer CH, Nishimura DG, Macovski A. Deblurring for non-2D Fourier transform magnetic resonance imaging. Magn Reson Med. 1992;25(2):319–33.
25. Man LC, Pauly JM, Macovski A. Multifrequency interpolation for fast off-resonance correction. Magn Reson Med. 1997;37(5):785–92.
26. Schomberg H. Off-resonance correction of MR images. IEEE Trans Med Imaging. 1999;18(6):481–95.

Three-Dimensional Ultrashort Echo Time (3D UTE) Imaging

Michael Carl, Hyungseok Jang, Yajun Ma, Maggie Fung, and Jiang Du

Introduction

Conventional magnetic resonance imaging (MRI) techniques allow direct imaging of species with relatively long transverse relaxation times (T_2s). Spatial localization is achieved by using three orthogonal magnetic field gradients for slice selection (G_z), phase encoding (G_y), and frequency encoding (G_x), respectively [1]. The G_z gradient, together with a radiofrequency (RF) pulse, rotates proton magnetization to form a thin slice for two-dimensional (2D) imaging, or to form a thick slab for three-dimensional (3D) imaging. The G_y gradient enables the protons to gain or lose different phase increments according to their location on the y-axis. Meanwhile, the G_x gradient allows proton magnetizations to rotate at different frequencies according to their locations on the x-axis. Cartesian sampling is typically used to acquire the phase and frequency encoding data. Inverse Fourier Transformation (FT) of the k-space data reconstructs the final 2D or 3D MR images. Many MR techniques have been developed to generate high spatial resolution MR imaging of soft tissues in the body. Most sequences are either T_1-weighted or T_2-weighted and utilize spin echo or gradient

echo acquisitions. A spin echo is usually generated by a 90° pulse followed by a 180° pulse, whereas a gradient echo is usually generated by a single low flip angle RF pulse in conjunction with gradient reversal. The echo time (TE), defined as the time between the end of the RF pulse and the beginning of the read gradient, and the repetition time (TR), defined as the time between successive pulse sequences applied to the same slice or slab, are two key imaging parameters. Gradient echo sequences typically have much shorter TEs and TRs than spin echo sequences.

Conventional MR sequences cannot directly image tissues with short- and ultrashort-T_2s due to the fast decay of their transverse magnetizations to near zero before the spatial encoding gradients are applied and the signal is detected [2]. As a result, short- and ultrashort-T_2 tissues appear as signal voids on conventional clinical MR images. The lack of signal also means that conventional MRI techniques are often of little value for morphological and quantitative assessment of short- and ultrashort-T_2 tissues. Their MR relaxation times (e.g., T_1, T_2, T_2^*, and $T_{1\rho}$) and other tissue properties (e.g., magnetization transfer, perfusion, diffusion, and susceptibility) are often not well-characterized [3, 4]. These properties can include early biochemical changes such as proteoglycan depletion, collagen degradation, and changes in water content. They may play critical roles in early diagnosis and treatment monitoring at stages of disease progression where little or no morphological change has occurred.

Ultrashort echo time (UTE) sequences enable direct visualization of short- and ultrashort-T_2 tissues that are otherwise low to zero signal in clinical MR imaging [2]. This is usually achieved by acquiring the free induction decay (FID) of the MR signal as soon after the end of the RF excitation pulse as possible in combination with a radial center-out k-space trajectory and data sampling of a few hundred ms. Typical minimum TE values (defined as the time between the end of the RF pulse and the beginning of the read gradient) for clinical scanners range between a few tens and a few hundred ms. Volumetric 3D UTE techniques have gained higher popularity in recent years compared to 2D techniques, in part due to

M. Carl (✉)
GE Healthcare, San Diego, CA, USA
e-mail: Michael.Carl@ge.com

H. Jang · Y. Ma
Department of Radiology, University of California, San Diego, La Jolla, CA, USA
e-mail: h4jang@health.ucsd.edu; yam013@health.ucsd.edu

M. Fung
GE Healthcare, New York, NY, USA
e-mail: Maggie.Fung@med.ge.com

J. Du
Department of Radiology, University of California, San Diego, La Jolla, CA, USA

Department of Bioengineering, University of California, San Diego, La Jolla, CA, USA

VA San Diego Healthcare System, San Diego, CA, USA
e-mail: jiangdu@health.ucsd.edu

© The Author(s), under exclusive license to Springer Nature Switzerland AG 2023
J. Du, G. M. Bydder (eds.), *MRI of Short- and Ultrashort-T₂ Tissues*, https://doi.org/10.1007/978-3-031-35197-6_4

the greater availability of anisotropic resolution and field of view (FOV) capability for 3D UTE imaging [5–7]. In addition, applying slab selection (along with 3D k-space encoding) is less sensitive to gradient imperfections such as eddy current delays than relying solely on 2D slice selection in the z-direction. The introduction of novel contrast mechanisms provides an excellent depiction of short-T_2 tissues [5]. The development of quantitative UTE imaging techniques also provides systematic evaluation of MR relaxation times and tissue properties, which are not possible with conventional sequences [3].

Data Acquisition

UTE sequences are generally based on gradient echo acquisitions with TEs much shorter than those used in spin echo or fast spin echo acquisitions. There are several factors affecting the minimal achievable TE in regular gradient echo imaging. First, there is a delay after the initial RF excitation when the slice-selection gradient is needed to rephase the MR signal. Second, an extra delay is introduced due to the need for the phase encoding gradient. Third, the initial dephasing lobe of the frequency encoding gradient and the data acquisition before the center of k-space further delay TE. Finally, the use of a relatively long excitation RF pulse, usually of sinc shape required for slice or slab excitation,

further delays TE which is more accurately defined as the time between the peak of the RF pulse and the acquisition of the k-space center. As a result, conventional gradient echo sequences typically have TEs of the order of several ms or longer.

In order to significantly reduce TE, it is important to eliminate the time needed for slice/slab selection, phase encoding, and dephasing/rephasing of the frequency encoding gradient and to minimize the time for RF excitation and frequency encoding. A 3D UTE sequence can meet all these requirements by employing a short nonselective rectangular pulse (duration of the order of 10–100 μs) for volumetric excitation, followed by 3D radial ramp sampling with k-space traversed radially from $k = 0$ outwards [7]. Radial mapping of 3D k-space rather than conventional Cartesian k-space sampling eliminates the requirement for phase encoding. Radial ramp sampling also eliminates the need for dephasing and rephasing lobes of the frequency encoding gradient. A short rectangular pulse eliminates the time needed for slice encoding and minimizes the time needed for signal-excitation. Eddy currents associated with the slice/slab-selective gradients are also eliminated, although ramp sampling is still subject to eddy currents. Figure 4.1a–c shows the pulse sequence diagram for 3D UTE radial imaging, as well as different k-space sampling trajectories.

In radial sampling, N_p projections are acquired with N_r-acquired data points along each projection. This results in

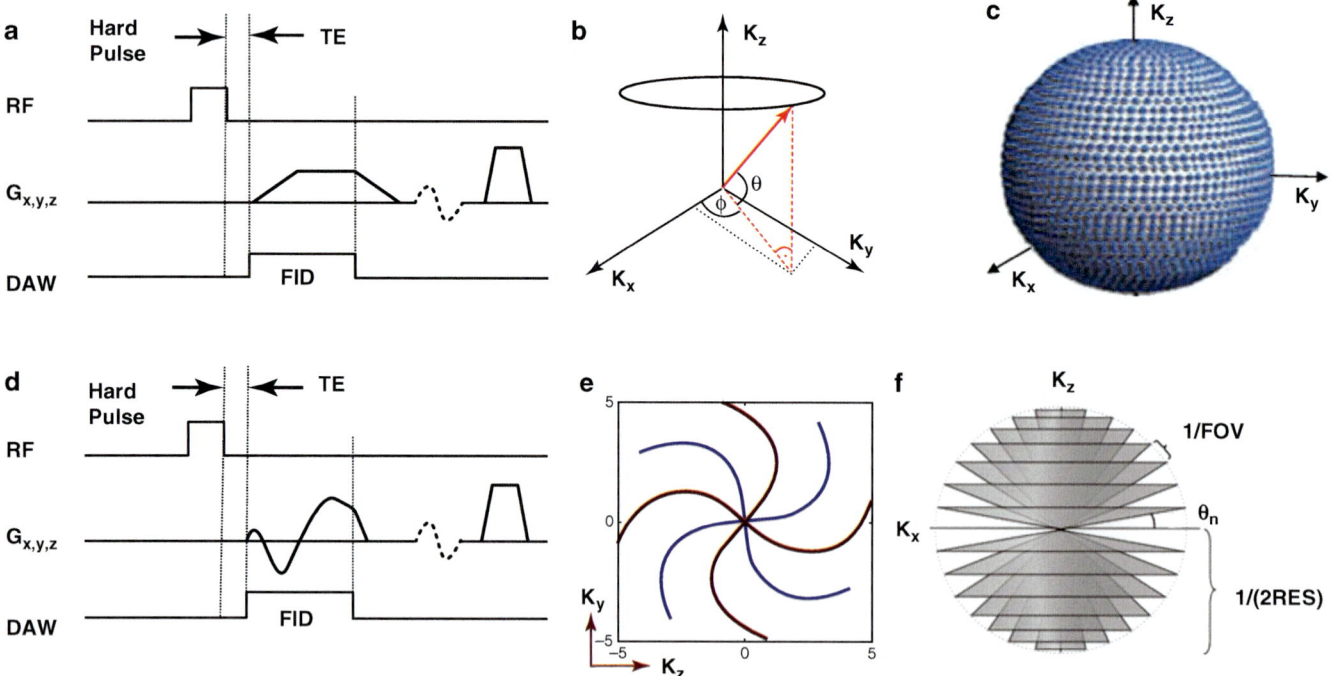

Fig. 4.1 Diagrams of the 3D radial UTE sequence (**a**) which employs a short rectangular pulse (hard pulse) excitation followed by 3D radial ramp sampling (**b**) with koosh ball trajectories (**c**), and the 3D spiral UTE (3D Cones) sequence (**d**) which employs a short rectangular pulse excitation followed by twisted radial sampling (**e**) with conical view ordering (**f**)

nonuniform sampling density with overweighted low spatial frequencies. The radial sampling supports an alias-free reconstruction when N_p equals π times N_r and 2D projection reconstruction (PR) is used. To get one image with isotropic in-plane spatial resolution, Fourier encoding spin-warp imaging requires N_r phase encoding lines. Therefore, radial ramp sampling PR acquisition is a factor of π less efficient than 2D spin-warp imaging. This decrease in sampling efficiency is due to the oversampling of central k-space, especially for 3D PR imaging. The PR acquisition is more sensitive to magnetic field inhomogeneity, susceptibility, chemical shift effects, and eddy currents. However, projection imaging also provides some desirable properties, including more robustness to bulk motion because of the averaging effects from repeated sampling of the low spatial frequencies, diffuse aliasing patterns that allow scan time reduction through undersampling, and FID acquisition for short-T_2 imaging with a minimal TE [3].

There have been several k-space trajectories employed for 3D UTE imaging, such as radial-out PR [8], acquisition-weighted stack of spirals (AWSOS) [9], twisted projection imaging (TPI) [10], variable echo time (vTE) [11], and Cones [12]. The radial trajectory can be extended for twisted projection imaging (TPI), or further twisted for more efficient 3D Cones imaging (Fig. 4.1d–f) [6, 12]. The Cones trajectory is a generalization of the 3D radial trajectory in which spokes twist around one of the axes, resulting in longer readout time per TR (higher duty cycle) and increased signal-to-noise ratio (SNR) efficiency. More twisting can be added to the Cones trajectory to further increase readout time and reduce the total number of readouts required for full sampling. Thus, the 3D Cones trajectory provides the flexibility to reduce total scan time while increasing SNR efficiency at the cost of an increased sampling window [12], which eventually leads to increased spatial blurring. The Cones trajec-

tory design requires consideration of slew rate limitations imposed by typical gradient hardware, proper adjustment of the sampling density, and careful consideration of the relationship between cones to minimize aliasing artifacts inside the specified FOV [12]. Special reconstruction techniques are needed to generate 3D UTE images from radial or Cones sampling.

Reconstruction

In conventional MRI, Cartesian sampling is typically used to collect phase and frequency encoding data in k-space. The final MR images are reconstructed using inverse FT of the 2D or 3D k-space data [1]. Radial or spiral UTE data sets do not fall on a regular Cartesian grid in spatial frequency space. Figure 4.2 shows schematic 2D k-space data sampled with the radial trajectory (Fig. 4.2a), spiral trajectory (Fig. 4.2b), and regridding reconstruction (Fig. 4.2c). A 3D radial UTE k-space is very similar to Fig. 4.2a but with a 3D koosh ball or similar sampling pattern. 3D Cones UTE k-space is similar to Fig. 4.2b but with conical view ordering of 3D spiral data [12]. There are many options for the reconstruction of non-Cartesian data, including back-projection, conjugate phase reconstruction, and regridding. The most popular way is to resample the radial or spiral data to a Cartesian grid, followed by inverse FT of re-gridded Cartesian k-space data to reconstruct the final UTE images. Figure 4.2c shows the basic idea of regridding, where data points lie along the sampled k-space trajectory. Each k-space data point is convolved with a gridding kernel. After every data point along each k-space trajectory is processed, a final Cartesian grid is produced [13]. A 3D inverse FT is then performed to generate the final UTE images.

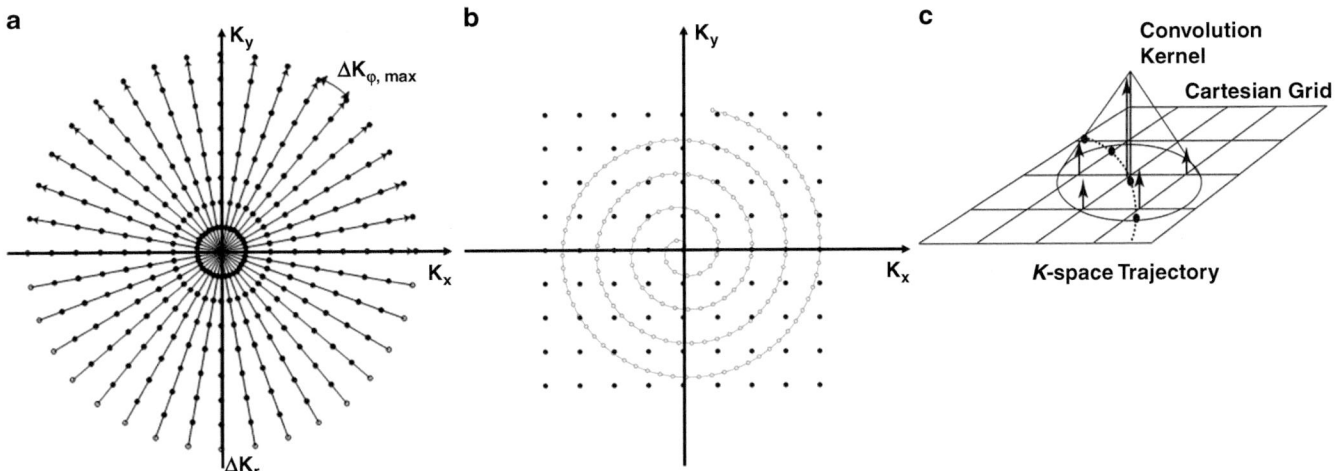

Fig. 4.2 Diagrams of k-space data with radial acquisition (**a**), and spiral acquisition (**b**), as well as regridding reconstruction (**c**)

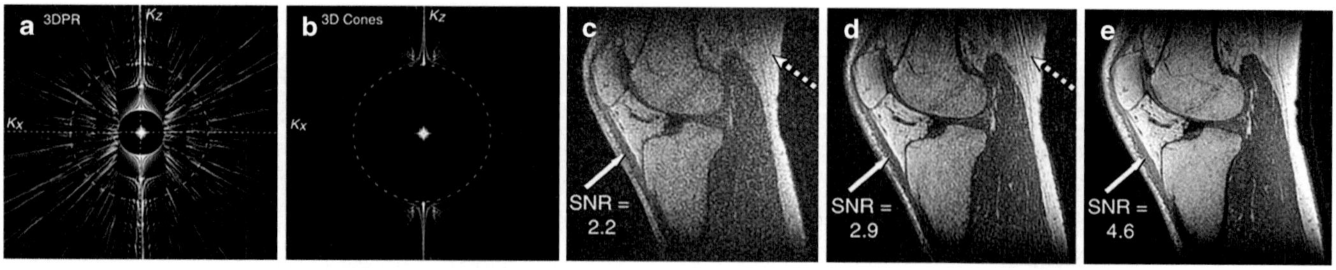

Fig. 4.3 Slice through the x–z plane of the PSFs for a 3D radial trajectory (**a**) and a 3D Cones trajectory (**b**), as well as a sagittal slice through the 3D UTE data set acquired with the high (**c**) and low (**d**) bandwidth 3D radial trajectories, and the 3D Cones trajectory (**e**). The PSF for the 3D Cones trajectory performs much better inside the prescribed FOV than the 3D radial trajectory. A significantly higher SNR was achieved for the patellar tendon (solid arrow) with the 3D Cones trajectory (SNR = 4.6) than with the 3D radial trajectory using a high bandwidth (SNR = 2.2) or a low bandwidth (SNR = 2.9). (Reproduced with permission from Ref. [12])

Figure 4.3 shows the point spread functions (PSFs) for undersampled radial trajectories (a) and 3D Cones (b), as well as an example of 3D UTE imaging of the knee joint in a healthy volunteer (c–e) [12]. The PSFs are symmetric about the z-axis, with much better performance observed with the 3D Cones trajectory than with the undersampled 3D radial trajectory. The 3D Cones trajectory has a highly diffuse, low-amplitude aliasing pattern in the x–y plane outside of the prescribed FOV allowing substantial undersampling in these directions to further speed up data acquisition. In contrast, there is a relatively coherent aliasing pattern along the z-axis outside the prescribed FOV due to the 3D Cones acquisition symmetry around the z-axis [12]. Therefore, undersampling in this direction should be avoided. A slab-select excitation in the z-direction can be used to limit the acquired FOV to the prescribed FOV for reduced artifacts (more details about this technique will be discussed in the section "Slab-Selective Excitation"). The advantage of the 3D Cones trajectory over the radial trajectory was demonstrated by calculating SNRs for the patellar tendon in the volunteer's knee joint. The 3D Cones trajectory provides a significantly higher SNR than the 3D radial trajectory with either a high or low bandwidth (BW) [12]. Similar results were achieved for the patella.

Figure 4.4 shows a more systematic study of the PSFs generated for four different trajectory lengths, ranging from a pure radial trajectory (readout duration 624 μs), trajectories with more twist (readout duration 680–1600 μs), to a more spiral-like trajectory with many full turns within one spoke (readout duration 4000 μs). The last trajectory only serves

for the purpose of comparison since such long trajectories introduce undesired T_2^* blurring of short-T_2 tissues. The designated k-space trajectories are designed to achieve a fixed short scan time of 55 s, FOV = 24 cm, and isotropic spatial resolution = 1 mm. Indicated in Fig. 4.4a are the undersampling factors required to achieve the same scan time. The PSFs are shown in Fig. 4.4b at twice the FOV (48 cm) of the reconstructed images (indicated by the dashed boxes) to show the region outside the supported area. The high undersampling for the radial trajectory results in only a small region of support surrounded by diffuse radial streaks, while the longer trajectories result in a larger region of FOV support but have a more coherent aliasing signal just outside that region. A standard-resolution phantom was imaged using a clinical 3T MRI system. Acquisition parameters included BW = ±125 kHz, isotropic FOV = 24 cm and spatial resolution = 1 mm, TE = 30 μs, and total scan time of 55 s. The native symmetry direction of the Cones design was along the z-axis, which was perpendicular to the axial images shown in Fig. 4.4c, d. These images were also reformatted into the coronal plane, as shown in Fig. 4.4e, f, which lies in the same plane as the PSFs. Two distinct artifacts can be observed. The images generated by the very short radial trajectory and the highest degree of undersampling show visible streak artifacts (red oval). At the other extreme, the image using a very long readout trajectory (last row) results in less visible aliasing artifacts with some blurring near the edge of the phantom (see also Fig. 4.4g). The trajectory in the second row shows reduced artifact compared to pure radial sampling without

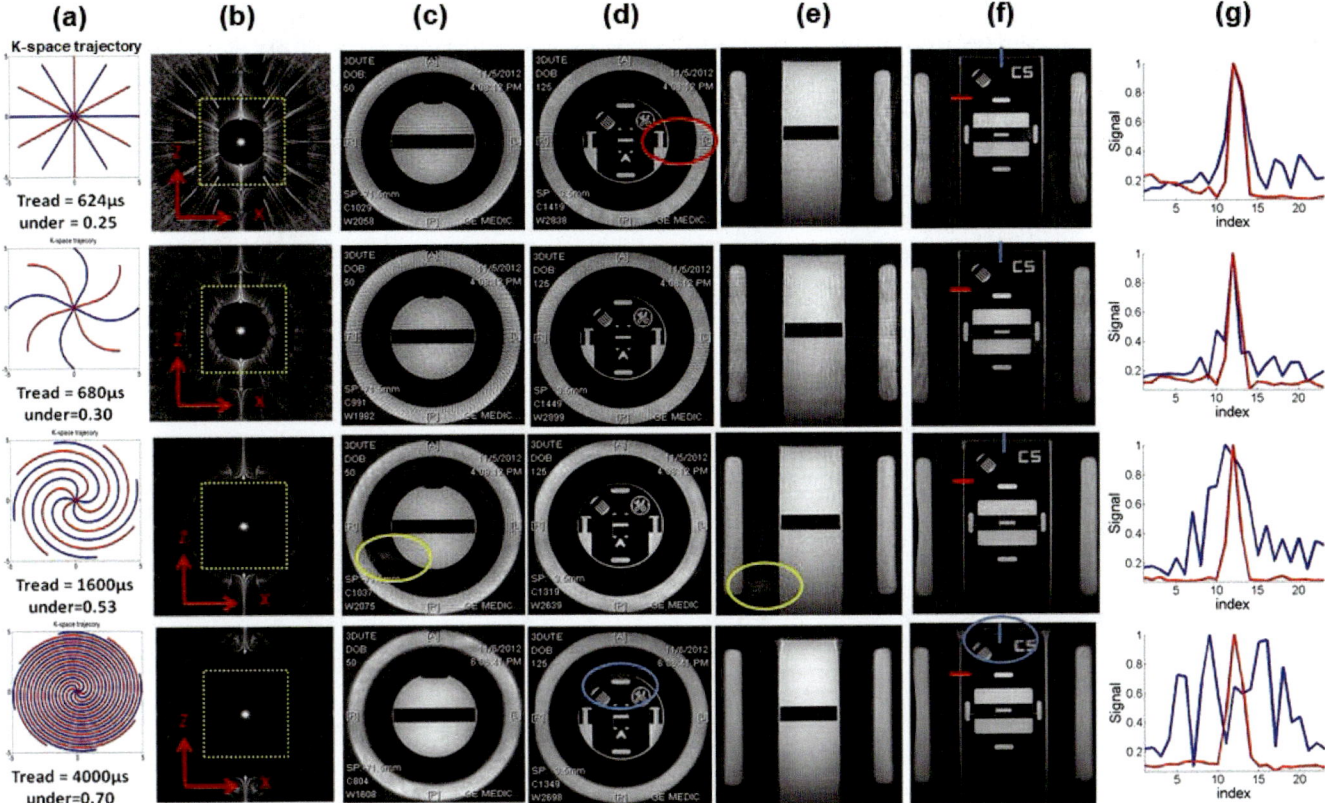

Fig. 4.4 *K*-space trajectories with various readout durations and curvatures (**a**). Corresponding PSFs for the *x–z* plane (**b**). Two axial slices (**c**, **d**). Two reformatted coronal slices. Image artifacts are highlighted by ovals (**d**, **e**). Many of these artifacts are less severe for the trajectory in the second row (Tread = 680 μs). 1D lines through two walls of the phantom (as indicated in **f**), showing increased blurring for longer trajectories (**g**)

the significant blurring seen in the very long readout trajectory. Finally, as expected, the SNR in the images from the longer trajectories is visibly higher than that seen with the shorter ones.

RF Excitation

Transverse relaxation during RF excitation does not usually require consideration in conventional MR imaging of long-T_2 species, where T_2 is typically much longer than the RF pulse duration. However, the T_2^* relaxation may be significant in imaging of short-T_2 species where T_2^*s may be of the order of the pulse duration or much shorter. As a result, UTE imaging of short-T_2 species typically uses a short rectangular pulse for more efficient excitation. However, the nonselective short hard pulse may produce undesired aliasing arti-

facts, which may be reduced by using a slab-selective excitation pulse as there is a relatively coherent aliasing pattern along the *z*-axis outside of the prescribed FOV in 3D UTE imaging. Water excitation pulses have also been implemented to create high contrast for UTE imaging of short-T_2 tissues.

Hard RF Excitation

Efficient excitation of short-T_2 species requires a wide RF excitation BW since the spectral profile increases in tissues with short T_2. A short rectangular pulse with maximal B_1 power is therefore ideal for short-T_2 excitation. The short pulse duration maximizes RF pulse spectral BW and minimizes signal loss during excitation, which, together with a high B_1, maximizes the excitation efficiency. The excitation efficiency is greatly reduced when the RF pulse duration is increased and the pulse amplitude is decreased. Figure 4.5a shows the "critical" transverse relaxation rate, $T_2^{\text{crit}} = (2\gamma B_1)^{-1}$, during excitation without appreciable T_1 relaxation [14]. The RF pulse effect is not purely a rotation but a modification of

the magnetization amplitude if magnetization experiences non-negligible relaxation during the excitation pulse. The excitation efficiency, defined as $M_{xy}/\sin(\alpha)$, is a function of T_2 and α, which equals $\gamma B_1 p$ where p is the pulse duration. This T_2-dependent excitation can be used to create relaxation-

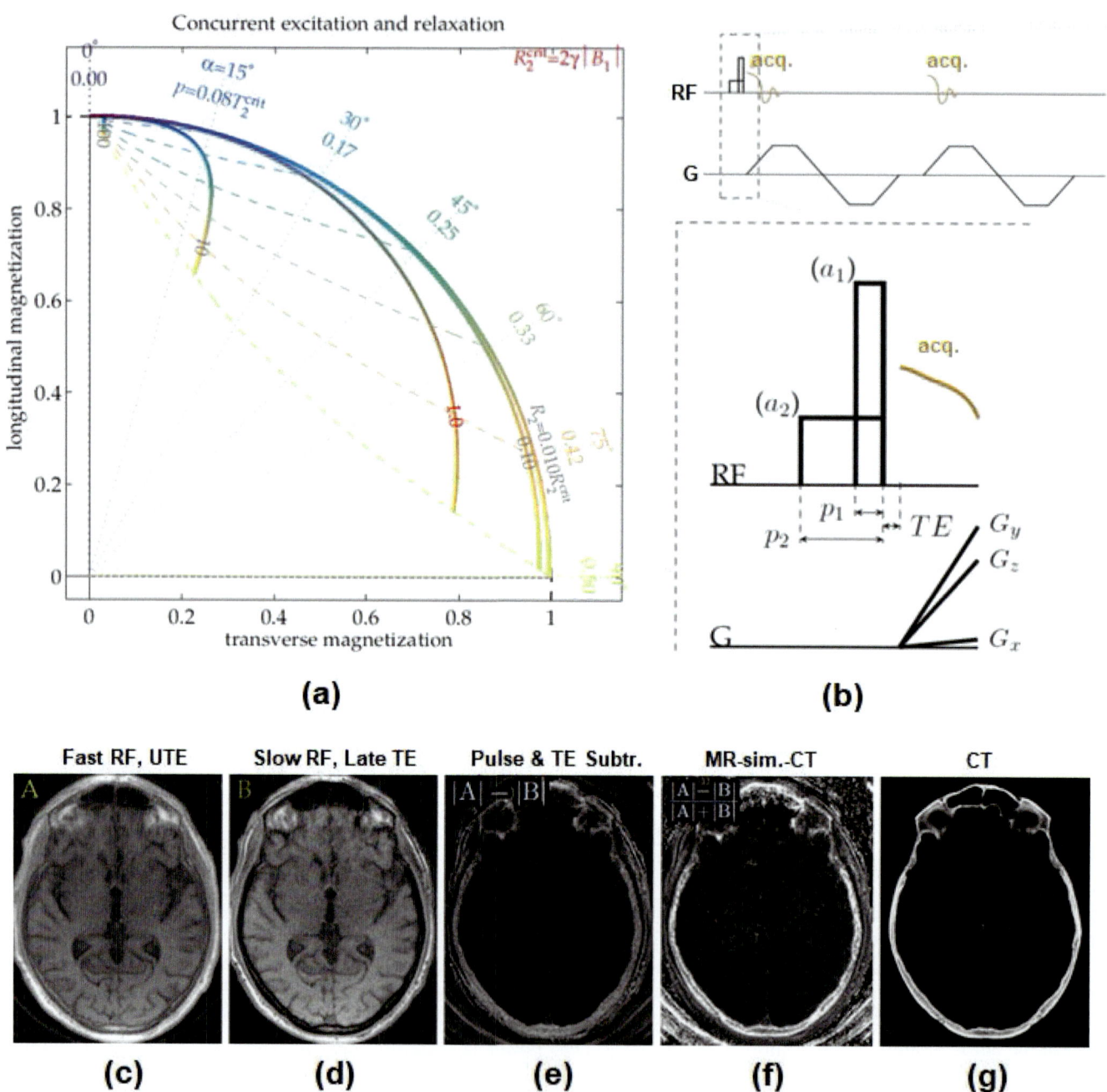

(a)   **(b)**

(c)   **(d)**   **(e)**   **(f)**   **(g)**

Fig. 4.5 Simulation of the short-T_2 excitation as a function of pulse duration p or nominal excitation angle $\alpha = \gamma B_1 p$ and R_2 (thick lines) (**a**). The relaxation-parameter contrast mechanism is based on two hard RF pulses with different durations but equal pulse areas to generate T_2-selective excitation (**b**). An example imaging of the skull is shown with 3D UTE pairing a fast excitation pulse with UTE (24.47 μT RF, 34 μs TE) (**c**) and a slow excitation pulse with a later echo (1.53 μT RF, 2 ms TE) (**d**). Subtraction of the two 3D UTE data sets (**b**) and (**c**) provides high-contrast imaging of the skull (**e**), which can be further improved by normalizing the difference to remove proton density weighting with contrast in the normalized difference MR-sim.-CT image (**f**) resembling that of an X-ray CT image (**g**) acquired from the same subject. (Reproduced with permission from Ref. [14])

parameter contrast that is compatible with UTE imaging of short-T_2 species such as cortical bone [14]. Figure 4.5a shows RF excitation pulse parameters selected to determine the extent of concurrent relaxation and excitation, where the pulse duration p and the amplitude are changed to adjust the relaxation dependence of the image contrast. Two pulse durations (i.e., p_1 and p_2) can be chosen to selectively detect signals from magnetization within a specific range of T_2 values. Subtraction of two UTE datasets with the same imaging parameters but different RF excitation pulses creates T_2-specific contrast. Figure 4.5c–f shows an example of imaging the skull of a healthy volunteer using 3D radial UTE. UTE with a short RF pulse detects all anatomical regions, including the skull (Fig. 4.5c). The second echo UTE image with a long-duration low-power pulse selectively avoids excitation and reception of signals from the skull (Fig. 4.5d). Subtraction of the two datasets provides high-contrast imaging of the skull (Fig. 4.5e). The normalized difference image (Fig. 4.5f) shows excellent positive contrast for the skull similar to that observed with X-ray CT (Fig. 4.5g) [14].

Slab-Selective Excitation

The 3D UTE sequence can apply a slice-selection gradient on the z-axis. This allows the application of slab selection to excite spins only from anatomies within the desired region (e.g., in sagittal spine imaging). This reduces the aliasing (or streak) artifacts commonly encountered with non-Cartesian imaging [15]. The simulation study by Gurney et al. demon-strates a relatively coherent aliasing pattern along the z-axis outside of the prescribed FOV in 3D Cones imaging which can be reduced by using a slab-select excitation in the z-direction [12]. As a result, the slab-selective pulse is expected to greatly reduce aliasing artifacts, especially when the slab coverage is narrow and the coil sensitivity is wide. Conventional slab selection in clinical MR sequences usually applies a symmetric sinc RF excitation pulse during the flattop portion of a slab-selection gradient, followed by a rewinder gradient of the opposite polarity. The required ramp-down and rewinder gradient usually push the minimum TE out to greater than 1 ms, making them impractical for UTE imaging. The rewinder time can be minimized by using a minimum-phase Shinnar–Le Roux (SLR) pulse [16] which concentrates most of the RF energy toward the end of the pulse (Fig. 4.6) and hence reduces the phase through which the slice needs to be rewound (i.e., reduced isodelay). Keeping the same excitation k-space deposition during the gradient ramp-down requires variable-rate selective excitation (VERSE) correction of the RF pulse [17].

Figure 4.7 shows slab profiles measured in a water bottle phantom. The slab profiles were obtained by imaging an approximately three times larger through-slice FOV than the slab-selective excitation and reformatting the data to image the slab profile shown in the top row. The second row shows averaged line profiles through the slabs. The last row shows the simulated profiles, including real (red) and imaginary (blue) parts. They agree well with the experimental profiles.

Figure 4.8 shows axial images of an ex vivo human brain using a hard pulse and the slab-selection pulse discussed

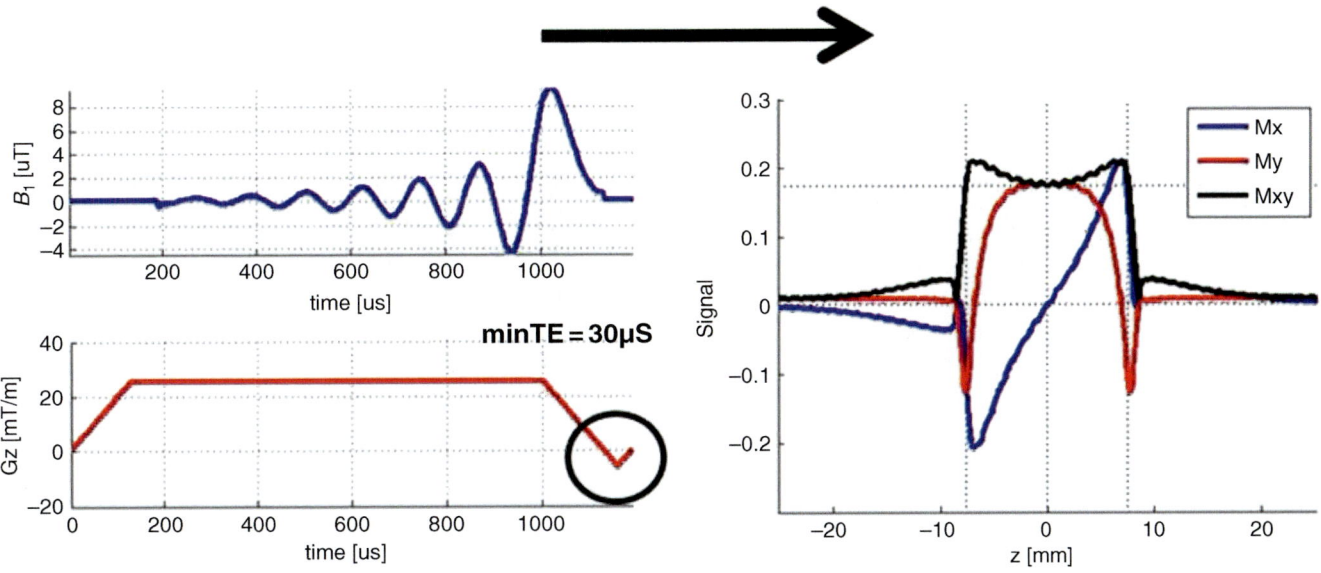

Fig. 4.6 SLR pulse with minor VERSE correction and only a small (optional) slab rewinder during the T/R switching time (30 μs). The resulting slab profile still has an imaginary signal and some signal outside of the nominal slab volume

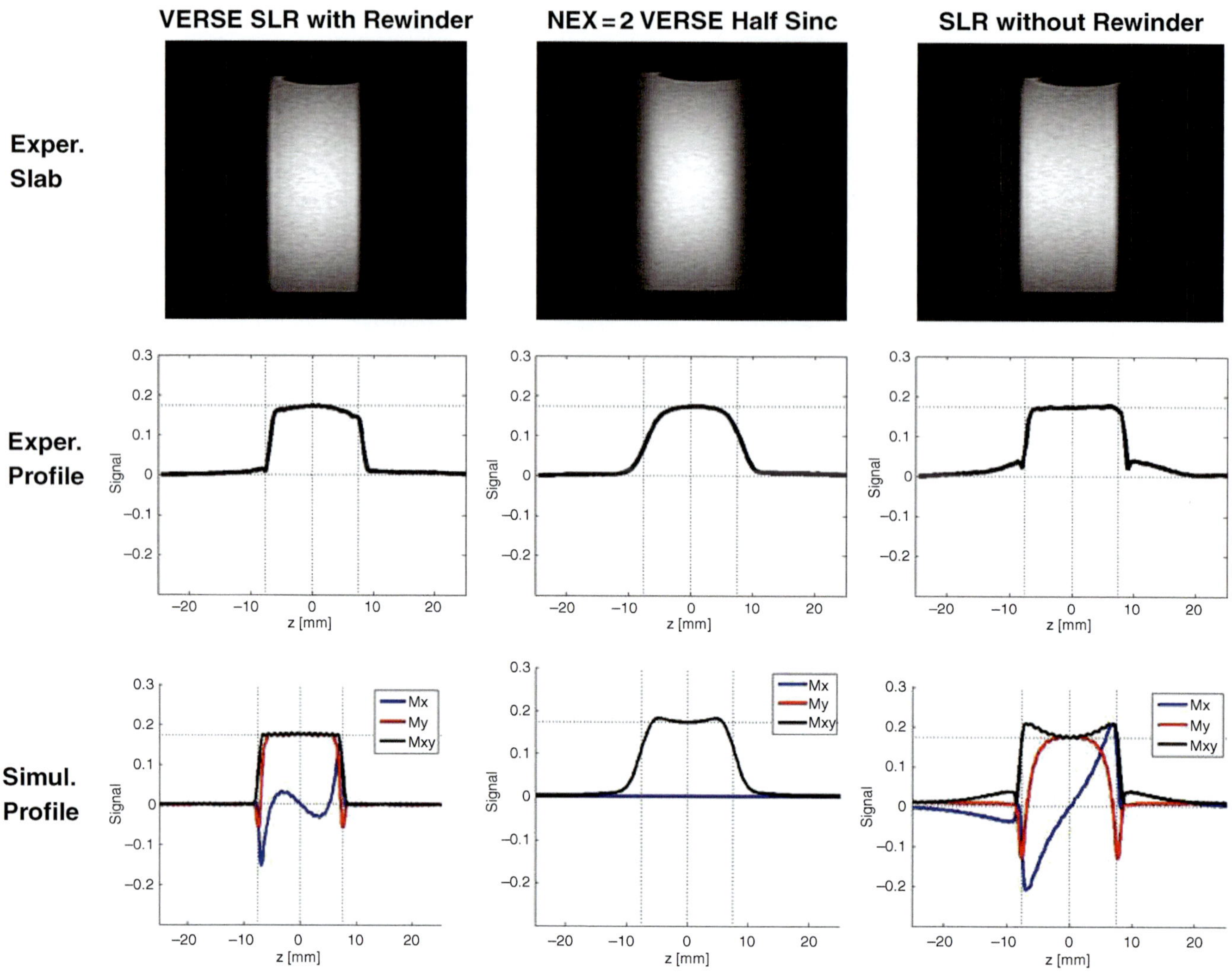

VERSE SLR with Rewinder
NEX = 2 VERSE Half Sinc
SLR without Rewinder
Exper. Slab
Exper. Profile
Simul. Profile
Signal
z [mm]
Mx
My
Mxy

Fig. 4.7 Experimental slab profiles measured in a water bottle phantom. These were obtained by imaging an approximately three times larger through-slice FOV than the slab-selective excitation and reformatting the data to image the slab profile (top row). Row two shows average line profiles through the slabs. For comparison, the last row shows the simulated profiles, including real (red), imaginary (blue), and magnitude (black) components, which agree well with the experimental profiles

a Localizer
b Hard Pulse
c Slab Selective

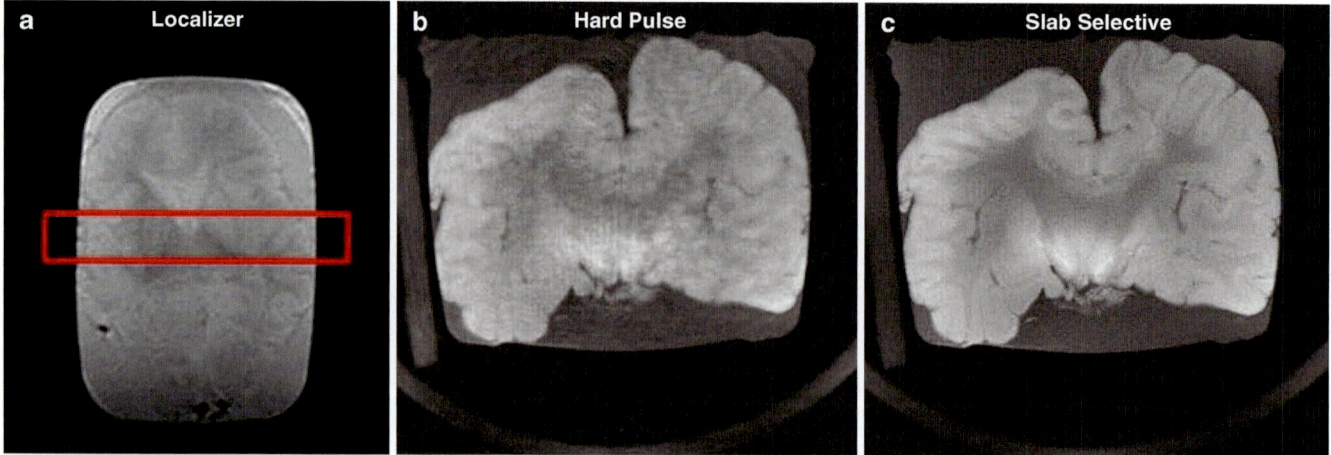

Fig. 4.8 A relatively thin imaging slab on the localizer of an ex vivo brain sample (**a**), the corresponding 3D UTE axial images using a hard pulse (b), and the slab-selection pulse (**c**). The hard pulse excitation shows through-slice artifacts because the through-slice length of the brain phantom (~20 cm) greatly exceeds the encoded volume in the slab direction (20 mm, red box on coronal localizer), causing aliasing artifacts. On the other hand, slab-selective imaging exhibits no visible major artifacts

above. The encoded volume in the slab direction was ten slices with 2 mm slice thickness (see red box on coronal localizer in Fig. 4.8a). The slab-selective imaging exhibits no major visible artifacts (Fig. 4.8c). On the other hand, the hard pulse excitation shows through-slice artifacts (Fig. 4.8b) because the through-slice length of the brain phantom (~20 cm) greatly exceeds the encoded volume in the slab direction (20 mm) and causes aliasing artifacts.

Water Excitation

Due to the minimal TE used, 3D UTE images are inherently low in image contrast. This contrast can be improved by suppressing signals from long-T_2 tissues such as fat. Although UTE is generally compatible with chemical shift suppression (chem-sat) techniques, this technique has the potential to significantly reduce short-T_2 signals of interest. As an alternative, direct water-selective excitation can be used to excite only water-based signals. This has the advantage that short-T_2 signals are not as directly affected as they are with chemical shift saturation techniques. Springer et al.

used a 1–1 double RF excitation pulse to selectively excite only water signals [18]. In this technique, a short RF pulse centered on the water resonance frequency is used to excite both fat and water at the same time. This is followed by a waiting period that allows fat signals to accumulate an off-resonance phase of 180° relative to water (e.g., 1.14 ms at 3 T). After this, a second identical on-water-resonance RF pulse is applied which tips the water signals again by the same flip angle while returning the fat magnetization back to the positive z-axis. As a consequence, it does not contribute to the imaging signals. The resulting images show excellent fat suppression on MSK images. Similarly, Ma et al. have developed an excitation scheme using a combination of a narrow BW soft RF pulse centered on the fat frequency, followed by a short hard pulse (with a wide BW covering both the fat and water signals) centered on the water frequency but using the opposite flip angle (Fig. 4.9a, b) [19]. The resulting excited transverse magnetization only contains water signals. The fat suppression quality is similar with either technique, but short-T_2 tissues (e.g., meniscus) are better preserved with the soft-hard composite excitation scheme (Fig. 4.9c–e).

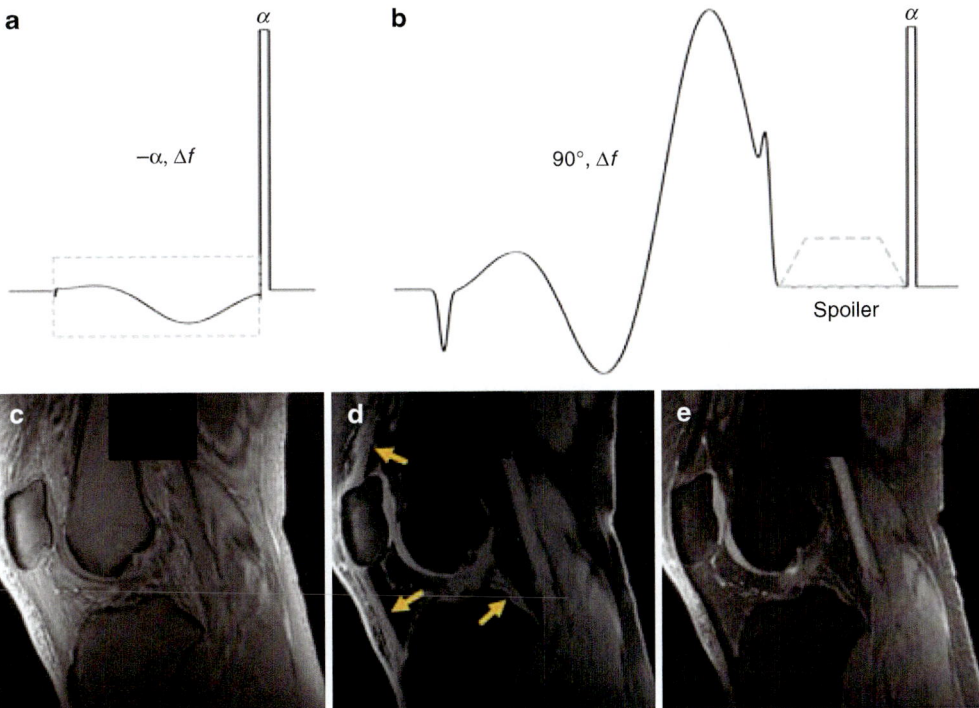

Fig. 4.9 The soft-hard composite pulse. This employs a soft RF pulse centered on fat on-resonance frequency (Δf) with a negative flip angle ($-\alpha$) which is used to flip only the fat magnetization. This is followed by a short hard pulse with a positive flip angle (α) which flips all the magnetizations (i.e., fat and water) in the opposite direction (**a**). The commonly used FatSat UTE pulse employs a 90° soft pulse centered on fat on-resonance frequency to flip and spoil the fat magnetization, followed by a hard pulse for water signal excitation (**b**). An example is shown on 3D UTE Cones imaging of the knee joint of a 24-year-old volunteer using excitations with a single hard pulse (**c**), the soft-hard water excitation pulse (**d**), and the conventional FatSat module (**e**). Fat was suppressed by both the soft-hard pulse and the FatSat module, but the short-T_2 signals are much better preserved with the soft-hard pulse (yellow arrows in **d**). (Reproduced with permission from Ref. [19])

Sampling Window

Imaging short-T_2 species requires consideration of transverse relaxation during the data acquisition window, as T_2 or T_2^* is of the order of the duration of the sampling window, or even shorter. Rahmer et al. investigated the effects of T_2^* decay during signal acquisition on the 1D, 2D, and 3D radial PSFs [7]. The impact of short-T_2^* relaxation on the PSF depends on the k-space trajectory. An exponential T_2^* decay in time corresponds to a centric exponential decay in k-space. The image space blurring function $P_{dec}(r)$ is just the 3D Fourier transform of this decay function. $P_{dec}(r)$ for 2D and 1D radial FID sampling can be derived in a similar way. Figure 4.10a–c shows the normalized blurring functions for the exemplary case in which the sampling window is four times longer than T_2^*. A smaller linewidth is observed in the 3D blurring function than in its 2D and 1D counterparts. Figure 4.10d–f shows an image of a short-T_2 phantom (rolled

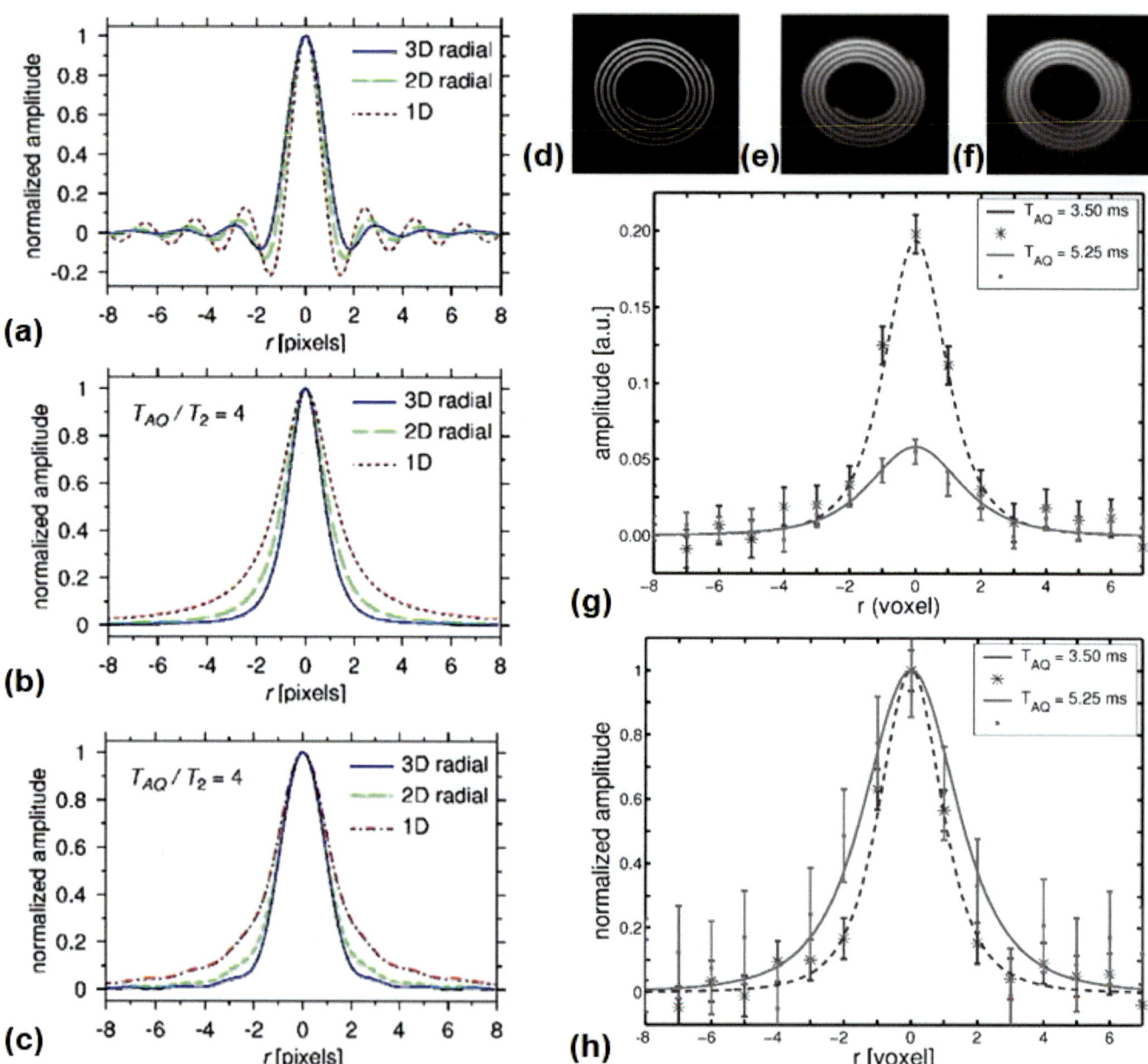

Fig. 4.10 Simulated PSF and blurring function for three sampling patterns, including unblurred PSF (**a**), normalized blurring functions for the exemplary case $T_{AQ}/T_2 = 4$ (**b**), and total PSFs for $T_{AQ}/T_2 = 4$ obtained from the convolution of (**a**) with (**b**) shown in (**c**). 3D UTE images of rolled rubberband ($T_2 = 660$ μs) with three different readout window durations T_{AQ} of 0.68 ms (**d**), 3.50 ms (**e**), and 5.25 ms (**f**).

Short-T_2 blurring function extracted from the image data by deconvolution of images (**e**) and (**f**) with (**d**), respectively (**g**). Solid lines correspond to simulated blurring functions. A normalized plot of the same data emphasizes the increase in linewidth with increasing T_{AQ} (**h**). (Reproduced with permission from Ref. [7])

rubber band with $T_2^* = 660$ μs) acquired using $T_{AQ} = 0.68$, 3.50, and 5.25 ms, respectively. The blurring function was extracted by deconvolution of the unblurred image (Fig. 4.10d) from the long-T_{AQ} images (Fig. 4.10e, f). Figure 4.10g shows the extracted blurring function. Figure 4.10h displays the same data scaled to unit amplitude to highlight the line broadening effect. The data were then modeled using the 3D blurring function for $T_2 = 660$ μs and respective sampling durations of $T_{AQ} = 3.50$ and 5.25 ms. Theoretical calculation suggests that the blurring function depends on T_2/T_{AQ} to the power of 3, while the fitted data show a power of 3.5 as the best fit. This is attributed to additional dephasing due to local off-resonances which is not compensated for by the applied single-frequency off-resonance correction. Aside from this effect, amplitude loss and line-broadening are both reproduced in the theoretical 3D blurring function. The theoretical and experimental results demonstrate that UTE imaging should aim at a short TE and optimize the readout-window duration to obtain high, well-resolved signals from short-T_2 species. According to the theoretically derived optimal T_{AQ} criterion for a given T_2 species, an optimal sampling window can be found that maximizes the SNR while introducing only slight blurring. Strong gradients and high reception bandwidths must be employed to meet the SNR criterion for short-T_2 species as the optimal window duration T_{AQ} is shorter than T_2 (e.g., $T_{AQ} = 0.69 T_2$ for 3D radial FID sampling) [7]. This theory also holds for 2D UTE sampling, where the optimal duration of the acquisition window is $T_{AQ} = 0.81 T_2$. However, the Rahmer study shows a somewhat simplified optimal sampling window. The sampling window is optimized only for SNR without considering spatial resolution maximization. Furthermore, for mathematical simplicity, a constant readout gradient is assumed to obtain a linear relationship between time and radial k value: $k(t) = \gamma G t$. In reality, UTE imaging is based on radial ramp sampling of the FID which significantly impacts the optimal sampling window. Ramp sampling leads to repeated sampling of low spatial frequency data. As a result, the optimal sampling window from the Rahmer study would produce low-resolution images of short-T_2 species such as cortical bone. With radial ramp sampling of UTE FID data, a longer window is needed to obtain improved spatial resolution of short-T_2 species. The simplified model works best for zero echo time (ZTE) type sequences, where k-space data points are sampled after gradients are fully ramped up [20].

Eddy Currents

UTE sequences acquire data with variable read gradients. The data points at and near the k-space center are acquired during the ramp-up period of the read gradients (ramp sampling). If there is a mismatch between the nominally designed gradients and the ones that actually occur in the scanner bore, this may result in gridding errors and image artifacts [21, 22]. These gradient imperfections may include gradient group delays or more general gradient amplitude distortions. For simple 3D UTE imaging, group delay corrections are often an effective way to compensate for gradient imperfections. These can be performed using specialized calibration sequences (especially if gradient-to-gradient delays need to be corrected as well), or simple manual tuning of the single overall group delay of the gradients relative to the data acquisition window (DAQ) [23–25]. For example, Addy et al. used an efficient linear time-invariant (LTI) characterization of the MR gradients to estimate trajectories achieved in the scanner [25]. Figure 4.11 shows phantom images of spiral, EPI, and 3D Cones reconstructions with and without trajectory correction. The corrected images show greatly improved image quality, as shown in Fig. 4.11b–d.

A similar but more automated/unsupervised method was developed by Herrman et al. [26]. In their work, a UTE sequence was utilized with each acquisition containing a quick calibration scan which utilized the phase of the readouts to detect the actual k-space center. Their approach used a short, integrated calibration scan which included a small pre-phase gradient applied just before the main readout gradient. Determining the maximum coherence of the phase information in the calibration scan allowed the determination of the actual k-space center. This information was then used to automatically correct the k-space trajectories of the imaging portion of the sequence. Figure 4.12 shows orthogonal phantom images with and without k-space correction. The corrected images show significantly reduced artifacts [26].

More complex waveform designs, such as Cones, may require a more thorough correction technique, for example, measuring individual gradient waveforms and applying correction during reconstruction. Duyn et al. have also developed a simple technique to accurately measure the actual k-space trajectory and to allow the correction of gradient hardware imperfections for arbitrary gradient waveforms [27].

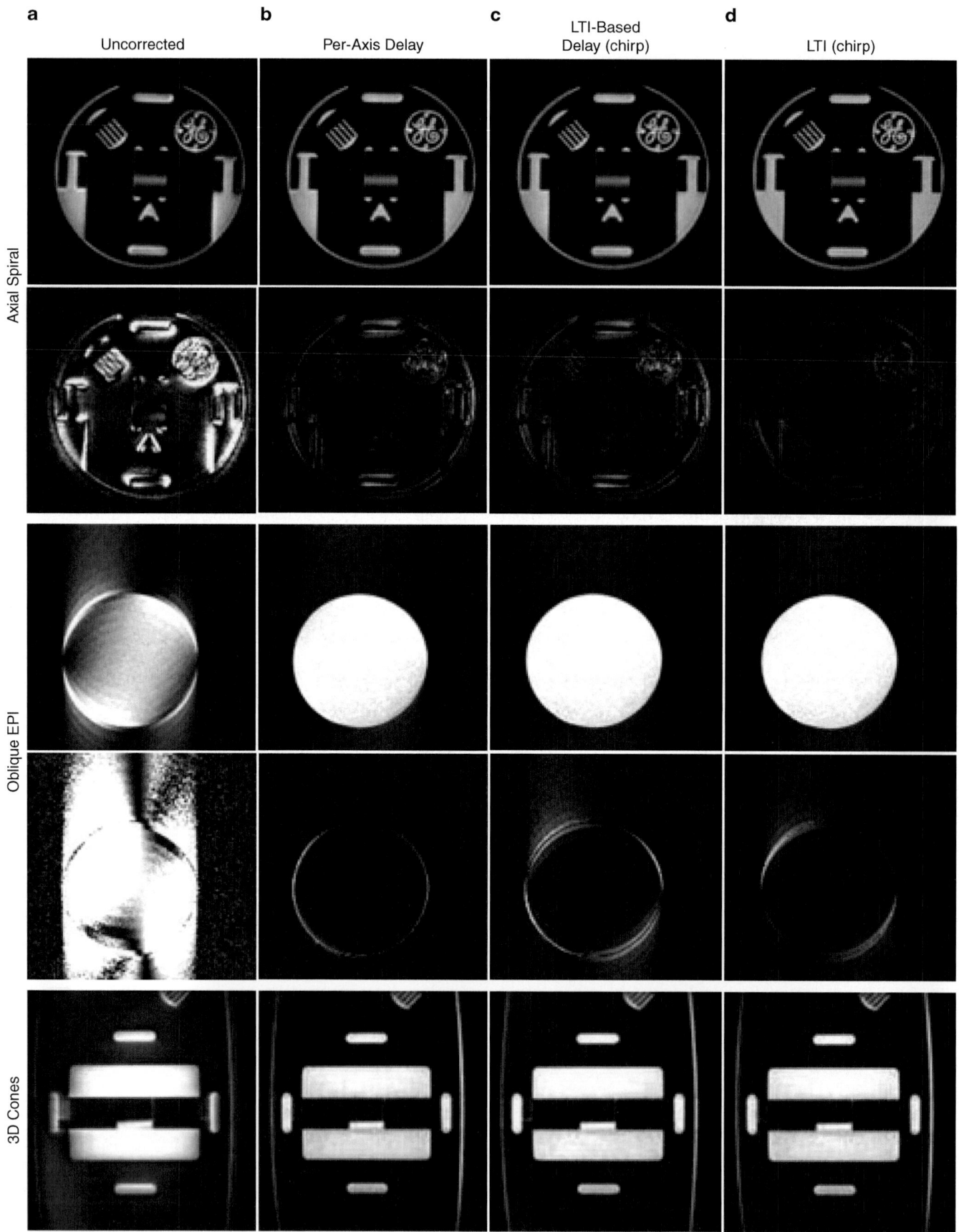

Fig. 4.11 Axial phantom images using spiral (top), oblique EPI (middle), and 3D Cones (bottom) reconstructions with the original trajectories (**a**), and trajectories estimated using the average delay (**b**), LTI-based delay (**c**), and full LTI-estimated (**d**) models. Difference images for spiral (second row) and EPI (fourth row) are made by comparison to a reference image reconstruction based on measured trajectories, and are scaled by 8×. (Reproduced with permission from Ref. [25])

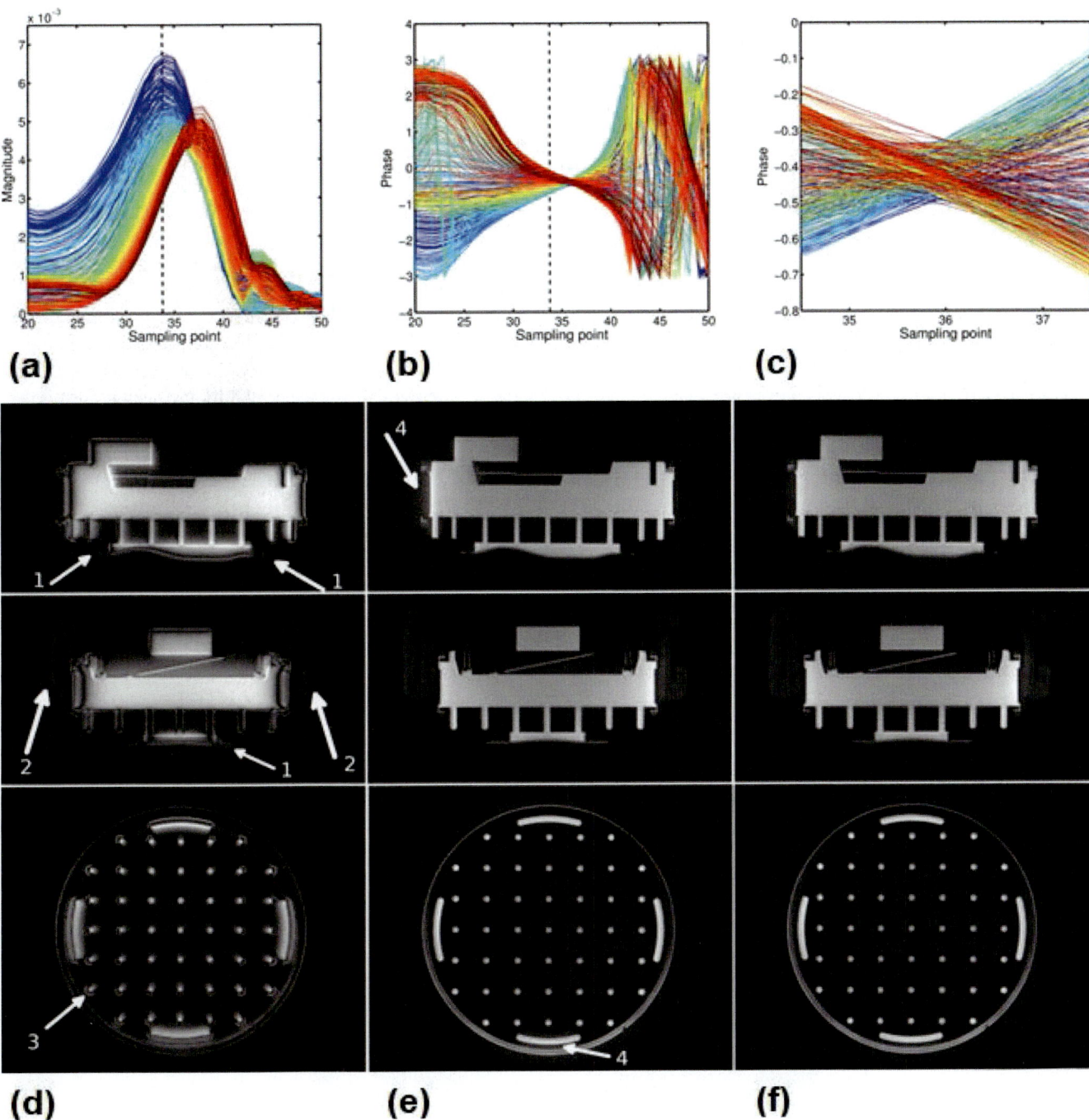

Fig. 4.12 Gradient delay calibration using 45 spokes of the measured calibration data from the x-y plane with the magnitude shown in (**a**), the phase in (**b**), and an enlarged central part of (**b**) shown in (**c**). The colors characterize the spoke index using a continous jet color map where blue is the first and red the last index. The dashed black line marks the expected position of the k-space center. The effect of delay correction is demonstrated through phantom images in three orthogonal planes of a structure phantom reconstructed without gradient delay correction (**d**), with global delay correction as extracted from the template (**e**), and with both global delay and axis-specific delays (**f**). (Reproduced with permission from Ref. [26])

Contrast Mechanisms

UTE sequences allow direct detection of signals from short-T_2 species; however, this does not necessarily mean that short-T_2 species will be obvious. Most short-T_2 species, such as bone and myelin, have lower proton densities than sur-

rounding or associated long-T_2 species [28, 29]. As a result, they may display much lower signals than long-T_2 species, making them relatively inapparent even with UTE sequences. A series of contrast mechanisms have been developed to improve the depiction of short-T_2 species, including fat suppression, dual-echo acquisition followed by echo subtraction

(ES) [7], long-T_2 saturation [30], inversion recovery (IR) [2], fat–water separation [31], and water excitation [18, 19]. A few major contrast mechanisms for 3D UTE imaging will be summarized here. Part II of this book provides more detail about short-T_2 contrast mechanisms.

UTE Imaging with Fat Saturation

The basic 3D UTE imaging sequence employs a short TR to reduce the total scan time. The short TR and short TE combination provides high T_1-weighting, leading to a high signal for fat with 3D UTE imaging of short-T_2 species. Besides, UTE imaging of short-T_2 species suffers from fat contamination due to partial volume effects and off-resonance artifacts induced by the non-Cartesian UTE acquisition [32]. Thus, fat suppression is very important for UTE imaging of musculoskeletal tissues. Figure 4.13 shows a cadaveric ankle specimen imaged with clinical T_1-weighted FSE and 3D UTE Cones sequences. Conventional clinical sequences show near-zero signal for the Achilles tendon and enthesis, while the 3D UTE Cones sequence shows high signal from both tissues [33].

Fat suppression pulses can saturate signals from short-T_2 species directly due to spectral overlap or indirectly due to

magnetization transfer [28, 34]. Chemical shift-based decomposition techniques such as the single- or multipoint Dixon approach and iterative decomposition of water and fat with echo asymmetry and least squares estimation (IDEAL) provide excellent water–fat signal separation for long-T_2 tissues [35]. These techniques can be combined with UTE, such as UTE-based IDEAL (UTE-IDEAL) [36], to preserve signals from short-T_2 species while providing high-contrast, water-only images, as well as T_2^* and fat fraction maps. The recently developed single-point Dixon-UTE technique allows fast water and fat separation [37]. Its combination with UTE is another promising approach for fast imaging of short-T_2 species without fat contamination [31, 38]. Chapters 15 and 16 provide more details about the various fat/water separation techniques used with UTE imaging of short-T_2 species.

UTE Imaging with Multi-echo Acquisition and Subtraction

Dual-echo 3D UTE data acquisition and subsequent ES are very effective for suppressing long-T_2 signals and providing high-contrast imaging of short-T_2 species [7]. Short-T_2 contrast is achieved by subtracting a second echo image from the

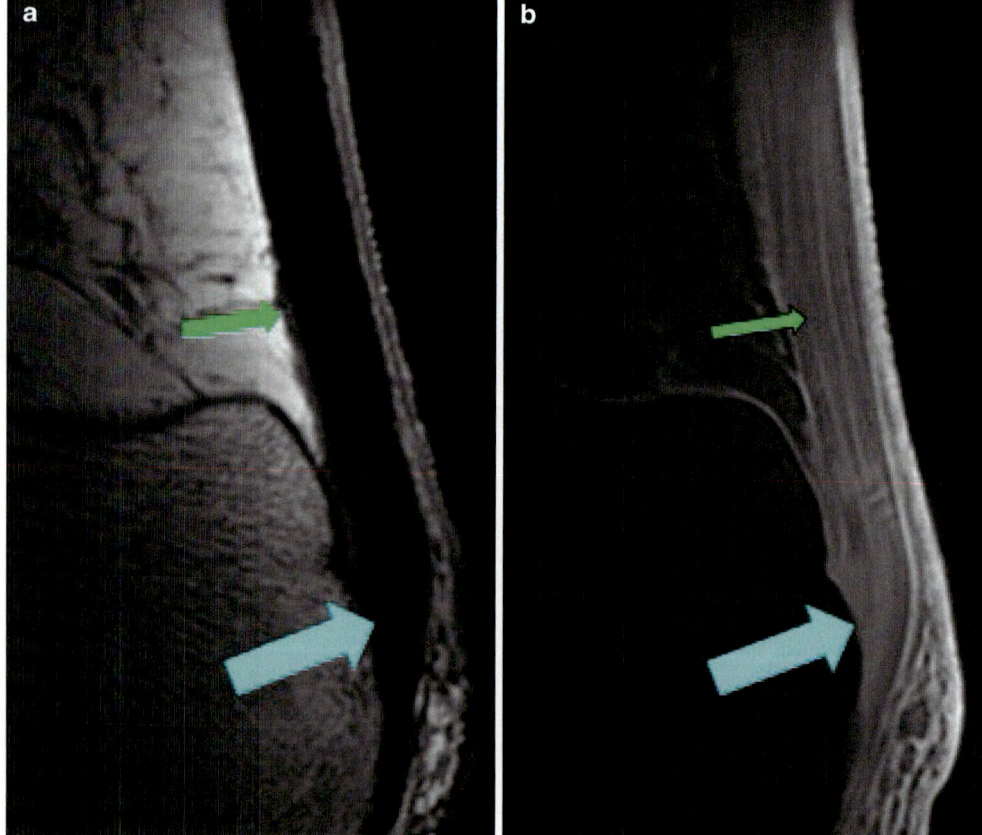

Fig. 4.13 Morphological imaging of a cadaveric human ankle specimen at 3 T using a clinical T_1-weighted FSE (**a**) and a 3D UTE Cones sequence with fat suppression (**b**). The Achilles tendon (thin arrow) and enthesis (thick arrow) are invisible with the clinical T_1-FSE sequence in (**a**), but show high signal and contrast with the fat-saturated 3D UTE Cones sequence in (**b**). (Reproduced with permission from Ref. [33])

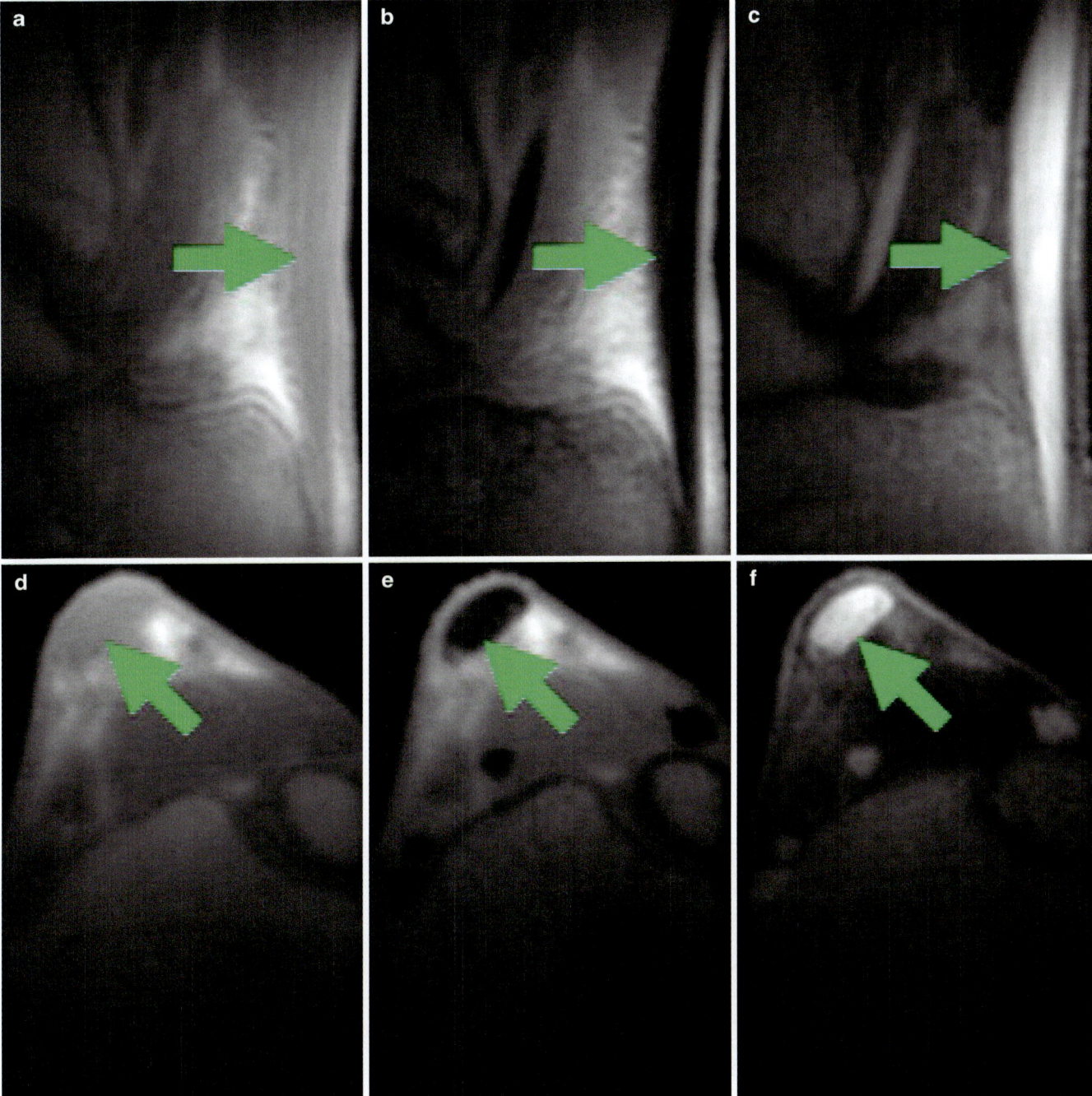

Fig. 4.14 Dual-echo 3D UTE imaging of the Achilles tendon of a volunteer with a TE of 8 μs (**a, d**) and 2.2 ms (**b, e**), and the corresponding ES (**c, f**). The MR "invisible" Achilles tendon shows a high signal and contrast on the 3D UTE ES images in the sagittal (**c**) and axial (**f**) planes. (Reproduced with permission from Ref. [5])

first FID image, a technique that is equivalent to T_2 bandpass filtering. Signals from long-T_2 species decay minimally by the time of the second echo, leading to a significant reduction in long-T_2 signals after ES. Signals from short-T_2 species decay significantly by the time of the second echo and are much less affected by ES. Figure 4.14 shows an example of 3D UTE Cones imaging of a healthy volunteer's Achilles tendon at the ankle joint. The UTE images (Fig. 4.14a, d)

show little contrast for the Achilles tendon due to the lack of T_2-weighting, while more contrast is seen on the later echo image (Fig. 4.14b, e). Dual-echo subtraction can be performed to highlight the short-T_2 Achilles tendon (Fig. 4.14c, f), which typically appears as a signal void with conventional clinical MR imaging [5]. Chapter 11 provides a more comprehensive summary of the various ES techniques used for high-contrast imaging of short-T_2 species.

Adiabatic Inversion Recovery UTE (IR-UTE)

Magnetization inversion is another method used in UTE MRI to generate contrast and selectively suppress certain signals in images, such as long-T_2 fat and water signals in muscle. Traditionally, one acquires a single *k*-space spoke after each application of a single inversion pulse (Fig. 4.15a) [2]. A more efficient approach is the collection of several *k*-space spokes (e.g., Np spokes) after application of a single inversion pulse

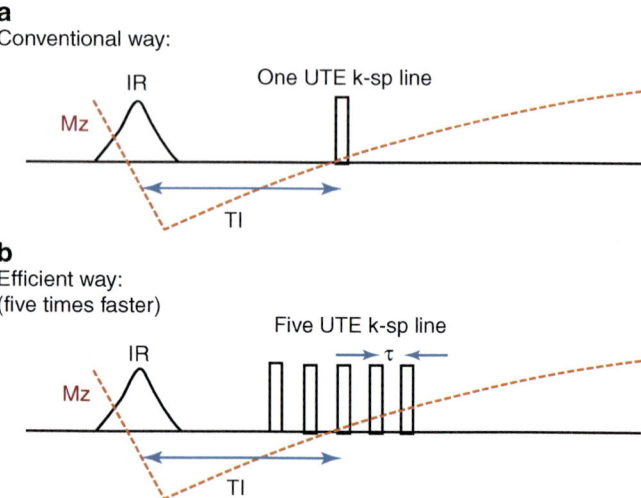

a
Conventional way:

b
Efficient way:
(five times faster)

Fig. 4.15 Diagram of an adiabatic IR preparation used with 3D UTE pulse sequences: conventional single-spoke IR (**a**), and more efficient multispoke design (**b**). (Reproduced with permission from Ref. [6])

(Fig. 4.15b for an example with Np = 5) [6]. This can reduce the total scan time by a factor of Np. The inversion pulse is repeated every TR period, during which Np *k*-space spokes are obtained. The spokes are separated by short time intervals τ. During each spoke, one UTE *k*-space line is acquired. The TI is defined as the time from the center of the inversion pulse to the center of the group of *k*-space spokes in the data acquisition, so that the sequence timing asymptotically approaches the conventional single-spoke case for small values of Np. In order to minimize the total scan time, TR should typically be chosen to be the minimum allowed value, as determined by specific absorption rate (SAR), gradient, and RF duty cycles, as well as sequence timing.

Figure 4.16 shows an axial scan of the tibia and a sagittal scan of the knee joint of a healthy volunteer using the 3D IR-UTE sequence. The adiabatic IR preparation provides excellent suppression of signals from bone marrow and muscle and provides high signal and contrast for cortical and trabecular bone as well as the patellar tendon. This figure also shows signal from coil elements and padding that contains short-T_2 materials.

In recent years, a series of adiabatic IR-prepared UTE techniques have been developed for high-contrast imaging of short-T_2 species, such as single adiabatic IR-UTE [39–41], dual adiabatic IR UTE (dual-IR-UTE) [42–44], double adiabatic IR UTE (double-IR-UTE) [45], adiabatic IR and fat saturation UTE (IR-FS-UTE) [46], double echo sliding IR UTE (DESIRE UTE) [47], and short TR adiabatic IR UTE (STAIR-UTE) [48]. These contrast mechanisms are most promising in large part because of the insensitivity of adia-

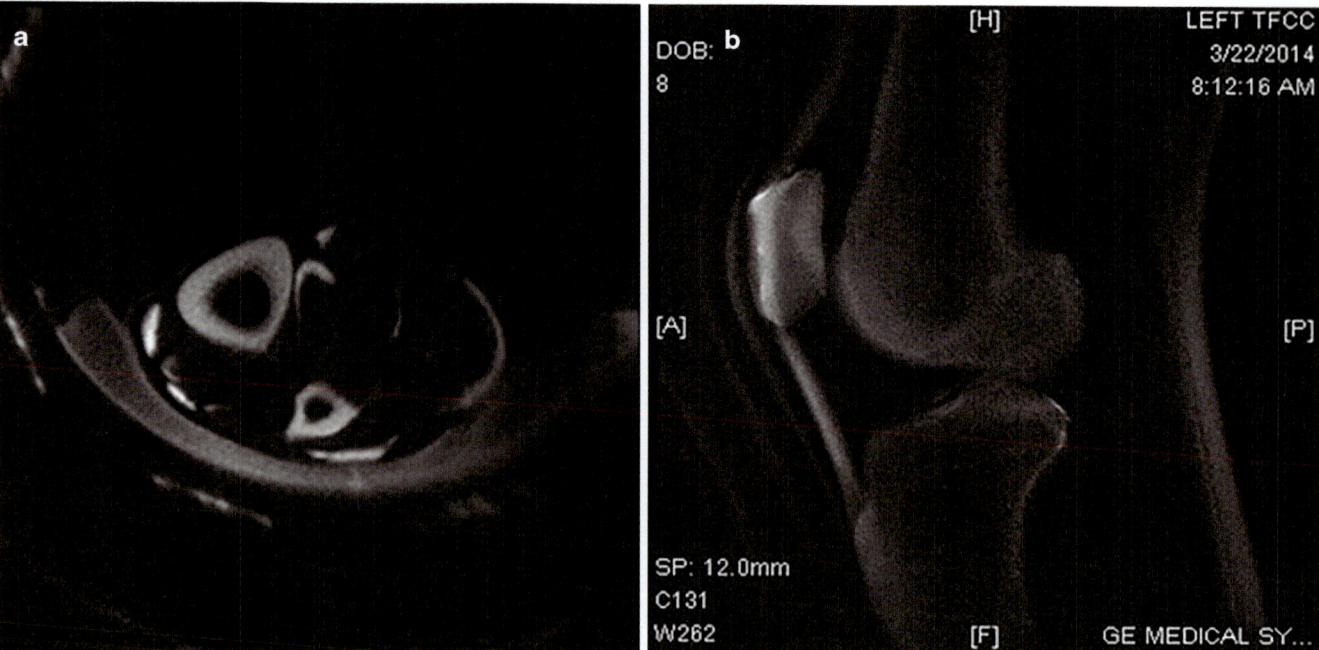

Fig. 4.16 3D IR-UTE Cones imaging of the tibial midshaft (**a**) and the knee joint (**b**) in a healthy volunteer. High signal and contrast are generated for the tibial cortex, patella, and tendons, as well as coil elements and padding

batic inversion pulses to B_1 and B_0 inhomogeneities [49]. Chapter 13 provides a systematic review of adiabatic IR-based UTE techniques for morphological and quantitative imaging of short-T_2 species.

Quantitative UTE Imaging

UTE sequences can also be used for quantitative imaging of short-T_2 species. This is important as quantitative imaging frequently allows early detection of tissue changes more effectively than morphological imaging, since morphological changes typically happen at later stages in disease progression. A variety of quantitative UTE techniques have been developed to measure MR relaxation times (i.e., T_1, T_2, T_2^*, $T_{1\rho}$) and other tissue properties (e.g., proton density, magnetization transfer ratio, magnetization transfer modeling of macromolecular proton fraction (MMF), perfusion, diffusion, and susceptibility) [3]. These techniques have great potential for improving diagnosis. A few quantitative 3D UTE imaging techniques will be described here. Part III of this book provides a systematic review of quantitative MRI techniques for short- and ultrashort-T_2 tissues.

T_2^* Quantification

T_2^* refers to the apparent transverse relaxation, which describes the exponential decay in M_{xy} following an RF excitation pulse as a function of time. T_2^* is an important tissue property that incorporates T_2 but is additionally affected by inhomogeneities in B_0 and susceptibility-induced field distortions produced by tissue, with the latter usually dominant in short-T_2 tissues. Conventional sequences cannot provide accurate T_2^* mapping for short-T_2 species due to the lack of detectable signals. UTE sequences solve this challenge. UTE-based T_2^* (UTE-T_2^*) mapping allows quantitative assessment of collagen fibril integrity and organization in short-T_2 species such as the deep articular cartilage, menisci, ligaments, and tendons [3]. UTE-T_2^* values have been shown to track cartilage extracellular matrix degeneration as determined by polarized light microscopy [50]. UTE-T_2^* values in deep articular cartilage are typically elevated with increased cartilage degeneration in subjects with osteoarthritis (OA) or anterior cruciate ligament (ACL) injury [50, 51]. UTE-T_2^* maps can be generated from a series of 3D Cones images acquired at a series of TEs (nonuniform spacing for more accurate T_2^* mapping) [12]. The Cones sequence samples MRI data starting at the center of k-space and twisting outwards along conical surfaces in 3D while allowing the use of anisotropic FOVs and resolution to speed up data acquisition. Two sets of interleaved 3D multi-echo UTE Cones data (e.g., set #1: TEs = 32 µs, 3.6, 7.2, 16.0 ms; set #2: TEs = 1, 4.7, 9.0, 12.7 ms) can be acquired for better detection of fast signal decay from short-T_2 species. Williams et al. applied the 3D UTE Cones T_2^* mapping technique to the study of alterations to the medial tibiofemoral subsurface cartilage matrix in human subjects 2 years after ACL reconstruction (ACLR) [52]. Their knee cartilage was found to be morphologically intact in 92% (35/38) of subjects (Fig. 4.17). In the

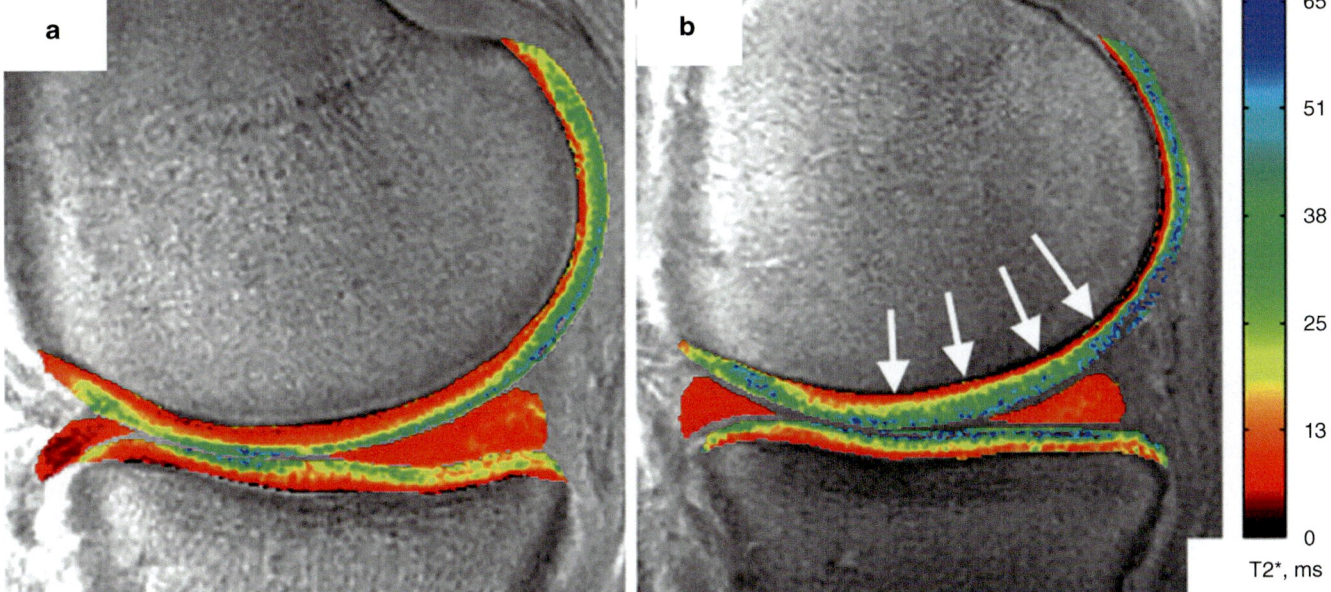

Fig. 4.17 UTE-T_2^* maps in an uninjured 29-year-old male control subject with typical laminar appearance to UTE-T_2^* values (**a**), and a 34-year-old male ACLR subject 2 years after reconstruction surgery, with no morphological evidence of medial cartilage (Outerbridge grade 0) or meniscus pathology (**b**). Elevations to UTE-T_2^* values throughout medial femorotibial cartilage, particularly in deep medial femoral cartilage (white arrows) were observed in the ACLR patient. (Reproduced with permission from Ref. [52])

medial compartment, 37% (14/38) of the subjects had intact and normal cartilage (grade 0), and 55% (21/38) showed intact cartilage with some areas of signal brightening (grade 1). Disruption to articular surfaces in the medial compartment (grade 2 partial-thickness defect) was seen in only 8% (3/38) of those subjects [52]. The results suggest that 3D Cones-based UTE-T_2^* mapping may be an efficient way of assessing degenerative changes in the knee joint.

Biological tissues frequently contain different water compartments with distinct T_2^* values. Quantifying different water components may be problematic with clinical MR sequences, as the initial TEs are usually too long to detect enough signals from shorter T_2 components. Signals from short-T_2 water components in short-T_2 tissues, such as tendons and bone, can be detected using UTE-based sequences. A multicomponent T_2^* analysis has been proposed to evaluate different water components in short-T_2 tissues [53, 54]. Single and multicomponent UTE-T_2^* analyses have been used to evaluate short-T_2 tissue degeneration [52, 55], iron deposition [56], temperature mapping [22], and soft tissue calcification [57]. Chapter 22 provides a systematic review of different T_2^* quantification techniques and clinical applications.

T_1 Quantification

Conventional T_1 quantification techniques based on inversion or saturation recovery are problematic for short-T_2 species due to significant signal decay during the relatively long duration inversion/saturation pulses used in clinical MR sequences. Variable repetition time (VTR) and variable flip angle (VFA) methods have been used for T_1 mapping [58, 59], but these methods are sensitive to B_1 field inhomogeneity. To overcome this limitation, an actual flip angle imaging (AFI) technique has been proposed for rapid B_1 mapping [60]. However, the AFI sequence is based on conventional MR data acquisitions and cannot be used for mapping the B_1 and T_1 of short-T_2 species due to a lack of detectable signal. Short-T_2 signal loss during the excitation process should also be considered for more accurate T_1 quantification. UTE-type sequences are needed for accurate quantification of the T_1 of short-T_2 species. The combination of UTE, AFI, and VFA techniques (3D UTE-AFI-VFA) can address all of the above challenges [61, 62]. Figure 4.18 shows excellent T_1 fitting for various knee joint tissues in a healthy volunteer. The T_1 values for long-T_2 species, such as cartilage ($T_1 = 1133 \pm 40$ ms at 3 T), muscle ($T_1 = 1406 \pm 63$ ms), and fat ($T_1 = 386 \pm 2$ ms), are largely consistent with the literature [59]. Relatively short-T_1 values are found in short-T_2 species, such as the meniscus ($T_1 = 832 \pm 18$ ms), quadriceps tendon ($T_1 = 779 \pm 7$ ms), patellar tendon ($T_1 = 637 \pm 16$ ms), and ACL ($T_1 = 870 \pm 13$ ms).

The T_1 values for short-T_2 species, such as the menisci, ligaments, and tendons, remain to be confirmed due to the lack of reference standard. T_1 is field strength dependent, with a longer T_1 expected at higher B_0 fields. Reference values can be derived from a spectrometer at 3 T where the strong RF and gradient systems allow accurate quantification of T_1 values for short-T_2 tissues, and the values can be used to validate UTE-measured T_1s obtained with a whole-body clinical 3T MR scanner. There are several UTE-based T_1 quantification techniques that have been developed in recent years, including saturation recovery UTE (SR-UTE) [2, 40], adiabatic IR-UTE [63], UTE-VTR [61], UTE-VFA [62], and their combinations. The advantages and disadvantages of each technique are summarized in Chap. 21.

$T_{1\rho}$ Quantification

$T_{1\rho}$ is the time constant for spin-lattice relaxation in the rotating frame in the presence of an external spin-lock pulse [64]. $T_{1\rho}$ reflects slow interactions between motion-restricted water molecules and their local macromolecular environment, thereby providing unique biochemical information in the low-frequency region ranging from a few hundred Hz to a few kHz [64]. Changes to the extracellular matrix, such as proteoglycan loss, may be reflected in measurements of $T_{1\rho}$ and $T_{1\rho}$ dispersion ($T_{1\rho}$ values as a function of the spin-locking field) [65]. $T_{1\rho}$ has been employed to assess the properties of the macromolecular environment inside tissues, such as loss of proteoglycan in musculoskeletal tissues [66]. However, conventional $T_{1\rho}$ imaging sequences cannot evaluate short-T_2 species due to the lack of detectable signal. UTE-based $T_{1\rho}$ (UTE-$T_{1\rho}$) sequences have been developed to evaluate macromolecular changes in short-T_2 species [67, 68]. In this technique, a continuous wave spin-lock pulse is used for magnetization preparation, with the magnetization stored along the z-axis subsequently detected by UTE data acquisition. This technique enables $T_{1\rho}$ imaging of various short-T_2 species such as the Achilles tendon, ligaments, and menisci. Figure 4.19 shows 3D Cones-based UTE-$T_{1\rho}$ imaging of the Achilles tendon in a healthy volunteer [68]. The conventional gradient echo-based $T_{1\rho}$ sequence shows little signal from the Achilles tendon because of its relatively long TE. The 3D Cones UTE-$T_{1\rho}$ sequence shows a much higher signal in the Achilles tendon and provides excellent single-component exponential fitting with a short mean $T_{1\rho}$ of 3.07 ± 0.35 ms. The 3D UTE-$T_{1\rho}$ sequence can potentially assess proteoglycan loss in both long-T_2 and short-T_2 species in the musculoskeletal system.

Conventional $T_{1\rho}$ imaging shows a significant magic angle effect [69]. $T_{1\rho}$ values can be doubled when collagen fibers are reoriented from 0° to near 54° (the magic angle) relative

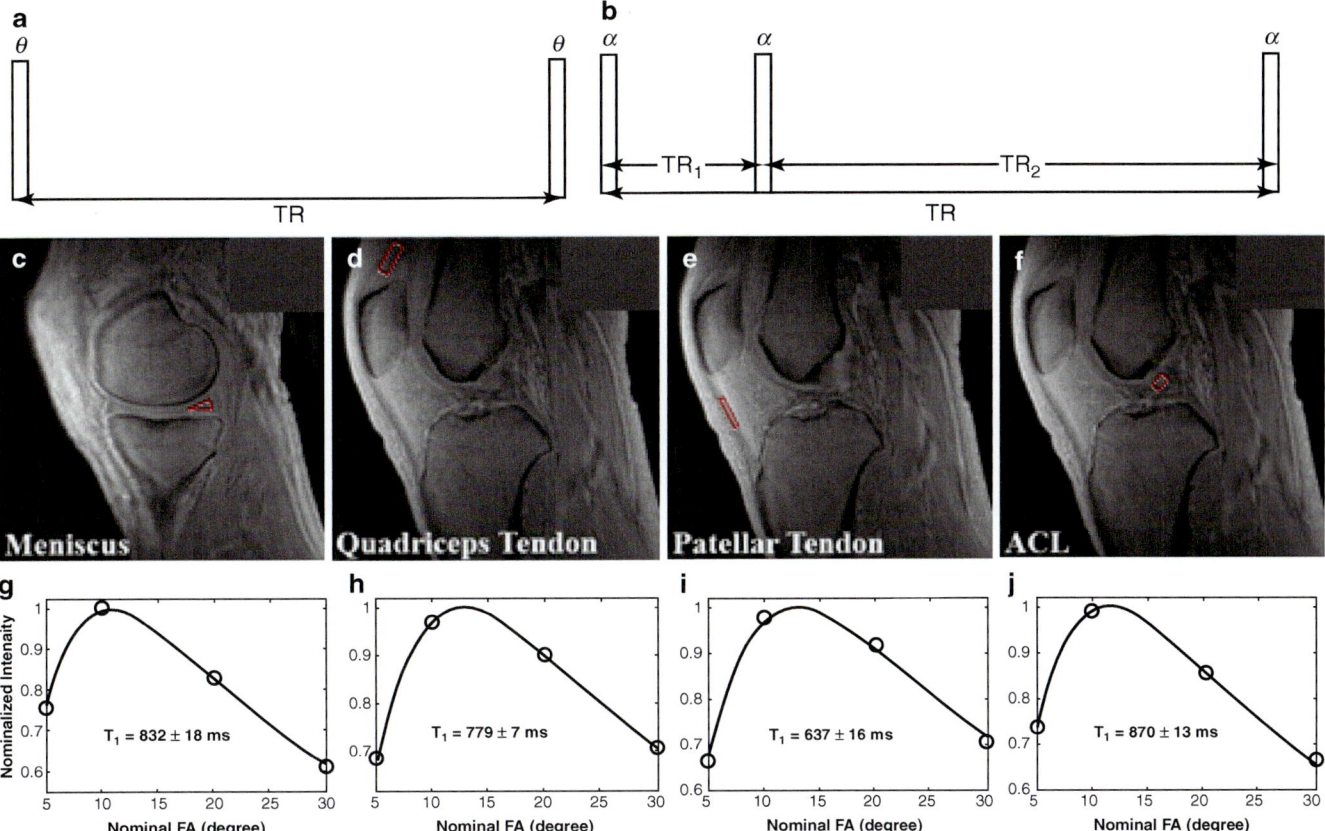

Fig. 4.18 The 3D UTE Cones sequence with a single TR can be used for T_1 measurement with the variable flip angle (VFA) method (**a**). The 3D UTE Cones actual flip angle imaging (AFI) sequence employs a pair of interleaved TRs for accurate B_1 mapping, which can be combined with the VFA method (UTE-AFI-VFA) to improve the accuracy of T_1 mapping (**b**). The 3D UTE-AFI-VFA method was applied to the knee joint of a 35-year-old volunteer to quantitatively image the meniscus (**c**), quadriceps tendon (**d**), patellar tendon (**e**), and ACL (**f**), as well as the corresponding T_1 fitting results, including a T_1 of 832 ± 18 ms for meniscus (**g**), 779 ± 7 ms for quadriceps tendon (**h**), 637 ± 16 ms for the patellar tendon (**i**), and 870 ± 13 ms for ACL (**j**). (Reproduced with permission from Ref. [62])

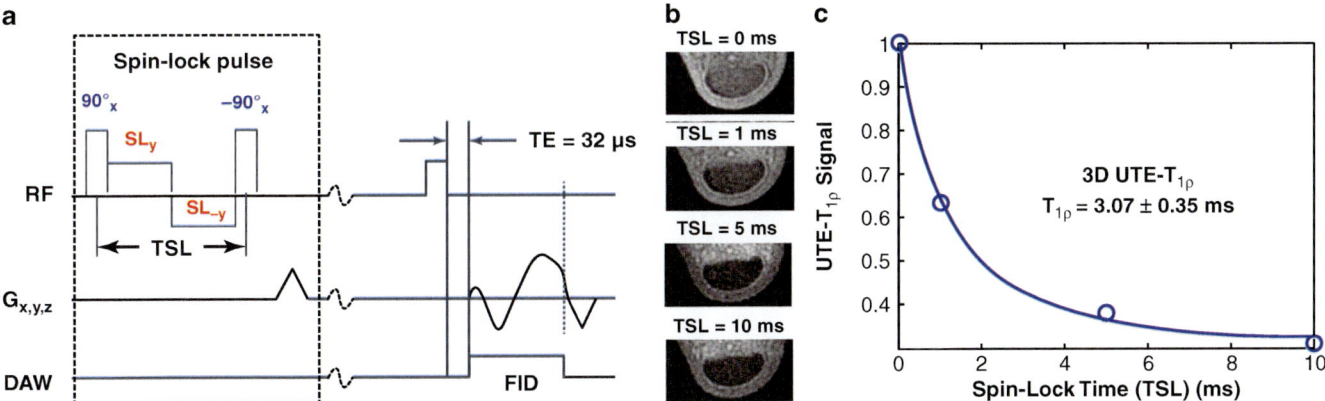

Fig. 4.19 The 3D UTE-$T_{1\rho}$ sequence employs a spin-lock preparation pulse followed by a Cones data acquisition (**a**). The preparation pulse consists of a rectangular 90° pulse followed by a composite spin-lock pulse and another −90° rectangular pulse. The phase of the second half of the composite spin-lock pulse is shifted 180° from the first half to reduce B_1 inhomogeneity-related artifacts. The Achilles tendon of a healthy volunteer was subject to fat-saturated UTE-$T_{1\rho}$ imaging with four spin-lock times of 0, 1, 5, and 10 ms (**b**). The excellent exponential curve fitting demonstrated a short $T_{1\rho}$ of 3.07 ± 0.35 ms for the Achilles tendon (**c**). (Reproduced with permission from Ref. [68])

to the B_0 field. Trains of adiabatic inversion pulses have been employed to measure adiabatic $T_{1\rho}$ (AdiabT$_{1\rho}$), which is less sensitive to the magic angle effect [70]. A UTE-based AdiabT$_{1\rho}$ (UTE-AdiabT$_{1\rho}$) sequence has been developed to provide orientation-independent $T_{1\rho}$ mapping of both short- and long-T_2 tissues on a clinical whole-body scanner [71].

$T_{1\rho}$ relaxation also depends on the power of the spin-lock pulse. A stronger spin-lock pulse tends to "lock" the transverse magnetization more efficiently along its direction, thereby producing a longer $T_{1\rho}$ value. This phenomenon is called $T_{1\rho}$ dispersion. The self-diffusion effect dominates at low spin-lock powers (i.e., $\omega_1 < 100$ Hz) while chemical exchange dominates at higher spin-lock powers (several hundred or thousand Hz) [72]. The UTE-$T_{1\rho}$ sequence provides reliable $T_{1\rho}$ mapping of short-T_2 species as well as the related $T_{1\rho}$ dispersion [67, 68, 73] and may be used to detect early changes in musculoskeletal tissues. A systematic review of the various $T_{1\rho}$ techniques and clinical applications is summarized in Chap. 23.

Magnetization Transfer Quantification

Magnetization transfer (MT) refers to the transfer of spin magnetization from macromolecular protons to water protons and has been introduced for quantitative evaluation of water and macromolecular proton pools in long-T_2 species [74]. A saturation pulse is placed at a frequency offset Δf away from the water peak to saturate macromolecular protons, which exchange with water protons either by chemical exchange or magnetization transfer, leading to a significant reduction in the detectable signal. As a result, MT imaging allows indirect assessment of macromolecules with restricted motion and extremely short T_2s (of the order of 10 μs). However, clinical MT sequences cannot assess short-T_2 species due to the lack of detectable signals. UTE-based MT (UTE-MT) sequences resolve this limitation and can be used to indirectly evaluate macromolecular protons in short-T_2 species such as cortical bone. Springer et al. first introduced the 3D UTE-MT sequence to calculate the MT ratio (MTR) in cortical bone [75]. MTR is semiquantitative and shows only a moderate correlation with the biomechanical properties of cadaveric human bone samples [76]. A two-pool MT model has been proposed to extract fundamental parameters describing a free pool composed of water protons and a semisolid pool composed of collagen protons in biological tissues [77]. This two-pool MT model can be combined with 3D UTE data acquisition, in which multiple spokes (N_{sp}) are acquired after each MT preparation to reduce the scan time by a factor of N_{sp} [78, 79]. Figure 4.20 shows the 3D Cones UTE-MT sequence, along with imaging of a bovine cortical bone sample. Excellent two-pool MT modeling and MT parameter mapping were achieved using a Gaussian line-shape fitting. Maps of macromolecular proton fraction (MPF), collagen backbone proton transverse relaxation (T_{2m}), exchange rate (RM_{0m}), and spin-lattice relaxation rate (R_{1w}) can be generated for cortical bone, which is "invisible" with conventional MR sequences.

UTE-MT techniques provide a panel of biomarkers, including MTR and MT modeling of macromolecular proton fraction, exchange, and relaxation rates for both short- and long-T_2 species [75, 80]. Furthermore, the UTE-MT biomarkers are much less insensitive to the magic angle effect than conventional T_2 and $T_{1\rho}$ [80] and may provide a more robust evaluation of tissue degeneration. Ex vivo studies have demonstrated the efficacy of this technique in detecting degenerative changes in musculoskeletal tissues [81, 82]. Decreased MMF and MTR were observed within cartilage

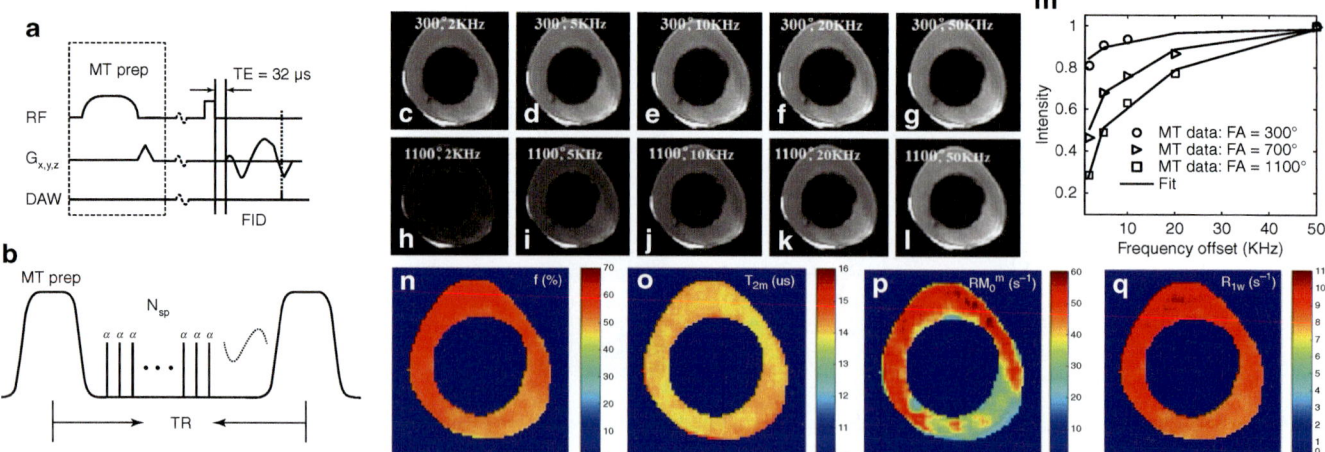

Fig. 4.20 The 3D UTE-MT sequence employs a Fermi pulse for MT preparation followed by Cones data acquisition (**a**). Multiple spokes (N_{sp}) are sampled after each Fermi pulse to speed up data acquisition (by a factor of N_{sp}) (**b**). Selected UTE-MT images of a bovine bone sample acquired with an MT power of 300° and five frequency offsets of 2 kHz (**c**), 5 kHz (**d**), 10 kHz (**e**), 20 kHz (**f**), and 50 kHz (**g**), as well as an MT power of 1100° and five frequency offsets of 2 kHz (**h**), 5 kHz (**i**), 10 kHz (**j**), 20 kHz (**k**), and 50 kHz (**l**). Excellent two-pool fitting is achieved (**m**), providing maps of macromolecular proton fraction (**n**), collagen backbone proton transverse relaxation T_{2m} (**o**), exchange rate RM_{0m} (**p**), and spin-lattice relaxation rate R_{1w} (**q**). (Reproduced with permission from Ref. [79])

and meniscus in mild and advanced OA compared to healthy subjects [83, 84]. A systematic review of the UTE-MT techniques and clinical applications is summarized in Chap. 25.

Conclusion

3D UTE is a powerful imaging tool to image short-T_2 species that would otherwise be invisible with conventional clinical MRI sequences. With recent advances in data acquisition, non-Cartesian image reconstruction, short-T_2 signal excitation, sampling window optimization, and eddy currents correction, 3D UTE has become an efficient technique with potential for widespread clinical adoption. 3D Cones, with its flexible k-space design, have the potential to further improve scan efficiency and reduce scan time [6, 12]. Various morphological UTE imaging techniques have been developed [3]. Among the different contrast mechanisms, dual-echo UTE with ES is the most time-efficient method, but it is sensitive to chemical shift, off-resonance, and susceptibility effects [3]. Adiabatic IR-based techniques are very promising as they are insensitive to B_1 and B_0 inhomogeneities [49]. A series of quantitative UTE imaging techniques have been developed for more robust assessment of short-T_2 tissue degeneration, such as collagen degradation (via UTE-T_2^*) [52], proteoglycan depletion (via UTE-$T_{1\rho}$) [82], and macromolecular changes (via UTE-MT modeling) [81]. All the major MR vendors have implemented UTE-type sequences on their equipment. With further development and optimization, 3D UTE MRI techniques can be used to improve the diagnosis of various diseases in the body's musculoskeletal, nervous, respiratory, gastrointestinal, and cardiovascular systems.

References

1. Plewes DB, Kucharczyk W. Physics of MRI: a primer. J Magn Reson Imaging. 2012;35(5):1038–54.
2. Robson MD, Gatehouse PD, Bydder M, Bydder GM. Magnetic resonance: an introduction to ultrashort TE (UTE) imaging. J Comput Assist Tomogr. 2003;27(6):825–46.
3. Afsahi AM, Ma Y, Jang H, Jerban S, Chung CB, Chang EY, et al. Ultrashort echo time magnetic resonance imaging techniques: met and unmet needs in musculoskeletal imaging. J Magn Reson Imaging. 2022;55(6):1597–612.
4. Ma Y, Jang H, Jerban S, Chang EY, Chung CB, Bydder GM, et al. Making the invisible visible-ultrashort echo time magnetic resonance imaging: technical developments and applications. Appl Phys Rev. 2022;9(4):041303.
5. Du J, Bydder M, Takahashi AM, Carl M, Chung CB, Bydder GM. Short T_2 contrast with three-dimensional ultrashort echo time imaging. Magn Reson Imaging. 2011;29(4):470–82.
6. Carl M, Bydder GM, Du J. UTE imaging with simultaneous water and fat signal suppression using a time-efficient multispoke inversion recovery pulse sequence. Magn Reson Med. 2016;76(2):577–82.
7. Rahmer J, Bornert P, Groen J, Bos C. Three-dimensional radial ultrashort echo-time imaging with T_2 adapted sampling. Magn Reson Med. 2006;55(5):1075–82.
8. Bergin CJ, Pauly JM, Macovski A. Lung parenchyma: projection reconstruction MR imaging. Radiology. 1991;179(3):777–81.
9. Qian Y, Boada FE. Acquisition-weighted stack of spirals for fast high-resolution three-dimensional ultra-short echo time MR imaging. Magn Reson Med. 2008;60(1):135–45.
10. Boada FE, Shen GX, Chang SY, Thulborn KR. Spectrally weighted twisted projection imaging: reducing T_2 signal attenuation effects in fast three-dimensional sodium imaging. Magn Reson Med. 1997;38(6):1022–8.
11. Song HK, Wehrli FW. Variable TE gradient and spin echo sequences for in vivo MR microscopy of short T_2 species. Magn Reson Med. 1998;39(2):251–8.
12. Gurney PT, Hargreaves BA, Nishimura DG. Design and analysis of a practical 3D cones trajectory. Magn Reson Med. 2006;55(3):575–82.
13. Beatty PJ, Nishimura DG, Pauly JM. Rapid gridding reconstruction with a minimal oversampling ratio. IEEE Trans Med Imaging. 2005;24(6):799–808.
14. Johnson EM, Vyas U, Ghanouni P, Pauly KB, Pauly JM. Improved cortical bone specificity in UTE MR imaging. Magn Reson Med. 2017;77(2):684–95.
15. Du J, Thornton FJ, Fain SB, Korosec FR, Browning F, Grist TM, et al. Artifact reduction in undersampled projection reconstruction MRI of the peripheral vessels using selective excitation. Magn Reson Med. 2004;51(5):1071–6.
16. Pauly J, Le Roux P, Nishimura D, Macovski A. Parameter relations for the Shinnar-Le Roux selective excitation pulse design algorithm [NMR imaging]. IEEE Trans Med Imaging. 1991;10(1):53–65.
17. Hargreaves BA, Cunningham CH, Nishimura DG, Conolly SM. Variable-rate selective excitation for rapid MRI sequences. Magn Reson Med. 2004;52(3):590–7.
18. Springer F, Steidle G, Martirosian P, Grosse U, Syha R, Schabel C, et al. Quick water-selective excitation of fast relaxing tissues with 3D UTE sequences. Magn Reson Med. 2014;71(2):534–43.
19. Ma YJ, Jerban S, Jang H, Chang EY, Du J. Fat suppression for ultrashort echo time imaging using a novel soft-hard composite radiofrequency pulse. Magn Reson Med. 2019;82(6):2178–87.
20. Weiger M, Pruessmann KP, Hennel F. MRI with zero echo time: hard versus sweep pulse excitation. Magn Reson Med. 2011;66(2):379–89.
21. Lu A, Daniel BL, Pauly JM, Pauly KB. Improved slice selection for R_2^* mapping during cryoablation with eddy current compensation. J Magn Reson Imaging. 2008;28(1):190–8.
22. Wansapura JP, Daniel BL, Pauly J, Butts K. Temperature mapping of frozen tissue using eddy current compensated half excitation RF pulses. Magn Reson Med. 2001;46(5):985–92.
23. Mason GF, Harshbarger T, Hetherington HP, Zhang Y, Pohost GM, Twieg DB. A method to measure arbitrary k-space trajectories for rapid MR imaging. Magn Reson Med. 1997;38(3):492–6.
24. Peters DC, Derbyshire JA, McVeigh ER. Centering the projection reconstruction trajectory: reducing gradient delay errors. Magn Reson Med. 2003;50(1):1–6.
25. Addy NO, Wu HH, Nishimura DG. Simple method for MR gradient system characterization and k-space trajectory estimation. Magn Reson Med. 2012;68(1):120–9.
26. Herrmann KH, Kramer M, Reichenbach JR. Time efficient 3D radial UTE sampling with fully automatic delay compensation on a clinical 3T MR scanner. PLoS One. 2016;11(3):e0150371.
27. Duyn JH, Yang Y, Frank JA, van der Veen JW. Simple correction method for k-space trajectory deviations in MRI. J Magn Reson. 1998;132(1):150–3.
28. Tyler DJ, Robson MD, Henkelman RM, Young IR, Bydder GM. Magnetic resonance imaging with ultrashort TE (UTE)

PULSE sequences: technical considerations. J Magn Reson Imaging. 2007;25(2):279–89.

29. Ma YJ, Jang H, Chang EY, Hiniker A, Head BP, Lee RR, et al. Ultrashort echo time (UTE) magnetic resonance imaging of myelin: technical developments and challenges. Quant Imaging Med Surg. 2020;10(6):1186–203.

30. Larson PE, Gurney PT, Nayak K, Gold GE, Pauly JM, Nishimura DG. Designing long-T_2 suppression pulses for ultrashort echo time imaging. Magn Reson Med. 2006;56(1):94–103.

31. Jang H, Carl M, Ma Y, Jerban S, Guo T, Zhao W, et al. Fat suppression for ultrashort echo time imaging using a single-point Dixon method. NMR Biomed. 2019;32(5):e4069.

32. Bydder M, Carl M, Bydder GM, Du J. MRI chemical shift artifact produced by center-out radial sampling of k-space: a potential pitfall in clinical diagnosis. Quant Imaging Med Surg. 2021;11(8):3677–83.

33. Chen B, Cheng X, Dorthe EW, Zhao Y, D'Lima D, Bydder GM, et al. Evaluation of normal cadaveric Achilles tendon and enthesis with ultrashort echo time (UTE) magnetic resonance imaging and indentation testing. NMR Biomed. 2019;32(1):e4034.

34. Carl M, Ma Y, Du J. Theoretical analysis and optimization of ultrashort echo time (UTE) imaging contrast with off-resonance saturation. Magn Reson Imaging. 2018;50:12–6.

35. Reeder SB, Pineda AR, Wen Z, Shimakawa A, Yu H, Brittain JH, et al. Iterative decomposition of water and fat with echo asymmetry and least-squares estimation (IDEAL): application with fast spin-echo imaging. Magn Reson Med. 2005;54(3):636–44.

36. Wang K, Yu H, Brittain JH, Reeder SB, Du J. k-space water-fat decomposition with T_2^* estimation and multifrequency fat spectrum modeling for ultrashort echo time imaging. J Magn Reson Imaging. 2010;31(4):1027–34.

37. Ma J. A single-point Dixon technique for fat-suppressed fast 3D gradient-echo imaging with a flexible echo time. J Magn Reson Imaging. 2008;27(4):881–90.

38. Kronthaler S, Boehm C, Feuerriegel G, Bornert P, Katscher U, Weiss K, et al. Assessment of vertebral fractures and edema of the thoracolumbar spine based on water-fat and susceptibility-weighted images derived from a single ultra-short echo time scan. Magn Reson Med. 2022;87(4):1771–83.

39. Larson PE, Conolly SM, Pauly JM, Nishimura DG. Using adiabatic inversion pulses for long-T_2 suppression in ultrashort echo time (UTE) imaging. Magn Reson Med. 2007;58(5):952–61.

40. Du J, Carl M, Bydder M, Takahashi A, Chung CB, Bydder GM. Qualitative and quantitative ultrashort echo time (UTE) imaging of cortical bone. J Magn Reson. 2010;207(2):304–11.

41. Horch RA, Gochberg DF, Nyman JS, Does MD. Clinically compatible MRI strategies for discriminating bound and pore water in cortical bone. Magn Reson Med. 2012;68(6):1774–84.

42. Du J, Takahashi AM, Bae WC, Chung CB, Bydder GM. Dual inversion recovery, ultrashort echo time (DIR UTE) imaging: creating high contrast for short-T(2) species. Magn Reson Med. 2010;63(2):447–55.

43. Bae WC, Dwek JR, Znamirowski R, Statum SM, Hermida JC, D'Lima DD, et al. Ultrashort echo time MR imaging of osteochondral junction of the knee at 3 T: identification of anatomic structures contributing to signal intensity. Radiology. 2010;254(3):837–45.

44. Du J, Carl M, Bae WC, Statum S, Chang EY, Bydder GM, et al. Dual inversion recovery ultrashort echo time (DIR-UTE) imaging and quantification of the zone of calcified cartilage (ZCC). Osteoarthr Cartil. 2013;21(1):77–85.

45. Ma YJ, Zhu Y, Lu X, Carl M, Chang EY, Du J. Short T2 imaging using a 3D double adiabatic inversion recovery prepared ultrashort echo time cones (3D DIR-UTE-Cones) sequence. Magn Reson Med. 2018;79(5):2555–63.

46. Ma YJ, Jerban S, Carl M, Wan L, Guo T, Jang H, et al. Imaging of the region of the osteochondral junction (OCJ) using a 3D adiabatic inversion recovery prepared ultrashort echo time cones (3D IR-UTE-cones) sequence at 3 T. NMR Biomed. 2019;32(5):e4080.

47. Ma YJ, Searleman AC, Jang H, Wong J, Chang EY, Corey-Bloom J, et al. Whole-brain myelin imaging using 3D double-echo sliding inversion recovery ultrashort echo time (DESIRE UTE) MRI. Radiology. 2020;294(2):362–74.

48. Ma YJ, Jang H, Wei Z, Cai Z, Xue Y, Lee RR, et al. Myelin imaging in human brain using a short repetition time adiabatic inversion recovery prepared ultrashort echo time (STAIR-UTE) MRI sequence in multiple sclerosis. Radiology. 2020;297(2):392–404.

49. Garwood M, DelaBarre L. The return of the frequency sweep: designing adiabatic pulses for contemporary NMR. J Magn Reson. 2001;153(2):155–77.

50. Williams A, Qian Y, Bear D, Chu CR. Assessing degeneration of human articular cartilage with ultra-short echo time (UTE) T_2^* mapping. Osteoarthr Cartil. 2010;18(4):539–46.

51. Chu CR, Williams AA, West RV, Qian Y, Fu FH, Do BH, et al. Quantitative magnetic resonance imaging UTE-T_2^* mapping of cartilage and meniscus healing after anatomic anterior cruciate ligament reconstruction. Am J Sports Med. 2014;42(8):1847–56.

52. Williams AA, Titchenal MR, Do BH, Guha A, Chu CR. MRI UTE-T_2^* shows high incidence of cartilage subsurface matrix changes 2 years after ACL reconstruction. J Orthop Res. 2019;37(2):370–7.

53. Du J, Diaz E, Carl M, Bae W, Chung CB, Bydder GM. Ultrashort echo time imaging with bicomponent analysis. Magn Reson Med. 2012;67(3):645–9.

54. Lu X, Jerban S, Wan L, Ma Y, Jang H, Le N, et al. Three-dimensional ultrashort echo time imaging with tricomponent analysis for human cortical bone. Magn Reson Med. 2019;82(1):348–55.

55. Jerban S, Lu X, Dorthe EW, Alenezi S, Ma Y, Kakos L, et al. Correlations of cortical bone microstructural and mechanical properties with water proton fractions obtained from ultrashort echo time (UTE) MRI tricomponent T_2^* model. NMR Biomed. 2020;33(3):e4233.

56. Krafft AJ, Loeffler RB, Song R, Tipirneni-Sajja A, McCarville MB, Robson MD, et al. Quantitative ultrashort echo time imaging for assessment of massive iron overload at 1.5 and 3 Tesla. Magn Reson Med. 2017;78(5):1839–51.

57. Du J, Corbeil J, Znamirowski R, Angle N, Peterson M, Bydder GM, et al. Direct imaging and quantification of carotid plaque calcification. Magn Reson Med. 2011;65(4):1013–20.

58. Deoni SC, Rutt BK, Peters TM. Rapid combined T_1 and T_2 mapping using gradient recalled acquisition in the steady state. Magn Reson Med. 2003;49(3):515–26.

59. Gold GE, Han E, Stainsby J, Wright G, Brittain J, Beaulieu C. Musculoskeletal MRI at 3.0 T: relaxation times and image contrast. AJR Am J Roentgenol. 2004;183(2):343–51.

60. Yarnykh VL. Actual flip-angle imaging in the pulsed steady state: a method for rapid three-dimensional mapping of the transmitted radiofrequency field. Magn Reson Med. 2007;57(1):192–200.

61. Ma YJ, Lu X, Carl M, Zhu Y, Szeverenyi NM, Bydder GM, et al. Accurate T_1 mapping of short T2 tissues using a three-dimensional ultrashort echo time cones actual flip angle imaging-variable repetition time (3D UTE-Cones AFI-VTR) method. Magn Reson Med. 2018;80(2):598–608.

62. Ma YJ, Zhao W, Wan L, Guo T, Searleman A, Jang H, et al. Whole knee joint T_1 values measured in vivo at 3T by combined 3D ultrashort echo time cones actual flip angle and variable flip angle methods. Magn Reson Med. 2019;81(3):1634–44.

63. Wei Z, Ma YJ, Jang H, Yang W, Du J. To measure T_1 of short T2 species using an inversion recovery prepared three-dimensional ultrashort echo time (3D IR-UTE) method: a phantom study. J Magn Reson. 2020;314:106725.

64. Sepponen RE, Pohjonen JA, Sipponen JT, Tanttu JI. A method for T_1 rho imaging. J Comput Assist Tomogr. 1985;9(6):1007–11.

65. Wang YX, Zhang Q, Li X, Chen W, Ahuja A, Yuan J. T_1rho magnetic resonance: basic physics principles and applications in knee and intervertebral disc imaging. Quant Imaging Med Surg. 2015;5(6):858–85.

66. Duvvuri U, Reddy R, Patel SD, Kaufman JH, Kneeland JB, Leigh JS. T_1rho-relaxation in articular cartilage: effects of enzymatic degradation. Magn Reson Med. 1997;38(6):863–7.

67. Du J, Carl M, Diaz E, Takahashi A, Han E, Szeverenyi NM, et al. Ultrashort TE T_1rho (UTE T_1rho) imaging of the Achilles tendon and meniscus. Magn Reson Med. 2010;64(3):834–42.

68. Ma YJ, Carl M, Shao H, Tadros AS, Chang EY, Du J. Three-dimensional ultrashort echo time cones T_1rho (3D UTE-cones-T_1rho) imaging. NMR Biomed. 2017:30(6). https://doi.org/10.1002/nbm.3709.

69. Shao H, Pauli C, Li S, Ma Y, Tadros AS, Kavanaugh A, et al. Magic angle effect plays a major role in both T_1rho and T_2 relaxation in articular cartilage. Osteoarthr Cartil. 2017;25(12):2022–30.

70. Hanninen N, Rautiainen J, Rieppo L, Saarakkala S, Nissi MJ. Orientation anisotropy of quantitative MRI relaxation parameters in ordered tissue. Sci Rep. 2017;7(1):9606.

71. Wu M, Ma YJ, Kasibhatla A, Chen M, Jang H, Jerban S, et al. Convincing evidence for magic angle less-sensitive quantitative T_1rho imaging of articular cartilage using the 3D ultrashort echo time cones adiabatic T_1rho (3D UTE cones-AdiabT_1rho) sequence. Magn Reson Med. 2020;84(5):2551–60.

72. Zu Z, Afzal A, Li H, Xie J, Gore JC. Spin-lock imaging of early tissue pH changes in ischemic rat brain. NMR Biomed. 2018;31(4):e3893.

73. Ma YJ, Carl M, Searleman A, Lu X, Chang EY, Du J. 3D adiabatic T1rho prepared ultrashort echo time cones sequence for whole knee imaging. Magn Reson Med. 2018;80(4):1429–39.

74. Henkelman RM, Huang X, Xiang QS, Stanisz GJ, Swanson SD, Bronskill MJ. Quantitative interpretation of magnetization transfer. Magn Reson Med. 1993;29(6):759–66.

75. Springer F, Martirosian P, Machann J, Schwenzer NF, Claussen CD, Schick F. Magnetization transfer contrast imaging in bovine and human cortical bone applying an ultrashort echo time sequence at 3 Tesla. Magn Reson Med. 2009;61(5):1040–8.

76. Chang EY, Bae WC, Shao H, Biswas R, Li S, Chen J, et al. Ultrashort echo time magnetization transfer (UTE-MT) imaging of cortical bone. NMR Biomed. 2015;28(7):873–80.

77. Sled JG, Pike GB. Quantitative interpretation of magnetization transfer in spoiled gradient echo MRI sequences. J Magn Reson. 2000;145(1):24–36.

78. Ma YJ, Tadros A, Du J, Chang EY. Quantitative two-dimensional ultrashort echo time magnetization transfer (2D UTE-MT) imaging of cortical bone. Magn Reson Med. 2018;79(4):1941–9.

79. Ma YJ, Chang EY, Carl M, Du J. Quantitative magnetization transfer ultrashort echo time imaging using a time-efficient 3D multi-spoke Cones sequence. Magn Reson Med. 2018;79(2):692–700.

80. Ma YJ, Shao H, Du J, Chang EY. Ultrashort echo time magnetization transfer (UTE-MT) imaging and modeling: magic angle independent biomarkers of tissue properties. NMR Biomed. 2016;29(11):1546–52.

81. Zhu Y, Cheng X, Ma Y, Wong JH, Xie Y, Du J, et al. Rotator cuff tendon assessment using magic-angle insensitive 3D ultrashort echo time cones magnetization transfer (UTE-Cones-MT) imaging and modeling with histological correlation. J Magn Reson Imaging. 2018;48(1):160–8.

82. Wan L, Cheng X, Searleman AC, Ma YJ, Wong JH, Meyer RS, et al. Evaluation of enzymatic proteoglycan loss and collagen degradation in human articular cartilage using ultrashort echo time-based biomarkers: a feasibility study. NMR Biomed. 2022;35(5):e4664.

83. Xue YP, Ma YJ, Wu M, Jerban S, Wei Z, Chang EY, et al. Quantitative 3D ultrashort echo time magnetization transfer imaging for evaluation of knee cartilage degeneration in vivo. J Magn Reson Imaging. 2021;54(4):1294–302.

84. Zhang X, Ma YJ, Wei Z, Wu M, Ashir A, Jerban S, et al. Macromolecular fraction (MMF) from 3D ultrashort echo time cones magnetization transfer (3D UTE-Cones-MT) imaging predicts meniscal degeneration and knee osteoarthritis. Osteoarthr Cartil. 2021;29(8):1173–80.

Zero Echo Time (ZTE) MRI

Markus Weiger and Klaas P. Pruessmann

Introduction

Generally, magnetic resonance imaging (MRI) of tissues or materials with rapid transverse relaxation needs to follow two fundamental principles [1]. First, to capture sufficient signal, gradient encoding and data acquisition must be started quickly after signal excitation. Second, to prevent resolution loss due to apodization in k-space, the time range after excitation during which all data is acquired, must be sufficiently small. Implementing these principles with different weighting and by using different conceptual approaches leads to four basic sequences dedicated to short-T_2 MRI, namely, constant time imaging (CTI) [2], single-point imaging (SPI) [3], ultrashort echo time (UTE) imaging [4], and zero echo time (ZTE) imaging [5–8]—which is the topic of the present chapter.

The ZTE sequence is shown in Fig. 5.1a. To efficiently capture and encode rapidly decaying signals, the sequence abstains from slice selection and phase encoding and covers 3D k-space with straight radial center-out trajectories. As a particular concept, only after setting the radial encoding gradient, radiofrequency (RF) excitation is performed. This is then immediately followed by data acquisition. This simple sequence scheme is the imaging analog of the pulse-acquire NMR experiment and was in fact used in the very first reported MRI scan [9]. It was only later identified and exploited as an approach particularly suitable for short-T_2 imaging.

The ZTE sequence is very effective at coping with rapidly decaying signals because it encodes fresh transverse magnetization immediately at full k-space speed and with zero

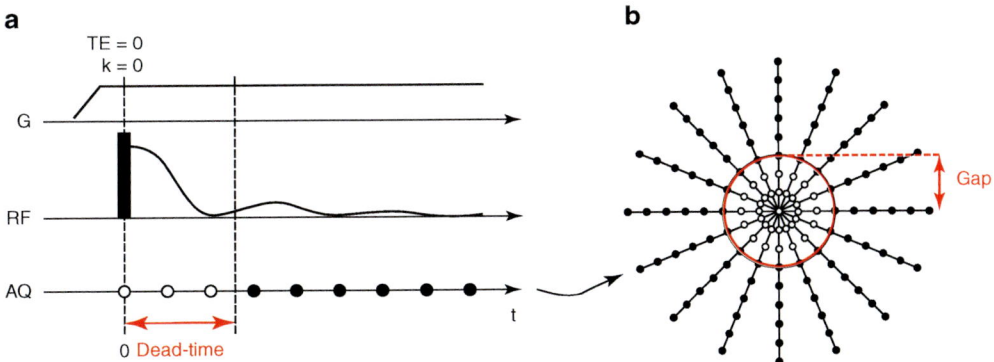

Fig. 5.1 The basic ZTE pulse sequence. (**a**) After setting the radial projection gradient (G) to full strength, an RF pulse of sufficient bandwidth is applied and the free induction decay signal is acquired (AQ) after the RF dead-time (black dots = acquired, white dots = missed). As gradient encoding starts immediately after signal creation, $k = 0$ is met inside the pulse, and TE is effectively zero. (**b**) 1D spokes are collected in a center-out radial fashion in order to fill the 3D-k-space volume of interest (one central plane is shown). The data missed during the dead-time translate into a gap in k-space, which leads to a spherical void in the k-space center. (Adapted with permission from Ref. [21])

M. Weiger (✉) · K. P. Pruessmann
Institute for Biomedical Engineering, ETH Zurich and University of Zurich, Zurich, Switzerland
e-mail: weiger@biomed.ee.ethz.ch

delay. All fresh magnetization leaves the center of k-space at the exact time at which it is created, leading to the notion of zero TE in analogy to the earlier UTE technique. This desirable capability comes with the challenge of keeping pace at the level of signal detection and starting data acquisition equally rapidly. With common MRI systems this is not quite possible due to the finite time required for switching RF chains from transmit to receive operation. This dead-time results in a gap in k-space which appears as a spherical void at the center of k-space (Fig. 5.1b), which needs to be addressed with additional measures specific to the ZTE approach (see sections "The Dead-Time Gap" and "Image Reconstruction").

Another challenge arises from excitation during the readout gradient, requiring RF pulses with corresponding high bandwidths, which can be substantially greater than those used in other modes of imaging. Suitably high bandwidths can be achieved with sufficiently short hard pulses or, for larger flip angles, with frequency-modulated pulses (see section "Excitation").

Conversely, the encoding gradient in the ZTE sequence does not need to be switched on and off; it only requires adjustment of its direction between successive excitations. This renders scanning relatively silent and minimizes gradient slew rate requirements as well as eddy currents. Moreover, with only minimal sequence overhead for excitation and spoiling, very short, sub-millisecond repetition times (TRs) are feasible (see section "Further Sequence Aspects").

The principal difference between the ZTE sequence and its UTE counterpart is the temporal order of setting the encoding gradient and RF excitation. However, this swap is of considerable consequence. In addition to the opportunities and requirements mentioned above, ZTE imaging does not suffer from fidelity issues introduced by gradient ramping. On the other hand, it does not offer the freedom to adjust TE, which, in the UTE variant, provides control over T_2^* contrast and options for background signal suppression.

This chapter discusses ZTE imaging in detail, along with a number of other closely related techniques. The presentation covers sequence aspects, image reconstruction, hardware requirements, and applications.

The Dead-Time Gap

Both the key advantages and the main challenges of ZTE imaging are associated with RF excitation after the readout gradient has been switched on and is at full strength. It is this strategy that secures immediate gradient encoding at full k-space speed. However, it also renders the technique blind to the stretch of k-space covered during the RF pulse and to the period required to switch from RF transmission to signal reception. The different contributions to this dead-time are illustrated in Fig. 5.2. The RF pulse contribution amounts to the fraction of the pulse duration that extends beyond the magnetic center of the pulse, which is the actual center for symmetric waveforms of constant frequency. After the RF pulse, switching to receive mode requires either detuning the transmit coil and tuning the receive coil or, with a transmit-receive coil, redirecting the RF path by the use of a transmit-receive (T/R) switch. Beyond the immediate duration of these processes, spikes, and transients that corrupt the received signal often add to the dead-time. Finally, additional time is lost due to bandpass filtering for data decimation, which requires a lead-in time that is related to the net filter length.

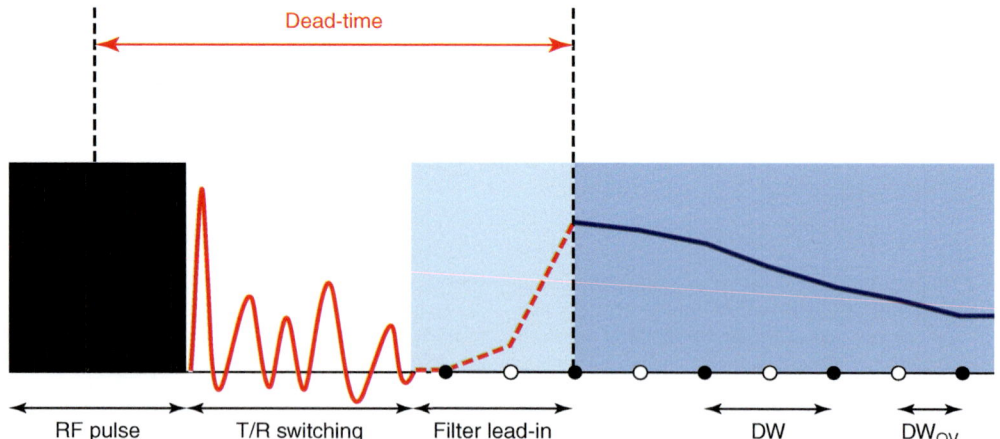

Fig. 5.2 Contributions to the initial RF dead-time of the ZTE sequence. For symmetric RF pulses of constant frequency, the magnetic center is located at the pulse center, so only half of its duration contributes to the dead-time. During transmit-receive (T/R) switching, the MR signal is corrupted by spikes and transients. Following these RF events, fully filtered and uncorrupted data are only available after the lead-in time of the digital filter, corresponding to half of its length in the case of a symmetric filter with a finite impulse response. The dwell time DW = 1/BW corresponds to the bandwidth (BW) in the target FOV, according to Nyquist, whereas DW_{OV} is smaller and associated with radial oversampling. (Adapted with permission from Ref. [1])

The total dead-time causes an initial gap in the acquired data, which, for the radial center-out ZTE encoding scheme, corresponds to a spherical void in the center of k-space (see Fig. 5.1b). The size of this gap is typically indicated in terms of Nyquist intervals $dk = 1/FOV$, where FOV is the field of view. With simple Fourier reconstruction, the k-space gap causes low-frequency artifacts in the reconstructed images. A variety of approaches have been developed to address these.

Minimizing Dead-Time

The first and natural strategy is to minimize each dead-time contribution. For a given flip angle, the duration of the RF pulse can only be reduced by increasing RF power, an approach constrained by hardware specifications and limits for specific absorption rate (SAR). Alternatively, the dead-time contribution of a long RF pulse can be greatly reduced by splitting the pulse into short sub-pulses interleaved with data acquisition as is done with the sweep imaging with Fourier transform (SWIFT) technique [10] (see section "Sweep Pulse"). As a third option, the dead-time contribution of continuous, long RF pulses can be avoided by using pulse-encoded ZTE [11], which involves slight variation of the pulse and algebraic reconstruction (see section "Sweep Pulse").

Decreasing the duration of T/R switching requires improvements in the electronics (see section "RF Chain") and, potentially, suppression of coil ringdown [12–15], depending on which transients are dominant.

The filter lead-in time can be minimized to a certain degree by means of filter design. In addition, it can be very effectively reduced by increasing the filter bandwidth and corresponding oversampling, albeit at the price of more data entering image reconstruction. This drawback can be greatly mitigated by multi-rate data acquisition [16], which limits oversampling to the vicinity of switching events.

For given dead-time, the size of the k-space gap scales linearly with the strength of the readout gradient. Hence, irrespective of dead-time, the gap can be reduced by scaling down the gradient. This, however, increases the time required to cover the desired k-space range, which should not exceed the shortest T_2 of interest to prevent image blurring due to signal decay [17].

Providing Missing Data

Common Fourier reconstruction is applicable only when the k-space gap is not more than $dk/2$, which limits the diameter of the central void in k-space to one dwell. This is frequently not possible using the measures listed above, and requires means for filling the void that are not part of regular scanning.

One option is to fill the center of k-space by algebraic reconstruction [18, 19]. Based on radial oversampling, this approach achieves filling of the gap by finite support extrapolation (see section "Algebraic ZTE"). However, it is limited to gaps up to approximately 3 dk.

For larger gaps, several techniques have been developed to obtain the missing data by complementary acquisitions at lower gradient amplitudes (Fig. 5.3). In water- and fat-suppressed projection proton MRI (WASPI) [20], a second set of radial acquisitions is performed with greatly reduced gradient strength. This approach is very time-efficient but results in a discontinuity in T_2* weighting at the boundary of the k-space gap, and this can impair depiction [21]. In point-wise encoding time reduction with radial acquisition (PETRA) [22], the data inside the gap are acquired in a single-point fashion on a Cartesian grid [23]. Continuous T_2* weighting gives it better depiction fidelity; however, this is at the expense of time with relatively inefficient single-point acquisition. Hybrid filling (HYFI) [24] is intermediate between these two options and combines a core of Cartesian single-point sampling with surrounding concentric shells, which are radially sampled.

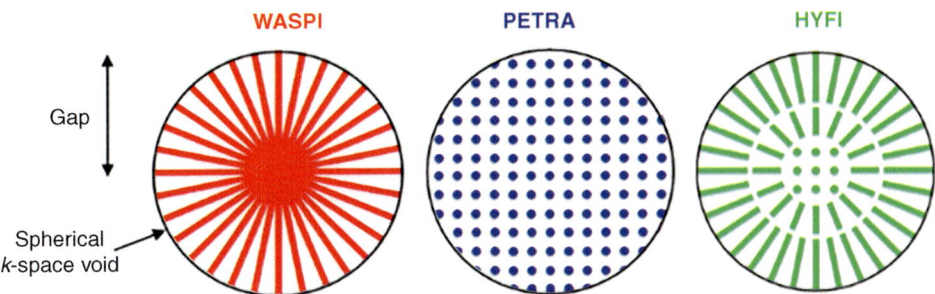

Fig. 5.3 Techniques to fill the spherical k-space void caused by the dead-time gap in ZTE data. WASPI, PETRA, and HYFI all provide the missing data using additional acquisitions at lower gradient strengths. However, these techniques differ in acquisition timing and geometry. In WASPI, a second set of radial acquisitions is performed with greatly reduced gradient strength. In PETRA, the k-space inside the gap is acquired single-pointwise on a Cartesian grid. HYFI consists of a Cartesian single-point core surrounded by several radially acquired shells. (Adapted with permission from Ref. [24])

Notably, single-point acquisition in central *k*-space as used by PETRA and HYFI implies a finite TE, with its lower limit determined by the minimum dead-time. This finite TE is associated with some loss in short-T_2 sensitivity, but it also introduces valuable contrast options (see section "Contrast").

Simultaneous RF Operation

In view of the effort required to address the *k*-space gap, an ideal solution would be to avoid the gap in the first place. To this end, efforts have been made to perform RF excitation and acquisition simultaneously, and thus remove the need for RF switching. One approach is based on sideband modulation [25], or, equivalently, two-photon excitation [26]. This permits spectral decoupling of the transmit and receive chains and has been successfully used for imaging with simultaneous excitation and acquisition [27, 28]. However, it comes with a trade-off in terms of transmit and receive efficiency and thus between SAR and signal-to-noise ratio (SNR). A second approach is decoupling by exact cancelation of cross-talk, which has also been used in imaging experiments [29–31] but it is challenging at regular transmitter power, particularly in vivo where motion and physiology can cause the coupling to fluctuate. Because of these constraints, simultaneous RF operation has not yet reached routine use.

Excitation

Another challenge posed by the ZTE sequence is the uniformity of RF excitation. The spectral selectivity of the excitation must be contained to prevent artifacts due to inconsistency of data obtained using different gradient directions [32]. To address this, the spectrum of the RF pulse must cover the band of Larmor frequencies induced by the readout gradient with sufficient uniformity. This requirement leads to a particular entanglement between signal bandwidth, flip angle, pulse duration, dead-time (see section "The Dead-Time Gap"), transmit power, and SAR.

Hard Pulse

The traditional ZTE sequence uses a hard pulse, i.e., a pulse with constant amplitude and frequency that is short enough to uniformly excite the imaged object (Fig. 5.4a). As a rule of thumb, for robust uniformity, the pulse duration should not exceed approximately DW/3 [33], where DW = 1/BW is the Nyquist dwell time and BW is the signal bandwidth across

a Hard pulse

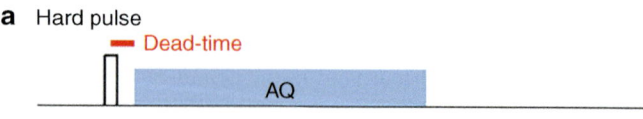

b Sweep pulse

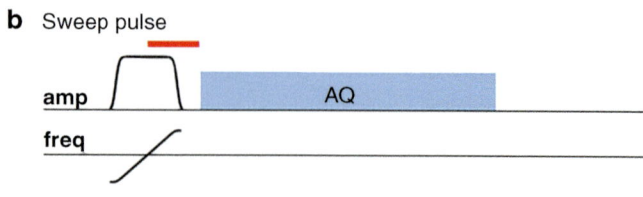

c Pulse encoding

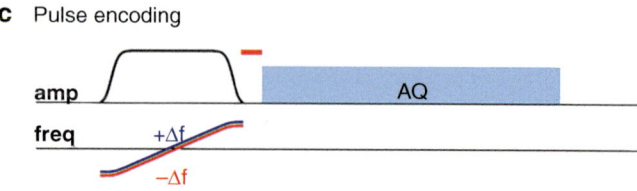

d SWIFT

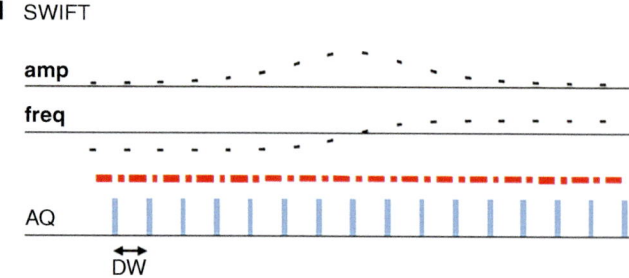

Fig. 5.4 Different excitation strategies for ZTE-type imaging. (**a**) The simplest, traditional approach is a hard pulse. It must be sufficiently short to excite the full bandwidth spanned by the readout gradient over the FOV that potentially limits the achievable flip angle. (**b**) Using a frequency-swept pulse instead renders the bandwidth independent of the pulse length, thus allowing larger flip angles. However, the pulse duration is limited by the acceptable total dead-time. (**c**) With pulse encoding, the contribution of the pulse to the dead-time can be eliminated, enabling much longer sweep pulses. This is achieved by employing slightly different pulses in successive excitations, e.g., with small frequency offsets. (**d**) Very long frequency-swept pulses are used with the SWIFT technique, where excitation and acquisition are performed quasi-simultaneously by alternating between the two modes of operation. A downside to this approach is that two dead-times occur for each pulse interval which reduces both the RF and the acquisition duty cycles. Furthermore, the switching rate is governed by the Nyquist dwell time DW, thus limiting the achievable bandwidth

the FOV. However, in practice durations up to about DW can also provide useful results although they may need appropriate correction during image reconstruction (see section "RF Pulses").

When shortening a hard pulse to meet bandwidth requirements, its power must be increased in proportion to the inverse square of its duration to maintain an optimal flip angle. With strong readout gradients this demand may exceed the power limits of the transmit chain. In this case, a feasible hard pulse may miss the optimal flip angle, resulting in a loss of SNR and/or T_1 contrast. In addition to hardware limits, SAR limits must be observed. At a fixed flip angle, the SAR of a block pulse increases in proportion to the inverse of its duration, which can become limiting in high-bandwidth applications (see section "High Bandwidth").

Sweep Pulse

The strict relationship between pulse duration and bandwidth is overcome by frequency modulation, particularly by pulses with a frequency sweep, which provide approximately uniform spreads of power in the time and spectral domains (Fig. 5.4b) [34, 35]. This enables the use of longer pulses to achieve higher flip angles. Notably, the SAR of frequency-swept pulses does not depend on the pulse duration but only on flip angle and bandwidth. However, increased pulse duration does add to the total dead-time, which may exceed the feasible range for algebraic reconstruction. It also increases the time required for filling the k-space gap by complementary acquisition (see section "Providing Missing Data").

One solution to this problem is to perform frequency-swept excitation and data acquisition in a rapidly interleaved fashion, as done in the SWIFT technique [10] (Fig. 5.4d). The rate of interleaving matches the pulse bandwidth, and each pair of pulse and acquisition intervals includes two RF switching operations. This approach reduces the pulse-related dead-time to half the duration of a sub-pulse and enables the use of sweep pulses of arbitrary length. As it involves frequent alternation between transmit and receive operation, it particularly benefits from rapid T/R switches, which favor both the achievable bandwidth and the net acquisition time [36].

For long, continuous sweep pulses the dead-time penalty has been addressed by pulse encoding [11], which uses an algebraic reconstruction framework and accounts for the full-pulse waveform (see section "RF Pulses"). The conditioning of this signal model benefits greatly from the successive use of two pulses that cover the same bandwidth but with different phase modulation, e.g., due to a small mutual frequency offset (Fig. 5.4c). Although at first sight this comes at the price of doubling the scan time, SNR efficiency is nevertheless maintained, and various sequence modifications are possible to circumvent this issue.

As an important note, rapid transverse relaxation during extended RF excitation does not entail signal loss if the pulse is appropriately taken into account during image reconstruction [11].

Reducing Gradient Strength

When the excitation bandwidth reaches power or SAR limits, it may be reduced by using a lower gradient strength during the application of the RF pulse and only ramping up the gradient to full strength thereafter. This intermediate sequence between ZTE and UTE has been suggested for gradient-modulated PETRA [37], ramped hybrid encoding (RHE) [38], and gradient-modulated SWIFT [39]. Its benefit in terms of excitation bandwidth comes with a certain trade-off against effective resolution at very short T_2 values, and potential eddy current effects due to gradient ramping. For high-bandwidth applications (see section "High Bandwidth"), even reduced ramp times may be too long. In these regards, too, the ramped approach covers a middle ground between ZTE and UTE imaging.

Image Reconstruction

Generally, image reconstruction amounts to inverting all relevant encoding that the recorded signal experienced, be it from dynamic gradient fields or fields of other spatial order, static fields, RF coil sensitivities, or RF pulses. In an algebraic formulation, the linear model $\mathbf{s} = \mathbf{E}\boldsymbol{\rho}$ describes how the signal $\mathbf{s}$ is obtained from spin density $\boldsymbol{\rho}$ by the application of the encoding matrix $\mathbf{E}$, assembling all the contributions mentioned above [40]. The image $\hat{\boldsymbol{\rho}} = \mathbf{Fs}$ is then obtained by the application of the reconstruction matrix, typically calculated as the pseudoinverse $\mathbf{F} = \mathbf{E}^+$.

The actual content of $\mathbf{E}$, as well as the particular algorithm used to calculate $\hat{\boldsymbol{\rho}}$ via $\mathbf{F}$, strongly depend on sequence design and experimental setup, and only those aspects that are specific for ZTE imaging are described below.

Algebraic ZTE

From data obtained with the basic ZTE sequence shown in Fig. 5.1, the algebraic approach enables reconstruction of artifact-free images for k-space gaps up to approximately 3 dk. To this end, oversampling is used during radial acquisition (Fig. 5.5a), and image reconstruction is based on the assumption that all signal originates strictly from inside the reconstructed FOV. Jointly with oversampling, this assumption enables so-called finite support extrapolation [41] into the k-space gap, as illustrated in Fig. 5.5b. At the level of encoding functions, it can be understood as the ability to approximate the missing low harmonics by linear combination of the harmonics associated with the actually acquired data, provided that it is oversampled.

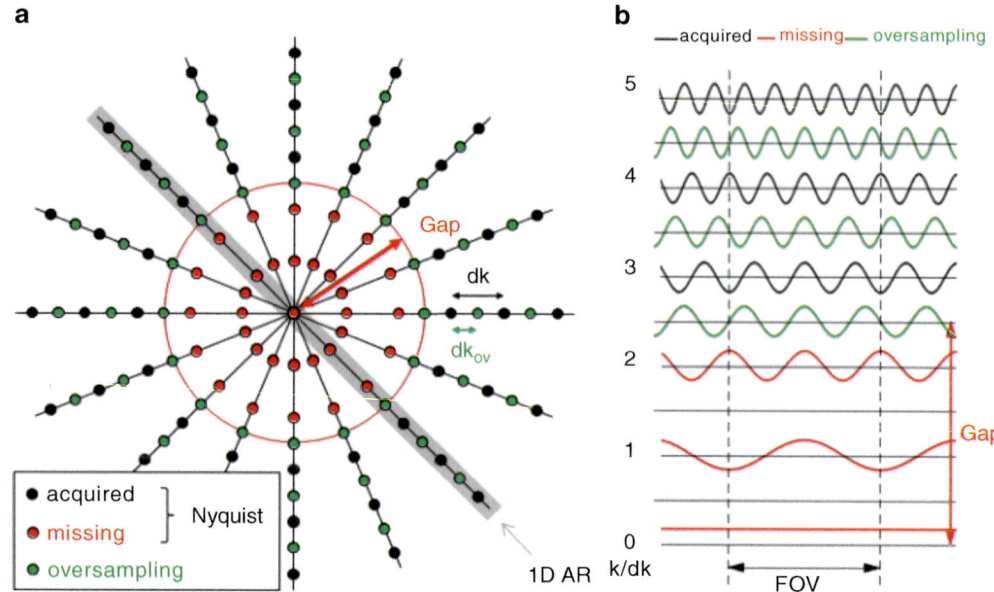

Fig. 5.5 Principles of algebraic reconstruction (AR) in ZTE imaging. (**a**) ZTE data acquisition scheme in 3D k-space, represented by a 2D plane through the center. Data points, as required according to the Nyquist criterion for the chosen FOV, are at distance apart dk. From these points, the acquired data are shown in black, while missing data are shown in red. Additional data points acquired due to radial oversampling by a factor ov (which is two in this case) are shown in green and result in an actual sampling distance dk_{ov} = dk/ov. The resulting gap in k-space leads to an empty central sphere, which has a radius of 2.5 dk in the case shown. The grey bar indicates all data points involved in the AR of a 1D projection. (**b**) Encoding functions involved in the acquisition and AR of a 1D ZTE projection. The k-values are given in units of Nyquist intervals dk. Each encoding function corre-

sponds to a data point in (**a**), while only the central part of the positive k-space half is shown. The continuous spatial representation is depicted in a range covering twice the FOV, corresponding to twofold oversampling. The encoding functions as actually employed during data acquisition and used for AR are shown in black and green. The red ones are missing due to the gap, and are implicitly replaced by the effective encoding functions during AR. It can be anticipated that within the FOV, the encoding functions added by oversampling are not orthogonal to the Nyquist set and are therefore able to serve for creating the missing functions by linear combination. Hence, the assumed band limitation of the signal and the applied oversampling are the basis for enabling AR of ZTE data, thus involving finite support extrapolation of the missing data [41]. (Adapted with permission from Ref. [44])

In principle, the described reconstruction could be directly applied to the complete ZTE data set, resulting in a 3D image. However, the associated matrices would usually be impractically large, prompting iterative approaches [42], yet with potentially slow convergence related to suboptimal conditioning introduced by the gap. Alternatively, in the present case of pure radial sampling, the finite support extrapolation can be limited to 1D treatment of two opposite k-space spokes. Hence, in the signal model, ρ describes a 1D projection of the 3D object, and **s** assembles data obtained with identical gradient strength but opposite polarities. In the encoding matrix **E**, each row holds the harmonic function associated with a data sample, initial rows are missing due to the dead-time gap, additional rows are inserted by oversampling, and the finite FOV is reflected by the length of the rows.

The complete ZTE reconstruction procedure is illustrated in Fig. 5.6, where the projections obtained by 1D algebraic reconstruction are Fourier-transformed back to k-space, followed by standard 3D gridding [43]. As 3D radial data have a highly nonuniform k-space density, an appropriate correction must be applied, and this is done efficiently using the rho filter [1].

Unfortunately, the algebraic approach is limited to gaps up to approximately 3 dk, as conditioning of the encoding

matrix deteriorates with increasing gap size. This strongly penalizes the presence of background signal and enhances noise [44].

In this context, parallel imaging can play an interesting supporting role, where the extent of the coil footprint in k-space is utilized to expand the maximum possible gap size [45].

ZTE with Gap-Filling

Reconstructing images for ZTE-based techniques using additional acquisitions to fill the k-space gap, such as WASPI, PETRA, and HYFI (see section "Providing Missing Data"), is more straightforward. As in the 3D part of algebraic ZTE, data are fed into a 3D gridding procedure. However, as the k-space patterns obtained with gap-filling are less regular than with pure radial sampling, more attention needs to be paid to density correction. In principle, the latter is performed inherently when using iterative gridding algorithms [42]. However, convergence can considerably be improved by including pre-calculated density correction functions [46].

1D × N   **3D**

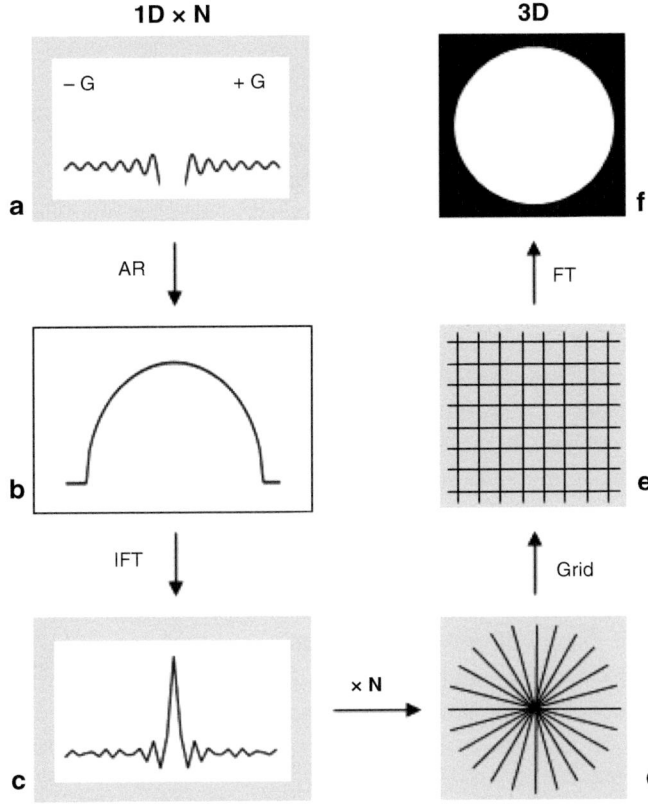

Fig. 5.6 Overview of algebraic reconstruction (AR) in ZTE imaging. One acquisition provides oversampled data with an initial gap. From two acquisitions of opposite gradient polarity (**a**), a 1D projection (**b**) is obtained by AR. The corresponding *k*-space data with both the gap and the oversampling removed (**c**) are obtained by inverse Fourier transform (IFT). *N* such *k*-space profiles with different projection directions are assembled (**d**) and interpolated onto a Cartesian grid (**e**) by a standard gridding procedure. The final 3D image (**f**) is obtained by 3D FT. The gray background indicates the *k*-space domain. (Adapted with permission from Ref. [19])

RF Pulses

As discussed in section "Excitation," RF excitation plays an unfamiliar role in ZTE imaging. In particular, it can affect signal encoding and may need to be considered in image reconstruction.

Hard pulses which are sufficiently short to provide largely uniform excitation can be neglected. However, longer hard pulses that introduce spatially dependent signal weighting need to be included in image reconstruction to limit errors arising from inconsistency in the data set [32].

Sweep pulses always have stronger encoding properties due to the typically approximately quadratic phase in their spectrum. They can either be directly included in the signal model [34, 35] or taken into account in the image domain by means of deconvolution [10].

For pulse-encoded ZTE [11], at least two different pulse shapes are assembled in one encoding matrix, thus combining gradient and pulse information during image reconstruction. In this way, pulse knowledge and finite support assumption are jointly used to enable generation of the data missing in the dead-time gap.

Purely radial encoding schemes (e.g., algebraic ZTE, WASPI, or SWIFT) offer the advantage that pulse-based image reconstruction can be limited to 1D before 3D gridding (cf. Fig. 5.6). For the less regular patterns of PETRA and HYFI, more involved approaches are necessary to combine pulse correction with 3D reconstruction [34].

Further Sequence Aspects

Apart from the main properties of the ZTE method, there are a few further aspects in which it differs from standard MRI techniques:

Gradients

One beneficial property of the ZTE sequence is that switching gradients on and off between TR intervals can be avoided, and only the subsequent radial direction must be prepared. In this way, acoustic noise is greatly reduced and eddy currents are minimized.

However, this mode of operation precludes the implementation of standard gradient spoiling where the same gradient integral per dimension in physical space is applied during each TR. Hence, the destruction of unwanted coherences must be achieved by extending the readout gradient and introducing randomization in the order of the radial directions.

Apart from the spoiling aspect, the selection and order of gradient directions also determine the angular distance between successive spokes and hence the required slew rate, which, in turn, affects the acoustic noise. Moreover, in some cases, interleaving of packages of equal *k*-space coverage is desired, e.g., for motion correction [47] or contrast preparation (see section "Contrast"). To serve these requirements, several selection algorithms have been proposed [48–52].

Repetition Time

The simple structure of the ZTE sequence without gradient switching, with a high acquisition duty cycle and usually short encoding durations, has the potential to achieve very short TRs, down to a few hundred microseconds [53]. This feature matches well the limitations with respect to achievable flip angles (see section "Excitation"), and so Ernst angle operation may still be feasible.

Notably, in this low flip angle, short TR regime, both SNR efficiency and SAR are independent of TR when the flip angle is adjusted accordingly [1].

Geometry

For pure radial frequency encoding, there is no particular readout dimension in which bandwidth-limited filtering can be applied to restrict the FOV. Hence, to avoid aliasing, the encoded FOV must cover the entire object, which may require more encoding effort than with conventional sequences.

For isotropic encoding, the 3D FOV of ZTE images is spherical, which may not be optimal for a given object shape or anatomy. As a simple solution, different gradient strengths may be selected per dimension, leading to an ellipsoidal FOV with anisotropic resolution. Alternatively, encoding may be designed to choose FOV and resolution independently [54].

Radial encoding also complicates imaging with an off-centered FOV, as frequencies need to be adapted for each gradient direction [19]. For excitation, this means that the carrier frequency of each RF pulse must be set independently. For data acquisition, the receiver frequency of each TR interval must be adapted accordingly, or, alternatively, radial oversampling can be performed and the off-center can be applied by data demodulation during image reconstruction.

Contrast

With zero TE and potentially small excitation flip angles (see section "Excitation"), there is limited intrinsic contrast in ZTE images, which often exhibit predominantly spin density weighting. Therefore, different ways of adding contrast to ZTE data have been developed [55].

Having TE = 0 means that $k = 0$ data—which dominate contrast—are obtained without any T_2^* weighting. However, k-values at increasing distance from the center do experience signal decay. Hence, by making gradients weaker and readouts longer, some T_2^* weighting can be introduced [19]; however, this is associated with increased blurring. As mentioned previously (see section "Providing Missing Data"), the ZTE variants with SPI-based gap-filling (PETRA and HYFI) have a finite TE, which also offers control of T_2^* weighting by increasing the dead-time above the technical minimum [24]. At unmodified gradient strength, this approach increases the k-space gap and thus scan time, which can be avoided by using weaker gradients, although this leads to longer readout durations. For longer TEs, it is more practical to create echo-based images by either inverting gradients [22, 56] or applying echo shifting [57]. Data with different TEs allow emphasizing short-T_2 components by image subtraction or model-based quantification of component T_2^* and amplitudes. As an example, Fig. 5.7 illustrates T_2^* mapping of samples with sub-millisecond T_2s.

Another approach is to create contrast using magnetization preparations, such as inversion recovery, long-T_2 signal suppression, diffusion weighting, or magnetization transfer [58]. As these preparations usually take much longer than a ZTE TR, multiple TR intervals should follow the preparation in a segmented fashion to make the sequence time-efficient. Figure 5.8 shows such an example, where long-T_2 suppression of water and/or fat signals is used to create positive short-T_2 contrast in musculoskeletal (MSK) MRI.

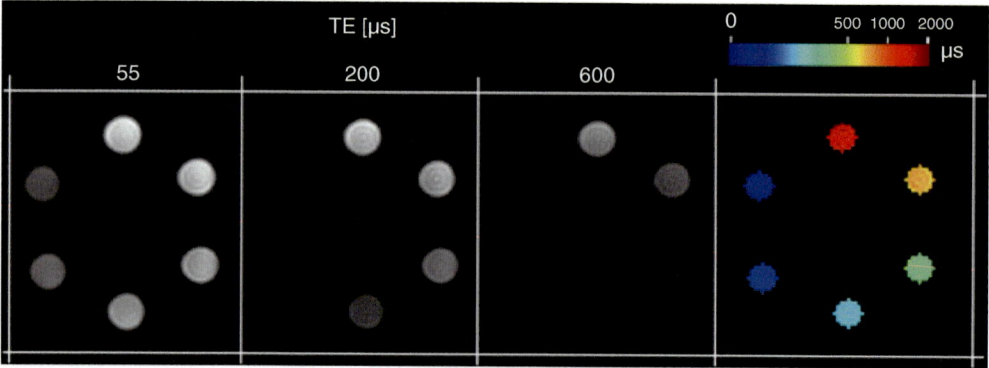

Fig. 5.7 T_2^* mapping in MnCl2 solutions with rapid transverse relaxation ($\approx$50–1500 μs). First three columns: series of HYFI images taken at different TE = dead-time of 55, 100, 200, 400, 600 μs (only a subset is displayed). Last column: maps of transverse relaxation times obtained by pixel-wise fitting the signal decay. (Adapted with permission from Ref. [24])

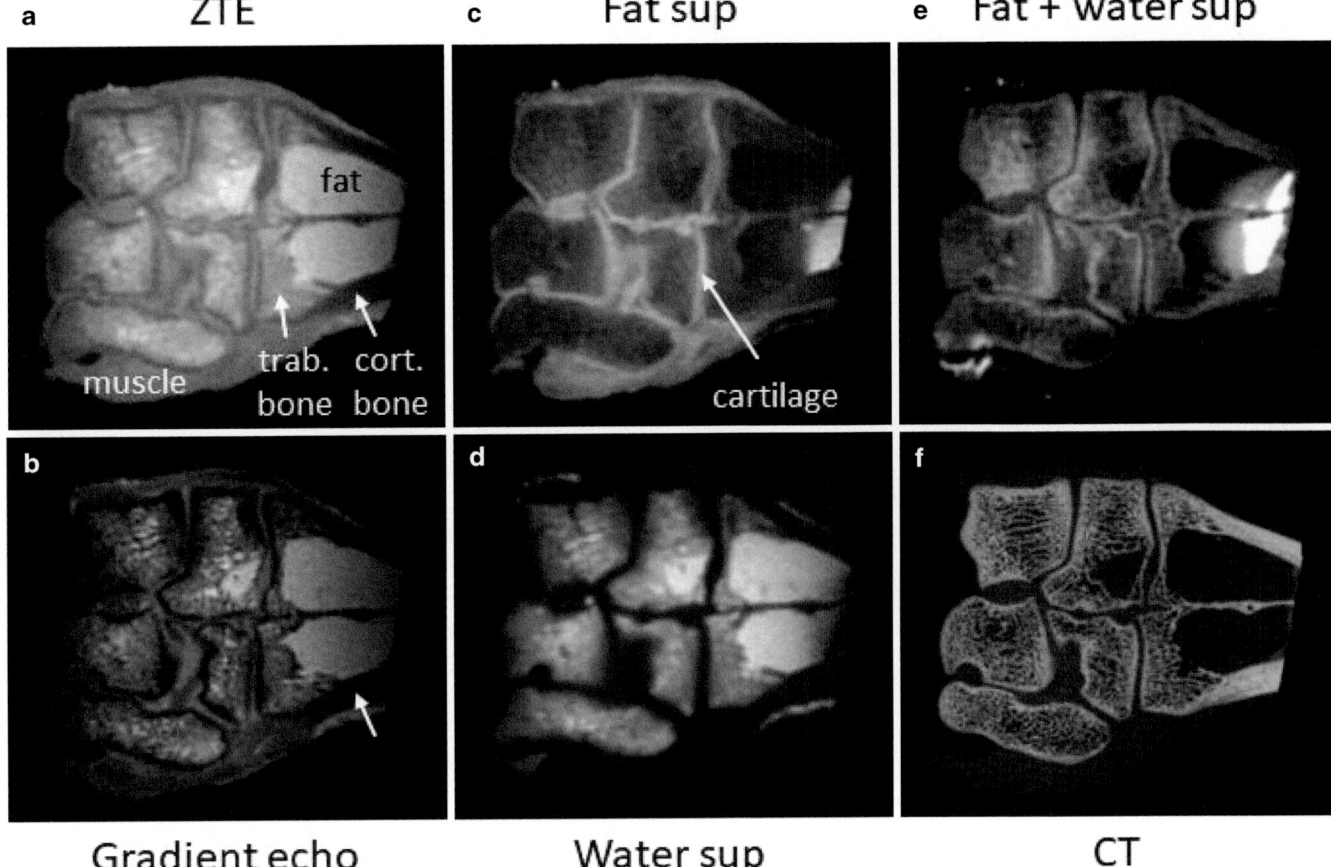

Fig. 5.8 Generating contrast in ZTE imaging by magnetization preparation demonstrated on an excised lamb joint. (**a**) Non-prepared ZTE image showing primarily proton density and some T_1 contrast. (**b**) In gradient echo imaging, signals from short-T_2 tissues are reduced, particularly those from cortical bone. (**c**) With ZTE imaging using fat suppression, both short- and long-T_2 water signals remain. (**d**) Selectively suppressing long-T_2 water in the ZTE images removes signals from cartilage and muscle, and fat signal dominates the image. (**e**) Suppressing both fat and long-T_2 water results in positive contrast for short-T_2 tissues, showing primarily trabecular and cortical bone. The remaining high fat signal (right) indicates its imperfect suppression due to local off-resonance. Note that also in trabecular bone, fat suppression may be imperfect due to local off-resonance at tissue interfaces, which could be improved by inversion recovery-based presaturation. (**f**) In the CT reference image, strong similarities with the MRI data in (**e**) are observed. (Adapted with permission from Ref. [66])

Hardware

Overall, the concept of setting the read gradient before RF excitation moves some of the demands on MRI hardware from the gradient system to the RF chain, but it also poses some specific challenges on the gradient side.

RF Chain

Minimizing the contribution of T/R switching to dead-time is key for successful and efficient ZTE imaging (see section "Minimizing Dead-time"). To this end, several designs that minimize spikes and transients have been developed to bring switching times down to the low microsecond range [59–61]. The particular need and challenge are to realize rapid switching at high power (i.e., in the kW range) and so enable sufficiently short RF pulses (see section "Excitation").

The ability to detect signals with very short T_2s also applies to the materials of the MR scanner, in particular components of, and near the RF coils (Fig. 5.9). To avoid associated artifacts and additional restrictions on the imaging protocol, ideally the materials used for coil construction should not contain the observed nucleus [62–64]. For proton-based MRI, suitable materials are nonmagnetic metals, glass, and fluorinated polymers.

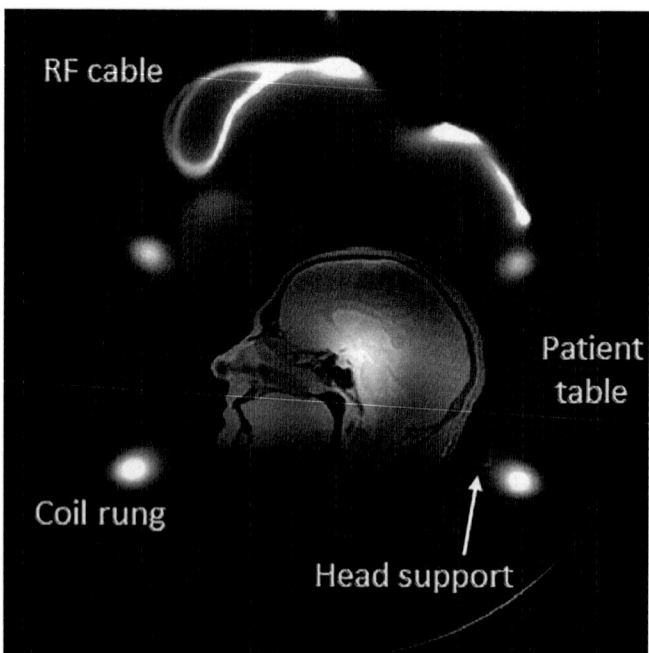

Fig. 5.9 Background signal in ZTE imaging. Images of a human head were acquired at 7 T using a T/R birdcage RF coil. Numerous extraneous signals were detected, including those from very short-T_2 materials of the RF coil and cables, the head support, and the patient table. The unwanted signals require encoding a large FOV to prevent aliasing, particularly with algebraic ZTE, where out-of-band signal can be strongly enhanced (see section "Algebraic ZTE"). Within the head, nonuniformities typical with 7 T imaging are observed. (Adapted with permission from Ref. [1])

Console

Short and possibly modulated RF pulses as well as tight sequence timing require sequence definition with temporal resolution in the microsecond range and below. This requirement may not be fulfilled on commercial MR systems but is enabled in more advanced devices [53].

On the receiver side, high acquisition bandwidths up to the MHz range are necessary to cover signals sampled at large gradient strength (see section "High Bandwidth") potentially with oversampling (see section "Providing Missing Data"). Moreover, in conjunction with high spatial resolution and array detection, 3D acquisition with oversampling yields very large quantities of data that need to be handled and stored. Furthermore, minimization of the dead-time contributed by digital filtering (see section "Minimizing Dead-time") benefits from improved performance and flexibility in the receiver system [16].

Gradient System

Unlike conventional MRI and UTE imaging, the quasi-continuous gradient operation with ZTE sequences means that slew rate is of ancillary importance and only affects the minimum possible TR. On the other hand, high gradient strength is crucial to achieving high spatial resolution for samples with short T_2s (see section "High Bandwidth"). Moreover, continuous operation requires a full duty cycle, which is a rather uncommon criterion for gradient systems but has been realized in a dedicated design [65].

Applications

The key parameter in application protocols is the signal bandwidth, as it affects both dead-time gap and RF excitation. The bandwidth is governed by the targeted spatial resolution and T_2 values according to BW $\approx$ M/2/T_2, where the temporal range of data acquisition is limited to approximately T_2 to contain blurring [1, 17], and the image matrix size M characterizes the resolution independent of object size. With this key role, bandwidth requirements can be used to assign applications to the two somewhat distinct groups described below.

Moderate Bandwidth

For many typical short-T_2 applications, the bandwidth amounts to a few hundred kHz. For example, with the rule of thumb given above, T_2 = 400 μs and M = 200 lead to BW $\approx$ 250 kHz. The necessary gradient strength is often available on commercial systems, even at full duty cycle. For the previous example, a FOV of 20 cm requires a gradient strength of 29 mT/m. Depending on the specifications of the RF chain, k-space gaps may be small enough to employ algebraic ZTE. Otherwise, gap-filling with relatively low overhead should be possible. Figure 5.10 shows four such applications from MSK, pulmonary, dental, and head MRI.

For applications in this category, usually UTE imaging can also be employed. Possible benefits of the ZTE techniques include improved short-T_2 sensitivity due to higher initial k-space speed, greater robustness against eddy currents, and much reduced acoustic noise.

High Bandwidth

With very short target T_2s (e.g., below 100 μs) and/or higher resolution, higher bandwidth is required reaching into the MHz range. Hence, a new regime is entered concerning hardware and methodological requirements, which are usually not provided on today's clinical systems. However, employing dedicated hardware such as high-performance gradients (see section "Gradient System") and rapid T/R switches (see section "RF Chain") as well as appropriate

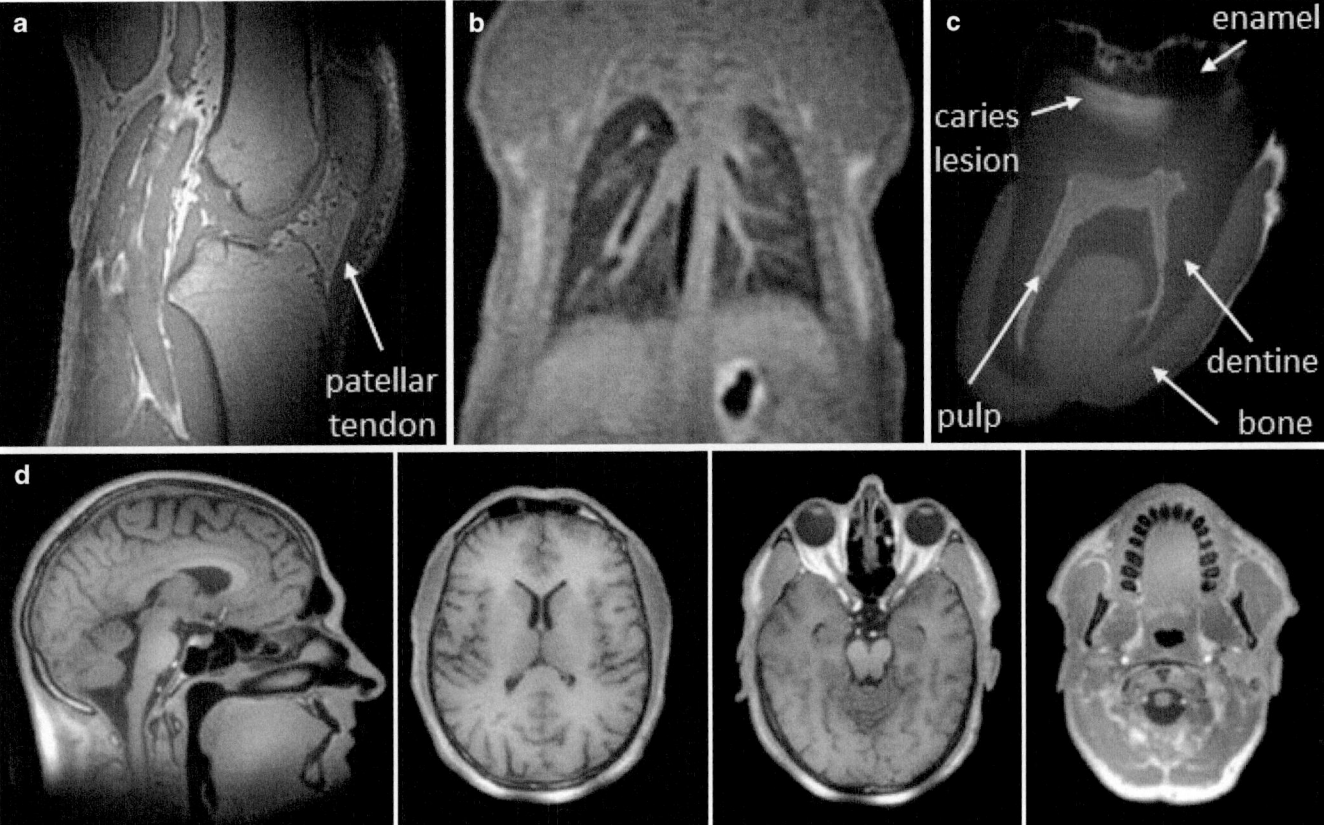

Fig. 5.10 Selected short-T_2 applications with moderate signal bandwidth (BW) obtained with algebraic ZTE MRI. (**a**) MSK: human knee acquired at 7 T with isotropic spatial resolution of 0.75 mm and BW = 250 kHz in 4 m 17 s. (Reproduced with permission from [64]). (**b**) Pulmonary: mouse lung acquired at 4.7 T with a spatial resolution of 0.31 mm and BW = 200 kHz in 4 m 30 s using respiratory gating. (Reproduced with permission from [67]). (**c**) Dental: excised human tooth acquired at 11.7 T with a resolution 0.13 × 0.13 × 0.18 mm³ and BW = 200 kHz in 21 m 18 s. (Reproduced with permission from [68]). (**d**) Head: Human head acquired at 3 T with a resolution of 1.04 mm and BW = 300 kHz in 19 m 28 s. T_1-weighting was achieved by employing pulse-encoded ZTE with a sweep pulse of 35 μs duration. (Adapted with permission from Ref. [11])

excitation (see section "Sweep Pulse") and efficient acquisition schemes (see section "Providing Missing Data") enables applications in this extreme regime. The benefits of using high bandwidths in short-T_2 MRI are illustrated in Fig. 5.11.

A particularly promising application in vivo is the direct depiction of the myelin bilayer where most of the signal has an ultrashort T_2 (see Chap. 41 "Myelin Bilayer Imaging"). The particular challenges of using high bandwidths in vivo are SAR limitations, which also ultimately constrain SNR.

Fig. 5.11 Selected short-T_2 applications with high signal bandwidth (BW) acquired at 3 T. (**a**) Materials: PMMA (polymethylmethacrylate) sample with $T_2 \approx 10\ \mu s$ acquired with isotropic spatial resolution of 0.7 mm, BW = 200|1000 kHz, and G = 40|200 mT/m. Actually, resolving the grid structure requires high bandwidth. (Adapted with permission from [69]). (**b**) Bone: portion of bovine tibia with $T_2 \approx 150\ \mu s$ acquired with resolution of 0.4 mm, BW = 158|766 kHz, and G = 41|200 mT/m. Fine details are only resolved at high bandwidth. (Adapted with permission from [69]). (**c**) Mummy: mummified foot specimen from about 1550–1100 BC acquired with resolution of 0.6 mm, BW = 1125 kHz, and G = 98 mT/m. (Adapted with permission from Ref. [70])

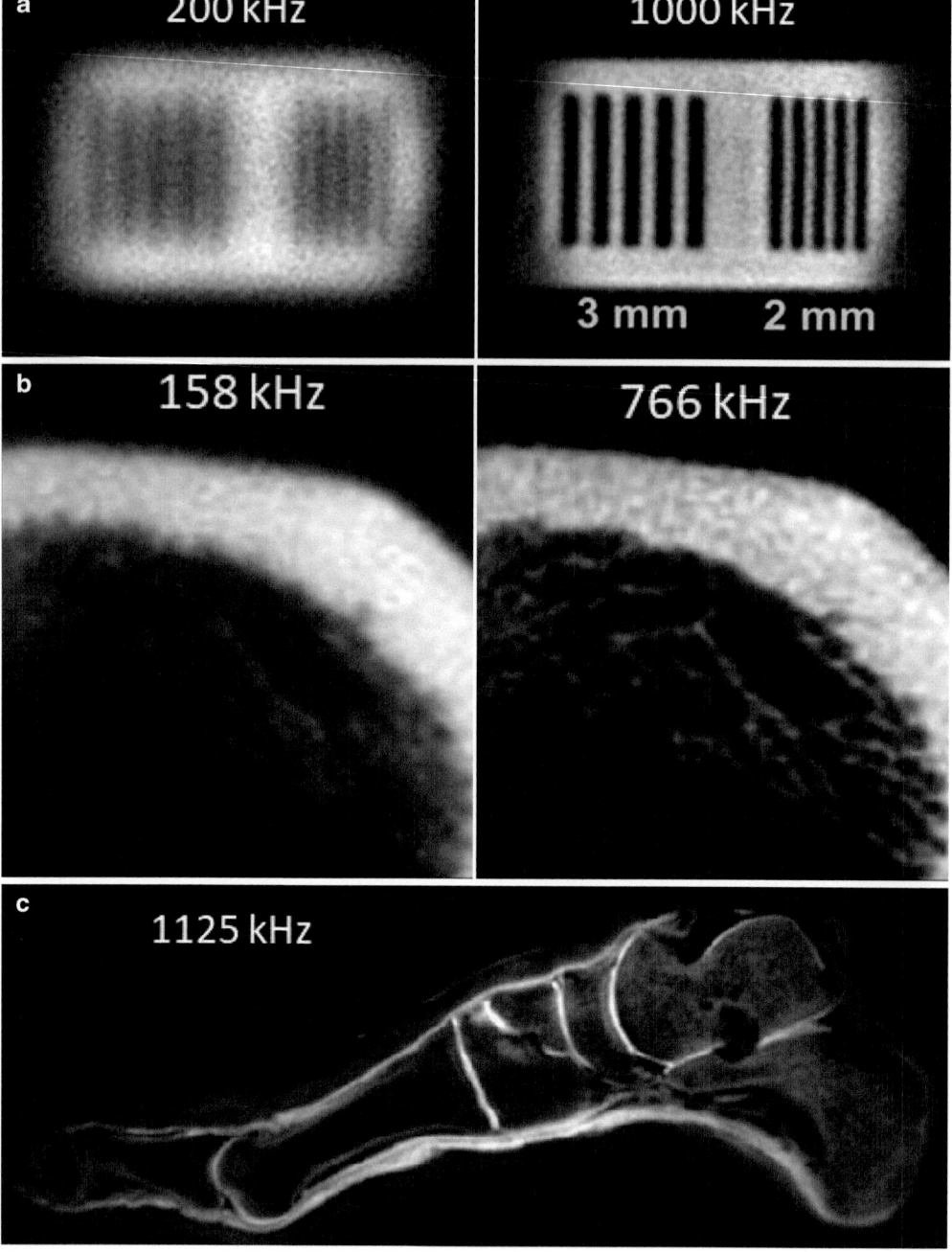

Conclusion

Overall, ZTE imaging plays an increasingly important role in short-T_2 MRI due to its particularly high sensitivity to the targeted species and its general robustness. The key to successful deployment has been developments which overcome specific methodological and hardware challenges. With these advances, applications that give MRI access to a new range of tissues and materials have become possible.

References

1. Weiger M, Pruessmann KP. Short-T_2 MRI: principles and recent advances. Prog Nucl Magn Reson Spectrosc. 2019;114–115:237–70.
2. Choi S, Tang XW, Cory D. Constant time imaging approaches to NMR microscopy. Int J Imag Syst Technol. 1997;8(3):263–76.
3. Emid S, Creyghton J. High resolution NMR imaging in solids. Physica B+C. 1985;128(1):81–3.
4. Glover GH, Pauly JM, Bradshaw KM. Boron-11 imaging with a 3-dimensional reconstruction method. J Magn Reson Imag. 1992;2(1):47–52.

5. Suits BH, White D. NMR imaging in solids. Solid State Commun. 1984;50(4):291–5.

6. Hafner S. Fast imaging in liquids and solids with the back-projection low-angle shot (BLAST) technique. Magn Reson Imag. 1994;12(7):1047–51.

7. Madio DP, Lowe IJ. Ultra-fast imaging using low flip angles and FIDs. Magn Reson Med. 1995;34(4):525–9.

8. Kuethe DO, Caprihan A, Fukushima E, Waggoner RA. Imaging lungs using inert fluorinated gases. Magn Reson Med. 1998;39(1):85–8.

9. Lauterbur PC. Image formation by induced local interactions: examples employing nuclear magnetic resonance. Nature. 1973;242(5394):190–1.

10. Idiyatullin D, Corum C, Park JY, Garwood M. Fast and quiet MRI using a swept radiofrequency. J Magn Reson. 2006;181(2):342–9.

11. Froidevaux R, Weiger M, Pruessmann KP. Pulse encoding for ZTE imaging: RF excitation without dead-time penalty. Magn Reson Med. 2022;87(3):1360–74.

12. Brunner DO, Pruessmann KP. Coil ringdown suppression by broadband forward compensation. In: Proc Intl Soc Mag Reson Med; 2014. p. 951.

13. Peshkovsky AS, Forguez J, Cerioni L, Pusiol DJ. RF probe recovery time reduction with a novel active ringing suppression circuit. J Magn Reson. 2005;177(1):67–73.

14. Borneman TW, Cory DG. Bandwidth-limited control and ringdown suppression in high-Q resonators. J Magn Reson. 2012;225:120–9.

15. Hoult DI. Fast recovery, high sensitivity NMR probe and preamplifier for low frequencies. Rev Sci Instrum. 1979;50(2):193–200.

16. Marjanovic J, Weiger M, Reber J, Brunner DO, Dietrich BE, Wilm BJ, et al. Multi-rate acquisition for dead time reduction in magnetic resonance receivers: application to imaging with zero echo time. IEEE Trans Med Imag. 2018;37(2):408–16.

17. Rahmer J, Bornert P, Groen J, Bos C. Three-dimensional radial ultrashort echo-time imaging with T_2 adapted sampling. Magn Reson Med. 2006;55(5):1075–82.

18. Kuethe DO, Caprihan A, Lowe IJ, Madio DP, Gach HM. Transforming NMR data despite missing points. J Magn Reson. 1999;139(1):18–25.

19. Weiger M, Pruessmann KP. MRI with zero echo time, eMagRes, vol. 1. Chichester, UK: Wiley; 2012. p. 311–22.

20. Wu YT, Ackerman JL, Chesler DA, Graham L, Wang Y, Glimcher MJ. Density of organic matrix of native mineralized bone measured by water- and fat-suppressed proton projection MRI. Magn Reson Med. 2003;50(1):59–68.

21. Froidevaux R, Weiger M, Brunner DO, Dietrich BE, Wilm BJ, Pruessmann KP. Filling the dead-time gap in zero echo time MRI: principles compared. Magn Reson Med. 2018;79(4):2036–45.

22. Grodzki DM, Jakob PM, Heismann B. Ultrashort echo time imaging using pointwise encoding time reduction with radial acquisition (PETRA). Magn Reson Med. 2012;67(2):510–8.

23. Halse M, Goodyear DJ, MacMillan B, Szomolanyi P, Matheson D, Balcom BJ. Centric scan SPRITE magnetic resonance imaging. J Magn Reson. 2003;165(2):219–29.

24. Froidevaux R, Weiger M, Rosler MB, Brunner DO, Pruessmann KP. HYFI: hybrid filling of the dead-time gap for faster zero echo time imaging. NMR Biomed. 2021;34(6):e4493.

25. Brunner DO, Pavan M, Dietrich BE, Rothmund D, Heller A, Pruessmann KP. Sideband excitation for concurrent RF transmission and reception. In: Proc Intl Soc Mag Reson Med; 2011:625.

26. Michal CA. Nuclear magnetic resonance noise spectroscopy using two-photon excitation. J Chem Phys. 2003;118(8):3451–4.

27. Brunner DO, Dietrich BE, Pavan M, Pruessmann KP. MRI with sideband excitation: application to continuous SWIFT. In: Proc Intl Soc Mag Reson Med; 2012:150.

28. Han V, Liu C. Multiphoton magnetic resonance in imaging: a classical description and implementation. Magn Reson Med. 2020;84(3):1184–97.

29. Davies GR, Lurie DJ, Hutchison JMS, McCallum SJ, Nicholson I. Continuous-wave magnetic resonance imaging of short T_2 materials. J Magn Reson. 2001;148(2):289–97.

30. Idiyatullin D, Suddarth S, Corum CA, Adriany G, Garwood M. Continuous SWIFT. J Magn Reson. 2012;220:26–31.

31. Özen AC, Bock M, Atalar E. Active decoupling of RF coils using a transmit array system. Magn Reson Mater Phys. 2015;28(6):565–76.

32. Grodzki DM, Jakob PM, Heismann B. Correcting slice selectivity in hard pulse sequences. J Magn Reson. 2012;214:61–7.

33. Idiyatullin D, Corum C, Moeller S, Garwood M. Gapped pulses for frequency-swept MRI. J Magn Reson. 2008;193(2):267–73.

34. Li C, Magland JF, Seifert AC, Wehrli FW. Correction of excitation profile in zero echo time (ZTE) imaging using quadratic phase-modulated RF pulse excitation and iterative reconstruction. IEEE Trans Med Imag. 2014;33(4):961–9.

35. Schieban K, Weiger M, Hennel F, Boss A, Pruessmann KP. ZTE imaging with enhanced flip angle using modulated excitation. Magn Reson Med. 2015;74(3):684–93.

36. Weiger M, Pruessmann KP, Hennel F. MRI with zero echo time: hard versus sweep pulse excitation. Magn Reson Med. 2011;66(2):379–89.

37. Kobayashi N, Goerke U, Wang L, Ellermann J, Metzger GJ, Garwood M. Gradient-modulated PETRA MRI. Tomography. 2015;1(2):85–90.

38. Jang H, Wiens CN, McMillan AB. Ramped hybrid encoding for improved ultrashort echo time imaging. Magn Reson Med. 2016;76(3):814–25.

39. Zhang J, Idiyatullin D, Corum CA, Kobayashi N, Garwood M. Gradient-modulated SWIFT. Magn Reson Med. 2016;75(2):537–46.

40. Pruessmann KP. Encoding and reconstruction in parallel MRI. NMR Biomed. 2006;19(3):288–99.

41. Jackson J, Macovski A, Nishimura D. Low-frequency restoration. Magn Reson Med. 1989;11(2):248–57.

42. Pruessmann KP, Weiger M, Bornert P, Boesiger P. Advances in sensitivity encoding with arbitrary k-space trajectories. Magn Reson Med. 2001;46(4):638–51.

43. Beatty PJ, Nishimura DG, Pauly JM. Rapid gridding reconstruction with a minimal oversampling ratio. IEEE Trans Med Imag. 2005;24(6):799–808.

44. Weiger M, Brunner DO, Tabbert M, Pavan M, Schmid T, Pruessmann KP. Exploring the bandwidth limits of ZTE imaging: spatial response, out-of-band signals, and noise propagation. Magn Reson Med. 2015;74(5):1236–47.

45. Oberhammer T, Weiger M, Hennel F, Pruessmann KP. Prospects of parallel ZTE imaging. In: Proc Intl Soc Mag Reson Med; 2011:2890.

46. Zwart NR, Johnson KO, Pipe JG. Efficient sample density estimation by combining gridding and an optimized kernel. Magn Reson Med. 2012;67(3):701–10.

47. Ljungberg E, Wood TC, Solana AB, Williams SCR, Barker GJ, Wiesinger F. Motion corrected silent ZTE neuroimaging. Magn Reson Med. 2022;88(1):195–210.

48. Wong ST, Roos MS. A strategy for sampling on a sphere applied to 3D selective RF pulse design. Magn Reson Med. 1994;32(6):778–84.

49. Kuethe DO, Adolphi NL, Fukushima E. Short data-acquisition times improve projection images of lung tissue. Magn Reson Med. 2007;57(6):1058–64.

50. Piccini D, Littmann A, Nielles-Vallespin S, Zenge MO. Spiral phyllotaxis: the natural way to construct a 3D radial trajectory in MRI. Magn Reson Med. 2011;66(4):1049–56.

51. Boucneau T, Fernandez B, Besson FL, Menini A, Wiesinger F, Durand E, et al. AZTEK: adaptive zero TE k-space trajectories. Magn Reson Med. 2021;85(2):926–35.

52. Nataraj G, Lustig M, editors. Tennisball: slew-efficient trajectory design for 3D-radial imaging. In Proc Intl Soc Mag Reson Med; 2022:1712.

53. Weiger M, Brunner DO, Dietrich BE, Muller CF, Pruessmann KP. ZTE imaging in humans. Magn Reson Med. 2013;70(2):328–32.

54. Larson PEZ, Gurney PT, Nishimura DG. Anisotropic field-of-views in radial imaging. IEEE Trans Med Imag. 2008;27(1):47–57.

55. Ljungberg E, Damestani NL, Wood TC, Lythgoe DJ, Zelaya F, Williams SCR, et al. Silent zero TE MR neuroimaging: current state-of-the-art and future directions. Prog Nucl Magn Reson Spectrosc. 2021;123:73–93.

56. Lee HM, Weiger M, Giehr C, Froidevaux R, Brunner DO, Rösler MB, et al. Long-T_2-suppressed zero echo time imaging with weighted echo subtraction and gradient error correction. Magn Reson Med. 2020;83(2):412–26.

57. Wiesinger F, Menini A, Solana AB. Looping star. Magn Reson Med. 2019;81(1):57–68.

58. Szeverenyi NM, Carl M. Contrast manipulation in MR imaging of short T_2 and T_2^* tissues, eMagRes, vol. 1. Chichester, UK: Wiley; 2012. p. 581–6.

59. Brunner DO, Furrer L, Weiger M, Baumberger W, Schmid T, Reber J, et al. Symmetrically biased T/R switches for NMR and MRI with microsecond dead time. J Magn Reson. 2016;263:147–55.

60. Schildknecht C, Weiger M, Froidevaux R, Pruessmann KP, editors. Rapid high power transmit-receive switching using a timed cascade of PIN diodes. In Proc Intl Soc Mag Reson Med; 2021:1411.

61. Schildknecht C, Weiger M, Froidevaux R, Pruessmann KP, editors. Gallium nitride MOSFETs enable transmit-receive switching in less than 100ns. In Proc Intl Soc Mag Reson Med; 2021:1407.

62. Horch RA, Wilkens K, Gochberg DF, Does MD. RF coil considerations for short-T_2 MRI. Magn Reson Med. 2010;64(6):1652–7.

63. Eichhorn T, Ludwig U, Fischer E, Grobner J, Gopper M, Eisenbeiss AK, et al. Modular coils with low hydrogen content especially for MRI of dry solids. PLoS One. 2015;10(10):e0139763.

64. Weiger M, Brunner DO, Schmid T, Froidevaux R, Rösler MB, Gross S, et al. A virtually 1H-free birdcage coil for zero echo time MRI without background signal. Magn Reson Med. 2017;78(1):399–407.

65. Weiger M, Overweg J, Rösler MB, Froidevaux R, Hennel F, Wilm BJ, et al. A high-performance gradient insert for rapid and short-T_2 imaging at full duty cycle. Magn Reson Med. 2018;79(6):3256–66.

66. Weiger M, Wu M, Wurnig MC, Kenkel D, Boss A, Andreisek G, et al. ZTE imaging with long-T_2 suppression. NMR Biomed. 2015;28(2):247–54.

67. Weiger M, Wu M, Wurnig MC, Kenkel D, Jungraithmayr W, Boss A, et al. Rapid and robust pulmonary proton ZTE imaging in the mouse. NMR Biomed. 2014;27(9):1129–34.

68. Weiger M, Pruessmann KP, Bracher AK, Kohler S, Lehmann V, Wolfram U, et al. High-resolution ZTE imaging of human teeth. NMR Biomed. 2012;25(10):1144–51.

69. Froidevaux R, Weiger M, Rosler MB, Brunner DO, Dietrich BE, Reber J, et al. High-resolution short-T_2 MRI using a high-performance gradient. Magn Reson Med. 2020;84(4):1933–46.

70. Baadsvik EL, Weiger M, Froidevaux R, Rosler MB, Brunner DO, Ohrstrom L, et al. High-resolution MRI of mummified tissues using advanced short-T_2 methodology and hardware. Magn Reson Med. 2021;85(3):1481–92.

Pointwise Encoding Time Reduction with Radial Acquisition (PETRA) MRI

David Grodzki

Introduction

As discussed in previous chapters in this book, there are two different general approaches to imaging of species with short T_2s. The first approach is UTE (ultrashort echo time) imaging in which radiofrequency (RF) pulses are applied initially, and then gradients are ramped up to a constant value during the readout. The second approach is ZTE (zero echo time) imaging in which the readout gradients are switched on initially, and after they are fully ramped up, the RF pulse is applied. This is the reverse order of what is used with UTE. During the readout, both approaches acquire k-space with radial center-out projections in order to acquire data as quickly as possible. With UTE imaging, there is a delay from the end of the RF pulse to the beginning of k-space encoding (which usually starts on the ramp-up of the gradients). With ZTE imaging, k-space encoding and data acquisition are not possible during the application of the RF pulse and the time required to switch from transmit to receive mode so that the central region of k-space (beginning at the middle of the RF pulse) is not mapped, and mapping of this is done algebraically or using an additional separate acquisition.

UTE acquisitions allow flexible TE settings, e.g., for T_2^* quantification and 2D acquisitions as well as flexible flip angles such as used with conventional sequences. On the other hand, since the gradients are already ramped up before the RF excitation, no time is lost during ramping of the gradients with ZTE, and encoding effectively starts in the middle of the RF pulse. Thus, looking at each k-space point, encoding times with ZTE are shorter, and less signal is lost due to T_2 decay during the acquisition. Also, potential gradient delays or eddy currents during gradient ramping, which can significantly decrease the robustness of UTE acquisitions, are not relevant with ZTE sequences. Nevertheless, ZTE scans are limited to 3D imaging and generally to very short hard RF pulses with limited flip angles.

Another aspect of ZTE imaging is the need for extremely short hardware switching times between the end of the RF pulse and the beginning of the readout (called T hardware [T_{HW}] in this chapter). As the encoding starts in the middle of the RF pulse, early k-space points during the readout are missed because of the time required for switching, as illustrated in Fig. 6.1. In any case, the first k-space point—which is at the center of k-space—cannot be acquired, because it would need to be measured in the middle of the RF pulse. As described in previous chapters of this book, algebraic reconstruction of the missing points can be used, but it becomes ineffective if the missing gap in k-space is larger than four points [1]. Thus, to allow algebraic reconstruction and imaging with ZTE, T_{HW} needs to be well below 10 μs with typical MR system settings.

On clinical scanners using standard coils, switching times as short as 10 μs are not usually achievable, so ZTE cannot be applied. To overcome this, the goal of the PETRA sequence [2] is to achieve the shortest possible encoding time given the hardware limitations of the MR system and to produce viable and robust scans on every MR scanner with every coil setup without need for fast hardware switching times.

D. Grodzki (✉)
Siemens Healthcare GmbH, Magnetic Resonance,
Erlangen, Germany

Department of Neuroradiology, Friedrich-Alexander-Universität
Erlangen-Nürnberg, Erlangen, Germany
e-mail: David.grodzki@siemens-healthineers.com

© The Author(s), under exclusive license to Springer Nature Switzerland AG 2023
J. Du, G. M. Bydder (eds.), *MRI of Short- and Ultrashort-T₂ Tissues*, https://doi.org/10.1007/978-3-031-35197-6_6

Fig. 6.1 Illustration of a ZTE repetition. T_{HW} describes the time that the hardware requires to switch from transmit mode (TX) to receive mode (RX). TE is defined as the time measured from the middle of the RF pulse to the beginning of the acquisition. Because encoding of spins effectively starts in the middle of the RF pulse, k-space points from there up until the end of T_{HW} are missed

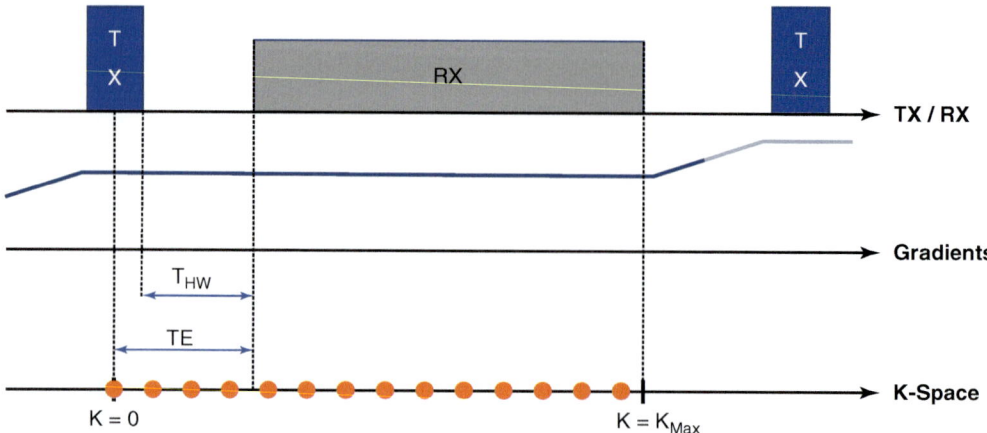

The Petra Acquisition

In order to completely fill the missing points of a ZTE acquisition independent of scanner switching times, the PETRA sequence utilizes a combination of radial and Cartesian acquisitions, as shown in Fig. 6.2.

The outer radial part of the sequence is similar to the ZTE sequence. The radial spokes are evenly distributed over a sphere in k-space as described by Saff and Kuijaars in reference [3] using the trajectory described by Nielles-Vallespin et al. in reference [4]. After the gradient ramp-up, a hard low flip angle pulse is applied and the readout is started at the earliest possible time, as indicated in Fig. 6.1. As with ZTE, the applied absolute gradient strength $|\vec{G}|$ is kept constant during the radial part, while the direction of $\vec{G}$ changes with each repetition. As encoding of spins starts at $t = 0$ at the middle of the RF pulse, k-space values with $|\vec{k}| < k^*$ where

$$k^* = \gamma |\vec{G}| \, TE \qquad (6.1)$$

cannot be measured because they would require data acquisition *before* the hardware is ready for this. The missing points in the middle of k-space are essential both for image reconstruction and to achieve high signal-to-noise (SNR) ratios.

With the PETRA approach, the missing points are acquired pointwise in the central Cartesian part of the sequence. In general, every Cartesian k-space value that lies within the sphere where $|k| < k^*$ is measured. The Cartesian measurement runs similar to single-point ramped imaging with T_1 enhancement (SPRITE) sequences as described in references [5–7]. In this part of the sequence, gradients are ramped up before the RF pulse is applied and one single point is acquired at $t = TE$. To measure a certain k-space point $\vec{k}$ with $|\vec{k}| \le k^*$, the gradient strength in each spatial direction is given by

$$\vec{G} = \frac{\vec{k}}{\gamma TE} \qquad (6.2)$$

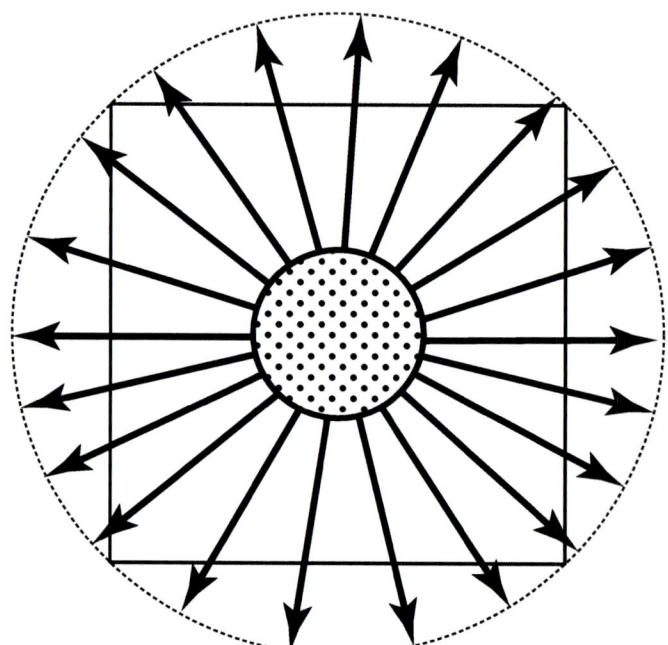

Fig. 6.2 Diagram of PETRA k-space mapping. The acquisition in the outer k-space parts is radial and is similar to a ZTE acquisition, while the acquisition in the inner k-space points is Cartesian and is acquired pointwise. (Reproduced with permission from Ref. [2])

All gradients are zero for $\vec{k} = 0$ and so a free induction decay (FID) signal is acquired at this point with $t = TE$.

While in the radial part of the sequence the absolute gradient strength $|\vec{G}|$ is kept constant, in the Cartesian part, the encoding time is kept constant. Equations 6.1 and 6.2 imply that the applied gradient strength in the Cartesian part of the sequence is always lower than the gradient strength used during the radial part of the sequence. In our implementation, only one k-space point is acquired at each Cartesian readout. Figure 6.3 illustrates the encoding times for the PETRA sequence. It is important to note that due to the combination of the Cartesian single-point acquisition with the radial acquisition, there is no discontinuity in the encoding time.

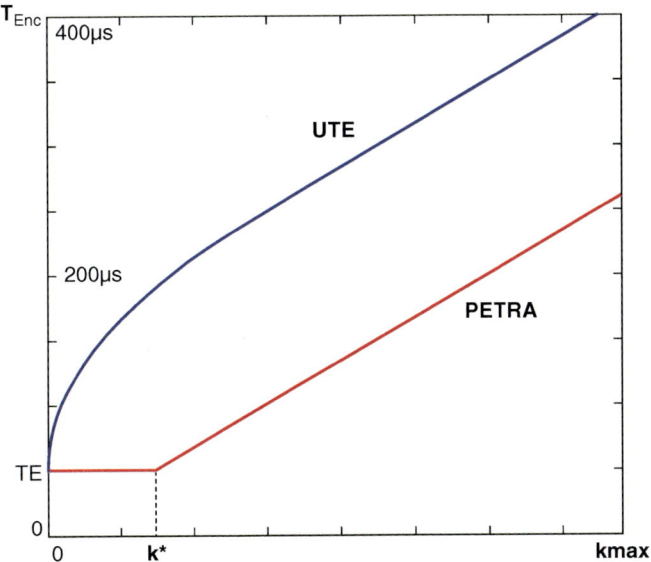

Fig. 6.3 Illustration of encoding time (T_{Enc}) vs k-space number for UTE and PETRA acquisitions. PETRA has shorter encoding times at every k-space point. The encoding time for PETRA is constant in the Cartesian part of the sequence for $k < k^*$ and increases linearly during the radial acquisition. (Reproduced with permission from Ref. [2])

This also means that the phase evolution is continuous which is different from methods like WASPI and is an important factor in ensuring robustness during PETRA acquisitions.

Due to the additional Cartesian acquisition part, the PETRA acquisition time is longer than the ZTE acquisition time. As an example, for a matrix size of 256^3, FOV = 300 mm, TE = 70 μs and a gradient strength of 8 mT/m, around 1400 points need to be acquired in the Cartesian part. This compares to usually around 50,000 spokes in the radial part and corresponds to an increase in scan time of less than 3%. To resolve faster relaxing signals, a higher gradient strength may be needed to shorten the total readout time in the radial part. In this case, more data points are missed in the center of k-space, and these need to be sampled in the Cartesian way which prolongs scan time.

In principle with PETRA, TE could be set to any value longer than T_{HW} plus half of the pulse duration. This is not possible with the ZTE sequence. For longer TEs with PETRA, more points need to be acquired in the Cartesian part of the sequence, and scan times can get significantly longer. For this reason, TE is usually set to the shortest possible value.

At the end of each repetition, spins need to be completely spoiled. The contrast resembles that of FLASH (fast low angle shot) and ranges from proton density to T_1, depending on the TR and flip angle. For a given tissue with known values of T_1 and proton density, signal arising from the tissue can be approximated by the Ernst equation.

In vivo there are usually different proton pools with a wide variety of different T_2^*s present in each voxel. To obtain an image that only contains signals from tissues with short T_2s, two methods have been proposed in the literature: firstly, use of T_2-selective pre-pulses to suppress tissues with longer T_2s [8–10]. In reference [11], an improved suppression method for the PETRA sequence is presented. The second option is to reverse the gradient after the readout and refocus the spins to produce a second echo at a second TE, TE_2. With this method, two images are produced in one measurement. The two images can be subtracted, leaving only signals from tissue with a short T_2. In reference [12], the subtraction method was found to be more reliable than the T_2-selective pre-pulse method. In our implementation, a second echo is acquired with the PETRA sequence. Gradient directions are inverted once the first half-projection is acquired, and spins are refocused from a gradient echo at $t = TE_2$. During the second readout, a full projection is acquired. It is possible to reconstruct the second echo with data acquired only from radial spokes, as no gap arises in the k-space with this echo.

Image Reconstruction

In its current implementation, central k-space is filled using a Cartesian grid. While the points acquired in the Cartesian part of the sequence can simply be filled in their corresponding positions, data handling for the radial part is more complex. Before the radial spokes are mapped onto the Cartesian grid, their values have to be weighted with a density matrix [13]. The density matrix needs to be adapted to the density of points in the Cartesian center of k-space. Also, if not enough radial spokes are acquired and k-space is radially undersampled, a certain level (or plateau) is reached in the outer part of the density matrix. This can improve image quality at the expense of image resolution. In our implementation, we use a density matrix that adapts to these needs using the methods described in reference [14].

According to the Nyquist criterion, the total number of radial spokes N_{Spokes} needed is given by $N_{Spokes} = 4\pi R^2$ [4], where R is the number of points acquired with each radial half-projection. A matrix size of $N = 256^3$ in which $R = 128$ points are acquired at every half-projection would therefore need $N_{Spokes} \approx 200,000$ radial spokes. In practice, a value of N_{Spokes} of around 50,000 is used. The level of the plateau of the density matrix is reached at point R_{Pl} of the readout. After the density matrices are applied to the radially sampled data, points are mapped onto the Cartesian grid using a Kaiser-Bessel-Window [15] with a width of 3.0 and ß = 4.2054, which was used in reference [4]. For receiver channel combinations, a weighted root-sum-of-squares algorithm is used for image reconstruction.

Correction of Unintended Slice Selectivity [1]

Many of the main sequences described in this book—including the PETRA, ZTE, SPRITE and WASPI sequences—apply a short hard pulse excitation while gradients are switched on for each k-space spoke or point that is acquired in the corresponding repetition. As an approximation, these pulses are assumed to be infinitesimally short and completely nonspatially selective so that effects of the pulse spectral profile can be ignored.

However, in reality, the RF pulses have a finite duration of, e.g., 3–20 μs, which is necessary to achieve sufficient excitation within potential RF power amplifier (RFPA) or SAR restrictions. This corresponds to a full width at half maximum (FWHM) of the sinc-shaped spectral profile of 60–300 kHz. In the current implementation of the PETRA sequence, a hard pulse with an effective duration of 14 μs is applied, allowing flip angles of up to 6–8°.

With a finite pulse duration, the spectral bandwidth and profile become important, and it becomes obvious that the excitation is not truly nonspatially selective. A slice that is defined by the spectral profile of the RF pulse and the gradient constellation is excited. The thickness of the excited slice scales inversely with readout gradient strength. Throughout the sequence, this excited slice not only rotates when different radial projections are acquired but also changes its thickness if the gradient strength is changed. The bandwidth of the excitation must be large enough to avoid unwanted slice selectivity in the object. For the SWIFT (sweep imaging with Fourier transformation) sequence, this means that the rectangular excitation shape must cover the entire object at the applied gradient strength. For hard pulse excitations, the FWHM should be as large as possible to ensure a homogeneous excitation. If the excitation bandwidth is not sufficient for the applied gradient strength and FOV, the excitation is not homogeneous over the object as demonstrated in the following Fig. 6.4.

The effect becomes more severe with higher readout gradient amplitudes. High gradient amplitudes, however, are required especially for acquisitions in which tissues with extremely fast-decaying signals need to be imaged with data acquired as rapidly as possible in order to reduce the signal decay over the acquired k-space spoke.

The following simulation in Fig. 6.5 demonstrates the effect of the slice selectivity with a PETRA sequence at different gradient strengths.

Assuming a one-dimensional object with the magnetization distribution $f(x)$ in image space, during an idealized MRI scan, k-space $F(k)$ is measured as

$$F(k) = \sum_x f(x) e^{ikx} \qquad (6.3)$$

To obtain an MR image, k-space is inverse Fourier-transformed to image space by

$$I(x) = \sum_k F(k) e^{-ikx} \qquad (6.4)$$

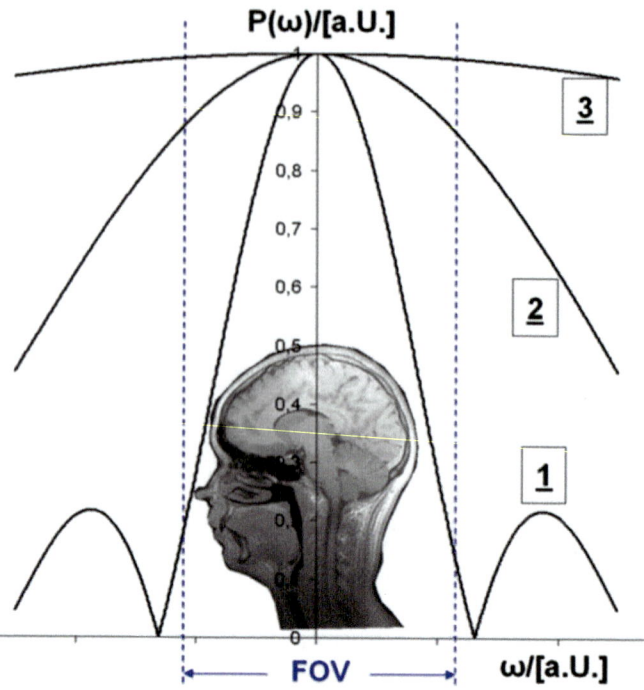

Fig. 6.4 Illustration of unwanted slice selectivity with hard RF pulse sequences. If the bandwidth of the excitation is not sufficient, the excitation is not homogeneous over the object, and a slice with a sinc-shaped profile is obtained. The minimum of the profile within the FOV, Pmin, is about 0.15 for line 1, 0.88 for line 2, and 0.98 for line 3. (Reproduced with permission from Ref. [16])

and the image $I(x) = f(x)$. The magnetization distribution $f(x)$ in Eq. 6.3 during nonselective excitation in the presence of gradients is superposed by the spectral shape of the excitation pulse $P(x)$, and it is given by the Fourier transform (FT) of the pulse shape in time domain $p(t)$. The hard pulse sequences use a rectangular excitation pulse $p(t)$:

$$p(t) = \begin{cases} B_1, \text{if } |t| < \tau/2 \\ 0, \text{elsewhere} \end{cases} \qquad (6.5)$$

with duration τ and RF excitation field B_1. In the frequency domain, this corresponds to a sinc-shaped spectral profile $P(\omega)$ with

$$P(\omega) = \frac{\sin(1/2\,\omega\tau)}{1/2\,\omega\tau} = \sin(1/2\,\omega\tau) \qquad (6.6)$$

and phase

$$\phi(\omega) = \exp\left(-i\frac{\omega}{2\pi}\frac{\tau}{2}\right) \qquad (6.7)$$

which is accounted for in the k-space values of the reconstruction. In the presence of gradient G, the resonance frequency ω is a function of the point x in image space, given by

$$\omega = 2\pi\,\gamma\,x\,G \qquad (6.8)$$

In the case of alternating gradients throughout the sequence, ω is also a function of the acquired k-space point k. The excitation profile of the pulse therefore can be expressed as $P(\omega) = P(\omega,k)$. The disturbed k-space $F'(k)$

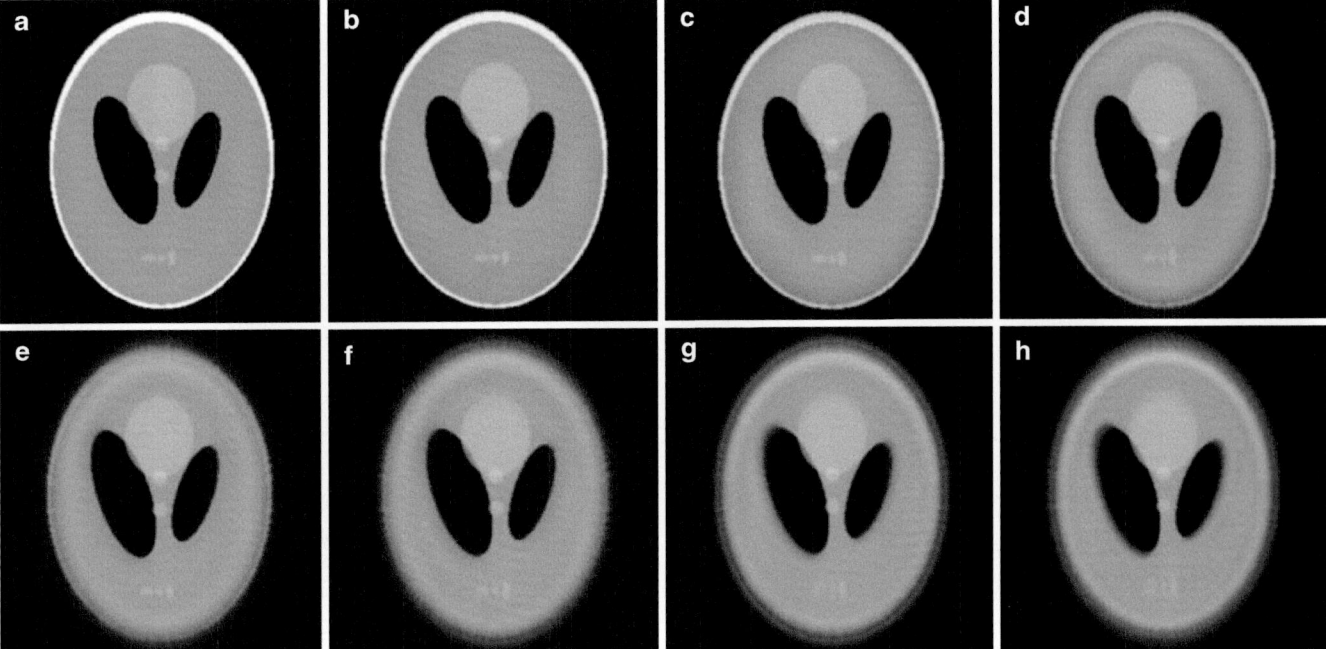

Fig. 6.5 PETRA simulation of a two-dimensional object $f(x,y)$ and the expected image perturbations of the original object in (**a**) $I'(x,y)$ with different gradient strengths (**b–h**). The maximum gradient strengths were 4, 8, 12, 16, 20, 30, and 40 mT/m from (**b**) to (**h**). Simulated FOV = 300 mm, $N = 250^2$, pulse duration $\tau = 14$ μs, and TE = 70 μs. The high signal outer boundary is progressively lost from (**b**) to (**e**) and becomes lower signal and biphasic in (**f–h**). (Reproduced with permission from Ref. [16])

$$F'(k) = \sum_x f(x) P(x,k) e^{ikx} \qquad (6.9)$$

is measured. If the disturbed k-space $F'(k)$ is inverse Fourier-transformed to image space using Eq. 6.4, the disturbed image $I'(x) \neq f(x)$ is calculated:

$$I'(x) = \sum_k F'(k) e^{-ikx} \qquad (6.10)$$

In the current implementation of the PETRA sequence, the influence of the excitation profile is solved by using matrix inversion instead of inverse FTs. Defining the matrix

$$D_{kx} = P(x,k) e^{ikx} \qquad (6.11)$$

with $N \times N = N^2$ elements, Eq. 6.9 can be rewritten as a matrix equation

$$F'_k = D_{kx} f_x \qquad (6.12)$$

F'_k is the perturbed k-space data measured on the MRI scan. The elements of D_{kx} are known and can be calculated. They depend on the gradient trajectories and timings of the specific sequence, pulse profiles, resolution, and FOV. The system of linear equations in Eq. 6.12 can be solved by the matrix inversion

$$f_x = I_x = D_{kx}^{-1} F'_k \qquad (6.13)$$

and the unaffected image $I_x = f_x$ is obtained.

With nonzero imaging gradients during the excitation, a slice defined by the gradient vector $\vec{G}$ and Eq. 6.6 is excited. During a repetition of the radial part of the PETRA sequence, the absolute gradient strength $|\vec{G}| = G_{Max}$ is kept constant. The direction of the gradient vector is altered for every repetition, and radial spokes that are evenly distributed over a sphere are acquired. The excited slices rotate with the direction of the projection or acquired k-space point as well. During the Cartesian part of the PETRA sequence or SPRITE acquisition, the gradient vector $\vec{G}$ is calculated according to the k-space point to be acquired; see Eq. 6.2. Inserting the k-space-dependent gradient strength $\vec{G}(\vec{k})$ and Eq. 6.8 into Eq. 6.6, we obtain

$$P(\omega) = P(\vec{r}, \vec{k}) = \mathrm{sinc}\left(\pi \gamma \tau \, \vec{r} \, \vec{G}(\vec{k})\right) \qquad (6.14)$$

The FWHM of this excitation profile on a projection through k-space is plotted in Fig. 6.6 (dashed line). The FWHM indicates the thickness of the slice selected during the excitation. While the slice thickness is constant in the radial part, it increases as it comes closer to the center of k-space in the Cartesian part.

We define $r_0 = (\gamma \tau G_{Max})^{-1}$ as the radius in image space, where the spectral profile has its first minimum using G_{Max}. If r_0 is outside of the FOV, P_{min} is the minimal value of $P(\vec{r}, \vec{k})$ during one measurement. P_{min} is reached at $|\vec{G}| = G_{max}$ and the outer edge of the FOV, where $|\vec{r}| = \text{FOV}/2$. P_{min} illustrates the excitation decrease at the outer edges of the FOV; see Fig. 6.4. The maximum value of the spectral profile is always situated in the center of the image and is normalized to 1.

$P(\vec{r}, \vec{k})$ is symmetric with respect to the origin for both the point in image space $\vec{r}$ and in k-space $\vec{k}$ and only depends

Fig. 6.6 Gradient strength of a complete line through k-space for the PETRA sequence. In the radial part with $|k| < k^*$ (see Eq. 6.1), $|G|$ equals G_{Max}. In the Cartesian part with $|k| \leq k^*$, gradients are stepped through according to Eq. 6.1 for each k-space point. The corresponding FWHM of the excitation bandwidth (dashed line) is inversely proportional to the gradient strength. It is constant in the radial part and rises closer to the center of k-space in the Cartesian part. (Reproduced with permission from Ref. [16])

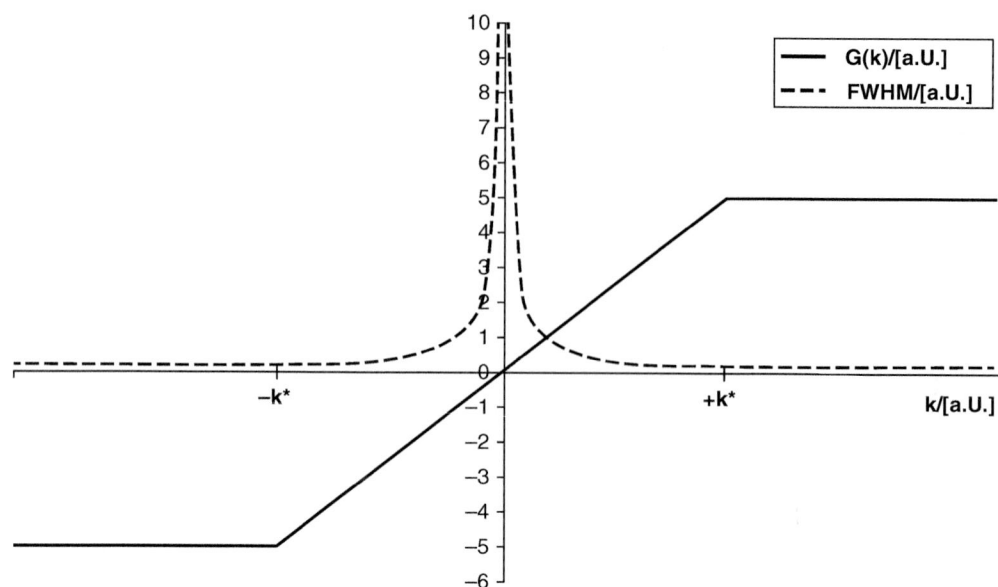

on the absolutes $\left|\vec{r}\right|$ and $\left|\vec{k}\right|$. This radial symmetry of the problem is used in the 3D data handling.

The correction approach presented above can in principle also be used in dimensions greater than one. The matrix size increases from N^2 to N^4 elements in 2D and N^6 elements in 3D, which would be approximately 2.8×10^{14} elements for a 256^3 matrix.

The radial symmetry of the spectral shape $P\left(\vec{r}, \vec{k}\right)$ allows us to avoid 3D correction with a large number of matrix elements and exceedingly long image reconstruction times. In the radial part of the sequence, half spokes through k-space are acquired. These 1D lines can be processed with Eq. 6.13. Due to the radial symmetry, the inverted matrix D_{kx}^{-1} only has to be calculated once during the entire reconstruction.

Using the Fourier slice theorem [17], the corrected image line $I_x = f_x$ can be processed in a three-dimensional projection or Radon reconstruction [18]. The PETRA sequence consists of radial and Cartesian acquisition parts. In order to correct and combine these two parts, we do not use projection reconstruction but Fourier transform the corrected line $I(x)$ back to k-space and apply a 3D gridding algorithm in k-space. This k-space line $F(k)$ is calculated from the corrected image $I(x)$ using the standard FT given in Eq. 6.3. This equation can be written in matrix form with the matrix elements $E_{kx} = e^{ikx}$. Using Eq. 6.13, it can be found that the perturbed k-space F'_k yields the unaffected k-space F_k as

$$F_k = E_{kx} D_{kx}^{-1} F'_k = C_{xk} F'_k \qquad (6.15)$$

Due to the radial symmetries, the matrix $C_{xk} = E_{kx} D_{kx}^{-1}$ also needs to be calculated only once during image reconstruction.

Because the number of Cartesian points is not too large—about $N = 10\text{--}25$ points per line—the Cartesian part of the sequence is processed with the correction algorithm in 3D. As an example, for $N = 20$ points, C_{xk} has $N^6 = 6.4 \times 10^7$

complex points. This can easily be handled with current standard reconstruction systems.

Depending on the RF power amplifier (RFPA) and the transmit chain of the scanner, a hard RF pulse does not usually have a perfectly rectangular shape. In order to determine the actual pulse shapes on different systems, pulses were measured in test scans with an oscilloscope connected to the RFPA of the scanner. FT of these measurements yields the actual spectral distribution of the excitation that is fed into the correction.

The PETRA sequence can be extended to acquire a second gradient echo. For the second echo, a complete projection through k-space is acquired without any gap arising in the middle of k-space. The absolute gradient strength does not change during this projection so that Eq. 6.14 loses its dependency on $\vec{k}$. Due to the radial symmetries, in this situation Eq. 6.9 describes a convolution and the perturbed image $I'(x)$ equals $I'(x) = f(x)P(x)$. Thus, for the second echo, the influence of the excitation profile can be either eliminated by division in image space or by using Eq. 6.13 for the acquired radial projections. This is also the case for a ZTE sequence that does not use a Cartesian acquisition and where $\left|\vec{G}\right|$ is constant throughout the acquisition. On the other hand, the SPRITE sequence uses different absolute gradient strengths for each k-space point, like the first echo of a PETRA acquisition. Thus, for SPRITE, the problem can be solved in a similar fashion to that presented here for the PETRA sequence.

Figures 6.7 and 6.8 show phantom and in vivo examples of the implemented approach, acquired with the PETRA sequence. The measurements confirm the simulations shown in Fig. 6.4, as well as the functionality of the correction algorithm. As can be seen on the images, even at low gradient strengths, where the first minimum is far outside the FOV,

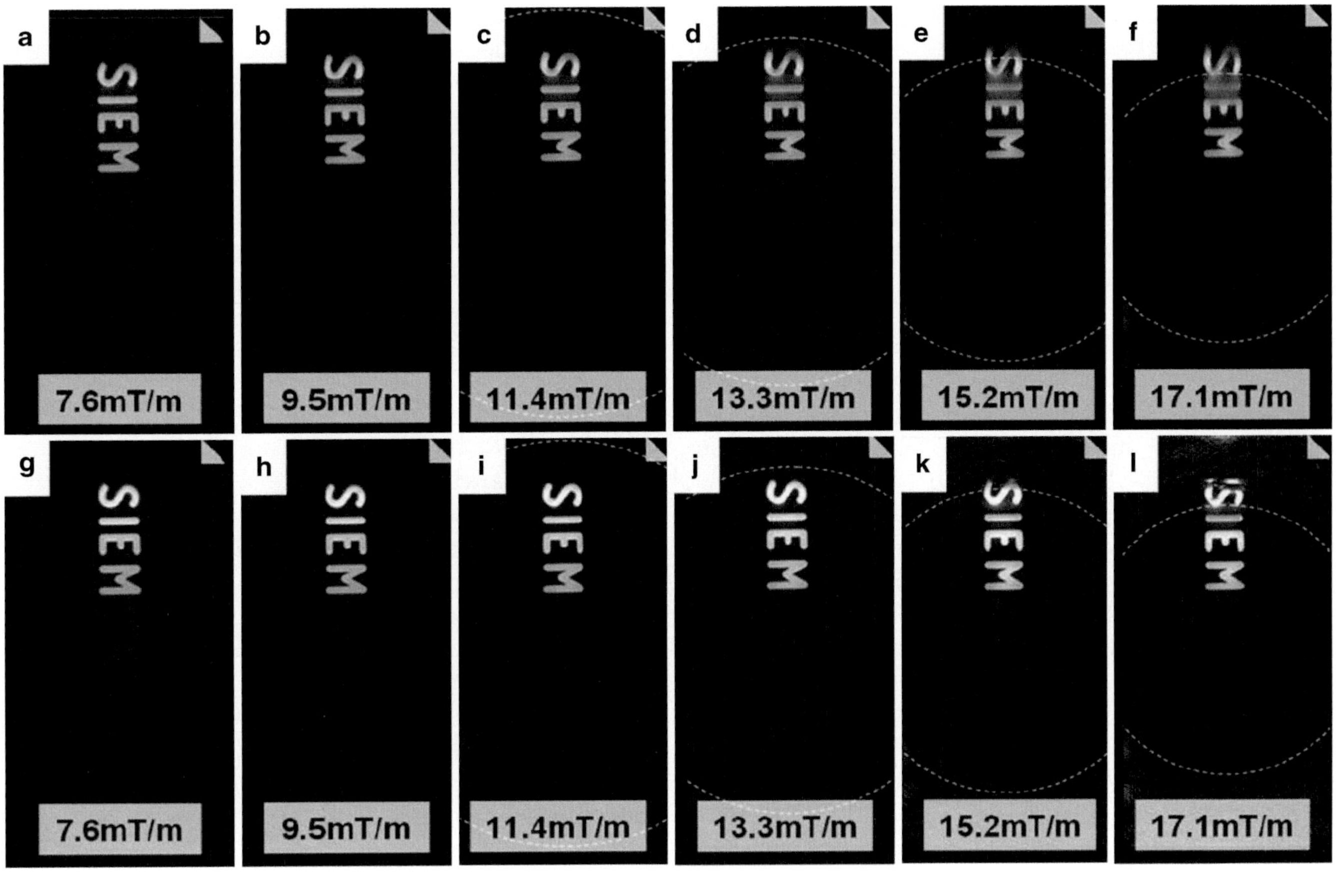

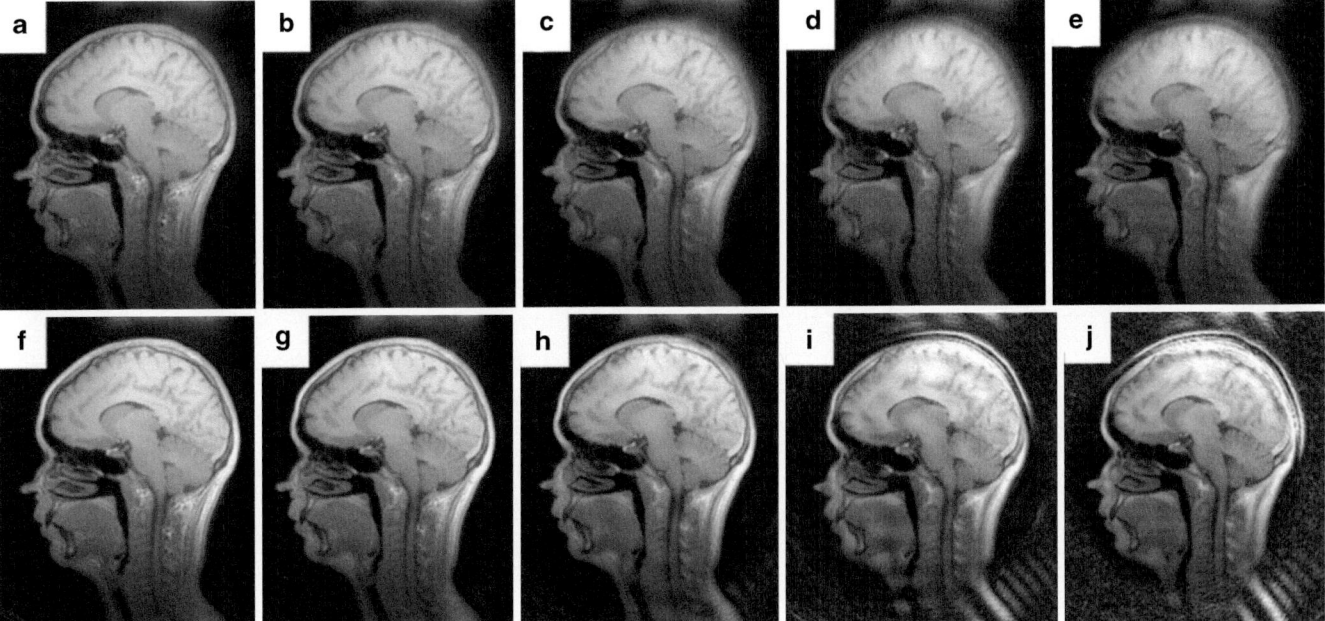

Fig. 6.7 Images of a structural phantom acquired with PETRA at different maximum gradient strengths without correction (**a–f**) and with correction (**g–l**). The dashed rings indicate r_0. Images have identical windowing scaled to the noise level. The FOV was 300 mm isotropic. The complete FOV is shown in the vertical direction. (Reproduced with permission from Ref. [16])

Fig. 6.8 In vivo head images acquired with PETRA at different maximum gradient strengths without correction (**a–e**) and with correction (**f–j**). The images have identical windowing. The FOV was 300 mm isotropic. The complete FOV is shown in the vertical direction. Gradient strengths were increasing from 8.6 mT/m to 17.2 mT/m with steps of 2.15 mT/m. (Reproduced with permission from Ref. [16])

intensity degradation is visible. For stronger gradients, where the selected slice becomes thinner, severe blurring occurs in the outer parts of the image. With smaller gradients, where the first minimum of the excitation is outside of the object, intensity errors in the outer parts as well as slight blurring are visible in both the phantom and the in vivo measurements; see Figs. 6.7a–f and 6.8a–e. Artifact-free imaging can be obtained if P_{min} is not less than 0.4, and imaging with only slight blurring at the edges of the FOV is still possible if P_{min} is not less than 0.25. If r_0 lies within the object, radial blurring and ringing artifacts occur, as can be seen in Figs. 6.7f and 6.8e. These artifacts arc due to insufficient excitation of the outer image part at high k-space frequencies, while for lower k-space frequencies, the excitation is more homogeneous.

The proposed correction algorithm restores the influence of the excitation pulse within the post-processing by matrix inversions in a fast image reconstruction time. Using this correction, the influence of the spectral excitation profile can be eliminated in the simulation experiments. In the MR measurements, the functionality is proven, but limitations of the approach are present. If the first minimum of the excitation is outside of the object, the corrected images show improved signal intensity homogeneity, and the blurring is eliminated. If the first minimum lies within the object, the algorithm is no longer able to compensate for the effects of the excitation away from the minimum. The noise levels outside of the first minimum are raised and the blurring cannot be eliminated. As a limitation for the correction algorithm, r_0 should be outside of the object as the noise level is increased close to minimal excitations. This increase in noise level and signal folded into the image can also lead to the appearance of radial ring artifacts. Inside of r_0, increased image quality is present, and blurring is eliminated.

Using the correction, it is possible to use a broader frequency range, and P_{min} can be lowered from about 0.4 to 0.0 for the PETRA sequence. With this, higher readout bandwidths are enabled allowing shorter encoding times and less T_2^* blurring than with UTE imaging. Furthermore, longer RF pulses can be used and these allow use of higher flip angles.

The correction algorithm presented here for the PETRA sequence can easily be adapted for other sequences with nonzero gradients during excitation such as ZTE, WASPI, and SPRITE. It can also be used for nonselective sequences with nonzero gradients during excitation such as the Burst sequence.

Discussion and Outlook

The PETRA sequence has been and is used in several clinical and nonclinical studies and applications. An example of a wrist image acquired with PETRA is shown in Fig. 6.9. For further reading, please consult the selected publications referenced here [19–25].

As explained in more detail in a later chapter in this book, a rather unintended benefit of the PETRA sequence is its quietness, which may produce significant increase in patient comfort and compliance. Due to the high social and commercial interest in this topic, the PETRA sequence was released as a medical product on Siemens Healthcare scanners from 2014 onwards.

Nevertheless, the main intention of the sequence is imaging of tissues with rapidly decaying signals. In reference [1], different approaches for filling the missing points in k-space with ZTE-like acquisitions are compared. Especially in situations in which more than four k-space points are missing, PETRA was found to generally achieve superior image qual-

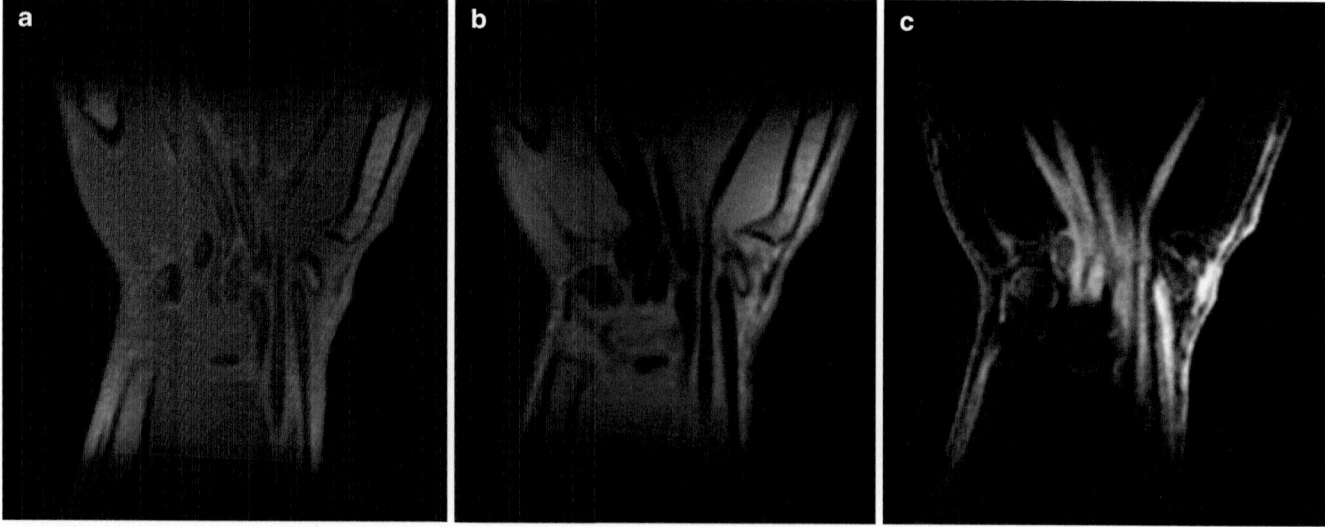

Fig. 6.9 Double echo PETRA imaging of a wrist. (**a**) displays the first echo with TE = 70 µs, (**b**) shows the second echo with a TE = 4.6 ms, and (**c**) shows the subtraction of (**a**) and (**b**) in which the flexor tendons are well seen. (Reproduced with permission from Ref. [2])

ity in comparison with other methods (all of which are included in this book).

For systems with very short switching times, the differences between ZTE and PETRA vanish. If transmit and receive cannot be performed simultaneously, ZTE always misses at least the central k-space point, because encoding starts in the middle of the hard pulse. Thus, with extremely short switching times, the only difference between PETRA and ZTE is that PETRA acquires the k-space center point with a single-point acquisition during an FID, while ZTE uses algebraic reconstruction to calculate this missing information.

Very fast-decaying signals in tissues need to be acquired as quickly as possible after excitation to avoid signal loss during the readout which is responsible for blurring in the image. In the community, this raises an immediate need for (a) shorter switching and TEs and (b) shorter readouts with higher bandwidths. However, these have some downsides that need to be considered, and the requirements vary depending on the application.

High readout bandwidths lead to faster acquisition of k-space projections and with this to decreased T_2 decay during the readout, and so blurring is reduced. Due to the shorter acquisition window, the minimum TR also decreases. On the other hand, higher readout bandwidths decrease the measured SNR, which is dependent to 1/sqrt (BW). Thus, short-T_2 species might have a better point spread function but become barely visible unless more repetitions are performed. Acquisition times then become longer and might not be acceptable for in vivo scanning.

Shorter switching times and TEs allow earlier acquisition of the decaying signal, and the acquired signal intensity of the first k-space points increases. Furthermore, with the PETRA sequence, the number of Cartesian points is reduced, resulting in faster scan times. On the other hand, loss of effective sharpness may be introduced in the images. Looking at Fig. 6.3 and Eq. 6.1, a shorter TE would move k^* closer to 0, and the flat top part would become smaller. As an example, considering a decrease in TE from 70 μs to 10 μs, the first k-space points of the line would be acquired with much shorter encoding time, while all points > 70 μs would still be acquired at the same encoding time. Thus, the relative signal difference for a fast-decaying signal between the k-space center and outer k-space would increase. This increased signal difference degrades the point spread function, leading to loss of image sharpness.

Thus, neither the need for higher bandwidth nor that for shorter switching times alone should dominate pulse sequence choice. Depending on the circumstances such as the minimum acceptable spatial resolution, available SNR of the tissue, scanner performance (e.g., field strength and coils), tolerated scan times, and, most importantly, the T_2^* of

the tissue of interest, parameters such as readout bandwidth and TE can be optimized. However, the readout bandwidth and TE need not necessarily be respectively as high, or as short, as possible. On clinical scanners, the gradient amplitude and available SNR are usually the main limitations for acquisition of extremely fast-decaying signals, e.g., in solid or semisolid species.

After the initial PETRA application in 2014, several approaches to improve the overall performance of the technique have been published. Gradient-modulated (GM) PETRA [26] is a method for reducing image blurring and SAR limitations or RF peak power. With this technique, gradients are lower during the excitation than during the readout itself, bringing the PETRA (and ZTE) sequence closer to the UTE approach. In reference [27], compressed sensing methods were applied to the PETRA sequence, yielding accelerated scan times while maintaining the image quality of the original non-accelerated scan. Another approach for reducing scan times, at least for some dedicated applications, is to move to 2D projection, in which no encoding is performed in the z-direction, but further research is needed to prove the usefulness of this technique. Considering future advances, reduction in scan time using machine learning techniques and parallel imaging could both benefit the PETRA sequence.

In conclusion, the PETRA sequence is a method for imaging tissues with very fast-decaying signals that generates robust images with the shortest possible encoding time. Unlike other techniques it does not require changes in conventional clinical MR system hardware to do this.

References

1. Froidevaux R, Weiger M, Brunner DO, Dietrich BE, Wilm BJ, Pruessmann KP. Filling the dead-time gap in zero echo time MRI: principles compared. Magn Reson Med. 2018;79(4):2036–45.
2. Grodzki DM, Jakob PM, Heismann B. Ultrashort echo time imaging using pointwise encoding time reduction with radial acquisition (PETRA). Magn Reson Med. 2012;67(2):510–8.
3. Saff EB, Kuijaars ABJ. Distributing many points on a sphere. Math Intell. 1997;19(1):5–11.
4. Nielles-Vallespin S, Weber MA, Bock M, Bongers A, Speier P, Combs SE, Wohrle J, Lehmann-Horn F, Essig M, Schad LR. 3D radial projection technique with ultrashort echo times for sodium MRI: clinical applications in human brain and skeletal muscle. Magn Reson Med. 2007;57(1):74–81.
5. Heid O, Deimling M. Rapid single Point (RASP) imaging. Proc Soc Mag Reson Med. 1995:684.
6. Balcom BJ, Macgregor RP, Beyea SD, Green DP, Armstrong RL, Bremner TW. Single-point ramped imaging with T_1 enhancement (SPRITE). J Magn Reson A. 1996;123(1):131–4.
7. Grodzki DM, Deimling M, Heismann B, Fautz HP, Jakob P. Single point sequences with shortest possible TE—GOSPEL. Proc Intl Soc Mag Reson Med. 2010:2977.
8. Sussman MS, Pauly JM, Wright GA. Design of practical T_2-selective RF excitation (TELEX) pulses. Magn Reson Med. 1998;40(6):890–9.

9. Larson PE, Gurney PT, Nayak K, Gold GE, Pauly JM, Nishimura DG. Designing long-T_2 suppression pulses for ultrashort echo time imaging. Magn Reson Med. 2006;56(1):94–103.

10. Du J, Takahashi AM, Bae WC, Chung CB, Bydder GM. Dual inversion recovery, ultrashort echo time (DIR UTE) imaging: creating high contrast for short-T(2) species. Magn Reson Med. 2010;63(2):447–55.

11. Li C, Magland JF, Zhao X, Seifert AC, Wehrli FW. Selective in vivo bone imaging with long-T_2 suppressed PETRA MRI. Magn Reson Med. 2017;77(3):989–97.

12. Rahmer J, Blume U, Bornert P. Selective 3D ultrashort TE imaging: comparison of "dual-echo" acquisition and magnetization preparation for improving short-T_2 contrast. MAGMA. 2007;20(2):83–92.

13. Pipe JG, Menon P. Sampling density compensation in MRI: rationale and an iterative numerical solution. Magn Reson Med. 1999;41(1):179–86.

14. Pipe JG. Reconstructing MR images from undersampled data: data-weighting considerations. Magn Reson Med. 2000;43(6):867–75.

15. Jackson JI, Meyer CH, Nishimura DG, Macovski A. Selection of a convolution function for Fourier inversion using gridding [computerized tomography application]. IEEE Trans Med Imaging. 1991;10(3):473–8.

16. Grodzki DM, Jakob PM, Heismann B. Correcting slice selectivity in hard pulse sequences. J Magn Reson. 2012;214(1):61–7.

17. Kak AC, Slaney M. Principles of computerized tomographic imaging. Society of Industrial and Applied Mathematics; 2001. ISBN:978-0-89871-494-4

18. Lim SJ. Two-dimensional signal and image processing. Englewood Cliffs, NJ: Prentice Hall; 1990. p. 42–5.

19. Ida M, Wakayama T, Nielsen ML, Abe T, Grodzki DM. Quiet T1-weighted imaging using PETRA: initial clinical evaluation in intracranial tumor patients. J Magn Reson Imaging. 2015;41(2):447–53.

20. Lee YH, Suh JS, Grodzki D. Ultrashort echo (UTE) versus pointwise encoding time reduction with radial acquisition (PETRA) sequences at 3 tesla for knee meniscus: a comparative study. Magn Reson Imaging. 2016;34(2):75–80.

21. Dournes G, Menut F, Macey J, Fayon M, Chateil JF, Salel M, Corneloup O, Montaudon M, Berger P, Laurent F. Lung morphology assessment of cystic fibrosis using MRI with ultrashort echo time at submillimeter spatial resolution. Eur Radiol. 2016;26(11):3811–20.

22. Aida N, Niwa T, Fujii Y, Nozawa K, Enokizono M, Murata K, Obata T. Quiet T_1-weighted pointwise encoding time reduction with radial acquisition for assessing myelination in the pediatric brain. AJNR Am J Neuroradiol. 2016;37(8):1528–34.

23. Hilgenfeld T, Prager M, Heil A, Schwindling FS, Nittka M, Grodzki D, Rammelsberg P, Bendszus M, Heiland S. PETRA, MSVAT-SPACE and SEMAC sequences for metal artefact reduction in dental MR imaging. Eur Radiol. 2017;27(12):5104–12.

24. Nozawa K, Niwa T, Aida N. Imaging of cystic lung lesions in infants using pointwise encoding time reduction with radial acquisition (PETRA). Magn Reson Med Sci. 2019;18(4):299–300.

25. Nishikawa A, Kakizawa Y, Wada N, Yamamoto Y, Katsuki M, Uchiyama T. Usefulness of pointwise encoding time reduction with radial acquisition and subtraction-based magnetic resonance angiography after cerebral aneurysm clipping. World Neurosurg X. 2020;9:100096.

26. Kobayashi N, Goerke U, Wang L, Ellermann J, Metzger GJ, Garwood M. Gradient-modulated PETRA MRI. Tomography. 2015;1(2):85–90.

27. Ilbey S, Jungmann PM, Fischer J, Jung M, Bock M, Özen AC. Single point imaging with radial acquisition and compressed sensing. Magn Reson Med. 2022;87(6):2685–96.

Hyungseok Jang, Soo Hyun Shin, Michael Carl, Yajun Ma,
and Jiang Du

Introduction

The MRI sequences designed to image short-T_2 tissues can be divided into two different classes based on their radiofrequency (RF) excitation and data encoding schemes, namely, zero echo time (ZTE) [1–5] and ultrashort echo time (UTE) [6–8]. The readout scheme in ZTE sequences employs fully ramped (or pre-ramped) constant readout gradients to quickly encode short-T_2 signals in 3D k-space during their rapid free induction decay (FID). Data encoding is performed only using the constant plateau of the gradient. UTE sequences are based on a different approach in which readout gradients are played out only after RF excitation is completed, and the subsequent RF dead-time (i.e., blind time preventing data readout due to the transmit to receive mode switching time) has elapsed. In this scheme, data readout is performed using both the ramping part and the constant plateau of the gradients.

In general, the strategy for UTE imaging provides flexible imaging and allows greater room for modifications of the sequence. For example, slice/slab-selection gradients and different encoding trajectories, such as spiral [9] and stack-of-stars [10], can be readily incorporated into UTE imaging. Moreover, UTE imaging allows flexible selection of imaging parameters such as flip angle (FA) and readout bandwidth (rBW). In contrast, ZTE sequences can be advantageous in achieving silent imaging since their gradient slew rate (i.e., speed of ramping) can be flexibly reduced to decrease acoustic noise without affecting encoding efficiency because the encoding scheme only uses the plateau of the gradient. Moreover, ZTE sequences can capture signals with ultrashort-T_2 decays more rapidly owing to its use of a fully ramped-up gradient that allows data readout with full encoding efficiency beginning at the near zero echo time (TE).

A downside of the ZTE-based approaches is that data are missing at the center of k-space due to the lack of data collection during RF excitation isodelay (i.e., the time between the peak and the end of RF pulse) as well as RF transmit-receives switching dead-time when the frequency encoding gradient is enabled. The k-space trajectory is missing from the origin of k-space to the beginning of the data acquisition, which is typically immediately after the RF dead-time, and this leaves a spherical hole at the center of k-space. Additional data acquisition is usually required to fill this gap in the missing data. Filling can be achieved by encoding data in a separate acquisition using a very low rBW (e.g., 8x lower rBW). This leaves a negligibly small region of missing data due to the low gradient amplitude. The approach is often called water- and fat-suppressed solid-state proton projection imaging (WASPI) [11]. Another approach is to use single-point imaging (SPI) to acquire data at the center of k-space. SPI is based on a traditional pure phase encoding scheme that acquires a single point in a k-space at a constant time delay [12]. SPI is free from missing data due to the RF dead-time because the k-space trajectory is controlled by scaling the phase encoding gradient. For example, zero amplitude of the phase encoding gradient leads to the center of k-space at any TE even after the RF dead-time. Combining the ZTE sequence with SPI is often called pointwise encoding time reduction with radial acquisition (PETRA) [5].

Another issue with ZTE sequences is selective excitation of undesirable and uncontrollable spins [13]. With ZTE sequences, a short hard pulse is typically used for RF excita-

H. Jang (✉) · S. H. Shin · Y. Ma
Department of Radiology, University of California, San Diego,
La Jolla, CA, USA
e-mail: h4jang@health.ucsd.edu; shs033@health.ucsd.edu;
yam013@health.ucsd.edu

M. Carl
GE Healthcare, San Diego, CA, USA
e-mail: Michael.Carl@ge.com

J. Du
Department of Radiology, University of California, San Diego,
La Jolla, CA, USA

Department of Bioengineering, University of California,
San Diego, La Jolla, CA, USA

VA San Diego Healthcare System, San Diego, CA, USA
e-mail: jiangdu@health.ucsd.edu

J. Du, G. M. Bydder (eds.), *MRI of Short- and Ultrashort-T_2 Tissues*, https://doi.org/10.1007/978-3-031-35197-6_7

tion to achieve a short TE. Due to the nonzero gradient turned on during the RF excitation, spins resonate at spatially varying Larmor frequencies, resulting in selective excitation (or slab selection). This unwanted selective excitation (or spatially varying flip angle) occurs in the readout direction and has a specific slice profile based on the shape of the applied RF pulse. Theoretically, a hard pulse results in a sinc-shaped excitation profile. This unwanted selection of spins may impair imaging if the main lobe of the slice profile is narrower than the desired field of view (FOV). The direction of the selective excitation varies from spoke to spoke due to the rotating readout gradient used in the 3D ZTE imaging, resulting in different slice profiles which modulate k-space data. This produces blurriness in the radial direction. To reduce the slice selectivity effect and thus minimize interference of ZTE imaging, a shorter RF pulse (i.e., lower flip angle) and a lower gradient amplitude (i.e., a lower rBW) should be used. However, this often limits signal-to-noise-ratio (SNR) and image contrast and exacerbates chemical shift artifacts due to the longer readout duration.

To address the two issues mentioned above (i.e., missing data and unwanted slice selectivity), a ramped hybrid encoding (RHE) technique has been proposed [14]. This benefits from the use of SPI and use of controlled gradient amplitudes during RF excitation. In this chapter, RHE and its applications are described.

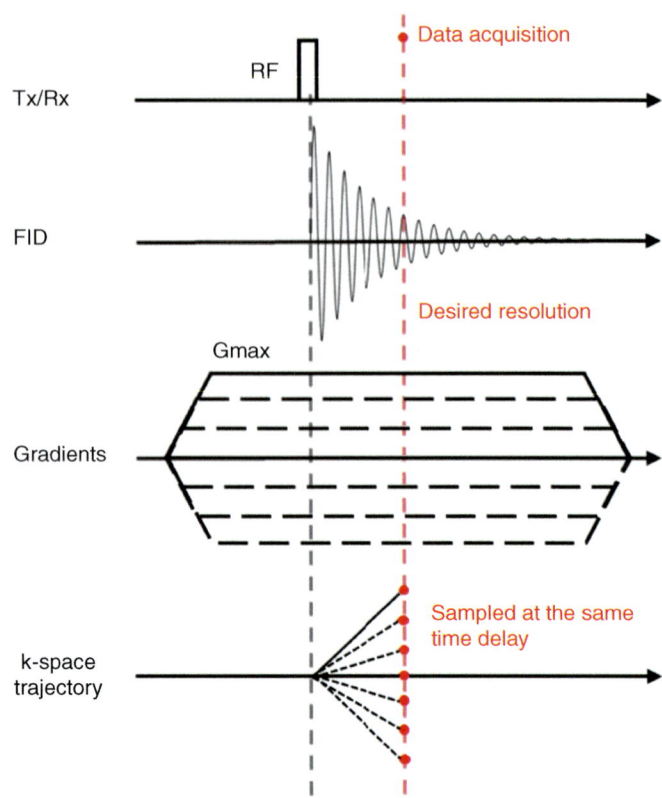

Fig. 7.1 Single-point imaging (SPI). SPI is a pure phase encoding technique in which a single data point is acquired at a constant TE during each TR. Different k-space data points are acquired using linearly scaled gradients

Single-Point Imaging (SPI)

SPI utilizes pure phase encoding to acquire the data at a single k-space coordinate in each TR [12, 15, 16]. As with conventional phase encoding, a k-space location is achieved using linearly scaled phase encoding gradients. Figure 7.1 shows a 1D example of SPI with seven phase encoding steps. Note that all data points are acquired with a constant time delay (red dotted line in Fig. 7.1). The FOV is determined by the number of phase encoding steps, N_p, the gradient waveform, G, and the encoding time delay, t_p, as shown in the following equation [17]:

$$FOV\left(t_p\right) = 2\pi N_p \left/ \left(\gamma \int_0^{t_p} G(t)dt \right) \right. \tag{7.1}$$

where γ is the gyromagnetic ratio. Thus, the spatial resolution (i.e., FOV/N_p) depends on the total gradient dephasing moment which is the integral of $G(t)$ over time from 0 to t_p.

3D SPI can be achieved by applying the phase encoding gradients in three orthogonal gradient directions and scaling the gradients one by one in a nested loop, resulting in a 3D cubical phase encoding pattern. The phase encoding points near the corner of the cube (i.e., outside of the inscribed sphere) are typically removed to reduce duty cycle demands on the gradient system and decrease scan time.

Slice Selectivity with ZTE Sequences

As mentioned above, ZTE-type sequences suffer from unwanted slice selectivity due to the effective gradient field present during RF excitation. The slice selectivity effect is also problematic in hybrid encoding schemes utilizing SPI such as PETRA. Figure 7.2a shows an example of a pulse sequence for PETRA. Figure 7.2b shows an example of the excitation profiles of a 24 μs hard RF pulse under various encoding gradient amplitudes (0, 7, 14, 20, and 30 mT/m). With radial sampling the unwanted slice selectivity occurs in the orientation of the net readout gradient, which is rotated over many TRs to cover 3D spherical k-space. In SPI, both the orientation and amplitude of the net phase encoding gradient are changed at each TR, which results in slice profiles with various line widths and directionalities. Consequently, the net effect of the slice selectivity artifact with hybrid encoding is contributed to by both the radial spokes and SPI encoded data modulated with different RF excitation profiles. This yields an exotic blurriness artifact, as shown in Fig. 7.2c. The longer RF pulse (e.g., a pulse width of 24 μs) with the higher gradient amplitude (e.g., 20 mT/m) worsens the slice selectivity artifact with PETRA. At the same time, frequency encoding-based UTE (FE-UTE) is not affected by these artifacts due to its nonselective RF excitation.

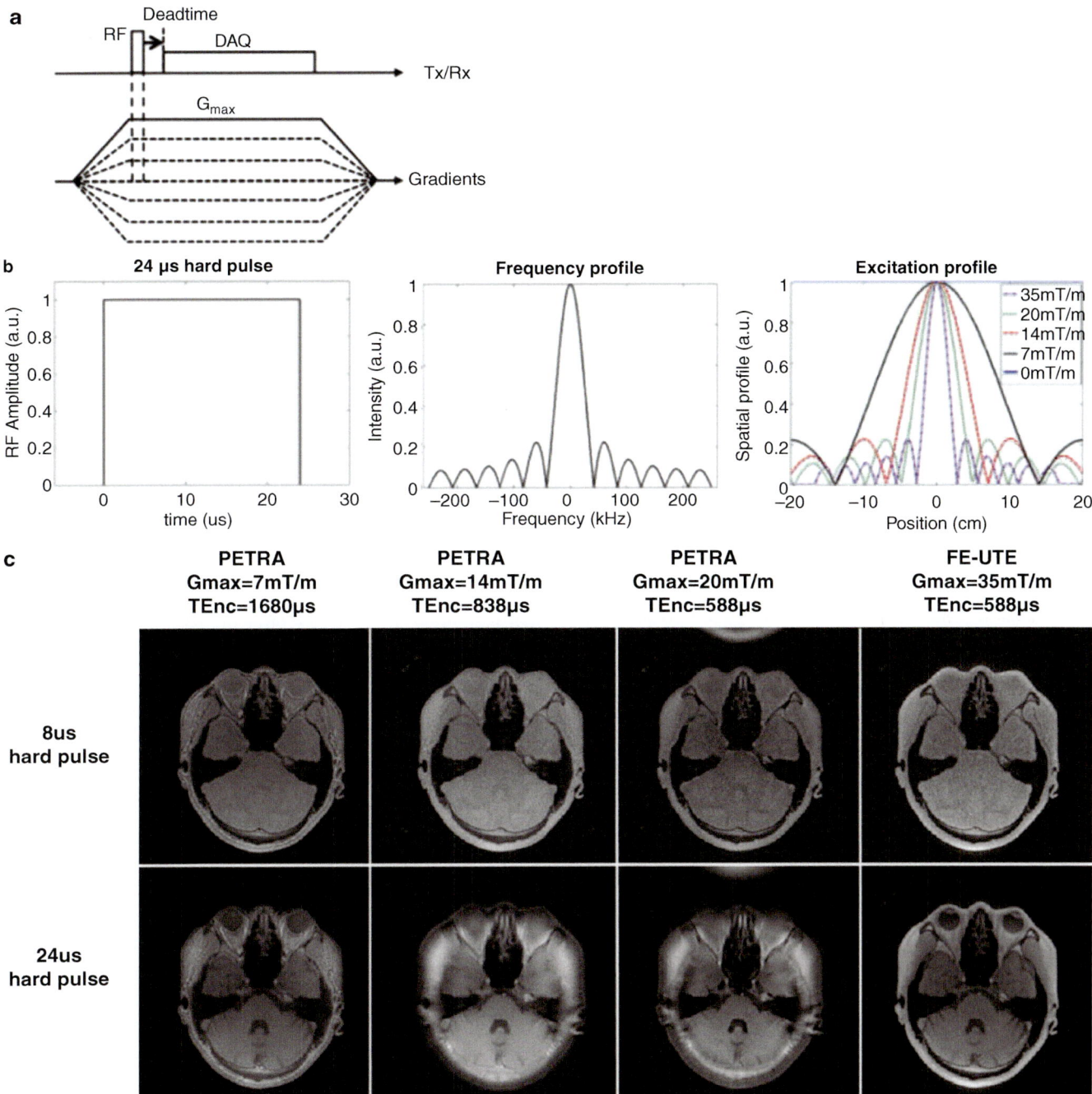

Fig. 7.2 Slice selectivity. (**a**) Pulse sequence diagram for PETRA imaging, (**b**) excitation profile of a 24 μs hard pulse and the resultant excitation profiles, and (**c**) slice selectivity with PETRA and FE-UTE (frequency encoding UTE). Note that the degree of slice selectivity artifact increases with the higher encoding gradient amplitude and pulse width used in PETRA imaging. FE-UTE shows no such artifact due to its nonselective excitation. (Adapted with permission from Ref. [14])

As demonstrated in Fig. 7.2, with hybrid encoding, the effective FOV under the slice selectivity effect is determined by the width of the RF excitation profile which becomes broader with shorter RF pulses (i.e., higher excitation bandwidths) and lower gradient amplitudes (i.e., lower readout bandwidths), and vice versa. Therefore, a shorter RF pulse and a lower rBW can be used with PETRA to alleviate unwanted slice selectivity artifacts and achieve the desired FOV without compromising image quality. Alternatively, phase-modulated RF pulses may be used to allow broader excitation bandwidths [18–20]. This approach achieves a larger effective FOV with ZTE sequences. However, the attainable peak FA with this approach is limited due to the use of frequency-swept excitation which requires a higher B_1

to achieve the same peak FA as a standard hard pulse. Another method to address the slice selectivity problem has been proposed. This is based on a post-processing technique in which the slice selection is demodulated after each k-space spoke [13]. To achieve this, prior information is required, such as the physical location of each pixel and the corresponding RF excitation profile in space. The downside of this approach is that noise can be amplified near zero-crossing regions in the slice profile (i.e., lower B_1 regions) during post-processing, where the data is divided by the slice profile. Moreover, it is not trivial to accurately estimate pixel locations and excitation profiles due to imperfections with MRI systems causing nonlinear distortions of the B_0, B_1, and gradient fields.

Ramped Hybrid Encoding (RHE)

RHE has been proposed by Jang et al., to control slice selectivity and achieve full encoding efficiency using fast ramp sampling. Figure 7.3a shows a pulse sequence diagram of RHE. With RHE, an effective gradient during RF excitation, G_{RF} is used to control the slice selectivity for a given FA and desired FOV. Immediately after the RF excitation, an encoding gradient is ramped up to maximum amplitude, G_{max}, to achieve full encoding efficiency. Data acquisition is performed after the RF dead-time. Figure 7.3b shows an example of the sampling pattern (or k-space trajectory) with

RHE. Similar to PETRA, SPI is performed to fill the missing data in the central area of k-space, while radial frequency encoding is performed to acquire data in outer k-space. Figure 7.3c shows an example of multi-echo RHE based on a gradient echo train using bipolar readout gradients.

In RHE, the minimum diameter of the SPI region required to avoid wrapping artifact is determined by the desired FOV, the TE, and the gradient shape using the following equation for N_{SPI}, the number of spokes:

$$N_{SPI} = \left[2\bar{\gamma} \, fov_D \left(G_{RF} t_D + 0.5 g_s t_D^2 \right) \text{ if } t_D \leq \left(G_{max} - G_{RF} \right) / g_s \right],$$
$$\left[2\bar{\gamma} \, fov_D \left(G_{max} t_D - 0.5 \left(G_{max} - G_{RF} \right)^2 / g_s \right) \text{ otherwise} \right]$$

(7.2)

where $\bar{\gamma}$ is the reduced gyromagnetic ratio, g_s denotes gradient slew rate, fov_D denotes the desired FOV, and t_D is the desired TE chosen after dead-time.

RHE can be regarded as a generalized technique encompassing both hybrid encoding (i.e., PETRA) and ramp sampled FE-UTE. If G_{RF} is set to G_{max}, RHE becomes equivalent to PETRA. If G_{RF} is set to zero, RHE becomes similar to FE-UTE, except for different timing of the readout gradient that is applied immediately after the RF pulse in RHE, not after the dead-time. Note that with FE-UTE the gradients begin to ramp up after RF dead-time to avoid missing data. In this case, RHE still achieves more efficient encoding with

Fig. 7.3 Ramped hybrid encoding (RHE). (**a**) Pulse sequence diagram, (**b**) 2D example of k-space trajectory, and (**c**) multi-echo RHE. RHE controls slice selectivity using a low G_{RF} and provides efficient encoding by using a high G_{max}. The ramped-up G_{RF} allows more efficient encoding than conventional UTE sequences at the cost of increased scan time due to the SPI encoding required to fill in the central missing data (Adapted with permission from Ref. [14])

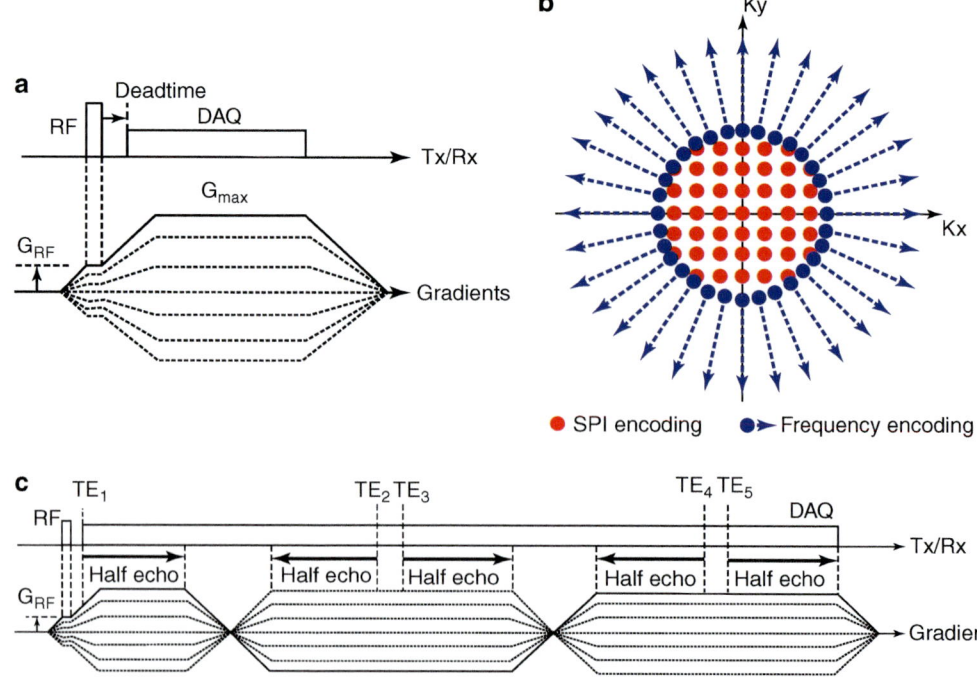

a shorter readout duration than FE-UTE, although it requires SPI to fill in the missing data.

Encoding Speed and T$_2$* Blurring with RHE

When imaging short-T$_2$* tissues, the data acquisition should be performed as fast as possible to minimize signal decay during readout which may cause unwanted signal modulation in k-space and time-varying signal weighting from the center to the outside of k-space. This is similar to low-pass filtering. This effect is often called T$_2$* blurring as it blurs the point spread function (PSF) and the resultant image. It is a function of encoding efficiency and speed (i.e., k-space trajectory encoding time compared to encoding time delays) and T$_2$* decay. Figure 7.4a shows simulated per-excitation encoding time plotted against k-space position with different encoding schemes, including PETRA, RHE, and FE-UTE. Figure 7.4b, c shows the corresponding 1D images simulated with two different T$_2$*s (100 and 500 μs). PETRA shows the most blurry images (i.e., the highest degree of short-T$_2$* blurriness effect) due to its long readout duration.

FE-UTE shows blurriness when the T$_2$* is very short (i.e., 100 μs), resulting from the inefficient sampling at the beginning of data acquisition where it takes a certain amount of time to ramp up the gradient to reach full encoding efficiency (i.e., maximum gradient amplitude). RHE overall shows the most robust imaging for all cases with T$_2$* of 100 and 500 μs at the cost of slight blurriness occurring at the peripheral FOV due to the unwanted slice selectivity effect which is exacerbated with higher values of G_{RF}.

Figure 7.5 shows results obtained using a LEGO phantom (Big Ben, item # 21013, a cowboy minifigure from Palace Cinema, item # 10232, and a white horse manufactured by LEGO, Billund, Denmark) and made of acrylonitrile butadiene styrene (ABS) with an approximate T$_2$* of 400–500 μs. PETRA with a low readout bandwidth (i.e., G_{max} = 7 mT/m) exhibits strong T$_2$* blurriness due to its long encoding time of 1680 us. PETRA with a higher readout bandwidth (i.e., G_{max} = 14 and 20 mT/m) improves the blurriness, but results in strong slice selectivity artifacts. FE-UTE exhibits no slice selectivity artifacts due to its nonselective RF excitation (i.e., G_{RF} = 0). RHE with G_{RF} of 7 mT/m shows good image quality with no strong slice selectivity. RHE shows improved

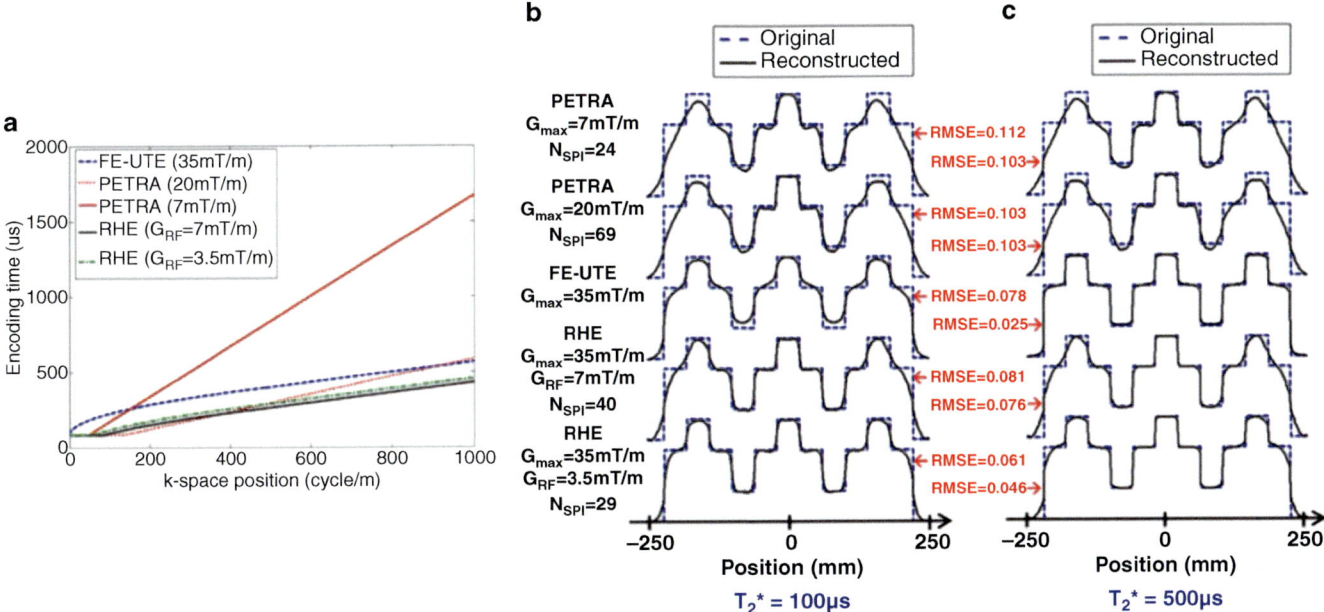

Fig. 7.4 Encoding efficiency (encoding time plotted against k-space position) for FE-UTE, PETRA, and RHE (**a**) and 1D images simulated with T$_2$* = 100 μs (**b**) and T$_2$* = 500 μs (**c**). PETRA with a gradient amplitude of 20 mT/m achieves fast encoding in an earlier encoding time (red dotted line) but produces a strong slice selectivity artifact.

FE-UTE exhibits good image quality, but with short T$_2$*s, it shows some blurriness due to inefficient sampling at the beginning of data acquisition. RHE achieves good image quality with controlled slice selectivity and the most efficient encoding. (Adapted with permission from Ref. [14])

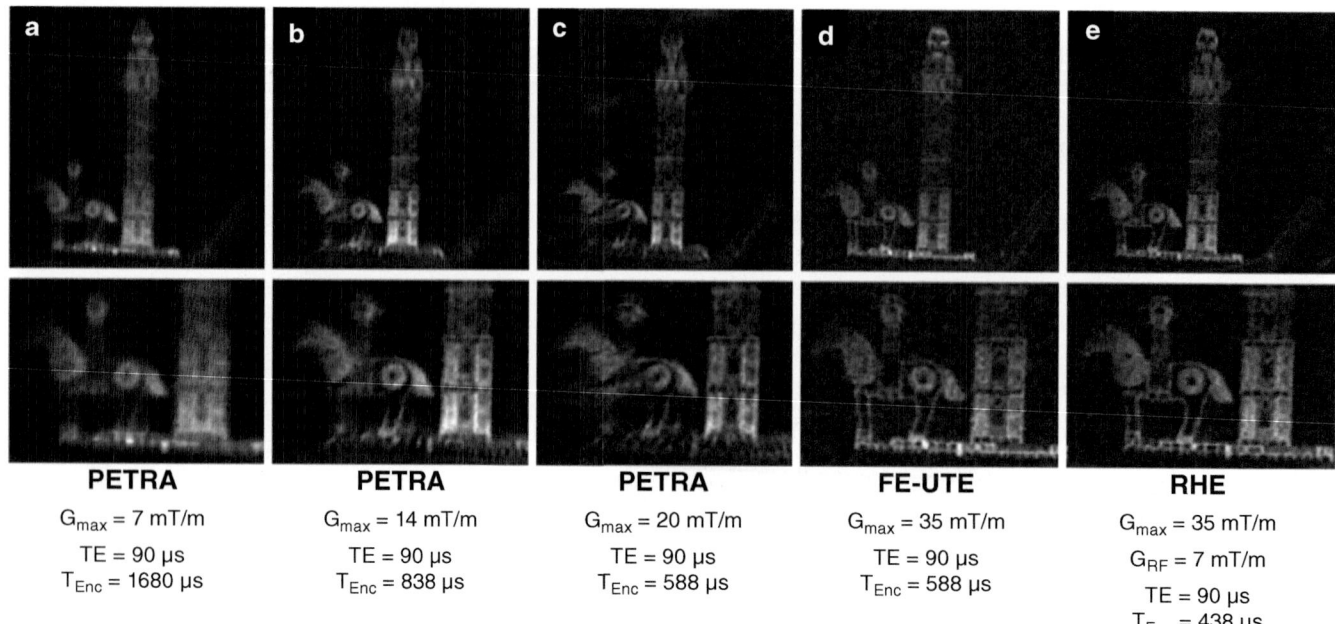

PETRA	PETRA	PETRA	FE-UTE	RHE
G_{max} = 7 mT/m	G_{max} = 14 mT/m	G_{max} = 20 mT/m	G_{max} = 35 mT/m	G_{max} = 35 mT/m
TE = 90 μs	TE = 90 μs	TE = 90 μs	TE = 90 μs	G_{RF} = 7 mT/m
T_{Enc} = 1680 μs	T_{Enc} = 838 μs	T_{Enc} = 588 μs	T_{Enc} = 588 μs	TE = 90 μs
				T_{Enc} = 438 μs

Fig. 7.5 Phantom experiment. PETRA with (**a**) G_{max} = 7 mT/m, (**b**) G_{max} = 14 mT/m, (**c**) G_{max} = 20 mT/m, (**d**) FE-UTE with G_{max} = 35 mT/m, and (**e**) RHE with G_{RF} = 7 mT/m and G_{max} = 35 mT/m. PETRA with a low gradient amplitude (7 mT/m) shows an overall blurry image due to short-T_2^* blurriness caused by its long readout duration (1650 μs). With PETRA, higher gradient amplitudes yield sharper images, but strong slice selectivity is exhibited. FE-UTE shows overall robust imaging with no slice selectivity artifact. RHE exhibits the best image quality with no slice selectivity and the best SNR due to its short readout duration (438 μs). (Adapted with permission from Ref. [14])

image quality with a higher SNR than FE-UTE, presumably due to improved encoding efficiency with a shorter encoding time of 438 μs compared to FE-UTE with a slightly longer encoding time of 588 μs.

The Efficacy of SPI in RHE

SPI in RHE plays a critical role in filling the missing data in the center of the k-space. SPI is expected to allow more robust imaging than WASPI because all the data are acquired at a constant TE with near-zero readout duration (i.e., there is no T_2^* decay or eddy current effect on the data filling the hole in k-space). Downsides of SPI are a longer acquisition time imposed by expensive single-point encoding and increased acoustic noise caused by rapidly changing phase encoding gradients.

The benefit of SPI in terms of image quality has been reported in the literature. In RHE, the relative size of the SPI encoded region in a k-space can be controlled by reconstructing data acquired at different TEs; a delayed TE results in larger size of SPI in k-space [21, 22]. SPI should be slightly oversampled to avoid aliasing artifacts at the delayed TE. A phantom experiment was performed to test the effect of different sizes of SPI in RHE (2, 3, and 4%) as well as 0% SPI (i.e., FE-UTE) (Fig. 7.6a). The images with larger SPI regions showed sharper boundaries and reduced signal bias inside the object [23]. Figure 7.6b shows myelin images from a human brain using adiabatic inversion recovery prepared RHE (IR-RHE) to suppress long-T_2 white and gray matter signals and achieve myelin specific contrast [24]. As shown, a larger SPI region dramatically improves the myelin contrast and improves signal suppression in the gray matter regions (green arrows), presumably due to the robustness of SPI to eddy current effects.

Similarly, multiple images can be reconstructed from the same dataset in RHE by applying higher degrees of overs-

Fig. 7.6 Efficacy of SPI in RHE. (**a**) Phantom experiment and (**b**) in vivo myelin imaging in a 30-year-old healthy volunteer. RHE with larger SPI reduces blurriness near the object boundary in the phantom experiment. In (**b**) the images with the larger SPI show improved myelin contrast with suppressed signal in gray matter (green arrows). R_{SPI} is the ratio of the radius of SPI to the radius at the maximum k-space location. (Adapted with permission from Refs. [23, 24])

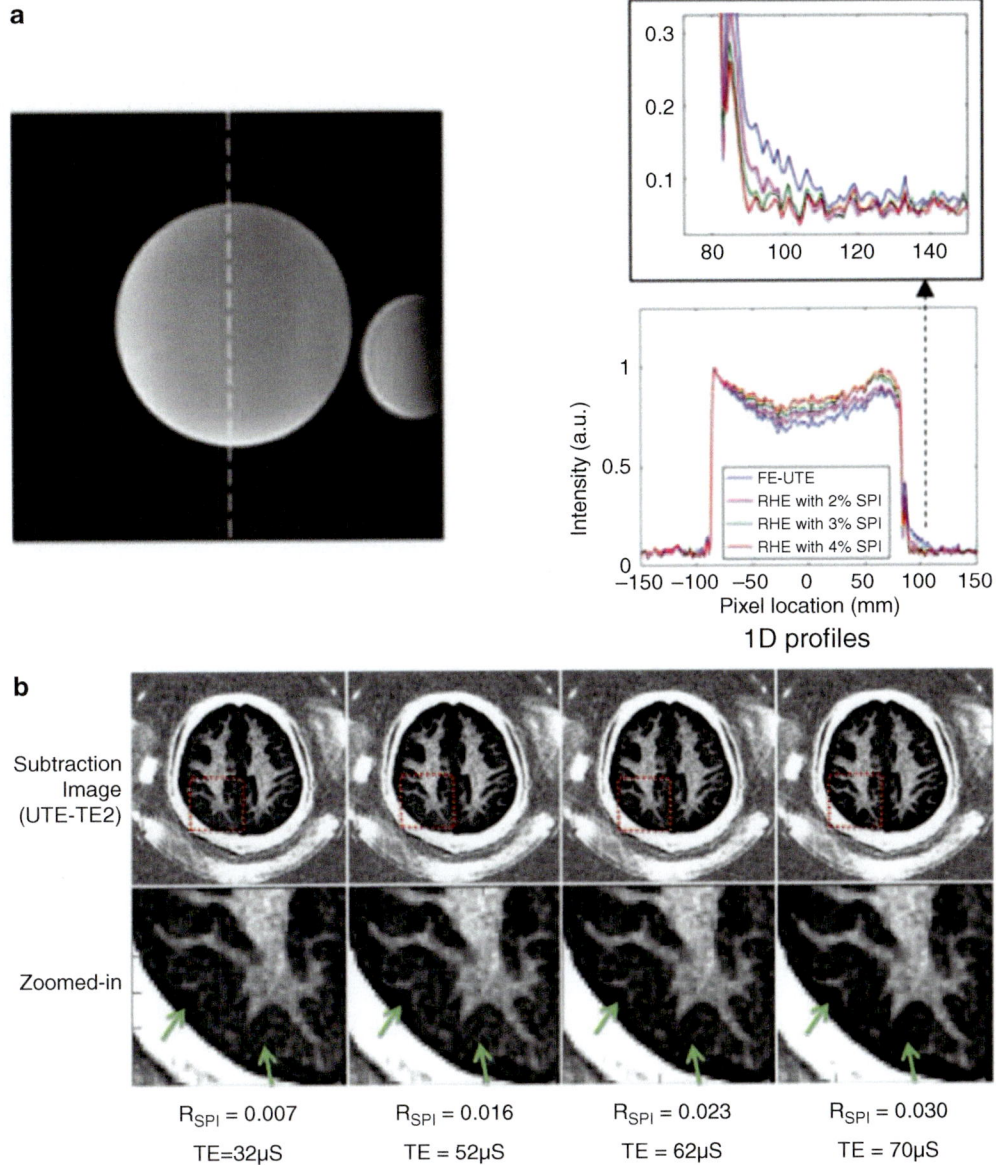

ampling in SPI and reconstructing images with delayed TEs. Jang et al. showed the efficacy of this strategy using 14 RHE images obtained in a single scan with oversampled SPI for head segmentation [23]. Their study also showed that multiple RHE images can be used to improve tissue segmentation.

Applications and Variants of RHE

The feasibility and efficacy of RHE in morphological and quantitative imaging have been demonstrated in several applications.

MR-Based Attenuation Correction

Jang et al. proposed a new MR-based attenuation correction (MRAC) technique for PET-MRI based on the use of rapid dual-echo RHE with oversampled SPI [23]. The rapid RHE scan acquires multiple images, including in-phase UTEs at 52, 54, 56, 58, 60, 62, 64, 66, 68, 70, 72, 74, 76, and 78 μs and an out-of-phase gradient recalled echo (TE = 1.1 ms) in a scan time of 35 s. This allows segmentation of the head into four tissue types (i.e., bone, air, brain, and fat) using a histogram-based approach and a two-point Dixon-based fat and water separation technique. The segmented tissue map was used to generate pseudo-CT images for subsequent attenua-

Fig. 7.7 RHE-based MRAC. Results with PET/MR system-based MRAC using LAVA-Flex (MRAC-1) (**a**) and atlas-based method (MRAC-2) (**b**), dual-echo RHE-based MRAC (dRHE-MRAC) (**c**), and ground truth CT-based attenuation correction (CTAC) (**d**). In contrast to MRAC-1 and MRAC-2, dRHE-MRAC achieves significantly reduced error in PET reconstruction showing errors below 1% in most brain regions. (Adapted with permission from Ref. [23])

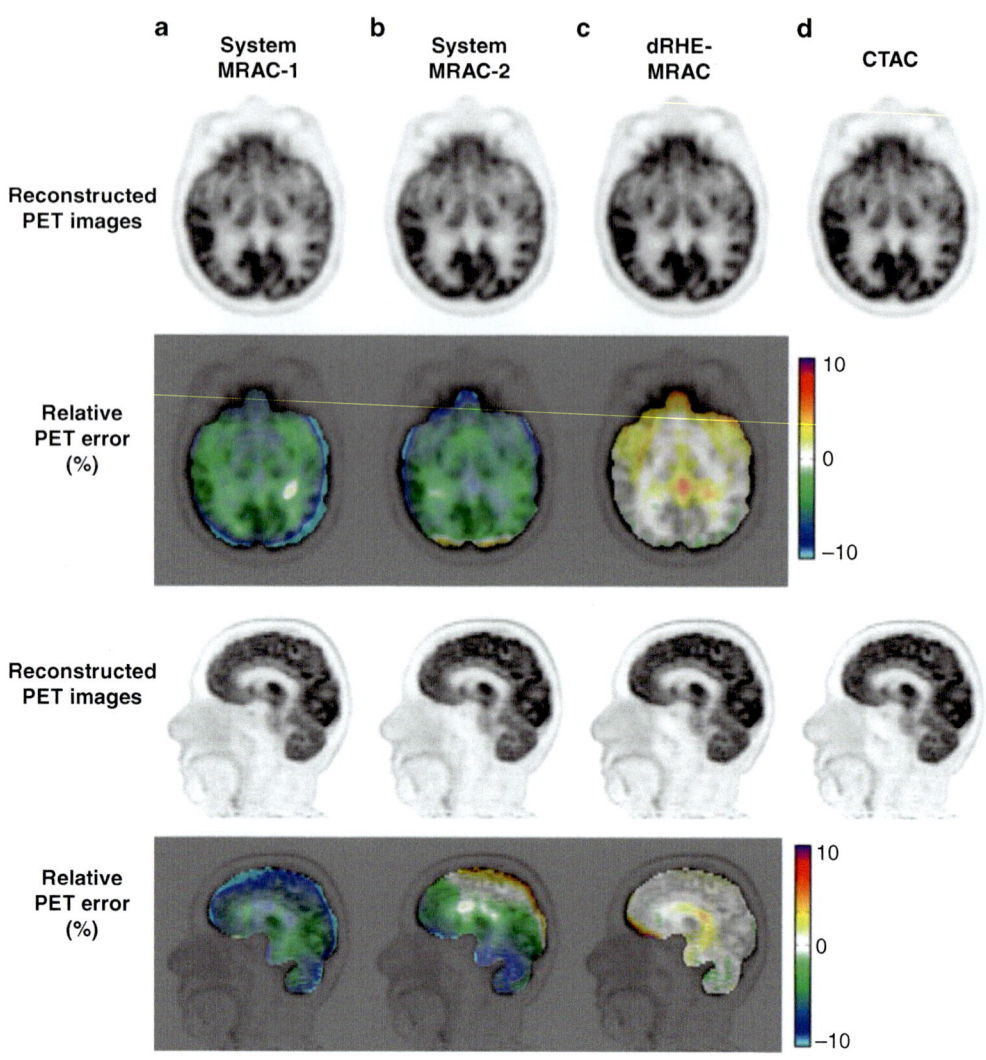

tion correction in PET reconstruction (Fig. 7.7). The same sequence has been used for deep learning-based MRAC [25]. The MRAC based on dual-echo RHE showed improved performance with a significantly reduced PET reconstruction error below 1% in most brain regions compared with conventional MRAC methods ($P < 0.05$).

Single-Scan Bicomponent T_2^* Mapping in the Knee

RHE has also been investigated in musculoskeletal (MSK) imaging. Jang et al. showed the feasibility of bicomponent T_2^* mapping in the human knee using a flyback echo train-based RHE sequence in which 16 echoes were acquired in a single scan [26]. In this study, the original version of RHE was modified to accommodate a selective Shinnar-Le Roux (SLR) pulse which was incorporated to achieve slab selec-

tion and fat saturation to suppress signals from adipose tissue. Similar to the study with MRAC where multiple RHE images were reconstructed with delayed TEs [23], two RHE images at TEs of 0.04 and 0.11 ms were acquired by utilizing an oversampled SPI technique (Fig. 7.8a). A total of 16 echoes were acquired between 0.04 ms and 30 ms, and these were used for biexponential fitting of knee joint tissues. Figure 7.8b shows estimated bicomponent T_2^* parameter maps in the patellar tendon, anterior cruciate ligament (ACL), posterior cruciate ligament (PCL), and meniscus. These showed parameter estimates similar to those reported in the literature.

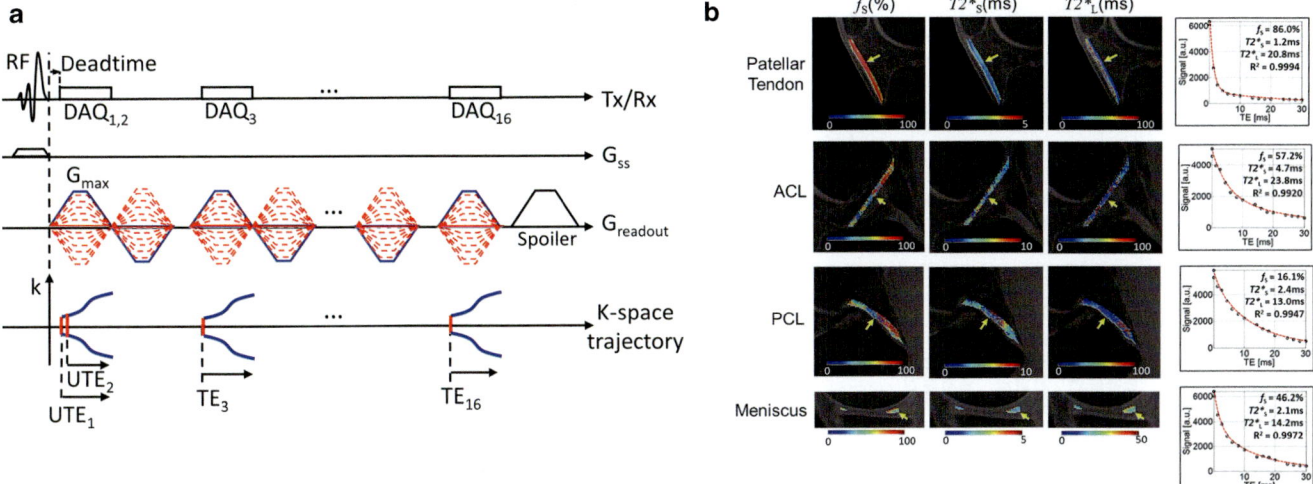

Fig. 7.8 Single-scan bicomponent T_2^* mapping of knee tissues using RHE. (**a**) Pulse sequence diagram and (**b**) results of bicomponent parameter mapping (f_s, the short-component fraction; T_2^*s, T_2^* of the short component; $T_{2\,L}^*$, T_2^* of the long component) in the patellar tendon, ACL, PCL, and meniscus. (Adapted with permission from Ref. [26])

Direct Myelin Imaging with Interleaved Hybrid Encoding

UTE imaging has been used frequently for direct myelin imaging [27–30]. RHE combined with adiabatic IR preparation has also been investigated for direct myelin imaging in the brain [24]. In this study, dual-echo RHE imaging was used to acquire two images (i.e., a UTE image and a gradient recalled echo image with a longer TE) at the nulling point for long-T_2 components in white matter. Echo subtraction yielded short-T_2 contrast which was specific for myelin.

For efficient 3D IR imaging, multiple spokes are usually encoded with each IR preparation [31–33], so that the scan time is shortened by the number of spokes acquired per preparation. With this approach, a group of spokes is acquired near the desired inversion time (TI). This results in the inclusion of spokes with shorter and longer TIs than the optimum, and imperfect nulling of signal which may result in compromised signal contrast due to the inclusion of data acquired with variable T_1-weighting, also called T_1 blurring. In direct myelin imaging based on adiabatic IR, this can be an issue too and may result in imperfect nulling of white matter. To alleviate this effect, a group of spokes is typically centered on a TI chosen so that spokes are acquired before and after the nulling point, and so produce both negative and positive signals. In this way, the signals from spokes with different polarities cancel, and this reduces the error [29, 34].

To further improve the image contrast with IR-RHE, Jang et al. have proposed interleaved hybrid encoding (IHE) [24]. In conventional PETRA and RHE, it is common to perform

SPI and radial encodings sequentially with SPI and radial frequency encoding performed one after another. However, this is not the optimal way for IR-RHE when SPI data in the central region of k-space has variable T_1-weighting (because it is obtained at different TIs). IHE benefits from reordered sampling with SPI acquisitions interleaved at TIs near the nulling point so that the central region of k-space is filled with data acquired at, or near, the desired TI (Fig. 7.9a). This approach allows the use of a high number of encoded spokes (~60 spokes) per IR preparation. The improved image quality with IR-IHE with an increased number of spokes per IR preparation was demonstrated by a computer simulation (Fig. 7.9b). Compared to conventional IR-prepared projection radial-based UTE (IR-PRUTE) and IR-prepared RHE with sequential sampling (IR-HE), IR-IHE exhibited much improved myelin contrast and accurate detection of demyelinated lesions with up to 61 spokes per IR preparation.

RHE with adiabatic IR and interleaved encoding (i.e., IR-IHE) showed the feasibility of in vivo direct myelin imaging in healthy controls and multiple sclerosis (MS) patients within a clinically acceptable scan time (6 min 54 s). In in vivo experiments with healthy volunteers, IR-IHE showed dramatically improved myelin contrast compared to IR-RHE using a sequential encoding scheme (Fig. 7.10a). In imaging of MS patients, IR-IHE achieved high quality myelin imaging in which normal myelin and demyelinating lesions in white matter were detected (red arrows in Fig. 7.10b).

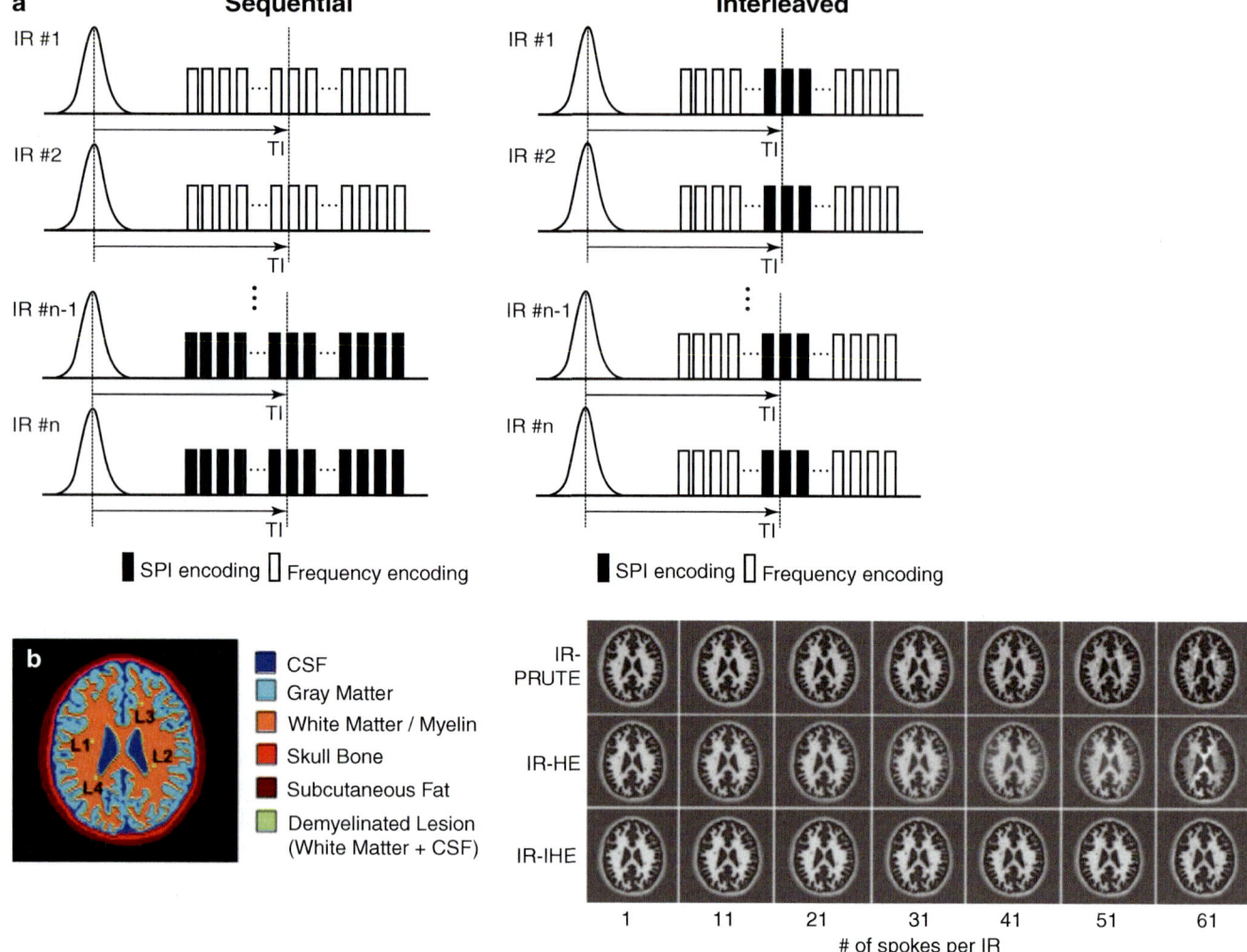

Fig. 7.9 Interleaved encoding for IR-prepared RHE. (**a**) Conventional sequential ordering of SPI, radial frequency encoding and interleaved encoding, and (**b**) computer simulation of the two encoding schemes (IR-HE, IR-based hybrid encoding with sequential encoding; IR-IHE, IR-based interleaved hybrid encoding) as well as IR-based projection radial UTE (IR-PRUTE). In the computer simulation, IR-IHE yielded dramatically improved myelin image quality with suppression of the streak artifacts that were obvious with IR-PRUTE and IR-HE when using a high number of spokes per IR preparation. (Adapted with permission from Ref. [24])

RHE-Based Sodium MRI

Sodium (^{23}Na) is an essential chemical element that plays a vital role in human physiology. Sodium is the second most abundant nucleus that provide endogenous MRI signal in the human body. It can be a biomarker for various diseases, including tumors [35–37], stroke [38, 39], neurodegenerative disease [40], and MSK disorders [41–43]. Despite its promise, sodium MRI suffers from two significant challenges. First, the ^{23}Na signal is very low compared to clinical proton MRI, resulting in low SNR. Second, ^{23}Na signals typically undergoes rapid biexponential T_2^* decay. Therefore,

UTE or ZTE sequences are likely to improve signal acquisition. Unfortunately, ZTE sequences are not a good option due to their limited FA, which is critical due to the low density of ^{23}Na. As a result, UTE imaging is typically used for sodium MRI.

Blunck et al. have recently utilized RHE for sodium MRI to take advantage of its efficient and rapid encoding (i.e., short readout duration) compared to conventional UTE imaging, and this reduces T_2^* blurring and increases SNR [44]. To allow use of a high FA of 90 degrees, G_{RF} was set to zero in this study, and the sequence was described as zero G_{RF} RHE (zG_{RF}-RHE). In their 1D computer simulation,

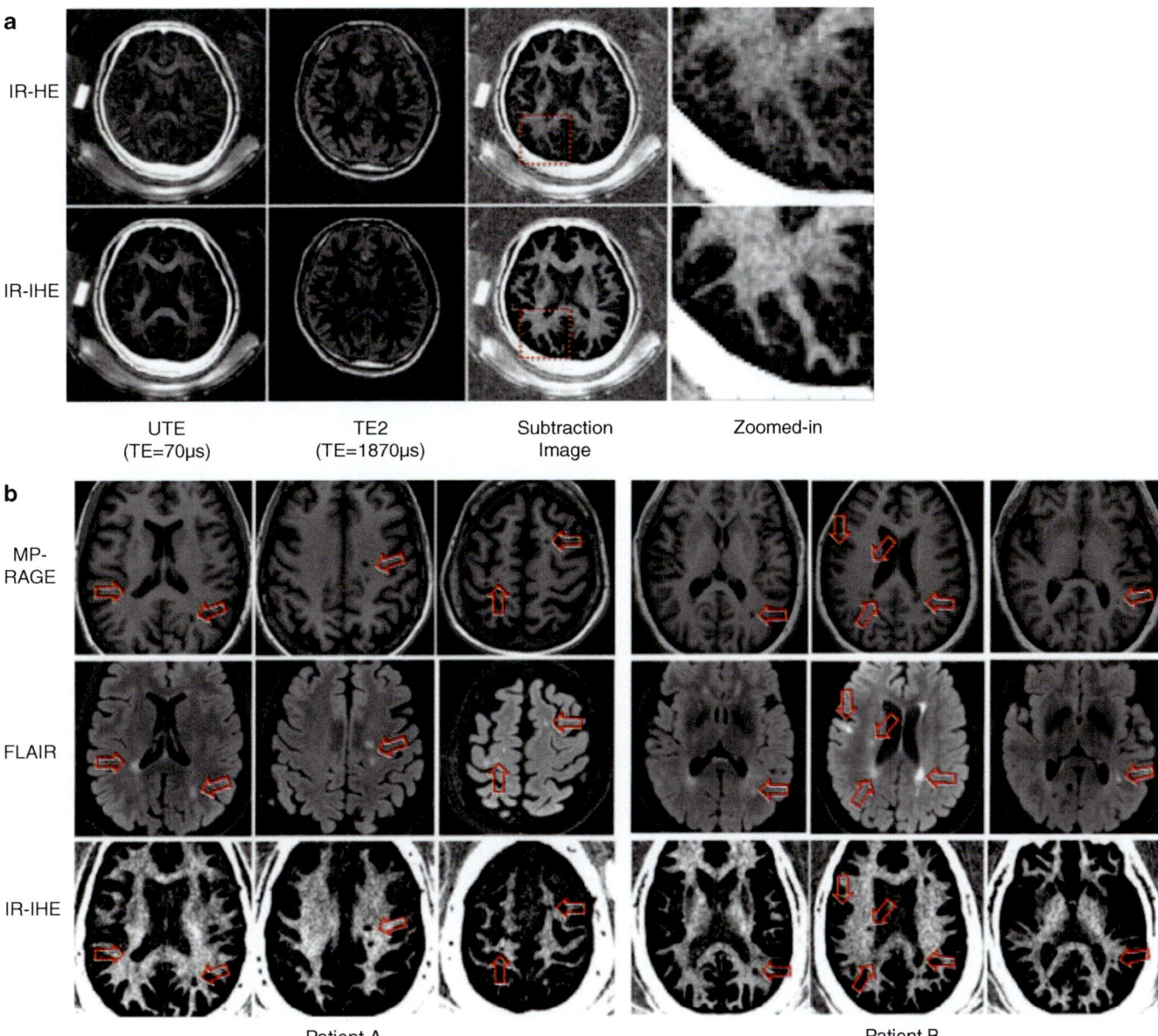

Fig. 7.10 In vivo myelin imaging. (**a**) Efficacy of interleaved encoding demonstrated in a healthy volunteer (30-year-old male) and (**b**) IR-IHE-based myelin imaging in MS patients compared with clinical MRI sequences (patient A, 59-year-old female; patient B, 51-year-old female). As shown in (**a**), IHE improves myelin contrast with reduced artifact in gray matter. In MS patients, IR-IHE provides direct morphological information on myelin and demyelinated lesions. (Adapted with permission from Ref. [24])

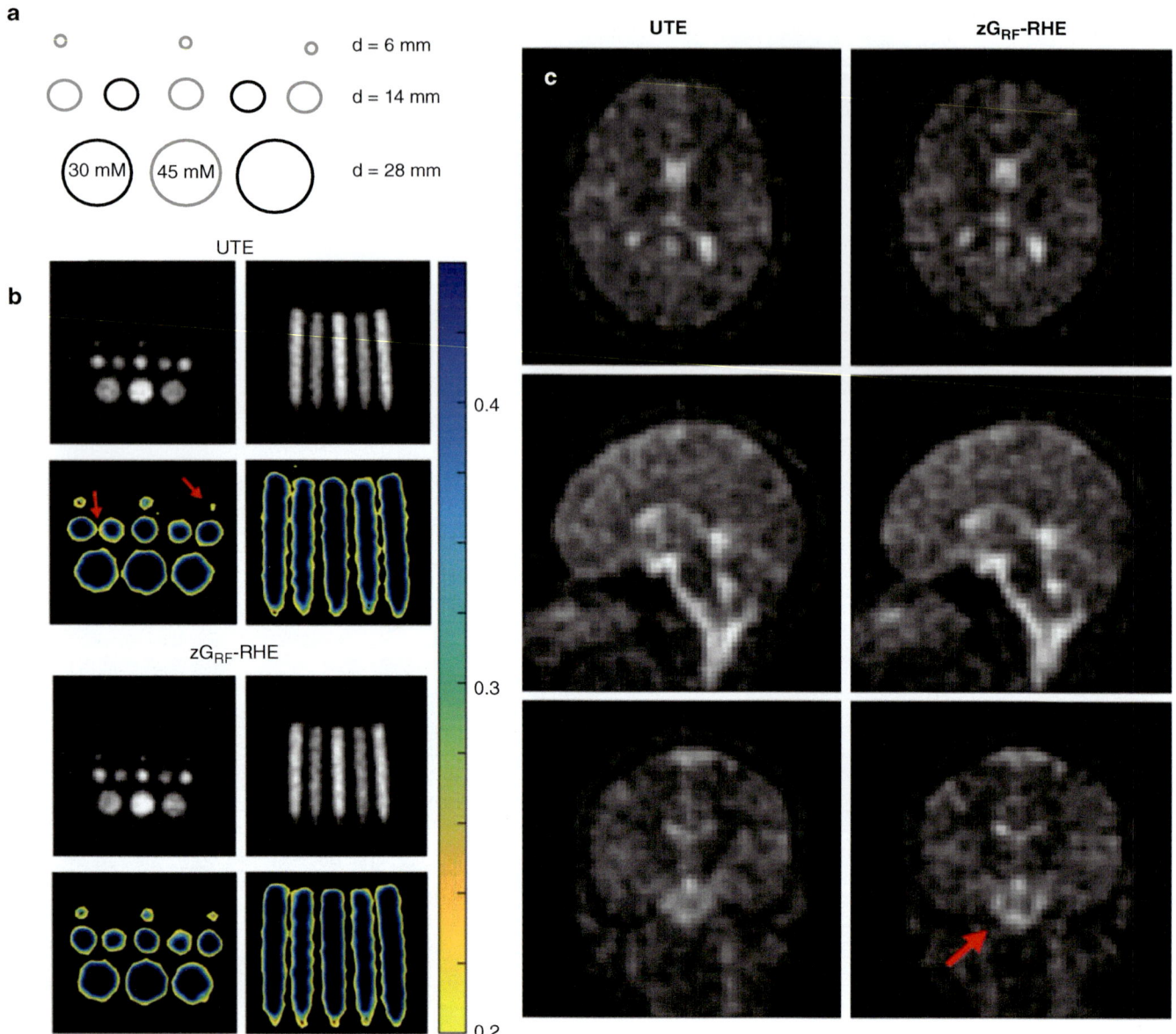

Fig. 7.11 Zero G_{RF} RHE (zG_{RF}-RHE) in sodium MRI. (**a**) Phantom design, (**b**) phantom images acquired with zG_{RF}-RHE and UTE, and (**c**) in vivo brain ^{23}Na MRI with UTE and zG_{RF}-RHE. The phantom experiment in (**b**) shows an improved contour profile with RHE (red arrows) compared with UTE. zG_{RF}-RHE in the in vivo sodium imaging also demonstrates improved image quality compared with UTE, with better demonstration of the brainstem (red arrow) and ventricular system. (Adapted with permission from Ref. [44])

RHE showed reduced T_2^* blurring with improved image quality. MRI experiments were performed using a research 7 T MRI scanner (Siemens Healthcare, Erlangen, Germany) with a transmit/receive dual-tuned 1H-^{23}Na head coil (QED, Mayfield Village, OH). For the phantom experiment, tubes with three different diameters (6, 14, and 28 mm) and two different saline concentrations (30 mM and 45 mM) were prepared (Fig. 7.11a). The resultant RHE images showed improved boundary profile (i.e., reduced T_2^* blurring) with better detection of small vials compared with the UTE image (Fig. 7.11b). In vivo experiments also showed improved image quality with RHE. In Fig. 7.11c, RHE exhibits improved detail around the brainstem region (red arrow) and in the corpus callosum compared with UTE.

Conclusion

RHE is an extended, generalized form of PETRA that benefits from use of a pre-ramped, controllable gradient during RF excitation (G_{RF}). As with PETRA, SPI is utilized to fill the missing data in the center of the k-space. The SPI encoding fills the missing data and contributes to improved image quality, due to its near-zero readout duration and its robustness to eddy current effects. In addition, more aggressive utilization of SPI demonstrated that it is based on oversampled SPI. This approach can be used to reconstruct multiple images using a single dataset acquired with a single scan. These multiple images can help improve brain segmentation [23] and allow biexponential fitting [26], as well as provide novel uses in direct myelin imaging [24] and sodium MRI [44].

RHE lies between ZTE and UTE imaging and benefits from their advantages such as pre-ramped-up gradient in ZTE and flexible imaging in UTE. A downside with RHE is the additional scan time required for SPI encoding. The size of the SPI encoding depends on the shape of the gradient waveform, including G_{RF}, G_{max} and slew rate, as well as RF deadtime. The scan time for SPI encoding is usually negligibly short with clinical MRI scanners unless oversampling is applied. It can be a more significant issue when high-performance gradient systems are used. To mitigate the additional scan time burden, the hybrid filling (HYFI) technique has been recently proposed [45]. HYFI utilizes mixed SPI and segmented radial frequency encoding to reduce the scan time. A downside expected with HYFI is compromise in image quality. Systematic comparison of the hybrid encoding family with standard UTE and ZTE techniques will be required to fully understand their advantages and disadvantages.

References

1. Weiger M, Pruessmann KP, Bracher A-K, et al. High-resolution ZTE imaging of human teeth. NMR Biomed. 2012;25(10):1144–51.
2. Weiger M, Pruessmann KP. MRI with zero echo time. Encycl Magn Reson. 2012;1:311–22. https://doi.org/10.1002/9780470034590. emrstm1292.
3. Wiesinger F, Sacolick LI, Menini A, et al. Zero TE MR bone imaging in the head. Magn Reson Med. 2016;75(1):107–14.
4. Weiger M, Brunner DO, Dietrich BE, Müller CF, Pruessmann KP. ZTE imaging in humans. Magn Reson Med. 2013;70(2):328–32.
5. Grodzki DM, Jakob PM, Heismann B. Ultrashort echo time imaging using pointwise encoding time reduction with radial acquisition (PETRA). Magn Reson Med. 2012;67(2):510–8.
6. Chang EY, Du J, Chung CB. UTE imaging in the musculoskeletal system. J Magn Reson Imaging. 2015;41(4):870–83.
7. Robson MD, Gatehouse PD, Bydder M, Bydder GM. Magnetic resonance: an introduction to ultrashort TE (UTE) imaging. J Comput Assist Tomogr. 2003;27(6):825–46.
8. Jerban S, Chang DG, Ma Y, Jang H, Chang EY, Du J. An update in qualitative imaging of bone using ultrashort echo time magnetic resonance. Front Endocrinol (Lausanne). 2020;11:555756.
9. Gurney PT, Hargreaves BA, Nishimura DG. Design and analysis of a practical 3D cones trajectory. Magn Reson Med. 2006;55(3):575–82.
10. Zhou Z, Han F, Yan L, Wang DJJ, Hu P. Golden-ratio rotated stack-of-stars acquisition for improved volumetric MRI. Magn Reson Med. 2017;78(6):2290–8.
11. Wu Y, Dai G, Ackerman JL, et al. Water- and fat-suppressed proton projection MRI (WASPI) of rat femur bone. Magn Reson Med. 2007;57(3):554–67.
12. Emid S, Creyghton JHN. High resolution NMR imaging in solids. Phys B+C. 1985;128(1):81–3.
13. Grodzki DM, Jakob PM, Heismann B. Correcting slice selectivity in hard pulse sequences. J Magn Reson. 2012;214(1):61–7.
14. Jang H, Wiens CN, McMillan AB. Ramped hybrid encoding for improved ultrashort echo time imaging. Magn Reson Med. 2016;76(3):814–25.
15. Jang H, Lu X, Carl M, et al. True phase quantitative susceptibility mapping using continuous single-point imaging: a feasibility study. Magn Reson Med. 2019;81(3):1907–14.
16. Balcom BJ, Macgregor RP, Beyea SD, Green DP, Armstrong RL, Bremner TW. Single-point ramped imaging with T_1 enhancement (SPRITE). J Magn Reson A. 1996;123(1):131–4.
17. Jang H, McMillan AB. A rapid and robust gradient measurement technique using dynamic single-point imaging. Magn Reson Med. 2017;78(3):950–62.
18. Li C, Magland JF, Seifert AC, Wehrli FW. Correction of excitation profile in zero echo time (ZTE) imaging using quadratic phase-modulated RF pulse excitation and iterative reconstruction. IEEE Trans Med Imaging. 2014;33(4):961–9.
19. Weiger M, Pruessmann KP, Hennel F. MRI with zero echo time: hard versus sweep pulse excitation. Magn Reson Med. 2011;66(2):379–89.
20. Schieban K, Weiger M, Hennel F, Boss A, Pruessmann KP. ZTE imaging with enhanced flip angle using modulated excitation. Magn Reson Med. 2015;74(3):684–93.
21. Kaffanke JB, Romanzetti S, Dierkes T, Leach MO, Balcom BJ, Jon SN. Multi-frame SPRITE: a method for resolution enhancement of multiple-point SPRITE data. J Magn Reson. 2013;230:111–6.
22. Jang H, Subramanian S, Devasahayam N, et al. Single acquisition quantitative single-point electron paramagnetic resonance imaging. Magn Reson Med. 2013;70(4):1173–81.
23. Jang H, Liu F, Bradshaw T, McMillan AB. Rapid dual-echo ramped hybrid encoding MR-based attenuation correction (dRHE-MRAC) for PET/MR. Magn Reson Med. 2018;79(6):2912–22.
24. Jang H, Ma Y, Searleman AC, et al. Inversion recovery UTE based volumetric myelin imaging in human brain using interleaved hybrid encoding. Magn Reson Med. 2020;83(3):950–61.
25. Jang H, Liu F, Zhao G, Bradshaw T, McMillan AB. Technical note: deep learning based MRAC using rapid ultrashort echo time imaging. Med Phys. 2018;45(8):3697–704.
26. Jang H, McMillan AB, Ma Y, et al. Rapid single scan ramped hybrid-encoding for bicomponent T_2^* mapping in a human knee joint: a feasibility study. NMR Biomed. 2020;33(11):e4391.
27. Sheth VR, Fan S, He Q, et al. Inversion recovery ultrashort echo time magnetic resonance imaging: a method for simultaneous direct detection of myelin and high signal demonstration of iron deposition in the brain—a feasibility study. Magn Reson Imaging. 2017;38:87–94.
28. Seifert AC, Li C, Wilhelm MJ, Wehrli SL, Wehrli FW. Towards quantification of myelin by solid-state MRI of the lipid matrix protons. NeuroImage. 2017;163:358–67.
29. Ma Y, Searleman AC, Jang H, et al. Volumetric imaging of myelin in vivo using 3D inversion recovery-prepared ultrashort echo time cones magnetic resonance imaging. NMR Biomed. 2020;33(10):e4326.
30. Jang H, Wei Z, Wu M, et al. Improved volumetric myelin imaging in human brain using 3D dual echo inversion recovery-prepared UTE with complex echo subtraction. Magn Reson Med. 2020;83(4):1168–77.
31. Nelson F, Poonawalla A, Hou P, Wolinsky J, Narayana P. 3D MPRAGE improves classification of cortical lesions in multiple sclerosis. Mult Scler. 2008;14(9):1214–9.

32. Ma Y, Jerban S, Carl M, et al. Imaging of the region of the osteochondral junction (OCJ) using a 3D adiabatic inversion recovery prepared ultrashort echo time cones (3D IR-UTE-cones) sequence at 3 T. NMR Biomed. 2019;32(5):e4080.

33. Jang H, Carl M, Ma Y, et al. Inversion recovery zero echo time (IR-ZTE) imaging for direct myelin detection in human brain: a feasibility study. Quant Imaging Med Surg. 2020;10(5):895–906.

34. Ma Y, Jang H, Lombardi AF, Corey-Bloom J, Bydder GM. Myelin water imaging using a short-TR adiabatic inversion-recovery (STAIR) sequence. Magn Reson Med. 2022;88(3):1156–69.

35. Schepkin VD. Sodium MRI of glioma in animal models at ultrahigh magnetic fields. NMR Biomed. 2016;29(2):175–86.

36. Nagel AM, Bock M, Hartmann C, et al. The potential of relaxation-weighted sodium magnetic resonance imaging as demonstrated on brain tumors. Investig Radiol. 2011;46(9):539–47.

37. Ouwerkerk R, Bleich KB, Gillen JS, Pomper MG, Bottomley PA. Tissue sodium concentration in human brain tumors as measured with 23Na MR imaging. Radiology. 2003;227(2):529–37.

38. Wetterling F, Gallagher L, MacRae IM, Junge S, Fagan AJ. Regional and temporal variations in tissue sodium concentration during the acute stroke phase. Magn Reson Med. 2012;67(3):740–9.

39. Tsang A, Stobbe RW, Asdaghi N, et al. Relationship between sodium intensity and perfusion deficits in acute ischemic stroke. J Magn Reson Imaging. 2011;33(1):41–7.

40. Inglese M, Madelin G, Oesingmann N, et al. Brain tissue sodium concentration in multiple sclerosis: a sodium imaging study at 3 tesla. Brain. 2010;133(3):847–57.

41. Zbýň Š, Mlynárik V, Juras V, Szomolanyi P, Trattnig S. Evaluation of cartilage repair and osteoarthritis with sodium MRI. NMR Biomed. 2016;29(2):206–15.

42. Marik W, Nemec SF, Zbýň Š, et al. Changes in cartilage and tendon composition of patients with type I diabetes mellitus. Investig Radiol. 2016;51(4):266–72.

43. Madelin G, Babb JS, Xia D, Chang G, Jerschow A, Regatte RR. Reproducibility and repeatability of quantitative sodium magnetic resonance imaging in vivo in articular cartilage at 3 T and 7 T. Magn Reson Med. 2012;68(3):841–9.

44. Blunck Y, Moffat BA, Kolbe SC, Ordidge RJ, Cleary JO, Johnston LA. Zero-gradient-excitation ramped hybrid encoding (zG RF -RHE) sodium MRI. Magn Reson Med. 2019;81(2):1172–80.

45. Weiger M, Froidevaux R, Baadsvik EL, Brunner DO, Rösler MB, Pruessmann KP. Advances in MRI of the myelin bilayer. NeuroImage. 2020;217:116888.

Acquisition-Weighted Stack of Spirals (AWSOS) MRI

Yongxian Qian and Fernando E. Boada

Introduction

This chapter is based on research about technical development and clinical applications of the acquisition-weighted stack of spirals (AWSOS) technique that we have published over the last decade [1–5]. Currently, AWSOS pulse sequences are routinely used in our research projects. In this chapter we integrate our latest experience with our earlier publications and organize the presentation so readers can easily understand the ideas and mathematics behind the technique and quickly learn how to implement it in practice.

In this chapter, ultrashort echo time (UTE) refers to an echo time less than 1.0 ms measured from the *center* of the radiofrequency (RF) excitation pulse to the start of data acquisition at the k-space center, rather than time measured from the *end* of the RF excitation pulse to the beginning of data acquisition which, instead of TE, is called the delay time. The main driving force for UTE techniques is clinical demand for noninvasive visualization of short-T_2 tissues such as cartilage (deep layers), menisci, ligaments, tendons, parts of muscles, cortical bones, and similar tissues [6]. These tissues are not visible using conventional MRI protocols with long TEs of >10 ms.

UTE imaging pulse sequences are specially designed to minimize signal decay caused by fast transverse relaxation (T_2 usually <10 ms). To do so, designs of pulse sequences aim to make three of their main components as short as possible, namely, RF excitation, delay time, and data acquisition. For instance, RF pulses are usually designed with power-efficient rectangular shapes (hard pulses) with a short duration of 0.05–1.0 ms. Delay times are usually as short as the hardware allows (e.g., 0.02 ms). The relevant hardware components include analog-to-digital converters (ADCs) and RF coils. Efforts in this direction have resulted in very short TEs of 0.6 ms or less on clinical MRI scanners [7, 8]. Data acquisition time (or ADC readout time, T_s) is associated with the sequence k-space trajectory which may be radial and consist of a straight line starting from the center of k-space and going out to its periphery. Radial trajectories of this type offer the shortest readout time of all k-space trajectories. However, it is highly challenging to take advantage of this short readout time while meeting clinical needs for limited total acquisition (TA) time, high spatial resolution, and high signal-to-noise ratio (SNR). Trade-offs have to be made among these needs for a pulse sequence to be clinically feasible and useful.

To minimize T_2-related signal decay, an ideal design of a pulse sequence is to combine a rectangular RF pulse with radial k-space acquisition, using the minimum (hardware limited) delay time. Use of a rectangular shape makes the RF pulse most power-efficient (thus shortest duration) among other shapes for a given flip angle. The radial trajectory makes data acquisition shortest among all types of k-space trajectories in order to minimize T_2-related signal decay. This ideal case, however, requires a relatively long scan time, such as 54 min for a typical three-dimensional (3D) isotropic image with a field of view (FOV) of 220 mm, matrix size 256×256, and repetition time (TR) 20 ms. This long scan time is not practical for clinical imaging and would limit UTE imaging to low spatial resolutions such as a matrix size of 64×64 for a clinically acceptable 3.5 min acquisition. Images with spatial resolution this low may not be clinically useful.

To reduce scan time while keeping spatial resolution high, the AWSOS technique employs a novel strategy inspired by the framework of acquisition-weighted data collections [6], in which 3D isotropic imaging is divided into 2D in-plane and 1D slice components. In this way, AWSOS not only dramatically reduces scan time for high in-plane resolution acquisitions but also increases SNR as the slice thickness is relatively large compared to the in-plane pixel size. To achieve this goal, the AWSOS sequence employs two measures. First, the slab-select gradient-refocusing lobe is sig-

Y. Qian (✉) · F. E. Boada
Department of Radiology, Center for Biomedical Imaging,
New York University Grossman School of Medicine,
New York, NY, USA
e-mail: Yongxian.Qian@nyulangone.org

nificantly reduced by lowering the amplitude of the slab-select gradient. Second, the in-plane phase and frequency encodings are replaced by fast spiral trajectories to substantially accelerate in-plane data collections. T_2-related signal decay during spiral readouts is minimized by properly selecting the number of spirals. The AWSOS technique acquires k-space data with a delay that varies with the duration of the slice encoding and is therefore referred to as acquisition-weighted stack of spirals, or AWSOS. There is independent selection of in-plane resolution and slice thickness. The AWSOS pulse sequence is able to generate high in-plane resolution (<1 mm) while keeping slice thickness unchanged (thus keeping total scan time short and SNR high).

This chapter is a summary based mainly on our previously published work [1–5], but is reorganized to simplify the description of the concepts, mathematics, and implementation. The chapter includes sections on the pulse sequence, mathematics, data acquisition, and technical tips, as well as exemplary images of the brain and knee at 1.5 T, 3 T, and 7 T to demonstrate the performance of the AWSOS sequence.

Pulse Sequence

The AWSOS pulse sequence has three principal features: selective excitation, variable-duration slice encoding, and movable spiral readout (Fig. 8.1a). The selective excitation is implemented using a frequency selective RF pulse, such as a sinc or Shinnar-Le Roux (SLR) pulse, combined with a slab-select gradient of low amplitude to allow use of a short refo-

cusing lobe. The special requirement for a short lobe highlights the need for highly selective RF pulses (i.e., with a narrow transition between passband and stopband) in order to attain a flat profile for the excited slab. This also creates a design challenge because low gradient amplitudes stretch the RF response and so enlarge the transition band which leads to a roll-off slab profile. Our experience suggests that a sinc pulse of cycle 1.5 or more is needed to reduce the transition band [1]. Another challenge in the design of the RF pulse is the concern about the specific absorption rate (SAR) when a short RF pulse (with a large B_1 value) is used to minimize TE. RF amplifier protection of MRI systems sets a limit on the maximum value of B_1 for certain types of coils (e.g., 25 μT for head coils) and thus restricts the minimum duration (or maximum flip angle) of RF pulses that is allowed. SAR issues attract more attention with short RF pulses than with long RF pulses, because peak power is inversely related to duration of the RF pulse. Volume-averaged SAR was calculated for the RF pulses used in AWSOS sequences using the formulas provided in Ref. [9]. Both B_1 and SAR restrictions were addressed in the design of the RF pulses. Optimization of RF pulse duration τ, slab thickness h, and TE was performed using the well-established relationship between them [9].

The slice encoding gradient, which partitions the slab into slices, was designed in such a way that the maximum slew rate (SR) of the MRI system (or the preset value in the protocol) was always used until the gradient amplitude reached the maximum value allowed by the system (or the protocol). Thus, the duration of the slice encoding gradient was minimized at each encoding step k_z and varied from one step to

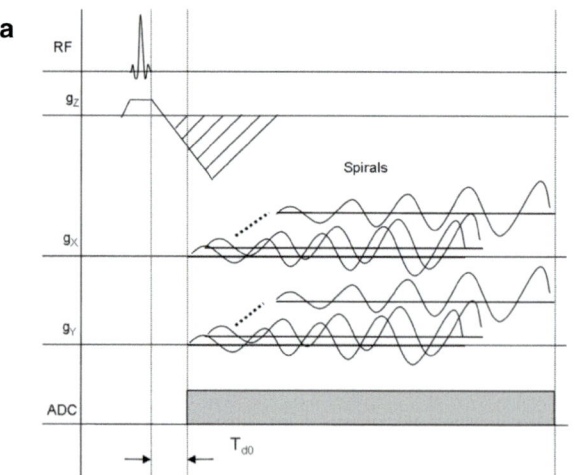
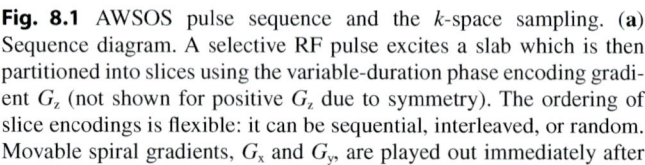
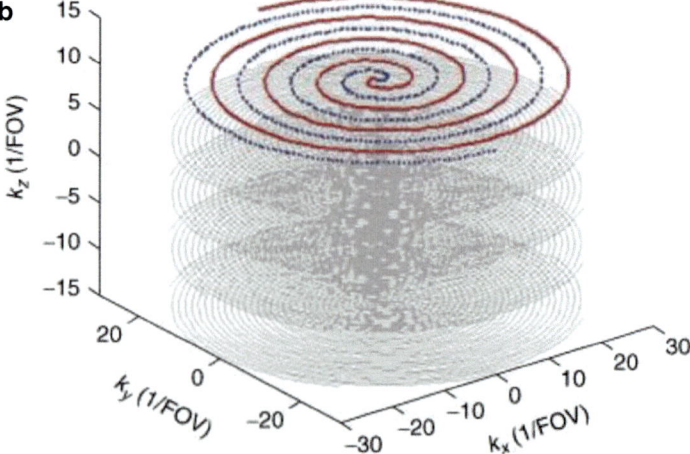

Fig. 8.1 AWSOS pulse sequence and the k-space sampling. (**a**) Sequence diagram. A selective RF pulse excites a slab which is then partitioned into slices using the variable-duration phase encoding gradient G_z (not shown for positive G_z due to symmetry). The ordering of slice encodings is flexible: it can be sequential, interleaved, or random. Movable spiral gradients, G_x and G_y, are played out immediately after

the slice encodings. ADC data acquisition starts at the beginning of spirals. A minimum delay of T_{d0} is required. This needs to be determined from the system hardware parameters, e.g., 20 μs in some MRI scanners. (**b**) A cylindrical volume in k-space is sampled by AWSOS data acquisitions via using interleaved spirals (red and blue). (Adopted with permission from Refs [1, 5])

another. In addition, the slice encoding gradient overlapped the refocusing lobe of slab-select gradient to reduce the total duration of the spatial encoding process.

Spiral readouts with the AWSOS pulse sequence start immediately after slice encoding, and data acquisition is performed in a plane perpendicular to the slab direction. To match the variable duration of the slice encoding, the starting time of the spiral gradients and readout is shifted, leading to movable spiral readout (Fig. 8.1a).

The AWSOS pulse sequence samples k-space in a cylindrical volume (Fig. 8.1b), with the symmetrical axis in the slab direction (defined as the k_z direction). The slice thickness, Δz, is determined by the maximum value of k_z, while the slab thickness, h, limits the increment, Δk_z, for full sampling under Nyquist sampling criteria. A disk-like area in the (k_x, k_y) plane is sampled using the spiral. The radius of the disk is determined by the in-plane spatial resolution Δx. Independent selection of in-place resolution from slice thickness offers the opportunity to increase in-plane resolution while keeping slice thickness unchanged and thus maintain a reasonable SNR.

Image reconstruction of raw data acquired with the AWSOS pulse sequence is the same as that for regular spiral k-space data sets [1]. First, fast Fourier transform (FFT) is performed along the slice encoding (k_z) direction to decompose the 3D AWSOS data sets into 2D. Then, a regridding algorithm [10, 11] is used to reconstruct images from the spiral data set on a slice-by-slice basis.

Mathematics

Slab-Select Gradient and Minimum TE

The amplitude G_0 of the slab-select gradient pulse is related to the slab thickness h,

$$G_0 = 4\eta_c / (\gamma h \tau_{rf}) \tag{8.1}$$

where γ is gyromagnetic ratio in Hz/T, η_c is the sinc cycle, and τ_{rf} is the duration of the RF pulse. The minimum echo time (TE$_{min}$) is associated with the RF excitation and given by Eq. 8.2:

$$\text{TE}_{min} = 0.5\tau_{rf} + t_1 + 2t_2 \tag{8.2a}$$

$$t_1 = G_0 / S_{max} \tag{8.2b}$$

$$t_2 = \sqrt{0.5 t_1 (t_1 + \tau_{rf})}, \text{with } t_2 S_{max} < G_{max} \tag{8.2c}$$

where G_{max} and S_{max} are the maximum amplitudes of the gradient and slew rate of the MRI system (or those allowed by the protocol), respectively. Optimization of RF duration τ_{rf}, slab thickness h, and minimum echo time TE$_{min}$ is implemented using Eqs. 8.1 and 8.2.

Slice Encoding Gradient

To make TE$_{min}$ as short as possible, the slice encoding gradient is overlapped with the refocusing lobe of the slab-select gradient (Fig. 8.1a), using slightly different waveforms for the positive and negative steps of k_z. In Fig. 8.3 of Ref. [2], under the slab-select gradient, area A is the area under the half constant segment, and area B is the area under the decay ramp. Area C is the refocusing area and is balanced by areas A and B. Waveforms of the slice encoding gradient are characterized using Eqs. 8.3, 8.4, and 8.5:

$$C = A + B = (1/2)G_0 (\tau_{rf} + \tau_{decay}) \tag{8.3}$$

where τ_{decay} is duration of the decay ramp. For a slice encoding step k_z, the corresponding area D is,

$$D = k_z / \gamma \tag{8.4}$$

If area D is smaller than area C, then the slice encoding waveform is switched. The total slice encoding area E is given in Eq. 8.5:

$$E = C + D, k_z < 0 \tag{8.5a}$$

$$E = C - D, k_z > 0 \text{ and } D \leq C \tag{8.5b}$$

$$E = D - C, k_z > 0 \text{ and } D > C \tag{8.5c}$$

The duration and amplitude of the resultant slice encoding gradient are calculated from the waveforms associated with area E.

Slice encoding (i.e., k_z) may be uniform or nonuniform within the limits $-k_{z,max} \leq k_z < k_{z,max}$, where the maximum value of k_z is determined by the slice thickness Δz (i.e., spatial resolution in the slice direction) and $k_{z,max} = 1/(2\Delta z)$. Slice-encoding step size Δk_z is determined by the slab thickness h and $\Delta k_z = 1/h$, when uniform sampling is implemented.

Spiral Encoding Gradients

The in-plane spiral encoding gradients (G_x, G_y) are designed using the analytical formula given by Glover [12] which generates the shortest readout time given the maximum gradient and slew rate and is efficiently computable in real time. However, the original version of Glover's spiral gradients has a risk of discontinuity at the transition between the constant slew rate segment and the constant amplitude segment when short duration spirals are used. This potential risk is avoided in the AWSOS pulse sequence by employing a modified spiral.

Spiral trajectories in the (k_x, k_y) plane are also calculated during the design of spiral gradients [13]. The number and readout time of the spiral interleaves required for Nyquist sampling are real-time evaluated for the AWSOS pulse sequence for given FOVs and matrix sizes (or in-plane resolutions). The optimal number of trajectories and readout times can then be determined for particular total acquisition times and tolerable levels of image blurring.

In addition to the use of analytical formulas, spiral trajectories and gradients can be computed in real time using numerical formulas [14] due to the tremendous improvement in computation power of MRI systems relative to that available two decades ago. The numerical computation also overcomes two pitfalls encountered in the analytical computation (i.e., discontinuity in gradients and overshoot in slew rate). The numerical computation uses the basic formula for a spiral trajectory and the relationship between gradient $g(t)$ and trajectory $k(t)$, under the constraints of maximum gradient G_{max} and maximum slew rate S_{max}, as described in Eqs. 8.6, 8.7, and 8.8:

$$k(t) = A\Theta(t)e^{j\theta(t)} \tag{8.6}$$

$$g(t) = \frac{\left(\frac{1}{\gamma}\right)dk(t)}{dt}, \text{ with } g(t) \le G_{max} \tag{8.7}$$

$$s(t) = \frac{dg(t)}{dt}, \text{ with } |s(t)| \le S_{max} \tag{8.8}$$

In Eq. 8.6, the constant A is determined by the number of spiral interleaves N_s and the FOV for full sampling in the k-space, $A = N_s/(2\pi \text{FOV})$. The time step Δt in $k(t)$ is limited to the raster time of the gradients or multiples (or fractions) of this under the constraints imposed by G_{max} and S_{max}.

Data Acquisition

MRI Systems

The AWSOS pulse sequence is applicable to clinical MRI scanners at 1.5 T, 3 T, and 7 T, with maximum gradient amplitudes of 40 mT/m and maximum slew rates of 150 T/m/s or higher. In principle, it is also applicable at low fields such as 0.5 T or lower, where it may have unique benefits in SNR resulting from the long readout time of spiral acquisitions. AWSOS pulse sequences have no extra requirement for RF transmit or receive coil performance and thus are compatible with standard coils and coil arrays for the head and body, as well as custom-built ones.

Optimization of RF Excitation

The RF excitation profile of the slab is critical for the quality of AWSOS images when the MRI system's body coil is employed for RF excitation to image a limited area of anatomy such as the head or knee. The slab profile is desired to be flat, but, in practice, it may be curved or even contaminated by wraparound artifacts when low values of the sinc cycle are used (Fig. 8.2). Use of sinc cycles of 1.0 and 1.5 can avoid wraparound artifacts, and the cycle of 1.5 produces a better profile (Fig. 8.2f, g). Use of a wide transition band in the slab profile decreases the intensity of four to five slices at each end of the slab, so that only two-thirds of the total number of slices is useful. This can be acceptable for imaging of the knee joint, but not for the head where higher and lower slices are as important as central ones. A nonselective hard pulse may be used to achieve a flat profile when a long slab is used, or a localized receive coil may be used. SLR pulses with linear or minimum phases were employed to try and achieve a flat profile, but this did not work out.

The minimum echo time (TE_{min}) achievable with the AWSOS pulse sequence depends on the RF pulse duration, slab thickness, and hardware limitations (e.g., maximum gradient G_{max} and slew rate S_{max}, coil switching time from transmit to receive mode, and pulse synchrony). TE_{min} decreases monotonically with increasing slab thickness. For instance, it is 0.98 ms at a slab thickness of 10 mm but 0.52 ms at a slab thickness of 150 mm when the RF pulse is 0.8 ms in duration. Notably, TE_{min} decreases substantially ($\sim$50%) when the slab thickness increases from 10 to 70 mm. Further increase in slab thickness does not reduce TE_{min} a lot (<20%), reflecting the small change in the duration of the refocusing gradient. TE_{min} is dominated by the duration of the refocusing gradient for short slabs but not by the duration of the RF pulse for long slabs. Therefore, decreasing the duration of RF pulse is an efficient way of producing a short TE_{min}, but this is limited by safety requirements on clinical MRI scanners. Short RF durations require large B_1 amplitudes, and the maximum B_1 is limited by the RF subsystem. Nevertheless, both RF duration and slab thickness can be adjusted to produce the shortest practical TE_{min} making careful choice of their values. For instance, to achieve a TE_{min} of 0.6 ms, the minimum slab thickness is 30 mm for an RF pulse of 0.6 ms duration, 60 mm for 0.8 ms, and 200 mm for 1.0 ms.

SAR concerns impose an extra constraint on the duration of RF pulses. SAR was estimated in our previous work [1] using volume averaging over a spherical head model via Eq. 27.43 in Haacke et al. [9]. With parameters $\sigma = 0.3$ S/m; $R = 200$ mm; $\theta = 90°$; $\rho = 1.0$ g/cm^3; TR = 100 ms; and $\tau_{rf} = 0.8$ ms, SAR was estimated as 0.165 W/kg at 1.5 T, 0.666 W/kg at 3 T, and 3.626 W/kg at 7 T, respectively. These estimates are within the IEC/FDA limit of 2 W/kg for whole body at normal operating mode [9, 15] for 1.5 T and 3 T but not for 7 T. Longer TRs (>200 ms) or smaller flip angles (<45°) are required on 7 T scanners to keep SAR within safety limits.

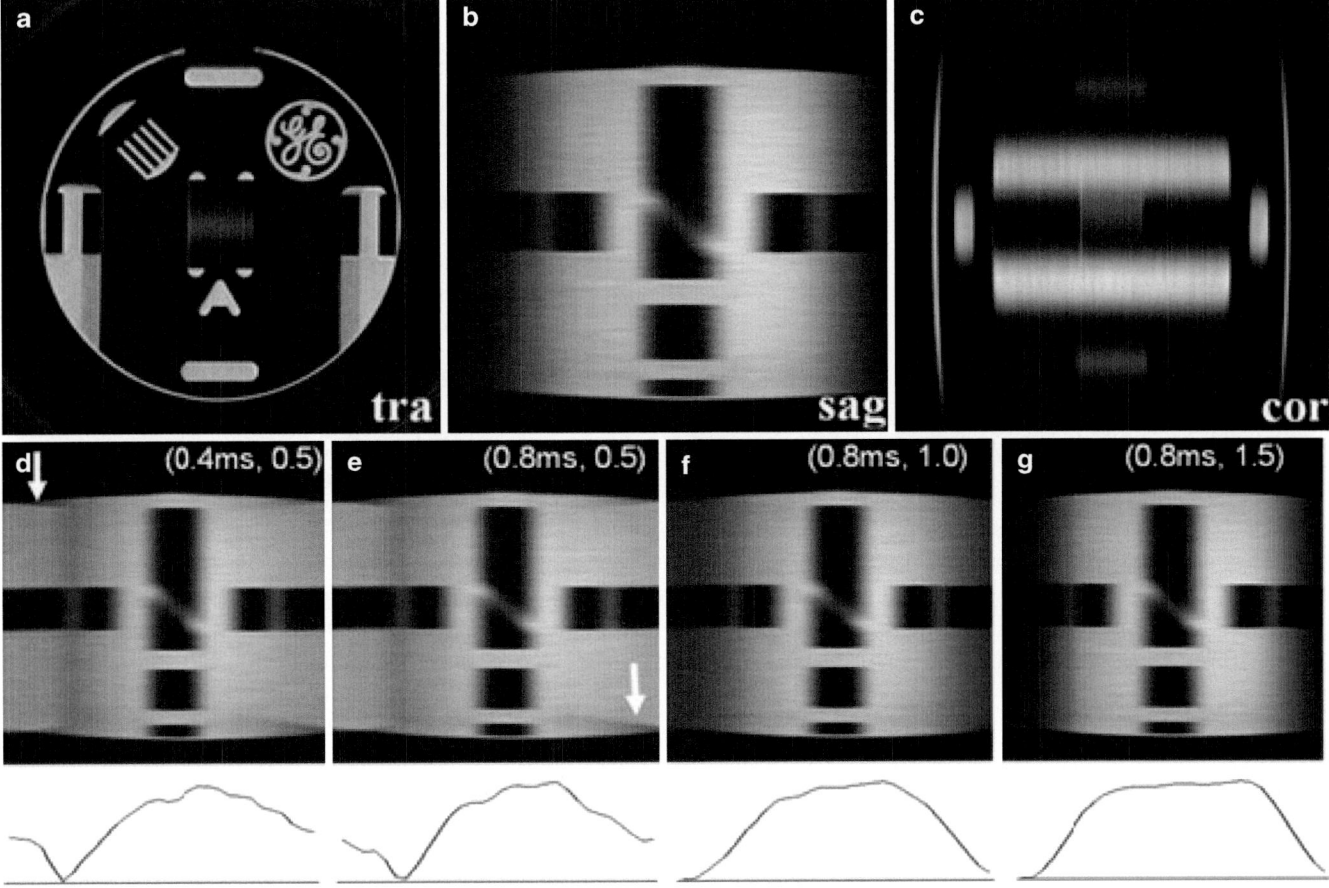

Fig. 8.2 AWSOS images of a phantom obtained at 1.5 T: (**a–c**) axial, sagittal, and coronal slices. The oblique comb bars in (**a**) are clearly visible with high in-plane resolution of 0.55 mm. (**d–g**) Sagittal images and slab profiles (below) at different durations and cycles of a sinc RF pulse. Short duration and small cycle (**d–f**) produce wrap-around arti-facts (arrows). A flat profile (**g**) is produced at 0.8 ms duration and 1.5 cycles. TE/TR = 0.608/100 ms; flip angle = 30°; FOV = 140 × 140 × 150 mm^3; matrix size = 256 × 256 × 30; and spiral interleaves = 36. (Adopted with permission from Ref. [1])

Optimal Parameters for Spiral Trajectories

The number of spiral interleaves determines the readout time of a spiral interleaf and total scan time. Use of a short read-out time means that a large number of spiral interleaves are needed. Thus, there is a trade-off between readout time and spiral number for acceptable total scan times. Given the fact that a readout time of two to three times the value of T_2 is acceptable in UTE MRI (e.g., 6–9 ms for a typical short T_2 of 3.0 ms), the optimal number of spirals is 2–4 for a matrix size of 64 × 64, 6–10 for a matrix size of 128 × 128, 18–30 for a matrix size of 256 × 256, and 60–120 for a matrix size of 512 × 512, at a FOV = 220 mm (Table 8.1) [1]. For a FOV of 140 mm as used in knee imaging, the numbers become 3–4 for a matrix size of 64 × 64, 8–12 for a matrix size of 128 × 128, and 24–40 for a matrix size of 256 × 256. The total scan time can be as short as 72 s for an in-plane FOV of 220 mm. The total scan time can be further reduced if fewer slice encodings are used.

Table 8.1 Optimal spiral gradient parameters for AWSOS sequences at G_{max} = 40 mT/m, S_{max} = 150T/m/s, and T_2 = 3 ms. (Adopted with permission from Ref. [1])

FOV (mm)	Matrix size	Resolution (mm)	Number of spirals	Readout time (ms)	Total acquisition time (s)[a]
220	64	3.44	2–4	10.120–5.064	6–12
	128	1.72	6–10	9.544–5.728	18–30
	256	0.86	18–30	9.352–5.784	54–90
	512	0.43	60–120	10.080–5.448	180–360
140	64	2.19	3–4	8.456–6.344	9–12
	128	1.09	8–12	9.088–6.160	24–36
	256	0.55	24–40	10.064–6.304	72–120

AWSOS acquisition-weighted stack of spirals, FOV field of view
[a]Calculated with TR = 100 ms and slice encoding number = 30 without signal averaging

Table 8.2 Efficiency of the AWSOS acquisitions for 3D imaging. (Adopted with permission from Ref. [1])

Sampling mode	Total shots	Ratio	Ratio at $N_{spiral} = 64$, $N_{slice} = N_{phase} = 256$
Cartesian/partial radial[a]	$N_{slice} \times N_{phase}$	1.0	1.0
Full radial	$\pi N_{phase} \times N_{phase}$	$\pi N_{phase}/N_{slice}$	3.14
AWSOS	$N_{slice} \times N_{spiral}$	N_{spiral}/N_{phase}	0.25

AWOS acquisition-weighted stack of spirals, 3D three-dimensional
[a]Partial radial sampling takes 32% (or $1/\pi$) of that for full radial projections. Isotropic resolution in the three spatial directions was used in the calculation

Typical MRI Scans of the Head and Knee

For scans of the human head at 1.5 T and 3 T, the following parameters are used in our practice: a sinc pulse of 0.8 ms duration and 1.5 cycles to excite a slab of 180 mm thickness to obtain 60 slices of 3 mm thickness (or 120 mm slab thickness for 60 slices of 2 mm thickness); axial slice orientation; TE/TR = 0.6/100 ms (with fat saturation); flip angle = 30°; in-plane square FOV of 220 mm; spiral interleaves = 24 at matrix size 256 × 256 (resolution = 0.86 mm), or 64 at matrix size 512 × 512 (resolution = 0.43 mm), or 512 at matrix size 1024 × 1024 (TR = 40 ms) (resolution = 0.22 mm). TR is adjustable to produce a total acquisition time within an acceptable range.

For scans of the human knee joint at 1.5 T and 3 T, we suggest similar parameters: i.e., a sinc pulse of 0.8 ms duration and 1.5 cycles to excite a slab of 120 mm thickness for 60 slices of 2 mm thickness; sagittal (coronal or axial) slice orientation; TE/TR = 0.6/80 ms (with fat saturation); flip angle = 30°; in-plane square FOV of 140 mm; spiral interleaves = 24 at matrix size 256 × 256 (resolution = 0.55 mm), or 64 at matrix size 512 × 512 (resolution = 0.27 mm), or 512 at matrix size 1024 × 1024 (with TR = 40 ms) (resolution = 0.14 mm).

For scans of the human head/knee at 7 T, the following parameters are changed: a sinc pulse of 1.0 ms duration and 1.5 cycles to excite a slab of 180 mm for 60 slices of 3 mm thickness (or 120 mm slab thickness for 60 slices at a 2 mm thickness); TE/TR = 0.6/100 ms (with fat saturation); and flip angle = 18–20°. Other parameters are the same as those used at 3 T.

Sampling Efficiency and SNR

The efficiency of AWSOS sampling is similar to that of conventional stack of spirals acquisitions [1, 16] and is measured using the total number of shots ($N_{slice} \times N_{spiral}$) needed for a Nyquist sampling. The SNR of AWSOS images is estimated by comparing image intensity computed using the point spread function (PSF) and its full width at half maximum (FWHM). This includes effects due to T_2 decay during slice encoding and spiral readout. The noise variance is computed using a formula for weighted multiple random vari-

ables (Eq. 8.29 as described by Liang and Lauterbur [17]). This gives the formulas shown in Eqs. 8.9 and 8.10:

$$SNR \propto psf(0)(FWHM)^2 \left(N_{slice} N_{spiral} N_{pts} \right)^{1/2} / \eta \quad (8.9)$$

$$\eta \equiv \left(N_{spiral} N_{pts} \sum_k w_k^2 \right)^{1/2} \quad (8.10)$$

where N_{pts} is data points per spiral interleaf, w_k is sampling-density weighting at each point, $\eta \approx 1.0$, and $N_{spiral}N_{pts} \approx N_{phase}N_{freq}$ for full spiral sampling and N_{phase} (N_{freq}) is the number of phase encodings (frequency encoding points). Thus, SNR in spiral sampling is almost the same as for Cartesian sampling, when T_2 decay is ignored.

Table 8.2 lists the efficiency of AWSOS sampling relative to Cartesian and radial sampling. Although UTE imaging needs more spirals than conventional long-TE imaging to minimize T_2 decay, AWSOS sampling is 4 times as fast as Cartesian or partial radial sampling, and 12 times as fast as full radial sampling. The SNR of a voxel on AWSOS images was found to be 91–97% of that without T_2 decay, at four tested ratios of sampling time T_s to T_2, i.e., $T_s/T_2 = 0.867$, 1.07, 1.93, and 3.21. Spiral readout time did not change SNR significantly (<10%).

Technical Tips

Positioning of Study Subjects

The AWSOS sequence employs a non-Cartesian data acquisition with a spiral trajectory, and so there is no simple relationship between the image domain object and k-space data in shifting FOVs. As a result, non-Cartesian sampling does not support shifting of the FOV on the display screen without additional adjustment [18]. Adding a phase term to the raw data is necessary to support FOV shifting during data acquisition via analog/digital conversion (ADC) or during image reconstruction through mathematically complex multiplication. Current approaches provided by MRI systems, such as phase modification to waveforms of spiral encoding gradients, allow operators to shift FOVs on the display screen, but this generates image distortion when large shifts are made (Fig. 8.3). To mitigate this type of distortion, our experience suggests positioning the area of interest (e.g., head or knee

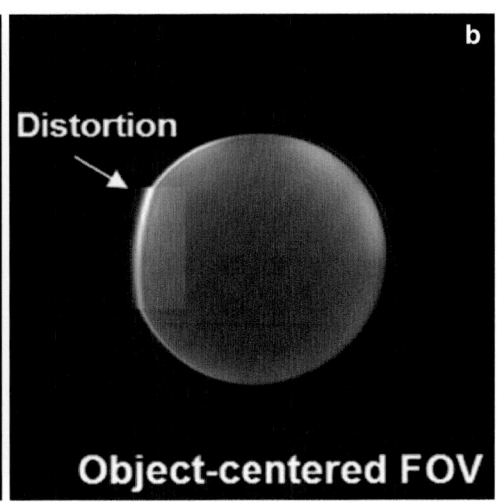

Fig. 8.3 AWSOS positioning and image distortion of a bottle phantom at 3 T: (**a**) isocenter and (**b**) off-isocenter positioning of the FOV. At the isocenter FOV in (**a**), there is no image distortion (arrow, magnified zone). At the off-isocenter FOV in (**b**), there is image distortion (arrow, magnified zone). The off-isocenter FOV in (**b**) was obtained with the object at the center of the prescribed FOV. TE/TR = 0.6/30 ms; $\theta = 15°$; FOV = 220 mm; and matrix size = 256. (Adopted with permission from Ref. [3])

joint) at the isocenter of the magnet, or as close as possible to this, and ideally within a small fraction of the FOV (<10% of FOV) [3]. In the slice direction, however, the AWSOS sequence allows free positioning as it uses uniform encoding.

Figure 8.3 demonstrates the effect of positioning on image blurring. A standard bottle phantom was scanned with and without centering the FOV (220 mm). When the FOV was placed at the isocenter of the magnet, the phantom image had no distortion as shown in the magnified zone in Fig. 8.3a. When the FOV was shifted away from the isocenter by distances of $\Delta x = 54.3$ mm and $\Delta y = 33.0$ mm, and repositioned at the center of the phantom, the image showed obvious distortion (Fig. 8.3b). However, no distortion was observed when the FOV was shifted distances less than 20 mm (not shown in the figure). Thus, isocenter positioning minimizes image distortion relative to off-center positioning.

B_0 Field Shimming

Spiral data acquisitions in the k-space are sensitive to inhomogeneity of the B_0 field, and this causes image blurring [19]. The blurring can be minimized by good shimming (linewidth <60 Hz at 3 T). This is achievable through manual shimming and frequency adjustment (a process that removes the constant and linear terms in the B_0 field inhomogeneity), as well as by use of a short spiral readout time [20]. Manual shimming, including frequency adjustment, usually needs three iterations and requires ~1.5 min to complete, which is

relatively long compared to auto shimming which requires ~0.5 min to complete.

Image Blurring Due to Off-Resonance Effects

Image blurring due to off-resonance is much larger than that due to T_2 decay and can range from 1–40 times pixel size [1, 13]. For instance, image blurring is 12 times pixel size with a readout duration of 9.352 ms and a small frequency offset of 1.0 ppm and 40 times pixel size at 3.4 ppm frequency offset (i.e., that of fat signals). As a result, fat signal suppression is critically important for AWSOS imaging. In addition, large scale blurring is accompanied by wide scattering of pixel energy, and this leads to pixel intensities as low as 20% of the original value, or even down to the level of background noise at high field (≥3 T). As a consequence of this, the spiral readout has an inherent ability to suppress off-resonance signals. More details about the spiral off-resonance effects and corrections can be found in work by Noll et al. [19] and Yudilevich and Stark [20].

Image Blurring Due to T_2^* Decay

T_2^* decay during spiral readout serves as a windowing function in k-space and causes image blurring which can be assessed by measuring the FWHM of the PSF. Blurring increases linearly with spiral readout time [1]. T_2^* relaxation adds 40–66% blurring to a pixel when the spiral readout is two to three times T_2^*. On average, 20% blurring is produced by each T_2^* period in the readout. Notably, even without T_2^* relaxation, spiral sampling itself contributes 23% to blurring because of its disk region in k-space. The pixel size at a readout time of three times T_2^* nearly doubles pixel size. In addition, pixel intensity, characterized by the PSF maximum, also decreases with spiral readout time. The intensity is reduced to 50–42% from its relaxation free value at readouts between two to three times T_2^*. Thus, T_2^* relaxation significantly increases image blurring when spiral readouts are used. However, this negative effect can be controlled by use of short spiral readouts, such as those about twice the duration of T_2^*. These are usually acceptable because the moderate image blurring is compensated for by a substantially reduced total acquisition time.

Examples: Brain Imaging

Figure 8.4 shows AWSOS head images of a healthy volunteer obtained at 1.5 T (GE Signa, Milwaukee, WI) with a maximum gradient amplitude of 40 mT/m and a maximum slew rate of 150 T/m/s. A GE standard birdcage head coil was used. The study was approved by our institutional review board (IRB). The slices were selected to show most of the excited slab centered at slice #15. A high in-plane nominal resolution of 0.86 mm was attained, clearly showing small structures in the nasal cartilages as well as in white and gray matter. The high spatial resolution also resulted in very little image blurring from inhomogeneity of the B_0 field. Measurement showed that fluctuation of the B_0 field during scanning was within 1.0 ppm.

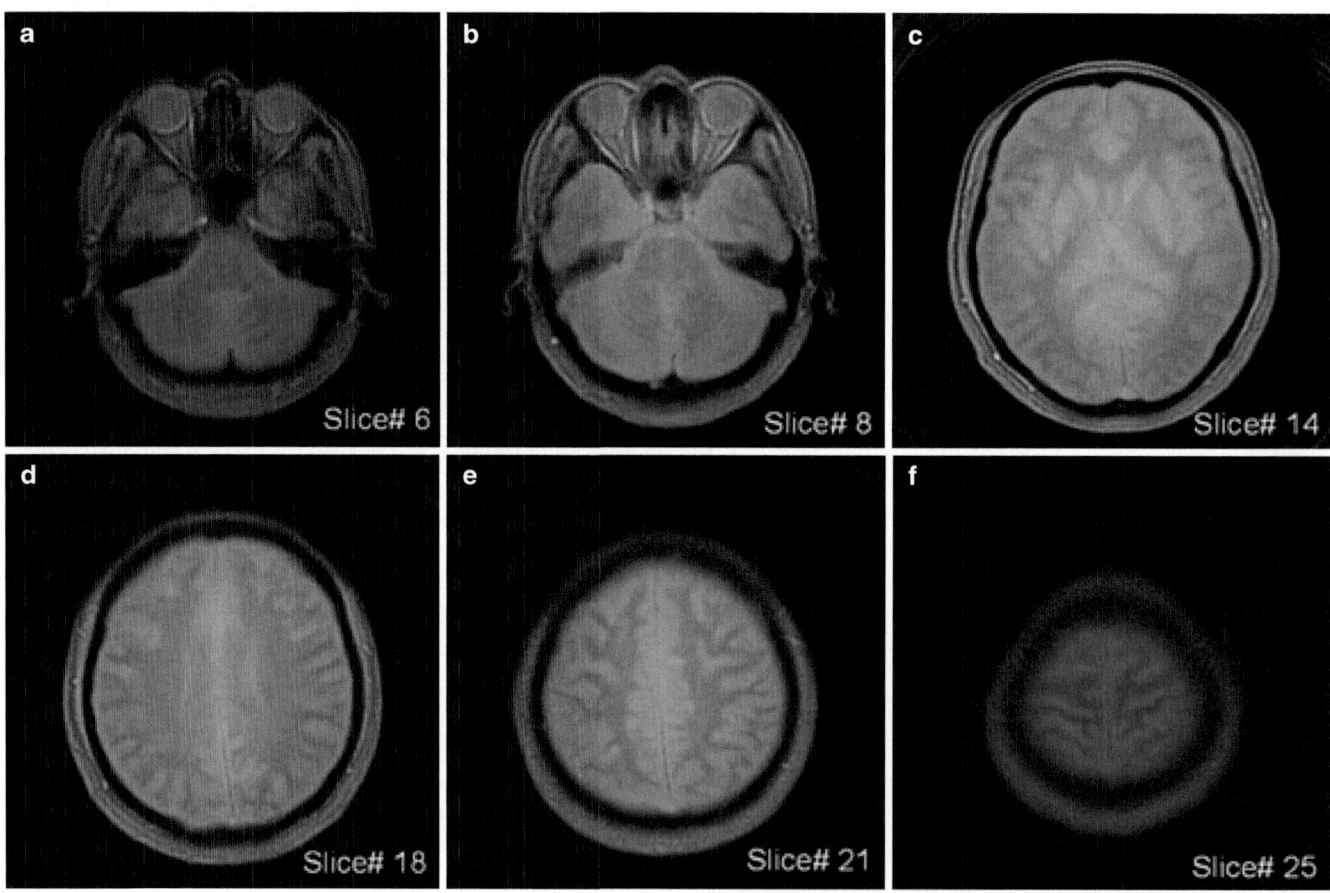

Fig. 8.4 AWSOS images of a healthy human brain at 1.5 T: (**a–f**) representative slices displayed at the same window width and level. The intensities of side slices #6 (**a**) and #25 (**f**) are decreased due to the transition band of the RF pulse. TE/TR = 0.608/500 ms; flip angle = 30°; FOV = 220 × 220 × 150 mm³; matrix size = 256 × 256 × 30; and sinc RF pulse of 0.8 ms duration and 1.5 cycles. (Adopted with permission from Ref. [1])

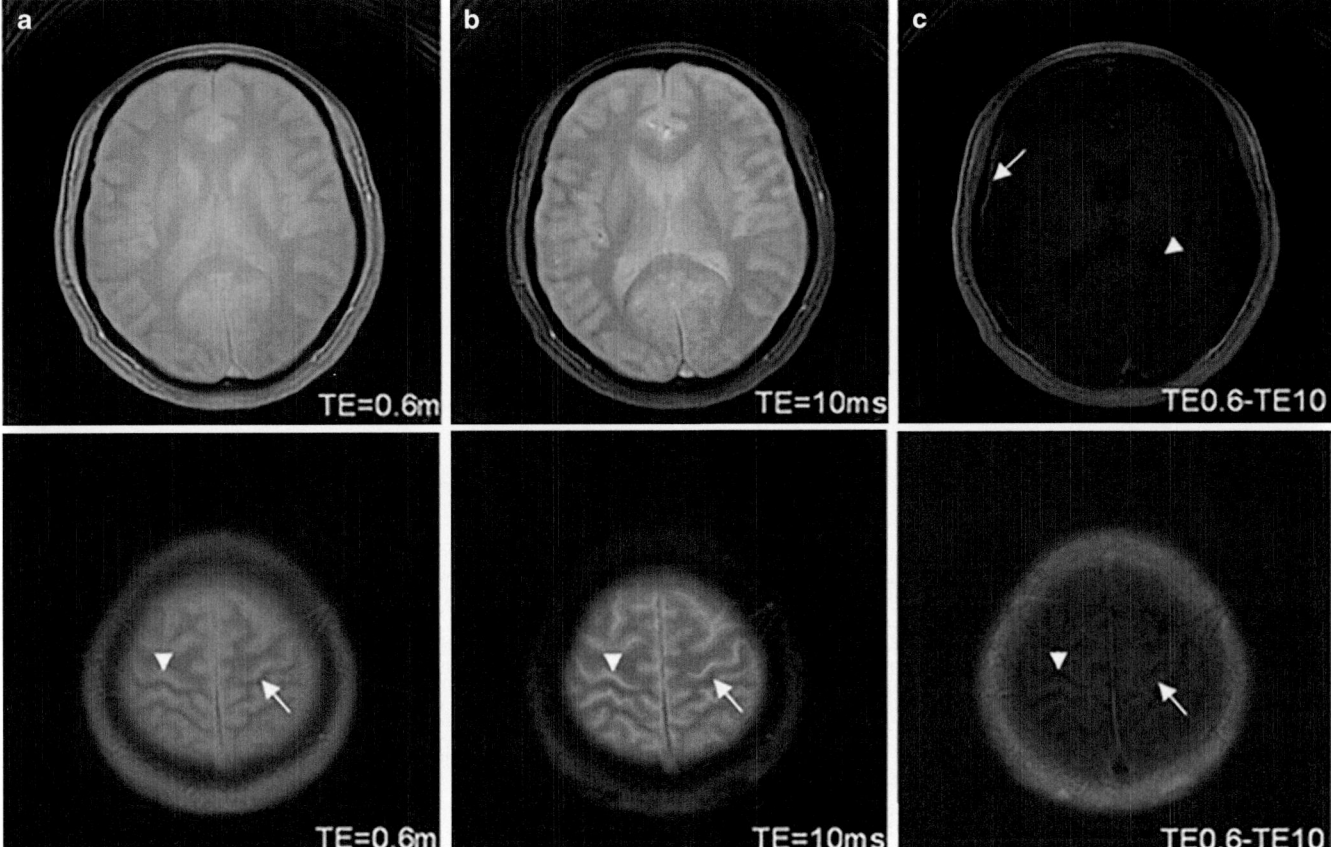

Fig. 8.5 AWSOS images of a healthy human brain at 1.5 T (two slices in the upper and lower rows): (**a**) UTE, (**b**) long TE, and (**c**) difference between (**a**) and (**b**). The difference images highlight meninges and parenchyma (arrows) but show low signal in CSF in the ventricles and in the parenchyma (arrowheads). (Adopted with permission from Ref. [1])

Figure 8.4 also demonstrates substantial signal from short-T_2 tissues. The nasal cartilage and optic nerve, which are rich in short-T_2 components, show high intensity on the UTE image (Fig. 8.4a). This high signal may be helpful in the diagnosis and monitoring of fractured nasal cartilages and disease of the optic nerve.

Figure 8.5 shows difference images between UTE (0.6 ms) and long TE (10 ms) images. In the top row, the meninges are highlighted on the difference image. Also shown is reduction of CSF signal in the lateral ventricles which may find applications in the imaging of adjacent disease of the brain. In the bottom row, the brain parenchyma is dominated by hyperintense CSF and blood vessels on both UTE and long TE images. In contrast, the difference image highlights the brain itself and depicts structures which may be helpful in disease diagnosis and treatment monitoring.

Examples: Knee Imaging

AWSOS knee imaging was implemented on a clinical 3T scanner (Magnetom Trio Tim, Siemens Medical Solutions, Erlangen, Germany) using an eight channel knee coil (In vivo, Gainesville, FL). The study protocols were approved by the authors' IRB [3].

Patellar Cartilage and Tendon Images

Figure 8.6 shows AWSOS images of the knee joint of a healthy subject. Figure 8.6 (top) shows patellar cartilage at two high resolutions of 0.28 mm and 0.14 mm, respectively. In Fig. 8.6a, patellar cartilage is fully visible but is only partially visible on conventional images obtained at a long TE ($\approx$10 ms). The zoom-in inset clearly presents hyperintensity

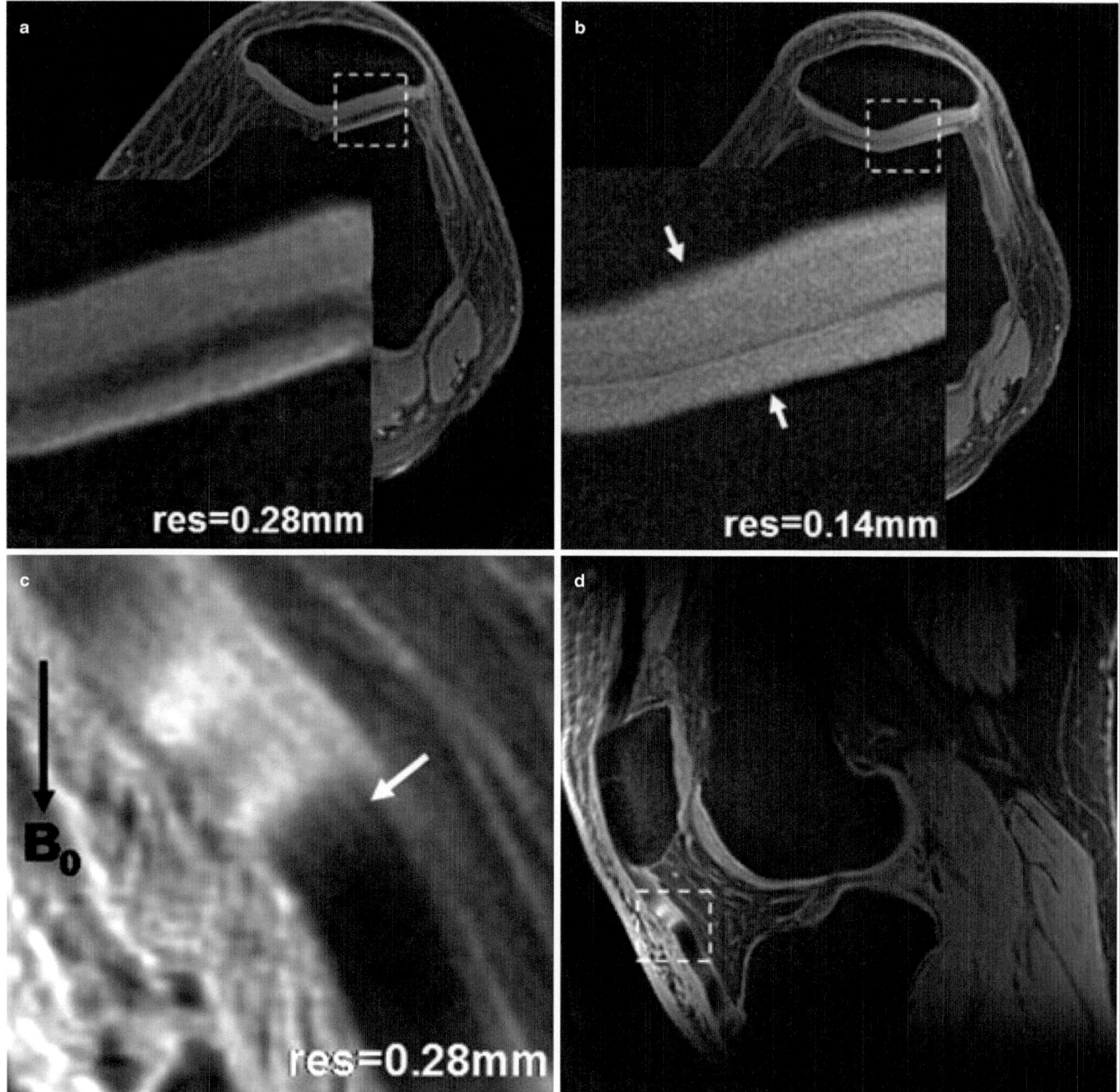

Fig. 8.6 AWSOS high-resolution UTE image of patellar cartilage and tendon in a healthy subject at 3 T. (**a**) high- and (**b**) ultrahigh resolution, with the inserts showing microstructure in cartilage (arrows). (**c**, **d**) Local and full views of the patellar tendon, clearly illustrating collagen bundles inside the tendon (arrow). B_0 indicates the direction of main magnetic field. The magic angle effect alters the intensity of the tendon in (**c**) and (**d**) and produces high signal leading to a bright and dark appearance. TE/TR = 0.6/80 ms; θ = 30°; FOV = 140 mm; slice thickness = 2 mm at matrix size = 512 (**a**); and 3 mm at matrix size = 1024 and TR = 60 ms (**b**). (Adopted with permission from Ref. [3])

across the entire depth of the cartilage, especially in the deep uncalcified cartilage. Even brighter signal is visible in the calcified layer adjacent to subchondral bone. Across the tissue, signal intensity increases from superficial to deep layers, reflecting T_1 values decreasing from superficial to deep tissue, as the UTE image is T_1-weighted (TE/TR = 0.6/80 ms).

In Fig. 8.6b, the higher-resolution image (0.14 mm) shows radial microstructure in the patellar cartilage next to the cartilage/bone interface and thus has the potential to detect microdamage in early osteoarthritis (OA).

Figure 8.6 (bottom) shows a patellar tendon image obtained at a high resolution of 0.28 mm, with clearly visible collagen structure inside, which is otherwise hypointense (dark) on conventional MRI at a long TE ($\approx$10 ms). The bright and dark areas in the tendon illustrate magic angle effects resulting from varying orientation of the collagen fibers to the static magnetic field. This is consistent with previous reports of the magic angle effect in tendons [21].

Meniscus, ACL, and PCL

Figure 8.7 demonstrates a meniscus in high-resolution transverse and sagittal views [3]. The transverse view clearly shows both the medial and lateral menisci (Fig. 8.7a, b), while the sagittal view demonstrates high signal intensity

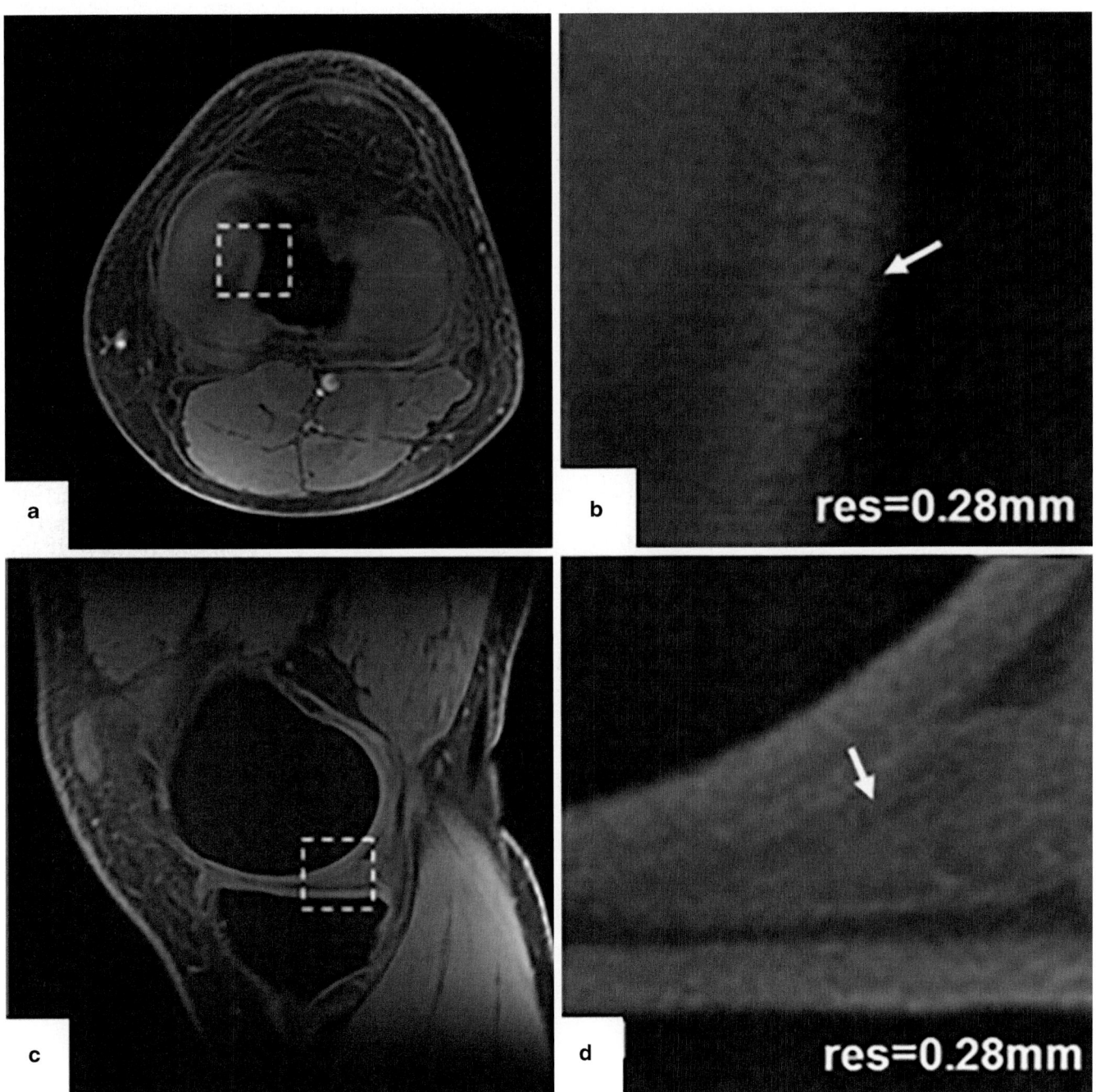

Fig. 8.7 AWSOS high-resolution UTE image of the meniscus in a healthy subject at 3 T. (**a**, **b**) Full and zoom-in views of in transverse orientation and (**c**, **d**) full and zoom-in views in sagittal orientation. In the zoom-in views (**b**, **d**), small fine structure in the meniscus is clearly visible (arrows). TE/TR = 0.6/80 ms; θ = 30°; FOV = 140 mm; matrix size = 512; and slice thickness = 2 mm. (Adopted with permission from Ref. [3])

throughout the meniscus (Fig. 8.7c, d). The zoom-in images illustrate fine structure in the medial edge of the meniscus (Fig. 8.7b) and central structures on the sagittal view (Fig. 8.7d). Figure 8.8 shows high-resolution UTE images of

the anterior cruciate ligament (ACL) and the posterior cruciate ligament (PCL). The ligaments appear hyperintense, in contrast to their hypointense appearance with long TE images. Ligaments and entheses are also clearly visible.

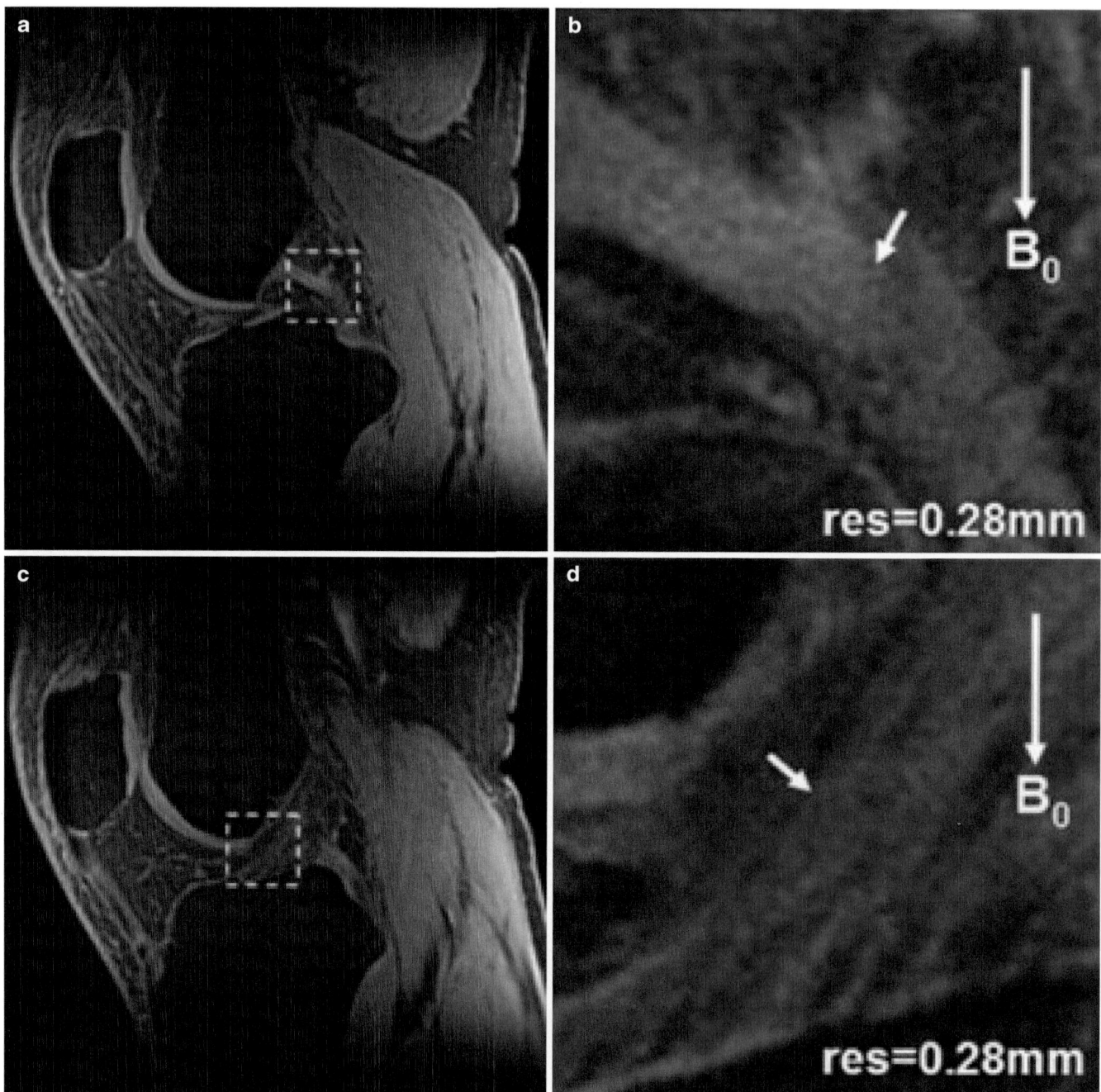

Fig. 8.8 AWSOS high-resolution UTE image of the PCL (**a**, **b**) and ACL (**c**, **d**) in a healthy subject at 3 T. B_0 indicates the direction of main magnetic field. Full (**a**, **c**) and zoom-in views (**b**, **d**) are shown. In the zoom-in views, PCL (**b**) and ACL (**d**) bundles (arrows) are clearly vis- ible (arrows). TE/TR = 0.6/80 ms; θ = 30°; FOV = 140 mm; slice thickness = 2 mm; and matrix size 512. (Adopted with permission from Ref. [3])

Examples: Imaging at 7 T

The 7T MRI has the potential to double the SNR of images relative to the 3 T. This is critically important when ultrahigh-resolution (0.14 mm) UTE imaging is pursued to detect subtle defects and alterations in key tissues of the knee joint, such as cartilage, meniscus, ligaments, tendons, and the chondro-osseous junction [22–24]. Osteoarthritis (OA), especially post-traumatic OA, in the knee joint involves multiple functional components of the joint. A comprehensive interaction among these functional tissues may be responsible for the onset and progression of OA [25, 26]. Use of 7T MRI could unleash the power of UTE imaging to detect disease onset and progression in OA.

A 7T whole-body MRI scanner (MAGNETOM 7T, Siemens) with a 28-channel Tx/Rx knee coil (QED, Ohio) was employed to study healthy subjects [4]. IRB approval and written informed consent were obtained. Data acquisition for AWSOS imaging was optimized using the following parameters: FOV = 140 × 140 × 120 mm^3; matrix size = 1024 × 1024 × 60; resolution = 0.14 × 0.14 × 2 mm^3; flip angle = 13°; fat saturation (Fatsat) = on; TE/TR = 0.6/53 ms; spirals = 250; spiral readout time T_s = 16.72 ms; and TA = 13 min 34 s. Image reconstruction was implemented offline (due to the limited computation capacity of the scanner, version VB17A) using a custom-developed program in C++ (MS Visual Studio 2019, Redmond, WA). SNR was measured on magnitude images by taking the ratio of the mean intensity in a region of interest (ROI) to the adjusted standard deviation (SD) of noise-only background [27], i.e., SNR = MEAN*0.656/SD.

Figures 8.9, 8.10, and 8.11 demonstrate AWSOS ultrahigh-resolution 7T UTE images and show the potential of the images to simultaneously visualize multiple functional connective tissues in the knee joint: femoral, tibial, and patellar cartilage as well as the chondro-osseous junction (Fig. 8.9); menisci (Fig. 8.10); ACL, PCL, and patellar tendon (Fig. 8.11). The measured SNR of these tissues was 22–34, which is high enough to visualize subtle alterations in morphology. The SNR in menisci across the male and female subjects was nearly constant (23.3 vs. 21.0), suggesting robustness and repeatability of the AWSOS technique.

AWSOS ultrahigh-resolution UTE imaging at 7 T provided in a single scan simultaneous visualization of multiple functional components of the knee joint. This advantage mainly resulted from matched combination of the AWSOS sequence, 7T magnet, and use of a dedicated knee coil. Without them, the power of ultrahigh-resolution UTE technique would not be revealed. The scan time (13 min 34 s) was acceptable. The studied subjects did not report complaints and were able to keep their knees still during the scan. SAR (specific absorption rate) was an issue that required a longer TR (53 ms) when fat saturation was used, compared with a shorter TR (20 ms), and thus a shorter scan time of 5 min 8 s when Fatsat was not used.

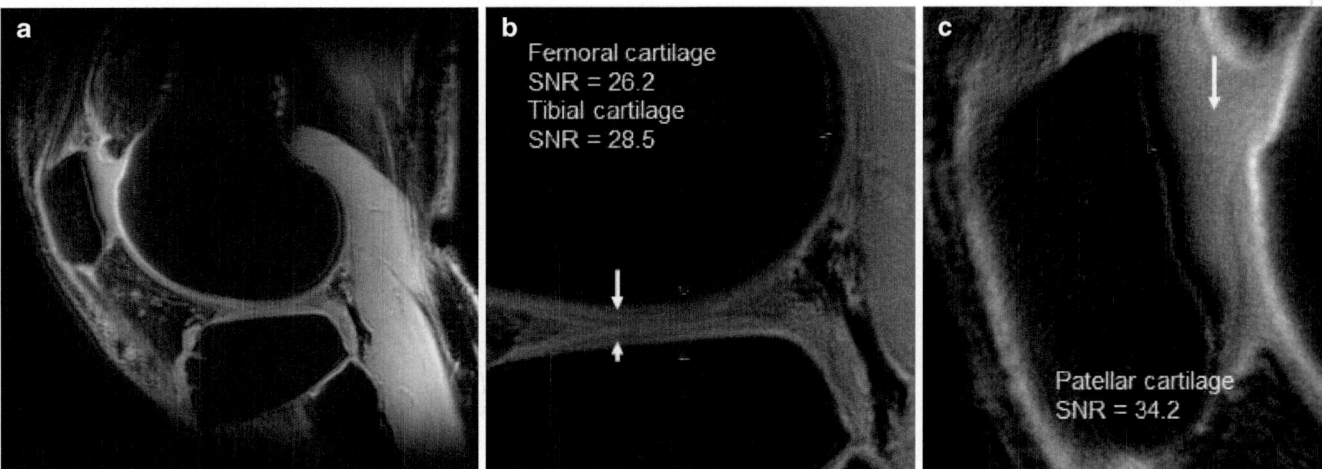

Fig. 8.9 AWSOS ultrahigh-resolution UTE image of femoral cartilage (long arrow), tibial cartilage (short arrow), patellar cartilage (long arrow), and chondro-osseous junction (red arrows, black region) in a 50-year-old healthy male, left knee at 7 T. (**a**) Full FOV; (**b**) local view of the femoral cartilage, tibial cartilage, and chondro-osseous junction; and (**c**) local view of the patellar cartilage. In-plane resolution 0.14 mm and slice thickness 2 mm. (Adopted with permission from Ref. [4])

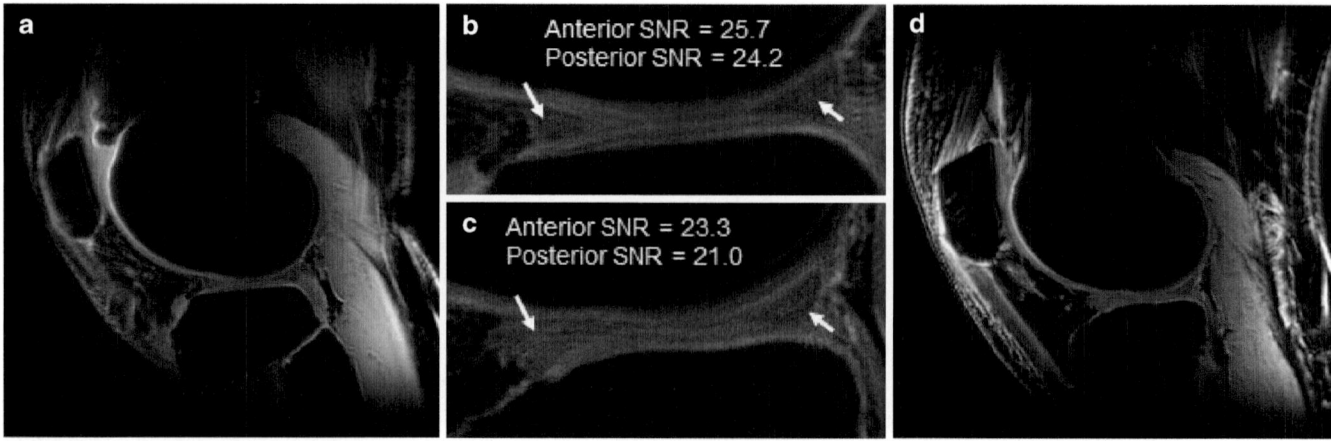

Fig. 8.10 AWSOS ultrahigh-resolution UTE image of anterior (long arrow) and posterior (short arrow) horns of a meniscus at 7 T. (**a, b**) Full and local views (healthy male, 50 years old, left knee), and (**c, d**) local and full views (healthy female, 47 years old, left knee). The meniscal tissue has nearly the same SNR and shows good repeatability of the ultrahigh-resolution UTE imaging at 7 T. In-plane resolution 0.14 mm and slice thickness 2 mm. (Adopted with permission from Ref. [4])

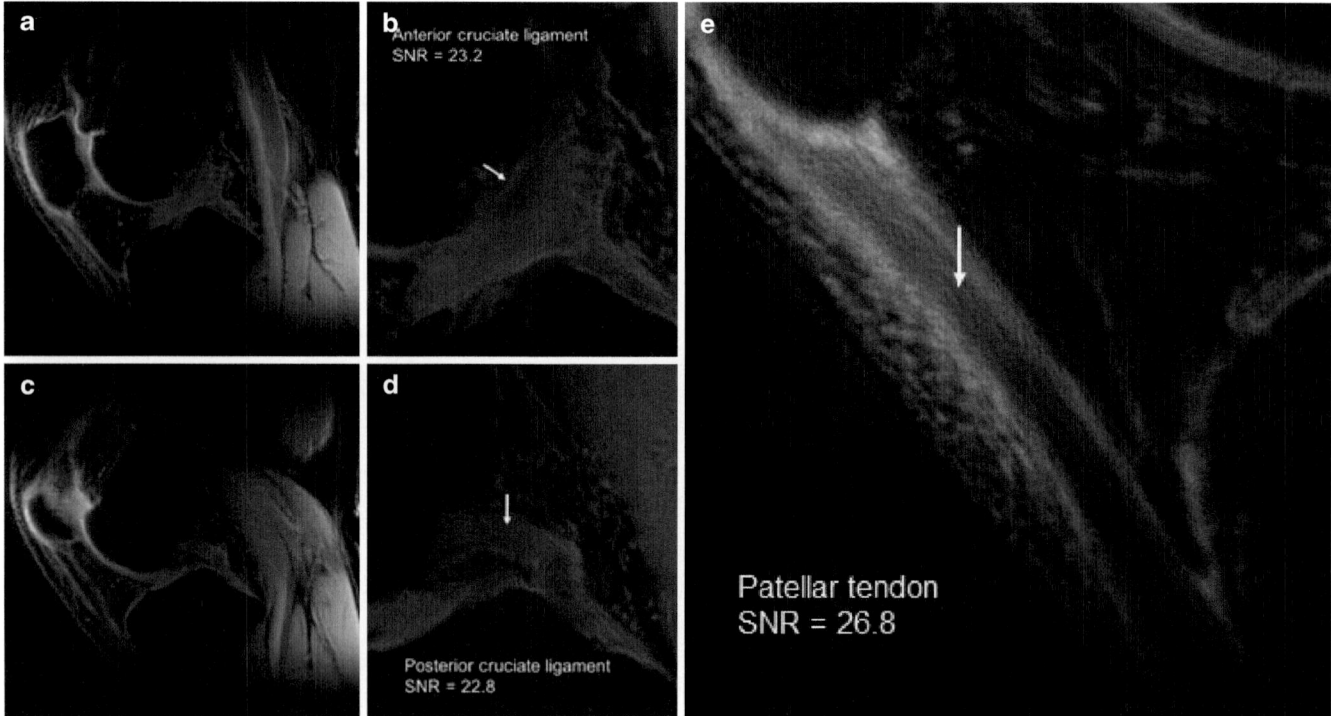

Fig. 8.11 AWSOS ultrahigh-resolution UTE image of a healthy subject (male, 50 years old, left knee) at 7 T. (**a, b**) Full and local views of the ACL. (**c, d**) Full and local views of the PCL. (**e**) Local view of the patellar tendon (arrow). In-plane resolution 0.14 mm and slice thickness 2 mm. (Adopted with permission from Ref. [4])

Discussion

AWSOS is an efficient pulse sequence for high-resolution UTE MRI of the human head and knee. The acquisition efficiency was attained by use of selective excitations and spiral data collections. The image SNR at high in-plane resolutions was preserved due to separation of in-plane resolution from slice thickness. The AWSOS pulse sequence is specifically suitable for imaging tissues with short T_2 values (1–10 ms). The minimum T_2 is limited by the use of slab-select excitation. This can be avoided by use of a nonselective or hard pulse for excitation when appropriate.

The number of slice encodings directly increases the total acquisition time with the AWSOS sequence. This number is determined by both slab length and slice thickness. When slice thickness is fixed (e.g., 2 mm), a shorter slab leads to fewer slice encodings. Another strategy to reduce the number of slice encodings is to use variable-density slice encoding with more encodings at the center of k-space than at the edge. This may reduce the encoding steps by as much as 60% but increases the complexity of image reconstruction (and thus the risk of unwanted image artifacts). Thus, short slabs and/or nonuniform slice encoding are options to improve the efficiency of AWSOS acquisitions.

Another major contribution to total acquisition time is the number of spiral interleaves. The minimum number is limited by tolerance to image blurring caused by long readout times. In our experience, a readout of $\sim 2 \times T_2$ is tolerable ($\sim 58\%$ blurring). Alternatively, the number of spirals can be reduced using parallel imaging with multiple coils without increasing readout times [28, 29]. When using the AWSOS pulse sequence with parallel imaging, it is convenient to skip spiral interleaves [29], but the image reconstruction is still time-consuming [28–33].

By sampling in a cylindrical volume in the k-space, the AWSOS sequence is able to separately select in-plane resolution and slice thickness and thus provides users with flexible choices of in-plane resolution while maintaining acceptable SNRs. For instance, at an in-plane FOV of 220 mm, users may select image matrix sizes of 64×64, 128×128, 256×256, 512×512, or 1024×1024 to produce nominal spatial resolutions of 3.4–0.22 mm, without changing slice thickness. On the other hand, slice thickness may be decreased or increased by changing the number of slice encodings, while the in-plane resolution remains unchanged.

There are no geometrical restrictions on the selection of slice direction in the AWSOS pulse sequence. It can be implemented in any part of the body on clinical MRI scanners with conventional coils using standard system parameters (e.g., field strength ≥ 1.5 T, maximum gradient ≥ 40 mT/m, and maximum slew rate ≥ 150 T/m/s). However, it is suggested that the slice direction should lie in the direction of lowest spatial resolution, such as use of axial slices in imaging the brain.

The AWSOS pulse sequence is applicable to multiple nuclei, including protons (^{1}H) and non-protons such as sodium (^{23}Na). Thus, there are no specific limitations to the type of nucleus with the AWSOS sequence. However, due to smaller gyromagnetic ratios, non-proton imaging may require larger gradient amplitudes and longer readout times. Optimal parameters for slab excitations and spiral readouts for non-proton imaging differ from those shown for proton imaging in this study.

Slab profile is a challenge with the AWSOS sequence due to the low amplitude of the slab-select gradient that is used. Approximately two-thirds of the slab is currently located within the passband of excitation, while one-third is in the transition band, decreasing the efficiency of the AWSOS imaging. In the future, RF pulses with narrower transition bands need to be developed to address this.

Summary

The images in this chapter show that the AWSOS sequence can perform 3D imaging with ultrashort TEs, high in-plane resolution, and short total scan times. These features result from variable-duration slice encodings, movable spiral data collections, and the separation of in-plane resolution from slice thickness.

Acknowledgments This work is based on previous work which was performed by colleagues and peers. The authors thank these people for their valuable advice and suggestions. They include Dr. V. Andrew Stenger, Department of Medicine, University of Hawaii, Honolulu, HI; Dr. Douglas C. Noll, Department of Biomedical Engineering, University of Michigan, Ann Arbor, MI; and Dr. Yi Wang, Weill Medical College of Cornell University, New York, NY. The authors also thank Dr. Michael Garwood, Center for Magnetic Resonance Research, University of Minnesota, Minneapolis, MN, and their former colleague, Dr. Edwin Nemoto, for their helpful discussions. The authors also wish to thank Dr. Zhenghui Zhang at GE Healthcare for his valuable assistance. The authors wish to express their special thanks to their former colleagues Dr. Constance R. Chu and Dr. Ashley A. Williams at Stanford University for their valuable collaborations with UTE knee imaging.

This work was financially supported in part by the National Institutes of Health (NIH) grants and by our former and current departments. The grants include NIH R01 CA106840, R01 AR052784, the Development Fund of the Department of Radiology at the University of Pittsburgh, and the General Research Fund of the Department of Radiology at the NYU Grossman School of Medicine.

References

1. Qian Y, Boada FE. Acquisition-weighted stack of spirals for fast high-resolution three-dimensional ultra-short echo time MR imaging. Magn Reson Med. 2008;60(1):135–45.
2. Qian Y, Boada FE. Method for producing a magnetic resonance image of an object having short T_2 relaxation time. US Pat. 7,750,632. 2010.
3. Qian Y, Williams AA, Chu CR, Boada FE. High resolution ultra-short echo time (UTE) imaging on human knee with AWSOS sequence at 3.0 tesla. J Magn Reson Imaging. 2012;35(1):204–10.
4. Qian Y, Chang G, Strauss E, Boada FE. Ultra-high resolution UTE imaging of the knee at 7T: simultaneous view of cartilage, meniscus, ligament, tendon, and the chondro-osseous junction. Proc Intl Soc Mag Reson Med. 2021:2973.
5. Qian Y, Boada FE. AWSOS pulse sequence and high-resolution UTE imaging. In: Encyclopedia of Magnetic Resonance. eMagRes. 2012;1:737–46.
6. Robson MD, Bydder GM. Clinical ultrashort echo time imaging of bone and other connective tissues. NMR Biomed. 2006;19(7):765–80.
7. Pauly JM, Nishimura DG. Magnetic resonance imaging of short T2 species. US Pat 5,025,216. 1991.
8. Young IR, Bydder GM. Magnetic resonance: new approaches to imaging of the musculoskeletal system. Physiol Meas. 2003;24(4):R1–23.
9. Haacke EM, Brown RW, Thompson MR, Venkatesan R. Magnetic resonance imaging-physical principles and sequence design. New York: John Wiley and Sons; 1999.
10. Jackson JI, Meyer CH, Nishimura DG, Macovski A. Selection of a convolution function for Fourier inversion using gridding. IEEE Trans Med Imaging. 1991;10(3):473–8.

11. Hoge RD, Kwan KS, Pike GB. Density compensation functions for spiral MRI. Magn Reson Med. 1997;38(1):117–28.
12. Glover GH. Simple analytic spiral k-space algorithm. Magn Reson Med. 1999;42(2):412–5.
13. Qian Y, Zhao T, Hue YK, Ibraham TS, Boada FE. High resolution spiral imaging on whole body 7T scanner with minimized image blurring. Magn Reson Med. 2010;63(3):543–52.
14. Zhao T, Qian Y, Hue Y-K, Ibrahim TS, Boada FE. Implementation of a 3D isotropic ultra-shot TE (UTE) sequence. Proc Intl Soc Mag Reson Med. 2009:2662.
15. International Electrotechnical Commission (IEC). International Standard IEC 60601-2-33 (2nd edition). 2002.
16. Irarrazabal P, Nishimura DG. Fast three-dimensional magnetic resonance imaging. Magn Reson Med. 1995;33(5):656–62.
17. Liang Z, Lauterbur PC. Principles of magnetic resonance imaging a signal processing perspective. New York: IEEE, Inc.; 2000.
18. Jung Y, Jashnani Y, Kijowski R, Block WF. Consistent non-cartesian off-axis MRI quality: calibrating and removing multiple sources of demodulation phase errors. Magn Reson Med. 2007;57(1):206–12.
19. Noll DC, Pauly JM, Meyer CH, Nishmura DG, Macovski A. Deblurring for non-2D Fourier transform magnetic resonance imaging. Magn Reson Med. 1992;25(2):319–33.
20. Yudilevich E, Stark H. Spiral sampling in magnetic resonance imaging: the effect of inhomogeneities. IEEE Trans Med Imaging. 1987;6(4):337–45.
21. Du J, Pak BC, Znamirowski R, et al. Magic angle effect in magnetic resonance imaging of the Achilles tendon and enthesis. Magn Reson Imaging. 2009;27(4):557–64.
22. Roemer FW, Kwoh CK, Hannon MJ, Hunter DJ, Eckstein F, Fujii T, Boudreau RM, Guermazi A. What comes first? Multitissue involvement leading to radiographic osteoarthritis, magnetic resonance imaging-based trajectory analysis over four years in the osteoarthritis initiative. Arthritis Rheumatol. 2015;67(8):2085–96.
23. Chu CR, Williams AA, West RV, Qian Y, Fu FH, Do BH, Bruno S. Quantitative magnetic resonance imaging UTE-T_2^* mapping of cartilage and meniscus healing after anatomic anterior cruciate ligament reconstruction. Am J Sports Med. 2014;42(8):1847–56.
24. Buckwalter JA, Brown TD. Joint injury, repair, and remodeling: roles in post-traumatic osteoarthritis. Clin Orthop Relat Res. 2004;423:7–16.
25. Lohmander LS. Articular cartilage and osteoarthritis. The role of molecular markers to monitor breakdown, repair and disease. J Anat. 1994;184(3):477–92.
26. Chu CR, Williams AA, Coyle CH, Bowers ME. Early diagnosis to enable early treatment of pre-osteoarthritis. Arthritis Res Ther. 2012;14(3):212.
27. Kellman P, McVeigh ER. Image reconstruction in SNR unit: a general method for SNR measurement. Magn Reson Med. 2005;54(6):1439–47.
28. Pruessmann KP, Weiger M, Bornert P, Boesiger P. Advances in sensitivity encoding with arbitrary k-space trajectories. Magn Reson Med. 2001;46(4):638–51.
29. Qian Y, Zhang Z, Stenger VA, Wang Y. Self-calibrated spiral SENSE. Magn Reson Med. 2004;52(3):688–92.
30. Yeh EN, McKenzie CA, Ohliger MA, Sodickson DK. Parallel magnetic resonance imaging with adaptive radius in k-space (PARS): constrained image reconstruction using k-space locality in radiofrequency coil encoded data. Magn Reson Med. 2005;53(6):1383–92.
31. Heberlein K, Hu X. Auto-calibrated parallel spiral imaging. Magn Reson Med. 2006;55(3):619–25.
32. Heidemann RM, Griswold MA, Seiberlich N, Kruger G, Kannengiesser SAR, Kiefer B, Wiggins G, Wald LL, Jakob PM. Direct parallel image reconstructions for spiral trajectories using GRAPPA. Magn Reson Med. 2006;56(2):317–26.
33. Qian Y, Zhang Z, Wang Y, Boada FE. Decomposed direct matrix inversion for fast non-Cartesian SENSE reconstructions. Magn Reson Med. 2006;56(2):356–63.

The Variable Echo Time (vTE) Sequence

Benedikt Hager, Vladimir Juras, Olgica Zaric,
Pavol Szomolanyi, Siegfried Trattnig, and Xeni Deligianni

Introduction

Conventional MRI sequences with long echo times (TEs) usually cannot adequately image tissues such as tendons and menisci because the transverse relaxation times (T_2s and T_2^*s) of these tissues are very short, and this results in low detectable signal. However, tissues with very short T_2s and T_2^*s are of great clinical importance, especially in musculoskeletal disease.

The variable echo time (vTE) sequence presented here uses very fast measurements with sub-ms TEs, to allow detection and measurement of tissue short T_2s and T_2^*s. The vTE sequence does not achieve TEs as short as those obtained with radial UTE sequences, but it requires a much shorter scan time for comparable protocols and is less susceptible to artifacts caused by system delays and eddy currents. As a result, the vTE sequence is more readily usable in clinical settings.

In this chapter, the general design of the vTE sequence, its various applications, and the differences between it and other short TE sequences are explained.

Sequence Description

Although it is difficult to pin down the exact origin of the vTE technique, it could be argued that the general concept underpinning it dates back to the technique of NMR Fourier zeugmatography described by Kumar, Welti, and Ernst in 1975 [1]. The latest version of the vTE sequence that we present here is, in addition, inspired by more recent work in which a vTE approach was used to study cortical bone water, the inner ear,

B. Hager · V. Juras
Department of Biomedical Imaging and Image-guided Therapy, High Field MR Centre, Medical University of Vienna, Vienna, Austria

CD Laboratory for MR Imaging Biomarkers (BIOMAK), Vienna, Austria

Austrian Cluster for Tissue Regeneration, Ludwig Boltzmann Institute for Experimental and Clinical Traumatology, Vienna, Austria

P. Szomolanyi
Department of Biomedical Imaging and Image-guided Therapy, High Field MR Centre, Medical University of Vienna, Vienna, Austria

CD Laboratory for MR Imaging Biomarkers (BIOMAK), Vienna, Austria

Austrian Cluster for Tissue Regeneration, Ludwig Boltzmann Institute for Experimental and Clinical Traumatology, Vienna, Austria

Department of Imaging Methods, Institute of Measurement Science, Slovak Academy of Sciences, Bratislava, Slovakia

O. Zaric
Department of Medicine, Faculty of Medicine and Dentistry,

Danube Private University GmbH (DPU), Krems an der Donau, Austria

Institute for Clinical Molecular MRI in the Musculoskeletal System, Karl Landsteiner Society, St. Pölten, Austria

S. Trattnig (✉)
Department of Biomedical Imaging and Image-guided Therapy, High Field MR Centre, Medical University of Vienna, Vienna, Austria

CD Laboratory for MR Imaging Biomarkers (BIOMAK), Vienna, Austria

Austrian Cluster for Tissue Regeneration, Ludwig Boltzmann Institute for Experimental and Clinical Traumatology, Vienna, Austria

Institute for Clinical Molecular MRI in the Musculoskeletal System, Karl Landsteiner Society, St. Pölten, Austria
e-mail: Siegfried.Trattnig@meduniwien.ac.at

X. Deligianni
Division of Radiological Physics, Department of Radiology, University of Basel Hospital, Basel, Switzerland

Research Coordination Team, Department of Radiology, University Hospital Basel, Basel, Switzerland

Basel Muscle MRI, Department of Biomedical Engineering, University of Basel, Allschwil, Switzerland

and the human skin with microscopic resolution (<100 μm) by Song et al., Techwiboonwong et al., and Ying et al. [2–4]. The core concept of the vTE technique is performing phase encoding by varying the duration of the phase encoding gradient rather than by varying its amplitude, which is the case with conventional clinical MRI sequences [5]. This principle and the fact that the signal contrast is determined by the lower spatial frequencies (which are located in the center of k-space) are exploited in vTE sequence schemes which achieve very short TEs at the center of k-space by using very short duration phase encoding pulses. Song and Wehrli extended the concept from two dimensions (2D) to three dimensions (3D) by varying phase encoding gradients to minimize the TE in both the z- and y-directions with 3D partial flip angle gradient and spin echo-based acquisitions [2].

The most recent application of the vTE concept described here is based on a 3D Cartesian spoiled gradient recalled echo (SPGR) sequence [6]. Employing a gradient echo sequence allows considerable reduction in total scan time, and this can be used to adapt protocols to the specific needs of short T_2 and T_2^* tissue imaging. Although the sequence was initially realized in 2D versions, 3D versions benefit most from the vTE concept. The first TE toward the center of k-space is minimized by dynamic adjustment while keeping the bandwidth constant (since the minimum TE depends strongly on the readout gradients) [2, 4, 6]. The TE is then minimized for each line of k-space toward the center where smaller gradient moments are required for phase and slice encoding. With minimal phase encoding, the TE is determined by the gradient moments for slice selection and frequency encoding which is the effective TE_{eff} (Fig. 9.1). The TE increases with increasing in-plane resolution for fixed readout bandwidths and a given slice thickness.

As the phase encoding moment increases, the TE_{eff} increases beyond the minimum TE (Fig. 9.1). The vTE sequence benefits greatly from increased gradient performance (i.e., maximum slew rate and amplitude) as well as switching times. The slew rates and maximum amplitude of

the gradient system greatly affect the minimum value that can be achieved for the first TE at a given readout bandwidth. As a result, the vTE sequence is particularly suitable for systems with small bores and strong gradient performance. Although interesting results have been shown at 1.5 T, the sequence generally performs better at high to very high static field strengths (3 T and 7 T).

The vTE scheme has been complemented by the addition of other new features in the latest version of the sequence. This provides efficient sub-millisecond (sub-ms) TE imaging [6]. The basic characteristics of the sequence, apart from the variable TE in the slice and phase directions, are a highly asymmetric readout, nonselective radiofrequency (RF) pulses for excitation, and 3D Cartesian k-space sampling.

The highly asymmetric partial echo readouts (i.e., typically 11–16%) with standard Cartesian sampling are of particular importance for the sequence, as they significantly reduce TEs. However, it is well known that partial echo data are prone to artifacts. Projection onto convex sets (POCS) has been successfully used to avoid these artifacts and improve image reconstruction.

Overall, the combination of these techniques reduces the effective TE to about 800 μs at spatial resolutions as high as 500 μm (see Table 9.1), thus providing a comprehensive protocol that is well suited for tissues with short T_2 and T_2^*s. If a longer TE is acceptable, higher resolution, greater coverage, and reduced scan times can be achieved.

RF Excitation

The basic excitation scheme for the sequence consists of short, nonselective RF pulses (<500 us), which allow very short TEs and so increased signal from short-T_2^* tissues. The excitation pulse duration may be decreased if the flip angle is decreased to meet the Ernst angle or contrast requirements.

The robust and fast sequence scheme also supports flexible addition of magnetization preparation modules, for

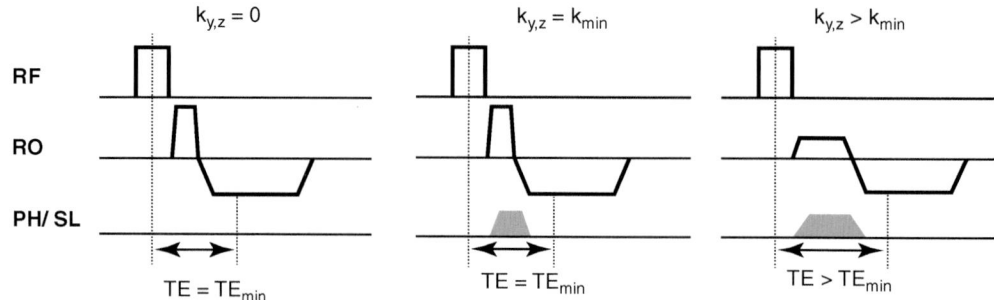

Fig. 9.1 The vTE sequence. The TE changes depending on the variable pre-phasing gradient moments k_y in the phase (PH) and k_z in the slice (SL) direction. A minimum TE is shown at the center of the k-space (left). This is primarily limited by the time acquired for excitation and frequency encoding along the readout (RO) direction. As long as the variable phase encoding moments k_y and k_z take less time than that for the excitation and frequency encoding, the minimum TE is maintained (center). After this, further increase in the phase encoding moments means that TE needs to increase (right) [6]

Table 9.1 Parameters for some exemplary vTE protocols used in previous studies [6–8]

TEs (ms)	Voxel resolution (mm³)/slices	Field strength (T)	Scan time (min)/averages	Region of interest
0.8/8.22	$0.55 \times 0.55 \times 2.5/52$	3 T – ^{1}H	2.4/1	Knee joint [6]
0.92/8.08	$0.36 \times 0.36 \times 1.0/120$	7 T – ^{1}H	7.5/1	Knee joint [6]
0.98/5.37	$0.6 \times 0.6 \times 5.0/12$	3 T^a – ^{1}H	5.4/7	Sciatic nerve [7]
1.02/–	$0.42 \times 0.42 \times 0.5/128$	7 T – ^{1}H	6.2/1	Achilles tendon [6]
1.22	$1.6 \times 1.6 \times 3/52$	7 T – ^{23}Na	25.1/28	Knee joint [8]

^{a}Wider bore clinical system

Table 9.2 Examples of sequence parameters used with interleaved echo acquisitions to perform T_2* mapping [10–12, 15, 16]

TEs (ms)	Voxel resolution (mm³)/slices	Field strength (T)	Scan time (min)/averages	Tissue of interest
0.8–20 (20 TEs)	$0.7 \times 0.7 \times 0.7/144$	3 T – ^{1}H	12.16/1	Achilles tendon [12]
0.4–12 ms (9 TEs)	$0.06 \times 0.06 \times 0.4/22$	7 T^a – ^{1}H	90/4	Menisci [10]
0.66–51.62 (40 TEs)	$0.098 \times 0.098 \times 0.4/72$	7 T^a – ^{1}H	96/1	Achilles and patellar tendon specimens [11]
0.75–22.42 (10 TEs)	$0.42 \times 1.02 \times 0.70/64$	3 T – ^{1}H	12.16/1	Menisci [15]
2.64–60.42 (10 TEs)	$4 \times 4 \times 15/12$	7 T – ^{23}Na	46:50/24	Kidneys [16]

^{a}Experiments with an additional MR microscopy system [10, 11]

example, to suppress fat signals [9, 10]. Fat signal suppression is especially important for visualizing short T_2 and T_2* components in clinical musculoskeletal (MSK) imaging and frequently improves the quality of images.

In the specific case of vTE schemes, fast spectral water excitation based on a short binomial excitation has been extensively studied and demonstrates excellent fat suppression in addition to an improved signal-to-noise ratio (SNR) [9]. Compared to conventional fat saturation (FAT-SAT) methods, binomial excitation offers greater time efficiency since little additional time is needed for magnetization preparation. In addition and in agreement with the simulations, a binomial pulse close to 90° was less sensitive to main magnetic field inhomogeneities, yielded minimum signal loss, and had comparable quality fat suppression to that obtained with a 180° inversion pulse. It should be underlined that, for short-T_2 and T_2* tissues, as well as operation at lower field strengths, the choice of the water–fat phase evolution time for binomial pulses is important.

Multiple Contrasts and Reconstruction

In the original form of the sequence, the first echo image is determined by the vTE scheme [6], while the subsequent second and other following images are fully sampled. Nevertheless, due to the flexibility of the sequence, alternative multi-echo sampling schemes with interleaved echo sampling have been developed [6, 10–13]. The second echo can be either fully or partially sampled. Partial sampling is used, for

example, with interleaved repetition of the variable echo [6]. Newer versions of the sequence are especially suitable for T_2* mapping of short T_2 and T_2* tissues, as the sampling and TEs are particularly flexible. Typically, TEs are rather densely distributed following the first TE and sparsely distributed at later TEs. However, this can be handled flexibly.

Online reconstruction of the double contrast (positive contrast) and reordering of the echoes have been programmed online with the IceLuva Plugin [14], which provides important initial feedback to the operator and makes the sequence suitable for clinical protocols.

Comparison with Other Short TE Sequences

In general, TEs of less than 1 ms down to a value of 0.4 ms can be achieved with vTE sequences [6, 10]. These TEs can be considered ultrashort by definition [17]. However, TEs in the ultrashort range of 0.2–0.3 ms, which are possible with non-Cartesian UTE and other ultrashort TE sampling techniques such as ZTE, cannot be achieved. vTE sequences benefit from the robustness of Fourier-encoding, offer high-resolution imaging, and have good SNRs which are achievable in clinically feasible scan times (Tables 9.1 and 9.2). Moreover, Cartesian sampling is more resistant to gradient imperfections than radial sampling. Another important point is that scanning is not restricted to positioning at the isocenter of the magnet or the use of isotropic voxels. Acceleration methods such as parallel imaging and partial Fourier acquisitions can also be readily used with vTE.

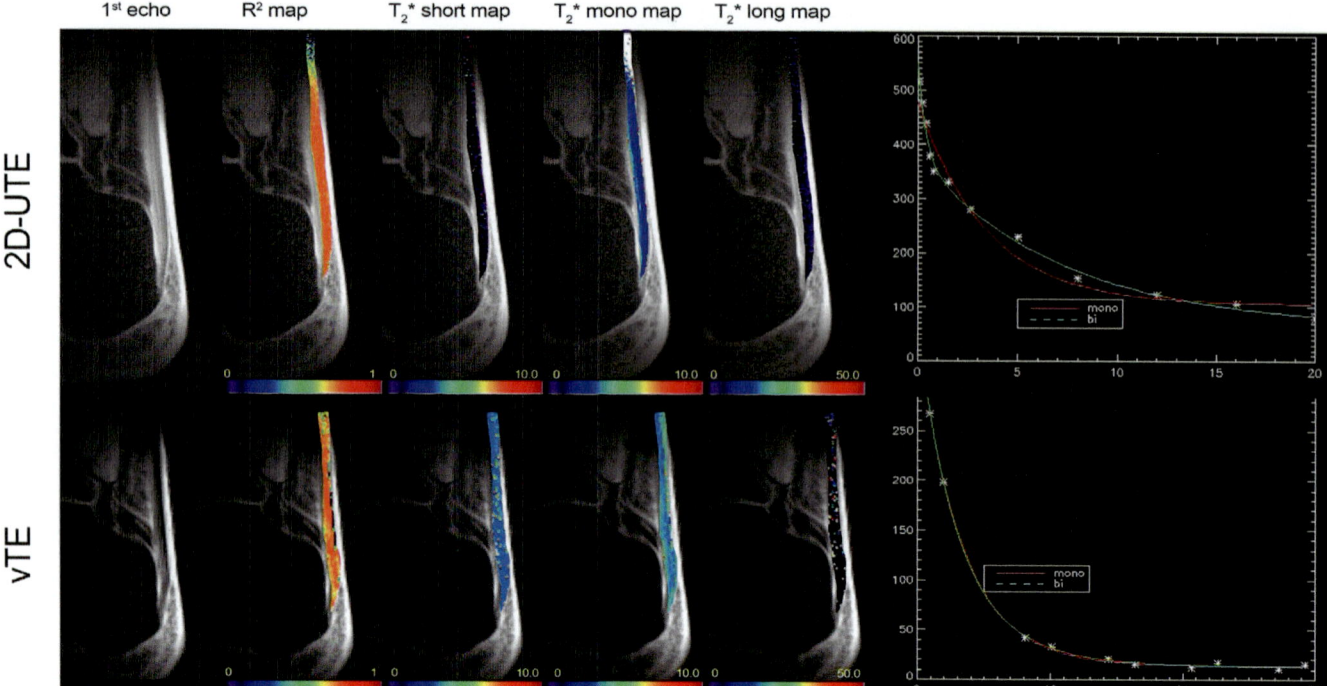

Fig. 9.2 Achilles tendon. Comparison of first echo, R_2 map, T_2^* short-component map, T_2^* single-component (mono) map, and T_2^* long-component map with plots of signal against time for the single-component (mono) maps and bicomponent maps (upper row) and the vTE images and corresponding plots (bottom row) [12, 20]. Signals in the shorter ultrashort-T_2 range are detected in the upper row but not in the lower row

In addition, due to their flexibility and robustness as well as the successful integration of interleaved schemes, vTE sequences are particularly suitable for T_2^* mapping of tissues with short-T_2 and T_2^* values [10–12, 15]. The echo spacing achieved with these sequence schemes is particularly well adapted to such tissues. This includes, for example, ^{1}H-imaging protocols with 20 echoes in vivo [12, 18] and 40 echoes ex vivo [11], as well as ^{23}Na imaging with 10 echoes in vivo [16] and 18 echoes ex vivo [19].

When comparing UTE with vTE in terms of T_2^* quantification, UTE-T_2^*, especially for bicomponent analysis performed at 3 T (see Fig. 9.2), provides more reliable results simply because there are more data points covering the ultrashort-T_2^* component. Images acquired with the vTE sequence, on the other hand, are more suitable for routine clinical use because of their higher resolution, faster acquisition, and lower vulnerability to blurring artifacts [12]. The robustness, insensitivity to gradient timing, and Cartesian k-space sampling of vTE provide considerable benefits with ultrahigh field MRI scanners. It was shown that the vTE-T_2^* results at both 3T and 7T scanners are comparable for most fast-relaxing MSK tissues; the only discrepancy found was with cartilage, but this was very likely due to the use of a suboptimal TE range which was not suitable for higher T_2^* values [12].

Outlook

For the study of tissues with short-T_2 and T_2^* values, protocols with not only short TEs but also very high spatial resolution are required. The vTE sequence described here allows very good compromises between TE, spatial resolution, and scan time. While it has been used for various applications, from imaging of cells labeled with superparamagnetic iron oxides [21], sciatic nerve imaging [7], and sodium imaging in the kidney [16], MSK applications, such as ^{1}H T_2^* mapping of menisci and tendons [11, 12, 15] and ^{23}Na imaging [8] are among the most successful.

MR Microscopy Using a vTE Sequence

To achieve very high spatial resolution, potentially even in the microscopic range (<100 μm), and to calculate accurate quantitative T_2^* maps with equally high spatial resolution, both hardware and sequence specific requirements must be met. In this context, SNR is a crucial measure. It compares the desired signal with the background noise. Acceptable voxel size in MRI is a function of machine SNR; higher SNR allows higher spatial resolution.

The following hardware features are crucial to achieving high SNR (and high spatial resolution):

Field strength: The higher the field strength, the higher the achievable SNR. A higher SNR allows higher spatial resolution and/or shorter measurement times. For higher field strengths ($B_0 > 0.5T$), the SNR is directly proportional to the field strength [22], i.e., SNR $\propto B_0$.

Coil diameter: A smaller coil absorbs less noise from a smaller volume and increases SNR. Thus, smaller coils show increased sensitivity, but the volume from which the coil can receive signals is also smaller. An inversely proportional relationship between coil diameter (d) and SNR has been reported for ordinary birdcage coils [23, 24], i.e., SNR $\propto$ 1/d.

Gradient strength: Another factor of importance in achieving high SNR is the gradient strength in millitesla per meter ($mT\,m^{-1}$). Stronger gradients are usually advantageous for achieving higher spatial resolution because they increase SNR efficiency. The achievable spatial resolution is approximately proportional to the gradient strength [25].

In addition to hardware, sequence specific properties are another important factor in measuring samples at microscopic resolution and using sub-ms TEs. For a classical radial center-out UTE sequence, the FID sampling starts directly at the k-space center, and therefore, the TE is commonly limited only by the length of the RF pulse and the capability of the hardware to switch between transmit and receive mode [26]. The possibilities offered by UTE sequences have already been outlined in other chapters in this book. However, it is worth noting again that tissues or materials with extremely short transverse relaxation times ($T_2^* < 0.1$ ms) cannot be directly imaged with these sequences using conventional clinical systems.

In contrast to radial UTE sequences, the vTE sequence, which is based on a spoiled GRE sequence, has a rectilinear sampling scheme [6]. As a result, it does not provide the same lower ultrashort TE values as UTE and ZTE sequences and hence cannot image tissues such as cortical bone. However, the use of the vTE technique in combination with an asymmetric readout and short, hard, nonselective pulses allows TEs of less than 1 ms using conventional whole-body MRI systems, and when very strong gradients are used (e.g., 750 $mT\,m^{-1}$), even TEs of around 0.4 ms are possible. This makes it particularly suitable for the study of highly ordered collagen-rich tissues, such as menisci and tendons [7]. The reason for these shorter TEs is that strong gradients and a slew rate of 7500 $mT\,m^{-1}\,ms^{-1}$, as was used in recent studies [10, 11], also lead to a more efficient asymmetric readout, i.e., the TE in outer k-space can also be significantly shortened. Moreover, the vTE approach can be performed more efficiently. Thus the TE at the k-space center can be shortened even further (compared to conventional clinical MRI systems), leading to the already mentioned effective TEs of as short as 0.4 ms.

Furthermore, the rectilinear sampling scheme of the vTE sequence offers advantages over radial UTE sequences in terms of k-space efficiency, provided that the Nyquist criterion is satisfied. Outer k-space contains the higher spatial frequencies that are important for image details, e.g., information about edges. While radial center-out UTE sequences allow use of extremely short TEs, to adequately sample the outer k-space, they must oversample the inner k-space and use many more radial readout spokes overall (when compared to the readout lines in Cartesian sequences such as the vTE sequence), resulting in a significantly longer measurement time for a similar spatial resolution. It should also be noted that a Nyquist criterion that is not met should be avoided, as it is usually manifested by streak artifacts and inadequate image quality with UTE sequences as a result of their radial acquisitions.

By meeting the hardware requirements described above and using the vTE sequence, ultrahigh spatial resolution, nearly blur free images can be obtained, and high-resolution T_2^* maps can be calculated. In publications by Hager et al., this combination was used to study menisci, Achilles tendons, and patellar tendons [10, 11]. Tissues were measured in vitro using an MR microscopy system with a gradient strength of 750 $mT\,m^{-1}$ (RRI, Billerica, Massachusetts, USA) and on a clinical 7T scanner (Siemens Magnetom Terra, Erlangen, Germany) using small 19- and 39-mm volume resonators (Rapid Biomedical, Würzburg, Germany).

The focus of these studies was to investigate the T_2^* characteristics and the orientation dependence of T_2^* in these tissues. Figure 9.3 shows (a) a representative T_2^* map of a degenerate human meniscus, (b) a comparison with a Picrosirius red-stained slice using polarized light, (c) a first echo image of the vTE sequence (TE = 0.4 ms), and (d) the eighth echo image (TE = 8 ms) obtained with the vTE sequence [10].

Transverse relaxation time anisotropy of the Achilles tendon and the patellar tendon was studied using the vTE sequence with in-plane microscopic resolution [11]. Figure 9.4 shows (a) a representative T_2^* map of one Achilles tendon measured at 11 angles ($0°, 10°, 20°, 30°, 40°, 50°, 55°, 60°, 70°, 80°,$ and $90°$), (b) the corresponding boxplot that shows how the T_2^* values change with the angle to B_0 and that the lowest values are obtained with fibers at $0°$ to B_0 and the highest values are in the range of the magic angle (fibers are $\approx 60°$ to B_0), (c) the position of the ROIs, and (d) the corresponding line plot for compartment-specific T_2^* analysis.

When comparing the fiber-to-field angles for the maximum and minimum of the dipolar interaction ($0°$ and $55°$), it was found that T_2^* values in the Achilles tendon and patellar

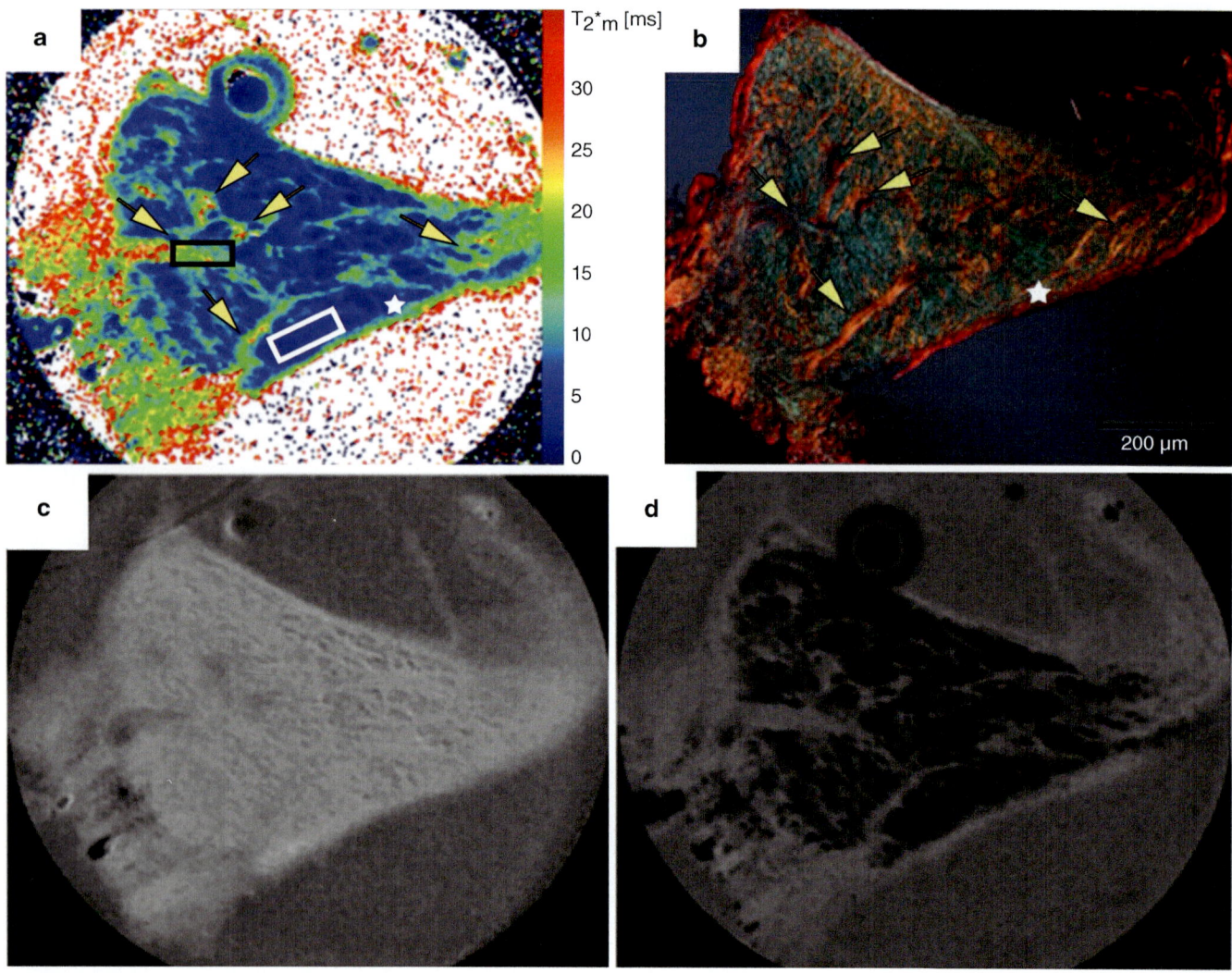

Fig. 9.3 (**a**) Representative T_2^* map of a degenerate human meniscus. (**b**) Corresponding Picrosirius red-stained slice obtained using a polarized light filter. The yellow arrows indicate fibrous tissue. (**c**) First echo (TE = 0.4 ms) of the vTE sequence. (**d**) Eighth echo (TE = 8 ms) of the vTE sequence. (Adapted with permission from Ref. [10])

tendon changed on average by factors of 15.5 and 16.0, respectively. For individual ROIs of fascicles, it was found that changing the angle from 0° to 55° increased T_2^* values by up to a factor of 80 from T_2^* (0°) = 0.43 ms to T_2^* (55°) = 34.21 ms. This study also suggests that regional T_2^* values are impacted by T_2^* orientation dependence as well as by the decay model (mono- or biexponential) which is preferred at specific angles to B_0 [11].

To summarize, microscopic MRI combined with a vTE sequence allows study of collagen-rich tissues with unprecedented detail and may lead to a deeper understanding of the relationship between T_2^* decay and T_2^* anisotropy and thus the complex, heterogeneous structure of these tissues.

Fig. 9.4 (**a**) T_2^* maps of an Achilles tendon measured at 11 different angles to B_0. (**b**) Boxplot showing the increase in T_2^* values from angles representing the maximum to the minimum of the dipolar interaction, i.e., 0 and 55°. (**c**) Position of ROIs. The blue and yellow ROIs mark polygonal fascicles. The red ROI is from the non-fascicular tissue. (**d**) The T_2^* values of the fascicular tissue change significantly from 0 to 55°. (Adapted with permission from Ref. [11])

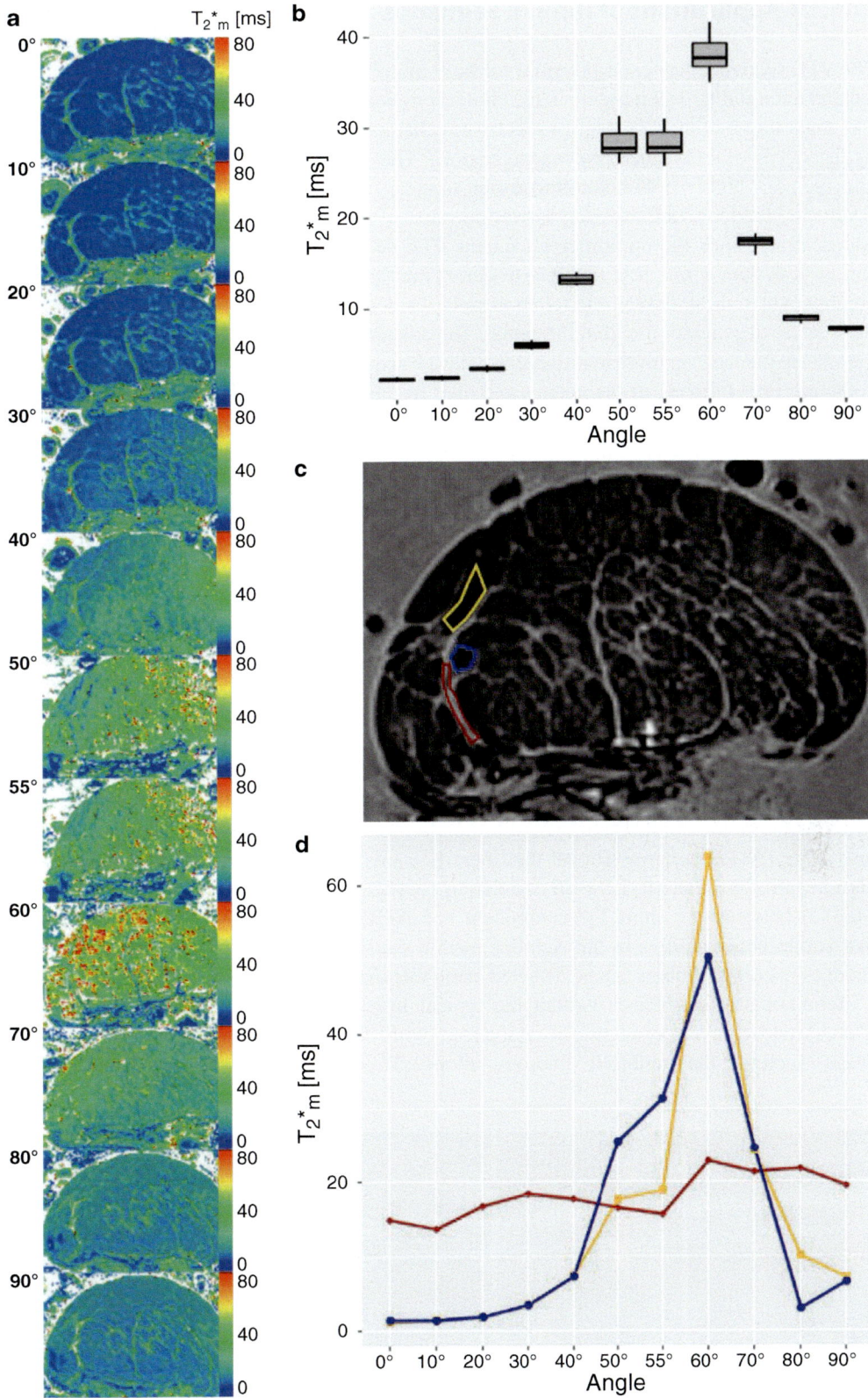

Clinical Applications of the vTE Sequence

The vTE sequence has great potential for both morphological and quantitative MR imaging in the clinical environment. The main target of the vTE sequence is tissues characterized by fast decay of their transverse magnetizations. This generally includes highly ordered, collagen-rich tissues, such as ligaments, tendons, and menisci, as well as parts of nerves and dentine. Since the minimum TE for the vTE sequence can be less than 1 ms, it is possible to detect multiple T_2^* components in these tissues and relate them to the degree of disorder or degeneration within the tissue. The advantage of the vTE sequence over more traditional radial UTE sequences is the minimal blurring of the images and their insensitivity to gradient timing errors, enabling robust and reliable pixel-by-pixel T_2^* analysis.

One of the possible clinical applications of T_2^* mapping is tendinopathy. Tendinopathy is a complex tendon pathology manifested by pain, deterioration in mobility, and reduced exercise tolerance. It is characterized by intratendinous collagen degeneration as well as neovascularization, and neoinnervation. There is a change in the mobility of water molecules near loosened collagen fibers which may be reflected in changes to T_2^* values. The relationship between vTE T_2^* values and clinically assessed tendinopathy has been studied by Juras et al. [12] (Fig. 9.5). A vTE sequence with a TE range from 0.8 ms to 20.0 ms was used to calculate short and long components of T_2^* and to find whether these correlated with the clinical score (Achilles tendon total rupture score (ATRS)). It was shown that there is a relatively high negative correlation (Pearson correlation coefficient of −0.846) between the short T_2^* component and ATRS and that subtle abnormalities in the Achilles tendon caused by changes in collagen fibers can be detected using this method.

Tendinopathy can occur without the typical history of overuse and can, for example, be associated with certain drugs, such as the antibiotic fluoroquinolone. The vTE sequence was used as part of a multiparametric study along with glycosaminoglycan chemical exchange saturation transfer (gagCEST) and sodium MRI, in which seven male volunteers were followed for 10 days and 5 months after ciprofloxacin treatment [27]. Although differences were found in the short- and long-T_2^* components at the two time points, these were not statistically significant. Glycosaminoglycan-specific methods, especially sodium MRI, showed a statistically significant reversible decrease in GAG content after treatment.

Tendon T_2^* values might serve as a biomarker for biomechanical alterations associated with tendinopathy and may reveal changes in collagen structure that are not visible with conventional MRI. Bachmann et al. studied artificially collagen degraded tendons [18] and found a significant negative correlation between tendon stress at 5% strain and T_2^* ($r = −0.74$) in degraded tendons suggesting that disruption of the collagen matrix has a considerable impact on the biomechanical properties of the tendon. On the contrary, T_1 values failed to distinguish between treated and non-treated tendons, which was attributed to the fact that T_1 reflects mostly extracellular fluid.

Another potential application of T_2^* mapping is the detection of meniscal degeneration. This is characterized by macroscopic changes in meniscal tissue and is accompanied by thinning and weakening of the meniscus. vTE-T_2^* mapping was used to classify meniscus degeneration using TEs ranging from 0.75 ms to 22.42 ms with both mono- and biexponential T_2^* analysis (Fig. 9.6) [15]. A hierarchical linear model revealed statistically significant differences in the short-T_2^* component between normal, degenerate, and torn menisci with T_2^* values of 0.82, 1.29, and 2.05 ms, respectively. Similarly, the mono-exponentially calculated T_2^* showed a similar trend with values for normal, degenerate, and torn menisci of 7.61, 9.54, and 14.59 ms, respectively (Fig. 9.6). At $0.47 \times 1.02 \times 0.7$ mm^3 resolution, it was also possible to determine regional differences within the menis-

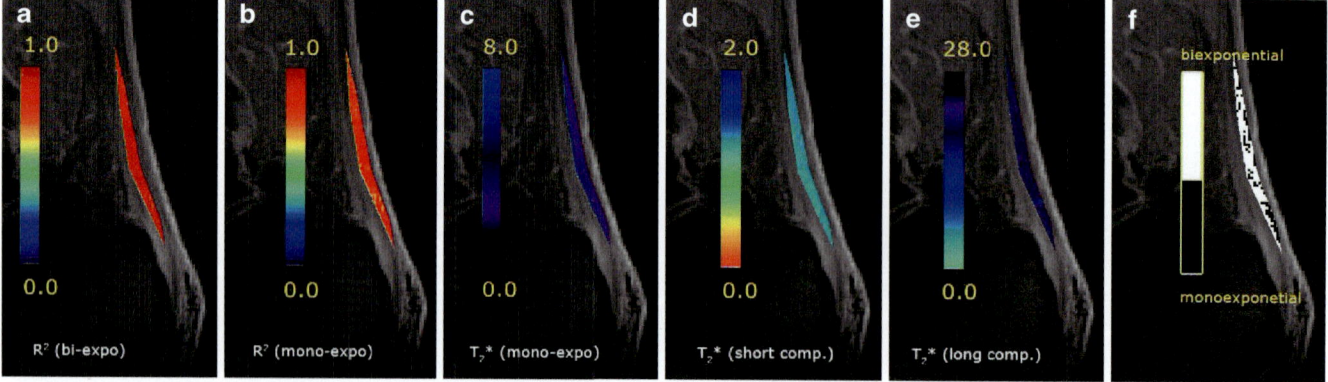

Fig. 9.5 T_2^* analysis of a healthy volunteer. (**a**) R_2 map (biexponential), (**b**) R_2 map (mono-exponential), (**c**) mono-exponential T_2^*, (**d**) short T_2^* component, (**e**) long T_2^* component, (**f**) binary map of mono- and biexponential pixels. (Adapted with permission from Ref. [12])

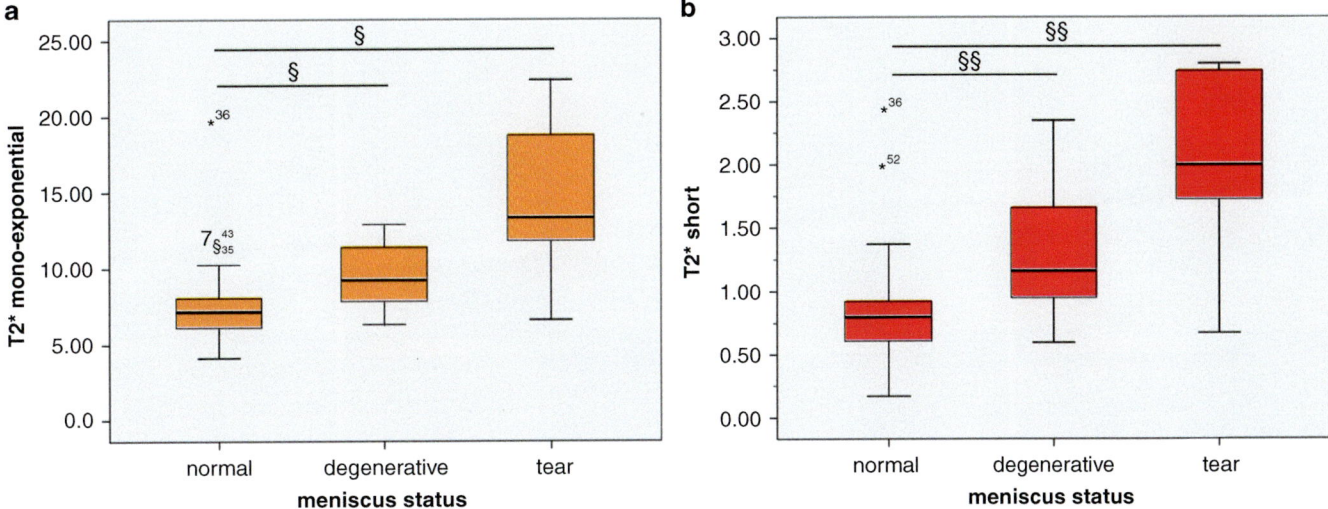

Fig. 9.6 Box plots of mono-exponential T_2^* (**a**) and short-T_2^* component (**b**) of the menisci acquired using a vTE sequence. (Adapted with permission from Ref. [15])

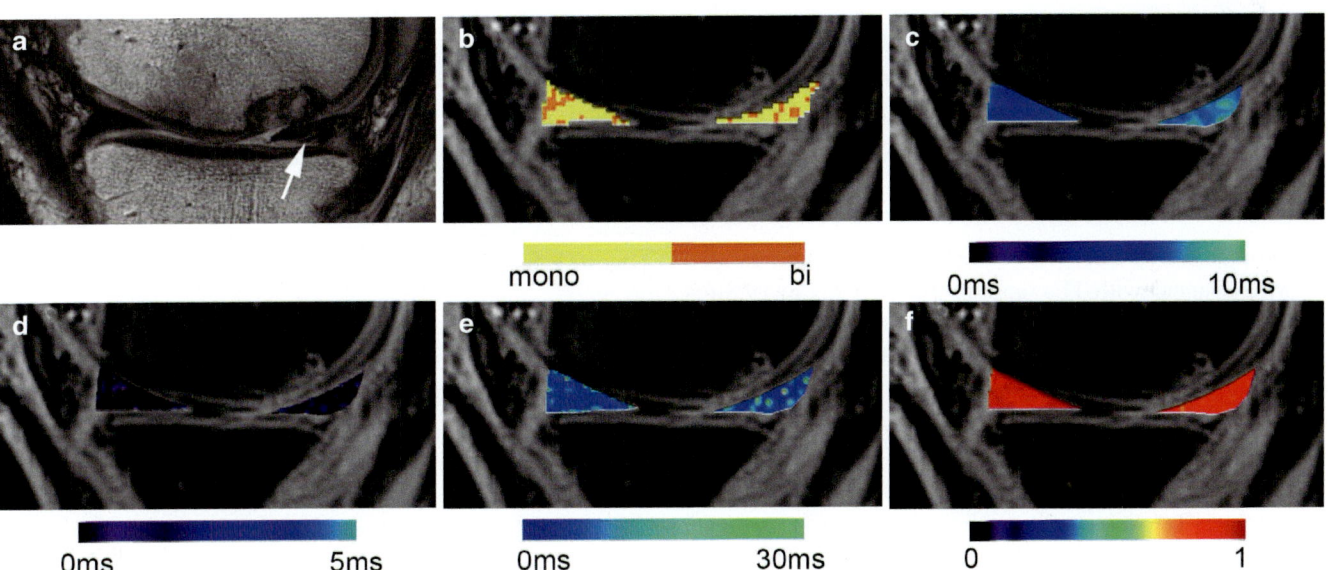

Fig. 9.7 A 45-year-old patient with a meniscal tear in the posterior horn of the medial meniscus (arrow). (**a**) Anatomical image; (**b**) binary map of pixels with biexponential (orange) and mono-exponential (yellow) fits; (**c**) mono-exponential T_2^* map; (**d**) short-T_2^* component map; (**e**) long T_2^* component map; and (**f**) R_2 map. (Adapted with permission from Ref. [15])

cus, between the red (vascular) and white (avascular) zones, as well as between the anterior and posterior horns (Fig. 9.7).

Noninvasive biochemical MRI can provide a perspective to determine functional processes. vTE has been used to study the changes of T_2^* in the human meniscus in vivo under continuous loading [13]. Four subjects were measured at four time points with a vTE sequence that had a total measurement time of 6:10 min. The vTE protocol had a resolution of $0.7 \times 0.7 \times 3.0$ mm³, and the TEs ranged from 0.8 ms to 10.1 ms. The anterior horn of the medial meniscus showed the strongest response to loading, with T_2^* increasing from 4.69 ms to 5.23 ms over the four time points. The T_2^* increase

under loading, contrary to that found with cartilage, was attributed to the changes in water distribution in the meniscus.

In another study, Stelzeneder et al. followed up patients with 7T MRI 3 and 6 months after meniscal repair using a vTE sequence with a resolution of $0.33 \times 0.29 \times 1.5$ mm³ and TEs ranging from 1.0 to 26.5 ms [28]. Using T_2^* mapping, meniscal regions with good healing and regions with limited healing could be identified.

The high-resolution and near artifact-free images allow these techniques to be applied to smaller structures. Dadour et al. used vTE-T_2^* mapping to identify patients with gluteal

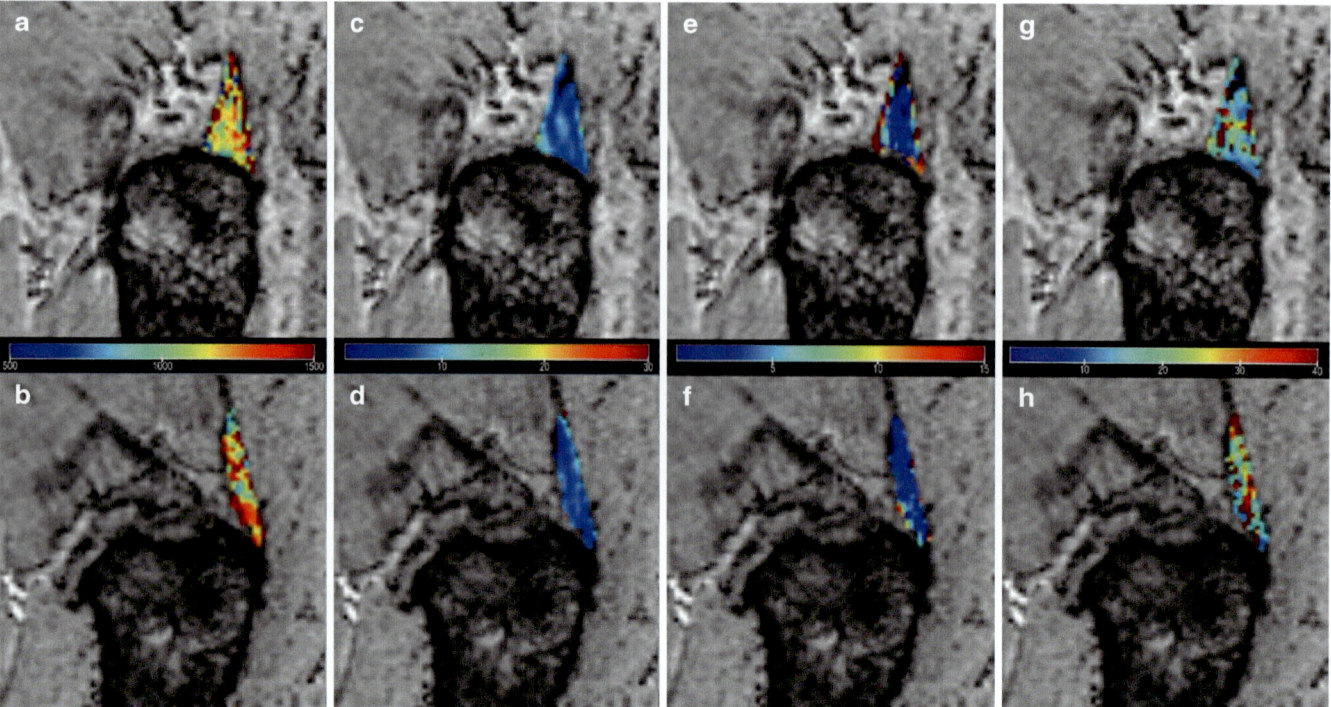

Fig. 9.8 Examples of T_1 maps (**a** and **b**) and T_2^* maps (**c** to **h**) in two subjects with gluteal tendons parallel to B_0: top row, a 70-year-old woman with gluteal tendinopathy, and bottom row, 64-year-old asymptomatic woman. (Adapted with permission from Ref. [29])

tendinopathy [29]. The vTE sequence was acquired using a 3T MRI scanner with TEs ranging from 1.1 ms to 19.8 ms and a resolution of $0.6 \times 0.8 \times 3$ mm³. Mono-exponential T_2^* and short-T_2^* component imaging demonstrated relatively high diagnostic accuracy, ranging from 0.80 to 0.89, and both parameters also showed a strong correlation with the clinical score. When imaging complex joints, the magic angle effect must be considered, as it has a significant impact on absolute T_2^* values. To minimize this effect, patients were positioned so that tendon fibers were parallel to the main magnetic field B_0 (Fig. 9.8).

Finally, the vTE sequence has also been used for quantitative imaging of intraneural connective tissues and myelin sheaths [7]. It was used with a resolution of $0.6 \times 0.6 \times 5.0$ mm³ and two TEs (0.98 and 5.37 ms) to compute apparent T_2^*s (aT_2^*s) by mono-exponential fitting. In addition, repeatability and reproducibility were determined. This study, involving 15 healthy volunteers, showed relatively good repeatability (dice indices of 0.68–0.7 and 0.70–0.72 for intra-rater and inter-rater, respectively), as well as good reproducibility (intra-inter reader ICC of 0.95–0.97). In the future, vTE may be useful for the assessment of peripheral nerve disorders.

The vTE Sequence for Sodium (^{23}Na) MRI

Sodium MRI (^{23}Na-MRI) is an advanced imaging modality that can be used for biochemical investigations of many clinical questions and can be applied to almost any part of the human body from cartilage to the brain [30].

Although sodium imaging offers very valuable information that is complementary to proton (^{1}H) MRI, the technique is challenging. ^{23}Na MRI is characterized by low sensitivity because, compared to ^{1}H imaging, it has a much lower SNR as a result of low sodium concentrations in vivo, a low gyromagnetic ratio, and much shorter relaxation times. In addition, ^{23}Na in tissue shows biexponential relaxation behavior, which means that most of the ^{23}Na signal is lost within a few ms [30]. One possibility to overcome these challenges is to develop pulse sequences that allow measurements with sub-ms TEs and very short signal readouts (sampling). A short TE is necessary to ensure that the sodium signal has not decayed to zero, or near zero, before the signal is sampled; also, a very short signal readout duration is required to minimize signal decay during signal sampling [31].

The vTE sequence developed by Deligianni et al. [6] and adapted for sodium imaging proved to be robust enough to

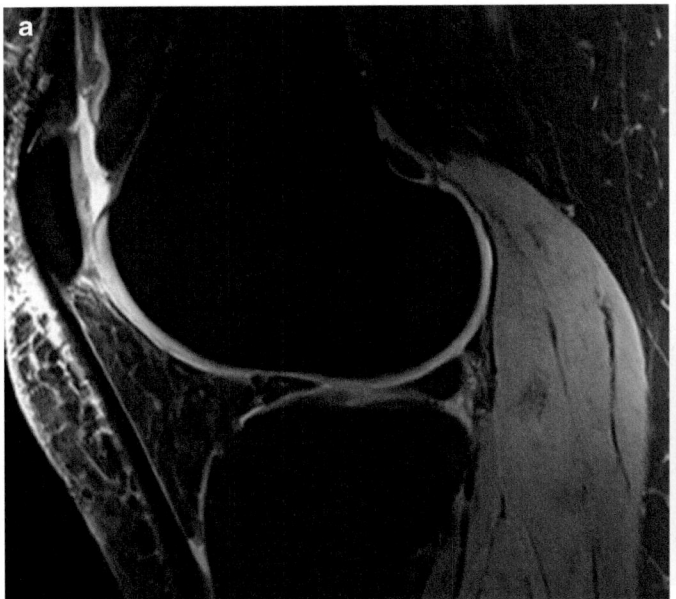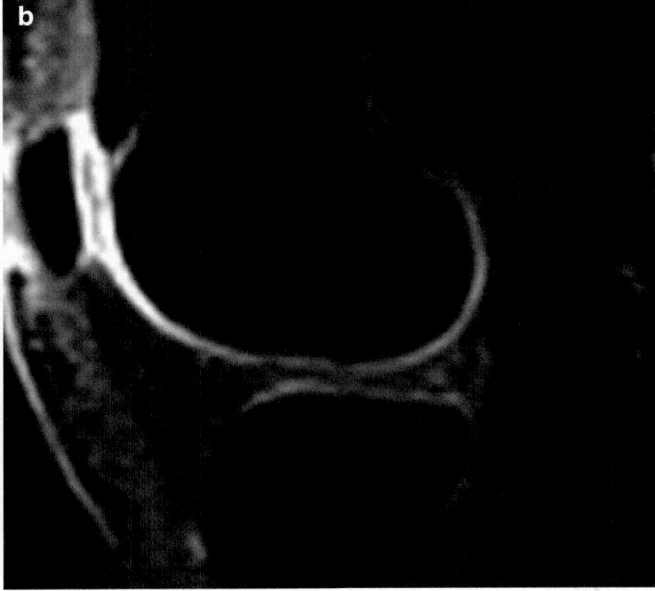

Fig. 9.9 Examples of knee images from a healthy volunteer acquired at 7 T. (**a**) Morphological proton density-weighted, 2D turbo spin echo image with fat suppression (resolution, $0.4 \times 0.4 \times 2.5$ mm³; acquisition time, 4:17 min). (**b**) Corresponding sodium vTE image (resolution, $1.4 \times 1.5 \times 3.0$ mm³; acquisition time, 28:14 min). (Adapted with permission from Ref. [32])

overcome the above mentioned challenges and has been successfully used in several published studies. As an example, Fig. 9.9 shows (a) a morphological proton density-weighted image and (b) the corresponding sodium vTE image of the knee joint of a healthy subject acquired at 7 T [32].

The vTE sequence was used for renal sodium MR imaging and investigation of the corticomedullary ^{23}Na gradient. The results of this study showed that ^{23}Na concentration increases from the cortex to the medullary pyramid [33].

The sequence was also applied to cartilage and tendon imaging; Marik et al. demonstrated the feasibility of using the vTE sequence to study changes in sodium content in cartilage in patients with diabetes mellitus I. The authors reported significantly lower mean normalized signal intensity (MNSI) values in cartilage ($P = 0.008$) and significantly higher values in tendons ($P = 0.025$) in patients compared to those parameters in healthy volunteers [34].

Zbyn et al. used the vTE sequence to assess low-grade focal cartilage lesions in the knee (baseline, 1 week, 3-month, and 6-month follow-up data) and found that the mean coefficients of variation of sodium corrected signal intensity (^{23}Na-cSI) values between the baseline and 1-week follow-up were 5.1% or less in all cartilage regions. At all time points, significantly lower ^{23}Na-cSI values were found in lesions than in weight-bearing and non-weight–bearing regions (all P values ≤ 0.002). Although a significant decrease in ^{23}Na-cSI values in the lesion from baseline was observed at the 3-month visit ($P = 0.015$), no significant change was observed at 6 months [8].

In addition, it was shown that ^{23}Na MRI data acquired with the vTE sequence can be used to determine the fixed charge density (FCD) distribution of knee joint cartilage. The results demonstrated that the decrease in FCD (the average decrease throughout the tibial cartilage was -17, -47, and -100%, in "early osteoarthritis (OA)," "advanced OA," and "no FCD" models, respectively) mainly as the result of fibril and axial strains. Compared to the "healthy" model, the largest differences in all the parameters observed were in the FCD. It was neglected in the "no FCD" models. The effect of FCD was more substantial in the lateral than in the medial tibial cartilage, particularly during the assessment of the loading response to stance [35].

Over the past few years, the vTE sequence has been shown to have great potential in clinical research. Further technical improvements may establish the vTE sequence as a reliable imaging tool for the study of the molecular properties of tissues, in addition to the clinical findings seen with standard diagnostic procedures.

References

1. Kumar A, Welti D, Ernst RR. NMR Fourier zeugmatography. J Magn Reson. 1975;18(1):69–83.
2. Song HK, Wehrli FW. Variable TE gradient and spin echo sequences for in vivo MR microscopy of short T_2 species. Mag Reson Med. 1998;39(2):251–8.
3. Techawiboonwong A, Song HK, Wehrli FW. In vivo MRI of submillisecond T_2 species with two-dimensional and three-dimensional

radial sequences and applications to the measurement of cortical bone water. NMR Biomed. 2008;21(1):59–70.

4. Ying K, Schmalbrock P, Clymer B. Echo-time reduction for sub-millimeter resolution imaging with a 3D phase encode time reduced acquisition method. Mag Reson Med. 1995;33(1):82–7.

5. Jeong EK, Parker DL, Tsuruda JS, Won JY. Reduction of flow-related signal loss in flow-compensated 3D TOF MR angiography, using variable echo time (3D TOF-VTE). Magn Reson Med. 2002;48(4):667–76.

6. Deligianni X, Bar P, Scheffler K, Trattnig S, Bieri O. High-resolution Fourier-encoded sub-millisecond echo time musculoskeletal imaging at 3 Tesla and 7 Tesla. Magn Reson Med. 2013;70(5):1434–9.

7. Felisaz PF, Belatti E, Deligianni X, Bergsland N, Santini F, Paoletti M, et al. Variable echo time imaging for detecting the short T_2* components of the sciatic nerve: a validation study. MAGMA. 2021;34(3):411–9.

8. Zbýň Š, Schreiner M, Juras V, Mlynarik V, Szomolanyi P, Laurent D, et al. Assessment of low-grade focal cartilage lesions in the knee with sodium MRI at 7 T: reproducibility and short-term, 6-month follow-up data. Investig Radiol. 2020;55(7):430–7.

9. Deligianni X, Bar P, Scheffler K, Trattnig S, Bieri O. Water-selective excitation of short T_2 species with binomial pulses. Magn Reson Med. 2014;72(3):800–5.

10. Hager B, Walzer SM, Deligianni X, Bieri O, Berg A, Schreiner MM, et al. Orientation dependence and decay characteristics of T_2* relaxation in the human meniscus studied with 7 tesla MR microscopy and compared to histology. Mag Reson Med. 2019;81(2):921–33.

11. Hager B, Schreiner MM, Walzer SM, Hirtler L, Mlynarik V, Berg A, et al. Transverse relaxation anisotropy of the Achilles and Patellar tendon studied by MR microscopy. J Magn Reson Imaging. 2022;56(4):1091–103.

12. Juras V, Apprich S, Szomolanyi P, Bieri O, Deligianni X, Trattnig S. Bi-exponential T2* analysis of healthy and diseased Achilles tendons: an in vivo preliminary magnetic resonance study and correlation with clinical score. Eur Radiol. 2013;23(10):2814–22.

13. Hornakova L, Juras V, Kubovy P, Hadraba D, Gerych D, Stursa P, et al. In vivo assessment of time dependent changes of T_2* in medial meniscus under loading at 3T: a preliminary study. J Appl Biomed. 2018;16(2):138–44.

14. Santini F, Patil S, Scheffler K. IceLuva: a scripting framework for MR image reconstruction based on free software. Concepts Magn Reson Part B Magn Reson Eng. 2011;39(1):1–10.

15. Juras V, Apprich S, Zbyn S, Zak L, Deligianni X, Szomolanyi P, et al. Quantitative MRI analysis of menisci using biexponential T_2* fitting with a variable echo time sequence. Magn Reson Med. 2014;71(3):1015–23.

16. Haneder S, Konstandin S, Morelli JN, Nagel AM, Zoellner FG, Schad LR, et al. Quantitative and qualitative 23Na MR imaging of the human kidneys at 3 T: before and after a water load. Radiology. 2011;260(3):857–65.

17. Bydder G. The Agfa Mayneord lecture: MRI of short and ultrashort T_2 and T_2* components of tissues, fluids and materials using clinical systems. Br J Rad. 2011;84(1008):1067–82.

18. Bachmann E, Rosskopf AB, Götschi T, Klarhöfer M, Deligianni X, Hilbe M, et al. T_1-and T_2*-mapping for assessment of tendon tissue biophysical properties: a phantom MRI study. Investig Radiol. 2019;54(4):212–20.

19. Zbyn S, Apprich S, Juras V, Szomolanyi P, Walzer S, Deligianni X, et al. Ex vivo mapping of sodium T_1 and T_2* relaxation times in human lumbar intervertebral discs at 7 Tesla. Proc Intl Soc Mag Reson Med. 2013:2473.

20. Juras V, Latta P, Kojan M, Starcuk Z, Deligianni X, Bieri O, et al. The comparison of two ultra-short echo time methods for T_2* mapping in Achilles tendon and enthesis. Proc Intl Soc Mag Reson Med. 2019:1399.

21. Deligianni X, Jirák D, Berková Z, Hájek M, Scheffler K, Bieri O. In vivo visualization of cells labeled with superparamagnetic iron oxides by a sub-millisecond gradient echo sequence. MAGMA. 2014;27(4):329–37.

22. Brown MA, Semelka RC, Dale BM. MRI: basic principles and applications. 5th ed. Hoboken, NJ: John Wiley & Sons/Blackwell; 2015.

23. Glover P, Mansfield P. Limits to magnetic resonance microscopy. Rep Prog Phys. 2002;65(10):1489.

24. Asher K, Bangerter NK, Watkins RD, Gold GE. Radiofrequency coils for musculoskeletal MRI. Top Magn Reson Imaging. 2010;21(5):315–23.

25. Froidevaux R, Weiger M, Rosler MB, Brunner DO, Dietrich BE, Reber J, et al. High-resolution short-T(2) MRI using a high-performance gradient. Magn Reson Med. 2020;84(4):1933–46.

26. Mastrogiacomo S, Dou W, Jansen JA, Walboomers XF. Magnetic resonance imaging of hard tissues and hard tissue engineered bio-substitutes. Mol Imaging Biol. 2019;21(6):1003–19.

27. Juras V, Winhofer Y, Szomolanyi P, Vosshenrich J, Hager B, Wolf P, et al. Multiparametric MR imaging depicts glycosaminoglycan change in the achilles tendon during ciprofloxacin administration in healthy men: initial observation. Radiology. 2015;275(3):763–71.

28. Stelzeneder B, Trabauer BM, Aldrian S, Stelzeneder D, Juras V, Albrecht C, et al. Evaluation of meniscal tissue after meniscal repair using ultrahigh field MRI. J Knee Surg. 2021;34(12):1337–48.

29. Dadour JR, Gilbert G, Lepage-Saucier M, Freire V, Bureau NJ. Quantitative MRI in patients with gluteal tendinopathy and asymptomatic volunteers: initial results on T_1-and T_2*-mapping diagnostic accuracy and correlation with clinical assessment. Skelet Radiol. 2021;50(11):2221–31.

30. Zaric O, Juras V, Szomolanyi P, Schreiner M, Raudner M, Giraudo C, et al. Frontiers of sodium MRI revisited: from cartilage to brain imaging. J Magn Reson Imaging. 2021;54(1):58–75.

31. Bangerter NK, Tarbox GJ, Taylor MD, Kaggie JD. Quantitative sodium magnetic resonance imaging of cartilage, muscle, and tendon. Quant Imaging Med Surg. 2016;6(6):699–714.

32. Zbýň Š, Mlynárik V, Juras V, Szomolanyi P, Trattnig S. Evaluation of cartilage repair and osteoarthritis with sodium MRI. NMR Biomed. 2016;29(2):206–15.

33. Haneder S, Juras V, Michaely HJ, Deligianni X, Bieri O, Schoenberg SO, et al. In vivo sodium (23Na) imaging of the human kidneys at 7 T: preliminary results. Eur Radiol. 2014;24(2):494–501.

34. Marik W, Nemec SF, Zbýň Š, Zalaudek M, Ludvik B, Riegler G, et al. Changes in cartilage and tendon composition of patients with type I diabetes mellitus: identification by quantitative sodium magnetic resonance imaging at 7 T. Investig Radiol. 2016;51(4):266–72.

35. Räsänen LP, Tanska P, Zbýň Š, van Donkelaar CC, Trattnig S, Nieminen MT, et al. The effect of fixed charge density and cartilage swelling on mechanics of knee joint cartilage during simulated gait. J Biomech. 2017;61:34–44.

Looping Star: Time-Multiplexed, Gradient Echo Zero TE MR Imaging

10

Florian Wiesinger and Ana Beatriz Solana

Introduction

Over the past few years, the rotating ultrafast imaging sequence (RUFIS) invented by Madio and Lowe in 1995 [1] has experienced a dramatic revival [2–7]. Its unique characteristics of zero nominal echo time (i.e., TE = 0) and silent MR imaging have stimulated exciting new clinical applications as well as novel technical refinements [2–6]. Nowadays, RUFIS is commonly referred to as Zero TE (ZTE).

Looping Star [7] is a new pulse sequence which extends ZTE toward gradient echo (GRE) imaging via a time-multiplexed gradient-refocusing mechanism. It provides a free induction decay (FID) image with a nominal TE = 0 (like standard ZTE) together with equidistant GRE images which contain additional T_2^* and susceptibility information. The name "Looping Star" reflects its self-refocusing (i.e., Looping) k-space trajectory and the use of 3D radial (i.e., Star) image encoding.

This chapter provides a detailed explanation of the Looping Star method with the focus on MR physics considerations and initial neuroimaging applications [7]. After first starting with a recap of ZTE and gradient refocusing, Looping Star is explained as a time-multiplexed, gradient-refocused ZTE sequence. Particular attention is paid to the so-called echo IN/OUT overlap artifact and various strategies to mitigate it. Coherence-resolved Looping Star [8] is then described as a recent refinement of the original Looping Star sequence which eliminates echo IN/OUT overlap via temporal separation within the pulse sequence. Subsequently, image reconstruction and further technical considerations are discussed. The chapter closes with a description of initial applications and future prospects.

F. Wiesinger (✉) · A. B. Solana
GE HealthCare, Munich, Germany

Center for Neuroimaging, Institute of Psychiatry, Psychology and Neuroscience (IoPPN), King's College London, London, UK

Recap of ZTE

Among the large zoo of existing MR pulse sequences, RUFIS-type ZTE [1] can be considered the simplest, at least in terms of radiofrequency (RF) and gradient waveform complexity. As illustrated in the ZTE section of Fig. 10.1, it consists of (i) very short, block-shaped RF hard pulses (colored vertical thick lines) for signal excitation, and (ii) constant amplitude readout gradients (gray horizontal line) for image encoding. This leads to 3D nonselective RF excitation followed by 3D center-out radial image encoding with a nominal echo time TE = 0 (i.e., image encoding starting at the time of RF excitation). While the readout gradient amplitude remains constant (i.e., $|G_{read}| = (G_x^2 + G_y^2 + G_z^2)^{1/2}$), the direction of this gradient changes between repetitions in such a way that the endpoints of the 3D center-out radial spokes follow a smooth spiral trajectory along the surface of the spherical 3D k-space (with uniform angular sampling density). As a consequence, gradient switching is reduced to a minimum (because of the small directional gradient updates), hence enabling virtually silent MR imaging clear of eddy currents. Besides its main characteristics of TE = 0 and silent imaging, ZTE also offers highly efficient sampling with exceptionally short repetition times (TRs) and robustness against eddy currents and patient motion.

Figure 10.1 also illustrates the excitation and temporal evolution of FID signal coherences in k-space (bottom subplot) in synchrony with the pulse sequence (top subplot). Each RF pulse excites a new signal coherence which then evolves in the presence of subsequent readout gradients. Each acquired k-space sample is the sum of the current FID signal (colored thick arrow) and previously excited coherences (colored thick lines). In standard ZTE, with only small directional readout updates between repetitions, earlier excited coherences quickly vanish in outer k-space due to gradient dephasing (i.e., gradient spoiling) and T_2^* signal decay, so that the acquired k-space samples primarily consist of the current FID (thick arrow). Accordingly, the measured signal (y_{FID}) originating from the FID magnetization distribution (i.e., the unknown image x_{FID}) is given by:

© The Author(s), under exclusive license to Springer Nature Switzerland AG 2023
J. Du, G. M. Bydder (eds.), *MRI of Short- and Ultrashort-T₂ Tissues*, https://doi.org/10.1007/978-3-031-35197-6_10

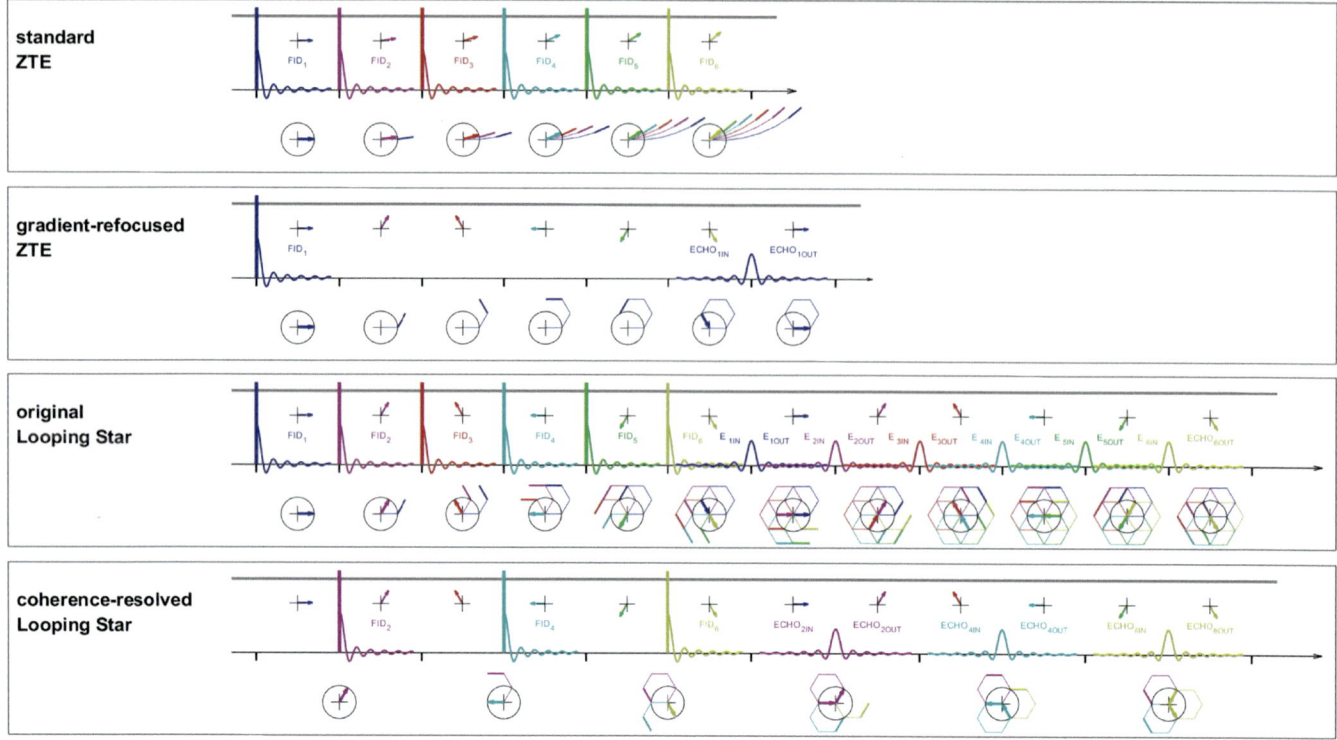

Fig. 10.1 Schematic showing standard ZTE (top), gradient-refocused ZTE (second row: $N_{SpkPerLoop} = 6$, $N_{Loop} = 2$), original Looping Star (third row: $N_{SpkPerLoop} = 6$, $N_{Loop} = 2$), and coherence-resolved Looping Star (bottom: $N_{SpkPerLoop} = 3$, $N_{Loop} = 2$). Each subplot illustrates the pulse sequence timing (top) and the corresponding creation and temporal evolution of signal coherences in k-space (bottom). The pulse sequence diagram exemplifies the short block-shaped RF pulses (colored vertical lines), the constant amplitude readout gradient (horizontal gray line), and the spoke readout direction (colored arrows) along the horizontal time axis, with ticks indicating the repetition time (TR). Each RF excitation (colored vertical lines) creates an FID signal coherence (colored sinc-shaped line) which, together with earlier excited coherences, evolves in k-space following the current spoke direction (colored arrow), with change in direction every TR. A gradient echo (colored sinc-shaped line) emerges whenever the cumulative k-space trajectory of a signal coherence refocuses back into the center of k-space. For educational purposes, the coloring of corresponding RF excitations, readout spokes, signal coherences, FID, and gradient echo signals, is matched. The black circle, with radius $k_{max} = M/2\ \Delta k$, indicates the event horizon beyond which signals are assumed to vanish due to gradient (and RF) spoiling. For simplicity, TR is assumed to be identical to the spoke readout duration (i.e., TR $= T_{Spk} = M/2\ \Delta t$)

$$y_{FID}\left(\mathbf{k}_{n,m}\right) = \int d^3 r\, x_{FID}\left(\mathbf{r}\right) e^{i\mathbf{k}_{n,m}\mathbf{r}} \left[1 + e^{-\frac{T_R}{T_2^*} + i\mathbf{k}_{n-1,END}\mathbf{r}} + \cdots + e^{-\frac{(n-1)T_R}{T_2^*} + i\left(\mathbf{k}_{1,END} + \cdots + \mathbf{k}_{n-1,END}\right)\mathbf{r}} \right]$$

$$\cong \int d^3 r\, x_{FID}\left(\mathbf{r}\right) e^{i\mathbf{k}_{n,m}\mathbf{r}}$$

(10.1)

where $\mathbf{k}_{n,m}$ describes the center-out 3D radial k-space encoding (i.e., $|\mathbf{k}_{n,m}| = m\ \Delta k$, with $\Delta k = \gamma\ |\mathbf{G}_{read}|\ \Delta t$, and Δt the dwell time), n is the spoke number (i.e., $n = 1 \ldots N_{spk}$), and m indexes the center-out sampling position along each spoke (i.e., $m = 0 \ldots M/2$). The thick arrows indicate $\mathbf{k}_{n,END}$ (i.e., the end-point of the nth spoke), and the black circle shows the nominal k-space radius $k_{max} = M/2\ \Delta k$. Assuming perfect gradient (and RF) spoiling, k_{max} can be considered an event horizon in the sense that only signals within k_{max} contribute to the measurement. Signal coherences outside k_{max} can still be rewound into the center of k-space via gradient refocus-ing and thereby generate a GRE signal (assuming that the rewinding occurs within the finite T_2^* signal lifetime). For educational purposes, let us consider a 3D imaging experiment with an imaging bandwidth BW = 100 kHz (corresponding to ±50 kHz) and imaging matrix size $M^3 = 256^3$ (cf. Figure 10.1 and Table 10.1). Under ideal conditions (i.e., neglecting transmit-receive switching and gradient update times), the repetition time (TR) is determined by the duration of the center-out readout spoke (T_{Spk}), according to TR $\cong T_{Spk} = M/2\ \Delta t = 1.28$ ms (i.e., $M/2 = 128$ samples acquired with a dwell time of $\Delta t = 1\,/\,$BW = 10 μs). The 3D

Table 10.1 Imaging example (i.e., $M^3 = 256^3$, BW = 100 kHz (= ±50 kHz)) to illustrate standard ZTE, gradient-refocused ZTE, original Looping Star, and coherence-resolved Looping Star pulse sequence parameters

	original ZTE	gradient-refocused ZTE	original Looping Star	coherence-resolved Looping Star
(given) image matrix: M^3	$M^3 = 256^3$			
(given) imaging bandwidth: BW and dwell time: Δt	BW = 100 kHz (= ±50 kHz) $\Delta t = 1/\text{BW} = 10\ \mu s$			
(given) number of spokes per loop: $N_{\text{SpkPerLoop}}$ and number of loops: N_{Loop}	n.a. n.a.	$N_{\text{SpkPerLoop}} = 6$ (radial) $N_{\text{Loop}} = 2$		$N_{\text{SpkPerLoop}} = 3$ (diameter) $N_{\text{Loop}} = 2$
repetition time: TR and spoke readout duration: T_{Spk}	$TR \cong T_{\text{Spk}}$ $T_{\text{Spk}} = (M/2)*\Delta t = 1.28$ ms			$TR \cong T_{\text{Spk}}$ $T_{\text{Spk}} = M*\Delta t = 2.56$ ms
echo time spacing: ΔTE and echo times: TE	n.a. TE = 0	$\Delta\text{TE} = N_{\text{SpkPerLoop}}*T_{\text{Spk}} = 7.68$ ms TE = $[0 \ldots N_{\text{Loop}}\text{-}1]*\Delta\text{TE} = [0, 7.68]$ms		
max. RF pulse width: Δt_{RF} and max Flip angle: FA_{max} ($B_{1,\text{max}} = 20\ \mu T$)	$\Delta t_{\text{RF}} = \Delta t = 1/\text{BW} = 10\ \mu s$ $FA_{\text{max}} = \gamma*B_{1,\text{max}}*\Delta t_{\text{RF}} = 3°$			
avg. RF pulse spacing: ΔRF and Ernst angle: FA_{Ernst} ($T_1 = 1$ s)	$\Delta\text{RF} = T_{\text{Spk}} = 1.28$ ms $FA_{\text{Ernst}} = 2.9°$	$\Delta\text{RF} = [(N_{\text{Loop}}\text{-}1)*N_{\text{SpkPerLoop}} + 1]*$ $T_{\text{Spk}} = 8.96$ ms $FA_{\text{Ernst}} = 7.7°$	$\Delta\text{RF} = N_{\text{Loop}}*T_{\text{Spk}}$ = 2.56 ms $FA_{\text{Ernst}} = 4.1°$	$\Delta\text{RF} = N_{\text{Loop}}*T_{\text{Spk}} = 5.12$ ms $FA_{\text{Ernst}} = 5.8°$
scan time and sampling efficiency	84 s 100%	$[(N_{\text{Loop}}\text{-}1)*N_{\text{SpkPerLoop}} + 1]*$ 84 s = 588 s $[2*(N_{\text{Loop}}\text{-}1) + 1]/$ $[(N_{\text{Loop}}\text{-}1)*N_{\text{SpkPerLoop}} + 1] = 43\%$	$N_{\text{Loop}}*84$ s = 168 s 100%	$N_{\text{Loop}}*84$ s = 168 s $(N_{\text{Loop}}\text{-}0.5)/N_{\text{Loop}} = 75\%$

center-out radial acquisition results in a k-space sampling density which decreases with increasing distance from the k-space center. The sampling density at the periphery of k-space (i.e., $|\mathbf{k}_{n,\text{END}}| = M/2\ \Delta k$) is defined as the number of spokes divided by the enclosed spherical surface area, according to $N_{\text{spk}} / (4\ \pi\ |\mathbf{k}_{n,\text{END}}|^2) = N_{\text{spk}} / (\pi M^2\ \Delta k^2)$. The Nyquist sampling criterion requires at least one spoke per unit k-space surface area (i.e., Δk^2), which in turn determines the number of required spokes according to $N_{\text{Spk}} = M^2 = 65{,}536$ (including an undersampling factor of π, which is often considered acceptable in 3D radial imaging). With $TR \cong T_{\text{Spk}}$ the whole scan time (i.e., $N_{\text{Spk}}\ TR \cong 84$ s) is used for acquiring data resulting in a sampling efficiency of ~100%.

Gradient Refocusing Along Polygonal k-Space Trajectories

Gradient refocusing of a single FID coherence into a GRE signal can be achieved by choosing spokes so that their cumulative trajectory rewinds back into the center of k-space. The gradient-refocused ZTE section in Fig. 10.1 illustrates this for a single coherence (i.e., FID_1 excited in the first repetition) and number of spokes per loop $N_{\text{SpkPerLoop}} = 6$ with a relative angular increment of $\Delta\varphi = 2\pi / N_{\text{SpkPerLoop}} = 60°$. The excited FID coherence then follows a hexagonal trajectory and, after $TE = N_{\text{SpkPerLoop}}\ TR$, refocuses back from outer

k-space into its origin (i.e., $\sum_{l=1}^{N_{\text{SpkPerLoop}}} k_{l,\text{END}} = 0$) where it forms a GRE signal (y_{ECHO}) according to:

$$y_{\text{ECHO}}\left(\mathbf{k}_{n,m}\right) = \int d^3r\ x_{\text{FID}}\left(\mathbf{r},t\right)e^{i\left(\sum_{l=1}^{N_{\text{SpkPerLoop}}} k_{l,\text{END}}+\mathbf{k}_{n,m}\right)\mathbf{r}}$$
$$= \int d^3r\ x_{\text{ECHO}}\left(\mathbf{r}\right)e^{i\mathbf{k}_{n,m}\mathbf{r}} \quad (10.2)$$

The spatiotemporal evolution of the FID signal during the course of the refocusing introduces additional T_2^* weighting and $\Delta\omega$ off-resonance evolution in the echo image (x_{ECHO}), according to:

$$x_{\text{ECHO}}\left(\mathbf{r}\right) = x_{\text{FID}}\left(\mathbf{r},t = T_E\right) = x_{\text{FID}}\left(\mathbf{r}\right)e^{\left(-\frac{1}{T_2^*(\mathbf{r})}+i\Delta\omega(\mathbf{r})\right)T_E} \quad (10.3)$$

Because of short spoke readout durations (i.e., $TR < 2$ ms), spatiotemporal signal evolution within the acquisition is typically considered negligible.

It is important to note, that the original center-out, half-echo FID signal coherence (FID_1) refocuses into a full-diameter echo in-center-out GRE starting with the inward echo (i.e., $\text{ECHO}_{1,\text{IN}}$) followed by the outward echo (i.e., $\text{ECHO}_{1,\text{OUT}}$), each occupying one full TR. Repeating the readout spoke number of loops (N_{Loop}) times (along the hexagonal self-refocusing trajectory) produces one FID and ($N_{\text{Loop}} - 1$) GREs with equidistant TE spacing given by $\Delta\text{TE} = N_{\text{SpkPerLoop}}\ TR$.

Continuing with our example and assuming $N_{\text{SpkPerLoop}} = 6$ and $N_{\text{Loop}} = 2$ (cf. Figure 10.1 and Table 10.1), the TE spacing becomes $\Delta\text{TE} = N_{\text{SpkPerLoop}}\ TR = 7.68$ ms and the scan time increases to $[(N_{\text{Loop}} - 1) N_{\text{SpkPerLoop}} + 1]$ 84 s = 588 s. Gradient-refocused ZTE provides one FID image followed by $(N_{\text{Loop}} - 1)$ equidistant GRE images, with each GRE acquiring a full-diameter echo in-center-out spoke (compared to radius center-out spokes for the FID). Compared to the original ZTE sequence, the scan efficiency decreases to $[2 (N_{\text{Loop}} - 1) + 1] / [(N_{\text{Loop}} - 1) N_{\text{SpkPerLoop}} + 1] = 43\%$.

Looping Star

The gradient-refocused ZTE described above is inefficient, in the sense that only a fraction of the time is used for acquiring data. Looping Star improves this by time-multiplexing the gradient refocusing to $N_{\text{SpkPerLoop}}$ coherence pathways. As illustrated in the original Looping Star section of Fig. 10.1, RF excitation is now applied at each of the initial $N_{\text{SpkPerLoop}}$ repetitions, and each of the excited $N_{\text{SpkPerLoop}}$ FID coherences then traverses k-space along a hexagonal trajectory (with each signal pathway rotated by $2 \pi/N_{\text{SpkPerLoop}}$ relative to the previous one). By continuing the hexagonal trajectory during the refocusing phase (with the RF excitation turned off), GRE signals are obtained for each of the $N_{\text{SpkPerLoop}}$ FID coherences. In other words, $N_{\text{SpkPerLoop}}$ coherences excited one after the other during the initial FID excitation phase are refocused one after the other during the gradient-refocusing phase. In Looping Star, the refocusing criterion must be fulfilled for each of the $N_{\text{SpkPerLoop}}$ excited coherences according to $\sum_{r=1}^{N_{\text{SpkPerLoop}}} \mathbf{k}_{n+r,M} = 0, \forall n \in \{1 \ldots N_{\text{SpkPerLoop}}\}$. It is important to note that the refocusing criterion is not limited to straight spokes (as illustrated in Fig. 10.1) but can be extended toward twisted spokes including, e.g., out-of-plane rotations for higher sampling efficiency. In analogy to gradient echo ZTE, also Looping Star provides one FID and $(N_{\text{Loop}}-1)$ gradient echoes with equidistant echo time spacing of $\Delta\text{TE} = N_{\text{SpkPerLoop}}$ TR. For 3D spatial image encoding, the basic Looping Star building block (as illustrated in Fig. 10.1) must be repeated $N_{\text{Spk}}/N_{\text{SpkPerLoop}}$ times with the readout gradient waveform (and hence the k-space encoding) rotated in a 3D pseudorandom manner [7, 9, 10].

The illustrated Looping Star example with $N_{\text{SpkPerLoop}} = 6$ and $N_{\text{Loop}} = 2$ (Fig. 10.1 and Table 10.1) provides one FID and one GRE image with TE spacing $\Delta\text{TE} = N_{\text{SpkPerLoop}}$ TR = 7.68 ms. In comparison to gradient-refocused ZTE, the scan time is now much shorter N_{Loop} 84 s = 168 s with a sampling efficiency of ~100%.

Echo IN/OUT Overlap

The Looping Star sequence is highly efficient in the way it excites FID coherences and gradient refocuses them to form echo signals; it effectively allows continuous sampling of FID and gradient echo signals without dead-time gaps. However, the fact that each signal coherence produces an echo which extends over two TRs and leads to echo IN/OUT overlap of acquired k-space samples (within the event horizon k_{max}) during the refocusing phase. As can be seen in the original Looping Star section of Fig. 10.1, signal overlap primarily affects the echo signals (i.e., $\text{ECHO}_{1,\text{OUT}}$ overlaps with $\text{ECHO}_{2,\text{IN}}$, … $\text{ECHO}_{5,\text{OUT}}$ overlaps with $\text{ECHO}_{6,\text{IN}}$) but also mixes the last FID with the first incoming echo (i.e., FID_6 overlaps with $\text{ECHO}_{1,\text{IN}}$).

The echo IN/OUT overlap can be resolved by (i) k-space filtering, (ii) RF excitation phase cycling, (iii) model-based image reconstruction, and (iv) coherence-resolved Looping Star [7, 8, 11]. The first two methods (i.e., k-space filtering and phase cycling) aim to separate the data into ECHO_{OUT} and ECHO_{IN} components. More specifically, the first method (i.e., filtering) divides each readout into an ECHO_{OUT} signal (dominant at the beginning of the TR) and an ECHO_{IN} signal (dominant at the end of the TR) by applying a Fermi filter with a flat signal response for the respective regions and zero outside. This eliminates echo IN/OUT overlap at the expense of cutting off high spatial frequency information and hence a loss of spatial resolution. With the second method (i.e., RF excitation phase cycling), each loop is recorded twice, without (default) and with π RF phase cycling between consecutive RF excitations. Echo-in and echo-out signal components can then be separated by means of a simple linear combination at the cost of a longer scan time but without loss of spatial resolution. The remaining two methods (i.e., coherence-resolved Looping Star and model-based image reconstruction) are discussed in detail in subsequent sections.

Figure 10.2 which is explained in the image reconstruction section, illustrates the Looping Star echo IN/OUT overlap problem and its various mitigation strategies for a numerical 2D Shepp-Logan phantom.

Coherence-Resolved Looping Star

The echo IN/OUT overlap problem encountered in the original Looping Star implementation can also be resolved via temporal separation of the signal coherences in the pulse sequence [8]. As illustrated in Fig. 10.1, in coherence-resolved Looping Star, only every other FID signal coherence gets excited during the excitation phase thereby leaving sufficient temporal separation for each signal coherence to fully rewind during the refocusing phase without temporal echo IN/OUT overlap. The number of excited coherences is reduced by half, but each coherence still follows a hexagonal trajectory. Accordingly, coherence-resolved Looping Star provides radial center-out FID signals during the excitation phase (first loop) and uncontaminated diameter in-center-out GRE signals during the refocusing phase (subsequent loops).

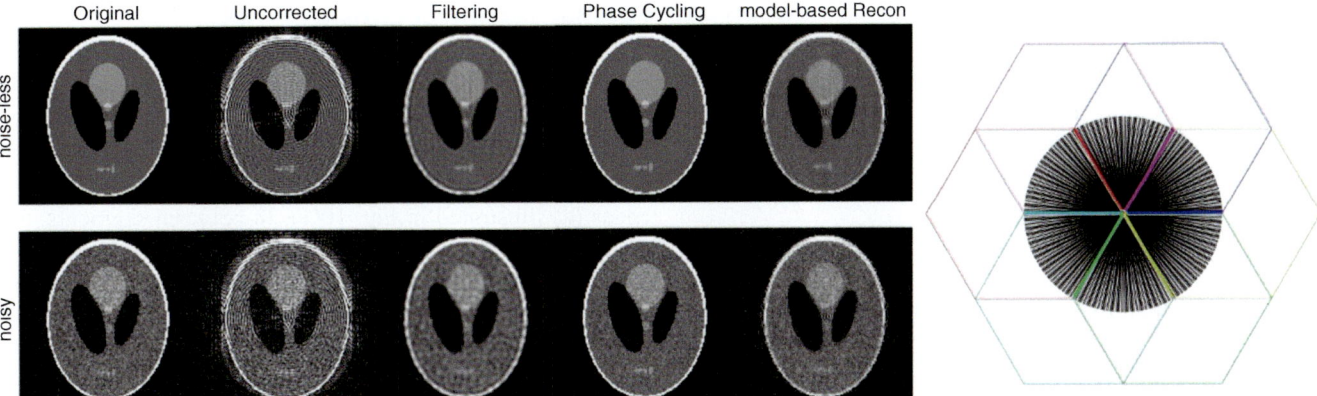

Fig. 10.2 2D Shepp-Logan Looping Star imaging simulation ($M^2 = 128^2$, $N_{\text{SpkPerLoop}} = 6$, $N_{\text{Spk}} = 408$) demonstrating echo IN/OUT artifact (second column) and various ways of mitigation including filtering (third column), phase cycling (fourth column), and model-based image reconstruction (fifth column). The figure illustrates results for both infinite (top) and finite (bottom) SNR scenarios

Conceptually the coherence-resolved Looping Star is analogous to the original Looping Star with k-space filtering. However, coherence-resolved Looping Star accounts for echo IN/OUT separation in the pulse sequence design and thereby maintains the echo spacing and image resolution of the echo images. Additionally, it leads to a cleaner and more symmetric pulse sequence design with the RF excitation and the resulting GREs centered in the middle of the now doubled repetition time. In this way, coherence-resolved Looping Star provides a full in-center-out diameter GRE, while the original Looping Star only permits time for echo-out radial sampling thereby causing echo IN/OUT overlap.

Extending our example from above, coherence-resolved Looping Star reduces the number of spokes per loop by half to $N_{\text{SpkPerLoop}} = 3$ and doubles the spoke duration $T_{\text{Spk}} = 2.56$ ms but maintains the same TE spacing (i.e., ΔTE = $N_{\text{SpkPerLoop}}$ TR = 7.68 ms). Importantly and unlike the earlier examples, coherence-resolved Looping Star acquires diameter spokes. These capture only half as many FID spokes during the excitation phase but sample the same spokes during the refocusing phase clear of echo IN/OUT overlap. Compared to the original Looping Star sequence, the scan duration is the same (i.e., N_{Loop} 84 s = 168 s), but the sampling efficiency decreases somewhat to ($N_{\text{Loop}} - 0.5$)/$N_{\text{Loop}} = 75\%$ because of the reduced number of FID spokes. By extending the readout during the excitation phase, the spatial resolution of the FID spokes (and accordingly the sampling efficiency) can be increased.

Image Reconstruction

Image reconstruction of the unknown image x($\mathbf{r}$) via the measured/known k-space data y($\mathbf{k}$) is based on a discretized signal model in which the 3D image-space position vector $\mathbf{r}_{u,v,w}$ and the 2D k-space spokes $\mathbf{k}_{n,m}$ are both flattened into 1D vectors, so that:

$$\mathbf{y}_{(n,m)} = \sum_{(u,v,w)} \mathbf{E}_{(n,m),(u,v,w)} \, \mathbf{x}_{(u,v,w)} \tag{10.4}$$

where $\mathbf{E}$ is the Looping Star image encoding matrix, modeling the forward encoding of the image $\mathbf{x}$ into corresponding k-space samples $\mathbf{y}$.

Conventional Looping Star aims to separate the measured data into echo-out (i.e, $\mathbf{y}^{\text{OUT}} = \mathbf{E}^{\text{OUT}}$ x) and echo-in (i.e., $\mathbf{y}^{\text{IN}} = \mathbf{E}^{\text{IN}}$ x) contributions via filtering, RF phase cycling, or coherence-resolved Looping Star, which translates into simple Fourier image encoding matrices for each echo contribution independent of the other one:

$$\mathbf{E}^{\text{OUT}}_{(n,m),(u,v,w)} = e^{i\mathbf{k}^{\text{OUT}}_{(n,m)}\mathbf{r}_{(u,v,w)}} = e^{i\mathbf{k}_{n,m}\mathbf{r}_{(u,v,w)}}$$
$$\mathbf{E}^{\text{IN}}_{(n,m),(u,v,w)} = e^{i\mathbf{k}^{\text{IN}}_{(n,m)}\mathbf{r}_{(u,v,w)}} = e^{i\left(-\mathbf{k}_{n,\text{END}} + \mathbf{k}_{n,m}\right)\mathbf{r}_{(u,v,w)}} \tag{10.5}$$

with $\mathbf{k}^{\text{OUT}}_{(n,m)} = \mathbf{k}_{n,m}$ the outward spoke trajectory and $\mathbf{k}^{\text{IN}}_{(n,m)} = -\mathbf{k}_{n,\text{END}} + \mathbf{k}_{n,m}$ the inward spoke trajectory. Equations 10.5 can be solved independently using standard 3D non-Cartesian gridding-based image reconstruction [7, 12–15].

For general Looping Star image reconstruction without prior echo IN/OUT separation, the measured k-space samples constitute a linear superposition of echo-out and echo-in contributions (i.e., $\mathbf{y} = \mathbf{y}^{\text{OUT}} + \mathbf{y}^{\text{IN}} = (\mathbf{E}^{\text{OUT}} + \mathbf{E}^{\text{IN}})$ x), which can be modeled via a joint encoding matrix, according to:

$$\mathbf{E}_{(n,m),(u,v,w)} = \mathbf{E}^{\text{OUT}}_{(n,m),(u,v,w)} + \mathbf{E}^{\text{IN}}_{(n,m),(u,v,w)}$$
$$= 2e^{-\frac{i\mathbf{k}_{(n,\text{END})}\mathbf{r}_{(u,v,w)}}{2}} \cos\left(\frac{\mathbf{k}_{(n,\text{END})}\mathbf{r}_{(u,v,w)}}{2}\right) \mathbf{E}^{\text{OUT}}_{(n,m),(u,v,w)} \tag{10.6}$$

using cos(z) = 1/2 [exp(+iz) + exp(−iz)]. Apparently, extending the echo-out model to include echo-in contributions results in an extra modulation (i.e., exp(−i $\mathbf{k}_{n,\text{END}}$ $\mathbf{r}$ / 2) cos ($\mathbf{k}_{n,\text{END}}$ $\mathbf{r}$/2)) with consequent dampening/zeroing of certain *k*-space samples and hence worsening of the overall conditioning of the inverse image reconstruction problem. The echo IN/OUT image reconstruction problem can be solved either by naively inverting the full encoding matrix (Eq. 10.6) using e.g., conjugate gradient [11], or by correcting the extra modulation for each individual spoke (via e.g., regularized division).

With simultaneous multicoil receive, the Fourier gradient encoding can be extended by additional coil sensitivity encoding (i.e., parallel imaging) to enhance overall image encoding efficiency [16, 17]. The resulting inverse image reconstruction problem can be solved using, e.g., non-Cartesian, conjugate gradient sensitivity encoding [15, 18]. Calibration of the coil sensitivity profiles can be achieved either using traditional methods [17, 19, 20] or simply using the single coil FID images as pseudo coil sensitivities. In addition to coil sensitivity calibration for parallel imaging, the latter also achieves intrinsic normalization of the reconstructed GRE images (i.e., corrected by the TE = 0 FID magnitude and phase) such that the obtained GRE images can be used directly for quantitative T_2^* and/or susceptibility mapping. Since Looping Star acquires FID and GRE data simultaneously and with identical spatial encoding, the FID pseudo coil sensitivity maps perfectly match the GRE images without being affected by spatiotemporal incongruity due to, e.g., motion, geometric distortions, or resampling errors.

Figure 10.2 illustrates Looping Star image reconstruction for a numerical 2D Shepp-Logan imaging phantom with $M^2 = 128^2$, $N_{Spk} = 408$, and $N_{SpkPerLoop} = 6$. The resulting image encoding matrices ($\mathbf{E}$, $\mathbf{E}^{IN}$, $\mathbf{E}^{OUT}$) are sufficiently small (i.e., $(N_{Spk} M / 2) \times M^2 = 26,112 \times 16,384$) such that they can be stored (i.e., ~3.2GB in single precision) and inverted using, e.g., truncated singular value decomposition (tSVD). The measured *k*-space signals are synthesized by forward application of the full encoding matrix on the flattened, numerical Shepp-Logan image vector (i.e., $\mathbf{y} = (\mathbf{E}^{OUT} + \mathbf{E}^{IN}) \mathbf{x}$). Neglecting echo-in signal contamination when solving the inverse signal model (i.e., $\mathbf{y} = \mathbf{E}^{OUT} \mathbf{x}$) demonstrates echo IN/OUT overlap artifacts in the reconstructed image (second column). Fermi-filtering $\mathbf{y}$ with a cutoff at half the spoke extent largely eliminates echo-in signal contamination at the cost of reduced image resolution (third column). RF phase cycling separates the measured signals into echo-out ($\mathbf{y}^{OUT}$) and echo-in ($\mathbf{y}^{IN}$) contributions and, hence, allows reconstruction of images without echo IN/OUT artifact (i.e., $\mathbf{y}^{OUT} = \mathbf{E}^{OUT} \mathbf{x}$, and $\mathbf{y}^{IN} = \mathbf{E}^{IN} \mathbf{x}$) at the cost of a twofold increase in scan time (fourth column). Finally, model-based image reconstruction (fifth column) (i.e., $\mathbf{y} = (\mathbf{E}^{OUT} + \mathbf{E}^{IN}) \mathbf{x}$) reduces but does not eliminate the echo IN/OUT artifact (right column).

Further Technical Considerations

For practical implementation, the Looping Star pulse sequence is structured in segments, with each segment containing the fundamental Looping Star building block in the form of RF excitation and refocusing of $N_{SpkPerLoop}$ coherences (as illustrated in Fig. 10.1). In between segments, the readout gradients are ramped down and back up again in a soft and unbalanced manner to minimize acoustic noise and eliminate (i.e., gradient spoil) residual coherences. To minimize gradient switching (and hence acoustic noise and eddy currents), the directional gradient updates are distributed along the spoke readout resulting in curved (vs. straight) 3D spokes. The number of required segments is determined according to $N_{Seg} = N_{Spk}/N_{SpkPerLoop}$. The segmented structure also provides flexibility for interleaving T_1 and/or T_2 magnetization preparations [21] similar to magnetization-prepared segmented ZTE imaging [22, 23]. Finite RF transmit-receive switching results in a central, spherical *k*-space gap in the acquired FID data (but not in the echo data). This so-called deadtime gap can be reacquired (at reduced readout gradient amplitude) and filled at the end with minimal scan time penalty [2–4, 24].

The regular polygonal geometry of Looping Star *k*-space trajectories offers a subtle but important difference between even and odd numbered spokes in terms of *k*-space encoding efficiency which is illustrated in Fig. 10.3 for $N_{SpkPerLoop} = 6$ (first column) and $N_{SpkPerLoop} = 5$ (second column). While an even number of $N_{SpkPerLoop}$ spokes produces incoming echoes (dashed lines) which overlap the outgoing ones (thick solid lines), an odd number of $N_{SpkPerLoop}$ spokes produces incoming echoes which end up in between the outgoing ones. For the example considered, with $N_{SkPerLoop} = 6$ there are only six unique spokes (with each echo-in spoke overlapping another echo-out spoke), while with $N_{SpkPerLoop} = 5$ there are ten unique spokes (without overlap of echo-in and echo-out spokes). Accordingly, odd $N_{SpkPerLoop}$ values provide overall improved angular sampling density for both conventional and coherence-resolved Looping Star. With curved spokes (third and fourth column), which are used in most implementations of Looping Star, this advantage is somewhat reduced but still apparent.

In order to achieve consistent volume excitation independent of the readout gradient, Looping Star (and similarly ZTE) uses extremely short, block-shaped RF pulses. More specifically, the requirement that the RF excitation bandwidth ($BW_{Tx} = 1/\Delta t_{RF}$) must encompass the full imaging frequency spectrum (i.e., $BW_{Tx} > BW$) limits the RF pulse duration to less than the dwell time ($\Delta t_{RF} < \Delta t$) and the maximum flip angle to $\alpha_{max} = \gamma B_{1,max} \Delta t$ [25]. The steady-state longitudinal magnetization ($M_{z,ss}$) of Looping Star (and similarly also of ZTE) is of spoiled gradient echo (SPGR) nature [6]:

$$M_{z,ss} = \frac{M_0 E_2^* (1 - E_1)}{1 - E_1 \cos(\alpha)} \cong \frac{M_0 E_2^*}{1 + \dfrac{T_1 \alpha^2}{T_R 2}}, \quad E_1 = e^{-\frac{T_R}{T_1}}, E_2^* = e^{-\frac{T_E}{T_2^*}}$$

(10.7)

with an SNR-optimal Ernst angle of $\alpha_{Ernst} = \mathrm{acos}(E_1) \cong \sqrt{\dfrac{2T_R}{T_1}}$. The indicated approximation (i.e., $\alpha \ll 1$ rad, and TR $\ll T_1$) is appropriate for Looping Star (and similarly ZTE). Since RF excitation does not occur at every TR, Looping Star requires definition of an average RF excitation repetition time (T_{RF}) as the ratio of the scan time to the total number of RF excitations. Compared to ZTE, Looping Star leads to a longer T_{RF} and correspondingly higher α_{Ernst} values (Table 10.1). For the example considered (i.e., BW = 100 kHz, $\Delta t = 1/\mathrm{BW} = 10\,\mu s$, and assuming a maximum RF excitation amplitude of $B_{1,max} = 20\,\mu T$), we obtain $\alpha_{max} = 3°$. While a maximum flip angle of 3° still allows SNR-optimal ZTE imaging (i.e., $\alpha_{Ernst} = 2.9°$), it is somewhat below the Ernst angle for conventional (i.e., $\alpha_{Ernst} = 4.1°$) and coherence-resolved (i.e., $\alpha_{Ernst} = 5.8°$) Looping Star (assuming $T_1 = 1$ s).

Initial Applications and Future Prospects

Looping Star offers unique MR imaging opportunities by enabling 3D multi-gradient echo imaging in a silent and yet efficient manner. In addition to equidistant GRE images, it also provides a TE = 0 FID image which can be used as pseudo coil sensitivity for parallel imaging and/or amplitude and phase referencing in multi-gradient echo T_2^* and/or QSM mapping experiments.

Since its invention in ~2016 [26], Looping Star has been investigated primarily for silent neuroimaging, including high-resolution T_2^* and susceptibility-weighted structural imaging as well as T_2^* BOLD functional MRI (fMRI). Enabling quiet T_2^* BOLD fMRI is a unique advantage of Looping Star compared to conventional GRE-EPI-based fMRI which generates sound levels up to 130 dB(A). This is known to cause discomfort and confound sensory stimulation [27–32], which is a specific problem for auditory, sleep and resting-state fMRI, as well as studies involving subjects sensitive to acoustic noise (i.e., hyperacusis) as frequently encountered in tinnitus, migraines, autism, and studies of children.

Figure 10.4 illustrates three protocols published in the original *Magnetic Resonance in Medicine* paper [7], including two for high-resolution and structural (left and middle) and one for functional (right) Looping Star MR imaging. The field of view FOV = $(192\ mm)^3$, the imaging bandwidth BW = ± 31.25 kHz and the flip angle FA = 2° were kept the same in all three experiments. The middle row illustrates the $N_{SpkPerLoop}$ curved spokes together with the cumulative looping k-space trajectory for one coherence. With the highest resolution (i.e., res = $(0.8\ mm)^3$, middle column) the readout spokes reach out furthest in k-space ($k_{max} = \pi/\mathrm{res}$), while for the highest number of spokes per loop (i.e., $N_{SpkPerLoop} = 32$, right column) the signal coherences traverse the largest orbit (relative to k_{max}). 3D spatial encoding is achieved by means of pseudorandom rotations (with the first five loops illustrated in the bottom row). For each protocol, the acoustic noise produced by the pulse sequence was only slightly above (i.e., <8.4 dB(A), <6.4 dB(C)) the ambient noise level (i.e., LAeq = 64.2 dB(A), LCpeak = 91.4 dB(C)) which ren-

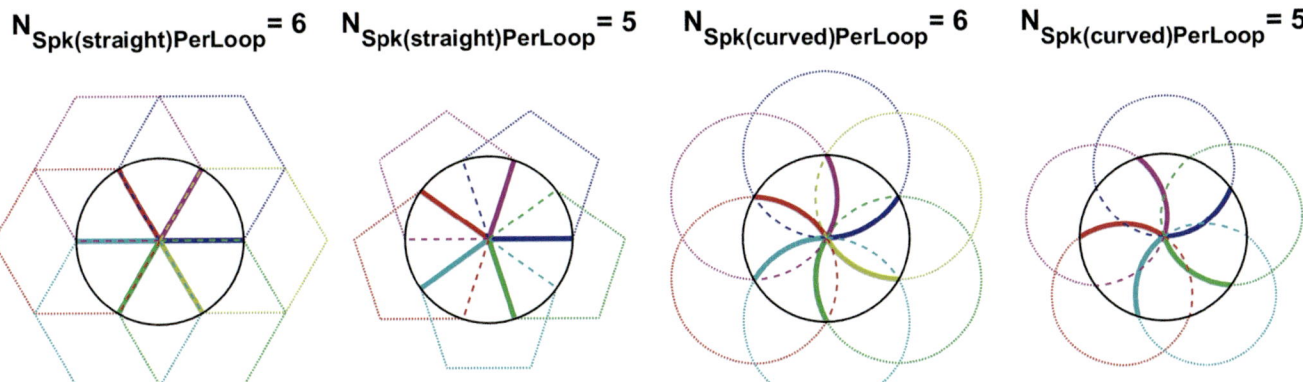

Fig. 10.3 Illustration of Looping Star k-space encoding and signal refocusing for even (i.e., $N_{SpkPerLoop} = 6$) and odd (i.e., $N_{SpkPerLoop} = 5$) numbers of spokes per loop. While for even $N_{SpkPerLoop}$, the incoming echo signals (i.e., $\mathbf{y}_{ECHO,IN}$ dashed lines) overlay the outgoing echo signals (i.e., $\mathbf{y}_{ECHO,OUT}$ solid lines); for odd $N_{SpkPerLoop}$ the incoming echo signals (i.e., $\mathbf{y}_{ECHO,IN}$ dashed lines) fill in additional k-space samples between outgoing echo signals (i.e., $\mathbf{y}_{ECHO,OUT}$ solid lines) and thereby improve overall k-space encoding efficiency. For curved spokes (illustrated on the right), the k-space sampling advantage for odd values of $N_{SpkPerLoop}$ is reduced but still apparent

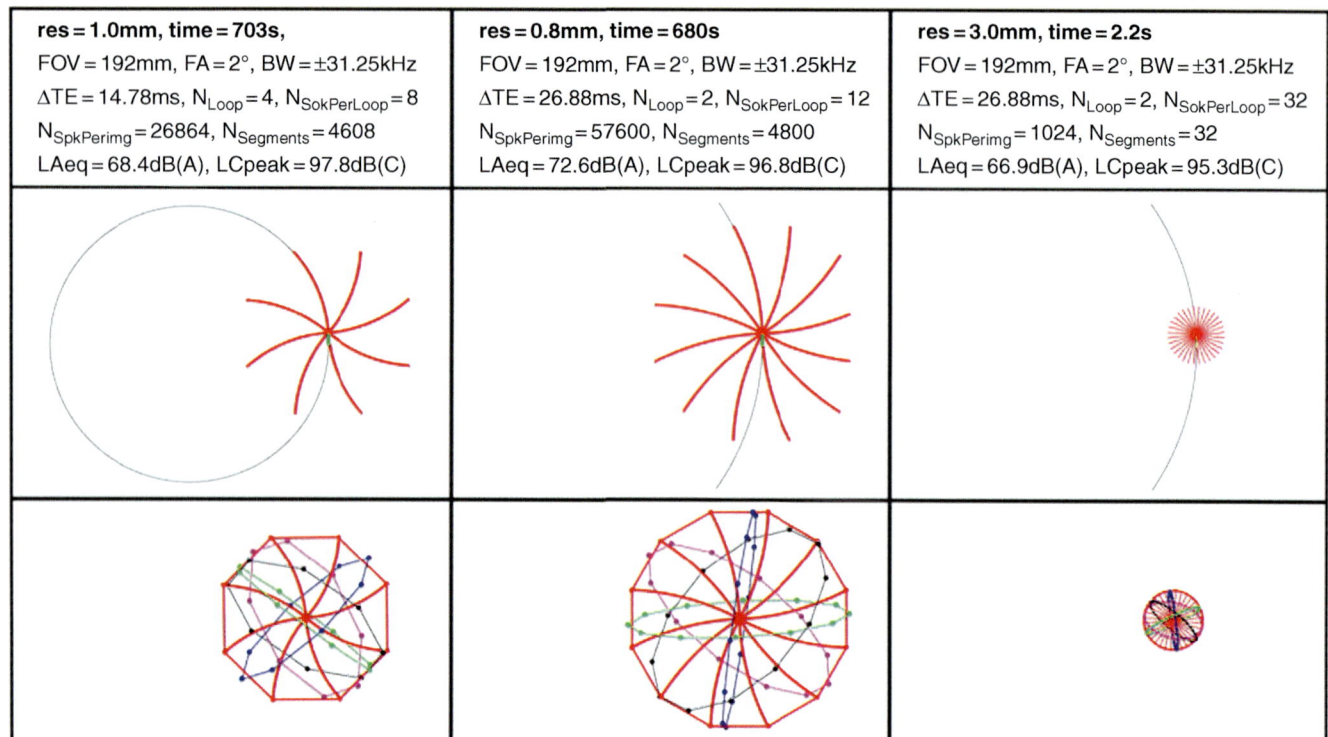

res = 1.0mm, time = 703s,	res = 0.8mm, time = 680s	res = 3.0mm, time = 2.2s
FOV = 192mm, FA = 2°, BW = ±31.25kHz	FOV = 192mm, FA = 2°, BW = ±31.25kHz	FOV = 192mm, FA = 2°, BW = ±31.25kHz
ΔTE = 14.78ms, N_{Loop} = 4, $N_{SokPerLoop}$ = 8	ΔTE = 26.88ms, N_{Loop} = 2, $N_{SokPerLoop}$ = 12	ΔTE = 26.88ms, N_{Loop} = 2, $N_{SokPerLoop}$ = 32
$N_{SpkPerimg}$ = 26864, $N_{Segments}$ = 4608	$N_{SpkPerimg}$ = 57600, $N_{Segments}$ = 4800	$N_{SpkPerimg}$ = 1024, $N_{Segments}$ = 32
LAeq = 68.4dB(A), LCpeak = 97.8dB(C)	LAeq = 72.6dB(A), LCpeak = 96.8dB(C)	LAeq = 66.9dB(A), LCpeak = 95.3dB(C)

Fig. 10.4 Parameter settings and acoustic noise measurements for the two structural (i.e., Fig. 10.5: res = (1.0 mm)³, 703 s, and Fig. 10.6: res = (0.8 mm)³, 680 s) and one functional fMRI (i.e., Fig. 10.7: res = (3.0 mm)³, 2.2 s/frame) Looping Star protocol. The background noise level was LAeq = 64.2 dB(A) and LCpeak = 91.4 dB(C). The curved $N_{SpkPerLoop}$ spokes and the cumulative 2D k-space trajectory (shown for the first spoke only) are illustrated in the middle row. 3D spatial encoding is achieved by means of pseudorandom rotations (with the first five segments illustrated in the bottom row). The varying k-space coverage reflects differences in the image resolution of the three tested protocols. (Reproduced with permission from Ref. [7])

ders Looping Star uniquely attractive for MR examinations involving subjects sensitive to acoustic noise.

Figure 10.5 illustrates multi-echo Looping Star (i.e., res = (1.0 mm)³, $N_{SpkPerLoop}$ = 8, N_{Loop} = 4, left protocol in Fig. 10.4) showing the FID image (left) together with the three equidistant GRE images at TE = 14.8 ms (second column), 29.6 ms (third column), and 44.4 ms (right). The different rows illustrate the effect of echo IN/OUT overlap. If uncorrected (top row), echo IN/OUT overlap results in a grainy salt and pepper like interference pattern overlaid on top of the echo images (but not the FID). Fermi-filtering (middle row) removes that artifact at the cost of image resolution. Phase cycling (bottom row) produces high-resolution images clear of echo IN/OUT overlap at the cost of a twofold increase in scan time. The GRE images demonstrate signal cancelation around air–tissue interfaces (e.g., sinuses, oral cavity, ear canal) induced by intravoxel B_0 off-resonance signal dispersion. This effect increases with TE and voxel size. On the other hand, off-resonance effects during the short readout period (typically <2 ms) are comparatively small/negligible (cf. FID image).

Figure 10.6 illustrates high-resolution Looping Star (i.e., res = (0.8 mm)³, $N_{SpkPerLoop}$ = 12, N_{Loop} = 2, middle protocol in Fig. 10.4) and shows the magnitude (left) and phase (right) of the FID (top) and GRE (middle row) images together with corresponding T_2^* (bottom, left) and QSM (bottom, right) maps. The GRE images (and particularly the QSM maps) highlight iron-rich, deep brain structures which are otherwise difficult to depict.

Figure 10.7 illustrates Looping Star T_2^*-BOLD fMRI (i.e., res = (3.0 mm)³, $N_{SpkPerLoop}$ = 32, N_{Loop} = 2, 2.2 s/frame, right protocol in Fig. 10.4) for finger-tapping motor activation in a single subject and shows the activation map overlaid on a high-resolution T_1-weighted anatomical scan (top row), the FID image (second row), and the Looping Star echo image (third row). The bottom row shows the signal time course for the peak z-value voxel in the left primary motor cortex which clearly follows the expected block-design activation with ~5% relative signal change, as expected for T_2^* BOLD fMRI. Looping Star fMRI has also been used for a variety of neuronal tasks including motor, auditory, working-memory, and resting-state fMRI [7, 33,

Fig. 10.5 Conventional multi-echo, structural Looping Star MR imaging (left protocol in Fig. 10.4 with res = (1.0 mm)³, ΔTE = 26.88 ms, 703 s, eight-channel brain coil) illustrating the echo IN/OUT artifact (top) together with filtering (middle) and phase cycling (bottom) as possible ways for mitigation of the artifact. (Reproduced with permission from Ref. [7])

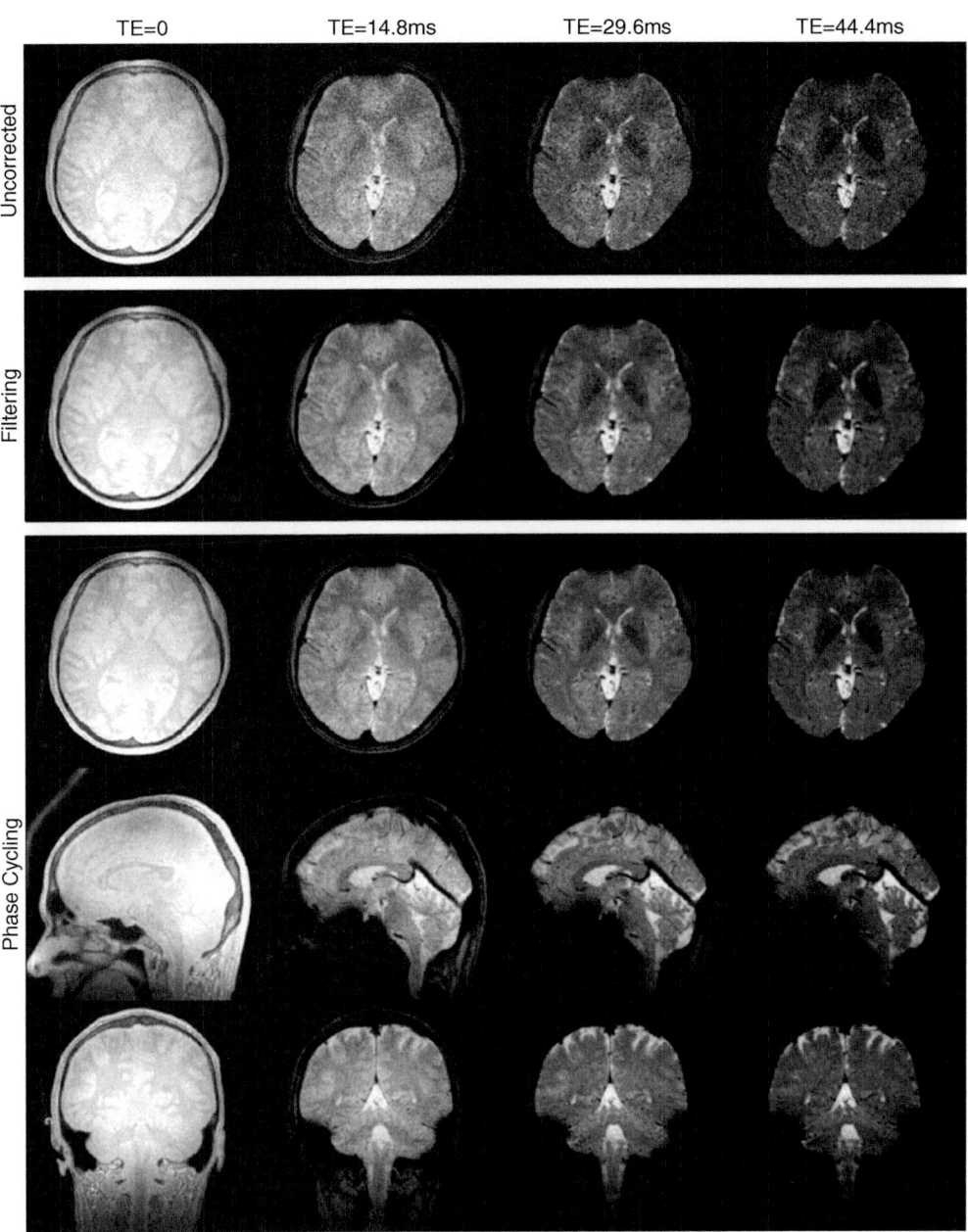

34]. The spatiotemporal resolution of Looping Star fMRI can be further enhanced using advanced image reconstruction methods based on parallel imaging [15, 18], compressed sensing [35], (multi-scale) low-rank [10, 36], or deep learning [37–39].

Besides neuroimaging, Eggers et al. [40] have utilized Looping Star for Dixon-type fat–water imaging, while Feddersen et al. [41] have used it for proton resonance frequency shift (PRFS) based MR thermometry. By increasing the number of echoes and decreasing the TE spacing, Looping Star can also be adapted for MR spectroscopic imaging (MRSI) [42, 43]. For example, Looping Star with $M^3 = 64^3$, BW = 167 kHz, $\Delta t = 1/BW = 6$ μs, $N_{SpkPerLoop} = 4$, and $N_{Loop} = 64$ provides a spectral bandwidth of $1/(2\Delta TE) = 651$ Hz with ~10 Hz frequency resolution, which is appropriate for 3T MRSI in the brain. The segmented pulse sequence structure allows incorporation of fat and/or water RF suppression pulses which are typically required for MRSI. Looping Star is also expected to benefit musculoskeletal MRI for the detection and characterization of short-T_2 tissues. The TE = 0 FID image enables structural depiction of cortical bone anatomy similar to CT [44–50], and the

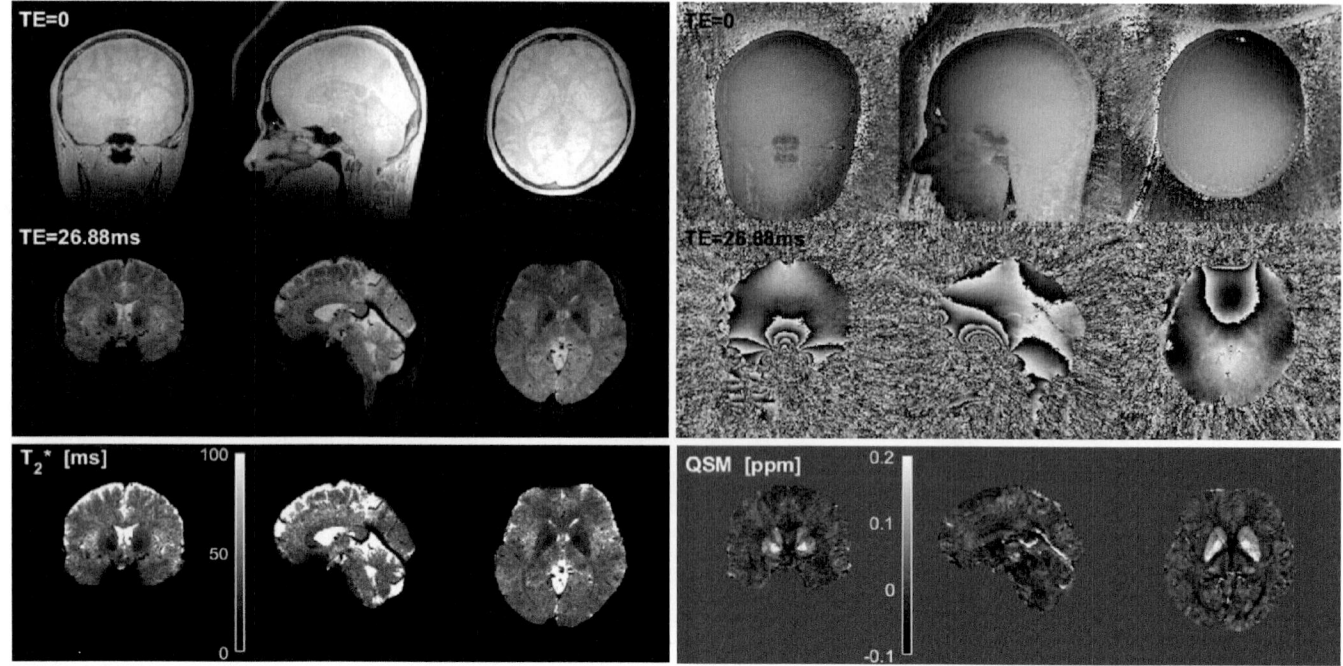

Fig. 10.6 Conventional submillimeter, structural Looping Star MR imaging (middle protocol in Fig. 10.4 with res = (0.8 mm)^3, ΔTE = 26.88 ms, 680 s, phase cycling, eight-channel brain coil) showing rooted-sum-of-square magnitude (left) and phase (single-channel, right) FID (top) and GRE (middle) images, together with corresponding T_2^* (bottom, left) and QSM (bottom, right) maps. (Reproduced with permission from Ref. [7])

GRE images (together with the FID image) provide detailed T_2^* and susceptibility characterization of musculoskeletal tissue [51, 52].

Looping Star shows interesting similarities with BURST-type imaging methods [53–59]. In both cases a set of signal coherences are excited by a train of low flip angle RF excitations (sometimes referred to as DANTE or BURST pulse train) followed by spin echo and/or gradient echo refocusing. However, in BURST imaging signal rephasing gets reversed in between consecutive echoes, leading to inconsistent TE contributions for odd echoes. More specifically, in BURST-type imaging the first FID gets refocused last and vice versa. In contrast Looping Star provides perfectly equidistant refocusing of each FID. Additionally, Looping Star provides a TE = 0 FID image, which is advantageous for normalization of the gradient echo images as required for, e.g., T2* and B_0 mapping.

In summary, Looping Star is a promising and still relatively new MR imaging method and, as such, provides ample opportunities for researchers interested in its further technical development (i.e., pulse sequence, image reconstruction, parameter mapping) and/or clinical evaluation.

Fig. 10.7 Conventional Looping Star fMRI (right protocol in Fig. 10.4 with res = (3 mm)^3, ΔTE = 26.88 ms, 2.2 s/frame, eight-channel brain coil) for a single subject, block-design, finger-tapping experiment. The statistical activation map overlaid on the high-resolution anatomical T$_1$-weighted image (top), the FID Looping Star image (TE = 0, second row), and the GRE Looping Star image (TE = 26.88 ms, third row). The temporal signal change (bottom) of the peak z-value voxel in the left primary motor cortex demonstrates a BOLD sensitivity of ~5%. (Reproduced with permission from Ref. [7])

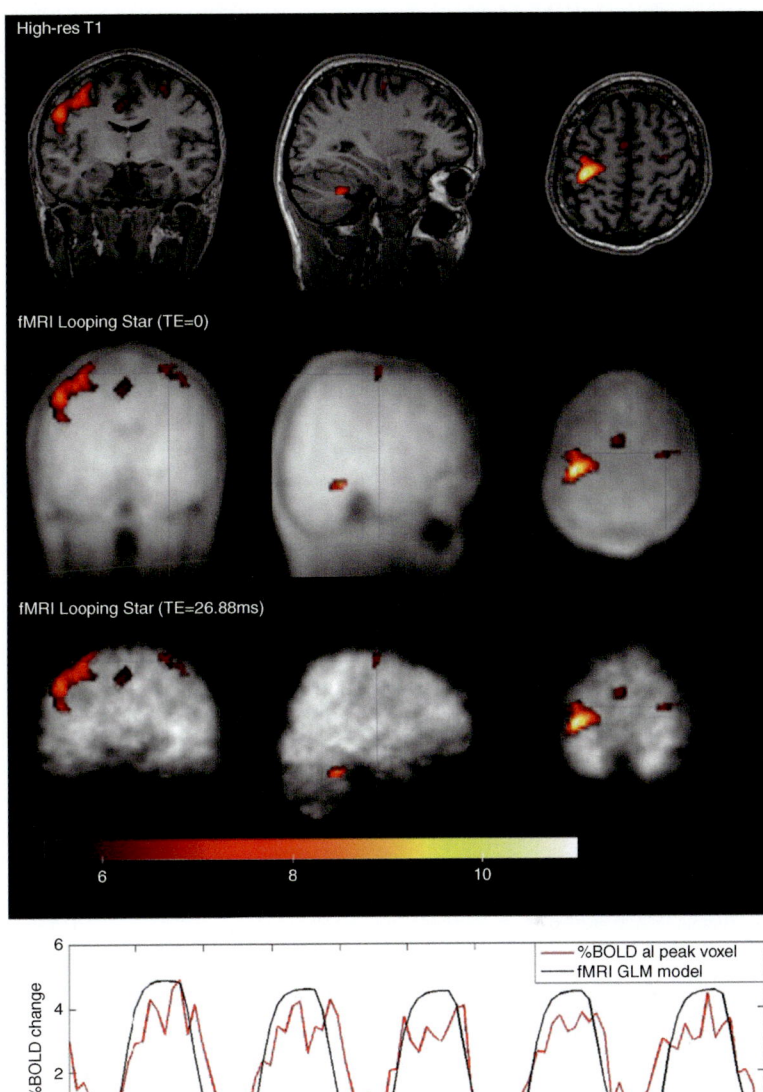

Acknowledgments The authors would like to acknowledge Anne Menini for joint development of Looping Star and the MR physics team at the Center for Neuroimaging at King's College London (i.e., Nikou Damestani, Tobias Wood, Emil Ljungberg, David Lythgoe, Fernando Zelaya, Gareth Barker, and Steven Williams) for fruitful collaboration and evaluation of Looping Star in the context of silent neuroimaging.

References

1. Madio DP, Lowe IJ. Ultra-fast imaging using low flip angles and FIDs. Magn Reson Med. 1995;34(4):525–9.
2. Kuethe DO, Caprihan A, Lowe IJ, Madio DP, Gach HM. Transforming NMR data despite missing points. J Magn Reson. 1999;139(1):18–25.
3. Wu Y, Dai G, Ackerman JL, et al. Water- and fat-suppressed proton projection MRI (WASPI) of rat femur bone. Magn Reson Med. 2007;57(3):554–67.
4. Grodzki DM, Jakob PM, Heismann B. Ultrashort echo time imaging using pointwise encoding time reduction with radial acquisition (PETRA). Magn Reson Med. 2012;67(2):510–8.
5. Weiger M, Pruessmann KP. Short-T_2 MRI: principles and recent advances. Prog Nucl Magn Reson Spectrosc. 2019;114-115:237–70.
6. Ljungberg E, Damestani NL, Wood TC, et al. Silent zero TE MR neuroimaging: current state-of-the-art and future directions. Prog Nucl Magn Reson Spectrosc. 2021;123:73–93.
7. Wiesinger F, Menini A, Solana AB. Looping star. Magn Reson Med. 2019;81(1):57–68.
8. Wiesinger F, Solana AB. Looping star: revisiting echo in/out separation. Proc Intl Soc Mag Reson Med. 2020;3733.
9. Chan RW, Ramsay EA, Cunningham CH, Plewes DB. Temporal stability of adaptive 3D radial MRI using multidimensional golden means. Magn Reson Med. 2009;61(2):354–63.
10. Leynes AP, Damestani NL, Lythgoe DJ, et al. Extreme looping star: quiet fMRI at high spatiotemporal resolution. Proc Intl Soc Mag Reson Med. 2021:458.
11. Xiang H, Fessler JA, Noll D. Model-based image reconstruction in looping-star MRI. Proc Intl Soc Mag Reson Med. 2022:2346.
12. Jackson JI, Meyer CH, Nishimura DG, Macovski A. Selection of a convolution function for Fourier inversion using gridding (computerised tomography application). IEEE Trans Med Imaging. 1991;10(3):473–8.
13. Beatty PJ, Nishimura DG, Pauly JM. Rapid gridding reconstruction with a minimal oversampling ratio. IEEE Trans Med Imaging. 2005;24(6):799–808.
14. Fessler JA. On NUFFT-based gridding for non-Cartesian MRI. J Magn Reson. 2007;188(2):191–5.
15. Wood TC, Ljungberg E, Wiesinger F. Radial interstices enable speedy low-volume imaging. J Open Source Softw. 2021;6:3500.
16. Sodickson DK, Manning WJ. Simultaneous acquisition of spatial harmonics (SMASH): fast imaging with radiofrequency coil arrays. Magn Reson Med. 1997;38(4):591–603.
17. Pruessmann KP, Weiger M, Scheidegger MB, Boesiger P. SENSE: sensitivity encoding for fast MRI. Magn Reson Med. 1999;42(5):952–562.
18. Pruessmann KP, Weiger M, Börnert P, Boesiger P. Advances in sensitivity encoding with arbitrary k-space trajectories. Magn Reson Med. 2001;46(4):638–51.
19. Walsh DO, Gmitro AF, Marcellin MW. Adaptive reconstruction of phased array MR imagery. Magn Reson Med. 2000;43(5):682–90.
20. Uecker M, Lai P, Murphy MJ, et al. ESPIRiT--an eigenvalue approach to autocalibrating parallel MRI: where SENSE meets GRAPPA. Magn Reson Med. 2014;71(3):990–1001.
21. Haase A. Snapshot FLASH MRI. Applications to T_1, T_2, and chemical-shift imaging. Magn Reson Med. 1990;13(1):77–89.
22. Alibek S, Vogel M, Sun W, et al. Acoustic noise reduction in MRI using silent scan: an initial experience. Diagn Interv Radiol. 2014;20(4):360–3.
23. Solana AB, Menini A, Sacolick LI, Hehn N, Wiesinger F. Quiet and distortion-free, whole brain BOLD fMRI using T_2-prepared RUFIS. Magn Reson Med. 2016;75(4):1402–12.
24. Froidevaux R, Weiger M, Rösler MB, Brunner DO, Pruessmann KP. HYFI: hybrid filling of the dead-time gap for faster zero echo time imaging. NMR Biomed. 2021;34(6):e4493.
25. Grodzki DM, Jakob PM, Heismann B. Correcting slice selectivity in hard pulse sequences. J Magn Reson. 2012;214(1):61–7.
26. Solana AB, Menini A, Wiesinger F. Looping star: A novel, self-refocusing zero TE imaging strategy. In proceedings of the 24th Annual Meeting of the International Society of Magnetic Resonance in Medicine, Singapore. 2016. p. 104.
27. Tomasi D, Caparelli EC, Chang L, Ernst T. fMRI-acoustic noise alters brain activation during working memory tasks. NeuroImage. 2005;27(2):377–86.
28. Talavage TM, Edmister WB, Ledden PJ, Weisskoff RM. Quantitative assessment of auditory cortex responses induced by imager acoustic noise. Hum Brain Mapp. 1999;7(2):79–88.
29. Cho Z-H, Chung S-C, Lim D-W, Wong EK. Effects of the acoustic noise of the gradient systems on fMRI: a study on auditory, motor, and visual cortices. Magn Reson Med. 1998;39(2):331–5.
30. Fjaeldstad AW, Nørgaard HJ, Fernandes HM. The impact of acoustic fMRI-noise on olfactory sensitivity and perception. Neuroscience. 2019;406:262–7.
31. Andoh J, Ferreira M, Leppert IR, Matsushita R, Pike B, Zatorre RJ. How restful is it with all that noise? Comparison of interleaved silent steady state (ISSS) and conventional imaging in resting-state fMRI. NeuroImage. 2017;147:726–35.
32. Han Q, Zhang Y, Liu D, Wang Y, Feng Y, Yin X, Wang J. Disrupted local neural activity and functional connectivity in subjective tinnitus patients: evidence from resting-state fMRI study. Neuroradiology. 2018;60(11):1193–201.
33. Dionisio-Parra B, Wiesinger F, Sämann PG, Czisch M, Solana AB. Looping star fMRI in cognitive tasks and resting state. J Magn Reson Imaging. 2020;52(3):739–51.
34. Damestani NL, O'Daly O, Solana AB, et al. Revealing the mechanisms behind novel auditory stimuli discrimination: an evaluation of silent functional MRI using looping star. Hum Brain Mapp. 2021;42(9):2833–50.
35. Lustig M, Donoho D, Pauly JM. Sparse MRI: the application of compressed sensing for rapid MR imaging. Magn Reson Med. 2007;58(6):1182–95.
36. Ong F, Zhu X, Cheng JY, et al. Extreme MRI: large-scale volumetric dynamic imaging from continuous non-gated acquisitions. Magn Reson Med. 2020;84(4):1763–80.
37. Hammernik K, Klatzer T, Kobler E, et al. Learning a variational network for reconstruction of accelerated MRI data: learning a variational network for reconstruction of accelerated MRI data. Magn Reson Med. 2018;79(6):3055–71.
38. Lebel RM. Performance characterization of a novel deep learning-based MR image reconstruction pipeline. ArXiv200806559 Cs Eess. 2020.
39. Hammernik K, Küstner T, Yaman B, et al. Physics-driven deep learning for computational magnetic resonance imaging. 2022; https://doi.org/10.48550/arXiv.2203.12215.
40. Eggers H, Nehrke K, Börnert P, van den Brink J. Quiet dixon imaging with looping star sequence. Proc Intl Soc Mag Reson Med. 2019:4638.
41. Feddersen T, Poot DHJ, Solana AB, et al. Silent PRFS MR thermometry based on looping star sequence. In: ESHO; 2019. p. L73.

42. Wiesinger F, Weidl E, Menzel MI, et al. IDEAL spiral CSI for dynamic metabolic MR imaging of hyperpolarized [1-13C]pyruvate. Magn Reson Med. 2012;68(1):8–16.

43. Lam F, Ma C, Clifford B, Johnson CL, Liang Z-P. High-resolution ^{1}H-MRSI of the brain using SPICE: data acquisition and image reconstruction. Magn Reson Med. 2016;76(4):1059–70.

44. Wiesinger F, Sacolick LI, Menini A, et al. Zero TEMR bone imaging in the head. Magn Reson Med. 2016;75(1):107–14.

45. Delso G, Wiesinger F, Sacolick LI, et al. Clinical evaluation of zero-echo-time MR imaging for the segmentation of the skull. J Nucl Med. 2015;56(3):417–22.

46. Wiesinger F, Bylund M, Yang J, et al. Zero TE-based pseudo-CT image conversion in the head and its application in PET/MR attenuation correction and MR-guided radiation therapy planning. Magn Reson Med. 2018;80(4):1440–51.

47. Breighner RE, Endo Y, Konin GP, Gulotta LV, Koff MF, Potter HG. Technical developments: zero echo time imaging of the shoulder: enhanced osseous detail by using MR imaging. Radiology. 2018;286(3):960–6.

48. Kaushik SS, Bylund M, Cozzini C, Shanbhag D, Petit SF, Wyatt J.J. Menze B. Region of interest focused MRI to synthetic CT translation using regression and segmentation multi-task network. Physics in Medicine & Biology. 2023;68(19):195003.

49. Engström M, McKinnon G, Cozzini C, Wiesinger F. In-phase zero TE musculoskeletal imaging. Magn Reson Med. 2020;83(1):195–202.

50. Wiesinger F, Ho M-L. Zero-TE MRI: principles and applications in the head and neck. Br J Radiol. 2022;95(1136):20220059.

51. Du J, Bydder GM. Qualitative and quantitative ultrashort-TE MRI of cortical bone. NMR Biomed. 2013;26(5):489–506.

52. de Mello R, Ma Y, Ji Y, Du J, Chang EY. Quantitative MRI musculoskeletal techniques: an update. AJR Am J Roentgenol. 2019;213(3):524–33.

53. Hennig J, Hodapp M. Burst imaging. Magma N Y N. 1993;1:39–48.

54. Lowe I, Wysong R. DANTE ultrafast imaging sequence (DUFIS). J Magn Reson. 1993;101:106–9.

55. Heid O, Deimling M, Huk WJ. Ultra-rapid gradient echo imaging. Magn Reson Med. 1995;33:143–9.

56. Zha L, Lowe IJ. Optimized ultra-fast imaging sequence (OUFIS). Magn Reson Med. 1995;33:377–95.

57. Doran SJ, Bourgeois ME, Leach MO. Burst imaging—can it ever be useful in the clinic? Concepts Magn Reson Part A. 2005;26A:11–34.

58. Jakob PM, Kober F, Haase A. Radial BURST imaging. Magn Reson Med. 1996;36:557–61.

59. Schulte RF, Buonincontri G, Costagli M, Menini A, Wiesinger F, Solana AB. Silent T_2^* and T_2 encoding using ZTE combined with BURST. Magn Reson Med. 2019;81:2277–87.

Part II

Contrast Mechanisms

Jiang Du, Sam Sedaghat, Hyungseok Jang, Yajun Ma, and Graeme M. Bydder

Introduction

Ultrashort echo time (UTE) sequences can generate high signals from short- and ultrashort-T$_2$ tissues, which display very fast transverse relaxation [1]. One of the challenges with UTE approaches is low contrast between short- and long-T$_2$ tissues, and methods for dealing with this need to be implemented to achieve useful direct imaging of various short-T$_2$ tissues. Echo subtraction is one of the most widely used contrast mechanisms to suppress signals from long-T$_2$ tissues and create high contrast for short-T$_2$ tissues [1–5]. This contrast mechanism relies on the substantial difference in T$_2$* signal decay between short- and long-T$_2$ tissues to maximize contrast. The difference in T$_2$ may produce little contrast at short echo times (TEs) but increased contrast between short- and long-T$_2$ tissues at longer TEs. By subtracting UTE datasets with longer TEs from those with short TEs, efficient suppression of long-T$_2$ signals can be obtained. To further improve short-T$_2$ contrast, the echo subtraction technique can be combined with other techniques such as fat saturation [2], long-T$_2$ saturation [6], off-resonance saturation [7],

long-T$_2$ inversion [8–12], specially designed radiofrequency (RF) pulse excitations [13], as well as dual-radiofrequency and dual-echo acquisitions [14]. In addition, complex echo subtraction may be used to enhance short-T$_2$ contrast [15]. Details of these different echo subtraction-based contrast mechanisms are presented below.

Dual-Echo UTE with Echo Subtraction

Dual-echo UTE data acquisition can be combined with subsequent echo subtraction to suppress long-T$_2$ signals, thereby producing high contrast imaging of short-T$_2$ tissues or tissue components [3]. In this contrast mechanism, short-T$_2$ contrast is acquired by subtracting a second echo image from a first echo image which is equivalent to T$_2$ bandpass filtering. Long-T$_2$ tissue signals experience minimal decay by the time of the second echo, while short-T$_2$ tissue signals undergo significant decay by the time of the second echo. As a result, long-T$_2$ tissues show a high signal in the second echo, while short-T$_2$ tissues show a signal void. Subtraction of the second echo image from the first echo image leads to suppression of long-T$_2$ signals, leaving short-T$_2$ tissues or tissue components unaffected. It is essential to minimize the RF pulse duration, the TE of the first image, and the readout window as far as possible to minimize T$_2$*-related signal loss [3]. The echo subtraction technique has been used for high contrast imaging of various short-T$_2$ tissues such as the patellar tendon, the Achilles tendon, menisci, ligaments, and the cartilaginous endplate, as well as graft material and fixation elements after surgical repair of tissue trauma [1–5]. Figure 11.1 shows the contrast mechanism and an example of the patellar tendon of a healthy volunteer imaged using a high contrast 3D UTE technique. Signals from long-T$_2$ tissues, such as muscle and articular cartilage, are well suppressed by echo subtraction, with short-T$_2$ signals in the patellar tendon highlighted. Cartilaginous endplate thickening and irregularity on subtracted 3D UTE images have also been described in the literature, where UTE-detected carti-

J. Du (✉)
Department of Radiology, University of California, San Diego, CA, USA

Department of Bioengineering, University of California, San Diego, CA, USA

VA San Diego Healthcare System, San Diego, CA, USA
e-mail: jiangdu@health.ucsd.edu

S. Sedaghat · H. Jang · Y. Ma
Department of Radiology, University of California, San Diego, CA, USA
e-mail: ssedaghat@health.ucsd.edu; h4jang@health.ucsd.edu; yam013@health.ucsd.edu

G. M. Bydder
Department of Radiology, University of California, San Diego, CA, USA

Mātai Medical Research Institute, Tairāwhiti, Gisborne, New Zealand
e-mail: gbydder@health.ucsd.edu

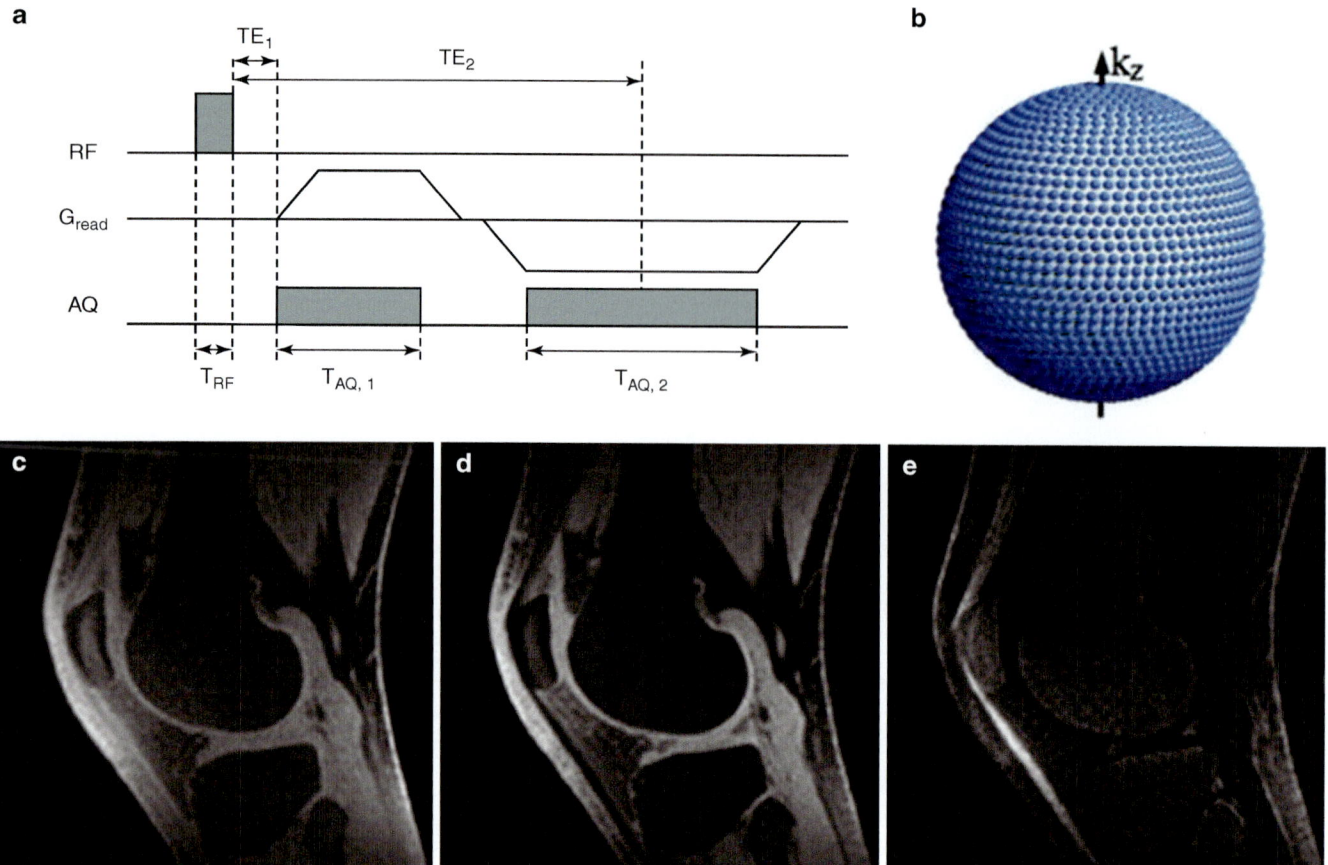

Fig. 11.1 Dual-echo 3D UTE sequence. This employs a nonselective excitation pulse (T_{RF}) followed by a half-echo ($T_{AQ,1}$) acquired at the echo time TE_1 and a later full gradient echo ($T_{AQ,2}$) acquired at TE_2, which is chosen to be the first water/fat in-phase TE (**a**). The first echo time (TE_1) is defined as the interval between the end of the RF excitation pulse and the beginning of the half-echo sampling window. The distribution of radial profiles in 3D *k*-space is shown in (**b**). A central slice of the fat-suppressed dual-echo 3D UTE dataset of the left knee of a healthy volunteer, including the first free induction decay (FID) image at TE = 100 µs, is shown in (**c**). There is high signal in the patellar tendon and menisci in (**c**). The image acquired at TE = 2.3 ms is shown in (**d**). The subtracted image highlighting short-T_2 components in the patellar tendon, quadriceps tendon, and menisci is shown in (**e**). (Reproduced with permission from Ref. [3])

laginous endplate abnormalities are significantly correlated with the Miyazaki grade [4]. A significant limitation of this contrast mechanism is its high sensitivity to susceptibility, B_0 field inhomogeneity, and chemical shift effects, all of which may significantly reduce the short-T_2 contrast.

Dual-Echo UTE with Rescaled Echo Subtraction

The combination of dual-echo UTE imaging with rescaled subtraction provides high contrast for short-T_2 tissues such as the cortical bone, tendons, and menisci [2, 16]. Simple subtraction of the second echo image from the first FID image may yield strong residual signal from long-T_2 tissues such as fat, which has at least six distinct spectral peaks at different resonance frequencies (i.e., at 0.9, 1.3, 2.1, 2.75, 4.2, and 5.3 ppm), leading to short-T_2^* relaxation [17, 18]. Fat signal decay during the time between echoes may be significant, given that fat has a much higher proton density than many short-T_2 tissues (e.g., cortical bone) and lead to reduced short-T_2 contrast. In the rescaled subtraction technique, the first UTE FID image is scaled down, resulting in a lower signal from long-T_2 tissues in the first compared to the second echo. In the subtracted images, long-T_2 signals become negative, while short-T_2 signals remain positive. UTE with a

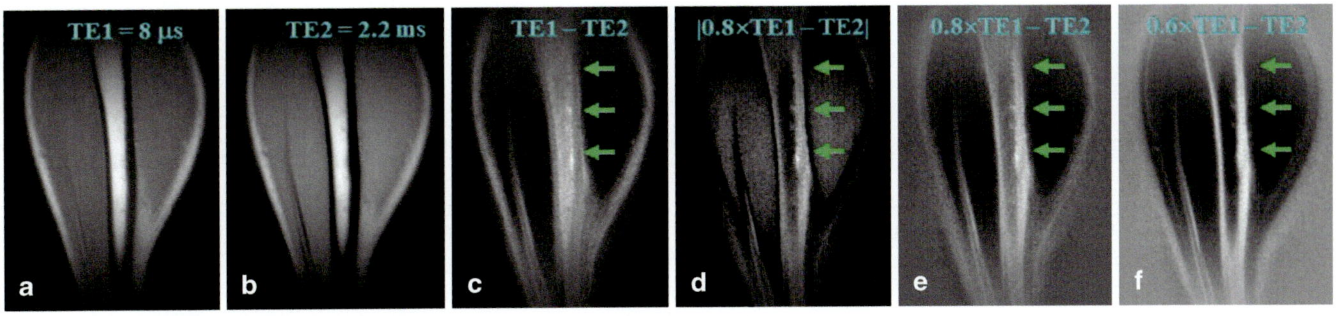

Fig. 11.2 Dual-echo 3D UTE imaging of the tibia of a healthy volunteer with the first TE of 8 μs (**a**) and the second TE of 2.2 ms (**b**). Subtraction of the second echo from the first UTE FID image shows limited contrast for cortical bone due to a high signal from marrow fat (**c**). Increased bone contrast is achieved by scaling down the UTE FID image by a factor of 0.8 and using absolute pixel intensity in the subtraction image (**d**). Bone contrast can be further improved by allowing negative signal intensity in long-T_2 tissues (**e**). (Reproduced with permission from Ref. [2])

rescaled subtraction technique works efficiently in creating high positive contrast for short-T_2 species, especially cortical bone, which has a much lower mobile proton density than surrounding muscle or fat. Regular unscaled echo subtraction may significantly reduce bone contrast due to residual signals from marrow fat. Figure 11.2 shows an example of 3D dual-echo UTE imaging with rescaled subtraction applied to the tibia of a healthy volunteer. Conventional 3D UTE imaging provides a relatively high signal but negative contrast for the tibia due to much higher signal from the surrounding muscle and marrow fat (Fig. 11.2a). Echo subtraction presents positive contrast between bone and muscle but a negative contrast between cortical bone and fat, as fat has a short T_2^* (Fig. 11.2c). The contrast between bone and fat/muscle increases using the UTE rescaled subtraction technique (Fig. 11.2d–f).

Dual-Echo UTE with Fat Saturation and Echo Subtraction

Fat is a major confounding factor in morphological imaging of short-T_2 tissues using the echo subtraction contrast mechanism due to its high proton density and short T_1, leading to high residual signal intensity on subtracted images. Each of the six major resonance peaks in the fat ^{1}H MR spectrum represents a structurally distinct proton moiety, and interactions between these cause loss of coherence with a short-T_2^* [17, 18]. As a result, subtraction of the second echo from the UTE FID may produce a strong signal from fat, which can be significantly higher than that from water-based short-T_2 tissues, such as the osteochondral junction and cortical bone. A combination of dual-echo subtraction with chemical shift-based fat saturation can be an efficient way to suppress fat signals and increase short-T_2 contrast. Figure 11.3 shows this in a cadaveric human patellar sample imaged using fat-saturated dual-echo UTE imaging. Echo subtraction provides excellent contrast demonstration of the osteochondral junction, with efficient suppression of signals from the superficial layers of articular cartilage and bone marrow fat using the chemical shift-based fat saturation approach. This technique can also be applied to short-T_2 tissues such as the Achilles tendon, menisci, ligaments, and cartilaginous endplate.

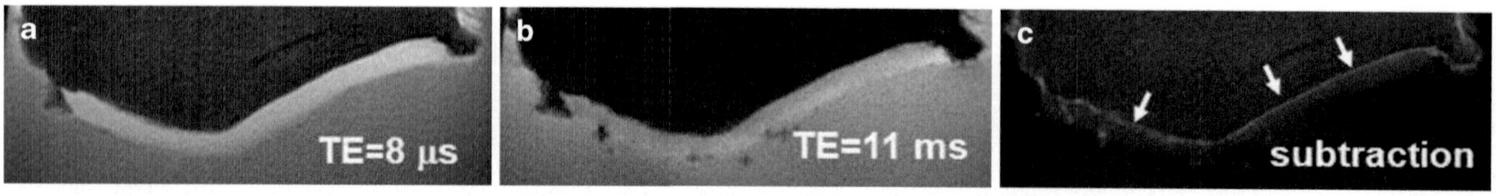

Fig. 11.3 Fat-saturated dual-echo UTE imaging of a cadaveric human patellar sample. This shows a high signal from the superficial layers of articular cartilage and the osteochondral junction but a low signal from bone marrow fat at TE = 8 μs (**a**) and a high signal from the superficial layers of articular cartilage but a low signal from the osteochondral junction and bone marrow fat at TE = 11 ms (**b**). The corresponding echo subtraction image depicts the osteochondral junction with excellent contrast (arrows) (**c**)

Dual-Echo UTE with Long-T$_2$ Saturation and Echo Subtraction

As short-T$_2$ tissues such as cortical bone may have much lower signals than surrounding long-T$_2$ tissues (e.g., muscle and bone marrow fat), generating high contrast images of them can be technically challenging. In addition, residual signals from long-T$_2$ tissues may be equal to or higher than those from the cortical bone. A combination of long-T$_2$ signal suppression and echo subtraction helps decrease long-T$_2$ signals further and increase short-T$_2$ contrast. Long-T$_2$ saturation pulses are employed to suppress long-T$_2$ tissue signals [6, 19]. For example, a 90° pulse with a relatively long duration and a low amplitude can rotate the longitudinal magnetization of long-T$_2$ tissues into the transverse plane, where a large spoiling gradient can subsequently dephase the transverse magnetization. However, short-T$_2$ tissues are not excited by this pulse as the decay rate of these tissues exceeds the excitation rate. Thus, a long 90° pulse can be used with a large spoiling gradient to suppress long-T$_2$ tissues, leaving short-T$_2$ tissues to be subsequently detected by UTE data acquisition after excitation. However, long duration 90° pulses have a narrow spectral bandwidth and are sensitive to B_1 and B_0 field inhomogeneities [6]. Therefore, a long pulse with a broader spectral profile is preferred to a long rectangular pulse as it is more tolerant of B_0 inhomogeneity. Figure 11.4 shows an example of long T$_2$ signal suppression using a long Gaussian pulse followed by UTE imaging to detect signals from the tibia in a healthy volunteer. Long-T$_2$ muscle signal is very well suppressed, but bone marrow fat shows a high signal. Subtraction of the second echo from the UTE FID image significantly increases the bone contrast. T$_2$ selective RF excitation (TELEX) is designed to increase short-T$_2$ contrast by using a long π/2 pulse, routinely interrupted by refocusing pulses to improve the off-resonance characteristics of the suppression [20]. Dual-band long-T$_2$ suppression pulses further improve the suppression of signals from long-T$_2$ water and fat components. However, residual long-T$_2$ signals due to B_1 and B_0 inhomogeneities may still compromise short-T$_2$ contrast [21].

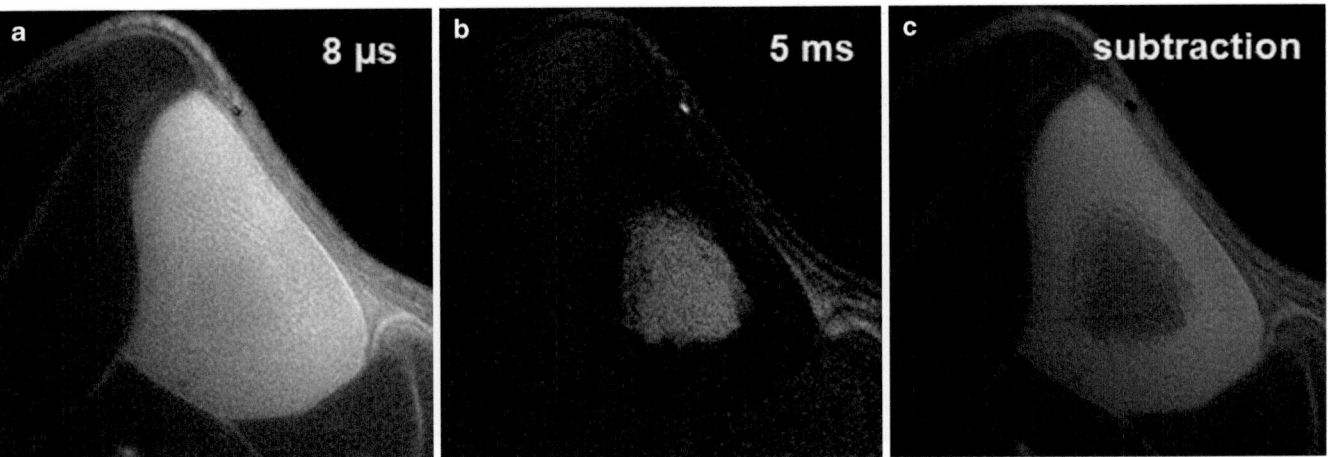

Fig. 11.4 Long-T$_2$ saturated dual-echo UTE imaging of the tibia of a healthy volunteer with a TE = 8 μs (**a**) and TE = 5 ms (**b**), and the corresponding echo subtraction image (**c**), which depicts cortical bone at the tibial midshaft with excellent contrast

UTE with Off-Resonance Saturation Contrast

Short-T$_2$ tissues, such as the osteochondral junction, tendons, ligaments, menisci, and cortical bone, have much broader absorption line shapes than long-T$_2$ tissues, such as articular cartilage, muscles, and synovium. Short-T$_2$ tissues are, therefore, more sensitive to off-resonance RF radiation. In UTE imaging with off-resonance saturation contrast (UTE-OSC) [7], a high-power saturation pulse is placed a few kHz off the water peak to preferentially saturate signals from short-T$_2$ tissues, leaving long-T$_2$ water and fat signals largely unaffected. Subtraction of UTE images with off-resonance saturation from basic UTE images can effectively suppress long-T$_2$ water and fat signals and create high contrast for short-T$_2$ tissues, as shown in Fig. 11.5a–c. UTE

images in the axial plane of the Achilles tendon of a healthy volunteer with and without the off-resonance saturation pulse are shown in Fig. 11.5d, e. A Fermi pulse with a duration of 16 ms and flip angle of 2400° placed +1 kHz away from the water peak effectively suppresses signals from the Achilles tendon, with only a small effect on muscle and fat. Subtraction of UTE images with and without the Fermi saturation pulse provides excellent depiction of the tensile tendon (Fig. 11.5g). Some signal in Fig. 11.5g comes from the skin, likely due to susceptibility effects, which may shift the skin resonance frequency toward the saturation pulse, resulting in increased direct saturation and increased contrast on the subtraction image. Overall, UTE-OSC provides much better contrast for the tensile tendon than conventional dual-echo UTE subtraction (Fig. 11.5h).

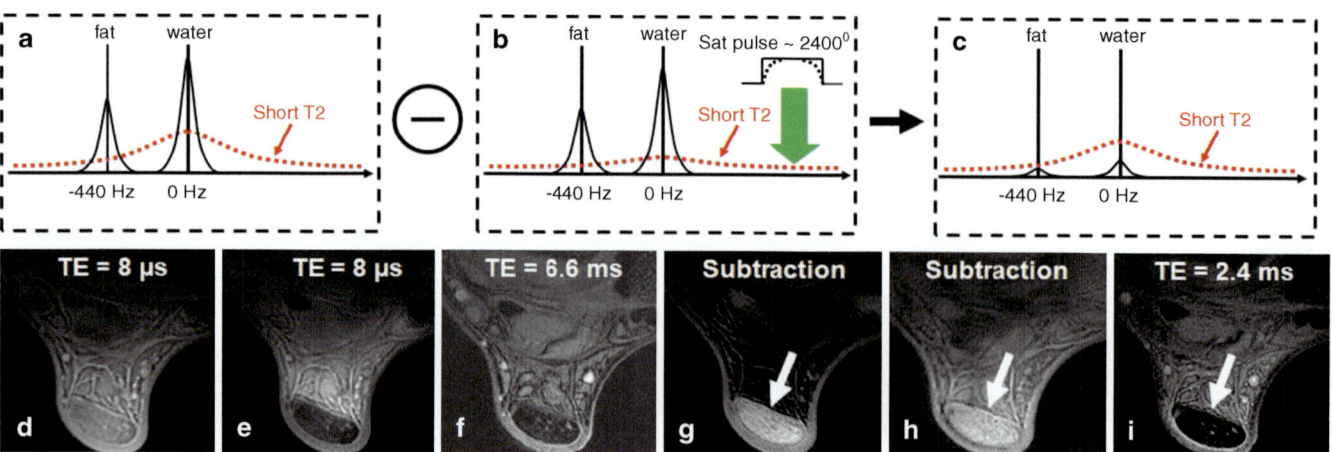

Fig. 11.5 UTE-OSC employs two UTE acquisitions without (**a**) and with (**b**) an off-resonance saturation pulse, followed by subtraction of the two datasets to create short-T_2 contrast (**c**). An example is shown in the Achilles tendon of a 54-year-old normal subject to axial UTE imaging without (**d**) and with (**e**) a 2400° Fermi pulse placed 1 kHz off the water peak, a later gradient echo (**f**), UTE-OSC subtraction (**g**), regular dual-echo subtraction (**h**), and clinical gradient echo imaging (**i**). UTE-OSC subtraction (**g**) provides much better contrast than regular dual-echo subtraction (**h**) (arrows). Clinical GRE shows a signal void for the Achilles tendon (arrow) (**i**). (Reproduced with permission from Ref. [7])

UTE with Adiabatic Inversion and Echo Subtraction

Adiabatic inversion recovery (IR) pulses have been utilized to uniformly invert the longitudinal magnetization of long T_2 components [22–24]. The combination of an IR-prepared UTE (IR-UTE) sequence and a dual-echo acquisition with echo subtraction has been used for selective imaging of non-aqueous myelin protons [8–11]. The long adiabatic inversion pulse is used to invert the longitudinal magnetizations of long-T_2 white matter (WM_L) and gray matter (GM_L). Myelin has an extremely short-T_2^* relaxation time (much shorter than the duration of the adiabatic pulse), and its longitudinal magnetization is not inverted but saturated due to the fast transverse relaxation during the long adiabatic inversion process. UTE data acquisition starts at an inversion time (TI), when the inverted WM_L reaches its null point, leaving signals from myelin and residual GM_L to be detected during the UTE FID data acquisition. The second echo acquires signals from non-nulled long-T_2 tissues (mainly GM_L). The myelin signal decays to near zero in the second echo. Subtraction of the second echo from the first UTE FID provides selective myelin imaging in the white matter. Figure 11.6a–b describes this contrast mechanism. At the null point, the gray matter myelin presents a positive longitudinal magnetization, while the GM_L has a negative longitudinal magnetization. At the second echo (e.g., TE ~ 2 ms), the myelin signal decays to zero, while the GM_L signal barely decays due to its long-T_2 and short echo spacing. As a result, the net signal of gray matter is higher at the second echo than at the initial FID. Echo subtraction produces a positive signal for myelin in white matter and a negative signal for myelin in gray matter. This creates very high contrast (Fig. 11.6e) [24].

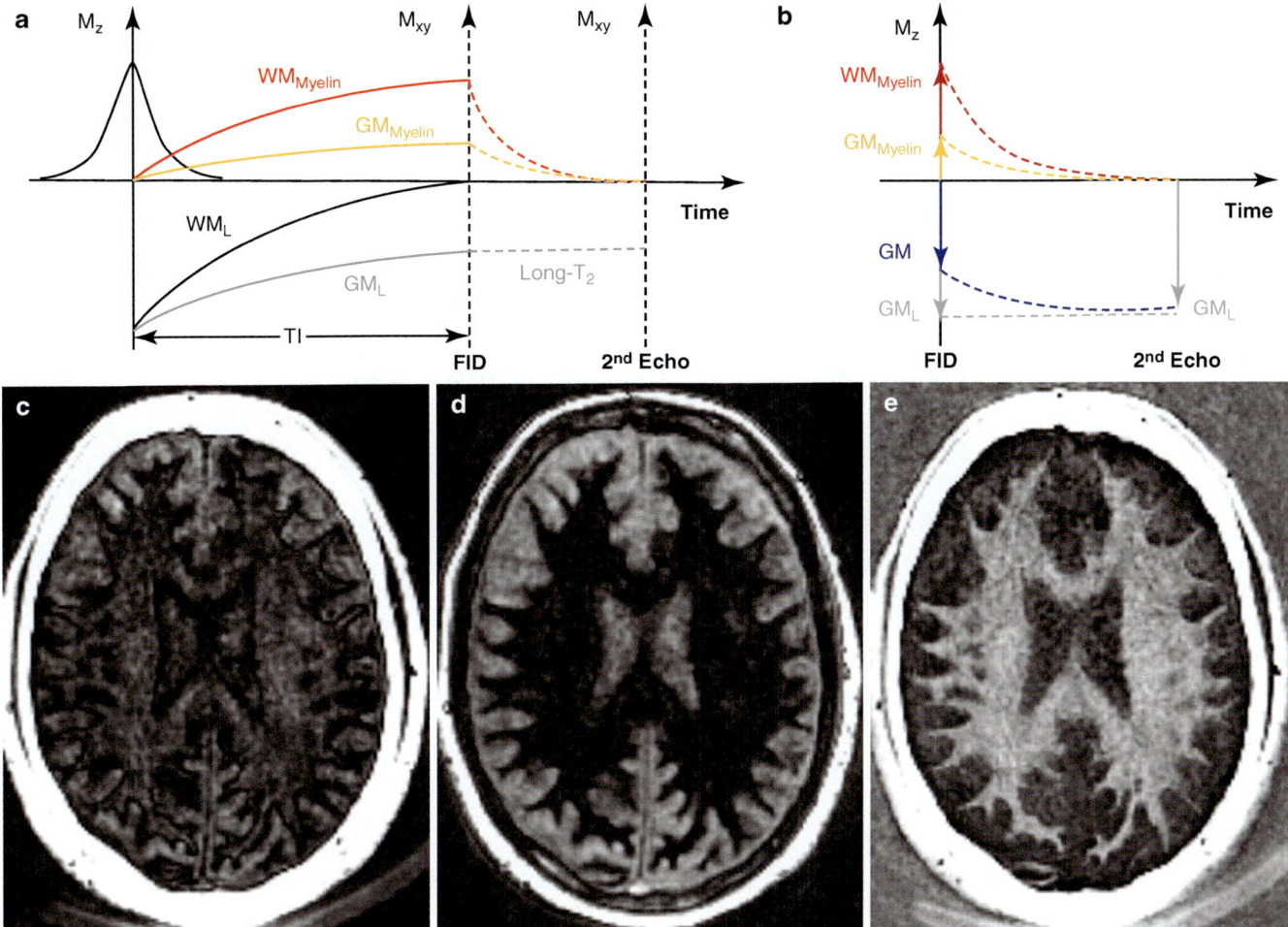

Fig. 11.6 Myelin imaging using on the IR-UTE dual-echo subtraction technique. This employs a long adiabatic inversion pulse to invert the longitudinal magnetizations of long-T$_2$ white matter (WM$_L$) and gray matter (GM$_L$), with myelin in white matter (WM$_{Myelin}$) and gray matter (GM$_{Myelin}$) largely saturated due to fast transverse relaxation during the long adiabatic inversion process (**a**). UTE FID acquisition starts at the inversion time (TI) when the inverted WM$_L$ reaches its null point, where the magnetizations of WM$_{Myelin}$ and GM$_{Myelin}$ are positive, but that of GM$_L$ is negative. At the second echo, the myelin signal decays to zero, and only the signal from GM$_L$ is imaged. Subtraction of the second echo from the UTE FID provides a positive signal for WM$_{Myelin}$ but a negative signal for myelin in gray matter (**b**). An example is shown on IR-UTE imaging of the brain of a volunteer with a TE = 32 µs (**c**) and TE = 2.2 ms (**d**). Echo subtraction provides excellent WM$_{Myelin}$ contrast in (**e**)

UTE with Adiabatic Inversion and Complex Echo Subtraction

Both magnitude and complex subtraction have been widely used in MRI, although magnitude subtraction is more popular. Complex subtraction has been reported to improve the detection of blood vessels compared to magnitude subtraction in MR angiography [25, 26]. Complex echo subtraction has also been used to estimate fat signal and fraction in conventional Dixon-based fat and water separation techniques [27, 28]. While IR-UTE with magnitude echo subtraction provides excellent contrast for myelin in the brain's white matter, as demonstrated by Fig. 11.6, contamination from residual long-T$_2$ signals remains due to variation in the T$_1$ of

white matter resulting in incomplete signal nulling and other factors. Recent research suggests that complex subtraction can reduce long-T$_2$ signal contamination and improve short-T$_2$ contrast [15]. In dual-echo IR-UTE myelin imaging, recovering the targeted myelin signal S$_m$(t$_1$) by magnitude subtraction is only possible if the short-T$_2$ white matter signal has a zero phase after RF excitation. The longitudinal magnetization of myelin remains positive after applying an adiabatic inversion pulse.

In contrast, the longitudinal magnetization of long-T$_2$ components can be positive or negative, depending on their T$_1$s. A phase offset may also be caused by phase evolution during the RF pulse or data acquisition and by imperfect image reconstruction [29]. In contrast to magnitude subtrac-

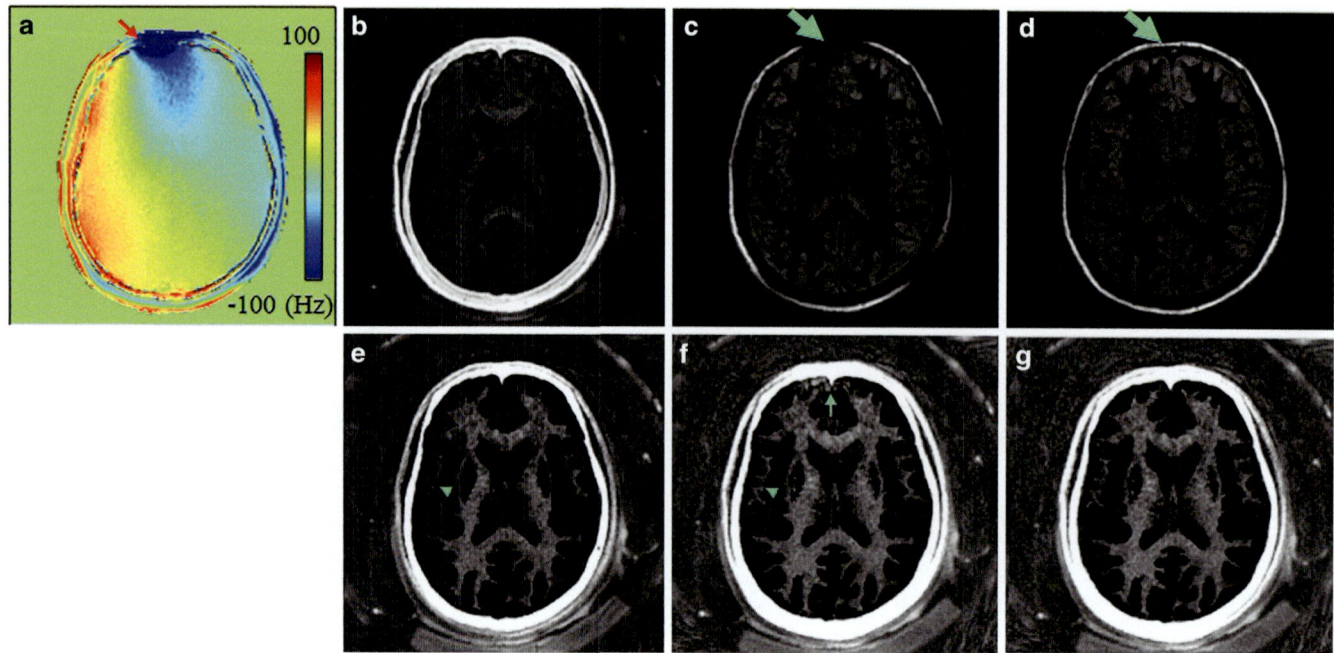

Fig. 11.7 Dual-echo IR-UTE imaging of a 29-year-old female volunteer showing the field map (**a**), the real part of UTE image at TE = 32 μs (**b**) and TE = 2.2 ms before (**c**) and after (**d**) correction for the additional phase errors caused by field inhomogeneity. The myelin image was obtained using magnitude subtraction (**e**), complex subtrac-tion without (**f**), and with (**g**) correction for the phase error induced by B_0 inhomogeneity using the field map. Complex subtraction shows morphological detail of myelin in the white matter with signal bias arti-facts (green arrows) suppressed by correcting the phase error induced by B_0 inhomogeneity. (Reproduced with permission from Ref. [15])

tion, which potentially underestimates the myelin signal, complex subtraction is not affected by the initial phase of myelin and long-T_2 signals. Instead, complex subtraction helps correct the phase offset induced by B_0 field inhomoge-neity and other factors [15]. Figure 11.7 shows correspond-ing results obtained from a 29-year-old volunteer, including an estimated field map (Fig. 11.7a), a UTE image (Fig. 11.7b), an image of the real part of the image at the second TE with and without phase correction for field inhomogeneity (Fig. 11.7c, d), and the corresponding myelin images with

magnitude subtraction and complex subtraction (Fig. 11.7e–g). The phase error due to strong B_0 field inhomogeneity results in artifactually biased signal in the myelin image in Fig. 11.7f, as indicated by the green arrows. This artifact is suppressed by correcting the phase error in Fig. 11.7g. Magnitude subtraction may cause an underestimation of the myelin signal in white matter regions with longer T_1s. Complex subtraction is less susceptible to T_1 variation than the magnitude subtraction [15].

UTE with Interleaved Adiabatic Inversion and Subtraction

Theoretically, a single adiabatic IR pulse may only be able to selectively null long-T$_2$ tissues with a particular T$_1$ [23]. Additionally, excitation of long-T$_2$ tissues is much easier to achieve than excitation of short-T$_2$ tissues, which decay relatively rapidly when excited using an RF pulse with a relatively long duration and low amplitude. It is, therefore, desirable to use an adiabatic inversion pulse with a long duration and minimal power (but still satisfying the adiabatic condition) to invert long-T$_2$ magnetization but minimize short-T$_2$ signal attenuation. However, long duration pulses typically have narrow spectral bandwidths and thus are sen-

sitive to off-resonance effects, and are thus incapable of covering both long-T$_2$ water and fat signals. UTE with interleaved adiabatic inversion and subtraction has been proposed to suppress signals from both long-T$_2$ water and fat, creating high contrast for short-T$_2$ tissues [23]. This technique includes two UTE acquisitions with adiabatic inversion magnetization preparation pulses applied to the water peak to generate a long-T$_2$ water-inverted image on the one hand and applied to the fat peak to generate a fat-inverted image on the other hand (Fig. 11.8a). Short-T$_2$ contrast is created by summing the two images.

However, long-T$_2$ components are not entirely suppressed by this technique. Relaxation during the adiabatic inversion pulses decreases the total magnetization, and an additional

Fig. 11.8 UTE imaging with the interleaved adiabatic inversion and subtraction technique. This acquires fat- and water-inverted images separately, followed by a scaled addition of these to create short-T$_2$ contrast (**a**). Axial imaging of the lower leg is shown, including a water-inverted magnitude image (**b**), a fat-inverted magnitude image (**c**), a water-inverted corrected phase image (**d**), a fat-inverted corrected phase image (**e**), the sum of water-inverted and fat-inverted images (**f**), and the scaled sum of water-inverted and fat-inverted images (**g**). The scaled sum of water- and fat-inverted images shows excellent contrast for the cortical bone in the tibia (long, thin arrow in **g**). The signals in the skin, around the vessels, as well as between muscles and fascicles (short, wider arrows in **g**), probably arise from short-T$_2$ components or signal suppression failure due to off-resonance or partial volume effects. (Reproduced with permission from Ref. [23])

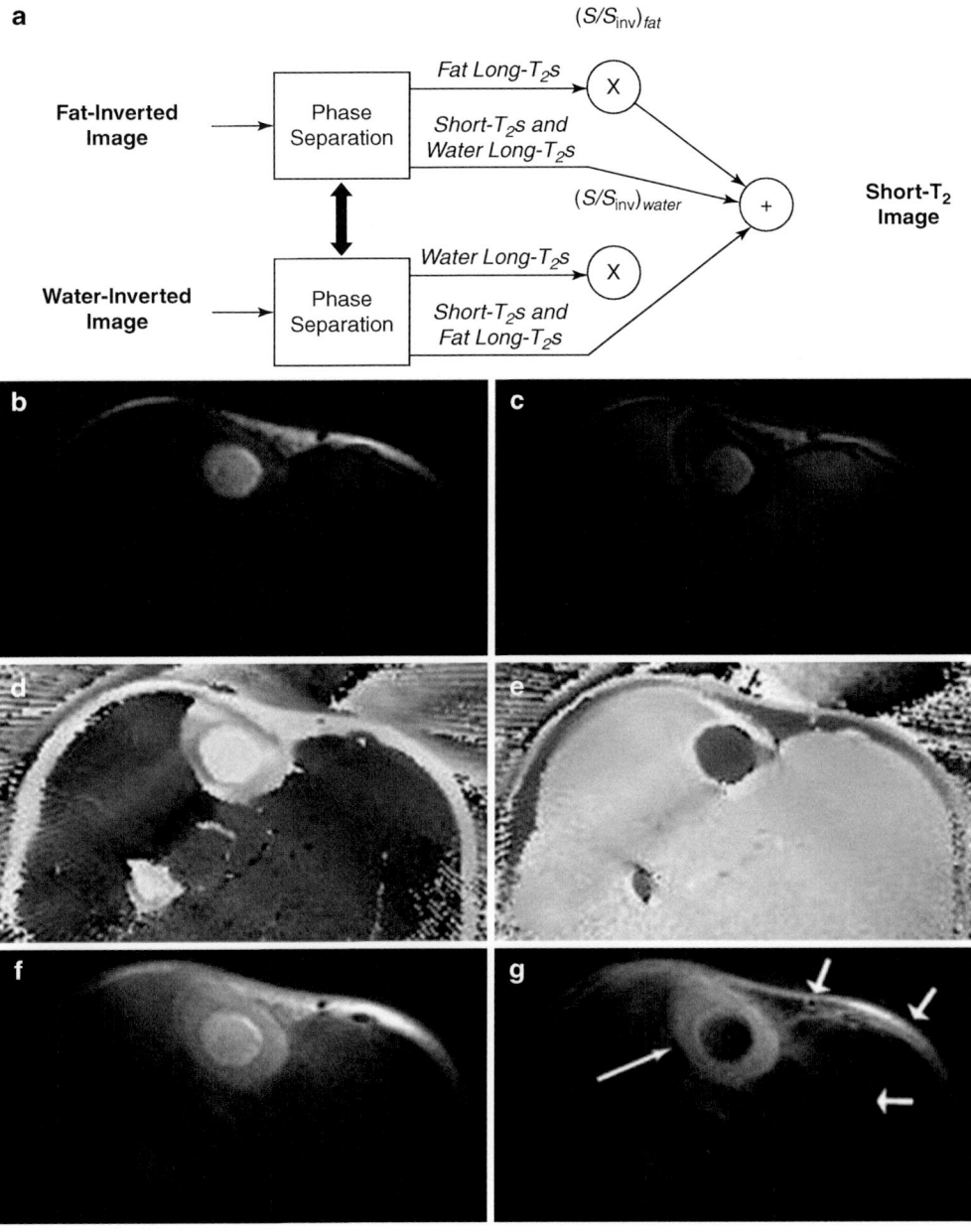

scaling factor is required to compensate for this effect and so improve the long-T_2 signal suppression. The scaling factors for water- and fat-inverted images can be predicted based on Bloch equation simulations. A phase separation process scales the inverted components in their respective images. The phase separation requires removal of the linear phase from each image. The linear phase is estimated by a least squares fit of the phase in the object, followed by the addition of a constant phase shift to unwrap phase discontinuities [23]. Thresholding the difference between the corrected phases helps in conducting phase separation, which is performed before the two scaling factors are applied to the inverted components in their respective images, eventually canceling out long-T_2 tissue signals at both the water and fat resonances. Figure 11.8b–i shows an example of imaging cortical bone in the tibia [23]. Only the muscle is inverted in the image phase when the inversion pulse is centered at the water resonance peak (Fig. 11.8d).

Fat next to skin and in bone marrow is inverted in image phase when the inversion pulse is centered at the fat resonance peak (Fig. 11.8e). However, the inverted components are not fully inverted, as indicated by their reduced signal on the magnitude images (Fig. 11.8b, c). The scaled sum (Fig. 11.8g) provides better cortical bone contrast than the unscaled sum (Fig. 11.8f), both of which are better than the UTE image alone (image not shown). This UTE technique with interleaved adiabatic inversion and subtraction can also be used for high contrast imaging of tendons and other short-T_2 tissues with robustness to variation in B_1 [23].

UTE with Relaxation-Parameter Contrast and Subtraction

While UTE-type pulse sequences are often implemented with short duration maximum power RF excitations, UTE data acquisition can be combined with relaxation-parameter contrast for short-T_2 imaging [13]. The relaxation-parameter contrast exploits the sensitivity of bone proton magnetization to both T_2 and RF pulse duration. RF excitation pulse parameters are selected to determine the extent of concurrent relaxation and excitation (Fig. 11.9a) [13]. The excitation RF pulse dimensions can be adjusted independently, or in combination with other sequence parameters such as flip angle or TE, to match a particular T_2 relaxation rate and improve short-T_2 contrast. The RF pulse duration p and the amplitude a may be changed to adjust the relaxation dependence of the image contrast. Nutation is T_2-dependent if the flip angle or pulse duration is tuned to balance the competing effects of relaxation and excitation for any particular RF amplitude [23]. In other words, the pulse duration p can be adjusted to match the desired T_2 sensitivity and improve short-T_2 contrast. To selectively detect signals from magnetization within a specific range of T_2 values, two RF pulse durations (i.e., p_1 and p_2) are chosen so that the sensitivity transition between them brackets the range of interest. Two UTE datasets with the same imaging parameters except for different RF excitation pulses are then acquired. Subtraction of the two UTE images creates T_2-specific contrast and highlights spins relaxing within a chosen range of T_2 relaxation times. Figure 11.9b–h shows an example of the skull of a healthy volunteer on 3D UTE images. UTE with a short RF pulse duration detects all anatomical regions (Fig. 11.9b), including the skull. The soft tissue signal is much higher due to its higher proton density compared to cortical bone. A longer echo UTE with a longer RF pulse selectively avoids excitation and reception of signals from the skull (Fig. 11.9c). Subtraction of the two datasets provides high contrast imaging of the skull with improved long-T_2 signal suppression compared to regular dual-echo UTE imaging with a short RF pulse followed by echo subtraction (Fig. 11.9f vs. g). This novel subtraction technique also captures more signal from bone than the pulse only difference image (i.e., UTE with the fast pulse minus UTE with the slow pulse) (Fig. 11.9f vs. h) [13].

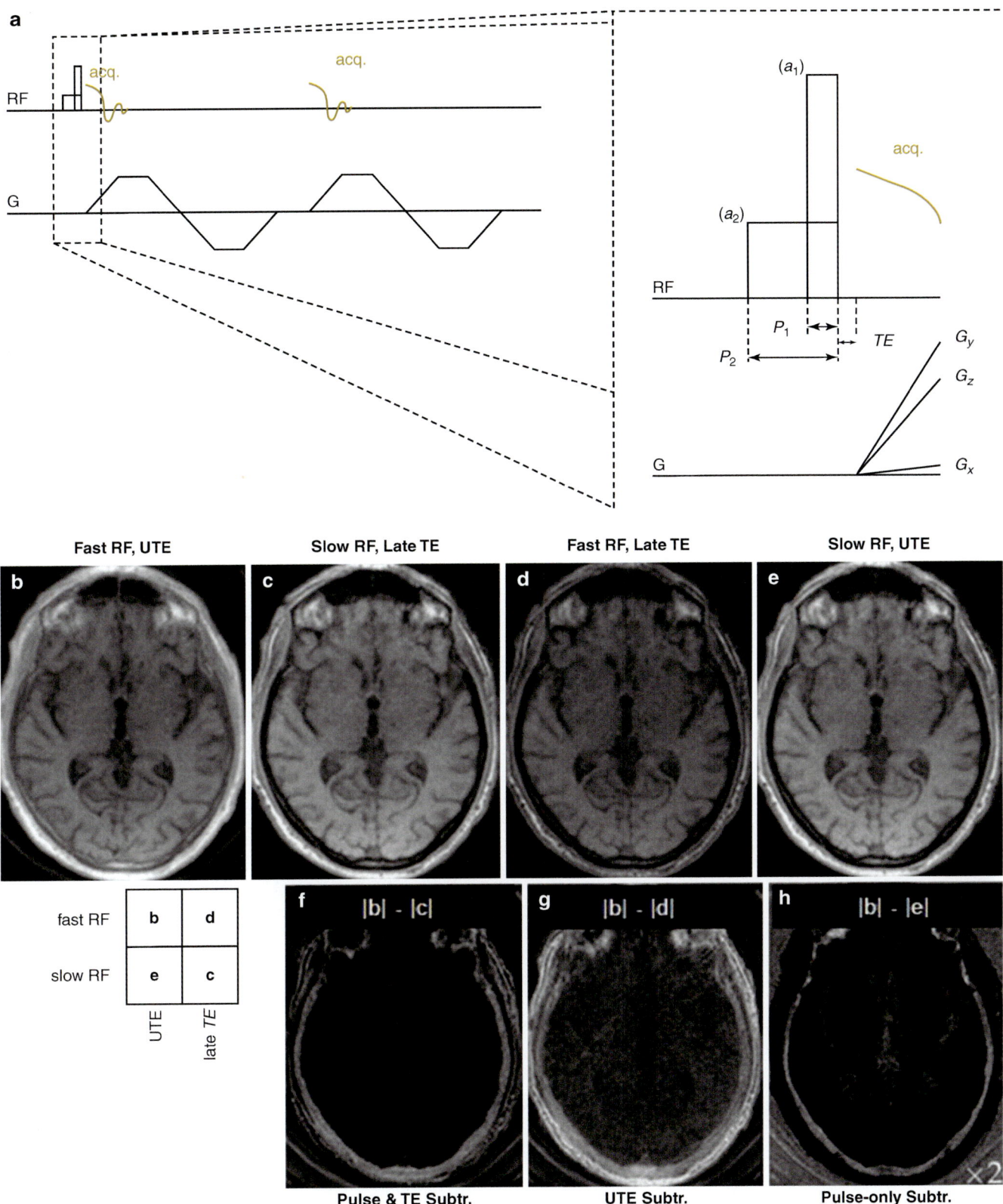

Fig. 11.9 The relaxation-parameter contrast mechanism. This is based on two hard RF pulses with different durations but equal pulse areas to generate T$_2$-selective excitation (**a**). The mechanism can be combined with single or dual-echo UTE using two RF amplitudes (a_1 and a_2) and pulse durations (p_1 and p_2) with equal pulse areas. The technique was applied to a volunteer's skull, including UTE with a short RF pulse (peak field 24.47 µT) and an ultrashort TE = 34 µs (**b**), UTE with long RF pulse (peak field 1.53 µT) and a longer TE = 2.0 ms (**c**), UTE with short RF pulse and a longer TE = 2.0 ms (**d**), and UTE with a long RF pulse and an ultrashort TE = 34 µs (**e**). The |b|–|c| difference image (**f**) depicts cortical bone more specifically than the conventional UTE subtraction |b|–|d| difference image (**g**). (**g**) is also more sensitive to the components of cortical bone than the pulse duration subtraction, |b|–|e| difference image (**h**). (Reproduced with permission from Ref. [13])

Dual-Radiofrequency and Dual-Echo (DURANDE) UTE with Subtraction

While relaxation-parameter contrast-based UTE enhances the discrimination of bone signals and yields a higher level of bone specificity than a standard dual-echo UTE sequence, the total scan time is doubled due to the use of two different RF interleaves with identical k-space coverage [13, 14]. Lee et al. proposed a rapid bone MR imaging method utilizing a 3D dual-radiofrequency and dual-echo (DURANDE) UTE pulse sequence together with bone-selective image reconstruction [14]. This technique acquires two dual-echo UTE datasets following short and long RF pulses, with encoding gradients varying continuously along the entire pulse train to reduce the total imaging time by a factor of two (Fig. 11.10a). The 3D DURANDE UTE sequence employs two hard RF pulses (RF_1 and RF_2), differing in duration and amplitude, but having the same pulse area applied alternately in successive TR periods along the entire pulse train. Two echoes at a short TE (TE_1) and a long TE (TE_2) are collected from the beginning of the gradient ramp-up within each TR. As a result, four echoes are produced, including $ECHO_{11}$, $ECHO_{12}$, $ECHO_{21}$, and $ECHO_{22}$, in which the subscripts represent the corresponding RF and TE indices. The four echoes are combined via a view-sharing (VS) approach to generate two independent k-space datasets during image reconstruction (Fig. 11.10b). Substantially accelerated UTE bone imaging can be achieved by using the sparsity of bone voxels in the corresponding subtraction images. This produces isotropic high-resolution volumetric craniofacial images in only 3 min. Figure 11.10c–e shows a volunteer study with three sets of images ($|I_1|$, $|I_2|$, and I_{Bone}) obtained by relaxation-parameter contrast-based UTE (Fig. 11.10c; $N_p = 50,000$ each for $ECHO_{11}$ and $ECHO_{22}$, respectively, imaging time = 12 min) and an accelerated version with an undersampling factor of two, without (Fig. 11.10d; $N_p = 25,000$ each for $ECHO_{11}$ and $ECHO_{22}$, 6 min scan time) and with (Fig. 11.10e; $N_p = 25,000$ each for all four echoes, 6 min scan time) using VS reconstruction. Figure 11.10f displays a line profile of I_{Bone} for each method, showing that the VS-DURANDE UTE technique provides a visually similar quality of images in under half the total scan time [14].

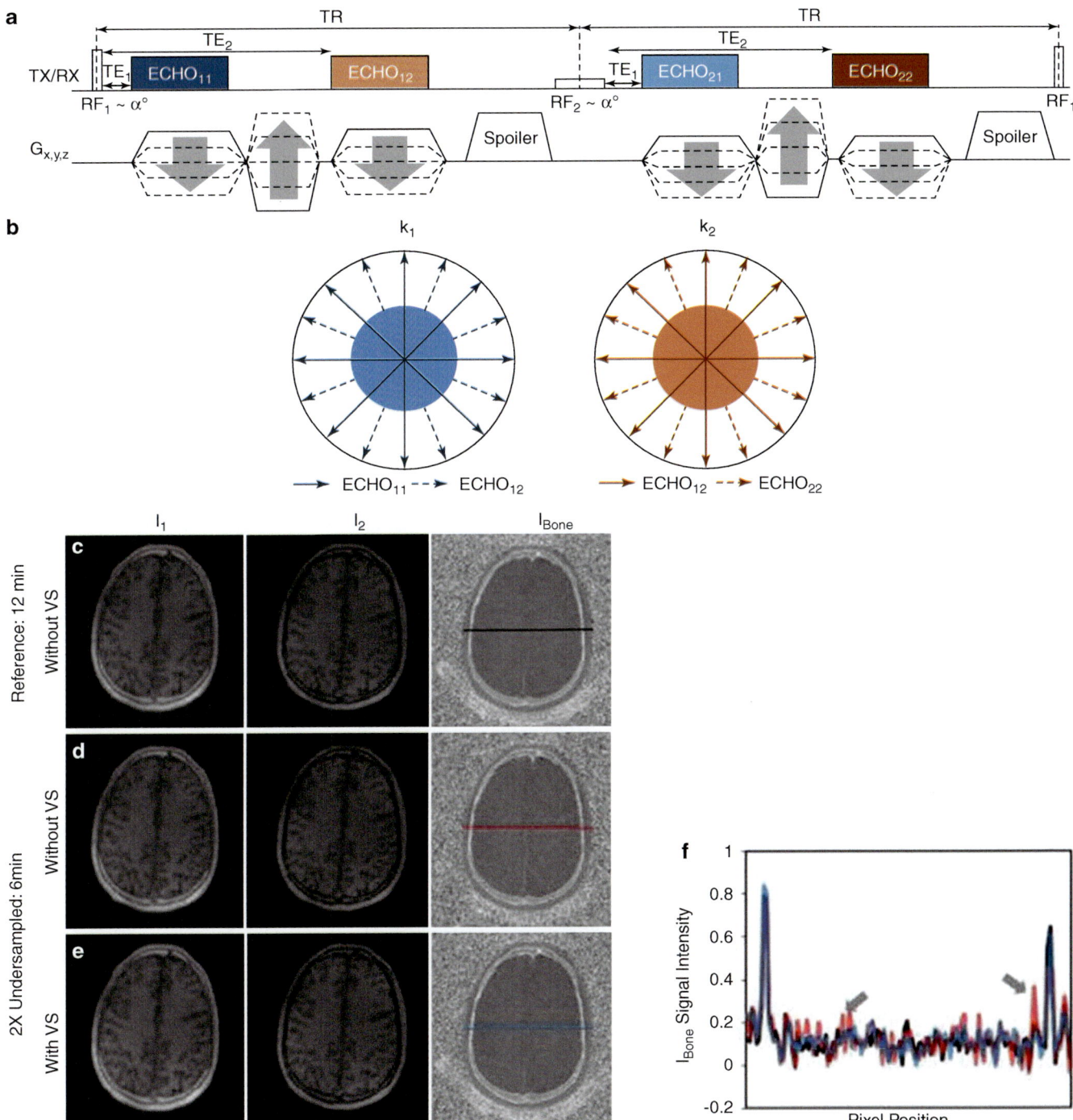

Fig. 11.10 The VS-DURANDE UTE sequence. This employs two RF pulses, RF$_1$ (short ~40 μs) and RF$_2$ (long ~520 μs), alternately followed by dual-echo acquisition to produce four independent datasets: ECHO$_{11}$, ECHO$_{12}$, ECHO$_{21}$, and ECHO$_{22}$ (**a**). A schematic of the *k*-space construction with VS between ECHO$_{11}$ and ECHO$_{21}$ (k_1) and between ECHO$_{12}$ and ECHO$_{22}$ (k_2) is shown in (**b**). Varying gradients (radial view angles) on a TR basis allows use of the VS approach to halve the total scan time. The central portions of k_1 and k_2 are composed only of ECHO$_{11}$ and ECHO$_{22}$, respectively, to maximize differences in bone signals between the two corresponding images. The 3D DURANDE UTE technique was applied in a volunteer to produce three sets of images ($|I_1|$, $|I_2|$, I_{Bone}), reconstructed with relaxation-parameter contrast (using only ECHO$_{11}$ and ECHO$_{22}$), with 50,000 (**c**; 12 min) and 25,000 (**d**; 6 min) radial views for each echo, and the VS scheme that utilizes all four echoes with 25,000 views each (**e**; 6 min). Signal profiles of I_{Bone}, corresponding to the colored lines in (**c–e**), are shown in (**f**). When compared with the reference (**c**), VS-DURANDE (**e**) suffers no appreciable loss in image quality, while undersampling-induced noise amplifications (arrows in **d**) are suppressed. (Reproduced with permission from Ref. [14])

Conclusion

Transverse magnetization decays exponentially in time following T_2^* relaxation in UTE imaging. The difference between two sets of UTE and later echo images acquired with different TEs provides T_2 sensitivity. A "band-selective" sensitivity in T_2^* is achieved by appropriately selecting TE and ΔTE. The most straightforward technique is to acquire two echoes using UTE FID as the first echo and a second echo. Subtraction of these provides high contrast imaging of short-T_2 tissues in a time-efficient way. A drawback of this technique is marked sensitivity to off-resonance effects and contamination from fat, which has a high proton density, short-T_1, and a long-T_2 but a relatively short-T_2^* [1–5]. Using fat-suppressed dual-echo UTE with echo subtraction improves the short-T_2 contrast for imaging of the osteochondral junction [2]. Long-T_2 saturation and an adiabatic inversion preparation can also be combined with dual-echo UTE data acquisition for improved short-T_2 contrast. UTE-based off-resonance saturation creates high contrast for short-T_2 tissues with the efficiency and artifact level closely related to the properties of the saturation pulse [7]. Adiabatic inversion preparation is robust for long-T_2 signal suppression, as it is insensitive to B_1 inhomogeneity once the adiabatic condition is met and insensitive to B_0 inhomogeneity when using a relatively broad spectral bandwidth [19]. Complex subtraction may further improve long-T_2 signal suppression, especially for tissue components subject to imperfect nulling due to T_1 variations [15]. UTE with an interleaved adiabatic inversion and subtraction allows high-contrast imaging of short-T_2 tissues such as cortical bone. However, the optimal contrast depends on the scaling factors, which are tissue dependent and may compromise clinical applications [23]. UTE with relaxation-parameter contrast followed by subtraction works well in highlighting ultrashort-T_2 tissues such as cortical bone in the skull [13]. The VS-DURANDE UTE technique is based on relaxation-parameter contrast. It uses view-sharing reconstruction and the sparsity of bone voxels to produce bone images in under half the usual scan time [14]. These different subtraction-based techniques may also be combined with other UTE-type sequences, such as zero echo time (ZTE) [30] and pointwise encoding time reduction with radial acquisition (PETRA) [31] for high contrast imaging of short-T_2 tissues.

References

1. Robson MD, Gatehouse PD, Bydder M, Bydder GM. Magnetic resonance: an introduction to ultrashort TE (UTE) imaging. J Comput Assist Tomogr. 2003;27(6):825–46.

2. Du J, Bydder M, Takahashi AM, Carl M, Chung CB, Bydder GM. Short T_2 contrast with three-dimensional ultrashort echo time imaging. Magn Reson Imaging. 2011;29(4):470–82.

3. Rahmer J, Bornert P, Groen J, Bos C. Three-dimensional radial ultrashort echo-time imaging with T_2 adapted sampling. Magn Reson Med. 2006;55(5):1075–82.

4. Kim YJ, Cha JG, Shin YS, Chaudhari AS, Suh YJ, Hwan Yoon S, et al. 3D ultrashort TE MRI for evaluation of cartilaginous endplate of cervical disk in vivo: feasibility and correlation with disk degeneration in T_2-weighted spin-echo sequence. AJR Am J Roentgenol. 2018;210(5):1131–40.

5. Rahmer J, Bornert P, Dries SP. Assessment of anterior cruciate ligament reconstruction using 3D ultrashort echo-time MR imaging. J Magn Reson Imaging. 2009;29(2):443–8.

6. Larson PE, Gurney PT, Nayak K, Gold GE, Pauly JM, Nishimura DG. Designing long-T_2 suppression pulses for ultrashort echo time imaging. Magn Reson Med. 2006;56(1):94–103.

7. Du J, Takahashi AM, Bydder M, Chung CB, Bydder GM. Ultrashort TE imaging with off-resonance saturation contrast (UTE-OSC). Magn Reson Med. 2009;62(2):527–31.

8. Waldman A, Rees JH, Brock CS, Robson MD, Gatehouse PD, Bydder GM. MRI of the brain with ultra-short echo-time pulse sequences. Neuroradiology. 2003;45(12):887–92.

9. Du J, Ma G, Li S, Carl M, Szeverenyi NM, VandenBerg S, et al. Ultrashort echo time (UTE) magnetic resonance imaging of the short T_2 components in white matter of the brain using a clinical 3T scanner. NeuroImage. 2014;87:32–41.

10. Du J, Sheth V, He Q, Carl M, Chen J, Corey-Bloom J, et al. Measurement of T_1 of the ultrashort T_2^* components in white matter of the brain at 3T. PLoS One. 2014;9(8):e103296.

11. Wilhelm MJ, Ong HH, Wehrli SL, Li C, Tsai PH, Hackney DB, et al. Direct magnetic resonance detection of myelin and prospects for quantitative imaging of myelin density. Proc Natl Acad Sci U S A. 2012;109(24):9605–10.

12. Ma YJ, Searleman AC, Jang H, Fan SJ, Wong J, Xue Y, et al. Volumetric imaging of myelin in vivo using 3D inversion recovery-prepared ultrashort echo time cones magnetic resonance imaging. NMR Biomed. 2020;33(10):e4326.

13. Johnson EM, Vyas U, Ghanouni P, Pauly KB, Pauly JM. Improved cortical bone specificity in UTE MR imaging. Magn Reson Med. 2017;77(2):684–95.

14. Lee H, Zhao X, Song HK, Zhang R, Bartlett SP, Wehrli FW. Rapid dual-RF, dual-echo, 3D ultrashort echo time craniofacial imaging: a feasibility study. Magn Reson Med. 2019;81(5):3007–16.

15. Jang H, Wei Z, Wu M, Ma YJ, Chang EY, Corey-Bloom J, et al. Improved volumetric myelin imaging in human brain using 3D dual echo inversion recovery-prepared UTE with complex echo subtraction. Magn Reson Med. 2020;83(4):1168–77.

16. Lee YH, Kim S, Song HT, Kim I, Suh JS. Weighted subtraction in 3D ultrashort echo time (UTE) imaging for visualization of short T_2 tissues of the knee. Acta Radiol. 2014;55(4):454–61.

17. Bydder M, Yokoo T, Hamilton G, Middleton MS, Chavez AD, Schwimmer JB, et al. Relaxation effects in the quantification of fat using gradient echo imaging. Magn Reson Imaging. 2008;26(3):347–59.

18. Hamilton G, Yokoo T, Bydder M, Cruite I, Schroeder ME, Sirlin CB, et al. In vivo characterization of the liver fat (1)H MR spectrum. NMR Biomed. 2011;24(7):784–90.

19. Du J, Carl M, Bydder M, Takahashi A, Chung CB, Bydder GM. Qualitative and quantitative ultrashort echo time (UTE) imaging of cortical bone. J Magn Reson. 2010;207(2):304–11.

20. Sussman MS, Pauly JM, Wright GA. Design of practical T_2-selective RF excitation (TELEX) pulses. Magn Reson Med. 1998;40(6):890–9.

21. Li C, Magland JF, Rad HS, Song HK, Wehrli FW. Comparison of optimized soft-tissue suppression schemes for ultrashort echo time MRI. Magn Reson Med. 2012;68(3):680–9.

22. Garwood M, DelaBarre L. The return of the frequency sweep: designing adiabatic pulses for contemporary NMR. J Magn Reson. 2001;153(2):155–77.

23. Larson PE, Conolly SM, Pauly JM, Nishimura DG. Using adiabatic inversion pulses for long-T$_2$ suppression in ultrashort echo time (UTE) imaging. Magn Reson Med. 2007;58(5):952–61.

24. Ma YJ, Jang H, Chang EY, Hiniker A, Head BP, Lee RR, et al. Ultrashort echo time (UTE) magnetic resonance imaging of myelin: technical developments and challenges. Quant Imaging Med Surg. 2020;10(6):1186–203.

25. Wang Y, Johnston DL, Breen JF, Huston J 3rd, Jack CR, Julsrud PR, et al. Dynamic MR digital subtraction angiography using contrast enhancement, fast data acquisition, and complex subtraction. Magn Reson Med. 1996;36(4):551–6.

26. Naganawa S, Ito T, Iwayama E, Fukatsu H, Ishiguchi T, Ishigaki T, et al. Magnitude subtraction vs. complex subtraction in dynamic contrast-enhanced 3D-MR angiography: basic experiments and clinical evaluation. J Magn Reson Imaging. 1999;10(5):813–20.

27. Coombs BD, Szumowski J, Coshow W. Two-point Dixon technique for water-fat signal decomposition with B$_0$ inhomogeneity correction. Magn Reson Med. 1997;38(6):884–9.

28. Jang H, Carl M, Ma Y, Jerban S, Guo T, Zhao W, et al. Fat suppression for ultrashort echo time imaging using a single-point Dixon method. NMR Biomed. 2019;32(5):e4069.

29. Carl M, Chiang JT. Investigations of the origin of phase differences seen with ultrashort TE imaging of short T$_2$ meniscal tissue. Magn Reson Med. 2012;67(4):991–1003.

30. Weiger M, Pruessmann KP, Hennel F. MRI with zero echo time: hard versus sweep pulse excitation. Magn Reson Med. 2011;66(2):379–89.

31. Grodzki DM, Jakob PM, Heismann B. Ultrashort echo time imaging using pointwise encoding time reduction with radial acquisition (PETRA). Magn Reson Med. 2012;67(2):510–8.

T₂ Relaxation During Radiofrequency (RF) Pulses

Peder Larson

Introduction

Radiofrequency (RF) pulses are a critical part of every MRI pulse sequence and must be specifically designed for ultrashort echo time (UTE) and zero echo time (ZTE) acquisitions. When considering the behavior of RF pulses, most often longitudinal T_1 or transverse T_2 relaxation are assumed to be negligible during the RF pulses themselves. This is usually valid with conventional sequences since most tissue T_1s and T_2s are much longer than typical RF pulse durations. However, when imaging tissues that have transverse relaxation times that are of the order of, or shorter than, the RF pulse duration, as is often the case with UTE and ZTE MRI, then relaxation during the pulse must be considered. This chapter covers the theory of T_2/T_2^* relaxation during an RF pulse and the implications as well as applications of this for imaging of short- and ultrashort-T_2^* species.

Theory

To determine the effect of relaxation during an RF pulse, we simply need to use the Bloch equations. However, solutions of the Bloch equations used in RF pulse simulation and design, such as the Shinnar-Le Roux (SLR) transform, cannot be used since they neglect relaxation. Numerical solutions to the Bloch equation can be used to provide the most accurate simulations of RF pulse profiles.

However, to gain insight into the interaction between an RF pulse including longitudinal and transverse relaxations, the following approximate solution to the Bloch equation for the longitudinal magnetization, M_Z, is useful:

$$M_Z\left(T_2\right) \approx M_0\left(1 - T_2 \int_{-\infty}^{\infty} \left|\Omega_1\left(f\right)\right|^2 \mathrm{d}f\right) \qquad (12.1)$$

Here, M_0 is the equilibrium magnetization, T_2 is the transverse relaxation time, f is frequency, and $\Omega_1(f)$ is the Fourier transform, or frequency spectrum, of the RF pulse. This result was derived assuming T_2 is short relative to fluctuations in the RF pulse shape and using a small-tip approximation [1]. This shows that there is a trade-off between total RF spectral power (e.g., pulse bandwidth) and short-T_2 signal attenuation.

The effect of RF pulses on short-T_2 components can also be understood in terms of spectral linewidths (Fig. 12.1). T_2 is inversely proportional to the linewidth, meaning that short-T_2 species have broad linewidths and long-T_2 species have narrow linewidths. The overlap between the spectrum of the RF pulse and the tissue spectrum determines the approximate degree of excitation. The narrow spectrum of long-T_2 species is more easily covered by the RF spectrum, and thus they are easily excited [2]. Broad short-T_2 species require a wide bandwidth RF pulse to be fully excited. Thus, a narrow bandwidth RF pulse can fully excite longer T_2 species but only partially excites shorter T_2 species (Fig. 12.1).

This intuitive understanding can be extended to off-resonance situations. For example, magnetization transfer (MT) applies RF pulses far from the water resonance frequency, which only leads to excitation of very broad linewidth ultrashort-T_2 components. Fat suppression pulses are also applied at the lipid resonance frequencies with relatively narrow bandwidths in order to selectively excite fat but not long-T_2 water.

P. Larson (✉)
Department of Radiology and Biomedical Imaging, University of California, San Francisco, CA, USA
e-mail: Peder.Larson@ucsf.edu

Fig. 12.1 Illustration of how spectral linewidth (proportional to T_2) and RF pulse bandwidth determine excitation. (**a**) Narrow bandwidth (dashed line) RF pulse that overlaps the majority of the long-T_2 spectrum but only a small fraction of the short-T_2 spectrum. The long-T_2 species is excited more by the pulse than the short-T_2 species. (**b**) Wide bandwidth (dashed line) RF pulse that overlaps both the long- and short-T_2 spectra, thus exciting both. (**c**) This also applies to MT pulses, which are applied off-resonance primarily to excite ultrashort-T_2 species. (Reproduced with permission from Ref. [1])

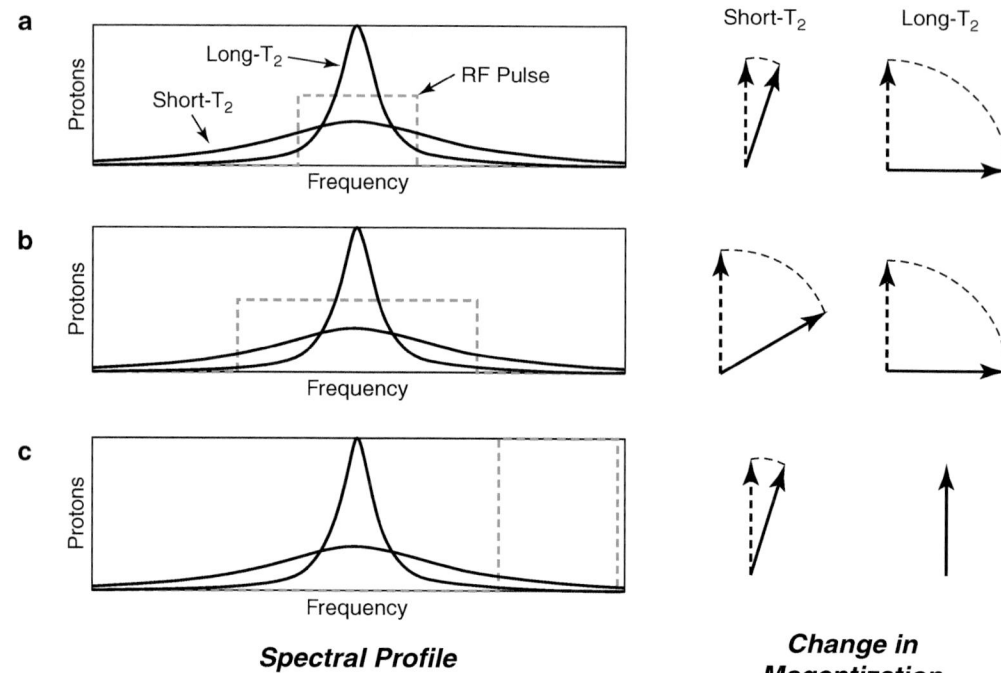

Excitation and T_2 Relaxation

The purpose of excitation is to generate transverse magnetization for imaging. When imaging ultrashort-T_2 species, the major consideration is to ensure there is an adequate flip angle applied to the rapidly decaying component. As shown in Fig. 12.2, the flip angle decreases with shorter T_2s, causing noticeable decreases when T_2 is of the order of, or shorter than, the pulse duration. Also note that shorter T_2s also lead to blurring of the slice profile.

To achieve sufficient excitation of an ultrashort-T_2 component, the intuition from Fig. 12.1 tells us that RF pulses should be designed to have as large a bandwidth as possible, as shown in Fig. 12.3. Equivalently, for a given pulse shape, the RF pulse should be as short as possible, since bandwidth scales inversely with duration. Ultimately, shortening the RF pulse is limited by the MR system peak B_1 amplitude and peak gradient strength (when performing slice selection).

Changes in excitation as a function of T_2 have also been exploited to improve the contrast for short-T_2 components [5]. This approach uses an acquisition with a short RF pulse, which has high signal from both long- and short-T_2 components, and an acquisition with a long RF pulse, which has high signal only from long-T_2 components. The long-T_2 component signal can then be suppressed by subtracting these two images, leading to improved short-T_2 contrast (Fig. 12.4).

Short-T_2 component excitation has also been combined with fat suppression in a soft-hard composite pulse approach

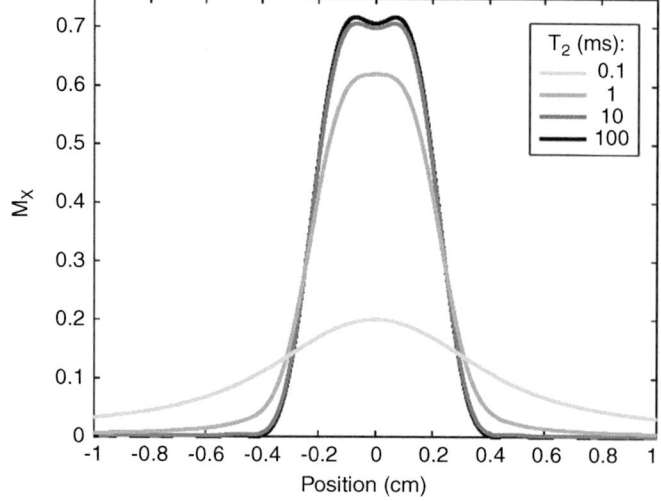

Fig. 12.2 Bloch equation simulated slice profile versus T_2 for a 1 ms, 45° half pulse [3, 4]. T_2 relaxation during the pulse blurs the desired 5 mm slice profile and decreases the flip angle for the shortest T_2 values

[6]. In this approach, the composite pulse contains a narrow bandwidth soft pulse centered on the fat peak with a small negative flip angle ($-\alpha$) and a short rectangular pulse with a small positive flip angle (α). The fat magnetization experiences both tipping down and tipping back with an identical flip angle and thus returns to its equilibrium state, leaving only the water magnetization excited. This avoids short-T_2 component saturation that happens during conventional fat saturation RF pulses (Fig. 12.5).

Fig. 12.3 Simulated half-pulse slice profiles for 45°, 2 ms pulses with bandwidths of 1.2 kHz (black), 1.8 kHz (dark gray), and 2.4 kHz (light gray line). As expected, the increasing bandwidth increases the short-T_2 excitation flip angle (**a**) but only changes the profile sharpness of long-T_2 components (**b**)

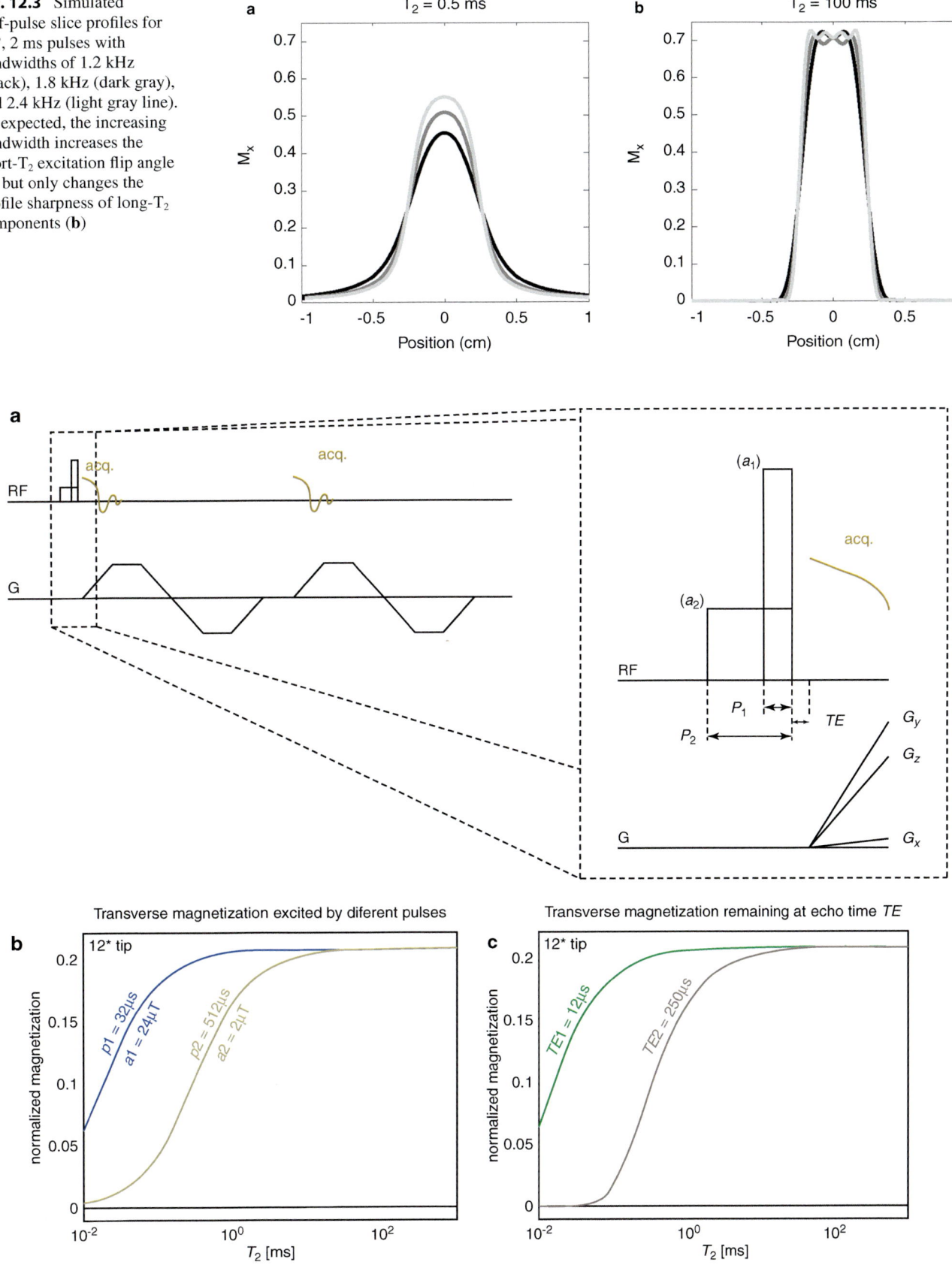

Fig. 12.4 RF excitation pulses of different lengths (**a**) can be used to create T_2 selectivity (**b**). For comparison, the T_2 selectivity at different TEs is also shown. The images (**d–j**) show how the fast and slow RF pulse images as well as different TE images can be subtracted to create short-T_2 contrast, in this case providing excellent depiction of cortical bone in the skull which has a $T_2^* \sim 0.3$ ms. (Adapted with permission from Ref. [5])

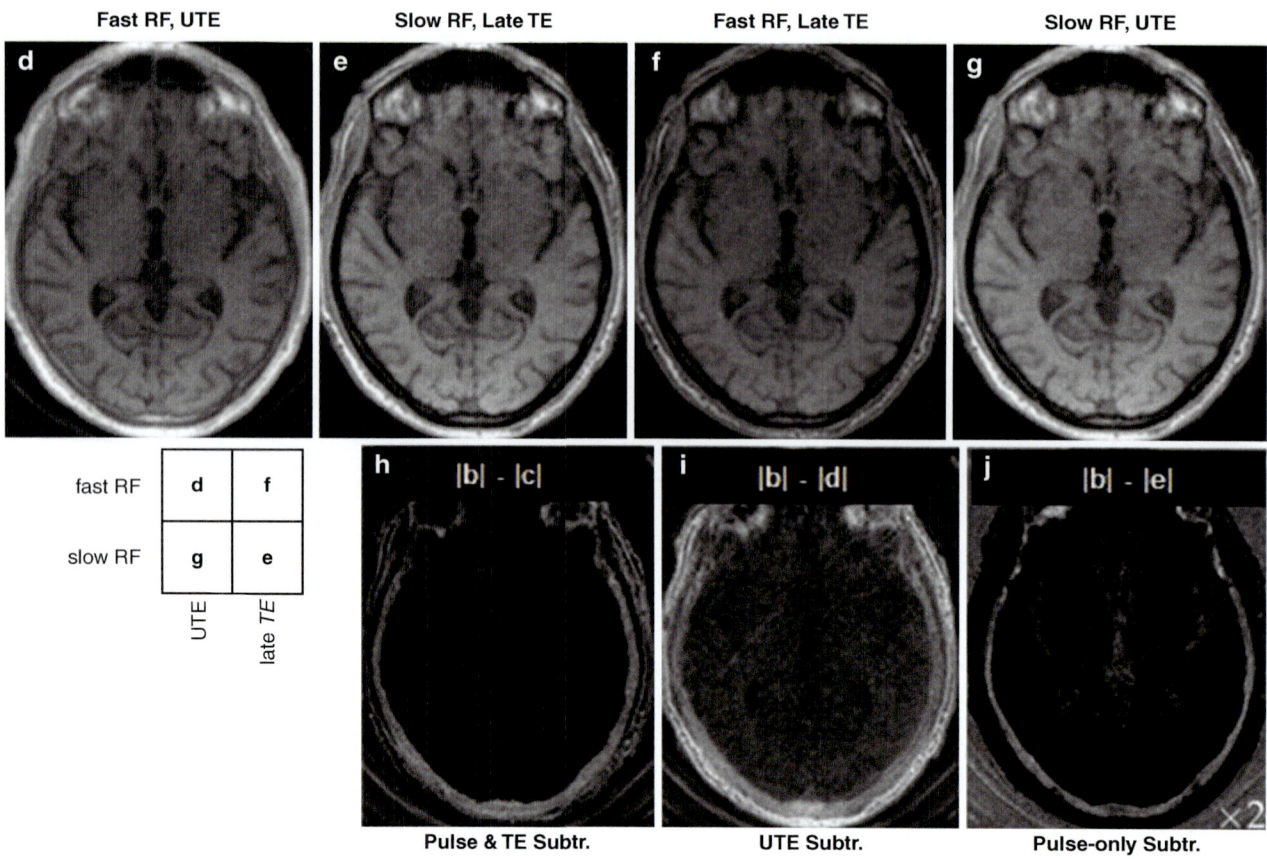

Fig. 12.4 (continued)

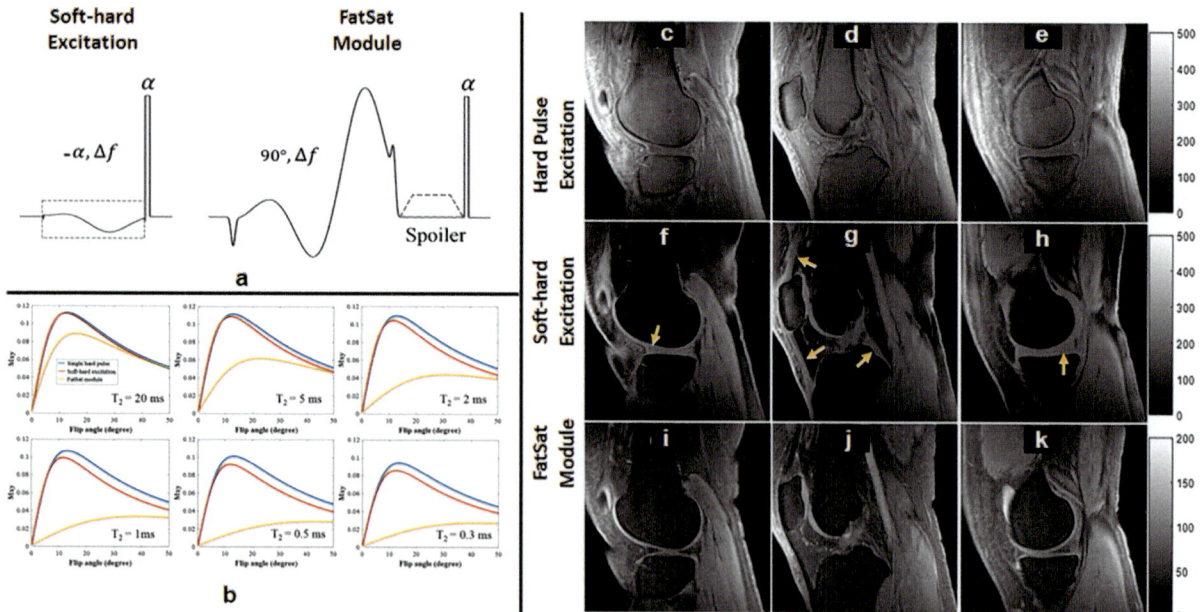

Fig. 12.5 Short-T_2 selective excitation can be achieved with a composite soft-hard excitation. (**a**) This consists of a narrow bandwidth negative flip angle ($-\alpha$) pulse followed by high bandwidth pulse with a positive flip angle ($+\alpha$) of the same magnitude. The simulations (**b**) and in vivo knee imaging results (**c–k**) show that this strategy creates improved short-T_2 component contrast without fat signal compared to standard 3D UTE with hard pulse excitation and also has less suppression of water short-T_2 components compared to use of a FatSat module as highlighted by the orange arrows pointing to meniscus, ligaments, and tendons. (Adapted with permission from Ref. [6])

Saturation and T$_2$ Relaxation

The T$_2$ selectivity of RF pulses has also been exploited to design saturation pulses intended to selectively saturate long-T$_2$ components and provide improved contrast for short-T$_2$ components. One challenge in imaging short-T$_2$ components is that they often have smaller signals due to relaxation and/or lower proton density compared to long-T$_2$ components. This problem can be overcome by designing low bandwidth 90° flip angle RF pulses, which are followed by a spoiling gradient to suppress spins excited by the pulse. Using the intuition in Fig. 12.1a, these low bandwidth pulses overlap the entire long-T$_2$ linewidth, causing full 90° excitation, while short- and ultrashort-T$_2$ components have smaller or incomplete excitation and thus will not be suppressed by the resulting spoiler gradient (Fig. 12.6).

The disadvantages of long-T$_2$ suppression pulses are that they are inherently sensitive to off-resonance, as they rely on use of a narrow pulse bandwidth for contrast, and, like other suppression pulse schemes, are sensitive to RF field inhomogeneities that lead to imperfect flip angles.

The principles of long-T$_2$ suppression pulses can also be applied with fat suppression, which is especially important for musculoskeletal applications where short-T$_2$ tissues such as tendons, ligaments, cartilage, and bone are often adjacent to fat. One approach that can be used is to create "dual-band" RF pulses, a single RF pulse which includes relatively narrow saturation bandwidths at both fat and water resonances to selectively excite long-T$_2$ components at these two resonances [1].

Another approach is to use separate 90° saturation pulses at both the fat and water resonances, as illustrated in Fig. 12.7. This approach also includes low bandwidth refocusing 180° pulses on alternate scans. These are included to correct for imperfections in the flip angle of the 90° saturation pulses, which is a challenge for 90° RF pulse-based saturation schemes. By using low bandwidth pulses, only the long-T$_2$ components experience this refocusing (Fig. 12.8).

T$_2$ selective suppression can also be achieved in a manner similar to MT by applying off-resonance contrast ("UTE-OSC") RF pulses [9]. Following the off-resonance RF pulse, only the short-T$_2$ components are excited (Fig. 12.1c), and these are suppressed by a spoiler gradient. The off-resonance saturated image is then subtracted from an unsuppressed image, leading to improved contrast of short-T$_2$ components. This approach is the inverse of long-T$_2$ suppression pulses (Fig. 12.9).

Fig. 12.6 Simulation results for longitudinal magnetization remaining after suppression pulses of different bandwidths for various T$_2$ values. As the pulse bandwidth increases, the signal remaining after suppression decreases. As T$_2$ increases, the signal also decreases. This simulation is consistent with the intuition shown in Fig. 12.1. (Reproduced with permission from Ref. [1])

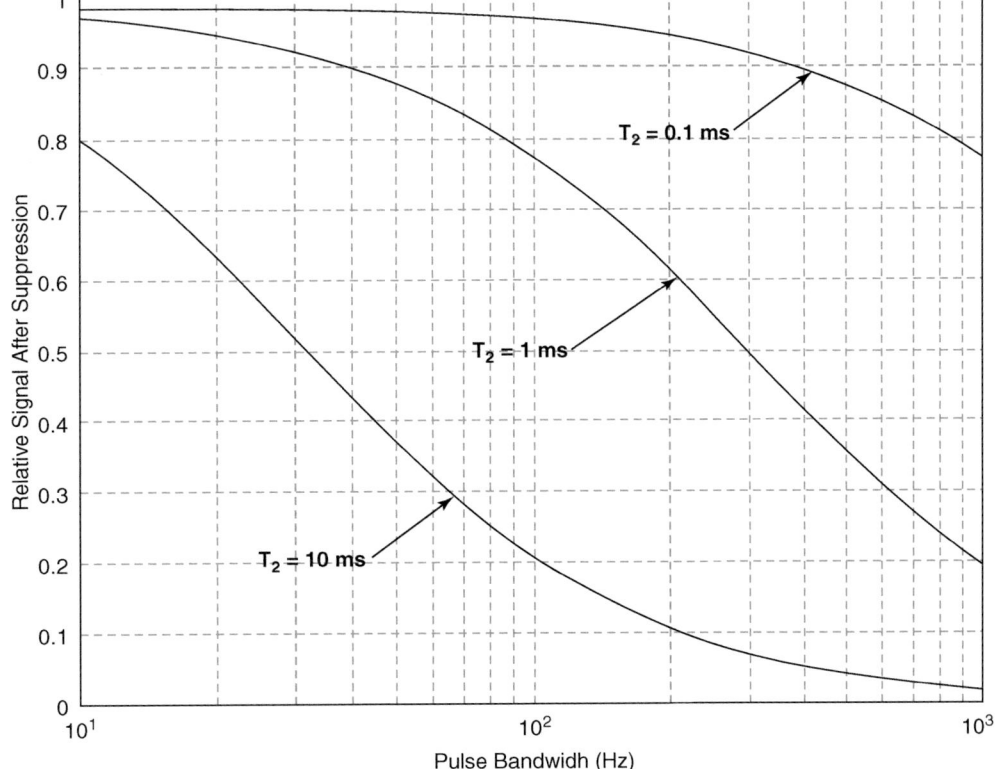

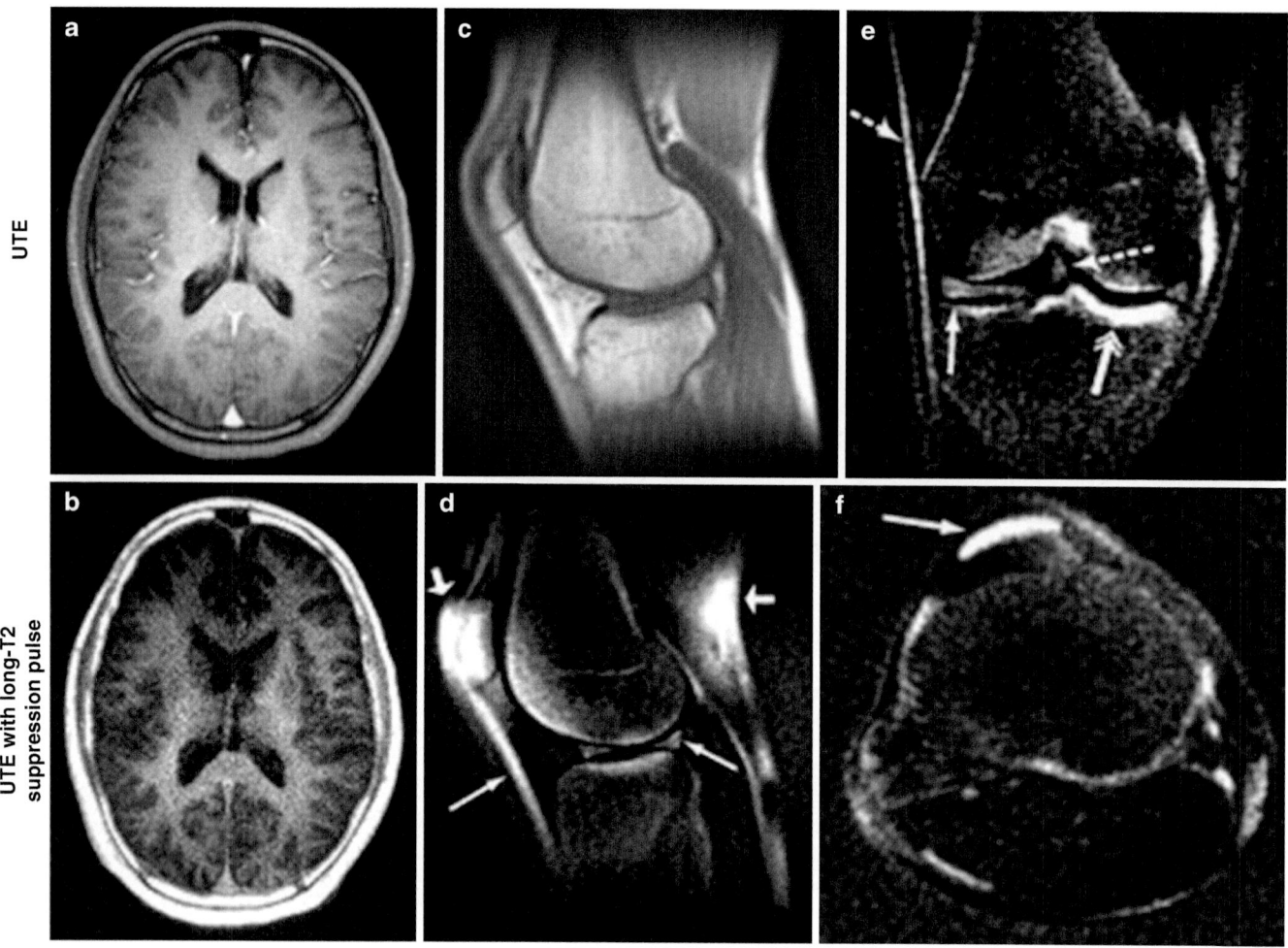

Fig. 12.7 Long-T$_2$ signal suppression pulse results in vivo. (**a**, **b**) In the brain, a low bandwidth saturation pulse applied at the water resonance frequency creates improved contrast for short-T$_2$ components in myelin as well as connective tissue and cortical bone compared to UTE without long-T$_2$ signal suppression. (**c–f**) 3D UTE results in the knee show greatly improved contrast of short-T$_2$ structures when using a dual-band suppression pulse (**d–f**) to suppress long-T$_2$ water and fat components compared to no suppression in (**c**). This provides excellent visualization of the menisci, patellar tendon, iliotibial band, and anterior cruciate ligaments, as well as the thickened tibial cortex. There are some fat suppression failures (short arrows in **d**) due to B_0 field inhomogeneity. (Adapted with permission from Ref. [1])

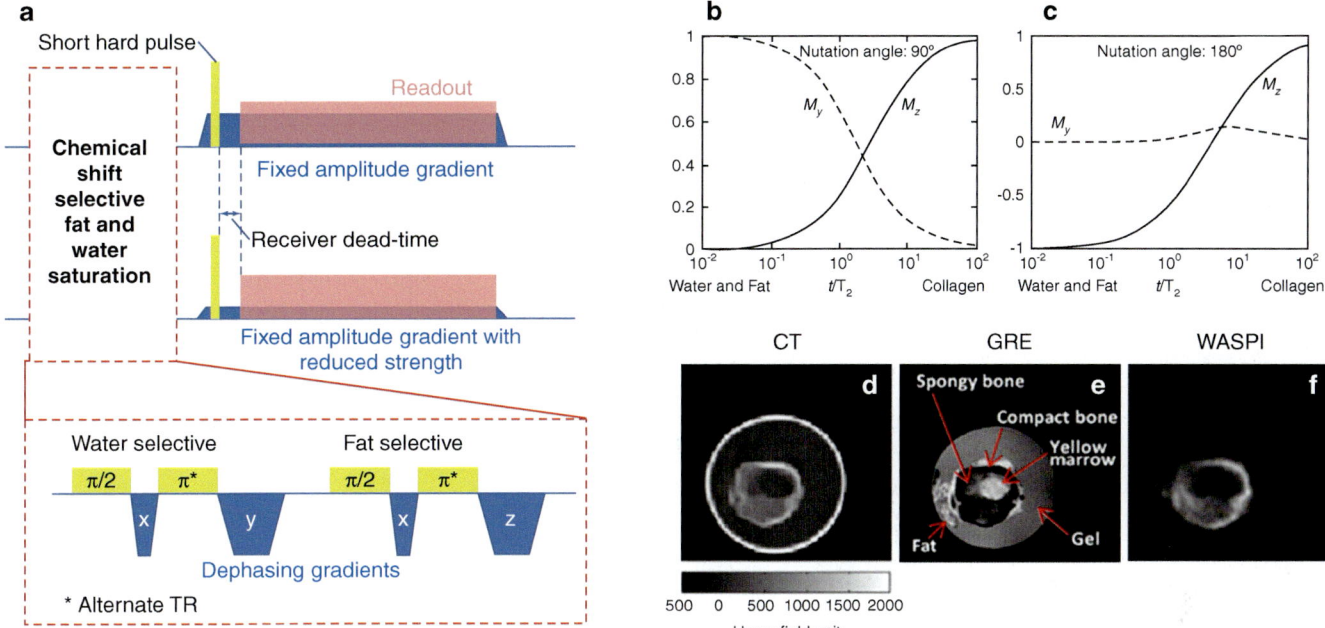

Fig. 12.8 (**a**) The water- and fat-suppressed proton projection imaging (WASPI) sequence. This uses separate water and fat selective low bandwidth suppression pulses prior to a ZTE readout to selectively suppress long-T$_2$ components at both fat and water resonances. The 180° pulses provide robustness to flip angle errors. (Top right) Simulated magnetization vs. t/T$_2$ following perfect rectangular RF pulses. (**b**) For low bandwidth 90° pulses, only the long-T$_2$ components are rotated into the transverse plane. (**c**) Similarly, for the low bandwidth 180° pulses, only the long-T$_2$ components are inverted. (**d–f**) Using this tissue suppression scheme, the long-T$_2$ water gel and long-T$_2$ fat components are suppressed, leaving a selective image of cortical bone with contrast similar to CT. (Adapted with permission from Refs. [7, 8])

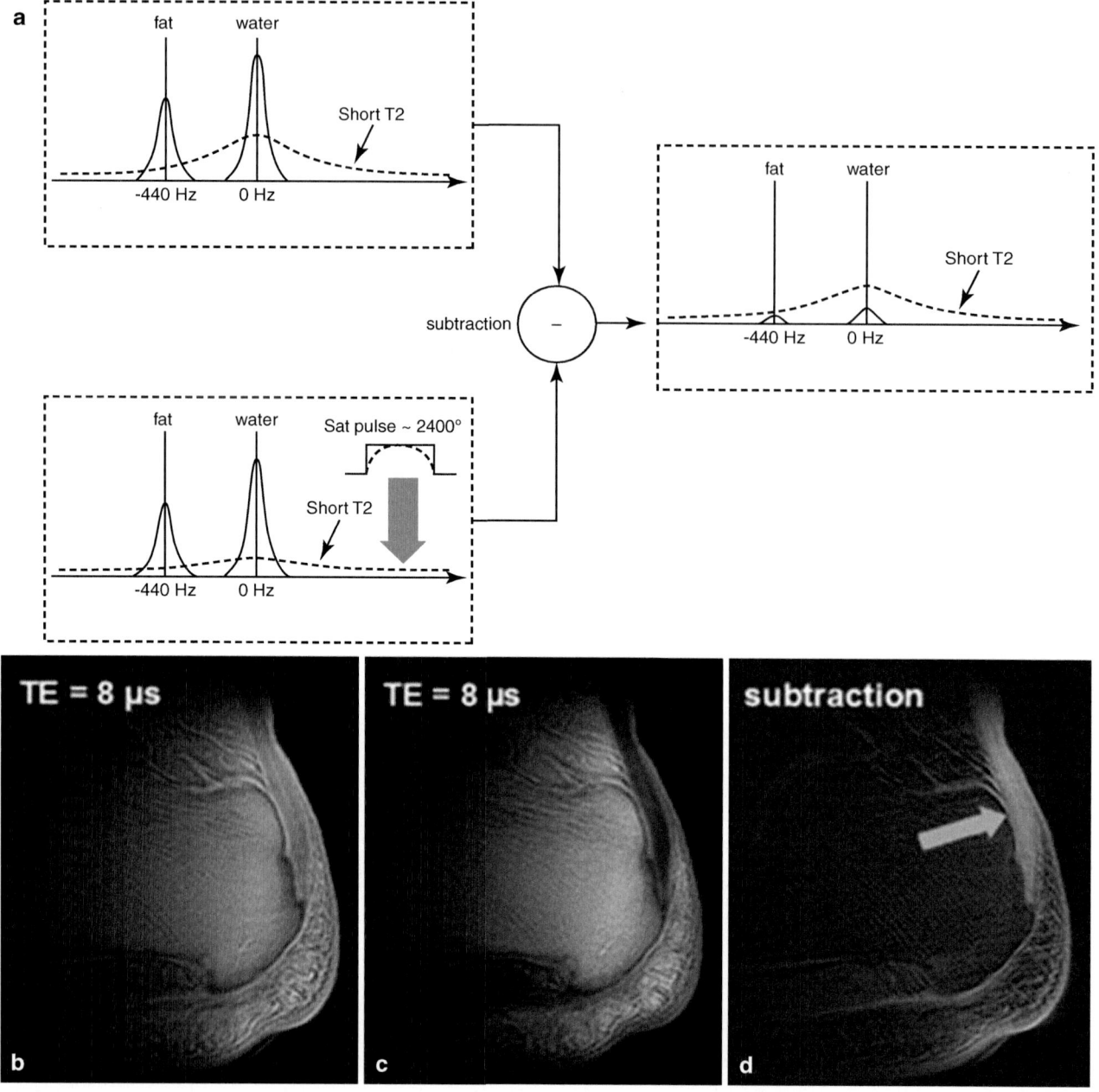

Fig. 12.9 (**a**) UTE with off-resonance saturation contrast (UTE-OSC). This includes two acquisitions with and without an off-resonance saturation pulse. The saturation pulse was placed +1 to +2 kHz away from the on-resonance water peak to minimize its spectral overlap with those of long-T_2 water and fat. Short-T_2 species have a broad spectrum and are suppressed by the saturation pulse. Subtraction of UTE images with and without off-resonance saturation pulse suppresses long-T_2 water and fat signals, leaving high contrast for short-T_2 species. (**b–d**) This is clearly shown in the ankle UTE imaging result, which shows unsaturated (**b**) and off-resonance saturated (**c**) images, from which subtraction leads to high-contrast visualization of the Achilles' tendon (arrow in **d**). (Adapted with permission from Ref. [9])

Inversion and T_2 Relaxation

Inversion pulses are valuable tools that are typically used to create T_1 contrast by including a time delay after a 180° pulse, also known as inversion recovery (IR). Using the principles in this chapter, we can also integrate T_2 selectivity into inversion pulses for short-T_2 imaging applications.

One approach is to use low bandwidth inversion pulses to prepare the magnetization and then combine with non-inverted images [10]. Since the low bandwidth pulses primarily invert long-T_2 components, they are suppressed in the combined images and provide improved short-T_2 contrast. This strategy can also be extended to include fat suppression by combining long-T_2 fat-inverted and long-T_2 water-inverted images (Fig. 12.10).

Fig. 12.10 (**a**) Adiabatic inversion pulses can create T₂ selective contrast. Simulations were performed for 30 ms Lorentz pulses. When the two images are combined, the long-T₂ species at both resonances are suppressed. The short-T₂ species, while attenuated, have significantly improved contrast. For the values shown, the short-T₂ to long-T₂ contrast is increased by a factor of 10. (**b**) For fat and water long-T₂ suppression, fat-inverted and water-inverted images are acquired and then separated into inverted and noninverted components based on the corrected phase. (**c–h**) Axial images at the middle of the lower leg: (**c**) water-inverted magnitude image; (**d**) fat-inverted magnitude image; (**e**) water-inverted phase image, corrected; (**f**) fat-inverted phase image, corrected; (**g**) sum of (**c**, **e**) and (**d**, **f**); (**h**) scaled sum of (**c**) and (**d**), showing improved contrast of cortical bone as well as skin and signal between muscles and fascicles. (Adapted with permission from Ref. [10])

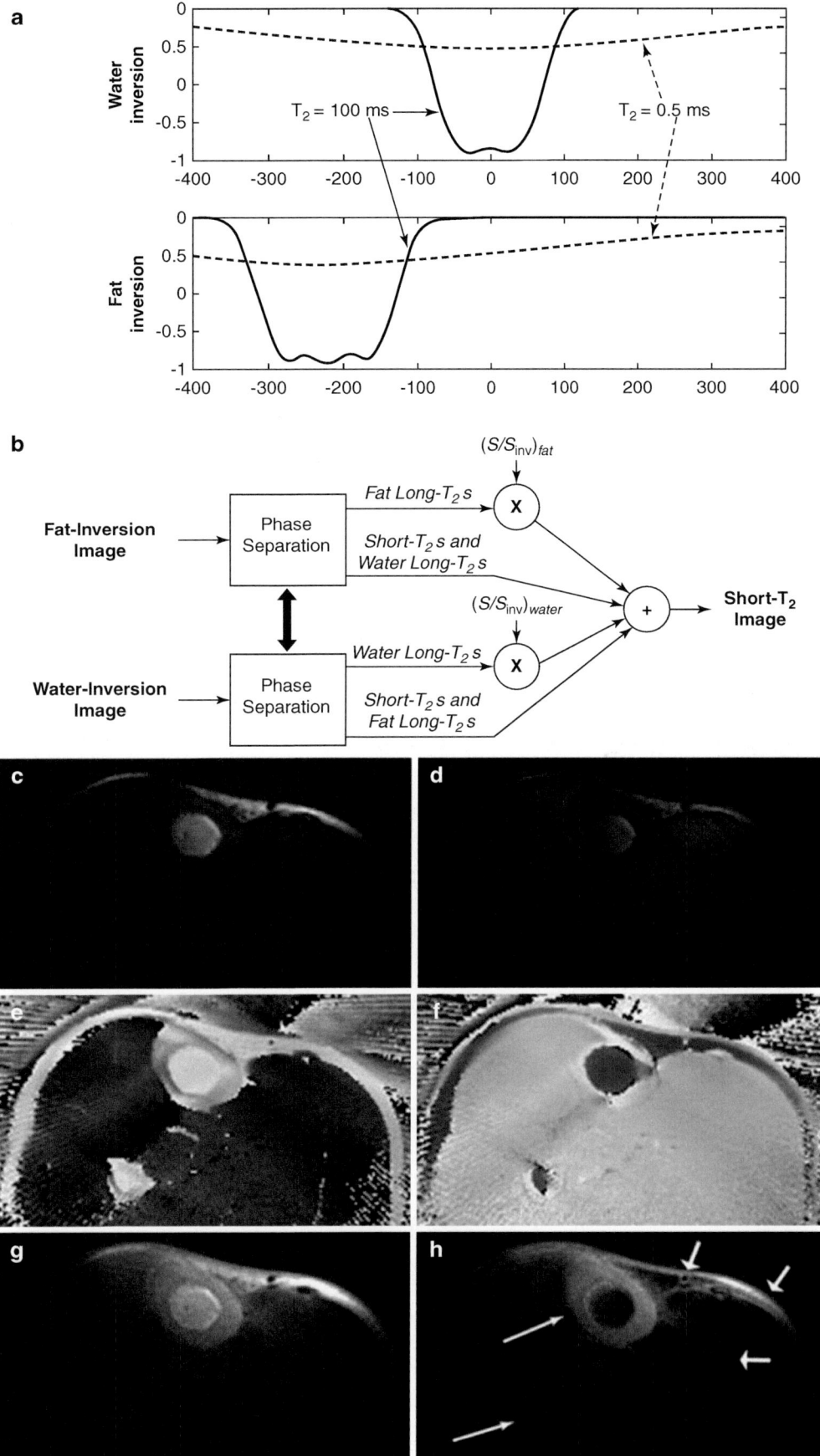

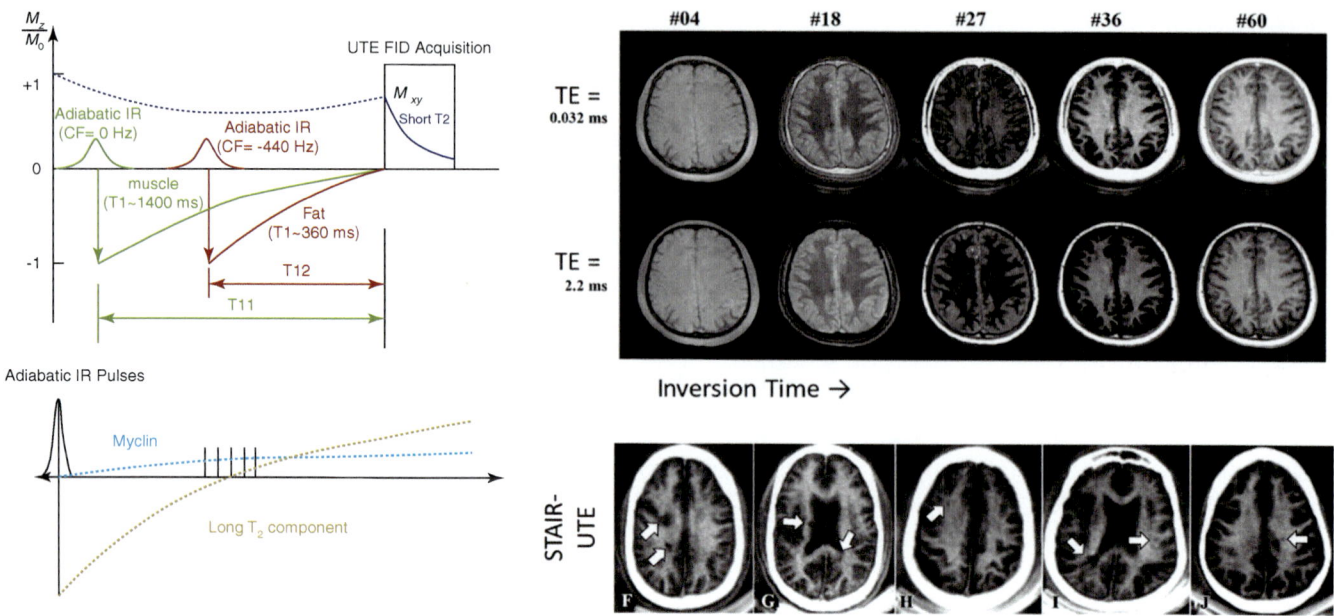

Fig. 12.11 (Left) Two examples of the expected signal response in IR-UTE. The short-T_2 components (e.g., myelin protons) are partially tipped by the inversion pulse, whereas the long-T_2 components are fully inverted. At the chosen TI, the long-T_2 components are nulled while the short-T_2 components have experienced T_1 recovery. (Right) Example results of IR UTE in the brain show how the contrast varies with TI and TE. Combining echo subtraction with a well-chosen TI leads to short-T_2 selective images of myelin, shown using the STAIR-UTE method in a multiple sclerosis patient with demyelinating lesions (arrows). (Adapted with permission from Refs. [12–14])

Short-T_2 imaging can also be combined with IR to suppress long-T_2 components [11]. This can simply be based on T_1 selectivity, but by designing reduced bandwidth inversion pulses, this can improve the contrast for short-T_2 components. This has been successfully applied with both single and dual IR (DIR) UTE sequences [12–15]. As illustrated in Fig. 12.11, the low bandwidth inversion pulses in these approaches aim to invert long-T_2 component longitudinal magnetization while minimally perturbing short-T_2 component magnetization. TIs are then chosen to null long-T_2 components based on their T_1s (Fig. 12.11).

Conclusion

For short-T_2 imaging with UTE and ZTE MRI pulse sequences, it is important to understand the effects of T_2 relaxation during RF pulses. This becomes significant when T_2 is of the order or shorter than the RF pulse duration. The main intuition presented in this chapter is that the T_2 selectivity is determined by the overlap of the signal component linewidths with the RF pulse frequency profile. The linewidth is inversely proportional to T_2, while the RF profile is determined by the pulse bandwidth and frequency offset. This chapter shows how to ensure adequate excitation of short-T_2 components as well as methods for improving short-T_2 component contrast through the use of T_2 selective excitation, saturation, and inversion RF pulses. The chapter also describes how fat suppression can be integrated and optimized for short- and ultrashort-T_2 imaging.

References

1. Larson PEZ, Gurney PT, Nayak K, Gold GE, Pauly JM, Nishimura DG. Designing long-T_2 suppression pulses for ultrashort echo time imaging. Magn Reson Med. 2006;56(1):94–103.
2. Sussman MS, Pauly JM, Wright GA. Design of practical T_2-selective RF excitation (TELEX) pulses. Magn Reson Med. 1998;40(6):890–9.
3. Pauly JM, Conolly SM, Nishimura DG, Macovski A. Slice-selective excitation for very short T_2 species. Proc Soc Mag Reson Imaging. 1989:28.
4. Nielsen HTC, Gold GE, Olcott EW, Pauly JM, Nishimura DG. Ultra-short echo-time 2D time-of-flight MR angiography using a half-pulse excitation. Magn Reson Med. 1999;41(3):591–9.
5. Johnson EM, Vyas U, Ghanouni P, Pauly KB, Pauly JM. Improved cortical bone specificity in UTE MR imaging. Magn Reson Med. 2017;77(2):684–95.
6. Ma YJ, Jerban S, Jang H, Chang EY, Du J. Fat suppression for ultrashort echo time imaging using a novel soft-hard composite radiofrequency pulse. Magn Reson Med. 2019;82(6):2178–87.
7. Wu Y, Ackerman JL, Chesler DA, Graham L, Wang Y, Glimcher MJ. Density of organic matrix of native mineralized bone measured by water- and fat-suppressed proton projection MRI. Magn Reson Med. 2003;50(1):59–68.
8. Huang C, Ouyang J, Reese TG, Wu Y, El Fakhri G, Ackerman JL. Continuous MR bone density measurement using water- and

fat-suppressed projection imaging (WASPI) for PET attenuation correction in PET-MR. Phys Med Biol. 2015;60(20):N369–81.

9. Du J, Takahashi AM, Bydder M, Chung CB, Bydder GM. Ultrashort TE imaging with off-resonance saturation contrast (UTE-OSC). Magn Reson Med. 2009;62(2):527–31.

10. Larson PEZ, Conolly SM, Pauly JM, Nishimura DG. Using adiabatic inversion pulses for long-T$_2$ suppression in ultrashort echo time (UTE) imaging. Magn Reson Med. 2007;58(5):952–61.

11. Gatehouse PD, Bydder GM. Magnetic resonance imaging of short T2 components in tissue. Clin Radiol. 2003;58(1):1–19.

12. Du J, Takahashi AM, Bae WC, Chung CB, Bydder GM. Dual inversion recovery, ultrashort echo time (DIR UTE) imaging: creating high contrast for short-T(2) species. Magn Reson Med. 2010;63(2):447–55.

13. Ma YJ, Searleman AC, Jang H, Wong J, Chang EY, Corey-Bloom J, Bydder GM, Du J. Whole-brain myelin imaging using 3D double-echo sliding inversion recovery ultrashort echo time (DESIRE UTE) MRI. Radiology. 2019;294(2):362–74.

14. Ma YJ, Jang H, Wei Z, Cai Z, Xue Y, Lee RR, Chang EY, Bydder GM, Corey-Bloom J, Du J. Myelin imaging in human brain using a short repetition time adiabatic inversion recovery prepared ultrashort echo time (STAIR-UTE) MRI sequence in multiple sclerosis. Radiology. 2020;297(2):392–404.

15. Li S, Ma L, Chang EY, Shao H, Chen J, Chung CB, Bydder GM, Du J. Effects of inversion time on inversion recovery prepared ultrashort echo time (IR-UTE) imaging of bound and pore water in cortical bone. NMR Biomed. 2015;28(1):70–8.

Jiang Du, Yajun Ma, Hyungseok Jang, Michael Carl, and Graeme M. Bydder

Introduction

Ultrashort echo time (UTE) sequences allow direct magnetic resonance imaging (MRI) of species in the body with very short-T$_2$s [1–4]. However, many of these "short-T$_2$ species," such as cortical bone and myelin, also have relatively low proton densities, rendering them "invisible" even with the use of UTE sequences if the imaging is not accompanied by suppression of signals from the higher proton density long-T$_2$ species associated with the short-T$_2$ species [4–7]. Residual signals resulting from incomplete suppression of long-T$_2$ species may be higher than those from short-T$_2$ species and significantly compromise short-T$_2$ contrast even when short-T$_2$ signals are successfully detected. These considerations put a high premium on efficient long-T$_2$ signal suppression, which should be insensitive to B_0 and B_1 inhomogeneities. Contrast mechanisms such as UTE dual-echo acquisition followed by echo subtraction [8–10], long-T$_2$ saturation [11], chemical shift-based fat saturation [12, 13], and off-resonance saturation [14] are sensitive to B_1 and/or B_0 inhomogeneities. As a result, these techniques may only provide limited contrast when performing UTE imaging of short-T$_2$ species such as myelin and trabecular bone [6, 15].

Myelin and trabecular bone are examples of two short-T$_2$ species in the body that are challenging for direct imaging. Myelin accounts for only a small fraction of the total UTE signal in white matter of the brain and an even smaller fraction in gray matter [16]. Trabecular bone imaging is complicated by its low proton density and the fact that it is surrounded by marrow fat and water, which have much higher proton densities. In addition, there are strong susceptibility artifacts at the bone marrow interfaces. Thus, low proton density, ultrashort-T$_2$*s, surrounding high signal from long-T$_2$ species, local susceptibility effects, and chemical shift effects make direct imaging of trabecular bone extremely challenging. There is a clear need for targeted, robust long-T$_2$ suppression mechanisms that are insensitive to B_1 and B_0 inhomogeneities to address these problems.

Adiabatic fast passage inversion pulses (Silver-Hoult) are an exceptional group of radiofrequency (RF) pulses that facilitate robust and uniform inversion of the longitudinal magnetizations of long-T$_2$ species [17–20]. Not only are the pulses insensitive to inhomogeneities in the B_1 field when the RF field amplitude is greater than the adiabatic threshold [17], but also single and multiple adiabatic inversion pulses can be combined with other contrast mechanisms such as fat suppression, echo subtraction, off-resonance saturation, and/or a special combination of repetition time (TR) and inversion time (TI) to generate robust long-T$_2$ signal suppression. This group of techniques allows high contrast UTE imaging of both short- and ultrashort-T$_2$ species, including myelin and trabecular bone. The theoretical background and technical details underpinning the use of different adiabatic inversion pulse-based contrast mechanisms are described below.

J. Du (✉)
Department of Radiology, University of California, San Diego, CA, USA

Department of Bioengineering, University of California, San Diego, CA, USA

VA San Diego Healthcare System, San Diego, CA, USA
e-mail: jiangdu@health.ucsd.edu

Y. Ma · H. Jang
Department of Radiology, University of California, San Diego, CA, USA
e-mail: yam013@health.ucsd.edu; h4jang@health.ucsd.edu

M. Carl
GE Healthcare, San Diego, CA, USA
e-mail: Michael.Carl@ge.com

G. M. Bydder
Department of Radiology, University of California, San Diego, CA, USA

Mātai Medical Research Institute, Tairāwhiti, Gisborne, New Zealand
e-mail: gbydder@health.ucsd.edu

Theory

Modern MR scanners allow continuous modulation of RF pulse amplitude and phase. As a result, tissue bulk magnetization can be excited by sweeping the effective B_1 magnetic field B_{eff} either slowly or adiabatically [17]. During this process, the bulk magnetization vector stays approximately collinear with B_{eff}, and excitation is accomplished over a broad range of resonant frequencies with a high degree of tolerance to B_1 field inhomogeneity. Adiabatic passage is performed by sweeping the RF pulse frequency $\omega_1(t)$ through a range of frequencies. Adiabatic rotations must be carried out rapidly relative to T_1 and T_2, a process termed "adiabatic rapid passage," to be useful in contemporary MR applications [17]. One of the most widely used adiabatic pulses has B_{eff} chosen to produce a rotation of 180° and is described as "adiabatic full passage" (AFP) or an "adiabatic inversion pulse." The adiabatic inversion pulse uniformly inverts tissue longitudinal magnetizations when the RF field amplitude is greater than the adiabatic threshold and the pulse duration is much shorter than the relevant tissue T_1 and T_2 values [17]. However, rotated longitudinal magnetization may experience significant transverse relaxation during the long adiabatic inversion process if its T_2 is of the order, or shorter than, the pulse duration τ [18]. Bloch equation simulations show that T_2 relaxation during an adiabatic hyperbolic secant (sech) pulse can forestall complete inversion of the longitudinal magnetization and create T_2-dependent contrast [18]. The T_2 contrast created by an RF pulse is determined by its spectral bandwidth and the tissue T_2. RF pulse-induced, T_2-dependent contrast can be understood conceptually by knowing that it is much easier to excite long-T_2 species such as muscle, white matter, gray matter, and cerebrospinal fluid (CSF) than to excite short-T_2 species such as bone and myelin [18]. While long-T_2 species are excited by the RF pulse, the transverse magnetization of short- and ultrashort-T_2 species leads to rapid decay of the magnetization. Figure 13.1a, b shows a numerical simulation of longitudinal magnetization increasing as a function of inversion pulse bandwidth [18]. The inversion is more effective as bandwidth increases and less effective as T_2 decreases. Theoretically, a long-duration adiabatic inversion pulse with low power and narrow spectral bandwidth would be ideal to invert long-T_2 species and not affect the longitudinal magnetization of short-T_2 species. However, a very narrow spectral bandwidth can increase sensitivity to B_0 field inhomogeneities to an intolerable degree. In practice, a hyperbolic secant Silver-Hoult pulse with a duration of ~8.64 ms and a spectral bandwidth of ~1.5 kHz provides uniform inversion of long-T_2 species, while displaying minimal sensitivity to B_1 and B_0 field inhomogeneities [19–21]. The combination of a long adiabatic inversion pulse of this type with a UTE (IR-UTE) free induction decay (FID) data acquisition can therefore provide selective imaging of short-T_2 species (Fig. 13.1c). There are also a variety of other adiabatic IR-based UTE techniques that have been developed to provide more robust imaging of short-T_2 species, such as those needed for trabecular bone and myelin [15, 21–31].

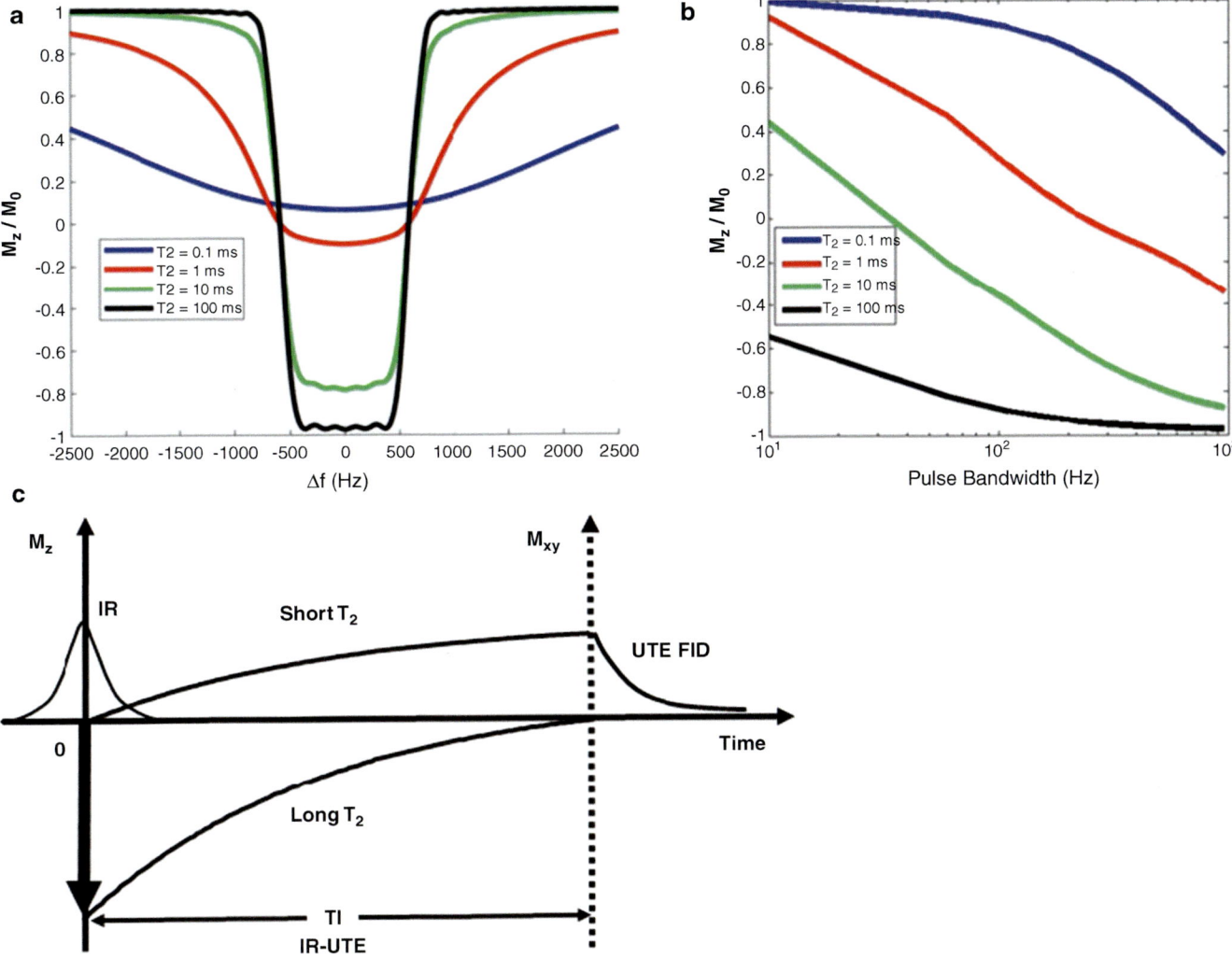

Fig. 13.1 Simulated off-resonance profiles of a Silver-Hoult adiabatic inversion pulse with a duration of 8.64 ms and a bandwidth of ~1 kHz applied at the water resonance frequency for tissue T$_2$s of 0.1 1, 10, and 100 ms (**a**) and simulated longitudinal magnetization after the adiabatic inversion pulses with different bandwidths for various values of T$_2$ (**b**). As the pulse bandwidth increases, M_z decreases, and the inversion becomes more complete (**b**). Longer T$_2$ species are inverted more than shorter T$_2$ species (**a**). This can be used to create short-T$_2$ contrast with the adiabatic inversion pulse prepared UTE (IR-UTE) sequence, where long-T$_2$ species are inverted and nulled using an appropriately chosen inversion time (TI). Short-T$_2$ species are selectively detected by the UTE data acquisition (**c**)

Single Adiabatic Inversion Recovery UTE (IR-UTE)

With the single adiabatic inversion recovery UTE (IR-UTE) contrast mechanism (Fig. 13.2a), a single adiabatic inversion pulse is used to invert the longitudinal magnetizations of long-T$_2$ water (e.g., muscle) and long-T$_2$ fat [1, 20]. The duration of the adiabatic inversion pulse is set to be much longer than the duration of tissue ultrashort-T$_2$s; as a result, the longitudinal magnetizations of long-T$_2$ water and long-T$_2$ fat are fully inverted, while those of ultrashort-T$_2$ species are not inverted but are largely saturated during the long adia-

batic inversion process [20]. The UTE data acquisition starts at values of TI and TR designed to allow the inverted long-T$_2$ magnetizations to approach the null points as closely as possible, leading to selective imaging of ultrashort-T$_2$ species. Because the adiabatic inversion pulse with a relatively broad spectral bandwidth is insensitive to B_1 and B_0 inhomogeneities, the IR-UTE technique provides uniform inversion of long-T$_2$ magnetizations when the pulse amplitude is above the adiabatic threshold, making the IR-UTE sequence a robust mechanism for high-resolution and high contrast imaging of ultrashort-T$_2$ species such as cortical bone [7]. Figure 13.2b, c shows representative clinical fast spin echo

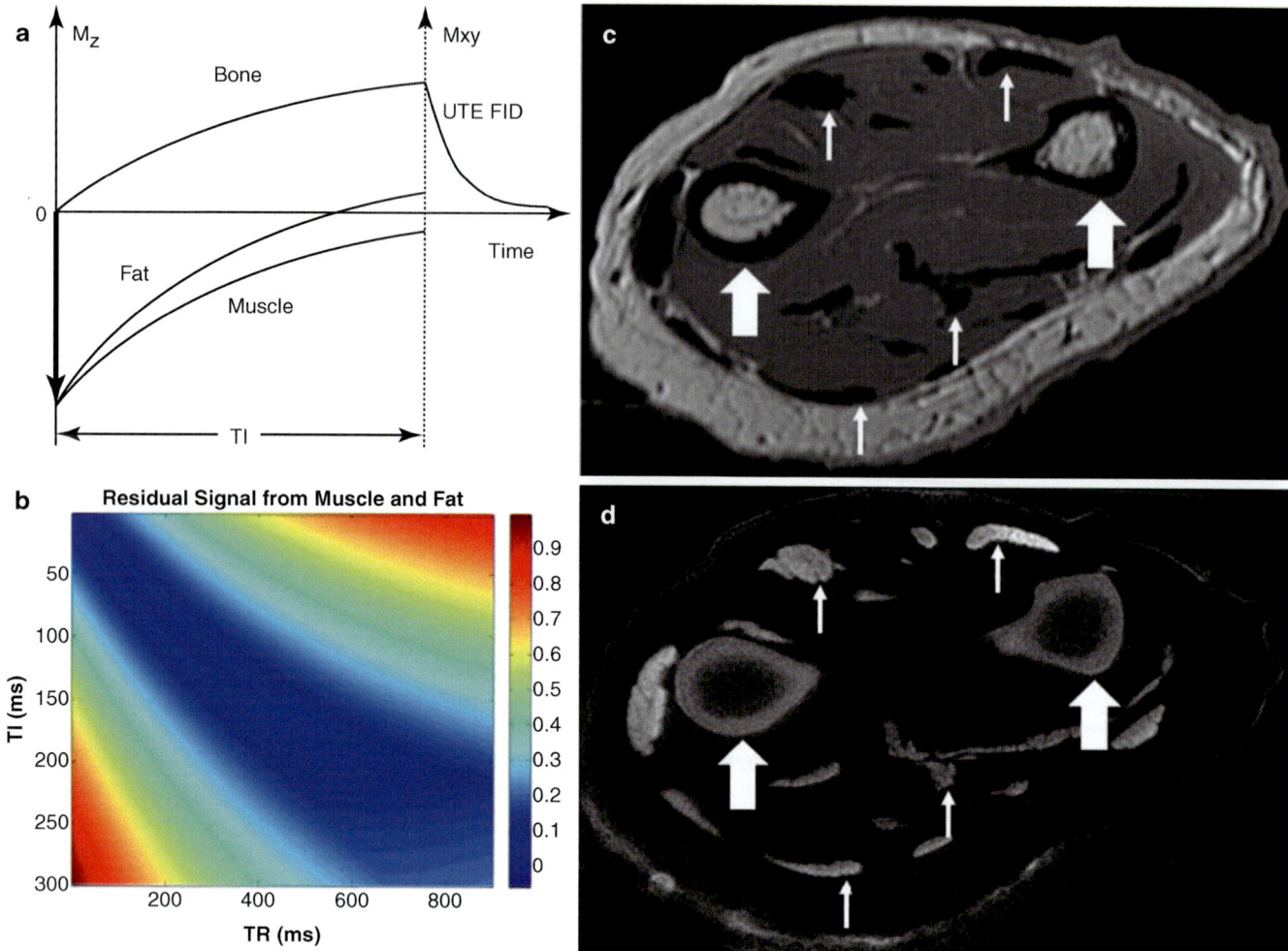

Fig. 13.2 The IR-UTE sequence employs a long adiabatic inversion pulse to invert the longitudinal magnetizations of long-T_2 species (e.g., muscle and fat), and this is followed by UTE acquisition with TI and TR adjusted so that the inverted long-T_2 magnetizations reach their null points as closely as possible (**a**). The longitudinal magnetizations of short-T_2 species (e.g., bone) are not inverted but are largely saturated and recover during TI after which they are selectively imaged by the UTE data acquisition. Simulation of the total residual signal from muscle and fat as a function of TI and TR shows that well-selected combinations of TR and TI can efficiently suppress signals from long-T_2 muscle and long-T_2 fat (**b**). Conventional clinical fast spin echo (FSE) imaging of the forearm shows near-zero signal for cortical bone (thick arrows) as well as tendons and aponeuroses (thin arrows) (**c**). In contrast, the IR-UTE sequence shows high signal and contrast in these tissues (**d**). (Reproduced with permission from Ref. [20])

(FSE) and IR-UTE images of cortical bone in the forearm with excellent image contrast and high signal-to-noise ratio (SNR). This sequence also creates high contrast for other short-T_2 and ultrashort-T_2 species, such as the osteochondral junction, menisci, ligaments, tendons, and aponeuroses [9].

Single Adiabatic Inversion Recovery UTE with Echo Subtraction (IR-UTE-ES)

One limitation of the single IR-UTE technique described above is its sensitivity to T_1 variation. Theoretically, a single adiabatic inversion pulse can invert and null only one par-

ticular T_1 of a specific long-T_2 species by use of an optimized TI. The longitudinal magnetizations of long-T_2 species with different T_1s will not reach the null point simultaneously although some compensation for this is possible by judicious choice of TR. After the UTE FID data acquisition, short- and ultrashort-T_2 signals decay quickly to noise or near-noise levels. A dual-echo acquisition followed by echo subtraction can be used to suppress residual long-T_2 signals further and thereby improve short-T_2 contrast. Single adiabatic inversion recovery UTE imaging with echo subtraction (IR-UTE-ES) is shown in Fig. 13.3a. This technique can create very high contrast imaging of short-T_2 species such as myelin in the white matter of the brain [6]. In this example, the adiabatic

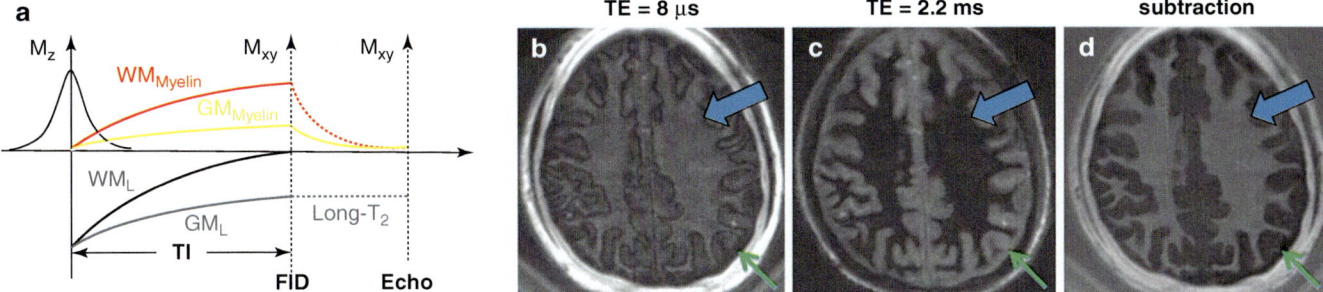

Fig. 13.3 The contrast mechanism for IR-UTE-ES imaging of myelin in white matter (WM$_{myelin}$) (**a**). The UTE data acquisition starts at a TI which is adjusted to null long-T₂ white matter (WM$_L$). At this TI, the longitudinal magnetization of the long-T₂ gray matter (GM$_L$) is negative due to its longer T₁. The adiabatic inversion pulse largely saturates the excited myelin magnetization because its T₂ is much shorter than the duration of the adiabatic inversion pulse. At the null point, the UTE FID signal for gray matter includes the positive myelin (GM$_{Myelin}$) and negative GM$_L$, which partially cancel. At the second echo, the gray matter myelin signal decreases to zero, while the GM$_L$ signal remains essentially unchanged. Subtraction of the magnitude of the second echo from the magnitude of the first UTE FID produces high positive contrast for WM$_{myelin}$ but negative contrast for gray matter. This is shown in the brain of a healthy volunteer with a TE = 8 µs (**b**) and 2.2 ms (**c**), as well as the corresponding echo subtraction image, which shows positive signal for white matter myelin (thick arrow) and negative signal for gray matter myelin (thin arrow) (**d**)

inversion pulse inverts the longitudinal magnetizations of long-T₂ white matter (WM$_L$) and gray matter (GM$_L$). In distinction, the longitudinal magnetizations of myelin in white matter (WM$_{myelin}$) and gray matter (GM$_{myelin}$) are saturated due to their ultrashort-T₂s [24–30, 32, 33]. UTE data acquisition starts at the TI necessary for the inverted longitudinal magnetization WM$_L$ to reach its null point. Because gray matter has a much longer T₁ than white matter, its longitudinal magnetization remains negative at the TI, which nulls WM$_L$. During TI, the saturated WM$_{myelin}$ and GM$_{myelin}$ magnetizations recover quickly due to myelin's short T₁ [25]. As a result, the UTE FID acquisition captures signals from WM$_{myelin}$ and GM$_{myelin}$, as well as from GM$_L$ (Fig. 13.3b). The second gradient echo acquires signal mainly from GM$_L$, which only decays slightly during the short time between the FID and the gradient echo. There is near-zero signal from myelin at the second echo due to its fast transverse relaxation (Fig. 13.3c). Subtraction of the second echo image from the first FID image suppresses signals from GM$_L$ and creates high contrast for myelin (Fig. 13.3d). The partial cancellation between positive longitudinal magnetization from GM$_{myelin}$ and negative longitudinal magnetization from GM$_L$ makes the overall signal lower on the UTE FID image than it is on the second echo image [6]. Echo subtraction of the magnitude of these signals, therefore, generates positive signal for myelin in white matter but negative signal for gray matter. This results in high contrast and creates a sharp boundary between myelin in white matter (positive signal) and myelin in gray matter (negative signal) (Fig. 13.3d).

Adiabatic Inversion Recovery Fat Saturation UTE (IR-FS-UTE)

In the adiabatic inversion recovery fat saturation UTE (IR-FS-UTE) contrast mechanism (Fig. 13.4a), an adiabatic inversion preparation is combined with chemical shift-based fat saturation for efficient suppression of long-T₂ water and fat signals [23]. The significant differences in T₁ between long-T₂ water and fat may lead to a strong residual signal with conventional IR-UTE imaging. The use of an adiabatic inversion pulse to suppress the long-T₂ water signal and a fat saturation pulse to suppress the fat signal provides high contrast for short-T₂ species, such as the cartilaginous endplate (CEP) of the spine [34–36]. In 3D IR-FS-UTE imaging of the CEP, a long adiabatic inversion pulse is used to invert the longitudinal magnetizations of long-T₂ components, such as the nucleus pulposus (NP) in the intervertebral disc. This pulse only partially inverts the longitudinal magnetizations of the CEP, which has a short T₂ [36]. Because the TI is not chosen to null fat, the fat signal is only partially suppressed by the adiabatic inversion pulse. Therefore, an additional chemical shift-based fat saturation pulse is applied to suppress the fat signal before the acquisition of UTE data. This leads to improved CEP contrast. After each pair of adiabatic inversion and fat saturation pulses, a series of spokes is acquired to speed up UTE data acquisition. Figure 13.4b–d compares conventional clinical and 3D IR-FS-UTE imaging of the lumbar spine in a patient. The IR-FS-UTE images show a small incipient Schmorl's node on the vertebral body

Fig. 13.4 The contrast mechanism for 3D IR-FS-UTE imaging (**a**) where an adiabatic inversion pulse and chemical shift-based fat saturation are followed by UTE data acquisition to provide high contrast imaging of short-T_2 species such as the cartilaginous endplate (CEP). The initial adiabatic inversion pulse inverts and nulls signal from the nucleus pulposus (NP) in the intervertebral disc. A later chemical shift-based fat saturation pulse is used to suppress the signal from fat. A multispoke 3D UTE acquisition is employed and provides high contrast imaging of the CEP. The spine (T11-L5) of a 38-year-old male volunteer is shown using conventional 2D T_2-FSE (**b**), 2D T_1-FSE (**c**), and 3D IR-FS-UTE (**d**) sequences. The 3D IR-FS-UTE sequence (arrow in **d**) shows high contrast for the CEP in comparison with the clinical T_2-FSE and T_1-FSE sequences (arrows in **b** and **c**). The preserved CEP around Schmorl's node in the superior endplate of L2 can only be seen with the 3D IR-FS-UTE sequence (**a–d**) (arrows). (Reproduced with permission from Ref. [36])

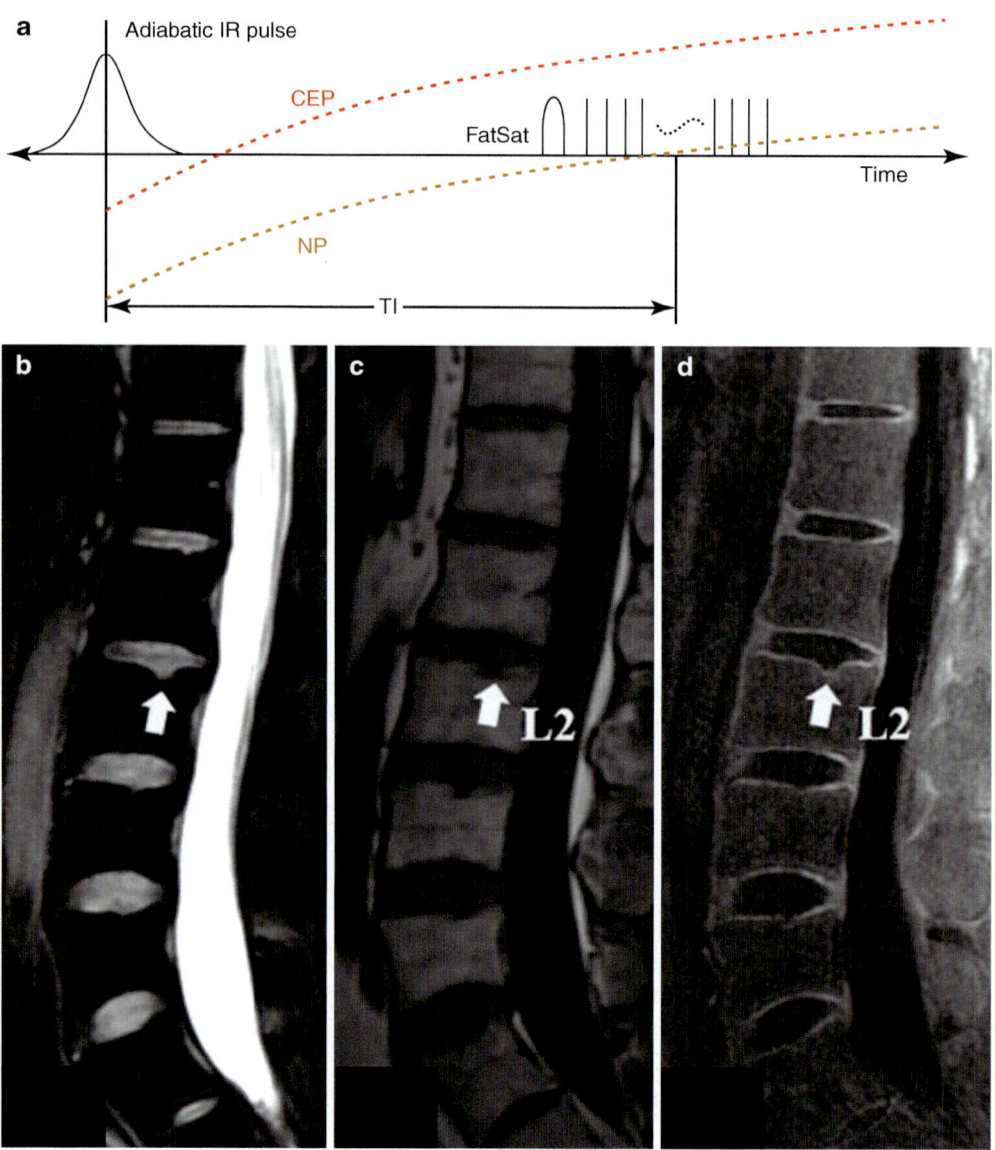

superior endplate with a preserved thin cartilaginous end-plate (arrow in Fig. 13.4d), which is not apparent on the conventional clinical T_1-FSE and T_2-FSE images (Fig. 13.4b, c). This result shows the use of the 3D IR-FS-UTE sequence for high contrast imaging of the CEP and its potential for diagnosing early degenerative changes in the intervertebral disc [36].

The 3D IR-FS-UTE sequence can also be used to depict other short-T_2 species, such as the osteochondral junction (OCJ), menisci, tendons, ligaments, and bone [23]. Furthermore, the IR-FS preparation module can be combined with other UTE-type sequences, such as zero echo time (ZTE), for selective imaging of short-T_2 species [37]. The 3D IR-FS-UTE sequence is insensitive to inhomogeneities in the B_1 and B_0 fields and provides significantly higher

image contrast for the CEP, OCJ, and other short-T_2 species than echo subtraction and long-T_2 saturation techniques [8–11].

Dual Adiabatic Inversion Recovery UTE (Dual-IR-UTE)

With the dual adiabatic inversion recovery UTE (dual-IR-UTE) contrast mechanism (Fig. 13.5a), two long adiabatic inversion pulses are used to invert the longitudinal magnetizations of long-T_2 water and long-T_2 fat, respectively [38, 39]. In distinction, the short-T_2 magnetization is only partly inverted or saturated. Attenuation of short-T_2 signals is reduced by using longer duration pulses with narrower spec-

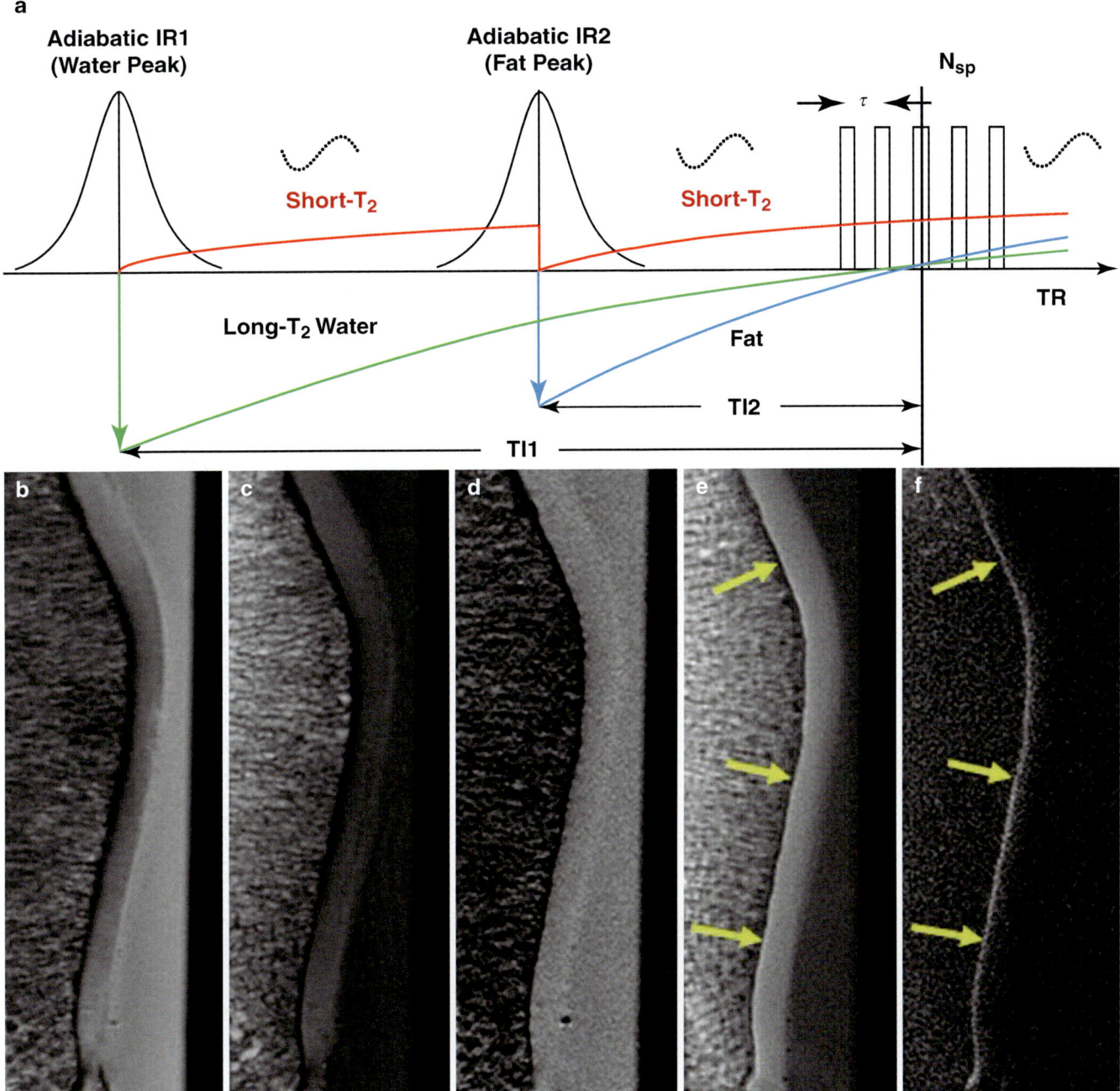

Fig. 13.5 The dual-IR-UTE contrast mechanism (**a**), where two long adiabatic inversion pulses are used to invert and null long-T$_2$ water and long-T$_2$ fat signals, respectively. This is followed by a UTE acquisition to selectively detect signals from short- and ultrashort-T$_2$ species. A cadaveric human patellar sample was imaged with conventional clinical proton density-weighted FSE (PD-FSE) (**b**), T$_1$-FSE (**c**), GRE (**d**), UTE (**e**), and dual-IR-UTE (**f**) sequences. The deep radial and calcified layers of cartilage are only visible with the UTE-type sequences (**e, f**). The dual-IR-UTE sequence selectively suppresses signals from the long-T$_2$ superficial layers of cartilage and bone marrow fat and shows a linear, well defined high signal region (arrows) (**f**). (Reproduced with permission from Ref. [39])

tral bandwidths (e.g., <440 Hz at 3 T) [38]. The first adiabatic inversion pulse is centered on the water peak to selectively invert long-T$_2$ water magnetization (e.g., muscle), and the second adiabatic inversion pulse is centered on the fat peak to invert fat longitudinal magnetization. The water longitudinal magnetization is inverted first because it has a longer T$_1$ and therefore requires a longer time delay TI$_1$ to reach the null point. Long-T$_2$ fat has a much shorter T$_1$ and requires a shorter time delay TI$_2$ to reach the null point. A proper combination of TI$_1$, TI$_2$, and TR allows robust and efficient suppression of long-T$_2$ water and long-T$_2$ fat signals. Figure 13.5b–f shows conventional FSE and gradient echo (GRE) imaging, UTE imaging, and dual-IR-UTE imaging of a cadaveric human patellar sample [39]. The deep radial and calcified layers of articular cartilage are "invisible" with conventional clinical sequences and visible, albeit with limited contrast when imaged with basic UTE or UTE with fat saturation. In contrast, the dual-IR-UTE sequence demonstrates excellent contrast for the thin deep radial and calcified layers of articular cartilage (arrows).

Double Adiabatic Inversion Recovery UTE (Double-IR-UTE)

With contrast mechanism for double adiabatic inversion recovery UTE sequence (double-IR-UTE) (Fig. 13.6a), two identical adiabatic inversion pulses (duration of ~6 ms) with

the same center frequency are used to sequentially invert the longitudinal magnetizations of long-T_2 species [22]. Multiple k-space spokes (N_{sp}) with an equal time interval τ are acquired after the double IR preparation to increase the acquisition efficiency. In each TR period, the two adiabatic inversion pulses are applied with specific inversion times TI_1, defined as the time between the centers of the two adiabatic inversion pulses, and TI_2, defined as the time from the center of the second adiabatic inversion pulse to the center spoke of the multispoke acquisition. The multispoke acquisition scheme produces robust long-T_2 suppression by timing the center spoke at the null point. Long-T_2 transverse magnetizations before the null point are of opposite polarity to those acquired after the nulling point, leading to cancellation in the regridding process during image reconstruction and, therefore, long-T_2 signal suppression. The short-T_2 magnetizations are

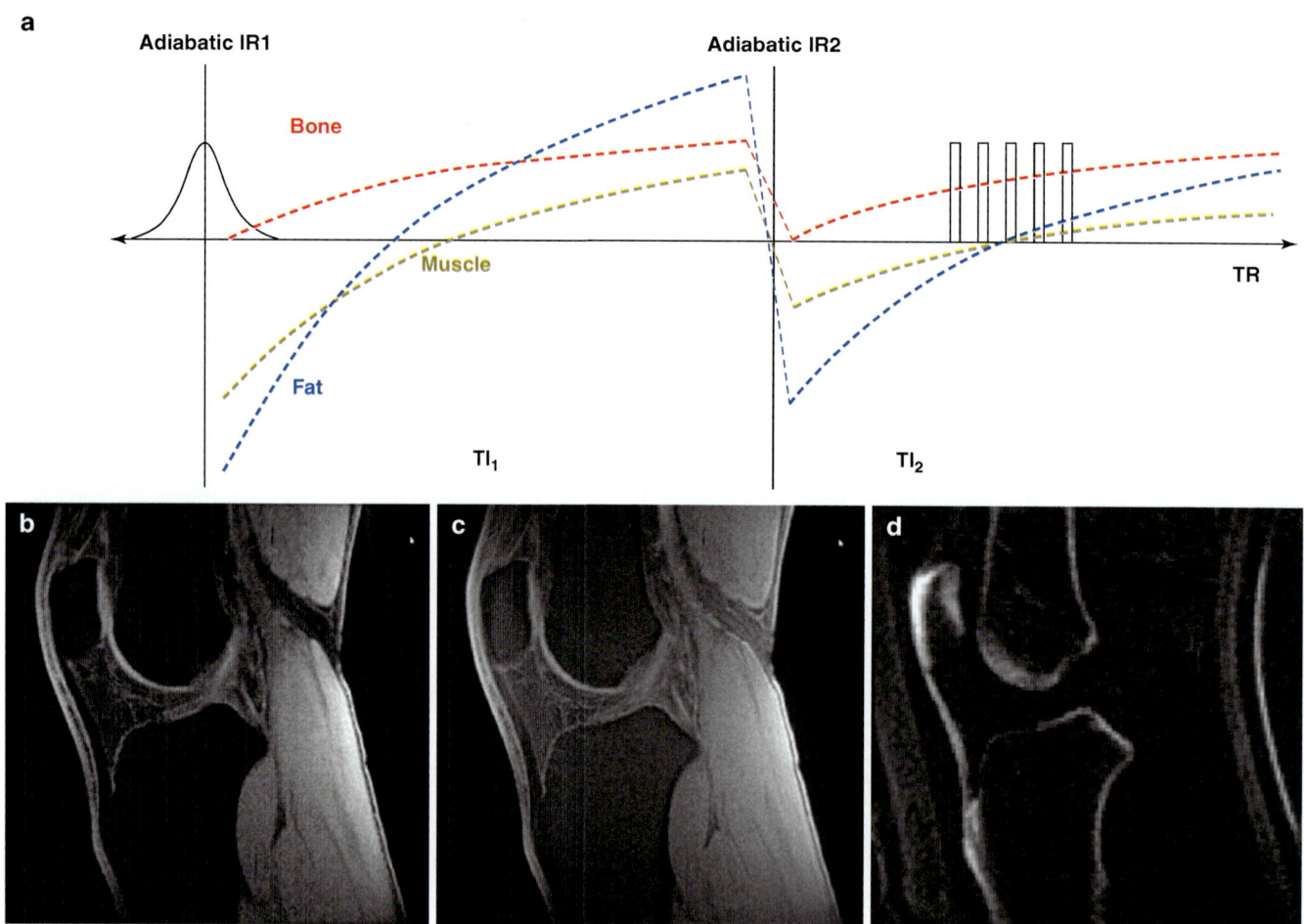

Fig. 13.6 The double-IR-UTE contrast mechanism (**a**), in which two identical adiabatic inversion pulses are used for simultaneous suppression of two long-T_2 species with different T_1s, such as muscle and fat. This is followed by 3D UTE data acquisition to produce high-contrast imaging of short- and ultrashort-T_2 species. To demonstrate its efficacy, the knee joint of a 31-year-old male volunteer was subject to clinical GRE (**b**), fat-saturated UTE (**c**), and double-IR-UTE (**d**) imaging. The GRE sequence shows a signal void for the patellar tendon and cortical bone (**b**). The fat-saturated UTE sequence shows low signal from cortical bone and the patellar tendon (**c**). The double-IR-UTE sequence shows simultaneous suppression of muscle and marrow fat and provides high signal imaging of the patellar tendon and cortical bone (**d**). (Reproduced with permission from Ref. [22])

not inverted but saturated mainly by the two adiabatic inversion pulses. They recover to produce positive longitudinal magnetization after the second TI_2, and are subsequently detected by UTE data acquisition. In this technique, species with a broad range of T_1s, such as fat and muscle, can be nulled simultaneously using specific TIs. The double-IR-UTE sequence is insensitive to inhomogeneities in the B_1 and B_0 fields. Figure 13.6b–d shows conventional clinical, UTE, and double-IR-UTE imaging of the knee joint in a healthy volunteer. The clinical fat-saturated GRE sequence provides high-signal, high-contrast imaging of long-T_2 species, such as femoral and tibial cartilage and muscle, but little or no signal from the patellar tendon and cortical bone. The conventional fat-saturated 3D UTE sequence shows similar

results, with little signal from the patellar tendon and cortical bone. The 3D double-IR-UTE sequence shows high signal from short- and ultrashort-T_2 species, such as the patellar tendon and cortical bone, with excellent suppression of muscle and marrow fat signals [22].

Double Echo Sliding Inversion Recovery UTE (DESIRE-UTE)

With the double echo sliding inversion recovery UTE (DESIRE-UTE) contrast mechanism (Fig. 13.7), a single adiabatic inversion recovery pulse is used to invert the longitudinal magnetizations of long-T_2 species while saturating

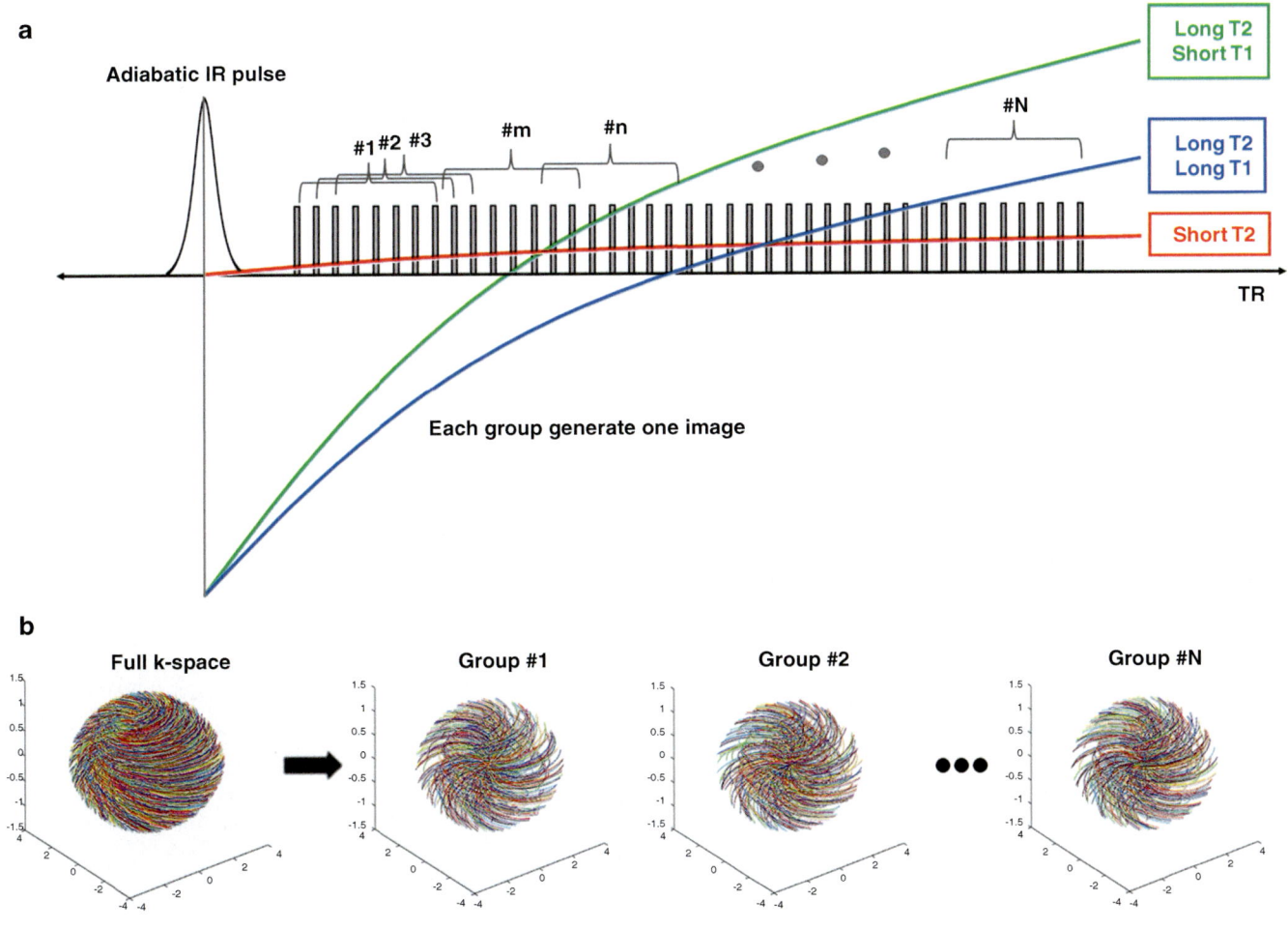

Fig. 13.7 The DESIRE-UTE contrast mechanism (**a**), in which a single adiabatic inversion pulse is followed by a train of 3D dual-echo UTE spokes (*N* spokes). A sliding window reconstruction technique is used to generate a series of images with increasing TIs. Spokes within a window size are used to create a single image. The window starts at the beginning and slides forward one spoke each time to generate a new image. The spokes are randomly ordered for data sampling to ensure that each group of spokes is uniformly distributed in *k*-space (**b**). (Reproduced with permission from Ref. [28])

the longitudinal magnetization of short- and ultrashort-T_2 species [28]. The long-T_2 species may have very different T_1s. For example, WM_L and GM_L have very different T_1s of ~1000 ms and ~1800 ms, respectively, at 3 T [40]. After an adiabatic inversion pulse, fat recovers much faster than WM_L, and WM_L recovers more quickly than GM_L. A wide range of TIs is needed to provide the optimal nulling times for all species with their different T_1s and so produce comprehensive signal nulling. This is a significant technical challenge. The DESIRE-UTE technique overcomes the problem by using a series of 3D dual-echo UTE acquisitions (e.g., the total number of spokes N_{sp}) following each adiabatic inversion pulse [28]. By sequentially acquiring a train of continuous image spokes (up to 71 or more), a wide range of TIs is covered, including all potential nulling points for long-T_2 species in health and disease corresponding to a wide range of T_1s. Random gradient encoding is employed to ensure that any arbitrary number of spokes uniformly covers 3D k-space (Fig. 13.7b). This allows use of a sliding-window image reconstruction technique to generate a series of images corresponding to the continuously increasing TIs (Fig. 13.7a). The window size (N_w) is adjustable, while the sliding step size is kept minimal (i.e., 1) to maximize the number of TIs. During image reconstruction, a window with a size of N_w spokes starts sliding from the shortest TI to the longest TI, generating a total number (N) of groups of images where N equals $N_{sp} - N_w + 1$. This sliding window generates a series of images with N different TIs, including those necessary to cover the optimal nulling points for WM_L, which has a shorter T_1, and for GM_L, which has a longer T_1, as well as the T_1s, which may be encountered in disease. The voxel-based TI_{null} can be determined based on the signal intensity of the second echo, where a minimum signal means the long-T_2 signal is effectively nulled. This way, accurate long-T_2 signal nulling can be achieved regardless of normal variation in T_1, or variation in T_1 due to disease (e.g., edema and iron deposition) [28].

The robustness of the DESIRE-UTE contrast mechanism for long-T_2 signal suppression was tested on a series of water phantoms with different T_1s. Six syringes of water were doped with gadobenate dimeglumine (i.e., MultiHance, Spectrum Chemical Mfg. Corp., Los Angeles, CA) with concentrations of 0.075, 0.125, 0.175, 0.225, 0.275, and 0.325 mM and placed in parallel in a cylindrical container filled with 1% agarose gel. The phantoms had T_1s of 513, 565, 678, 854, 1069, 1484, and 2880 ms, respectively, as measured by a 3D UTE actual flip angle imaging and variable flip angle technique [41, 42]. The DESIRE-UTE technique generated 76 images with different TIs, as shown in Fig. 13.8. The best nulling point for each phantom was found

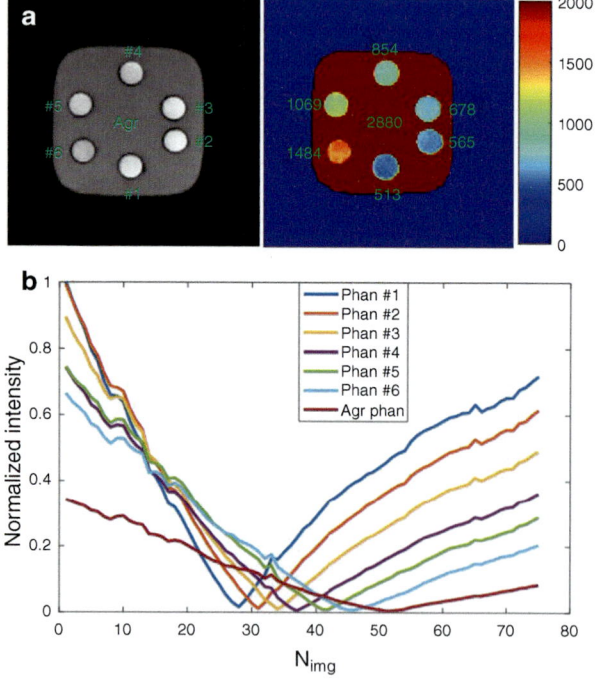

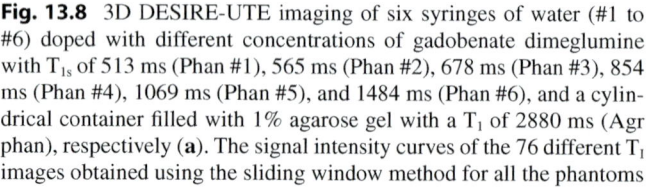

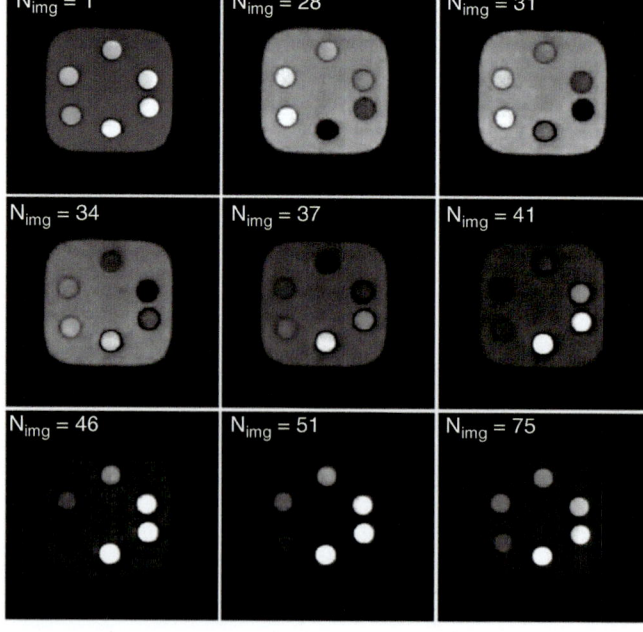

Fig. 13.8 3D DESIRE-UTE imaging of six syringes of water (#1 to #6) doped with different concentrations of gadobenate dimeglumine with T_1s of 513 ms (Phan #1), 565 ms (Phan #2), 678 ms (Phan #3), 854 ms (Phan #4), 1069 ms (Phan #5), and 1484 ms (Phan #6), and a cylindrical container filled with 1% agarose gel with a T_1 of 2880 ms (Agr phan), respectively (**a**). The signal intensity curves of the 76 different T_1 images obtained using the sliding window method for all the phantoms are shown in (**b**). DESIRE-UTE images reconstructed at the best nulling point are shown for each phantom (**c**). The image numbers N_{img} for nulling are $N_{img} = 28$ for phantom #1, $N_{img} = 31$ for phantom #2, $N_{img} = 34$ for phantom #3, $N_{img} = 37$ for phantom #4, $N_{img} = 41$ for phantom #5, $N_{img} = 46$ for phantom #6, and $N_{img} = 51$ for the agarose phantom (**c**). (Reproduced with permission from Ref. [28])

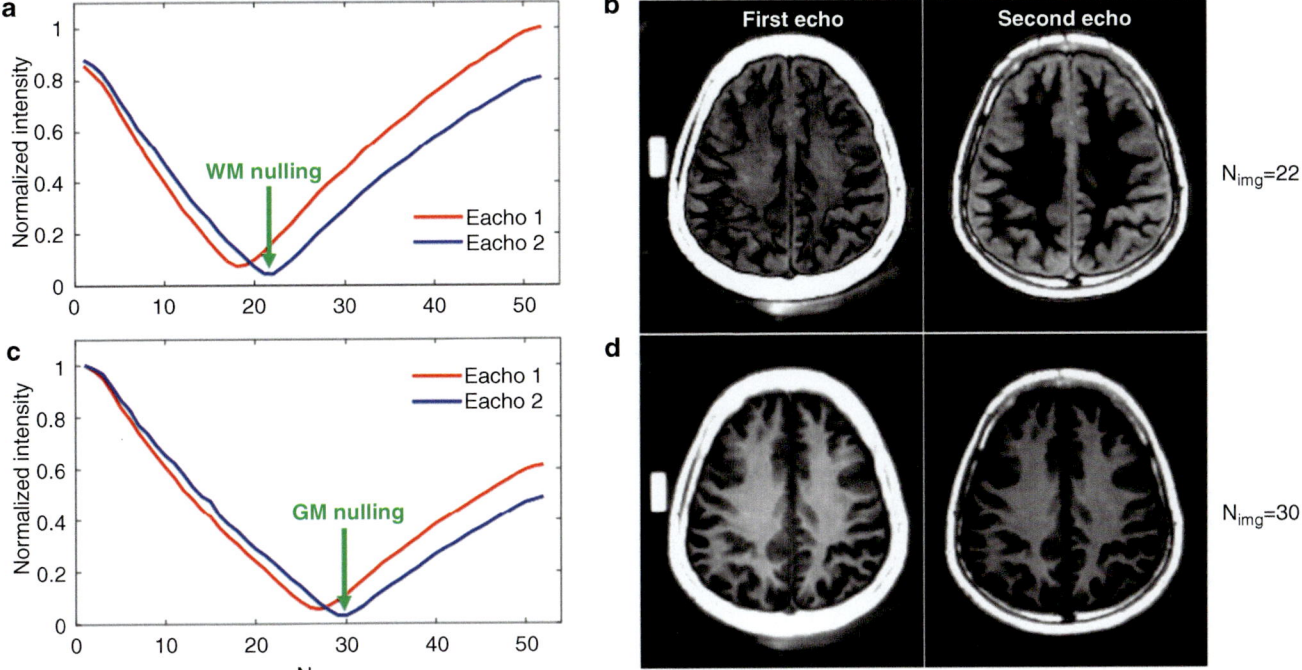

Fig. 13.9 Representative normalized signal intensity curves for the first echo (red curve) and the second echo (green curve) as a function of the reconstructed DESIRE-UTE image numbers (corresponding to different TIs) for an ROI in white matter (**a**) and gray matter (**c**) in a 49-year-old male volunteer measured from 52 sliding images. The long-T_2 white matter signal is nulled on the 22nd image (N_{img} = 22) where myelin shows a high signal in the first echo but pure noise on the second echo (**b**). The long-T_2 gray matter signal is nulled at the 30th image (N_{img} = 30) (**d**). The higher image number is due to the longer T_1 of gray matter

by choosing the TI with the lowest second echo signal intensity based on the signal intensity versus the TI curve for each phantom (Fig. 13.8b). This shows longer TI_{null} values for phantoms with longer T_1s. The DESIRE-UTE data can generate images with near perfect nulling of each phantom despite their very different T_1s.

The DESIRE-UTE sequence can generate whole-brain myelin maps of both white and gray matter with minimal water signal contamination. Figure 13.9 shows DESIRE-UTE imaging of the brain in a healthy volunteer. Representative normalized second echo signal intensity curves for a small ROI drawn in white and gray matter are shown to explain how the optimal nulling times are determined. Subtraction of the second echo from the first UTE FID image can be used to produce optimal long-T_2 signal suppression. A voxel-based optimal TI can be constructed, providing robust long-T_2 signal suppression and therefore selective mapping of myelin in the whole brain.

Short TR Adiabatic Inversion Recovery UTE (STAIR-UTE)

In the contrast mechanism for short TR adiabatic inversion recovery UTE (STAIR-UTE) (Fig. 13.10a, b) sequence, 3D IR-UTE data are acquired with a short TR, and a high flip angle within specific absorption rate (SAR) limits for clinical imaging [15, 29, 43]. The short TR and TI combination is selected to achieve robust suppression of signal from long-T_2 species with a broad range of T_1 values above a certain minimum value. Multiple spokes are then acquired for efficient volumetric imaging of short-T_2 species such as bone and myelin. The spokes from long-T_2 species acquired before and after the null point (center spoke) have opposite longitudinal magnetizations leading to signal cancellation and additional suppression of long-T_2 signal.

The efficiency of this signal suppression was demonstrated through numerical simulation of STAIR imaging with different TRs of 50, 100, 150, 200, 250, 500, and 800 ms, respectively. The simulated T_1s of the long-T_2 components ranged from 20 to 2500 ms, which was a broad enough selection to cover T_1s for typical long-T_2 species such as fat, muscle, white matter, and gray matter. The optimal TIs for signal suppression were determined by minimizing the average signals from long-T_2 water components with T_1s ranging from 250 to 1500 ms [29]. Contrast-to-noise (CNR) efficiency, defined by signal intensity difference between short- and long-T_2 components normalized by TR, was used to evaluate the contrast efficiency of the STAIR-UTE sequence with different TRs. The mean CNR efficiency is calculated by averaging the CNR efficiency for T_1s between 300 and 1500 ms. For simplicity, the short-T_2 com-

Fig. 13.10 Diagram of the contrast mechanisms in IR-UTE imaging with a longer TR (**a**) and a shorter TR (i.e., STAIR-UTE) (**b**). The distributions of TIs for long-T_1 and short-T_1 species approach each other as TR is shortened. Numerical simulation was performed to investigate the effect of TR and flip angle on long-T_2 signal suppression (**c**), CNR efficiency (**d**, **e**, and **f**), and SAR (**g**) in STAIR-UTE imaging of species with different TRs ranging from 50 to 800 ms and a wide range of T_1s ranging from 20 to 2500 ms. The zoomed-in curves (**c**) only display T_1s ranging from 300 to 2000 ms. Higher CNR efficiency is achieved when a shorter TR is used (**d** and **e**). The RF power increases significantly with a shorter TR (**f**). Mean CNR efficiency changes with excitation flip angle (**g**). (Reproduced with permission from Ref. [29])

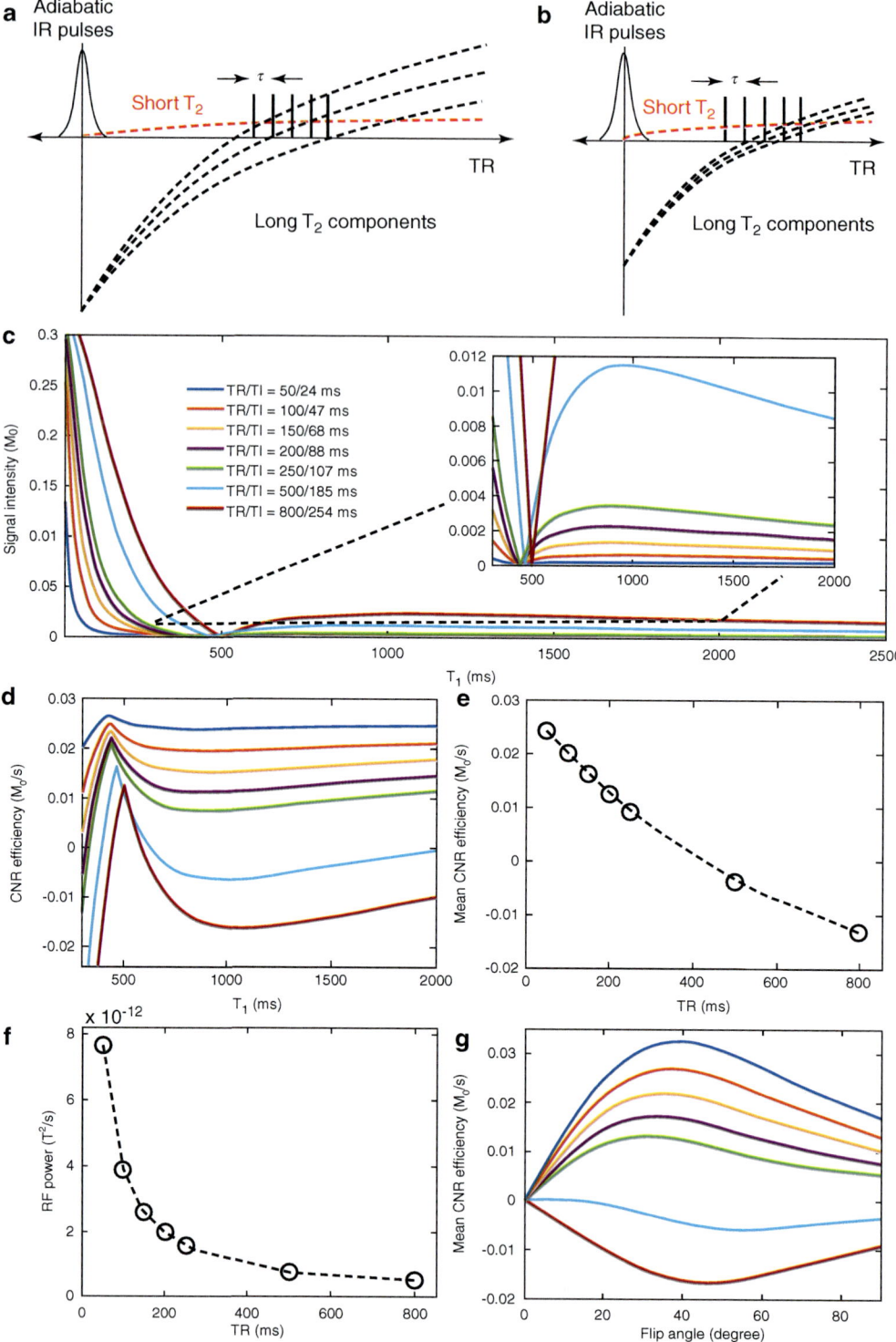

ponent was assumed to have a T_1 of 350 ms and a proton density of 6.5% (100% for long-T_2 components) [25, 44]. RF power was calculated by summing the squares of all the RF waveforms used in the sequence and normalizing this by the TR to assess the SAR of the STAIR-UTE sequence [29]. The CNR efficiency was investigated by varying the excitation flip angles from 0° to 90°.

Figure 13.10c–g shows the results of this numerical simulation, where a broad range of signals with different T_1s can be effectively suppressed when a TR of less than 250 ms is used. Improved long-T_2 signal suppression is achieved with shorter TRs. The simulated signal intensity takes the form of an asymmetric notch T_1 tissue property filter when using a linear X-axis [45]. Higher CNR efficiency over a broad range

Fig. 13.11 STAIR-UTE imaging of nine water phantoms doped with 0.0055, 0.01, 0.015, 0.0195, 0.0265, 0.0375, 0.085, 0.18, and 1.4828 g/L MnCl$_2$·4H$_2$O, with the corresponding T$_1$s of 2012, 1520, 1195, 1002, 801, 609, 299, 148, and 18 ms, respectively (**a**). The STAIR-UTE data were acquired with seven different TR/TI combinations of 50/24, 100/47, 150/68, 200/88, 250/107, 500/185, and 800/254 ms, respectively. The corresponding signal intensity vs. T$_1$ curves demonstrates that a shorter TR/TI combination is more efficient in suppressing long-T$_2$ signals with a broad range of T$_1$s than longer TR/TI combinations (**b**). (Reproduced with permission from Ref. [29])

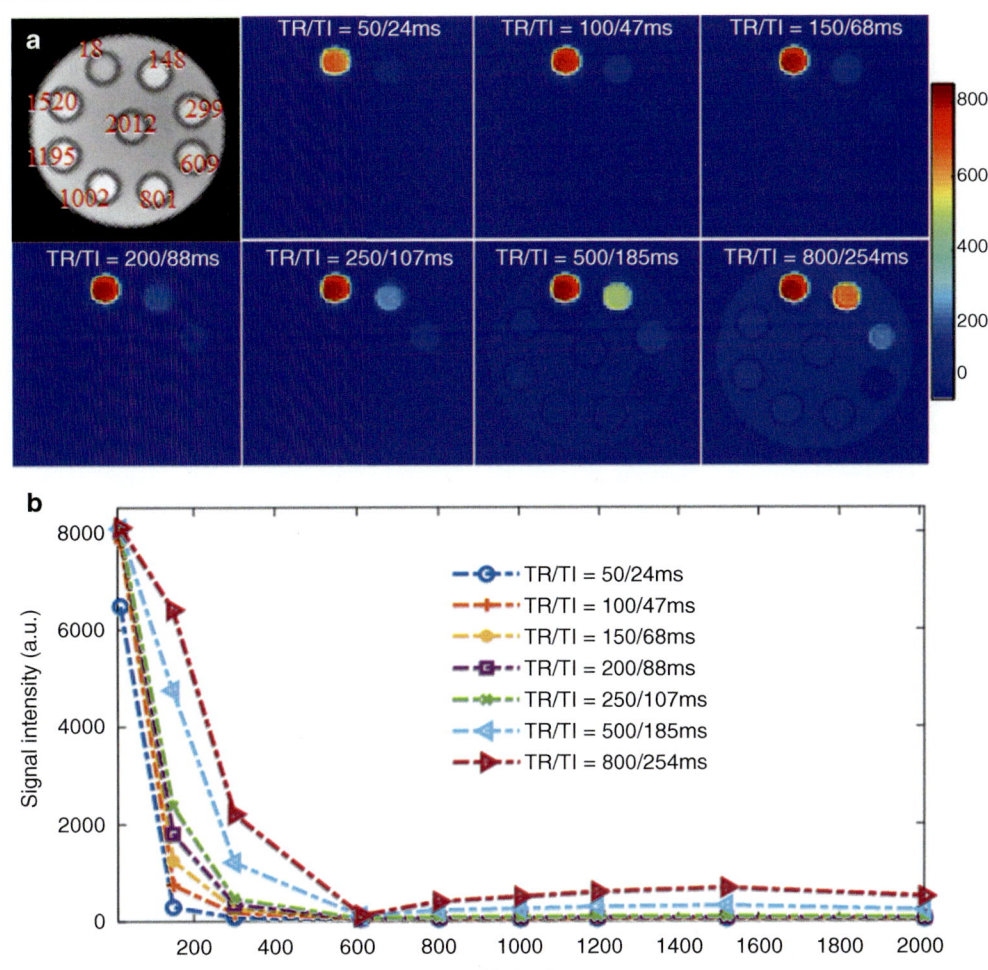

of T$_1$s (i.e., from 300 to 1500 ms) can be achieved when shorter TRs are used (Fig. 13.10c). However, RF power is substantially increased when shorter TRs are used (Fig. 13.10e). Mean CNR efficiency is also influenced by the excitation flip angle (Fig. 13.10f), with higher CNR efficiency achieved when using flip angles between 20° and 40° and a TR less than 250 ms. These numerical simulation results suggest that selective imaging of short-T$_2$ species can be achieved with 3D STAIR-UTE imaging using a TR of less than 150 ms. Even more efficient long-T$_2$ suppression can be achieved when TR is further decreased [29].

The STAIR-UTE sequence was used on a series of water phantoms with different T$_1$s to demonstrate its efficiency for long-T$_2$ suppression. The phantoms consisted of nine syringes of water doped with varying concentrations of MnCl$_2$·4H$_2$O (0.0055, 0.01, 0.015, 0.0195, 0.0265, 0.0375, 0.085, 0.18, and 1.4828 g/L), with T$_1$ values of 2012, 1520, 1195, 1002, 801, 609, 299, 148, and 18 ms, respectively. The syringes were placed in parallel in a cylindrical container filled with 1% agarose and then scanned using the 3D STAIR-UTE sequence with a series of TRs (50, 100, 150, 200, 250, 500, and 800 ms), and optimal TIs numerically

determined by minimizing the average signal from long-T$_2$ components with T$_1$ values ranging from 250 to 1500 ms. Figure 13.11 shows STAIR-UTE images in which signals in phantoms with T$_1$s greater than 299 ms are almost completely suppressed when TR is less than 250 ms. Signal intensities for all phantoms with different TRs are shown in Fig. 13.11b, demonstrating that improved long-T$_2$ signal suppression can be achieved with a shorter TR [29].

The clinical feasibility of the STAIR-UTE sequence was demonstrated by applying it to the brain of an MS patient, the hip of a healthy volunteer, and the lumbar spine of a healthy volunteer, as shown in Fig. 13.12. As can be seen, the clinical sequences only depict signals from long-T$_2$ species such as muscle, spinal cord, disc, and marrow fat (a, c, e). In contrast, the 3D STAIR-UTE sequence shows high contrast imaging of myelin in the brain (b), as well as cortical and trabecular bone (d, f), with excellent suppression of long-T$_2$ signals. Myelin loss in MS lesions was detected with excellent contrast using 3D STAIR-UTE imaging (b) [29].

Numerical simulation and phantom studies demonstrate that shorter TRs provide more effective long-T$_2$ signal suppression than longer TRs. In distinction, a higher flip angle

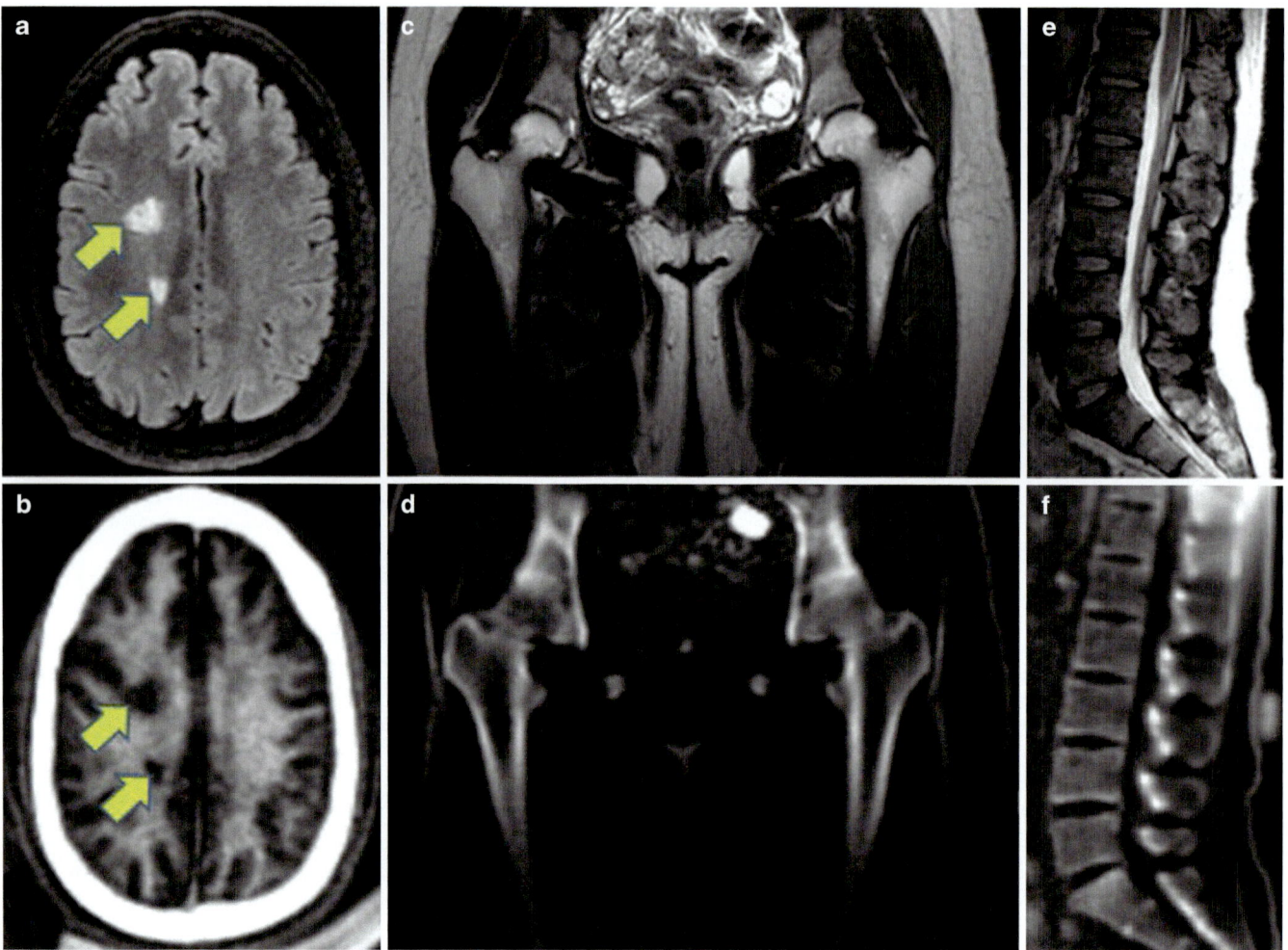

Fig. 13.12 Clinical and STAIR-UTE sequences in the brain of an MS patient (**a, b**), the hip of a volunteer (**c, d**), and the lumbar spine of a volunteer (**e, f**), respectively. Myelin loss in MS lesions is well depicted on the STAIR-UTE image (arrows) (**b**). Cortical bone and trabecular bone (**d, f**) are also depicted with excellent contrast using the STAIR-UTE sequence

provides more T_1-weighting, and this can benefit short-T_2 imaging because short-T_2 species typically have shorter T_1s than long-T_2 species [25, 46, 47]. As a result, STAIR-UTE provides more selective volumetric imaging of short-T_2 species when a shorter TR with a higher SAR can be used. The parallel transmission allows higher-power RF pulses with less SAR constraints [48], which is an excellent approach for STAIR-UTE imaging of myelin and other short-T_2 species. Recently, Weiger et al. reported the use of a high-performance gradient insert that provided a maximum gradient strength of 200 mT/m and a slew rate of 600 mT/m/ms, both of which are four to five times stronger than the typical gradient strengths and slew rates available on clinical scanners [49]. The combination of parallel transmission, gradient inserts, and STAIR-UTE imaging is expected to significantly improve the selective imaging of short-T_2 species.

Adiabatic Inversion Recovery UTE (AIR-UTE) and Double Adiabatic Full Passage UTE (DAFP-UTE)

The AIR-UTE and DAFP-UTE contrast mechanisms have been used to respectively image bound water and pore water in cortical bone [31]. In AIR-UTE imaging (Fig. 13.13a), an AFP pulse is added to a conventional UTE sequence, similar to the case with the IR-UTE contrast mechanism. The AFP pulse is used to largely invert and null pore water and to approximately saturate bound water in cortical bone when an appropriate TI is chosen to null pore water longitudinal magnetization. As a result, the final AIR-UTE signal is primarily from bound water. Bound water concentration (C_{bw}) can be estimated by comparing the AIR-UTE signal of cortical bone with a water calibration phantom after correction for relax-

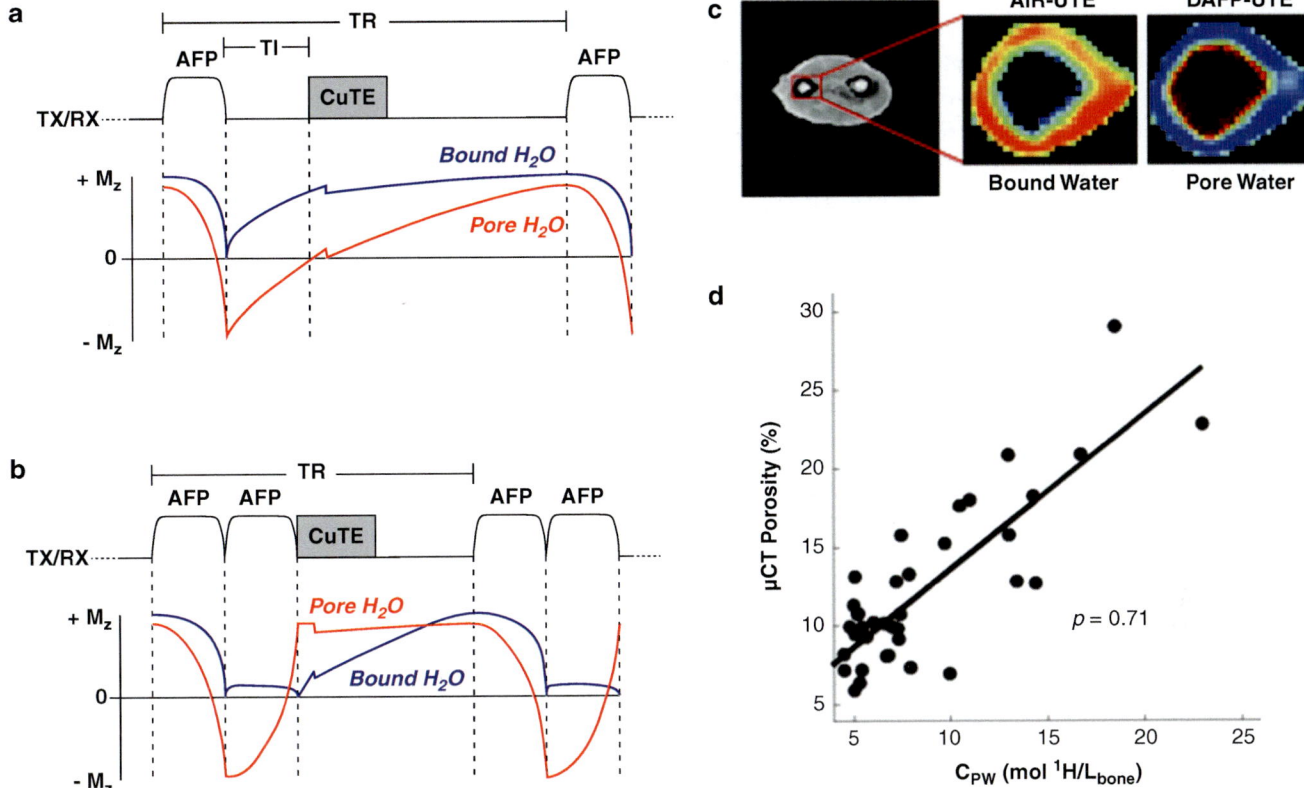

Fig. 13.13 Adiabatic inversion recovery (AIR) scheme. This employs an adiabatic full-passage pulse to saturate pore water and create a predominantly bound water signal which is subsequently detected with a conventional UTE data acquisition (**a**). The double adiabatic full-passage (DAFP) scheme employs two consecutive adiabatic full-passage pulses to saturate bound water longitudinal magnetization at the time of the readout and thus create signal dominated by pore water (**b**). Bound water and pore water maps were derived from AIR-UTE and DAFP-UTE imaging of a forearm specimen (**c**). An excellent linear correlation ($\rho - 0.71$) was observed between DAFP-UTE-measured C_{pw} and µCT-measured cortical porosity in 40 forearm specimens (**d**). TR repetition time, TI inversion time, G_R readout gradient, RF slice or volume excitation). (Reproduced with permission from Refs [31, 50])

ation effects and coil sensitivity. In DAFP-UTE imaging (Fig. 13.13b), a pair of sequential AFP pulses is used with a conventional UTE sequence. The DAFP pulse rotates long-T_2 pore water magnetization 360° while approximately saturating bound water. As a result, after RF excitation, the final DAFP-UTE signal is primarily from pore water. Pore water concentration (C_{pw}) can be estimated by comparing the DAFP-UTE signal of cortical bone with a water calibration phantom after correction for relaxation effects and coil sensitivity.

AIR and DAFP measurements of bound and pore water in cortical bone were validated on 40 fresh human cadaveric forearms (elbow to fingertip, ages 56–97, mean age 80 ± 9.5, 20 males, 20 females) [50]. Dual-energy X-ray absorptiometry (DXA) and MRI measures were first acquired on the intact arms, and then the radii were dissected and cut from the distal third of the bone 7.5 cm proximal to the wrist. After dissection, µCT imaging was performed on the radii with the

bone immersed in a phosphate-buffered saline (PBS) medium at pH 7.4 during the scan. All imaging measurements were performed at the distal third site of the radius. A short-T_2 reference phantom ($CuSO_4$-doped 10% H_2O:90% D_2O) was used to convert intensity into absolute concentration units (mol $^1H/L_{bone}$) [51]. Representative bound water and pore water maps are shown in Fig. 13.13c. The excellent correlation between DAFP-UTE-measured C_{pw} and µCT-measured cortical porosity shows that C_{pw} measurement is an indirect measure of porosity.

Conclusion

A series of adiabatic IR-based contrast mechanisms can be combined with 3D UTE data acquisition to generate high-contrast images of various short-T_2 species. Adiabatic inversion pulses from the hyperbolic secant family are frequently employed for robust long-T_2 signal suppression because of their insensitivity to inhomogeneities in the B_1 field. The performance of adiabatic inversion pulses may be significantly reduced at off-resonance frequencies, but this challenge can be addressed by using nonselective adiabatic inversion pulses with relatively broad spectral bandwidths. IR-based techniques typically use a relatively long TR to allow full recovery of longitudinal magnetization. This may significantly increase the total scan time. Multiple spokes are usually acquired after each adiabatic inversion pulse preparation to reduce scan time.

With the basic IR-UTE sequence, only one specific T_1 magnetization reaches the null point for each TR and TI combination, and this may result in significant residual long-T_2 signals from species with different T_1s [20]. More effective long-T_2 suppression of tissues with different T_1s can be achieved with more advanced adiabatic IR-based techniques, such as IR-UTE-ES [6], IR-FS-UTE [23, 36, 37], dual-IR-UTE [38, 39], double-IR-UTE [22], DESIRE-UTE [28], and STAIR-UTE [15, 29, 43]. DESIRE-UTE allows complete suppression of signals from long-T_2 species with widely different T_1s by selecting the optimal TI for each voxel and thereby providing genuinely voxel-based selective short-T_2 mapping (e.g., myelin mapping) [28]. However, DESIRE-UTE is time inefficient because many of the spokes are acquired at nonoptimal TIs. The STAIR-UTE sequence resolves this problem by acquiring 3D IR-UTE data with a short TR and as high a flip angle as possible within SAR limits, to minimize the long-T_2 signal and maximize the short-T_2 signal [15, 29, 43]. The SNR efficiency, in this case, is expected to be higher than other IR-based contrast mechanisms, although systematic comparison of the various IR-based contrast mechanisms remains to be done. Detailed clinical assessment of the newer techniques in musculoskeletal (e.g., osteoarthritis, osteoporosis) and neurological disease (e.g., MS, Alzheimer's disease, traumatic brain injury, Parkinson's disease) is awaited.

References

1. Gatehouse PD, Bydder GM. Magnetic resonance imaging of short T_2 components in tissue. Clin Radiol. 2003;58(1):1–19.
2. Robson MD, Gatehouse PD, Bydder M, Bydder GM. Magnetic resonance: an introduction to ultrashort TE (UTE) imaging. J Comput Assist Tomogr. 2003;27(6):825–46.
3. Reichert IL, Robson MD, Gatehouse PD, He T, Chappell KE, Holmes J, et al. Magnetic resonance imaging of cortical bone with ultrashort TE pulse sequences. Magn Reson Imaging. 2005;23(5):611–28.
4. Ma Y, Jang H, Jerban S, Chang EY, Chung CB, Bydder GM, et al. Making the invisible visible-ultrashort echo time magnetic resonance imaging: technical developments and applications. Appl Phys Rev. 2022;9(4):041303.
5. Afsahi AM, Ma Y, Jang H, Jerban S, Chung CB, Chang EY, et al. Ultrashort echo time magnetic resonance imaging techniques:

6. met and unmet needs in musculoskeletal imaging. J Magn Reson Imaging. 2022;55(6):1597–612.
6. Ma YJ, Jang H, Chang EY, Hiniker A, Head BP, Lee RR, et al. Ultrashort echo time (UTE) magnetic resonance imaging of myelin: technical developments and challenges. Quant Imaging Med Surg. 2020;10(6):1186–203.
7. Du J, Bydder GM. Qualitative and quantitative ultrashort-TE MRI of cortical bone. NMR Biomed. 2013;26(5):489–506.
8. Rahmer J, Bornert P, Groen J, Bos C. Three-dimensional radial ultrashort echo-time imaging with T_2 adapted sampling. Magn Reson Med. 2006;55(5):1075–82.
9. Du J, Bydder M, Takahashi AM, Carl M, Chung CB, Bydder GM. Short T_2 contrast with three-dimensional ultrashort echo time imaging. Magn Reson Imaging. 2011;29(4):470–82.
10. Kim YJ, Cha JG, Shin YS, Chaudhari AS, Suh YJ, Hwan Yoon S, et al. 3D ultrashort TE MRI for evaluation of cartilaginous endplate of cervical disk in vivo: feasibility and correlation with disk degeneration in T_2-weighted spin-echo sequence. AJR Am J Roentgenol. 2018;210(5):1131–40.
11. Larson PE, Gurney PT, Nayak K, Gold GE, Pauly JM, Nishimura DG. Designing long-T_2 suppression pulses for ultrashort echo time imaging. Magn Reson Med. 2006;56(1):94–103.
12. Ma YJ, Jerban S, Jang H, Chang EY, Du J. Fat suppression for ultrashort echo time imaging using a novel soft-hard composite radiofrequency pulse. Magn Reson Med. 2019;82(6):2178–87.
13. Jang H, Carl M, Ma Y, Jerban S, Guo T, Zhao W, et al. Fat suppression for ultrashort echo time imaging using a single-point Dixon method. NMR Biomed. 2019;32(5):e4069.
14. Du J, Takahashi AM, Bydder M, Chung CB, Bydder GM. Ultrashort TE imaging with off-resonance saturation contrast (UTE-OSC). Magn Reson Med. 2009;62(2):527–31.
15. Ma YJ, Chen Y, Li L, Cai Z, Wei Z, Jerban S, et al. Trabecular bone imaging using a 3D adiabatic inversion recovery prepared ultrashort TE cones sequence at 3T. Magn Reson Med. 2020;83(5):1640–51.
16. Fan SJ, Ma Y, Zhu Y, Searleman A, Szeverenyi NM, Bydder GM, et al. Yet more evidence that myelin protons can be directly imaged with UTE sequences on a clinical 3T scanner: Bicomponent T_2^* analysis of native and deuterated ovine brain specimens. Magn Reson Med. 2018;80(2):538–47.
17. Garwood M, DelaBarre L. The return of the frequency sweep: designing adiabatic pulses for contemporary NMR. J Magn Reson. 2001;153(2):155–77.
18. Larson PE, Conolly SM, Pauly JM, Nishimura DG. Using adiabatic inversion pulses for long-T_2 suppression in ultrashort echo time (UTE) imaging. Magn Reson Med. 2007;58(5):952–61.
19. Carl M, Bydder GM, Du J. UTE imaging with simultaneous water and fat signal suppression using a time-efficient multispoke inversion recovery pulse sequence. Magn Reson Med. 2016;76(2):577–82.
20. Du J, Carl M, Bydder M, Takahashi A, Chung CB, Bydder GM. Qualitative and quantitative ultrashort echo time (UTE) imaging of cortical bone. J Magn Reson. 2010;207(2):304–11.
21. Ma YJ, Jerban S, Jang H, Chang D, Chang EY, Du J. Quantitative ultrashort echo time (UTE) magnetic resonance imaging of bone: an update. Front Endocrinol (Lausanne). 2020;11:567417.
22. Ma YJ, Zhu Y, Lu X, Carl M, Chang EY, Du J. Short T2 imaging using a 3D double adiabatic inversion recovery prepared ultrashort echo time cones (3D DIR-UTE-cones) sequence. Magn Reson Med. 2018;79(5):2555–63.
23. Ma YJ, Jerban S, Carl M, Wan L, Guo T, Jang H, et al. Imaging of the region of the osteochondral junction (OCJ) using a 3D adiabatic inversion recovery prepared ultrashort echo time cones (3D IR-UTE-cones) sequence at 3 T. NMR Biomed. 2019;32(5):e4080.
24. Du J, Ma G, Li S, Carl M, Szeverenyi NM, VandenBerg S, et al. Ultrashort echo time (UTE) magnetic resonance imaging of the

short T$_2$ components in white matter of the brain using a clinical 3T scanner. NeuroImage. 2014;87:32–41.

25. Du J, Sheth V, He Q, Carl M, Chen J, Corey-Bloom J, et al. Measurement of T$_1$ of the ultrashort T$_2$* components in white matter of the brain at 3T. PLoS One. 2014;9(8):e103296.

26. Jang H, Ma Y, Searleman AC, Carl M, Corey-Bloom J, Chang EY, et al. Inversion recovery UTE based volumetric myelin imaging in human brain using interleaved hybrid encoding. Magn Reson Med. 2020;83(3):950–61.

27. Jang H, Wei Z, Wu M, Ma YJ, Chang EY, Corey-Bloom J, et al. Improved volumetric myelin imaging in human brain using 3D dual echo inversion recovery-prepared UTE with complex echo subtraction. Magn Reson Med. 2020;83(4):1168–77.

28. Ma YJ, Searleman AC, Jang H, Wong J, Chang EY, Corey-Bloom J, et al. Whole-brain myelin imaging using 3D double-echo sliding inversion recovery ultrashort echo time (DESIRE UTE) MRI. Radiology. 2020;294(2):362–74.

29. Ma YJ, Jang H, Wei Z, Cai Z, Xue Y, Lee RR, et al. Myelin imaging in human brain using a short repetition time adiabatic inversion recovery prepared ultrashort echo time (STAIR-UTE) MRI sequence in multiple sclerosis. Radiology. 2020;297(2):392–404.

30. Ma YJ, Searleman AC, Jang H, Fan SJ, Wong J, Xue Y, et al. Volumetric imaging of myelin in vivo using 3D inversion recovery-prepared ultrashort echo time cones magnetic resonance imaging. NMR Biomed. 2020;33(10):e4326.

31. Horch RA, Gochberg DF, Nyman JS, Does MD. Clinically compatible MRI strategies for discriminating bound and pore water in cortical bone. Magn Reson Med. 2012;68(6):1774–84.

32. Horch RA, Gore JC, Does MD. Origins of the ultrashort-T$_2$ 1H NMR signals in myelinated nerve: a direct measure of myelin content? Magn Reson Med. 2011;66(1):24–31.

33. Wilhelm MJ, Ong HH, Wehrli SL, Li C, Tsai PH, Hackney DB, et al. Direct magnetic resonance detection of myelin and prospects for quantitative imaging of myelin density. Proc Natl Acad Sci U S A. 2012;109(24):9605–10.

34. Bae WC, Statum S, Zhang Z, Yamaguchi T, Wolfson T, Gamst AC, et al. Morphology of the cartilaginous endplates in human intervertebral disks with ultrashort echo time MR imaging. Radiology. 2013;266(2):564–74.

35. Fields AJ, Han M, Krug R, Lotz JC. Cartilaginous end plates: quantitative MR imaging with very short echo times-orientation dependence and correlation with biochemical composition. Radiology. 2015;274(2):482–9.

36. Lombardi AF, Wei Z, Wong J, Carl M, Lee RR, Wallace M, et al. High contrast cartilaginous endplate imaging using a 3D adiabatic inversion-recovery-prepared fat-saturated ultrashort echo time (3D IR-FS-UTE) sequence. NMR Biomed. 2021;34(10):e4579.

37. Jang H, Ma Y, Carl M, Lombardi AF, Chang EY, Du J. Feasibility of an inversion recovery-prepared fat-saturated zero echo time sequence for high contrast imaging of the osteochondral junction. Front Endocrinol (Lausanne). 2021;12:777080.

38. Du J, Takahashi AM, Bae WC, Chung CB, Bydder GM. Dual inversion recovery, ultrashort echo time (DIR UTE) imaging: creating high contrast for short-T(2) species. Magn Reson Med. 2010;63(2):447–55.

39. Du J, Carl M, Bae WC, Statum S, Chang EY, Bydder GM, et al. Dual inversion recovery ultrashort echo time (DIR-UTE) imaging and quantification of the zone of calcified cartilage (ZCC). Osteoarthr Cartil. 2013;21(1):77–85.

40. Stanisz GJ, Odrobina EE, Pun J, Escaravage M, Graham SJ, Bronskill MJ, et al. T$_1$, T$_2$ relaxation and magnetization transfer in tissue at 3T. Magn Reson Med. 2005;54(3):507–12.

41. Ma YJ, Lu X, Carl M, Zhu Y, Szeverenyi NM, Bydder GM, et al. Accurate T$_1$ mapping of short T$_2$ tissues using a three-dimensional ultrashort echo time cones actual flip angle imaging-variable repetition time (3D UTE-cones AFI-VTR) method. Magn Reson Med. 2018;80(2):598–608.

42. Ma YJ, Zhao W, Wan L, Guo T, Searleman A, Jang H, et al. Whole knee joint T$_1$ values measured in vivo at 3T by combined 3D ultrashort echo time cones actual flip angle and variable flip angle methods. Magn Reson Med. 2019;81(3):1634–44.

43. Ma YJ, Jang H, Wei Z, Wu M, Chang EY, Corey-Bloom J, et al. Brain ultrashort T$_2$ component imaging using a short TR adiabatic inversion recovery prepared dual-echo ultrashort TE sequence with complex echo subtraction (STAIR-dUTE-ES). J Magn Reson. 2021;323:106898.

44. Boucneau T, Cao P, Tang S, Han M, Xu D, Henry RG, et al. In vivo characterization of brain ultrashort-T$_2$ components. Magn Reson Med. 2018;80(2):726–35.

45. Young IR, Szeverenyi NM, Du J, Bydder GM. Pulse sequences as tissue property filters (TP-filters): a way of understanding the signal, contrast and weighting of magnetic resonance images. Quant Imaging Med Surg. 2020;10(5):1080–120.

46. Chen J, Grogan SP, Shao H, D'Lima D, Bydder GM, Wu Z, et al. Evaluation of bound and pore water in cortical bone using ultrashort-TE MRI. NMR Biomed. 2015;28(12):1754–62.

47. Guo T, Ma Y, Jerban S, Jang H, Zhao W, Chang EY, et al. T$_1$ measurement of bound water in cortical bone using 3D adiabatic inversion recovery ultrashort echo time (3D IR-UTE) cones imaging. Magn Reson Med. 2020;84(2):634–45.

48. Zelinski AC, Angelone LM, Goyal VK, Bonmassar G, Adalsteinsson E, Wald LL. Specific absorption rate studies of the parallel transmission of inner-volume excitations at 7T. J Magn Reson Imaging. 2008;28(4):1005–18.

49. Weiger M, Froidevaux R, Baadsvik EL, Brunner DO, Rosler MB, Pruessmann KP. Advances in MRI of the myelin bilayer. NeuroImage. 2020;217:116888.

50. Manhard MK, Uppuganti S, Granke M, Gochberg DF, Nyman JS, Does MD. MRI-derived bound and pore water concentrations as predictors of fracture resistance. Bone. 2016;87:1–10.

51. Rad HS, Lam SC, Magland JF, Ong H, Li C, Song HK, et al. Quantifying cortical bone water in vivo by three-dimensional ultrashort echo-time MRI. NMR Biomed. 2011;24(7):855–64.

Ultrashort Echo Time Magnetic Resonance Imaging with Water Excitation

Yajun Ma, Saeed Jerban, Hyungseok Jang, Michael Carl, and Jiang Du

Introduction

Fat is commonly found in the musculoskeletal (MSK) system. For example, it is located in the marrow cavity of trabecular bone and accounts for ~70% of adult bone marrow volume [1]. Healthy muscle contains about 1.5% intramyocellular fat, including intramuscular fat between muscle groups and intramuscular fat within a muscle, and this can increase to over 5% in the obese [2]. Accumulation of fat in bone, liver, and muscle is a common feature of aging [3]. Fat shows a high signal with ultrashort echo time (UTE) imaging due to its short T_1, long T_2, and relatively high proton density. The high fat signal can significantly reduce imaging contrast for the tissue components of interest, such as muscle, cartilage, and cortical bone, with T_1-weighted UTE imaging [4].

Furthermore, UTE imaging is generally based on non-Cartesian k-space mapping, where fat produces strong off-resonance artifacts [5]. These artifacts are different from the chemical shift artifacts observed with conventional Cartesian MR imaging, where a spatial shift is observed in the frequency encoding direction due to misregistration of signal from fat and water molecules. UTE sequences employ center-out radial or spiral mapping of k-space, where chemical shift artifact from fat is manifested as spatial blurring due to its ring-shaped point spread function in all directions, leading to strong off-resonance and partial volume effects [5, 6]. The high fat signal also tends to reduce UTE image contrast and produces errors in quantitative UTE imaging [7]. Fat signal suppression is critical for high contrast morphological and accurate quantitative UTE imaging of MSK tissues.

There are several commonly used fat suppression techniques with UTE imaging, including classic chemical shift fat saturation (FatSat), inversion recovery (IR), and water excitation [8]. Unlike FatSat and IR techniques, no extra RF pulse preparation is needed for water excitation, which offers higher scan efficiency. Several comparative studies have demonstrated that water excitation provides better fat suppression than FatSat in terms of signal suppression homogeneity, presence of artifacts, conspicuity of lesions, and overall image quality [9–11]. Water excitation pulses can be combined with three-dimensional (3D) gradient echo sequences for accurate quantitative assessment of thin cartilage layers, including measurement of cartilage volume and thickness [9–11].

Recently, water excitation pulses have been applied to UTE imaging [12–15]. Advantages with water excitation have been found in fat signal suppression and/or water signal preservation in both morphological and quantitative UTE imaging. In this chapter, we describe the mechanisms that have been developed for water excitation pulses and their application in UTE imaging.

Y. Ma (✉) · S. Jerban · H. Jang
Department of Radiology, University of California, San Diego, CA, USA
e-mail: yam013@ucsd.edu; sjerban@health.ucsd.edu; h4jang@health.ucsd.edu

M. Carl
GE Healthcare, San Diego, CA, USA
e-mail: Michael.Carl@ge.com

J. Du
Department of Radiology, University of California, San Diego, CA, USA

Department of Bioengineering, University of California, San Diego, CA, USA

VA San Diego Healthcare System, San Diego, CA, USA
e-mail: jiangdu@health.ucsd.edu

Binomial Water Excitation Pulses

As can be seen in Fig. 14.1, a 1–1 binomial water excitation pulse can be used for signal excitation with a 3D UTE sequence [12]. The 1–1 binomial water excitation pulse includes two identical short rectangular pulses with the same duration T_{RF} but separated by T_{int}. Following signal excitation by the first rectangular pulse, the transverse magnetization of fat precesses with a resonant frequency difference of

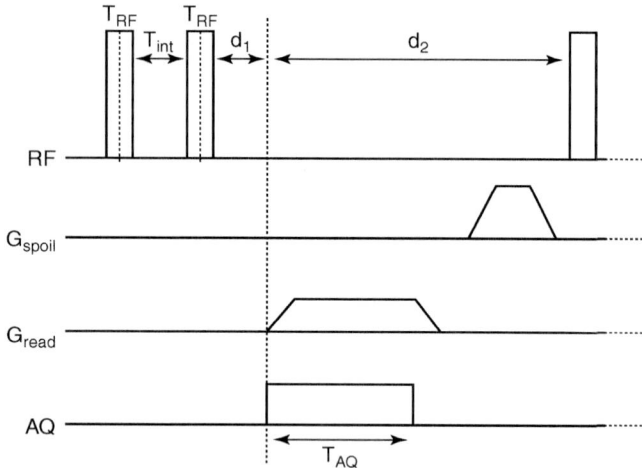

Fig. 14.1 The UTE imaging sequence. This employs a 1–1 binomial pulse for water excitation followed by 3D radial ramp sampling. The 1–1 binomial pulse consists of two identical rectangular pulses (duration = T_{RF}) separated by T_{int}. The effective TE is calculated as $T_{RF} + T_{int}/2 + d_1$, where d_1 is the time interval between the end of the second RF pulse and the beginning of ramp sampling. (Reproduced with permission from Ref. [12])

around −440 Hz relative to that of water at 3 T. After free precessing for a period T_{sat}, where $T_{sat} = T_{int} + T_{RF}$, the off-resonance fat magnetization has the opposite phase (i.e., 180°) to that of on-resonance water magnetization in the transverse plane. Because of this, the second rectangular pulse continues to tip the water magnetization down but tips the fat magnetization back to its original state. Therefore, after the second rectangular pulse, there is theoretically no fat transverse magnetization, while the water transverse magnetization is efficiently created. This is the basic mechanism for water excitation with simultaneous fat suppression. The 1–1 pulse allows use of a shorter TE than other binomial pulses, such as the 1–2–1 pulse. As a result, the 1–1 pulse is the primary choice among the different types of binomial water excitation pulses for high-contrast UTE imaging of MSK tissues [12].

Springer et al. were among the first to study UTE imaging of short-T_2 tissues with water excitation [12]. Numerical simulations were utilized to investigate the water excitation efficacy and fat suppression capability of 1–1 binomial pulses. As can be seen in Fig. 14.2a, the signal yield of the water excitation sequence is generally lower than that of the regular hard pulse excitation sequence when comparable imaging parameters are used. In addition, the Ernst angle is slightly increased with water excitation because the water

excitation efficiency of the water excitation pulse is generally lower than that with a regular hard pulse due to its relatively narrow excitation bandwidth. The water excitation efficiency is significantly reduced when the tissue T_2 is shorter than 2 ms (Fig. 14.2b). This is not surprising since the effective TE of this 1–1 type water excitation sequence is around 0.7 ms, which is about ten times longer than that of a regular UTE sequence. The FatSat module has a broader fat signal suppression band than the water excitation pulse (Fig. 14.2c), which means that the FatSat module used for fat suppression is less sensitive to the B_0 inhomogeneity than the water excitation pulse. On the other hand, the water excitation pulse shows better water signal preservation than the FatSat module, especially for short-T_2 tissues with T_2s of around 1 ms or less (Fig. 14.2d). This is because the FatSat module may directly saturate short-T_2 tissues with broad spectra. Figure 14.3 shows representative 3D UTE water excitation images of a finger and a knee joint. Fat signals are efficiently suppressed, and tendons and ligaments are clearly depicted with positive contrast in these images [12].

Deligianni et al. performed a similar study of water-selective excitation with binomial pulses in UTE imaging of short-T_2 species at 3 T and 7 T [13]. They also utilized the 1–1 binomial pulse for water excitation. This study aimed to compare and explore a series of short water excitation pulse schemes for efficient short-T_2 imaging. Figure 14.4a shows the RF pulse diagrams. The interval between the two rectangular pulses with the 1–1 water excitation pulse is determined by the precessional phase difference between the water and fat transverse magnetizations. Three different phases were considered in this study, namely, 45°, 90°, and 180°. Figure 14.4b shows the simulated signal loss ratio curves between water excitation and hard pulse excitation at 3 T and 7 T, respectively. For all the water excitation pulses, signal loss increases dramatically with decreasing T_2, especially when T_2 is shorter than 2 ms. The signal loss from water excitation is lowest with a 90° phase difference and highest with a 45° phase difference. This means that the 90° phase difference provides a good balance between the effect of increasing TE in reducing signal level and the effect of improving water signal excitation efficiency with the 1–1 binomial pulse. Figure 14.5 shows UTE water excitation images of a knee joint. The water excitation pulses with phase differences suppress fat signal effectively. Consistent with the simulation results in Fig. 14.4b, the water excitation pulse with a 90° phase difference performs best for water signal excitation and fat signal suppression.

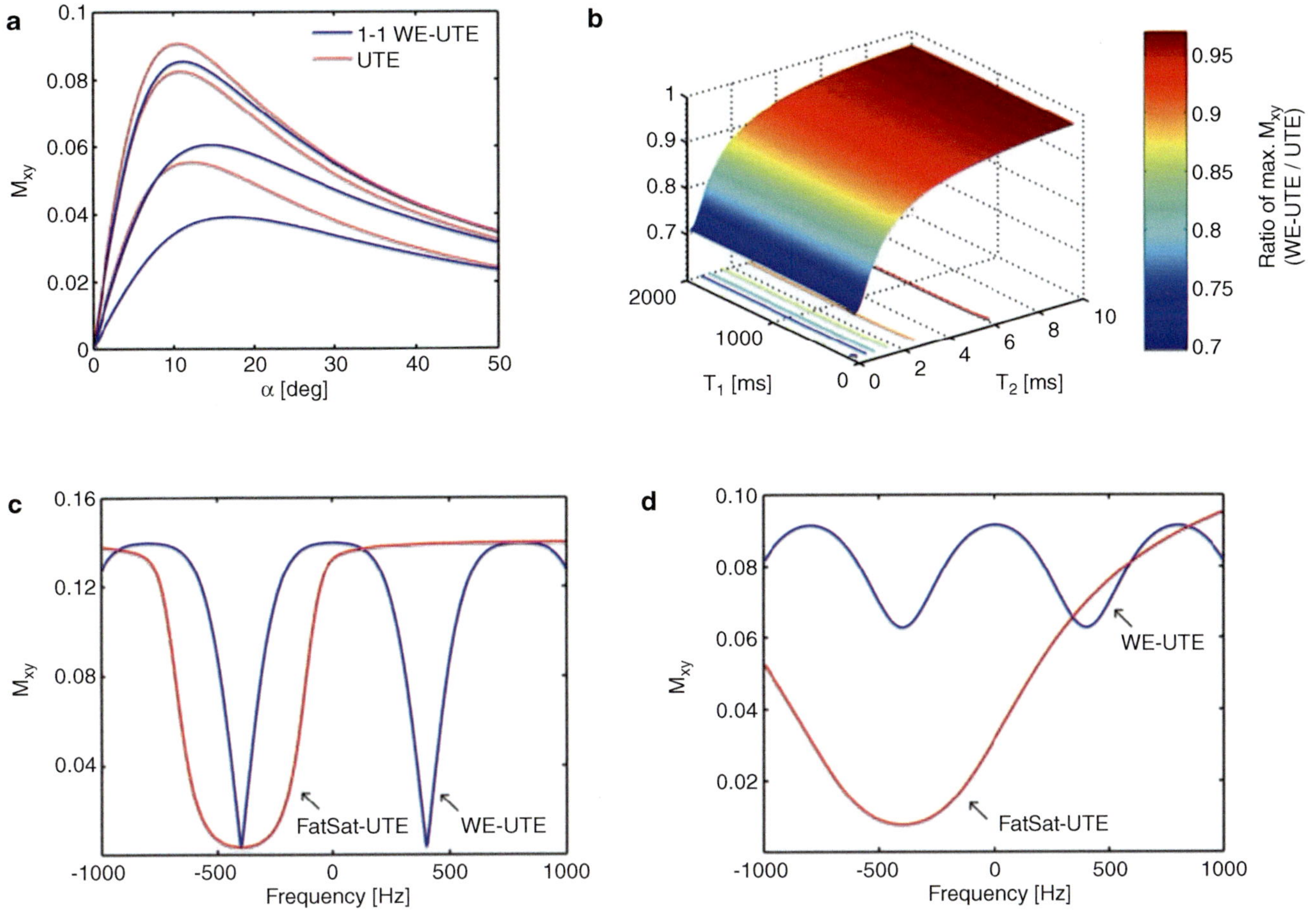

Fig. 14.2 Numerical simulations of water excitation efficiency and fat suppression capability of the 1–1 binomial pulse with TR = 10 ms; T_{RF} = 0.1 ms; d_1 = 0.02 ms; T_1 = 500 ms. The UTE with 1–1 water excitation (1–1 WE-UTE) sequence (blue line) has a lower signal yield than the regular UTE sequence (red line) for three different transverse relaxation times of 0.5, 2, and 10 ms (from lower to upper), respectively (**a**). The ratio of maximal achievable signal yield of WE-UTE and regular UTE sequences over a broad range of T_1 and T_2 values suggests that the signal excitation efficiency of the 1–1 binomial pulse is significantly reduced when the tissue T_2 is shorter than 2 ms (**b**). The FatSat module has a broader fat signal suppression band than the water excitation pulse (**c**), but it also attenuates more water signal from short-T_2 tissues (e.g., with T_2 = 1 ms used in this simulation) (**d**). (Reproduced with permission from Ref. [12])

Fig. 14.3 Representative UTE images of a finger in the sagittal (**a**) and axial (**b**) planes, as well as a knee joint shown in the sagittal plane (**c**) using a 1–1 binomial water excitation pulse. Flexor tendons of the fingers and the posterior cruciate ligament of the knee joint are clearly depicted with positive contrast. (Reproduced with permission from Ref. [12])

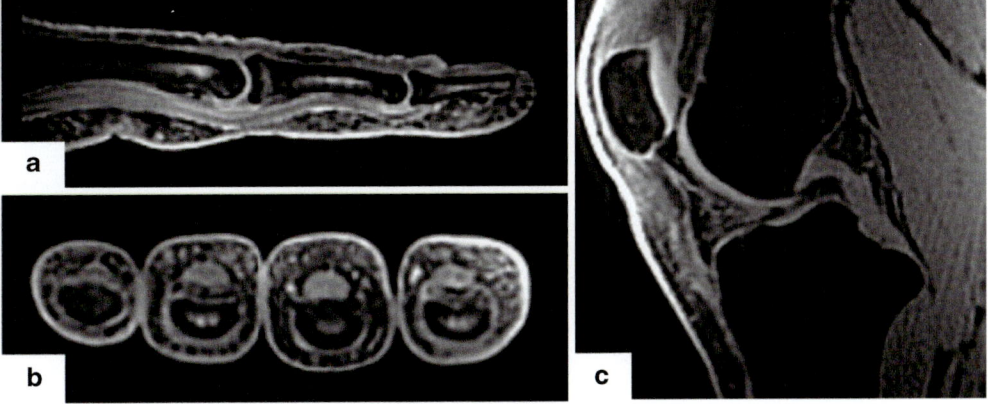

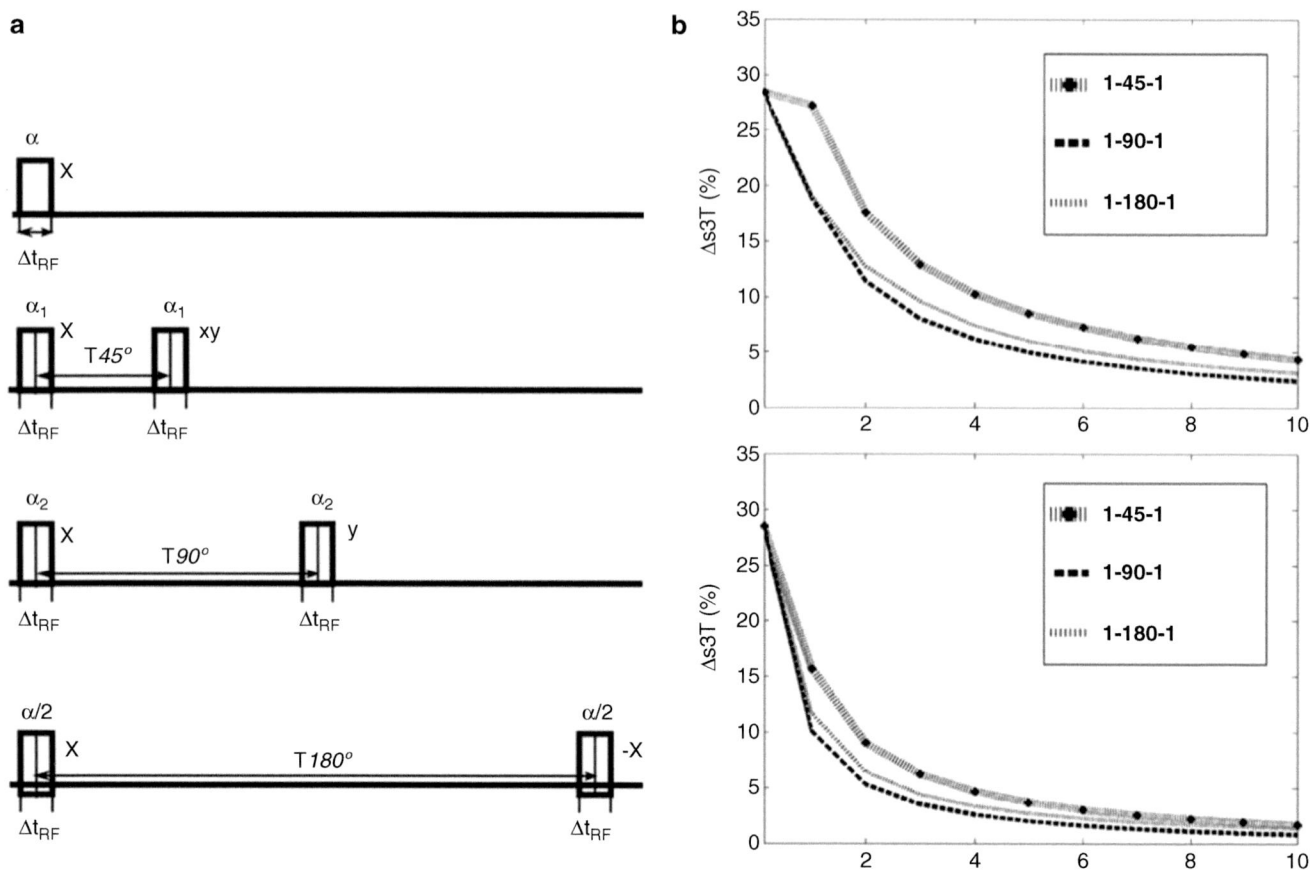

Fig. 14.4 RF pulse diagrams (**a**) and signal loss ratio curves (**b**). Four RF pulse diagrams are shown, including a single hard pulse (first row in a) and three 1–1 binomial water excitation pulses with different precessional phases (i.e., 45°, 90°, and 180°) (second to fourth rows in **a**). The signal loss ratio curves between water excitation and hard pulse excitation are simulated for field strengths of 3 T (right top) and 7 T (right bottom), respectively (**b**). (Reproduced with permission from Ref. [13])

Fig. 14.5 Representative UTE images of a knee joint with four different excitation schemes (**a**): (I) single hard pulse, (II) 1–1 water excitation with a phase of 45°, (III) 1–1 water excitation with a phase of 90°, and (IV) 1–1 water excitation with a phase of 180°. This is followed by the measured average signal with the different excitation schemes, normalized to the signal of the hard pulse excitation for each ROI for the respective regions (circles in a) (**b**). (Reproduced with permission from Ref. [13])

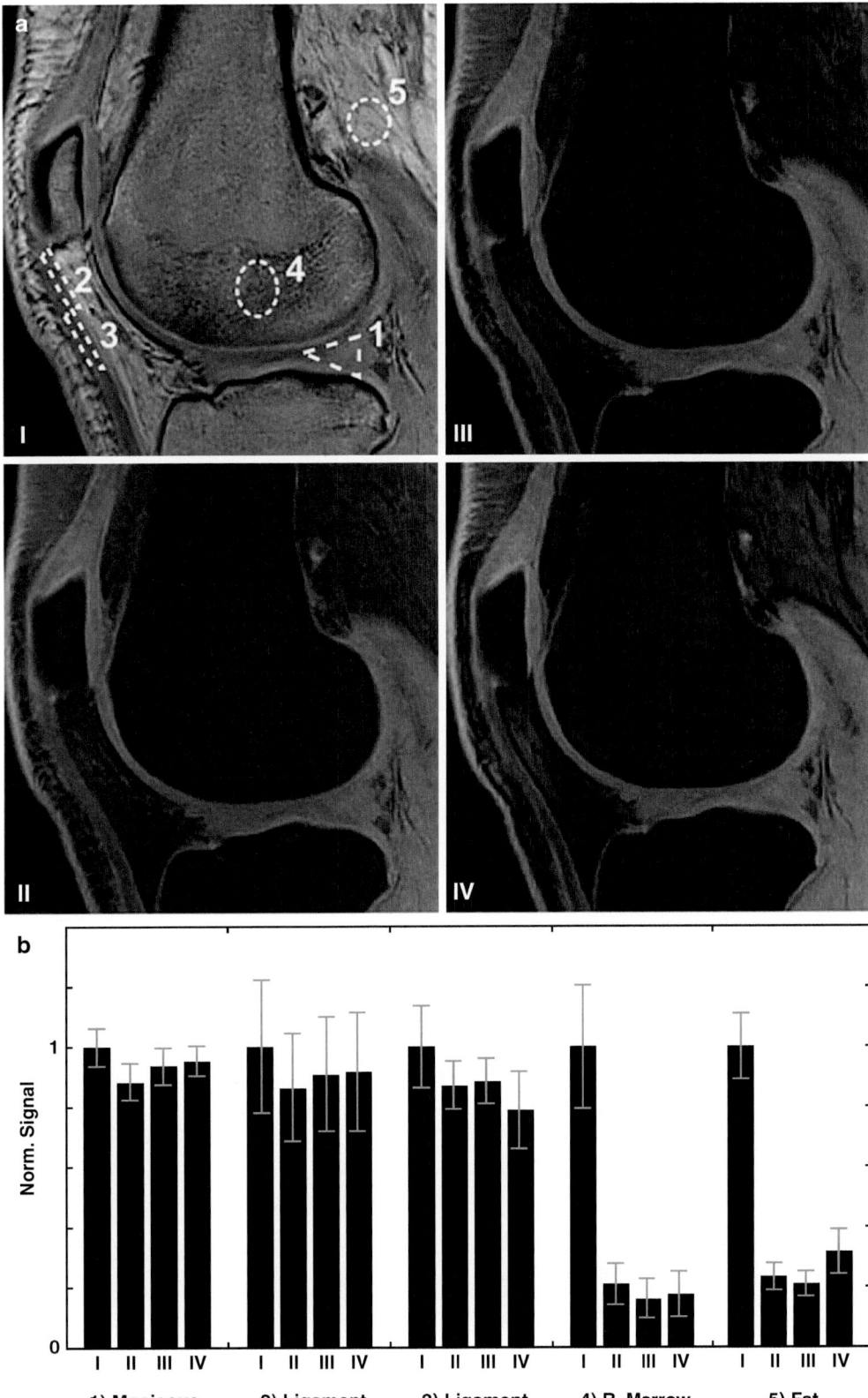

Soft-Hard Water Excitation Pulses

As seen in the above two studies by Springer et al. [12] and Deligianni et al. [13], the binomial water excitation pulse is very effective for fat suppression in UTE imaging of short-T_2 tissues. However, the water signal also suffers from attenuation due to the relatively long effective TE and the limited water excitation efficiency, especially when the tissue T_2 is very short. Thus, conventional binomial pulses may not be ideal for short-T_2 imaging.

Ma et al. have recently designed a new soft-hard water excitation pulse specifically for high contrast short-T_2 water imaging with simultaneous fat suppression [14]. Figure 14.6a shows the RF pulse diagrams. The new soft-hard excitation pulse consists of a low-power soft pulse and a high-power short rectangular pulse (first column in Fig. 14.6a). The two RF pulses have the same flip angles but opposite excitation phases. The excitation frequencies of the soft and hard pulses are centered on the fat and water peaks, respectively. A minimum-phase Shinnar–Le Roux (SLR) algorithm is used to design the soft pulse which

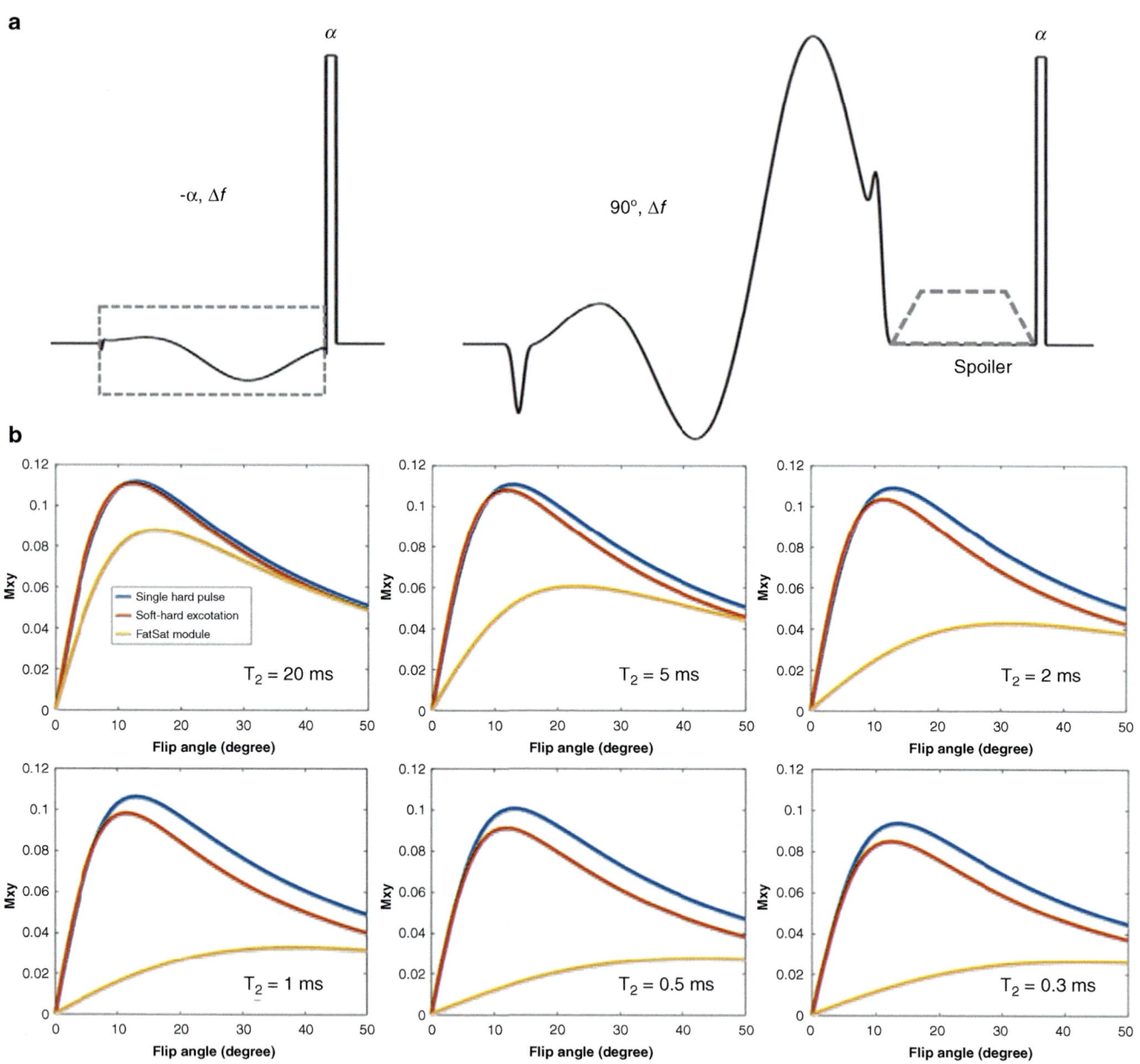

Fig. 14.6 RF pulse diagrams for soft-hard water excitation (first column) and a FatSat module (second column) (**a**) and numerical simulations of UTE imaging signal intensities for different tissues (T_2s of 20, 5, 2, 1, 0.5, and 0.3 ms) with three different excitation schemes: single hard pulse excitation, soft-hard water excitation, and single hard pulse excitation with FatSat preparation (**b**). A constant T_1 of 800 ms was used in all simulations. (Reproduced with permission from Ref. [14])

has a relatively narrow spectral bandwidth of around 500 Hz and a relatively long duration of around 4.4 ms to reduce signal saturation of short-T_2 tissues during excitation. With this soft-hard pulse design, the fat magnetization is first excited by the off-resonance soft pulse and then tipped back by the hard pulse. Thus, theoretically, no fat signals result. The water magnetization is almost entirely unaffected by the soft pulse excitation and efficiently excited by the following short hard pulse. The commonly used FatSat module is also shown in the second column of Fig. 14.6a for comparison.

Figure 14.6b shows numerical simulation results for UTE imaging with a single hard pulse excitation, a soft-hard pulse excitation, and a FatSat preparation for tissues with different T_2s. The signal intensity with soft-hard excitation is slightly reduced compared with single hard pulse excitation when T_2 is less than 2 ms. In comparison, the short-T_2 water signal is much lower in FatSat-prepared UTE imaging compared to UTE imaging with either a single hard pulse excitation or soft-hard pulse excitation. Due to the strong direct saturation of short-T_2 tissues, this water signal attenuation becomes more dramatic with FatSat-prepared UTE imaging of shorter T_2 tissues.

Figure 14.7 shows representative in vivo knee images using UTE imaging with a single hard pulse excitation, a soft-

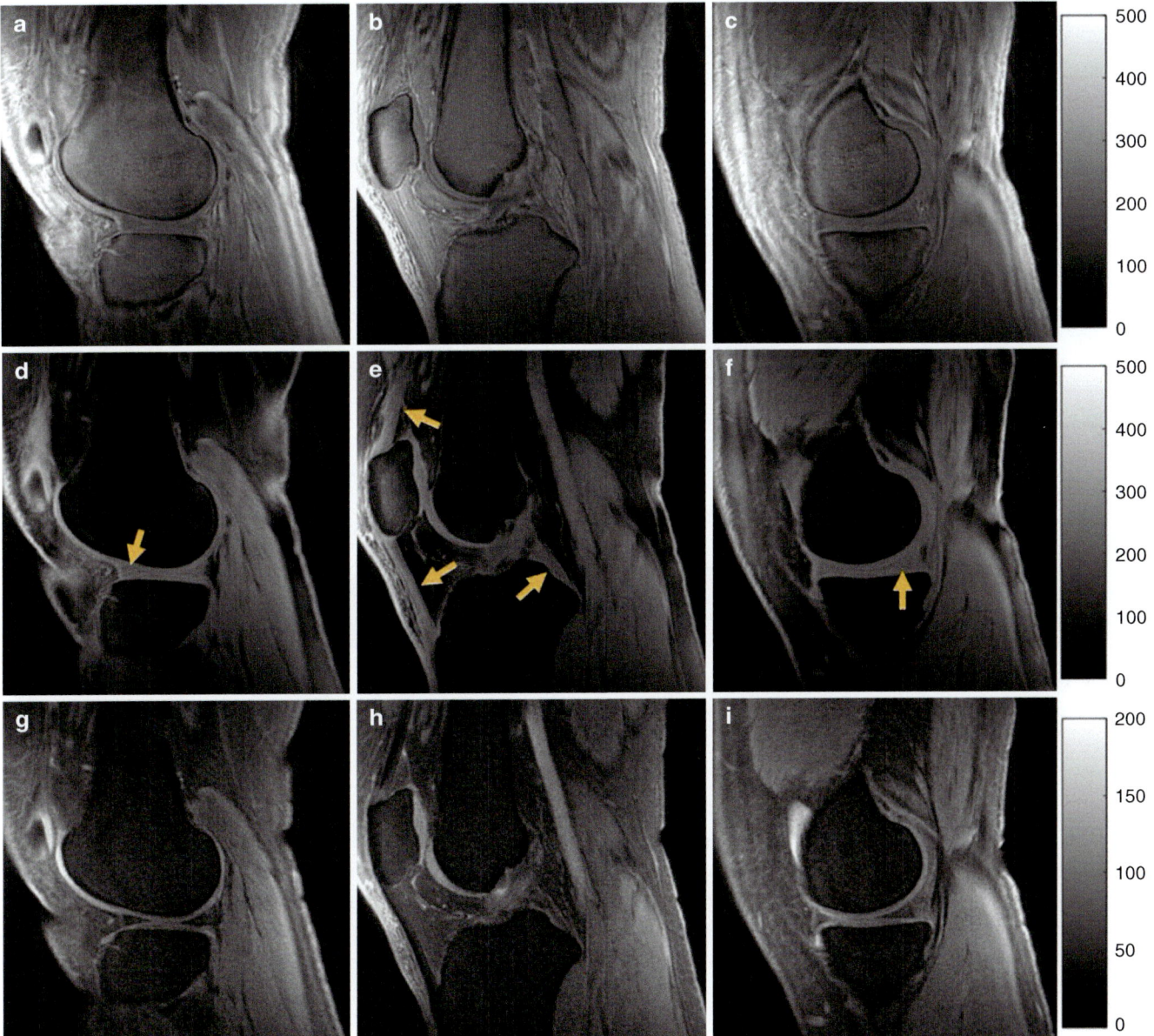

Fig. 14.7 Representative knee joint UTE imaging using excitations with a single hard pulse (**a–c**), the soft-hard water excitation pulse (**d–f**), and the FatSat module (**g–i**). Fat signal is well suppressed by both the soft-hard pulse and the FatSat module. The short-T_2 signals (yellow arrows) are much better preserved in UTE images with the soft-hard excitation pulse (**d–f**) than with the FatSat module (**g–i**). UTE images with the soft-hard water excitation show the best image contrast. (Reproduced with permission from Ref. [14])

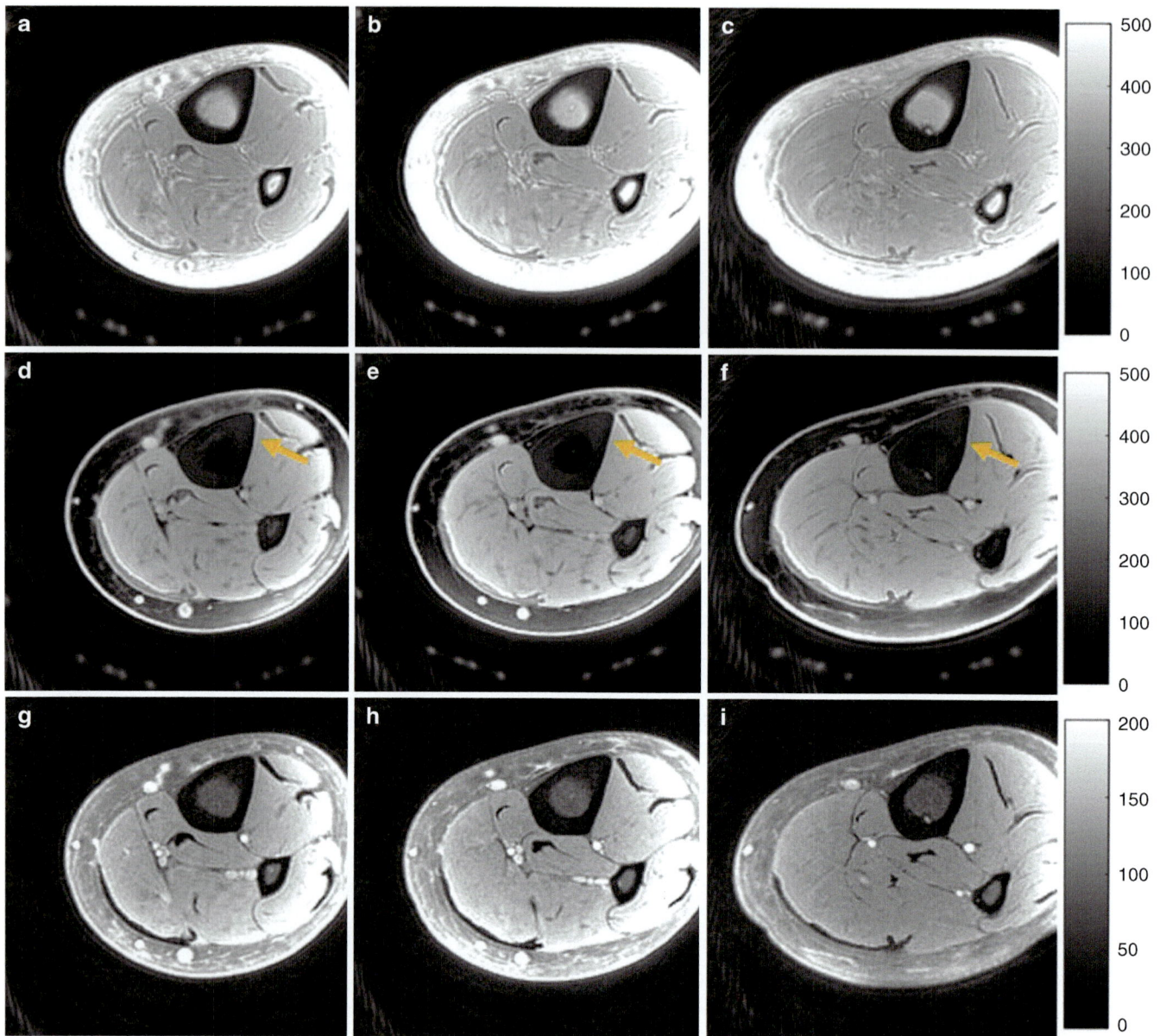

Fig. 14.8 Representative tibia UTE imaging using excitations with a single hard pulse (**a–c**), the soft-hard water excitation pulse (**d–f**), and the FatSat module (**g–i**). Fat signal is well suppressed by both the soft-hard pulse and the FatSat module. The short-T_2 signals (yellow arrows) are much better preserved on UTE images with the soft-hard excitation pulse (**d–f**) than with the FatSat module (**g–i**). UTE images with soft-hard water excitation show the best bone contrast. (Reproduced with permission from Ref. [14])

hard pulse excitation, and a FatSat preparation, respectively. Fat signals are well suppressed with both the soft-hard pulse and the FatSat module. However, water signals, especially those of short-T_2 tissues such as tendons and ligaments, are much lower with FatSat preparation than with soft-hard water excitation. Significantly better short-T_2 contrast is achieved in UTE images with soft-hard pulse excitation.

Figure 14.8 shows representative in vivo tibial midshaft UTE images with single hard pulse excitation, soft-hard pulse excitation, and FatSat preparation. Both subcutaneous and bone marrow fat are well suppressed on UTE images with soft-hard water excitation, and cortical bone is depicted

with excellent contrast. In comparison, the bone signal with FatSat-prepared UTE images is almost completely saturated by the FatSat module. In addition, short-T_2 coil elements can only be seen on UTE images with single hard pulse excitation and soft-hard pulse excitation. This further demonstrates that the FatSat module saturates short-T_2 species (e.g., cortical bone and coil elements), while the soft-hard water excitation pulse preserves short-T_2 signals very well.

The soft-hard water excitation pulse has also been applied to quantitative bicomponent imaging of cortical bone [15]. As shown in Fig. 14.9, excellent bicomponent curve fitting can be achieved using multi-echo UTE images with soft-

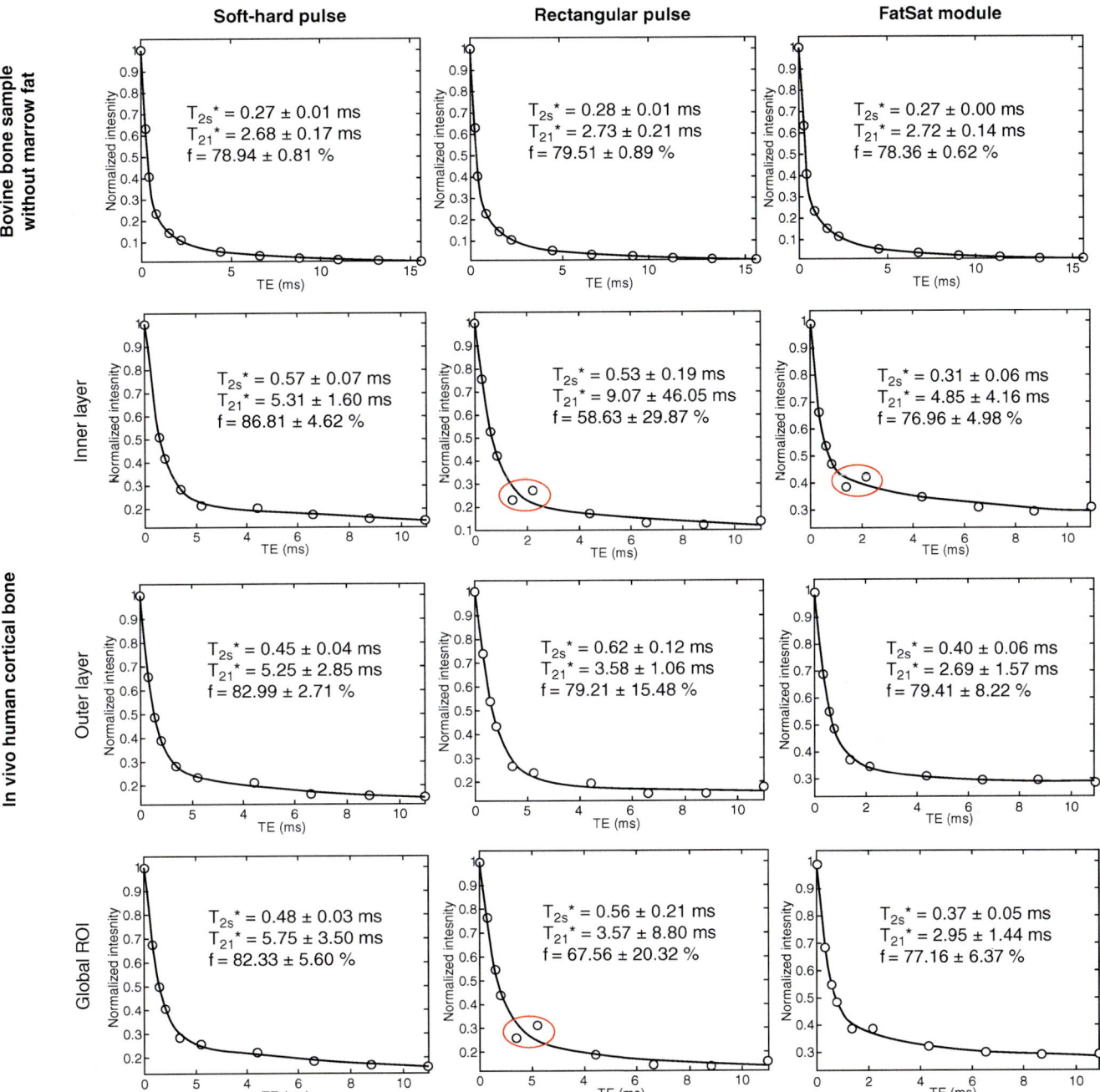

Fig. 14.9 Bicomponent analysis results of a bovine bone sample with marrow fat removed (the first row) and the tibial midshaft of a healthy volunteer (second to fourth rows) acquired using UTE sequences with the soft-hard excitation pulse (first column), the single hard pulse without (second column), and with the FatSat module (third column), respectively. When bone marrow fat is removed from the bovine bone sample, all three excitation schemes work equally well with little difference (first row). For the in vivo case, the signal oscillation due to fat contamination (as indicated by the red ellipses) is eliminated with the soft-hard pulse but is seen with the regular pulse which shows more marked oscillation in the inner layer (second row) than in the outer layer (the third row). (Reproduced with permission from Ref. [15])

hard water excitation for cortical bone measurements in both ex vivo and in vivo studies at 3 T. In comparison, fat contamination produces signal oscillation on UTE images with single hard excitation when TEs are close to 2 ms. This leads to a substantially reduced bound water fraction. The signal oscillation pattern is also found with FatSat-prepared UTE images. In this case, the FatSat module significantly attenuates the bone signal and thus reduces it to a level comparable to the residual fat signal. The inner layer of the tibial cortex is subject to significant partial volume and off-resonance artifacts. As a result, the water and fat spins go in and out of phase as a function of TE, leading to signal oscillation and this causes further quantification errors. This study demonstrates that the soft-hard pulse can sufficiently suppress fat signal and preserve bone signal for more accurate bicomponent fitting than the regular short rectangular pulse without, or with, a FatSat module [15].

Conclusion

Water excitation RF pulses provide effective fat suppression and preserve short-T_2 signals much better than the regular FatSat module in UTE imaging. Theoretically, the soft-hard pulse provides better preservation of short-T_2 signals than the 1–1 binomial water excitation pulse. The water excitation pulse minimizes errors in UTE bicomponent analysis of bound and pore water in cortical bone. It may also improve the accuracy of UTE-based quantitative magnetization transfer imaging [16], T_1 mapping [4], $T_1\rho$ mapping [17], and quantitative susceptibility mapping [18].

References

1. Fazeli PK, Horowitz MC, MacDougald OA, et al. Marrow fat and bone-new perspectives. J Clin Endocrinol Metab. 2013;98(3):935–45.
2. Addison O, Marcus RL, LaStayo PC, Ryan AS. Intermuscular fat: a review of the consequences and causes. Int J Endocrinol. 2014;2014:309570.
3. Kirkland JL, Tchkonia T, Pirtskhalava T, Han J, Karagiannides I. Adipogenesis and aging: does aging make fat go MAD? Exp Gerontol. 2002;37(6):757–67.
4. Ma Y, Zhao W, Wan L, et al. Whole knee joint T_1 values measured in vivo at 3T by combined 3D ultrashort echo time cones actual flip angle and variable flip angle methods. Magn Reson Med. 2019;81(3):1634–44.
5. Bydder M, Carl M, Bydder GM, Du J. MRI chemical shift artifact produced by center-out radial sampling of k-space: a potential pitfall in clinical diagnosis. Quant Imaging Med Surg. 2021;11(8):3677–83.
6. Gatehouse PD, Bydder GM. Magnetic resonance imaging of short T_2 components in tissue. Clin Radiol. 2003;58(1):1–19.
7. Chen Y, Li L, Le N, Chang EY, Huang W, Ma Y-J. On the fat saturation effect in quantitative ultrashort TE MR imaging. Magn Reson Med. 2022;87(5):2388–97.
8. Del Grande F, Santini F, Herzka DA, et al. Fat-suppression techniques for 3-T MR imaging of the musculoskeletal system. Radiographics. 2014;34(1):217–33.
9. Graichen H, Springer V, Flaman T, et al. Validation of high-resolution water-excitation magnetic resonance imaging for quantitative assessment of thin cartilage layers. Osteoarthr Cartil. 2000;8(2):106–14.
10. Glaser C, Faber S, Eckstein F, et al. Optimization and validation of a rapid high-resolution T_1-w 3D FLASH water excitation MRI sequence for the quantitative assessment of articular cartilage volume and thickness. Magn Reson Imaging. 2001;19(2):177–85.
11. Heudorfer L, Hohe J, Faber S, Englmeier KH, Reiser M, Eckstein F. Precision MRI-based joint surface and cartilage density analysis of the knee joint using rapid water-excitation sequence and semi-automatic segmentation algorithm. Biomed Tech (Berl). 2000;45(1):304–10.
12. Springer F, Steidle G, Martirosian P, et al. Quick water-selective excitation of fast relaxing tissues with 3D UTE sequences. Magn Reson Med. 2014;71(2):534–43.
13. Deligianni X, Bär P, Scheffler K, Trattnig S, Bieri O. Water-selective excitation of short T_2 species with binomial pulses. Magn Reson Med. 2014;72(3):800–5.
14. Ma Y-J, Jerban S, Jang H, Chang EY, Du J. Fat suppression for ultrashort echo time imaging using a novel soft-hard composite radiofrequency pulse. Magn Reson Med. 2019;82(6):2178–87.
15. Li L, Chen Y, Wei Z, et al. 3D UTE bicomponent imaging of cortical bone using a soft–hard composite pulse for excitation. Magn Reson Med. 2021;85(3):1581–9.
16. Ma Y-J, Chang EY, Carl M, Du J. Quantitative magnetization transfer ultrashort echo time imaging using a time-efficient 3D multispoke cones sequence. Magn Reson Med. 2018;79(2):692–700.
17. Ma Y, Carl M, Searleman A, Lu X, Chang EY, Du J. 3D adiabatic $T_1\rho$ prepared ultrashort echo time cones sequence for whole knee imaging. Magn Reson Med. 2018;80(4):1429–39.
18. Lu X, Jang H, Ma Y, Jerban S, Chang EY, Du J. Ultrashort echo time quantitative susceptibility mapping (UTE-QSM) of highly concentrated magnetic nanoparticles: a comparison study about different sampling strategies. Molecules. 2019;24(6):1143.

UTE–Dixon Fat–Water Imaging

Sophia Kronthaler, Georg Feuerriegel, Philipp Braun,
Kilian Weiss, Alexandra Gersing,
and Dimitrios C. Karampinos

Introduction

Fat is abundant throughout the human body, including locations within and between organs. It produces an important magnetic resonance (MR) signal component in diagnostic imaging that often needs to be either suppressed or separated from water-containing species when quantifying the MR properties of mixtures of different chemically shift species. An MRI of short-T_2 tissues often requires the suppression of signals from other long-T_2 water-containing tissues to improve the contrast in the depiction of the short-T_2 tissues. Suppression of long-T_2 fat signals is often also required. In addition, fat needs to be included in the assessment of tissue water properties such as proton density, particularly in the presence of partial volume effects.

Nowadays, fat–water imaging is a state-of-the-art imaging methodology, which is used to separate fat and water signals. It is performed either qualitatively, typically to suppress the fat signal, or quantitatively to derive biomarkers of tissue fat concentration. Fat–water imaging relies on encoding the chemical shift difference between fat and water using multi-echo acquisitions and is formally referred to as chemical shift encoded (CSE) water–fat separation or more frequently as Dixon imaging.

Fat–water imaging is combined with techniques for imaging short-T_2 tissues, especially ultrashort echo time (UTE) techniques. Techniques combining both UTE and Dixon imaging are described as UTE–Dixon imaging and are used both to suppress the fat signal with UTE acquisitions and to determine tissue proton density and other properties. This chapter aims to highlight the advantages of UTE–Dixon imaging. Here, the most important technical aspects of UTE–Dixon imaging are reviewed, including the most frequently employed data acquisition techniques and appropriate water–fat separation algorithms. Current applications of UTE–Dixon imaging are also described.

Dixon Imaging for Fat Suppression with UTE Acquisitions

Magnetization preparation techniques are most commonly used for fat suppression in clinical protocols due to the simplicity of their implementation and their compatibility with the majority of MR imaging sequences. Common magnetization preparation techniques are fat saturation, water excitation, short tau inversion recovery (STIR), spectral presaturation with inversion recovery (SPIR), and spectral adiabatic inversion recovery (SPAIR). Even though fat suppression techniques based on magnetization preparation are extremely useful for morphological and quantitative imaging, the use of conventional fat suppression methods is challenging with UTE imaging. Chemical shift-based fat saturation techniques lead to undesired loss of signal from short-T_2 tissues in addition to the loss of signal from fat. Compared to magnetization preparation techniques, CSE methods are more robust to B_0 and B_1 field inhomogeneities and have lower specific absorption rate (SAR) values. The major limitations of CSE-based methods are the increased scan time required for them and the need for post-processing methods to separate the detected signal into fat and water components.

Data Acquisition Techniques for UTE–Dixon Imaging

Dixon techniques utilize the phase evolution of the different chemical species during multiple echo times (TEs) for water- and fat-separated image reconstruction. The acquisition of

S. Kronthaler · G. Feuerriegel · P. Braun · A. Gersing ·
D. C. Karampinos (✉)
Department of Diagnostic and Interventional Radiology, Klinikum rechts der Isar, TUM School of Medicine, Technical University of Munich, Munich, Germany
e-mail: dimitrios.karampinos@tum.de

K. Weiss
Philips GmbH, Hamburg, Germany

J. Du, G. M. Bydder (eds.), *MRI of Short- and Ultrashort-T2 Tissues*, https://doi.org/10.1007/978-3-031-35197-6_15

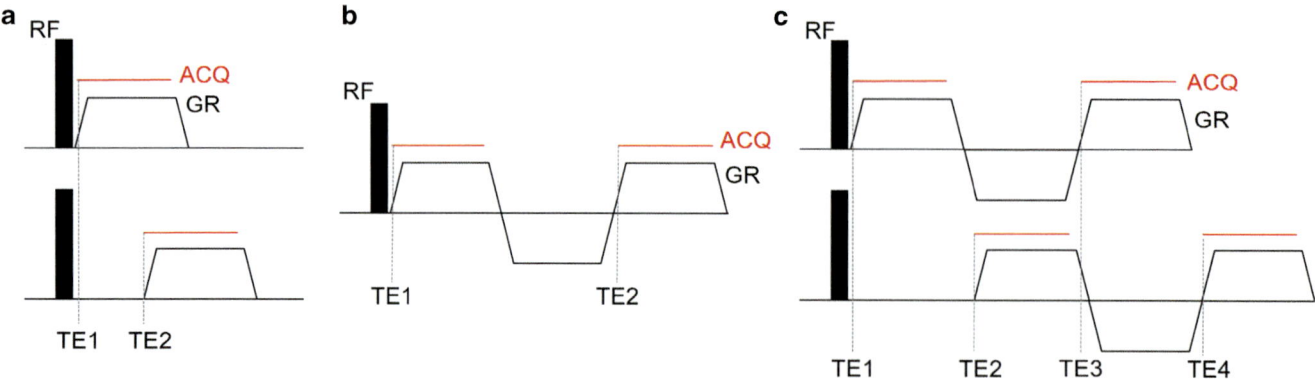

Fig. 15.1 Schematics of multi-TE UTE–Dixon acquisitions. (**a**) UTE–Dixon multi-acquisition for a dual-echo sequence: multiple TEs are acquired in consecutive repetitions. Although this allows high flexibility in choosing TEs, it comes at the cost of reduced scan time efficiency. (**b**) Multi-echo UTE–Dixon acquisition for a dual-echo sequence: multiple gradient echoes are acquired in each repetition. This approach has greater scan time efficiency compared to that of multi-acquisition UTE–Dixon. However, the need for optimal TEs for Dixon processing poses restrictions on the achievable echo spacing and the spatial resolution of the sequence. (**c**) Interleaved multi-echo UTE–Dixon. This combines the multi-echo and multi-acquisition UTE–Dixon approaches. In each sequence repetition, multiple echoes are acquired. Additionally, the TEs are shifted between multiple acquisitions to allow a more flexible choice of TEs. It combines the increased scan time efficiency of the multi-echo Dixon approach with increased flexibility in the choice of TEs

multiple TEs is necessary for UTE–Dixon imaging. Different approaches have been developed to allow multi-TE UTE–Dixon imaging [1]. The most straightforward method to acquire multi-TE UTE–Dixon data is by separate acquisition of multiple images, each with a different TE (multi-acquisition UTE–Dixon, Fig. 15.1a). Although this approach allows high flexibility in selecting individual TEs, it is associated with low scan time efficiency due to the need to repeat the sequence at each TE. Because of the sequential mode of acquiring data with multi-acquisition approaches, physiological variations and motion can impact the various TEs differently and may influence the quality of water–fat image reconstructions. Temporal interleaving of the different acquired TEs within one scan can alleviate the impact of physiological variations and motion; however, low scan time efficiency remains a limitation with the multi-acquisition approach.

To address the low scan time efficiency of multi-acquisition UTE–Dixon methods, methods acquiring multiple TEs with one repetition of the UTE sequence have been developed (multi-echo UTE–Dixon, Fig. 15.1b). In this approach, multiple gradient echoes (GREs) are acquired after each radiofrequency (RF) pulse excitation. To avoid problems with phase errors caused by hardware imperfections such as eddy currents or delays in the gradient chain activation, approaches with monopolar readouts, starting at the center of the k-space for the first echo, are often preferred. However, to achieve optimal TEs for Dixon processing, multi-echo UTE–Dixon poses limitations on the maximum achievable spatial resolution, especially at higher magnetic fields such as 3 T.

To combine increased scan time efficiency and high spatial resolution, approaches combining multi-acquisition and multi-echo UTE–Dixon have been developed. In these approaches, multiple gradient echoes are acquired with a single repetition of the UTE sequence, and the UTE sequence is repeated with a small shift in the gradient echo train. All acquired echoes are then interleaved in the reconstruction process. This interleaved multi-echo UTE–Dixon approach combines high flexibility in selecting the echo spacing of the TEs and long readout lengths for high spatial resolution (Fig. 15.1c).

While, in most cases, UTE–Dixon approaches are based on spoiled gradient echo sequences with radial center-out k-space sampling, the UTE–Dixon acquisition approaches described above can be combined with other sequence types and sampling strategies. For example, multi-acquisition UTE–Dixon sampling was used in the ultrashort echo time double echo steady-state (UTEDESS) sequence, to provide combined quantitative mapping of T_2 and CSE-based water–fat separation [2]. In another work, a UTE Cones k-space trajectory was combined with a multi-echo UTE sequence using bipolar sampling [3]. However, only the second TE was used for single-TE water–fat separation. Water-separated UTE images were then reconstructed using a weighted subtraction of the single-TE fat-separated images from the second TE. Furthermore, both approaches, UTEDESS and single-TE Dixon–UTE cones, were combined [4].

While the above approaches are based on multi-TE or single-TE CSE-based water–fat separation, multiple echoes still need to be acquired for water–fat separation. To this end, a single-TE Dixon approach has been developed, allowing direct water–fat separation based on single-echo UTE data [5]. No special acquisition strategies are necessary with this reconstruction to provide CSE-based water–fat separation.

Water–Fat Separation Methods

CSE algorithms are commonly used in routine clinical practice to suppress fat signals, generate water- and fat-separated images, and perform fat quantification on data acquired with the acquisition approaches outlined in the previous section. CSE techniques usually require the acquisition of multiple images at different TEs [6–9] and are generally associated with prolonged scan times. The CSE algorithms used in UTE imaging are described below.

Theory of Signal Models for Water–Fat Separation

It is important to have a clear understanding of the signal models used in the processing and interpretation of CSE images. In general, the time evolution of the complex MR signal $s(t_n)$ within a single voxel can be written as [10]:

$$s\left(t_n\right) = \sum_{p=0}^{P} \rho_p e^{-i\phi_p} e^{\left(i\omega_p - R_{2,p}^*\right)t_n} \tag{15.1}$$

where t_n is the time at the nth echo, ρ_p is the magnitude of the pth chemical species, ϕ_p is the phase after the RF excitation, ω_p is the resonance frequency, and $R_{2,p}^*$ is the transverse relaxation rate. To reduce the number of model parameters, and thus the number of required echoes, most CSE algorithms make the fundamental assumption that water and fat are the only two chemical species contributing to the object to be imaged. Furthermore, all peaks, including water, are assumed to decay with the same relaxation rate R_2^*. With these assumptions in CSE-MRI, a multipeak single-R_2^* model results as follows:

$$s\left(t_n\right) = \rho_0 e^{-i\phi_0} e^{\left(i\omega_0 - R_2^*\right)t_n} + \sum_{p=1}^{P} \rho_p e^{-i\phi_p} e^{\left(i\omega_p - R_2^*\right)t_n} \tag{15.2}$$

$$= \left(\rho_0 e^{-i\phi_0} + \sum_{p=1}^{P} \rho_p e^{-i\phi_p} e^{i\left(\omega_p - \omega_0\right)t_n}\right) e^{\left(i\omega_0 - R_2^*\right)t_n} \tag{15.3}$$

with $f_B = \dfrac{\omega_0}{2\pi}$; $W = \rho_0 e^{-i\phi_0}$; $c\left(t_n\right) = \sum_{p=1}^{P} \alpha_p e^{i\delta\omega_p t_n}$

$$s\left(t_n\right) = \left(W + c\left(t_n\right)F\right) e^{\left(i2\pi f_B - R_2^*\right)t_n} \tag{15.4}$$

where W and F denote the complex water and fat signals, respectively, f_B is the real-valued field map, which accounts for phase accumulated because of off-resonance effects due to B_0 main field inhomogeneity, α_p is the pth relative fat peak amplitude, and $\delta\omega_p$ is the chemical shift frequency difference between water and the pth fat peak in the fat spectral model that is used.

Water–Fat Separation in Multi-TE Dixon Imaging: The Methodology

The first water–fat separation algorithm developed by Dixon was based on the acquisition of two TEs and is often referred to as the "two-point Dixon method" [6, 11]. In this chapter, it is referred to as the two-TE Dixon method. To solve for W and F, two TEs are acquired when the fat and water signals are in phase (IP) ($c_{n=1} = +1$) and out of phase (OP) ($c_{n=2} = -1$). Under the assumption that $f_B = 0$, a single fat peak model and neglecting R_2^* decay effects ($R_2^* \to \infty$), real-valued W and F can be determined by adding and subtracting the IP and OP MR images. Because the original two-TE Dixon method has no field map terms, the water–fat separation is problematic in regions with large B_0 field inhomogeneities.

The three-TE Dixon technique, which requires three TEs acquired at IP and OP TEs, was introduced to account for B_0 field variations [8]. The off-resonance-induced phase map is computed and is used to calculate water- and fat-separated images. Similarly, in an extended two-TE technique, the magnitude-based method was replaced using the complex IP and OP images, which allows calculation of the off-resonance-induced phase map [12]. By accounting for f_B, the three-TE Dixon and the extended two-TE Dixon methods can improve the accuracy of fat–water separation [11, 13]. Most early two- and three-TE methods have the limitation of assuming a single fat peak, which only accounts for a portion of the fat signal and results in an underestimation of the fat content. Although the fat–water separation image quality improves when the field map is estimated, a water–fat swap can occur in areas with large phase variations due to B_0 field inhomogeneities. In addition, the early methods did not account for additional confounding factors such as T_1 or T_2^* bias, which need to be included to achieve accurate fat quantification.

Beyond the two- and three-TE Dixon water–fat separation methods, alternative methods have been proposed to solve the water–fat problem, which is a non-convex, nonlinear problem due to the field map term. Another approach to solving the water–fat problem is the iterative decomposition of water and fat with echo asymmetry and the least squares estimation (IDEAL) method [9]. The IDEAL approach uses a matrix formulation and iteratively linearizes the nonlinear problem to solve for the parameters in the signal model, which includes water and fat. The IDEAL technique allows use of arbitrary TEs and thus more flexible acquisitions, which may potentially improve the signal-to-noise ratio

(SNR) for signal fitting. However, the IDEAL technique relies on good initialization of the field map. Another approach to solving the water–fat problem relates to reformulating the problem to decouple estimation of the water and fat signals from the estimation of the field map using the variable projection (VARPRO) method [14]. For fat quantification, the IDEAL and VARPRO methods can be extended to account for confounding factors such as the multipeak fat spectrum and T_2^* bias [15]. A generalized formulation for multi-echo, gradient echo-based chemical species separation for all MR signal models described by a weighted sum of complex exponentials with linear phases with TEs has also been recently introduced [10].

To improve fat–water separation in the presence of B_0 field inhomogeneities, Dixon water–fat separation methods are combined with commonly used phase unwrapping techniques such as region-growing [16, 17], polynomial fitting [18], and solving Poisson's equations [19]. All phase unwrapping methods assume that the B_0 field varies smoothly across the image [11]. Specifically, because the fitting problem has multiple local minima, the solution for the field map in the water–fat separation problem depends on the initial guess [11, 20]. Region-growing algorithms [21] or advanced complex fitting algorithms, such as graph-cut approaches [22–25], are required to improve field map estimation, particularly in regions with low SNRs or rapid, spatially varying fields where water–fat swaps might occur.

Water–Fat Separation in Multi-TE UTE–Dixon Imaging of Tissues with Short T_2s

Different approaches to separate fat signal from water signal in the imaging of short-T_2 tissues have been investigated. One approach is to combine UTE with spectroscopic imaging (UTESI) [26, 27], which has been successful in separating different chemical species (primarily water and fat). However, the UTESI approach suffers from distortion of the slice profile and errors in radial k-space trajectories, including chemical shift and off-resonance artifacts.

Another approach extends the IDEAL algorithm with correction for the effects of R_2^* decay, using a k-space formulation and accurate multipeak spectral modeling [1]. The combined UTE–IDEAL method provided high contrast imaging of the short-T_2 tissues with robust fat–water separation. A major limitation of the UTE–Dixon methods is the assumption that water is present in a single-T_2 compartment in the imaged voxel, which may not be true, for example, in cartilage, tendon, or meniscus where long- and short-T_2^* water species are present. One possible approach to this includes incorporating prior knowledge of the multiple water compartments in the signal model, similar to multifrequency modeling of the fat spectrum; however, this requires a large number of echoes and a high SNR. The above assumptions imply that the T_2^* obtained by the proposed model is an average value of all the species and all the compartments within a voxel. Beyond water–fat imaging, the UTE–Dixon technique has been used to suppress long-T_2 components, which is beneficial for pseudo-CT imaging and attenuation map generation [28–32].

Water–Fat Separation in Single-TE Dixon Imaging: The Methodology

Single-TE Dixon methods directly decompose fat and water components from a single complex MR image [33]. Because only one complex TE image is required, single-TE Dixon methods have shorter acquisition times than multi-TE methods and were thus first investigated for dynamic imaging [33]. In the original single-echo Dixon method [33], data are acquired with fat in the imaginary channel and water in the real channel by choosing a TE when the phase between water and fat components is $\theta(t) = \pi/2$. It should be noted that $\theta(t)$ is defined by

$$\theta(t) = \angle(c(t_n))$$ (15.5)

Neglecting T_2^* decay effects, Eq. 15.4 can be rewritten as:

$$s(t_n) = (|W| + |F|c(t_n))e^{i\phi_{bulk}(t_n)}$$ (15.6)

Here, ϕ_{bulk} accounts for all the phase terms that water and fat experience as a common phase term. ϕ_{bulk} comprises contributions from spatially dependent field B_0 inhomogeneities $(2\pi f_B)$ [20], eddy currents, signal delays in the receiver chains, and phase contributions due to the B_1 transmit/receive phase [34].

Under the assumption that ϕ_{bulk} is zero, which implies a homogeneous B_0 field map, water and fat can be estimated by taking the real and imaginary parts of Eq. 15.6 so that

$$|F| = \frac{I\{s(t_n)\}}{\sin(\theta(t_n))}$$ (15.7)

$$|W| = R\{s(t_n)\} - |F|\cos(\theta(t_n))$$ (15.8)

The noise performance is optimal when the relative phase of the water and fat signals is $\pi/2$. Flexible TEs can be achieved if phase errors are corrected using a region-growing algorithm [34].

In practice, the assumption of a homogeneous B_0 field map is not valid and pre-calibration of the field map (e.g., using multi-TE Dixon) is required. To remove unwanted phase terms, different techniques have been reported . These use additional reference scans [3, 33], a region-growing algorithm to estimate the unwanted phase terms [34], or solve the smoothness-constrained inverse water–fat problem directly [5]. The acquisition of additional reference scans results in longer scan times and errors due to patient motion and other sources of inconsistency.

Water–Fat Separation in Single-TE UTE–Dixon Imaging of Tissues with Short T_2s

In the context of short-T_2^* imaging, different single-TE Dixon methods have been presented for fat suppression [3, 4], long-T_2 signal suppression [4], and water–fat imaging [4, 5]. Jang et al. [3] combined a single-TE Dixon method with a dual-echo UTE acquisition. Phase errors were corrected with an additional field map. A fat map was then estimated with single-TE Dixon processing of the non-UTE image. The fat image obtained from the non-UTE image was used to suppress the fat signal in the UTE image. The single-TE Dixon method demonstrated reliable fat and water separation unaffected by the short-T_2^* signal decay. Jang et al. demonstrated that the two-TE Dixon method incorrectly estimated fat and water signals in the tendons due to short-T_2^* signal decay. The advantage of their single-TE Dixon technique with dual-UTE acquisition is the high degree of flexibility it has in selecting the TE of the second echo. Echo spacing with the conventional two-TE Dixon method is limited by imaging parameters such as spatial resolution and field of view (FOV).

Recent work by Jang et al. [4] has shown UTE fat-suppressed images of the osteochondral junction, tendons, menisci, and ligaments in the knee joint as well as cortical bone and aponeuroses in the lower leg utilizing a UTE–Cones–DESS sequence and single-TE Dixon processing. The free induction decay (FID)-like S$^+$ image showed typical UTE image contrast with T_1-weighting. The echo-like S$^-$ image showed more T_2-weighting due to its longer TE. Here, the initial ϕ_{bulk} was calculated from the intrinsic signal properties of the S$^+$ and S$^-$ images, before separating the water and fat of both the S$^+$ and S$^-$ images with single-TE Dixon processing. The method yielded efficient fat suppression in both the S$^+$ and S$^-$ images without requiring additional acquisitions or preparation pulses. However, if there are strong B_0 field inhomogeneities that cannot be compensated for B_0 shimming, ϕ_{bulk} may become so large that an additional reference scan is required to avoid significant errors with the single-TE Dixon processing.

Another approach, presented by Kronthaler et al. [5], avoids the additional B_0 calibration measurement by formulating the problem as a smoothness-constrained nonlinear inverse water–fat problem. They showed that at UTE TEs (<0.14 ms at 3 T), phase contributions due to B_0 inhomogeneities are expected to be small as a result of the ultrashort TE. Such B_0 terms originate from magnetic inhomogeneity, the shim field, object-based susceptibility, and residual terms from background fields [20]. It should be noted that the UTE phase contains a strong contribution from the B_1 phase, which varies slowly in the axial plane (Fig. 15.2) and is the dominant term in UTE phase maps with TE = 0.14 ms when scanning the lumbar spine at 3 T. The B_1 phase is caused by the electrical conductivity of the tissue and has an approxi-

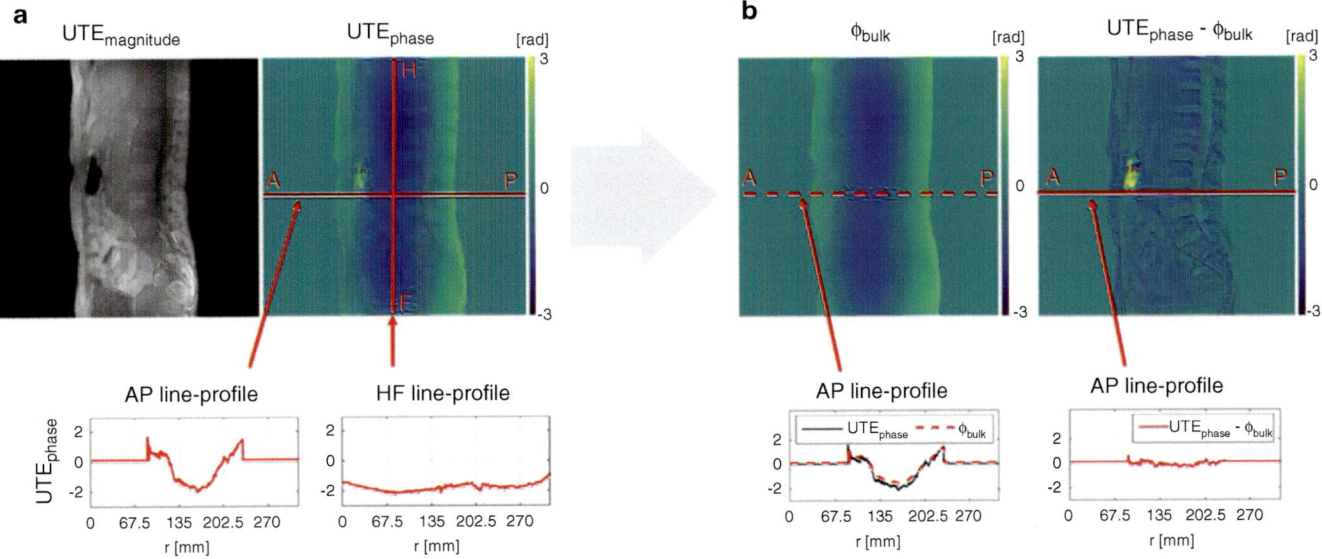

Fig. 15.2 (a) The UTE phase that includes contrast from the B_1 phase, which varies along the anterior-posterior (AP) and right-left (RL) (x–y plane) directions of the thoracic and lumbar spine. (b) The phase error ϕ_{bulk} is estimated after solving the smoothness-constrained inverse water–fat problem. Unwanted phase components, including the B_1 phase contribution, are removed in the corrected UTE phase (UTE$_{phase}$ − ϕ_{bulk}) shown in panel (b). UTE$_{magnitude}$ refers to the magnitude UTE image

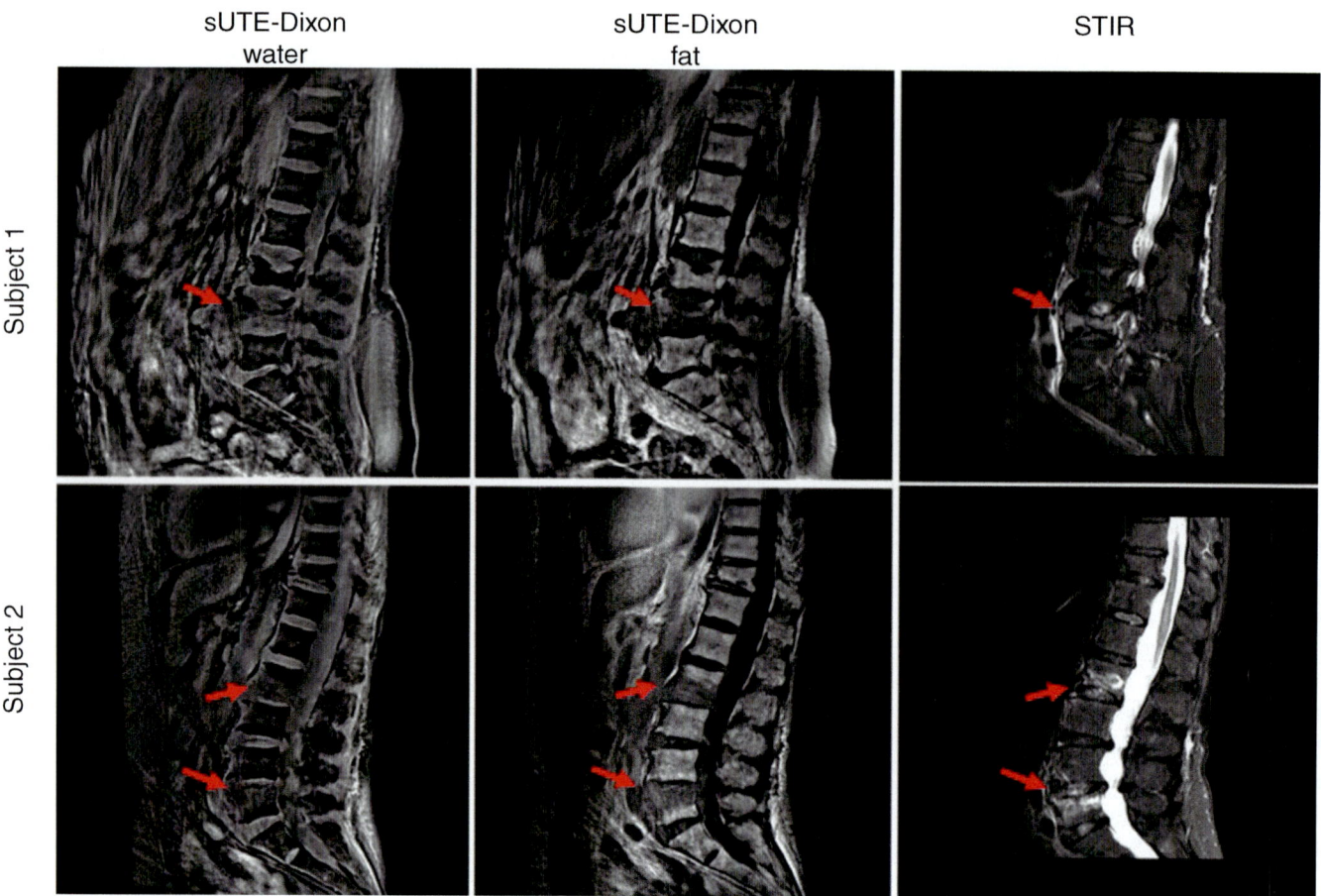

Fig. 15.3 Sagittal UTE thoracic and lumbar spine images from two patients with acute vertebral fractures (red arrows). The fluid buildup in the edema shows a high signal in the STIR images. The edema and fracture line are clearly visible in the single UTE–Dixon water–fat images

mately parabolic shape according to Maxwell's equations [35–37]. The proposed methodology assumes that the unwanted phase terms primarily consist of the B_1 phase, which varies smoothly over the FOV and is thus accounted for with a smoothness constraint. Their study, which included patients with lumbar spine vertebral fractures, demonstrated that the proposed methodology removed the unwanted low-frequency background phase and separated water–fat signals using a single-echo UTE image. The proposed method enabled simultaneous assessment of vertebral fractures and edema of the thoracolumbar spine using a single MR sequence (Fig. 15.3). In an extended study, the method was evaluated at different anatomical locations (Figs. 15.4, 15.5, and 15.6), on two different scanners, with various coils and varying TEs. A good depiction of short-T_2 components and good water–fat separation was achieved in all cases. In particular, in the cervical spine, large changes in B_0 inhomogeneity were successfully demodulated (Fig. 15.4). For the knee scans (Fig. 15.5), a transmit–receive coil was used, resulting in a different B_1 transmit-receive phase when compared to receive-only coils. Despite this additional challenge, the methodology provided high quality water- and fat-separated images. The method has the advantage of removing unwanted phase terms, whether caused by B_1 or B_0, without the need for an additional calibration scan. The post-processing is fully automated, which is superior to filtering approaches that require the kernel size and filter type to be defined for each subject.

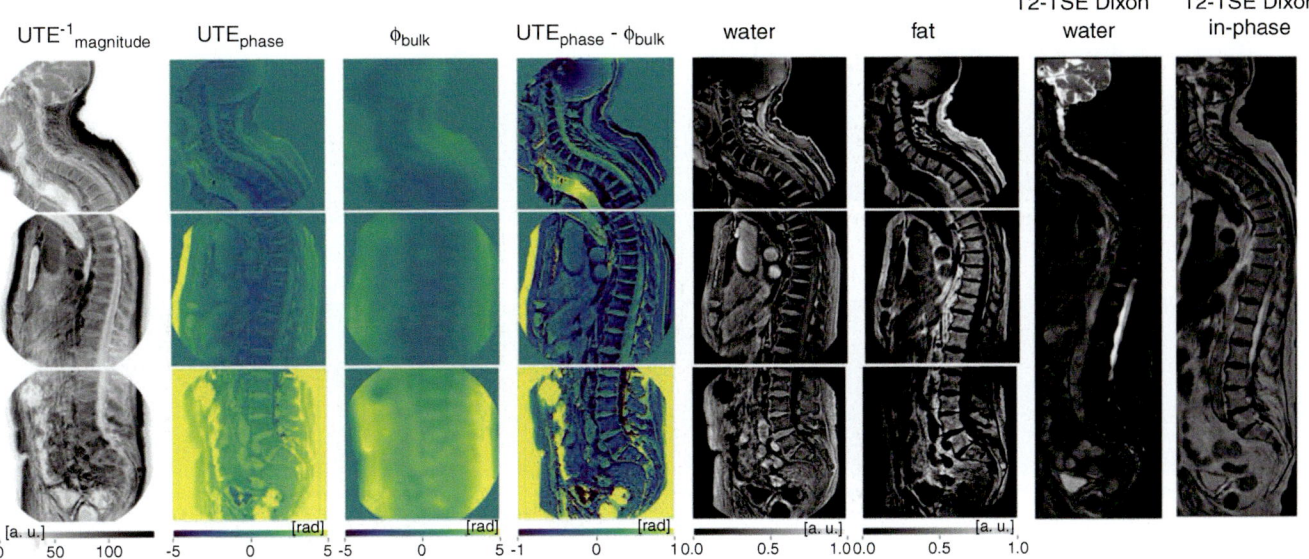

Fig. 15.4 High-resolution full spine scans of a patient. Three separate single-TE UTE scans were performed to obtain images from the cervical, thoracic, and lumbar spine. As a reference, T_2-weighted TSE Dixon water and in-phase images are presented. The ϕ_{bulk} image of the cervical spine shows significant phase contributions as a result of B_0 field inhomogeneities caused by the concave/convex anatomy of the spine. The anterior subcutaneous fat region is prone to errors due to respiratory motion. UTE$^{-1}_{magnitude}$ refers to the inverted magnitude UTE image

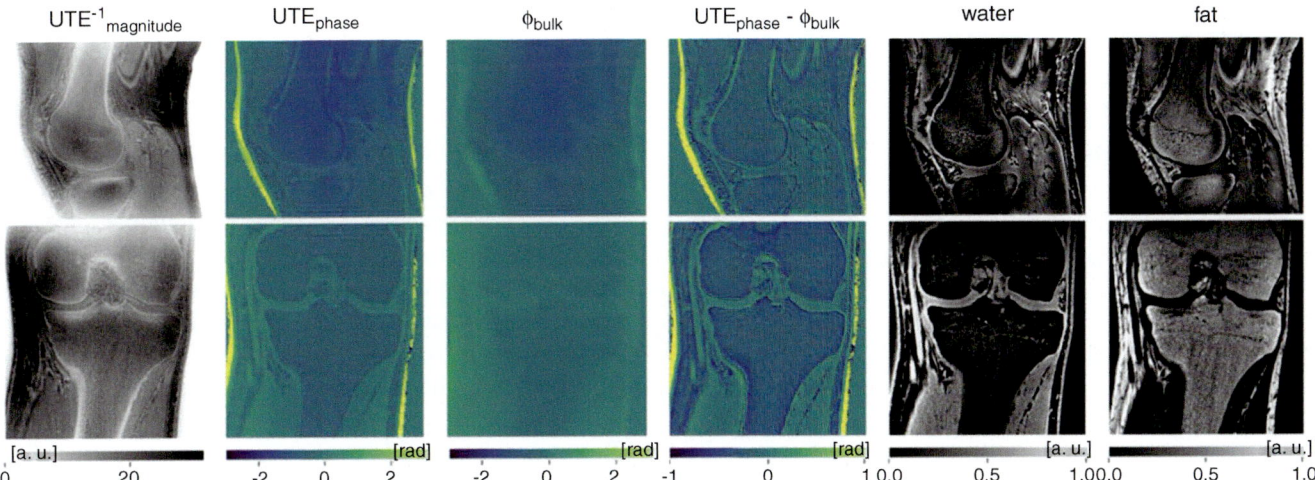

Fig. 15.5 High-resolution coronal and sagittal single-TE UTE scans of the knee in a healthy volunteer. Thin cortical bone structures are visible on the inverted UTE magnitude images. Phase modulations caused by B_0 inhomogeneities are seen in the ϕ_{bulk} images, particularly in the sagittal scans. These are corrected in the UTE$_{phase}$ − ϕ_{bulk} image. UTE$^{-1}_{magnitude}$ refers to the inverted magnitude UTE image

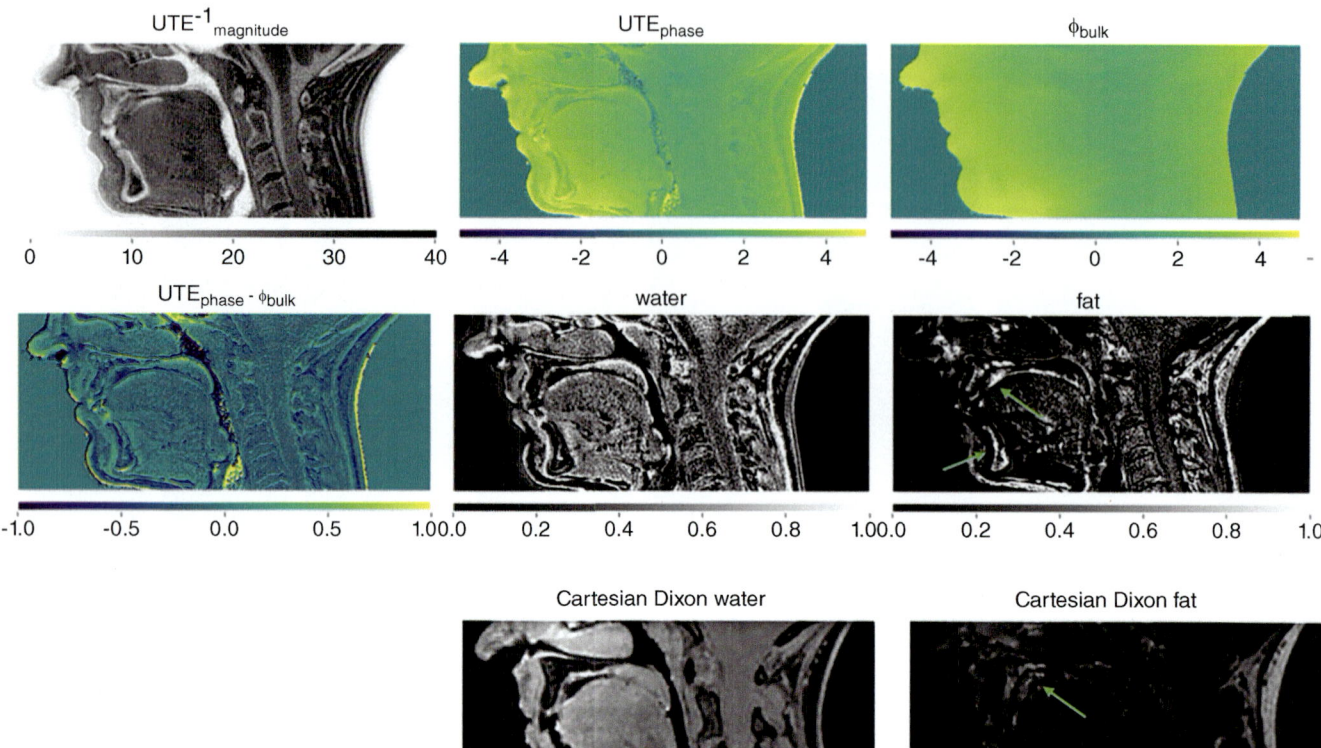

Fig. 15.6 A three-dimensional (3D) isotropic single-TE UTE scan of the mandible of a healthy volunteer. Compared to the Cartesian multi-echo Dixon fat-separated imaging, fat in the bone marrow of the man-dible is well depicted (green arrows). UTE$^{-1}_{magnitude}$ refers to the inverted magnitude UTE image

Clinical Applications

The clinical applications of water–fat UTE imaging are widespread and are being constantly expanded.

PET Attenuation Correction

In nuclear medicine, positron emission tomography (PET) combined with MRI is an emerging modality due to the excellent soft tissue contrast that it provides. This allows a detailed depiction of the anatomical structures and provides functional and molecular information. Reliable PET attenuation correction using MRI is difficult and time-consuming due to the complex MR signal, which is determined by tissue proton density and relaxation properties. Different methods are used for attenuation correction, including MR image segmentation for each tissue type to create attenuation maps as well as the production of attenuation maps based on co-registration of the acquired MR images with preexisting templates generated from CT. A combined multi-echo UTE–Dixon acquisition has been successfully implemented to simultaneously acquire signals from fat, water, and bone in a single acquisition for the estimation of linear attenuation coefficients (LACs). This method integrates a multi-echo Dixon method for robust water–fat separation as well as UTE imaging for tissues with short- and ultrashort-T2s (e.g., depiction of bone) into a single acquisition, which provides a continuous distribution of the attenuation coefficients in combination with a typical atlas-based segmentation. In order to reduce quantifications errors of the atlas-based approach, recently, a deep-learning-based convolutional neural network (CNN) together with a UTE multi-echo Dixon method has been used, and this showed significantly lower quantification errors than conventional atlas-based methods [30, 38–40].

Improved Tissue Delineation of Short-T$_2$ Tissues in Musculoskeletal Imaging

Conventional clinical MR imaging mainly relies on the detection of normal or abnormal long-T$_2$ signals. The assessment of tissues with short T$_2$/T$_2^*$'s such as the ligaments, menisci, tendons, cartilage, and bone mainly relies on indirect changes due to an increase or decrease in signals from tissues with longer T_2s (i.e., fat and water). UTE imaging methods are able to visualize short-T_2 signals and therefore allow direct assessment of short-T_2/T_2^* tissues. Fat saturation is typically performed in conventional UTE imaging to achieve the best possible contrast of short-T_2 tissues. The broad spectral width of short-T_2 tissues makes conventional chemical shift-based fat saturation problematic, and, therefore, different UTE–Dixon methods have been proposed. In the clinical setting, the enhanced UTE contrast allows better assessment and discrimination of various short-T_2^* tissues. Lombardi et al. [41] have been able to create high-resolution images of the vertebral body cartilaginous endplate, which is not possible using conventional MRI sequences due to its short T_2/T_2^*. The assessment helps with understanding intervertebral disc degeneration and may allow better evaluation of subtle abnormalities in the longitudinal ligaments and intervertebral foramina. Jang et al. [4] showed the application of a single-TE Dixon method for fat suppression of UTE images in the ankle and knee. They significantly improved the contrast-to-noise ratio for the Achilles, patella, and quadriceps tendons. This may help better assess degenerative changes and acute pathologies [1–3, 41, 42].

Water-Separated Images for Assessment of Edema in Musculoskeletal Imaging

Water–fat UTE imaging is mostly used to enhance the contrast of tissues with short T_2/T_2^* focusing on bone, menisci, ligaments, and cartilage. Quantification of tissue water content has been examined in several studies and has been shown to be feasible and reliable, albeit time-consuming, when assessing the menisci, deep radial calcified cartilage, and bone. Recently, Kronthaler et al. [5] have proposed a method for fat–water separation in order to assess bone marrow edema (BME) in the vertebral bodies of patients with acute vertebral fractures. Their method showed results comparable to conventional MR imaging in a study of 30 patients with spine fractures [43]. Conventional MRI relies on the acquisition of STIR and T_1-weighted sequences to assess BME and the fatty component of the bone marrow. The proposed method is based on single-TE Dixon processing, which solves the smoothness-constrained nonlinear inverse water–fat problem and allows fast reconstruction using an iterative reconstruction algorithm. The simultaneous examination of bone marrow edema and fat content of bone marrow with a single acquisition may help in the assessment of various pathologies of the spine, including acute and chronic fractures, bone marrow-infiltrating tumors, and osteoporotic fractures, while using significantly reduced scan times [5, 26, 44, 45].

Proton Density Fat Fraction (PDFF) Quantification

Osteoporosis is a systemic skeletal disease with a high socioeconomic burden, which is characterized by a loss of bone mass and microarchitectural deterioration. It predisposes to fragility fractures. Accurate bone marrow assessment is needed for therapy and fracture prevention. The utilization of quantitative MRI for assessment of the fracture risk and therapy monitoring has received increasing attention in recent years. Bone marrow PDFF is also emerging as a useful biomarker in the study of bone matrix health. Bone marrow PDFF is defined as the ratio of the density of mobile protons from fat (triglycerides) to the total density of protons from mobile triglycerides and mobile water and can be measured using multi-echo CSE-MRI with water–fat separation. PDFF might prove to be a useful standardized MR-based biomarker for quantification of fat tissue concentration and may help in the assessment of fracture risk and monitoring therapy in patients with osteoporosis [46–51].

To account for the presence of bone matrix susceptibility effects, CSE-MRI relies on a water–fat model with a single exponential R_2^* decay and aims to simultaneously extract R_2^* and PDFF. There are several confounders in PDFF mapping, such as T_2^*, T_1, and the multispectral nature of fat as well as noise bias, which need to be addressed. Kronthaler et al. have recently shown that R_2^* could be underestimated and quantification errors can occur when using short TEs and a water–fat model with an exponential R_2^* decay model in multi-echo GRE acquisitions [47]. The assessment of bone marrow R_2^* quantification errors was based on a UTE–Dixon acquisition [47]. Thus, UTE–Dixon acquisitions can assist in better understanding MR biophysical signal modeling in tissues, including short-T_2^* signal components.

Conclusion

The basic methods for UTE–Dixon imaging are described using either single or multiple echoes. The technique has been applied to attenuation corrections in PET–MRI and to musculoskeletal imaging. However, UTE–Dixon imaging remains a relatively new research topic with a limited number of methodological and application reports published to date. The major challenge that UTE–Dixon imaging faces in wider adoption is the acquisition of multiple echoes, which is usually associated with increased scan times. Therefore, further developments are needed to accelerate UTE–Dixon imaging using efficient k-space trajectories, minimizing the number of acquired echoes, or combining this with the reconstruction of undersampled acquisitions. In addition, larger clinical studies are needed to evaluate the advantages of UTE–Dixon imaging in clinical applications, especially in the study of short-T_2 tissues in musculoskeletal disease.

Acknowledgments The authors acknowledge the research support from DAAD (Project number: 57514573) and Philips Healthcare.

References

1. Wang K, Yu H, Brittain JH, Reeder SB, Du J. K-space water-fat decomposition with T_2^* estimation and multifrequency fat spectrum modeling for ultrashort echo time imaging. J Magn Reson Imaging. 2010;31(4):1027–34.

2. Chaudhari AS, Sveinsson B, Moran CJ, McWalter EJ, Johnson EM, Zhang T, Gold GE, Hargreaves BA. Imaging and T_2 relaxometry of short-T_2 connective tissues in the knee using ultrashort echo-time double-echo steady-state (UTEDESS). Magn Reson Med. 2017;78(6):2136–48.

3. Jang H, Carl M, Ma Y, Jerban S, Guo T, Zhao W, Chang EY, Du J. Fat suppression for ultrashort echo time imaging using a single-point Dixon method. NMR Biomed. 2019;32(5):e4069.

4. Jang H, Ma Y, Carl M, Jerban S, Chang EY, Du J. Ultrashort echo time cones double echo steady state (UTE-cones-DESS) for rapid morphological imaging of short T_2 tissues. Magn Reson Med. 2021;86(2):881–92.

5. Kronthaler S, Boehm C, Feuerriegel G, Bornert P, Katscher U, Weiss K, Makowski MR, Schwaiger BJ, Gersing AS, Karampinos DC. Assessment of vertebral fractures and edema of the thoraco-lumbar spine based on water-fat and susceptibility-weighted images derived from a single ultra-short echo time scan. Magn Reson Med. 2021;87(4):1771–83.

6. Dixon WT. Simple proton spectroscopic imaging. Radiology. 1984;153(1):189–94.

7. Glover GH. Multipoint Dixon technique for water and fat proton and susceptibility imaging. J Magn Reson Imaging. 1991;1(5):521–30.

8. Glover GH, Schneider E. Three-point Dixon technique for true water/fat decomposition with B_0 inhomogeneity correction. Magn Reson Med. 1991;18(2):371–83.

9. Reeder SB, Wen Z, Yu H, Pineda AR, Gold GE, Markl M, Pelc NJ. Multicoil Dixon chemical species separation with an iterative least-squares estimation method. Magn Reson Med. 2004;51(1):35–45.

10. Diefenbach MN, Liu C, Karampinos DC. Generalized parameter estimation in multi-echo gradient-echo-based chemical species separation. Quant Imaging Med Surg. 2020;10(3):554–67.

11. Ma J. Dixon techniques for water and fat imaging. J Magn Reson Imaging. 2008;28(3):543–58.

12. Skinner TE, Glover GH. An extended two-point Dixon algorithm for calculating separate water, fat, and B_0 images. Magn Reson Med. 1997;37(4):628–30.

13. Kovanlikaya A, Guclu C, Desai C, Becerra R, Gilsanz V. Fat quantification using three-point Dixon technique: in vitro validation. Acad Radiol. 2005;12(5):636–9.

14. Hernando D, Haldar JP, Sutton BP, Ma J, Kellman P, Liang ZP. Joint estimation of water/fat images and field inhomogeneity map. Magn Reson Med. 2008;59(3):571–80.

15. Yu H, Shimakawa A, McKenzie CA, Brodsky E, Brittain JH, Reeder SB. Multiecho water-fat separation and simultaneous R_2^* estimation with multifrequency fat spectrum modeling. Magn Reson Med. 2008;60(5):1122–34.

16. Szumowski J, Coshow WR, Li F, Quinn SF. Phase unwrapping in the three-point Dixon method for fat suppression MR imaging. Radiology. 1994;192(2):555–61.

17. Coombs BD, Szumowski J, Coshow W. Two-point Dixon technique for water-fat signal decomposition with B_0 inhomogeneity correction. Magn Reson Med. 1997;38(6):884–9.

18. Zhi-Pei L. A model-based method for phase unwrapping. IEEE Trans Med Imaging. 1996;15(6):893–7.

19. Song SM-H, Napel S, Pelc NJ, Glover GH. Phase unwrapping of MR phase images using Poisson equation. IEEE Trans Image Process. 1995;4(5):667–76.

20. Diefenbach MN, Ruschke S, Eggers H, Meineke J, Rummeny EJ, Karampinos DC. Improving chemical shift encoding-based water-fat separation based on a detailed consideration of magnetic field contributions. Magn Reson Med. 2018;80(3):990–1004.

21. Yu H, Reeder SB, Shimakawa A, Brittain JH, Pelc NJ. Field map estimation with a region growing scheme for iterative 3-point water-fat decomposition. Magn Reson Med. 2005;54(4):1032–9.

22. Cui C, Wu X, Newell JD, Jacob M. Fat water decomposition using globally optimal surface estimation (GOOSE) algorithm. Magn Reson Med. 2015;73(3):1289–99.

23. Cui C, Shah A, Wu X, Jacob M. A rapid 3D fat–water decomposition method using globally optimal surface estimation (R-GOOSE). Magn Reson Med. 2018;79(4):2401–7.

24. Hernando D, Kellman P, Haldar JP, Liang Z-P. Robust water/fat separation in the presence of large field inhomogeneities using a graph cut algorithm. Magn Reson Med. 2010;63(1):79–90.

25. Boehm C, Diefenbach MN, Makowski MR, Karampinos DC. Improved body quantitative susceptibility mapping by using a variable-layer single-min-cut graph-cut for field-mapping. Magn Reson Med. 2021;85(3):1697–712.

26. Du J, Hamilton G, Takahashi A, Bydder M, Chung CB. Ultrashort echo time spectroscopic imaging (UTESI) of cortical bone. Magn Reson Med. 2007;58(5):1001–9.

27. Diaz E, Chung CB, Bae WC, Statum S, Znamirowski R, Bydder GM, Du J. Ultrashort echo time spectroscopic imaging (UTESI): an efficient method for quantifying bound and free water. NMR Biomed. 2012;25(1):161–8.

28. Su KH, Friel HT, Kuo JW, Al Helo R, Baydoun A, Stehning C, Crisan AN, Traughber MS, Devaraj A, Jordan DW, Qian P, Leisser A, Ellis RJ, Herrmann KA, Avril N, Traughber BJ, Muzic RF Jr. UTE-mDixon-based thorax synthetic CT generation. Med Phys. 2019;46(8):3520–31.

29. Qian P, Zheng J, Zheng Q, Liu Y, Wang T, Al Helo R, Baydoun A, Avril N, Ellis RJ, Friel H, Traughber MS, Devaraj A, Traughber B, Muzic RF. Transforming UTE-mDixon MR abdomen-pelvis images into CT by jointly leveraging prior knowledge and partial supervision. IEEE/ACM Trans Comput Biol Bioinform. 2021;18(1):70–82.

30. Gong K, Han PK, Johnson KA, El Fakhri G, Ma C, Li Q. Attenuation correction using deep learning and integrated UTE/multi-echo Dixon sequence: evaluation in amyloid and tau PET imaging. Eur J Nucl Med Mol Imaging. 2021;48(5):1351–61.

31. Su KH, Hu L, Stehning C, Helle M, Qian P, Thompson CL, Pereira GC, Jordan DW, Herrmann KA, Traughber M, Muzic RF Jr, Traughber BJ. Generation of brain pseudo-CTs using an undersampled, single-acquisition UTE-mDixon pulse sequence and unsupervised clustering. Med Phys. 2015;42(8):4974–86.

32. Leynes AP, Yang J, Shanbhag DD, Kaushik SS, Seo Y, Hope TA, Wiesinger F, Larson PEZ. Hybrid ZTE/Dixon MR-based attenuation correction for quantitative uptake estimation of pelvic lesions in PET/MRI. Med Phys. 2017;44(3):902–13.

33. Yu H, Reeder SB, McKenzie CA, Brau AC, Shimakawa A, Brittain JH, Pelc NJ. Single acquisition water-fat separation: feasibility study for dynamic imaging. Magn Reson Med. 2006;55(2):413–22.

34. Ma J. A single-point Dixon technique for fat-suppressed fast 3D gradient-echo imaging with a flexible echo time. J Magn Reson Imaging. 2008;27(4):881–90.

35. Katscher U, van den Berg CAT. Electric properties tomography: biochemical, physical and technical background, evaluation and clinical applications. NMR Biomed. 2017;30(8):nbm.3729.

36. Kim DH, Choi N, Gho SM, Shin J, Liu C. Simultaneous imaging of in vivo conductivity and susceptibility. Magn Reson Med. 2014;71(3):1144–50.

37. van Lier AL, Brunner DO, Pruessmann KP, Klomp DW, Luijten PR, Lagendijk JJ, van den Berg CA. B1(+) phase mapping at 7 T and its application for in vivo electrical conductivity mapping. Magn Reson Med. 2012;67(2):552–61.

38. Berker Y, Franke J, Salomon A, Palmowski M, Donker HC, Temur Y, Mottaghy FM, Kuhl C, Izquierdo-Garcia D, Fayad ZA, Kiessling F, Schulz V. MRI-based attenuation correction for hybrid PET/MRI systems: a 4-class tissue segmentation technique using a combined ultrashort-echo-time/Dixon MRI sequence. J Nucl Med. 2012;53(5):796–804.

39. Han PK, Horng DE, Gong K, Petibon Y, Kim K, Li Q, Johnson KA, El Fakhri G, Ouyang J, Ma C. MR-based PET attenuation correction using a combined ultrashort echo time/multi-echo Dixon acquisition. Med Phys. 2020;47(7):3064–77.

40. Yu H, Shimakawa A, Hines CD, McKenzie CA, Hamilton G, Sirlin CB, Brittain JH, Reeder SB. Combination of complex-based and magnitude-based multiecho water-fat separation for accurate quantification of fat-fraction. Magn Reson Med. 2011;66(1):199–206.

41. Lombardi AF, Wei Z, Wong J, Carl M, Lee RR, Wallace M, Masuda K, Chang EY, Du J, Ma YJ. High contrast cartilaginous endplate imaging using a 3D adiabatic inversion-recovery-prepared fat-saturated ultrashort echo time (3D IR-FS-UTE) sequence. NMR Biomed. 2021;34(10):e4579.

42. Robson MD, Bydder GM. Clinical ultrashort echo time imaging of bone and other connective tissues. NMR Biomed. 2006;19(7):765–80.

43. Feuerriegel GC, Kronthaler S, Boehm C, Renz M, Leonhardt Y, Gassert F, Foreman SC, Weiss K, Wurm M, Liebig T, Makowski MR, Schwaiger BJ, Karampinos DC, Gersing AS. Diagnostic value of water-fat-separated images and CT-like susceptibility-weighted images extracted from a single ultrashort echo time sequence for the evaluation of vertebral fractures and degenerative changes of the spine. Eur Radiol. 2022;33:1445. https://doi.org/10.1007/s00330-022-09061-2.

44. Kijowski R, Wilson JJ, Liu F. Bicomponent ultrashort echo time T_2^* analysis for assessment of patients with patellar tendinopathy. J Magn Reson Imaging. 2017;46(5):1441–7.

45. Shao H, Chang EY, Pauli C, Zanganeh S, Bae W, Chung CB, Tang G, Du J. UTE bi-component analysis of T_2^* relaxation in articular cartilage. Osteoarthritis Cartilage. 2016;24(2):364–73.

46. Sollmann N, Löffler MT, Kronthaler S, Böhm C, Dieckmeyer M, Ruschke S, Kirschke JS, Carballido-Gamio J, Karampinos DC, Krug R, Baum T. MRI-based quantitative osteoporosis imaging at the spine and femur. J Magn Reson Imaging. 2021;54(1):12–35.

47. Kronthaler S, Diefenbach MN, Boehm C, Zamskiy M, Makowski MR, Baum T, Sollmann N, Karampinos DC. On quantification errors of R_2^* and proton density fat fraction mapping in trabecularized bone marrow in the static dephasing regime. Magn Reson Med. 2022;88(3):1126–39.

48. Ma YJ, Chen Y, Li L, Cai Z, Wei Z, Jerban S, Jang H, Chang EY, Du J. Trabecular bone imaging using a 3D adiabatic inversion recovery prepared ultrashort TE cones sequence at 3T. Magn Reson Med. 2020;83(5):1640–51.

49. Reeder SB, Hu HH, Sirlin CB. Proton density fat-fraction: a standardized MR-based biomarker of tissue fat concentration. J Magn Reson Imaging. 2012;36(5):1011–4.

50. Assessment of fracture risk and its application to screening for postmenopausal osteoporosis. Report of a WHO study group. World Health Organ Tech Rep Ser. 1994;843:1–129.

51. Kuhn JP, Hernando D, Meffert PJ, Reeder S, Hosten N, Laqua R, Steveling A, Ender S, Schroder H, Pillich DT. Proton-density fat fraction and simultaneous R_2^* estimation as an MRI tool for assessment of osteoporosis. Eur Radiol. 2013;23(12):3432–9.

Ultrashort Echo Time Spectroscopic Imaging (UTESI) of Short-T_2 Tissues

16

Jiyo Athertya, James Lo, Chun Zeng, Jerban Saeed, Christine B. Chung, and Jiang Du

Introduction

Chemical shift imaging (CSI) or spectroscopic imaging combines the acquisition of spectral and spatial information in a single scan [1]. Images at a series of resonance frequencies are generated. These provide robust fat–water separation and are tolerant to field inhomogeneity and susceptibility effects. Eliminating fat saturation pulses helps maintain short-T_2 signal intensities by avoiding direct saturation and magnetization transfer effects. Because long-T_2 tissues have narrow spectral peaks and short-T_2 tissues have broad peaks, spectroscopic imaging can create high contrast between short- and long-T_2 tissues at frequencies away from the narrow peaks of long-T_2 species [2]. Spectroscopic imaging also provides quantitative information, including T_2^*, chemical shift, and mobile proton density, which can be used to characterize short-T_2 tissues.

In conventional CSI, spatial information is obtained with phase encoding, which is followed by free induction decay (FID) sampling to generate spectroscopic information. This spatial encoding scheme is time-consuming and makes it challenging to create high-resolution images in realistic times. In addition, a relatively long echo time (TE) (>10 ms) is usually used, which makes it impossible to image short-T_2 tissues directly. To date, two approaches have been proposed to overcome these problems. The first approach, proposed by Gold et al., employs radiofrequency (RF) half-pulse excitations combined with a projection reconstruction (PR) acquisition and variable TEs to generate imaging and spectroscopic information from short-T_2 tissues [2]. A minimum TE of 200 μs was used with 4–8 spectral interleaves and 511 half projections in a total scan time of 8 min with a moderate spatial resolution (voxel size = 1.25 × 1.25 × 5 mm^3). This produced a moderate spectral resolution of 61–120 Hz with a limited bandwidth (BW) coverage of 1330 Hz. Another approach, proposed by Robson et al., is based on the use of a variable TE Cartesian acquisition [3]. The phase encoding steps near the center of the k-space only require small gradient moments, which allows the use of a short TE of 170 μs. The outer regions of the k-space require larger gradient moments and increased TEs. This technique generates spectroscopic images of ^{23}Na and ^{31}P with a low spatial resolution (voxel size = 15 × 12 × 12 mm^3) and a moderate spectral resolution. Both methods provide a spatial resolution that is too low to resolve the fine structure of the deep layers of cartilage or that of menisci and tendons. In addition, both the spectral resolution and bandwidth coverage are limited. Both techniques also have significant time penalties associated with increasing spatial and spectral resolution.

J. Athertya · J. Saeed
Department of Radiology, University of California, San Diego, La Jolla, CA, USA
e-mail: jathertya@health.ucsd.edu; sjerban@health.ucsd.edu

J. Lo
Department of Bioengineering, University of California, San Diego, La Jolla, CA, USA
e-mail: j5lo@health.ucsd.edu

C. Zeng
Department of Radiology, University of California, San Diego, La Jolla, CA, USA

Department of Radiology, the First Affiliated Hospital of Chongqing Medical University, Chongqing, China
e-mail: c3zeng@health.ucsd.edu

C. B. Chung
Department of Radiology, University of California, San Diego, La Jolla, CA, USA

VA San Diego Healthcare System, San Diego, CA, USA
e-mail: cbchung@health.ucsd.edu

J. Du (✉)
Department of Radiology, University of California, San Diego, La Jolla, CA, USA

Department of Bioengineering, University of California, San Diego, La Jolla, CA, USA

VA San Diego Healthcare System, San Diego, CA, USA
e-mail: jiangdu@health.ucsd.edu

J. Du, G. M. Bydder (eds.), *MRI of Short- and Ultrashort-T_2 Tissues*, https://doi.org/10.1007/978-3-031-35197-6_16

It would be of great interest to generate spectroscopic images of the short-T_2 tissues with both high spatial and spectral resolution as well as broad spectral coverage, since short-T_2 tissues show broad spectral responses. Projection reconstruction can be more efficient at achieving high spatial resolution per unit time than Cartesian imaging. In addition, the total scan time can be further reduced through angular undersampling without significant degradation of spatial resolution, as has been widely used with contrast enhanced time-resolved magnetic resonance (MR) angiography [4–6]. Spectral resolution can also be increased by acquiring more images with longer TE delays using multi-echo acquisitions, as is used in spiral spectroscopic imaging [7]. Ultrashort echo time spectroscopic imaging (UTESI) is a versatile method for achieving high-resolution spatial and spectral imaging of short-T_2 tissues [8–11].

The UTESI Pulse Sequence

UTESI uses a combination of highly undersampled interleaved projection reconstruction with multi-echo UTE acquisitions at progressively increasing TEs to achieve high spatial resolution spectroscopic imaging within clinically acceptable scan times [8]. The two-dimensional (2D) UTESI sequence is illustrated in Fig. 16.1. It employs half-pulse excitations with radial mapping of the k-space from the center out, followed by another half-pulse excitation and repeated radial mapping with the polarity of the slice-selective gradient reversed. Data from the two half-pulse excitations are added to produce a single slice-selective radial line of the k-space. This process is typically repeated through 360° in multiple steps (e.g., 511 half projections). The complete set of projections is interleaved into multiple groups of highly undersampled projections, with each group having a progressively increased TE to

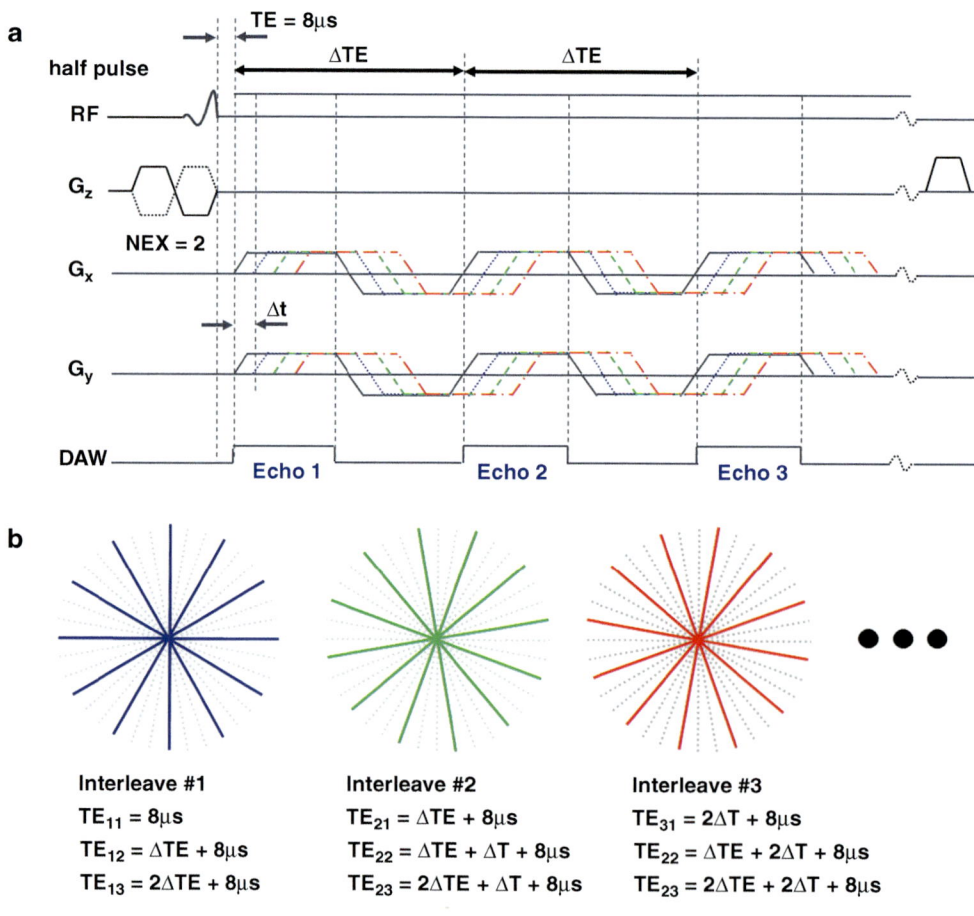

Fig. 16.1 (a) The 2D UTESI sequence. This employs a half-pulse for slice-selective excitation followed by multi-echo variable TE radial sampling with an echo spacing of ΔTE and a series of TE delays (a step size Δt). The UTESI sequence has a minimal achievable TE of 8 μs, enabling detection of short-T_2 species. (b) The data acquisition scheme: sets of half projections are interleaved into multiple groups, with each group sparsely but uniformly covering k-space with TE successively delayed by Δt while the echo spacing ΔTE is kept constant. Here, TE$_{ij}$ refers to the TE for interleave i at echo j. Spectroscopic information is generated through FT of the free induction decay (FID, called echo 1 for convenience) and multiple echo images. The highly undersampled interleaved projection reconstruction (PR) acquisition vastly reduces the scan time while generating streak-free water images since all streaks are shifted to high spectral frequencies. (Reproduced with permission from Du et al. [8])

reduce scan time. With multi-echo acquisitions, all the echoes are simultaneously shifted by Δt while keeping the echo spacing constant at ΔTE. The small number of projections in each group is sparsely but uniformly covered in the sample k-space. The interleaved groups of highly undersampled projections are ordered in such a way that the following three interleaved groups trisect the view angles of the first three; therefore, the high spatial frequency projection data from neighboring interleaves are uniformly spread through the k-space. Images corresponding to each TE are reconstructed from each group of projections, with some high-frequency projection data shared with the neighboring interleaved groups of projections to reduce streak artifacts. The interleaved projections produce oscillating streak artifacts among the multiple echo images, which are shifted to high temporal frequencies after Fourier transformation (FT) in the time domain, leaving streak artifact-free images near the water and fat resonance peaks, which are the regions of principal interest [8].

UTESI Image Reconstruction

In UTESI, the radial projections are highly undersampled and interleaved for each TE. The whole set of projections is interleaved into multiple groups (36–72), with each group at a progressively increased TE delay (Δt). Raw data from each echo are then mapped onto a Cartesian grid using a Kaiser–Bessel kernel and are reconstructed by 2D inverse FT. Spectroscopic images are generated through FT of the multi-echo images. The radial projections can be undersampled to reduce the total scan time. The 2D UTESI sequence is based on radial sampling, which tends to generate streak artifacts. Since the undersampled streaks are in alignment with the half projections, the oscillation pattern of the streaks can be controlled by adjusting the interleaving schedule. For simplicity, let us consider 9 interleaved groups, with each group having 45 projections sparsely but uniformly covering the k-space. We can sample the interleaved groups in the following way: 1, 4, 7, 2, 5, 8, 3, 6, 9. The high-frequency projection data uniformly cover the periphery of the k-space and can be shared to reduce streak artifacts using a tornado filter scheme. Figure 16.2 shows the UTESI images of a rubber band, demonstrating the efficacy of tornado filtering in streak artifact reduction in the time domain. The streaks periodically oscillate between every three groups, simulating a signal with a high temporal frequency. The FT of these multi-echo images shifts all the streaks to high temporal frequencies, leaving streak artifact-free images near the peak resonance frequencies.

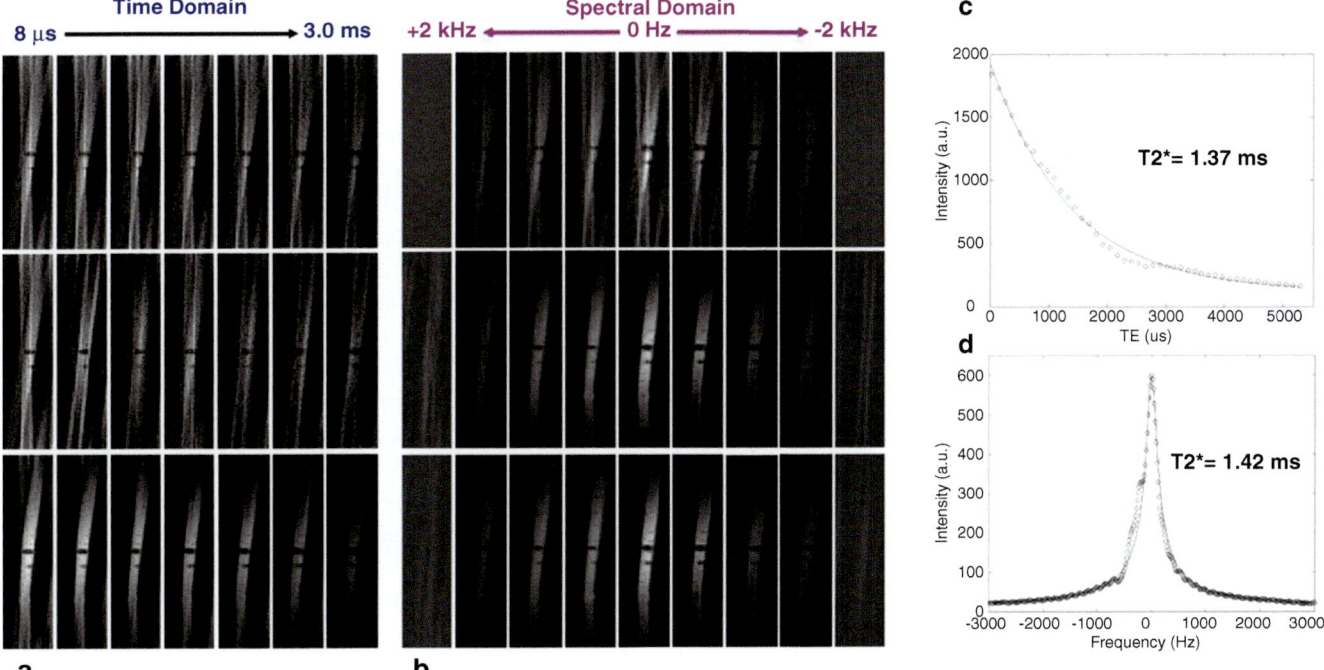

Fig. 16.2 UTESI imaging of a rubber band in the time domain (**a**) and spectral domain (**b**) without projection interleaving (first row), with projection interleaving but without view sharing (second row), and with (third row) view sharing. Streaks are reduced using the third approach in the time domain. In the spectral domain, streaks are shifted to high spectral frequencies, resulting in streak-free peak spectral images for both the second and third approaches. Similar T$_2$* values were derived from exponential fitting in the time domain and Lorentzian line shape fitting in the spectral domain (**c**). (Reproduced with permission from Du et al. [8])

UTESI Signal Processing

Following the UTESI data acquisition, raw data are transferred to a Linux computer for offline image reconstruction. The projection data are first re-gridded onto a 512 × 512 matrix before two-dimensional FT. These complex images with 180–864 TEs are zero-padded to 1024 in the time domain, and Fourier-transformed, yielding a spectroscopic imaging series with a matrix size of 512 × 512 × 1024. A complex image at time t can be described by the following equation:

$$s(\bar{r},t) = s_0(\bar{r})\exp(i2\pi f_0 t)\exp(-t/T_2^*) \tag{16.1}$$

where f_0 is the resonance frequency (for simplicity, a single component is assumed for each pixel), r is the position in image space, and $s_0(r)$ is the effective observable proton density distribution. Spectroscopic images can be generated through FT in the time domain, as shown in the following equation:

$$S(\bar{r},f) = \int_0^\infty s(\bar{r},t)\exp(-i2\pi ft)dt = \frac{s_0(\bar{r})\left[\dfrac{1}{\pi T_2^*} - i2(f-f_0)\right]}{\left(\dfrac{1}{\pi T_2^*}\right)^2 + 4(f-f_0)^2} \tag{16.2}$$

Typically, the real part in Eq. 16.2 is used for quantification, which is a Lorentzian line shape expressed by the following equation:

$$\text{Real}\left[S(\bar{r},f)\right] = \frac{\text{Real}\left[s_0(\bar{r})\right]\times\left(\dfrac{1}{\pi T_2^*}\right) + \text{Imag}\left[s_0(\bar{r})\right]\times 2(f-f_0)}{\left(\dfrac{1}{\pi T_2^*}\right)^2 + 4(f-f_0)^2} \tag{16.3}$$

Ideally, a real spectrum follows the Lorentzian line shape with the imaginary part of $s_0(r)$ being zero. However, $s_0(r)$ is typically complex due to eddy currents, B_0 field inhomogeneity, susceptibility, motion, and other factors. The phase shift results in spectral distortion, which must be corrected using algorithms such as principal component analysis or reference deconvolution [12, 13]. However, this process may be complicated with the UTESI sequence, which is more susceptible to eddy currents than conventional CSI sequences. An imperfect correction of phase errors may distort the real spectrum and thus produce significant errors in the quantification of T_2^* and proton density. Furthermore, UTESI data contain many spectra (typically 512 × 512 = 262,144) and may require excessively long processing times. The phase shift resulting from complex MR images can be avoided using a magnitude spectrum as described by Eq. 16.4, which is immune to phase errors, and significantly simplifies the process of quantification:

$$\left|S(\bar{r},f)\right| = \frac{\left|s_0(\bar{r})\right|}{\sqrt{\left(\dfrac{1}{\pi T_2^*}\right)^2 + 4(f-f_0)^2}} \tag{16.4}$$

A magnitude spectrum described by Eq. 16.4 is no longer Lorentzian and has a broader line width or full width at half maximum (FWHM) than a real spectrum. Magnitude spectra offer a significant advantage over real spectra in terms of robustness and simplicity, and the corresponding line broadening is considered acceptable for short-T_2 (broad) spectral processing.

Figure 16.3 shows selected UTESI images of three water tubes at a series of resonance frequencies. The signal from the long-T_2^* bottle rapidly drops away from that at the peak resonance frequency, whereas the short-T_2^* bottle maintains a higher signal over a broader spectral range. The spectrum from a small region of interest (ROI) is drawn in each bottle. T_2^* was measured with modified Lorentzian line shape fitting of the magnitude UTESI spectrum and mono-exponential signal decay fitting of images at different TEs. Both techniques showed T_2^* values of around 0.52 ms, 2.07 ms, and 14.41 ms, respectively. Image contrast between the short-T_2 ($T_2^* = 2.07$ ms) and long-T_2 bottles ($T_2^* = 14.41$ ms) had a negative value of −5.12 at the spectral peak, and this gradually increased to 11.78 at ±88 Hz and then dropped away with further increase of the off-resonance frequency. This demonstrated that high contrast between short- and long-T_2 components could be generated at off-peak resonance frequencies.

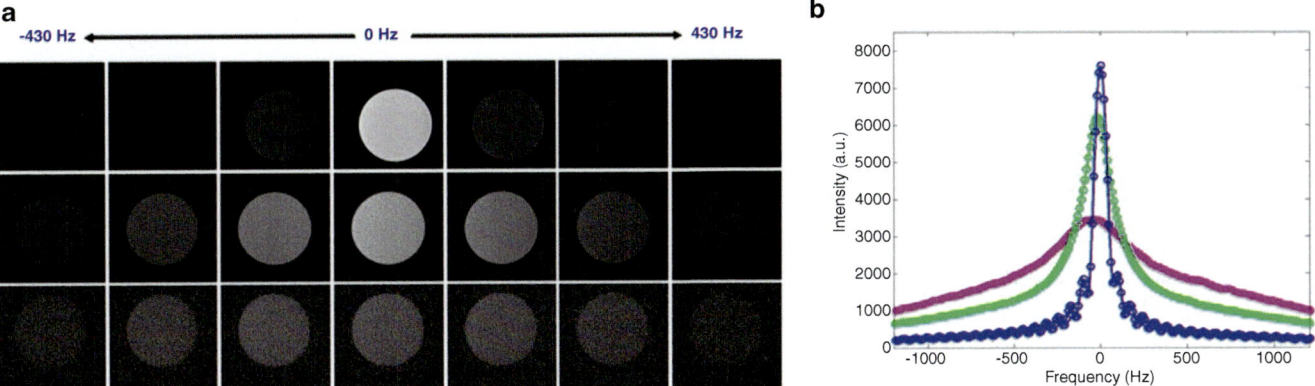

Fig. 16.3 UTESI images of water tubes doped with different levels of $MnCl_2$ with T_2*s of around 14.4 ms (first row), 2.07 ms (second row), and 0.52 ms (third row) (**a**). The UTESI spectrum of three water tubes (**b**). This shows that high contrast can be achieved for short-T_2 species at off-resonance frequencies where long-T_2 species have much lower signals

UTESI Image Quantification

Information on T_2*, chemical shift, mobile proton density, and frequency shift due to susceptibility effects can be derived from UTE-based spectroscopic images [8–11]. Details for each of these quantifications are provided below.

T_2* Quantification

There are two ways to quantify T_2*. The first approach is exponential signal decay fitting of the time-domain UTESI images at different TEs. The second approach is line shape fitting of magnitude UTESI spectra using Eq. 16.4. We validated the accuracy of magnitude spectra for T_2* quantification through numerical simulation and a rubber band phantom study. A phase error of 1 was introduced to an FID curve. A significant distortion was observed in the real spectrum, whereas the magnitude spectrum showed no distortion. FIDs of the rubber band can be generated on a clinical scanner using a short hard pulse (4 μs) with a low flip angle of 1.4° (due to RF power limitations), and a reference standard T_2* value can be calculated for comparison.

A meniscus sample was harvested from a cadaveric human knee specimen, and all soft tissues were removed. The sample was placed in a plastic container filled with phosphate-buffered saline (PBS) at the center of a 3-inch coil. Figure 16.4 shows UTESI images of the meniscus in the spectral domain. The imaging field of view (FOV) of 10 cm, readout of 512, and 2-mm slice thickness resulted in a high spatial resolution of $0.2 \times 0.2 \times 2.0$ mm³ (acquired voxel size) and excellent depiction of the internal meniscus structure [9]. Other acquisition parameters included: repetition time (TR) =150 ms, minimal TE = 8 μs, flip angle = 60°, BW = ±62.5 kHz, projections = 2025 (interleaved into 45

groups with a TE delay of 200 μs per interleave), and total scan time = 10 min. The corresponding exponential signal decay curve and spectra from a small ROI are also shown. There are some Gibbs ringing artifacts at high spectral frequencies, which can be suppressed by increasing the spectral resolution or low-pass filtering. The latter approach is used in conventional spectroscopy; however, this filtering leads to line broadening and increases errors in T_2 quantification. Line filtering was not used in our analysis. Excellent line shape fitting was achieved, providing a T_2* of 3.69 ± 0.16 ms, which was close to, but slightly longer than, the value of 3.58 ± 0.13 ms derived from exponential signal decay fitting.

Chemical Shift

A chemical shift, such as that from fat, can be directly quantified from UTESI images. A clinical single-voxel spectroscopic (point resolved spectroscopy (PRESS)) technique was used as the gold standard for evaluating the accuracy of UTESI spectroscopy with a uniform phantom containing pure plant oil [14]. Our results showed that the fat peak is typically shifted around −440 Hz away from the water peak, as expected at 3 T. Figure 16.5 shows axial UTESI images of the Achilles tendon with a 3-inch coil for signal reception. The imaging FOV of 10 cm, readout of 512, and 2-mm slice thickness produced a high spatial resolution of $0.2 \times 0.2 \times 2.0$ mm³ voxel size and provided excellent depiction of the tendon structure. The fat peak was shifted 476 Hz away from the water peak, providing robust fat–water separation. A high signal-to-noise ratio (SNR) was achieved for the Achilles tendon without signal degradation due to direct saturation or magnetization transfer, which is associated with fat saturation and preparation pulses. The water and fat

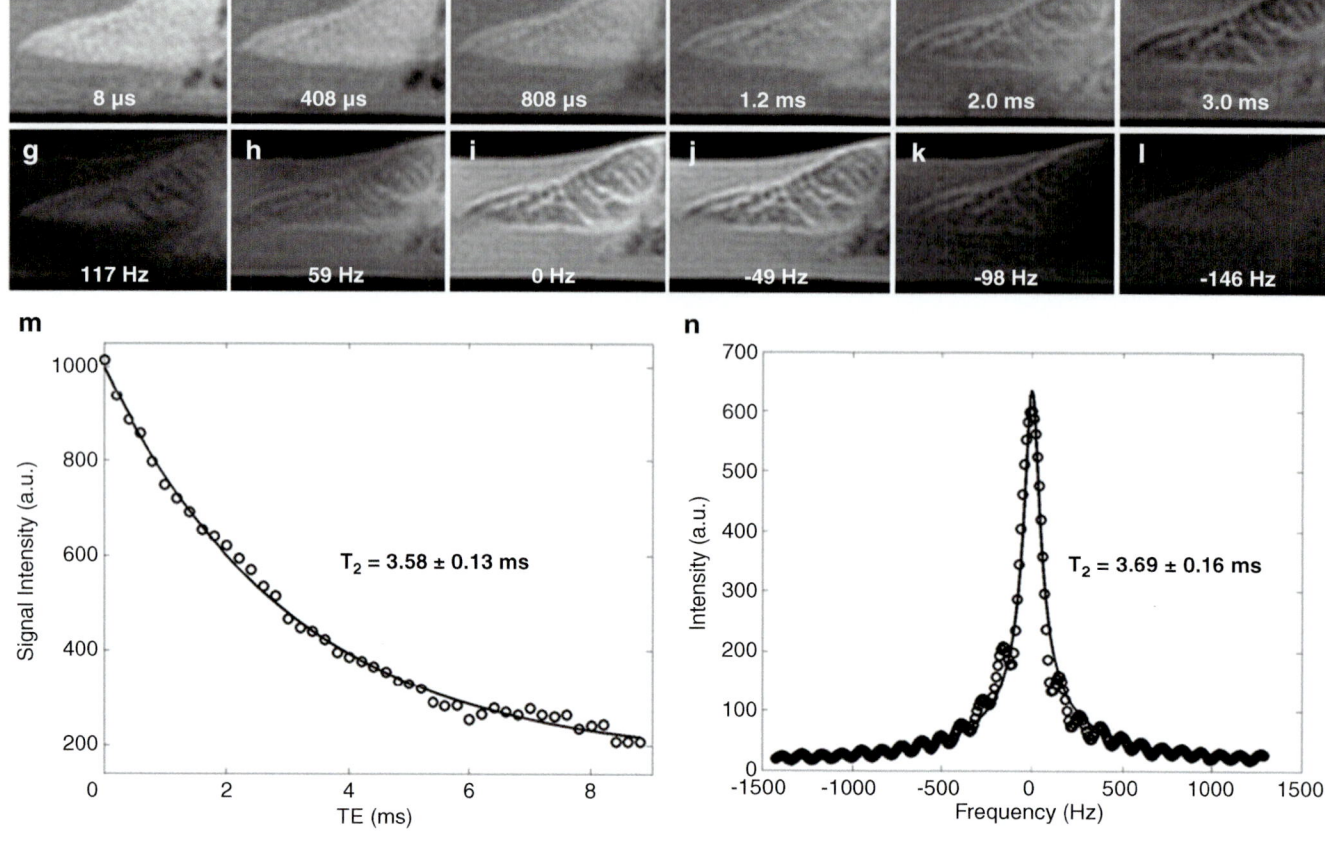

Fig. 16.4 Selected UTESI images of a meniscus sample in the time domain (**a–f**) and spectral domain (**g–l**). This shows excellent depiction of the meniscus structure with a high spectral resolution of 29 Hz and a broad spectral bandwidth overage of 5 kHz. T_2^* estimation of the meniscus sample using exponential signal decay fitting of the UTE images at variable TEs and line shape fitting of the magnitude spectrum show comparable results of 3.58 ± 0.13 ms (**m**) and 3.69 ± 0.16 ms (**n**), respectively. (Reproduced with permission from Du et al. [9])

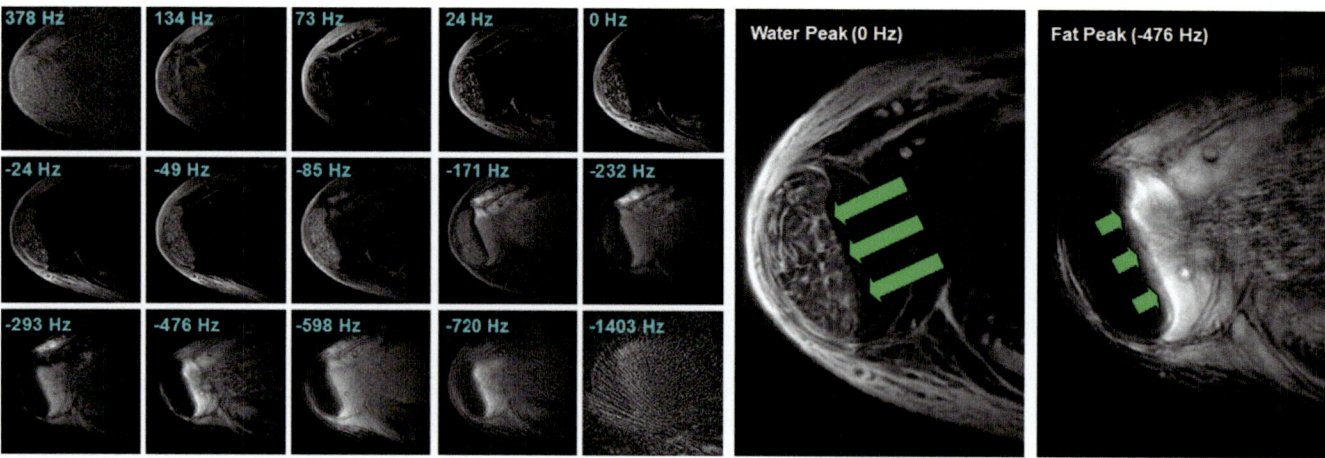

Fig. 16.5 Selected UTESI images of a cadaveric human ankle in the axial plane. This shows excellent depiction of the Achilles tendon (long arrows), including the fascicular pattern. Fat signals (short arrows) peaked at −476 Hz, and robust fat–water separation was achieved without tendon signal degradation

peaks of UTESI images of the tensile tendon are also shown. The fascicular pattern within the tensile tendon is depicted with high spatial resolution, high signal, and excellent contrast (robust fat–water separation).

Proton Density

Quantifying water content may provide a useful means of assessing tissue during aging, progression of osteoarthritis,

and response to treatment. Water content can be evaluated by comparing the UTESI spectral area of the short-T$_2$ tissue to a known water concentration reference sample. Relative water content and the resonance frequency shift due to bulk susceptibility can also be evaluated. Figure 16.6 shows UTESI imaging in a 29-year-old healthy volunteer. Both fat and muscle signals are well suppressed by the adiabatic inversion preparation pulse [15]. The cortical bone signal is high over a broad spectral range, consistent with its short T$_2$*. Oscillating streak artifacts in the time domain were shifted to

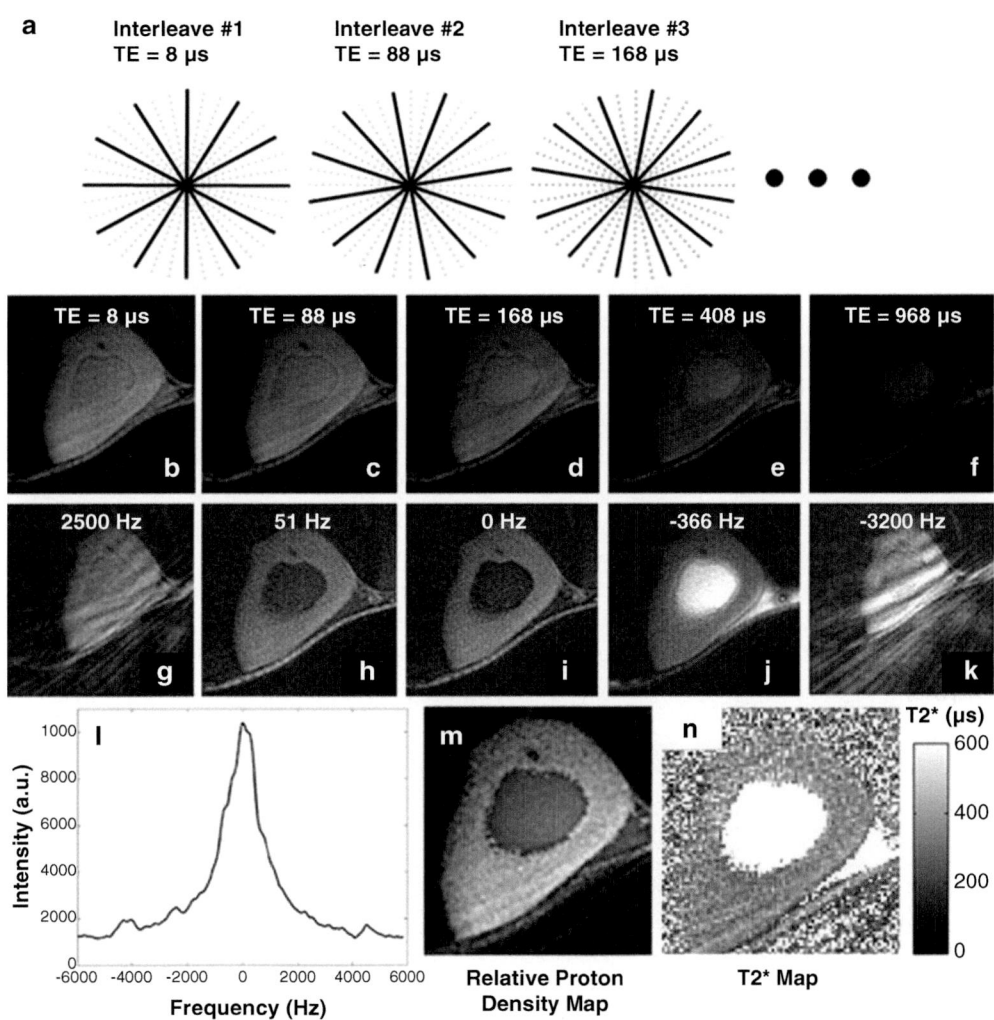

Fig. 16.6 UTESI. This employs highly undersampled interleaved variable TE acquisitions for fast high-resolution spectroscopic imaging. Each group of projections uniformly covers k-space with TE successively delayed by a selected time (e.g., 80 μs) (**a**). Selected UTESI images of a 29-year-old volunteer are displayed in the time domain with TEs of 8 μs (**b**), 88 μs (**c**), 168 μs (**d**), 408 μs (**e**), and 968 μs (**f**). A sliding window reconstruction algorithm is used to share high spatial frequency projection data among neighbor groups to reduce streak artifacts and in the spectrum domain with frequency offsets of 2500 Hz (**g**), 51 Hz (**h**), 0 Hz (**i**), −366 Hz (**j**), and −3200 Hz (**k**). Undersampling

streaks are shifted to high spectral frequencies, leaving streak-free water peak (**i**) and fat peak (**j**) images. An adiabatic inversion pulse was used to suppress long-T$_2$ water and fat signals. An UTE spectrum of a single pixel from the cortical bone (**l**), relative water proton density map (**m**), and T$_2$* map (**n**) are also displayed. Relative water content was calculated as the water peak area by fitting each spectrum using a modified Lorentzian line shape function, which also provides pixel-based T$_2$* values ranging from 300 to 500 μs. (Reproduced with permission from Du et al. [8])

high frequencies in the spectral domain, resulting in almost streak artifact-free images around the bone at on-resonance frequencies. Figure 16.6l–n shows the bone spectrum from a single pixel (l), relative water distribution (m), and T_2^* map (n). T_2^* values were derived through line shape fitting of the magnitude spectrum from each voxel and ranged from 300 to 500 μs. The UTESI sequence can generate spectroscopic images for many short-T_2 tissues, including the Achilles tendon, menisci, and deep cartilage [8–11]. The technique provides short-T_2 images with high spatial resolution, moderate spectral resolution, and minor streak artifacts in clinically acceptable scan times.

Bulk Susceptibility

Resonance frequency shifts due to bulk susceptibility are well known for bone and tendon [16, 17]. Wehrli et al. showed that bone has a resonance frequency shift of up to 2 ppm due to bulk magnetic susceptibility [17]. These authors' quantification was based on a powdered bone sample study using a small-bore spectrometer with 1-hour or longer scan time. UTESI can directly evaluate the bulk susceptibility-induced resonance frequency shift on a clinical scanner. Figure 16.7 shows an example using this approach with the following acquisition parameters: FOV = 16 cm, TR = 75 ms, TE = 8 μs, flip angle = 60°, BW = ±62.5 kHz, readout matrix = 128 × 128, projections = 2025 (interleaved into 45 groups with a TE delay of 80 μs per interleave), slice thickness = 8 mm, and scan time = 5 min. The UTESI sequence provides high-resolution and high contrast images of the tibia in a total scan time of only 5 min. Bone spectra, water maps, and T_2^* maps can be generated. Absolute water content maps can also be generated by comparing the spectral area of bone with that of a water phantom.

Fiber-Dependent Frequency Shift

Biological tissues may contain different groups of collagen fibers with distinct microstructures. For example, the knee joint meniscus consists of four major architectural subdivisions: the main body, the surface layer, the lamellar layer, and the cartilage-like inner portion [18–20]. The main body includes two major structural components: circumferentially oriented fascicles and radially oriented tie fibers. The surface layer is a group of meshwork fibers that cover meniscal surfaces. The lamellar layer has peripheral radially oriented fibers with more loosely organized collagen fibril bundles beneath the superficial network. The inner portion possesses similar, but not identical, traits to articular cartilage [20]. This highly organized fiber structure leads to strong dipole–dipole interactions and, subsequently, a short T_2 [21]. The organized system also affects the resonance frequency of each group of fibers. Figure 16.8 shows UTESI images of a cadaveric human meniscus sample in a plastic container filled with saline. UTESI depicts the internal fiber structure of the meniscus with high spatial and moderate spectral resolution. The radial, lamellar, and circumferential fibers have different T_2s and slightly different resonance frequency shifts due to susceptibility effects, which may be helpful in the evaluation of early meniscal degeneration.

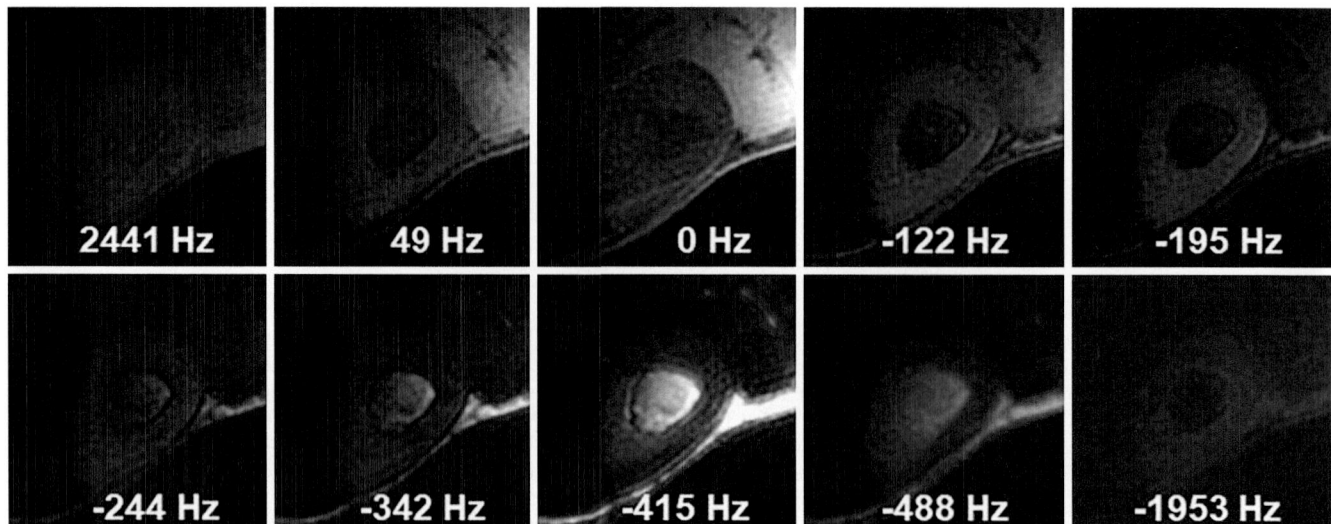

Fig. 16.7 UTESI imaging of the tibia in a 35-year-old healthy volunteer. Long-T_2 water and fat signals were suppressed using a long-duration 90° pulse followed by gradient dephasing. This shows clear definition of the cortical bone with a shift of −195 Hz relative to the muscle peak due to its greater diamagnetic susceptibility. (Reproduced with permission from Du et al. [8])

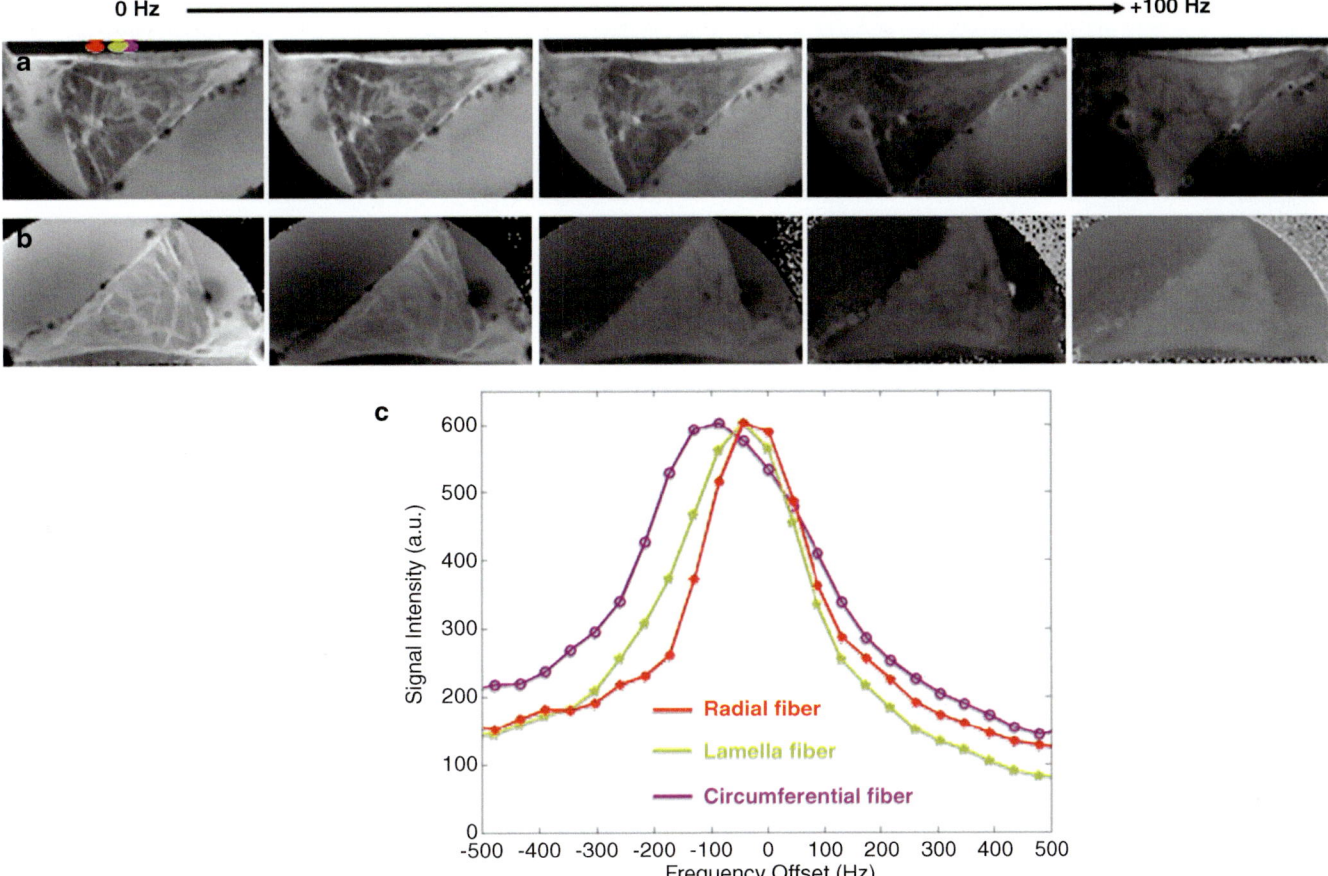

Fig. 16.8 Selected magnitude (**a**) and phase images (**b**) from UTESI imaging of a cadaveric human meniscus sample. The internal fiber structure is depicted with a high spatial and moderate spectral resolution. The radial, lamellar, and circumferential fibers display different FWHM or T_2 values and resonance frequency shifts as shown in panel (**c**)

Bicomponent T_2^* Analysis

Biological tissues usually contain multiple water components with distinct T_2 and/or T_2^* relaxation times and relative fractions [22]. Multicomponent T_2 fitting based on data acquired with the Carl–Purcell–Meiboom–Gill (CPMG) sequences is an effective method for separating the different water components [22–25]. However, multicomponent fitting is sensitive to the image SNR, the number of independent components, the minimum TE, the number of echoes, and the separation of the T_2 values [23]. Furthermore, CPMG sequences typically have initial TEs of 10 ms or longer on whole-body clinical MR scanners. These TEs are generally too long to image and quantify the fast-relaxing components found in a variety of biological tissues [26–28]. The UTESI sequence addresses these challenges by providing a large number of different TE images in a time-efficient manner [8–11]. It is significantly faster than the regular T_2^* mapping based on UTE acquisitions at progressively increasing TEs. The large number of different TE images can significantly reduce fitting errors, especially in bicomponent T_2^* fitting of bound and free water T_2^*s and relative fractions [29]. The

simulation results by Anastasiou and Hall suggest that the lower bounds increase dramatically when the T_2 values of the two components approach each other [30]. Our model considers only two components, the bound and free water components, with about an order of magnitude difference in their T_2^* values. The UTESI bicomponent T_2^* fitting model combines a short minimal TE, a large number of different echo images, and only two components with distinct T_2^* values, and thereby provides more reliable bound and free water evaluation. Figure 16.9 shows UTESI images of a bovine femur segment, which offers a relatively high SNR of 56 at a nominal TE of 8 µs. Bicomponent fitting of the UTESI images demonstrated an ultrashort T_2^* of 0.35 ± 0.01 ms and a longer T_2^* of 2.25 ± 0.02 ms with fractions of 75.7% and 24.3%, respectively. Most bone signal is from the ultrashort-T_2^* component or bound water. The fitting confidence is high in bicomponent T_2^* fitting as evidenced by the small fitting errors, largely because of the large number of different echo images generated by the UTESI sequence. Conventional clinical MRI sequences cannot detect signal from bound or free water in bovine bone because of their extremely short T_2^*s.

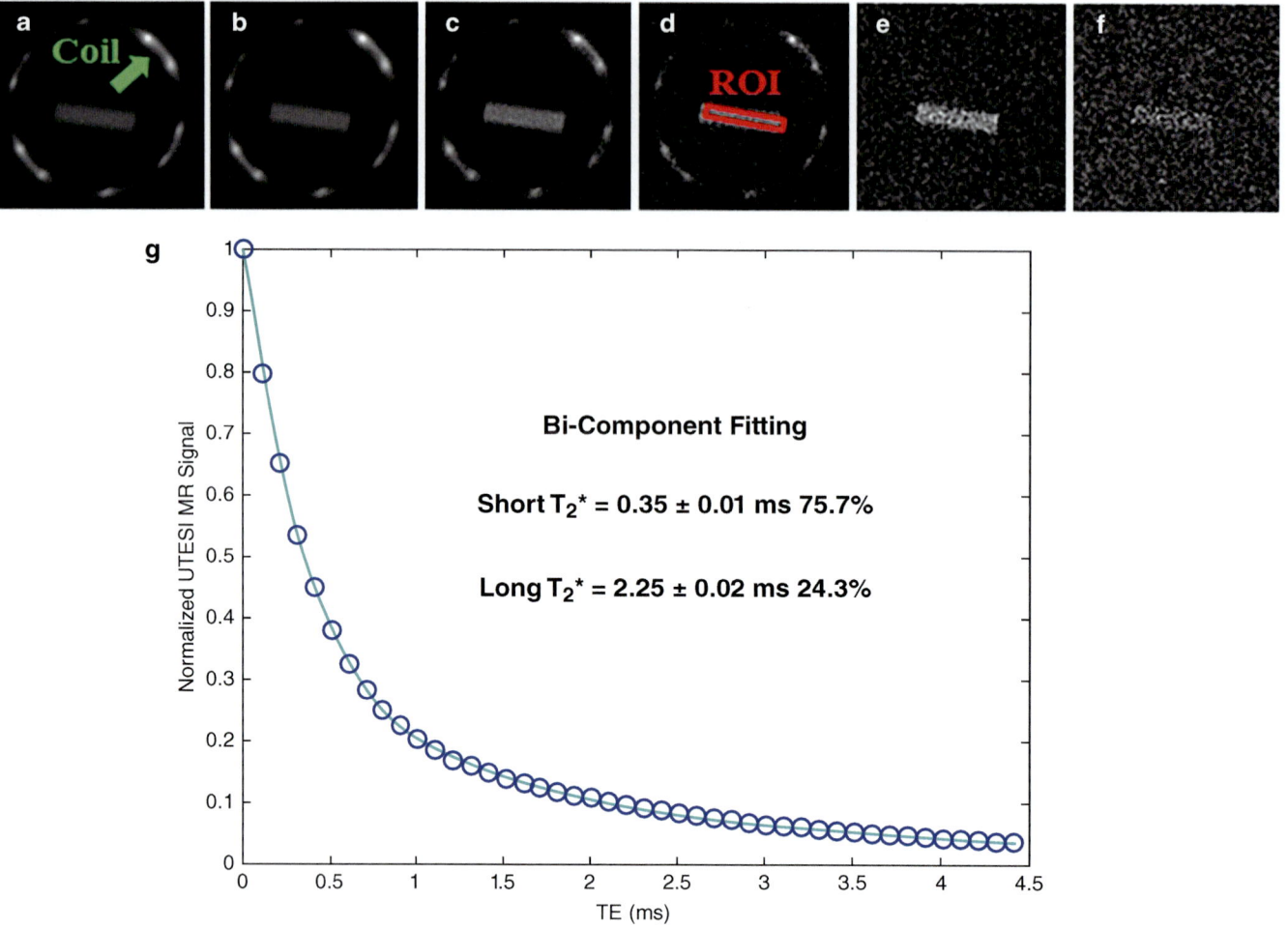

Fig. 16.9 UTESI images of a bovine femur segment (**a–f**) and bicomponent fitting of the UTESI images (**g**). The fitting shows an ultrashort T_2^* of 0.35 ± 0.01 ms and a long T_2^* of 2.25 ± 0.02 ms with fractions of 75.7% and 24.3%, respectively. (Reproduced with permission from Diaz et al. [29])

Conclusions

Spectroscopic imaging of short-T_2 tissues in the musculoskeletal (MSK) system can be performed with the UTESI sequence, which employs a multi-slice, multi-echo UTE acquisition combined with an interleaved variable TE acquisition scheme. This technique is time-efficient and uses undersampling without producing streak artifacts in water or fat images. The method provides images of short-T_2 tissues with a high spatial resolution and moderate spectral resolution as well as T_2^* estimation and robust fat–water separation in a single scan. It also provides a way of assessing bulk susceptibility effects in short-T_2 tissues in vivo using clinical MR systems. The UTESI sequence allows quantitative measurement of fiber-dependent frequency shifts in musculoskeletal tissues such as the meniscus and tendons. The time-domain UTESI images can be used for bicomponent T_2^* modeling of bound and free water components in ultrashort-T_2 tissues such as cortical bone. The broad range of

TEs and the large number of different echo images permit robust bicomponent fitting with significantly reduced quantification errors compared to conventional multicomponent T_2 or T_2^* analysis. Clinical applications of the UTESI technique in musculoskeletal disease remain to be investigated in larger studies.

References

1. Brown TR, Kincaid BM, Ugurbil K. NMR chemical shift imaging in three dimensions. Proc Natl Acad Sci U S A. 1982;79(11):3523–6.
2. Gold GE, Pauly JM, Macovski A, Herfkens RJ. MR spectroscopic imaging of collagen: tendons and knee menisci. Magn Reson Med. 1995;34(5):647–54.
3. Robson MD, Tyler DJ, Neubauer S. Ultrashort TE chemical shift imaging (UTE-CSI). Magn Reson Med. 2005;53(2):267–74.
4. Peters DC, Korosec FR, Grist TM, Block WF, Holden JE, Vigen KK, et al. Undersampled projection reconstruction applied to MR angiography. Magn Reson Med. 2000;43(1):91–101.
5. Du J, Carroll TJ, Brodsky E, Lu A, Grist TM, Mistretta CA, et al. Contrast-enhanced peripheral magnetic resonance

angiography using time-resolved vastly undersampled isotropic projection reconstruction. J Magn Reson Imaging. 2004;20(5):894–900.

6. Du J, Carroll TJ, Wagner HJ, Vigen K, Fain SB, Block WF, et al. Time-resolved, undersampled projection reconstruction imaging for high-resolution CE-MRA of the distal runoff vessels. Magn Reson Med. 2002;48(3):516–22.

7. Hiba B, Faure B, Lamalle L, Decorps M, Ziegler A. Out-and-in spiral spectroscopic imaging in rat brain at 7 T. Magn Reson Med. 2003;50(6):1127–33.

8. Du J, Hamilton G, Takahashi A, Bydder M, Chung CB. Ultrashort echo time spectroscopic imaging (UTESI) of cortical bone. Magn Reson Med. 2007;58(5):1001–9.

9. Du J, Takahashi AM, Chung CB. Ultrashort TE spectroscopic imaging (UTESI): application to the imaging of short T$_2$ relaxation tissues in the musculoskeletal system. J Magn Reson Imaging. 2009;29(2):412–21.

10. Wang K, Du J, O'Halloran R, Fain S, Kecskemeti S, Wieben O, et al. Ultrashort TE spectroscopic imaging (UTESI) using complex highly-constrained backprojection with local reconstruction (HYPR LR). Magn Reson Med. 2009;62(1):127–34.

11. Du J, Chiang AJ, Chung CB, Statum S, Znamirowski R, Takahashi A, et al. Orientational analysis of the Achilles tendon and enthesis using an ultrashort echo time spectroscopic imaging sequence. Magn Reson Imaging. 2010;28(2):178–84.

12. de Graaf AA, van Dijk JE, Bovee WM. QUALITY: quantification improvement by converting lineshapes to the Lorentzian type. Magn Reson Med. 1990;13(3):343–57.

13. Stoyanova R, Brown TR. NMR spectral quantitation by principal component analysis. III. A generalized procedure for determination of lineshape variations. J Magn Reson. 2002;154(2):163–75.

14. Bottomley PA. Spatial localization in NMR spectroscopy in vivo. Ann N Y Acad Sci. 1987;508:333–48.

15. Du J, Carl M, Bydder M, Takahashi A, Chung CB, Bydder GM. Qualitative and quantitative ultrashort echo time (UTE) imaging of cortical bone. J Magn Reson. 2010;207(2):304–11.

16. Krasnosselskaia LV, Fullerton GD, Dodd SJ, Cameron IL. Water in tendon: orientational analysis of the free induction decay. Magn Reson Med. 2005;54(2):280–8.

17. Wehrli FW, Song HK, Saha PK, Wright AC. Quantitative MRI for the assessment of bone structure and function. NMR Biomed. 2006;19(7):731–64.

18. Petersen W, Tillmann B. Collagenous fibril texture of the human knee joint menisci. Anat Embryol (Berl). 1998;197(4):317–24.

19. Andrews SH, Rattner JB, Abusara Z, Adesida A, Shrive NG, Ronsky JL. Tie-fibre structure and organization in the knee menisci. J Anat. 2014;224(5):531–7.

20. Makris EA, Hadidi P, Athanasiou KA. The knee meniscus: structure-function, pathophysiology, current repair techniques, and prospects for regeneration. Biomaterials. 2011;32(30):7411–31.

21. Du J, Carl M, Diaz E, Takahashi A, Han E, Szeverenyi NM, et al. Ultrashort TE T$_1$rho (UTE T$_1$rho) imaging of the Achilles tendon and meniscus. Magn Reson Med. 2010;64(3):834–42.

22. Graham SJ, Stanchev PL, Bronskill MJ. Criteria for analysis of multicomponent tissue T$_2$ relaxation data. Magn Reson Med. 1996;35(3):370–8.

23. Saab G, Thompson RT, Marsh GD. Multicomponent T$_2$ relaxation of in vivo skeletal muscle. Magn Reson Med. 1999;42(1):150–7.

24. Whittall KP, MacKay AL, Graeb DA, Nugent RA, Li DK, Paty DW. In vivo measurement of T$_2$ distributions and water contents in normal human brain. Magn Reson Med. 1997;37(1):34–43.

25. Reiter DA, Lin PC, Fishbein KW, Spencer RG. Multicomponent T$_2$ relaxation analysis in cartilage. Magn Reson Med. 2009;61(4):803–9.

26. Biswas R, Bae W, Diaz E, Masuda K, Chung CB, Bydder GM, et al. Ultrashort echo time (UTE) imaging with bi-component analysis: bound and free water evaluation of bovine cortical bone subject to sequential drying. Bone. 2012;50(3):749–55.

27. Du J, Diaz E, Carl M, Bae W, Chung CB, Bydder GM. Ultrashort echo time imaging with bicomponent analysis. Magn Reson Med. 2012;67(3):645–9.

28. Kijowski R, Wilson JJ, Liu F. Bicomponent ultrashort echo time T$_2$* analysis for assessment of patients with patellar tendinopathy. J Magn Reson Imaging. 2017;46(5):1441–7.

29. Diaz E, Chung CB, Bae WC, Statum S, Znamirowski R, Bydder GM, et al. Ultrashort echo time spectroscopic imaging (UTESI): an efficient method for quantifying bound and free water. NMR Biomed. 2012;25(1):161–8.

30. Anastasiou A, Hall LD. Optimisation of T$_2$ and M0 measurements of bi-exponential systems. Magn Reson Imaging. 2004;22(1):67–80.

UTE Phase Imaging

Michael Carl, Maggie Fung, Graeme M. Bydder, and Jiang Du

Introduction

In typical clinical gradient echo (GRE) or spin echo (SE) magnetic resonance imaging (MRI) with echo times (TEs) of the order of several milliseconds, short-T_2 tissues such as the tendons ($T_2 \approx 2$ ms), menisci ($T_2 \approx 4$–10 ms), ligaments ($T_2 \approx 4$–10 ms), and cortical bone ($T_2 \approx 0.5$ ms) appear as extremely low or zero signal intensity structures [1–5]. By acquiring the free induction decay (FID) of the MR signal, ultrashort echo time (UTE) imaging using a radial center-out k-space trajectory can capture these short-T_2 signals and produce magnitude images, which are usually reconstructed from re-gridded k-space data. In the particular case of UTE imaging, TE is defined as the time between the end of the radiofrequency (RF) pulse and the beginning of the readout gradient [6]. This nominal TE can be as short as a few to tens of milliseconds.

M. Carl (✉)
GE Healthcare, San Diego, CA, USA
e-mail: Michael.Carl@ge.com

M. Fung
GE Healthcare, New York, NY, USA
e-mail: Maggie.Fung@med.ge.com

G. M. Bydder
Department of Radiology, University of California, San Diego, La Jolla, CA, USA

Mātai Medical Research Institute, Tairāwhiti Gisborne, New Zealand
e-mail: gbydder@health.ucsd.edu

J. Du
Department of Radiology, University of California, San Diego, La Jolla, CA, USA

Department of Bioengineering, University of California, San Diego, La Jolla, CA, USA

VA San Diego Healthcare System, San Diego, CA, USA
e-mail: jiangdu@health.ucsd.edu

Phase imaging is an important source of contrast when studying the brain, body, and musculoskeletal systems. GRE sequences are typically used with TEs of 10–40 ms to allow time for appreciable phase evolution [7–9]. UTE imaging employs much shorter TEs to detect short-T_2 signals, limiting the time available to develop significant phase differences. Still, surprisingly, high phase contrast can be achieved with UTE sequences using TEs far shorter than those previously used for susceptibility-weighted imaging (SWI) [7–9].

Theory

With a standard GRE sequence, TE is a well defined quantity, starting at the center of the RF excitation pulse and ending at the center of the data acquisition window (DAQ), where $k = 0$ (see Fig. 17.1a). The phase evolution during a GRE sequence (Φ_{TE}) of a spin with off-resonance frequency $\omega_{off} = 2\pi f_{off}$ is simply given by

$$\Phi_{TE} = \omega_{off}\,\text{TE} \tag{17.1}$$

With a nominal TE of tens of microseconds, little or no phase evolution or phase contrast would be expected in UTE imaging. However, with a UTE sequence (see Fig. 17.1b), the nominal TE does not include the time available for phase evolution during excitation and readout. The phase accrual during the RF pulse (Φ_{RF}) and data acquisition (Φ_{DAQ}) need to be included. The combined phase in the final MR image, therefore, contains contributions from all three sources [10]:

$$\Phi = \Phi_{RF} + \Phi_{TE} + \Phi_{DAQ} = \Phi_{RF} + \omega_{off} \cdot TE + \Phi_{DAQ} \tag{17.2}$$

The theoretical equations are derived in detail in Carl and Jing-Tzyh [10] and Chiang et al. [11] and are summarized for three-dimensional (3D) UTE in Table 17.1 where, using a hard RF pulse of duration τ and amplitude B_1: $\omega_1 = \gamma B_1$, $\omega_2 = \sqrt{\omega_1^2 + \omega_{off}^2}$, G is the readout gradient strength, T_{ramp} is the readout gradient ramp-up duration, and L is the size of the structure/phantom. Although quantification is not the

Fig. 17.1 Pulse sequence diagrams: (**a**) GRE and (**b**) UTE. The defined TE is shown in both cases. (Reproduced with permission from Carl and Jing-Tzyh [10])

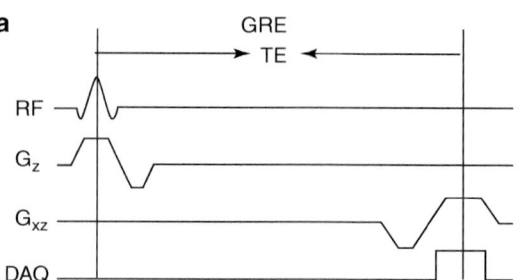

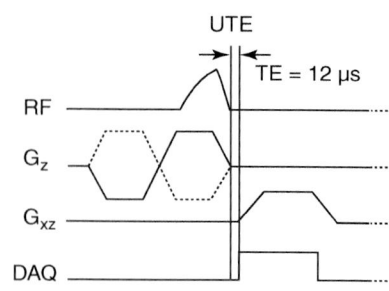

Table 17.1 Theoretical MR image phase accrual during the RF excitation and the data acquisition portion of UTE imaging

	RF (hard pulse)	DAQ
3D	$\Phi_{RF} = \operatorname{atan}\left(\dfrac{\omega_{off}\left[1-\cos\left(\omega_2\tau\right)\right]}{\omega_2\sin\left(\omega_2\tau\right)}\right)$	$\Phi_{DAQ} \approx \omega_{off}\left(\dfrac{3\pi}{4\gamma GL}+\dfrac{T_{ramp}}{2}\right)$

main objective of this chapter, Table 17.1 does highlight how an appreciable level of phase contrast can be generated in UTE imaging, even if the nominal TE is near zero.

Experimental Verification

Experiments were conducted on a clinical 3T MRI system on phantoms and various anatomies. Magnitude and phase images were obtained from the same datasets. The phantom setup was imaged in the scanner's coronal plane and contained 12 cylindrical containers approximately 10 cm in length with 3 groups of diameters L = 0.8 cm, 1.4 cm, and 2.6 cm. The four phantoms within each size group were filled with different chemical species (water, oil, CH_3CN, and dimethyl sulfoxide (DMSO)) to study the phase of the UTE images in the presence of different off-resonance frequencies. UTE images were obtained at different RF durations, readout gradient strengths, and slew rates. Figure 17.2 shows both magnitude (upper) and phase (lower) UTE images of the phantom setup for different readout gradient strengths and bandwidths (BWs). The typical ring-like artifact appearance around the magnitude images, especially with lower readout gradients, should be noted. Furthermore, unlike the situation when using GRE or spin echo (SE) sequences, the centers of the cylinders are not physically displaced with respect to each other.

Fig. 17.2 UTE phantom scans. Top: magnitude images; bottom: phase images. G = gradient strength. (Reproduced with permission from Carl and Jing-Tzyh [10])

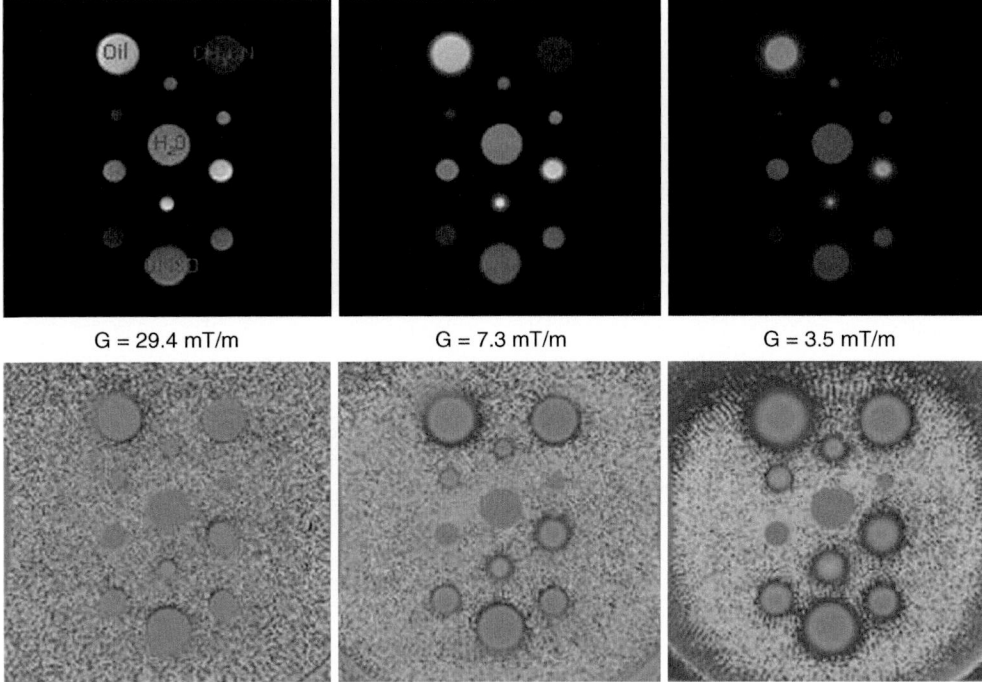

G = 29.4 mT/m   G = 7.3 mT/m   G = 3.5 mT/m

Specimen Study

Many connective tissues, such as the menisci, ligaments, and tendons, are rich in collagen fibers, which are highly organized and composed of fiber bundles of varying sizes. Petersen et al. studied the fibril texture of the human knee meniscus using electron microscopy and found three distinct layers: a meshwork of thin fibrils, a layer of lamella-like collagen fibril bundles, and central circumferential fibers [12]. The tendon has a highly ordered extracellular matrix in which collagen molecules assemble into filamentous collagen fibrils. Its multi-hierarchical structure contains collagen molecules arranged in fibrils, which are then grouped into fibril bundles, fascicles, and fiber bundles that are almost parallel to the long axis of the tendon and are named primary, secondary, and tertiary bundles, respectively [13]. Krasnosselskaia et al. investigated the dependence of FID on fiber orientation to B_0 in tendon [14]. They observed an angle-dependent multi-exponential FID decay, which they hypothesized was due to exchange between orientationally restricted water structured along the length of the collagen molecule and disordered water in cavities. Measured frequency and phase shifts were orientation-dependent and were interpreted as signatures of bulk magnetic susceptibility effects due to the geometry of cavities formed by adjacent gaps at the ends of the collagen molecules [14]. These findings suggested the potential for generating phase contrast within musculoskeletal tissue fibral structures.

To demonstrate UTE phase contrast in connective tissues, a human meniscus sample was cut into a 3-mm-thick slice, placed in a perfluorooctyl bromide (PFOB)-filled syringe, and imaged with UTE sequences. The circumferential cross section of the meniscus sample was oriented perpendicular to the scanner's B_0 field. Figure 17.3a shows a UTE magnitude image of the meniscus specimen. The corresponding phase image is shown in Fig. 17.3b. The phase image exhibits higher contrast between the different fiber groups than the magnitude image. This increased contrast can be attributed to the inverse relationship between the size of the UTE image phase and the object size L (see Table 17.1). Due to the minimal nominal TE used in UTE imaging, this phase evolution mainly stems from the excitation and acquisition portions of the sequence.

UTE phase imaging was further demonstrated in peripheral nerve in a clinical setting. The median nerve in a cadaveric human arm was scanned using a two-dimensional (2D) UTE sequence on a 3T clinical scanner. The arm specimen was placed parallel to the B_0 field. A body coil was used for signal excitation. An 1-inch loop coil was used for signal reception. The small surface coil provided extremely high signal-to-noise ratio (SNR) sensitivity, allowing ultrahigh spatial resolution imaging of the peripheral nerve structure. Figure 17.4 shows both magnitude and phase images of the peripheral nerve in situ. The fascicular pattern, the perineurium and epineurium, and the individual fascicles were extremely well depicted. UTE phase imaging provides

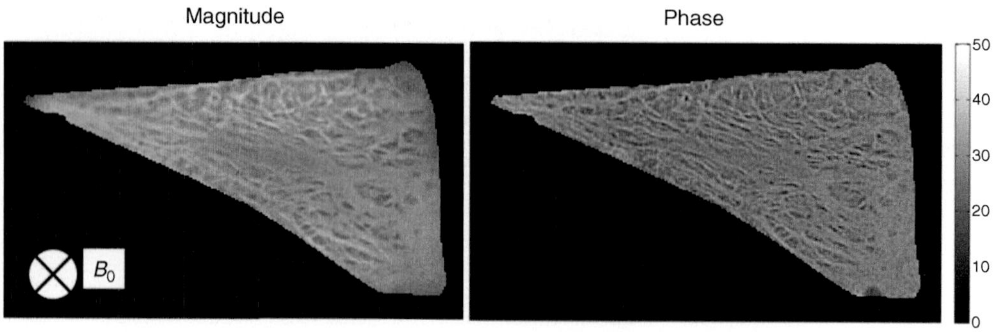

Fig. 17.3 UTE-based magnitude (left) and phase (right) images of a cadaveric human meniscus specimen. The internal fibers in the meniscus sample exhibit strong phase contrast. (Reproduced with permission from Carl and Jing-Tzyh [10])

Fig. 17.4 UTE-based magnitude (**a**) and phase (**b**) images of a cadaveric human forearm specimen. UTE phase imaging provides higher contrast than magnitude imaging for the peripheral nerve, especially for the perineurium of individual fascicles (arrow)

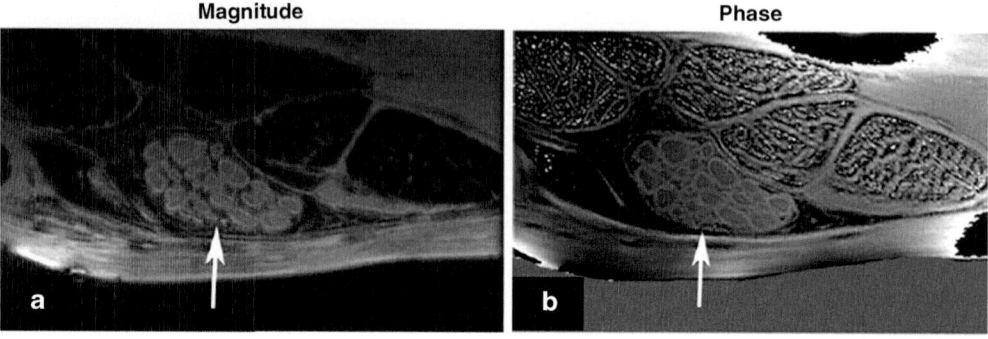

higher contrast for the perineurium than UTE magnitude imaging.

Biological tissues frequently contain multiple water components [15–17]. For example, cortical bone contains multiple water components, including pore water, which resides in the macroscopic pores of the Haversian and the lacunocanalicular systems, and bound water, which is loosely bound to the organic matrix [15]. While pore water and bound water both have extremely short T_2^*s (e.g., ~2 ms for pore water and ~0.3 ms for bound water at 3 T) [17], pore water has higher mobility and, therefore, a longer T_2^* than bound water. Adiabatic inversion pulses can be employed to partially invert and null the longitudinal magnetization of pore water [18]. During the inversion pulse, the longitudinal magnetization of bound water is largely saturated due to its extremely short T_2^*, which is much shorter than the duration of the adiabatic inversion pulse. Pore water nulling is important for accurately mapping bound water content, which correlates with cortical bone's organic matrix density. The degree of pore water inversion and nulling is determined by the inversion time (TI). The pore water magnetization is negative for a TI shorter than the nulling point and positive for a TI longer than the nulling point. A phase transition (~π) is expected before and after the nulling point [19]. Figure 17.5 shows the magnitude and phase images from IR-UTE imaging of a cadaveric human bone sample using a repetition time (TR) of 300 ms and a short TI of 20 ms. A positive phase was observed with TEs less than 0.4 ms (i.e., $\phi = 0.27$ for a TE of 8 μs and $\phi = 0.74$ for a TE of 0.4 ms) and a negative phase was observed with longer TEs in the range of 0.8–1.6 ms (i.e., $\phi = -2.47$ for a TE of 0.6 ms and $\phi = -2.03$ for a TE of 1.4 ms) [19]. The net IR-UTE signal is initially dominated by the positive bound water magnetization and by the negative pore water magnetization at longer TEs (Fig. 17.5a).

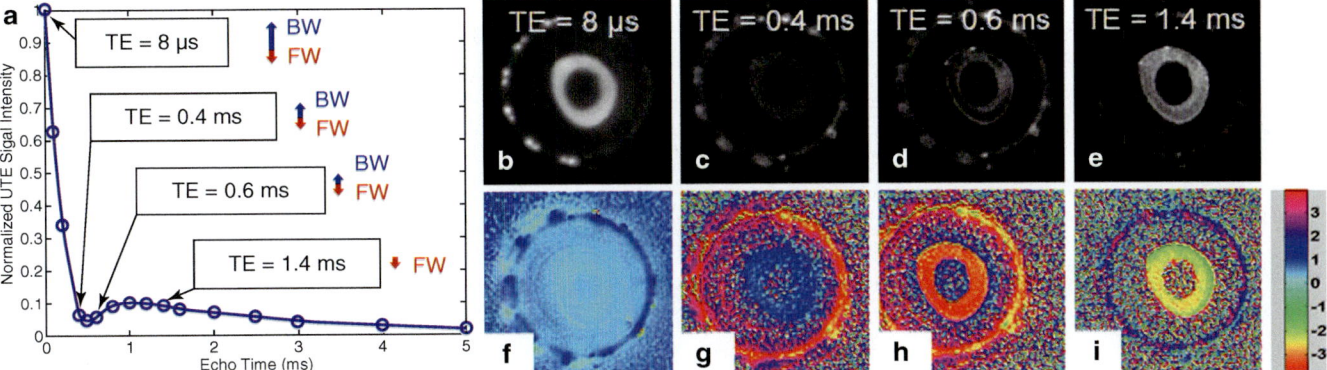

Fig. 17.5 Normalized magnitude signal decay for IR-UTE imaging of a human bone sample with a TR of 300 ms, a TI of 20 ms, and TEs ranging from 8 μs to 5 ms (**a**) and selected magnitude and phase images with a TE of 8 μs (**b** and **f**), 0.4 ms (**c** and **g**), 0.6 ms (**d** and **h**), and 1.4 ms (**e** and **i**). Schematic longitudinal magnetizations of bound water (BM) and free (pore) water (FW) at different TEs are shown in panel (**a**), where the positive signal from bound water dominates the IR-UTE signal at TEs < 0.6 ms. This signal decays quickly, and the negative signal from pore water slowly dominates the IR-UTE signal at longer TEs. The IR-UTE bone signals were of opposite phase before and after a TE of 0.5 ms (i.e., $\phi = 0.27$ for a TE of 8 μs and $\phi = 0.74$ for a TE of 0.4 ms, whereas $\phi = -2.47$ for a TE of 0.6 ms and $\phi = -2.03$ for a TE of 1.4 ms), consistent with a transition from positive to negative net magnetization at a TE of ~0.5 ms, the null point. (Reproduced with permission from Li et al. [19])

UTE Phase Imaging of the Lungs

Other applications of UTE phase imaging in the lungs and the knee joints were demonstrated by Lu et al. [20]. In their work, 3D UTE-based magnitude and phase images were combined in composite images (see Fig. 17.6), which aided simultaneous visualization of magnitude and phase information. For lung imaging, a total of 38,400 radial lines of *k*-space data were acquired with respiratory gating in a total scan time of about 7.5 min. Volumetric lung images were generated using gridding followed by complex Fourier transformation. A 3D low-pass filter was applied to the *k*-space data to reconstruct a set of low-resolution complex images. The final phase information was derived from the full resolution images multiplied by the conjugates of the low-resolution images. The magnitude images (Fig. 17.6a) depict lung parenchyma, large fissures, and vessels nicely, owing to the ultrashort TE used with the 3D UTE sequence. The phase images (Fig. 17.6b) show highly different contrasts, espe-

cially for lung parenchyma, and provide complementary information to the magnitude images. The vessel walls are depicted with excellent contrast, especially in the axial phase images, where blood signals appear dark, whereas the vessel wall signals appear light. The airways are also depicted with positive contrast likely due to the presence of tissues such as the hyaline cartilage. Large fissures are visible with negative contrast on the phase images (arrows in Fig. 17.6).

Furthermore, the corresponding UTE magnitude and phase images can be used as inputs to different color channels (e.g., magnitude image in cyan, phase image in magenta) to create composite color images. The dynamic range and contrast for each individual channel can be independently adjusted to achieve the desired composite image contrast. The composite UTE images provide easy visualization of the information contained within the magnitude and phase images (Fig. 17.6c), thereby adding important additional contrast and potentially widening the application of UTE MR phase information in a clinical setting.

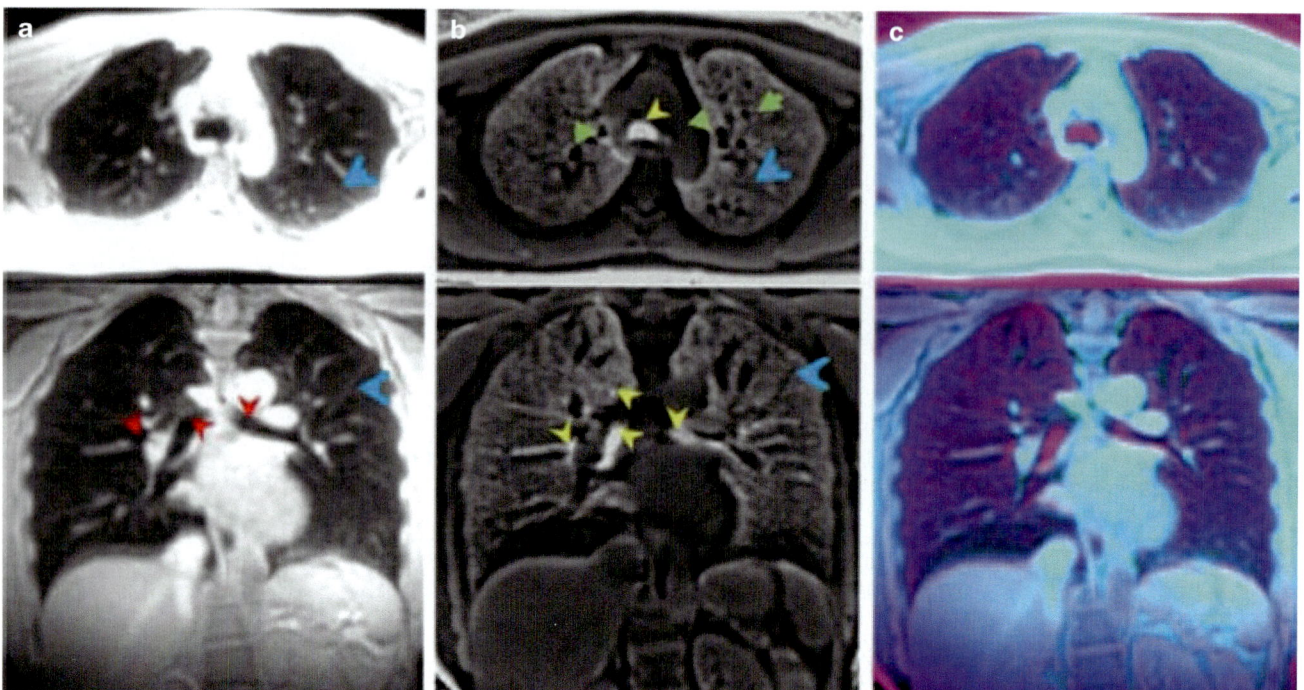

Fig. 17.6 3D images of UTE lungs: (**a**) magnitude, (**b**) phase, and (**c**) composite. (Images courtesy of Aiming Lu, Department of Radiology, Mayo Clinic, Rochester, Minnesota, USA)

UTE Phase Imaging in the Brain

Phase imaging of the brain is of considerable interest as it can provide greater contrast than magnitude images [21–23]. Almost all the studies to date have employed long TEs (of ~40 ms or longer) to create enough contrast between white and gray matter. The signal and contrast are mainly due to mobile water protons. The majority of myelin components have ultrashort T_2s and can only be visualized using UTE- and zero echo time (ZTE)-type techniques. The ultrashort-T_2 myelin components have much broader spectral absorption line shapes than the long-T_2 water components. They can be selectively affected by appropriately placed off-resonance radiofrequency (RF) irradiation. A high-power saturation RF pulse placed a few kilohertz away from the water peak can preferentially saturate signals from the short-T_2 components, leaving the long-T_2 water components largely unaffected. Off-resonance RF saturation can be used to create phase contrast for the short-T_2 myelin components. Recently, Wei et al. have reported the use of an off-resonance saturated 3D UTE sequence to enhance phase contrast in the brain (Fig. 17.7) [23]. In conventional MRI, the short-T_2 myelin components contribute minimally to phase contrast. Regular UTE images also do not show much phase contrast between gray and white matter. However, UTE imaging combined with off-resonance RF saturation can provide high phase contrast in the brain even at a nominal

TE of 106 μs [23]. UTE with off-resonance RF saturation provides reversed phase contrast between the gray and white matter. The magnitude and phase UTE images of the saturated components can be calculated using complex subtraction, providing a positive phase shift for the saturated signal component of the combined gray matter and cerebrospinal fluid (CSF), and a negative phase shift for the white matter. CSF has a similar positive phase shift in both UTE and GRE phase images, but white matter shows the opposite sign. UTE-based MRI phase images may improve the characterization of tissue microstructure in the brain by accessing short-T_2 myelin components, thereby providing a better way to demonstrate phase contrast [23].

Phase imaging can also be combined with other contrast mechanisms, such as adiabatic inversion recovery UTE (IR-UTE), for direct imaging of myelin in the brain [24–28]. Myelin has a much lower signal than long-T_2 water components in the white and gray matter of the brain. Efficient long-T_2 signal suppression is of critical importance in creating myelin contrast. Prior studies have demonstrated that the IR-UTE sequence allows selective myelin imaging on a clinical whole-body scanner [24, 26–28]. He et al. showed that high phase contrast could be generated from the rapidly decaying signal of the macromolecular components of myelin after the suppression of long-T_2 white matter components (Fig. 17.8) [29]. These methods can be readily translated for in vivo imaging. They concluded that the majority

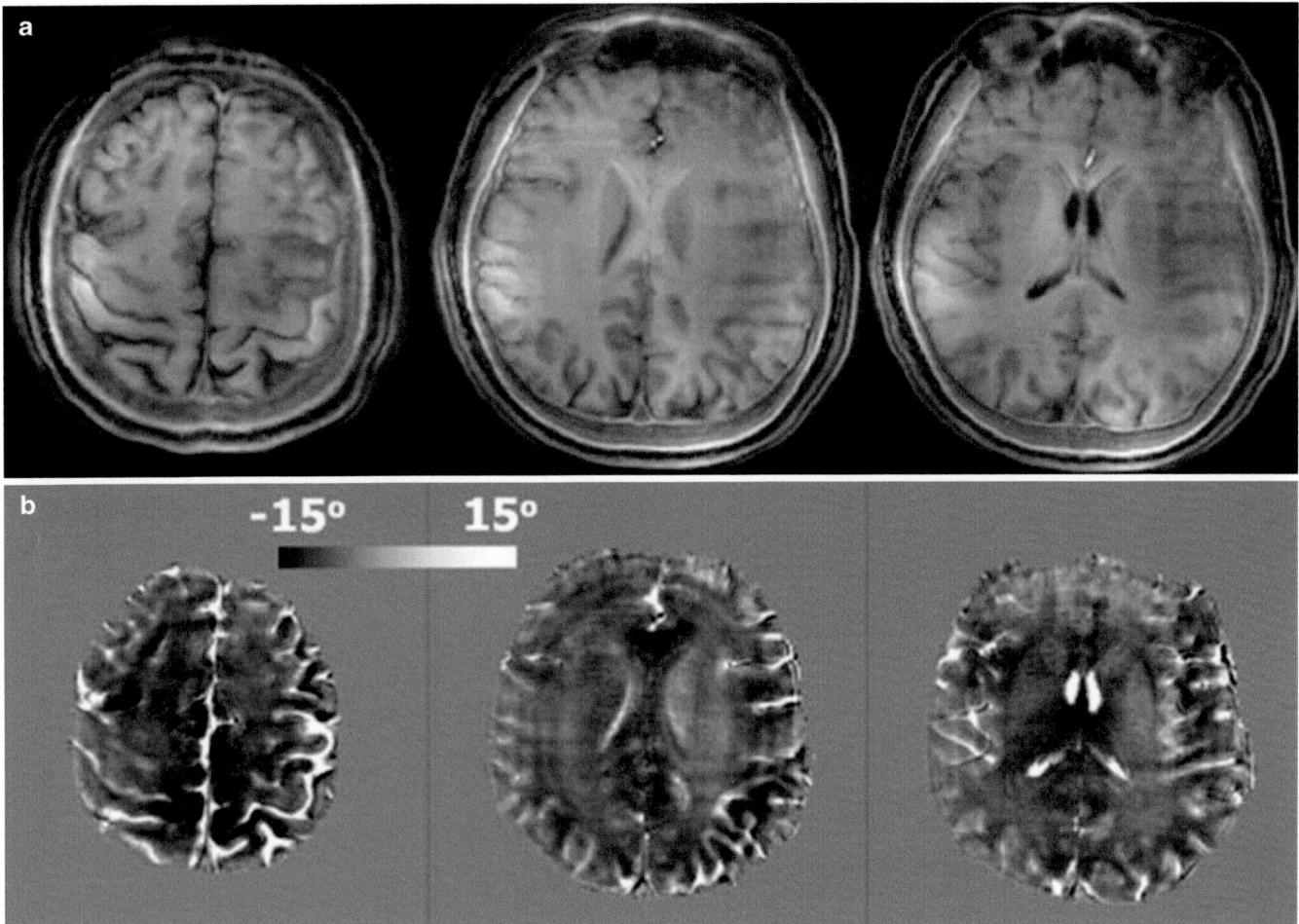

Fig. 17.7 Off-resonance saturated 3D UTE magnitude (**a**) and phase (**b**) imaging in the brain of a healthy volunteer with a TE of 0.106 ms and a saturation frequency of −1.2 kHz. Three representative axial magnitude images show high signal intensity in the white matter, indicating higher ultrashort-T_2 components (**a**). The corresponding phase images demonstrate negative phase shifts in the white matter and positive phase shifts in CSF (**b**). (Reproduced with permission from Wei et al. [23])

Fig. 17.8 IR-UTE brain imaging at a TE of 8 µs (**a**) and 4.4 ms (**b**). Echo subtraction provides high contrast for myelin (**c**). Adaptive phase reconstruction of the phased array data shows high myelin phase contrast (**d**). (Reproduced with permission from He et al. [29])

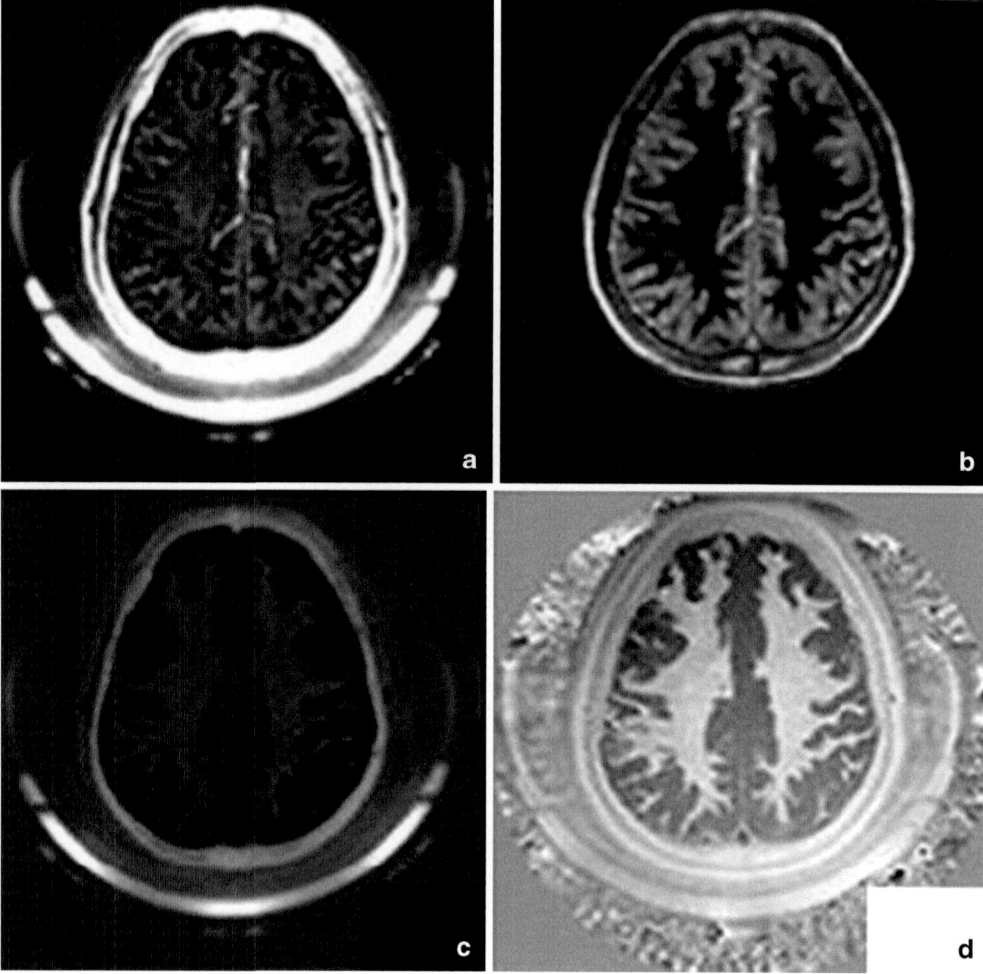

of myelin components demonstrate short-T_2 relaxation times and can be best visualized using UTE techniques. IR-UTE phase imaging may also improve the diagnosis and therapeutic monitoring of diseases that specifically target myelin (such as multiple sclerosis).

UTE Phase Imaging in the Vasculature

Kadbi et al. have used four-dimensional (4D) UTE phase imaging (with stack-of-stars) to study stenotic flow [30]. With conventional phase contrast (PC) imaging techniques, high velocities often lead to intravoxel dephasing and inaccurate flow quantification. Shortening TE using UTE sequences has a crucial impact on decreasing these effects. In their work, they used a rigid phantom model of vascular occlusion (Fig. 17.9). Their results show a good correlation between conventional and UTE sequences for measured flow at low and medium flow rates. However, at high flow rates of more than 250 mL/s, the UTE sequence resulted in more accurate flow quantification than the conventional sequences. In addition, they found that undersampling the number of UTE spokes by 50% still resulted in an acceptable trade-off between accuracy and scan time.

Fig. 17.9 (a) Velocity contours from conventional 4D flow MRI, showing intravoxel dephasing and signal loss. (b) 4D UTE flow MRI, showing reduced dephasing and signal loss. (Reproduced with permission from Kadbi et al. [30])

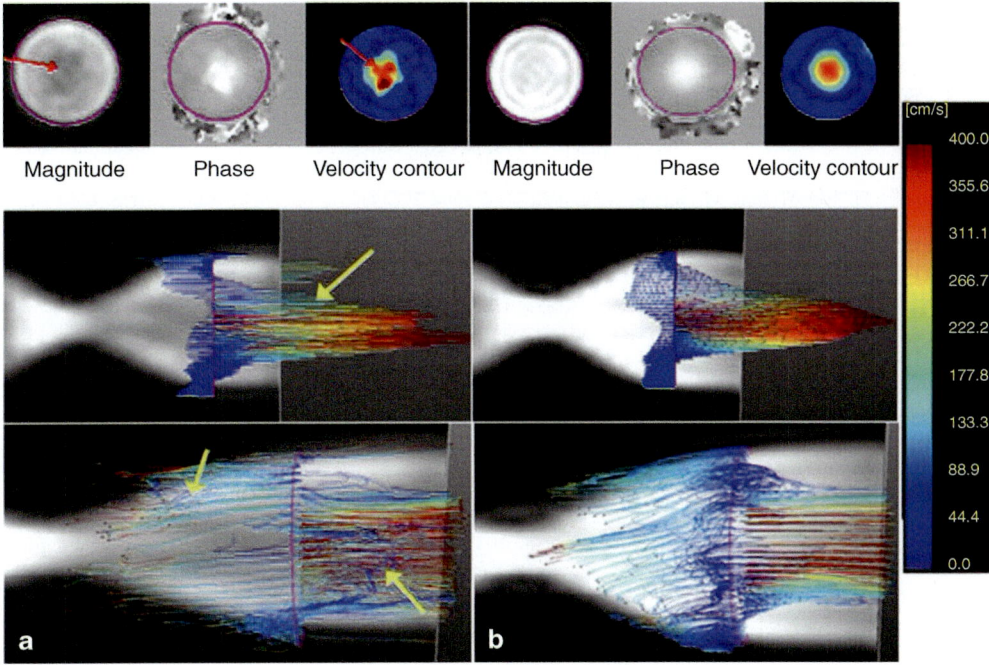

Conclusions

UTE phase imaging can provide high contrast visualization of short-T_2 tissues despite its ultrashort TE. These phase images can exhibit higher contrast for fiber structures than magnitude images, and highlight susceptibility differences between different tissue groups. Phase evolution with UTE imaging mainly occurs during RF excitation and data acquisition. The theoretical model shown in Table 17.1 was derived using an isolated object with simple geometry; there equations are only approximations of more complex structures. Other applications outside of the musculoskeletal system have also been explored, such as lung and myelin imaging, as well as improved accuracy of phase measurement in high velocity flow quantification.

References

1. Robson MD, Gatehouse PD, Bydder M, Bydder GM. Magnetic resonance: an introduction to ultrashort TE (UTE) imaging. J Comput Assist Tomogr. 2003;27(6):825–46.
2. Bergin CJ, Pauly JM, Macovski A. Lung parenchyma: projection reconstruction MR imaging. Radiology. 1991;179(3):777–81.
3. Gold GE, Pauly JM, Macovski A, Herfkens RJ. MR spectroscopic imaging of collagen: tendons and knee menisci. Magn Reson Med. 1995;34(5):647–54.
4. Gatehouse PD, Bydder GM. Magnetic resonance imaging of short T_2 components in tissue. Clin Radiol. 2003;58(1):1–19.
5. Ma Y, Jang H, Jerban S, Chang EY, Chung CB, Bydder GM, et al. Making the invisible visible-ultrashort echo time magnetic resonance imaging: technical developments and applications. Appl Phys Rev. 2022;9(4):041303.
6. Rahmer J, Bornert P, Groen J, Bos C. Three-dimensional radial ultrashort echo-time imaging with T_2 adapted sampling. Magn Reson Med. 2006;55(5):1075–82.
7. Haacke EM, Xu Y, Cheng YC, Reichenbach JR. Susceptibility weighted imaging (SWI). Magn Reson Med. 2004;52(3):612–8.
8. Rauscher A, Sedlacik J, Barth M, Mentzel HJ, Reichenbach JR. Magnetic susceptibility-weighted MR phase imaging of the human brain. AJNR Am J Neuroradiol. 2005;26(4):736–42.
9. Reichenbach JR, Venkatesan R, Yablonskiy DA, Thompson MR, Lai S, Haacke EM. Theory and application of static field inhomogeneity effects in gradient-echo imaging. J Magn Reson Imaging. 1997;7(2):266–79.
10. Carl M, Jing-Tzyh AC. Investigations of the origin of phase differences seen with ultrashort TE imaging of short T_2 meniscal tissue. Magn Reson Med. 2012;67(4):991–1003.
11. Chiang JT, Carl M, Bydder M, Du J, Mattrey RF, Bydder GM. Phase accrual during excitation in ultrashort TE (UTE) imaging: an alternate definition of TE for phase measurements. Proc Intl Soc Mag Reson Med. 2009:4546.
12. Petersen W, Tillmann B. Collagenous fibril texture of the human knee joint meniscus. Anat Embryol. 1998;197(4):317–24.
13. Franchi M, Trirè A, Quaranta M, Orsini E, Ottani V. Collagen structure of tendon relates to function. Sci World J. 2007;7:404–20.
14. Krasnosselskaia LV, Fullerton GD, Dodd SJ, Cameron IL. Water in tendon: orientational analysis of the free induction decay. Magn Reson Med. 2005;54(2):280–8.
15. Nyman JS, Ni Q, Nicolella DP, Wang X. Measurements of mobile and bound water by nuclear magnetic resonance correlate with mechanical properties of bone. Bone. 2008;42(1):193–9.

16. Reiter DA, Lin PC, Fishbein KW, Spencer RG. Multicomponent T$_2$ relaxation analysis in cartilage. Magn Reson Med. 2009;61(4):803–9.

17. Biswas R, Bae W, Diaz E, et al. Ultrashort echo time (UTE) imaging with bi-component analysis: bound and free water evaluation of bovine cortical bone subject to sequential drying. Bone. 2012;50(3):749–55.

18. Afsahi AM, Ma Y, Jang H, Jerban S, Chung C, Chang EY, Du J. Ultrashort echo time (UTE) MRI techniques: met and unmet needs in musculoskeletal imaging. J Magn Reson Imaging. 2022;55(6):1597–612.

19. Li S, Ma L, Chang EY, Shao H, Chen J, Chung CB, Bydder GM, Du J. Effects of inversion time on inversion recovery prepared ultrashort echo time (IR-UTE) imaging of free and bound water in cortical bone. NMR Biomed. 2015;28(1):70–8.

20. Lu A, Miyazaki M, Cheng O, Zhou X. Fusion of magnitude and phase images and its applications in ultra-short TE MR imaging. Proc Intl Soc Mag Reson Med. 2014:4233.

21. Duyn JH, van Gelderen P, Li TQ, de Zwart JA, Koretsky AP, Fukunaga M. High-field MRI of brain cortical substructure based on signal phase. Proc Natl Acad Sci U S A. 2007;104:11796–801.

22. Lee J, Hirano Y, Fukunaga M, Silva AC, Duyn JH. On the contribution of deoxy-hemoglobin to MRI gray-white matter phase contrast at high field. Neuroimage. 2010;49(1):193–8.

23. Wei H, Cao P, Bischof A, Henry RG, Larson PEZ, Liu C. MRI gradient-echo phase contrast of the brain at ultra-short TE with off-resonance saturation. Neuroimage. 2018;175:1–11.

24. Waldman A, Rees JH, Brock CS, Robson MD, Gatehouse PD, Bydder GM. MRI of the brain with ultra-short echo time pulse sequences. Neuroradiology. 2003;45(12):887–92.

25. Wilhelm MJ, Ong HH, Wehrli SL, Li C, Tsai PH, Hackney DB, Wehrli FW. Direct magnetic resonance detection of myelin and prospects for quantitative imaging of myelin density. Proc Natl Acad Sci U S A. 2012;109(24):9605–10.

26. Du J, Ma G, Li S, Carl M, Szeverenyi N, VandenBerg S, Corey-Bloom J, Bydder GM. Ultrashort TE echo time (UTE) magnetic resonance imaging of the short T$_2$ components in white matter of the brain using a clinical 3T scanner. Neuroimage. 2013;87:32–41.

27. Du J, Sheth V, He Q, Carl M, Chen J, Corey-Bloom J, Bydder GM, Du J. Measurement of T$_1$ of the ultrashort T$_2$* components in white matter of the brain at 3T. PLoS One. 2014;9(8):e103296.

28. Sheth V, Shao H, Chen J, VandenBerg S, Corey-Bloom J, Bydder GM, Du J. Magnetic resonance imaging of myelin using ultrashort echo time (UTE) pulse sequence: phantom, specimen, volunteers and multiple sclerosis patient studies. Neuroimage. 2016;136:37–44.

29. He Q, Ma Y, Fan S, Shao H, Sheth V, Bydder GM, Du J. Direct magnitude and phase imaging of myelin using ultrashort echo time (UTE) pulse sequences: a feasibility study. Magn Reson Imaging. 2017;39:194–9.

30. Kadbi M, Negahdar M, Cha JW, Traughber M, Martin P, Stoddard MF, Amini AA. 4D UTE flow: a phase-contrast MRI technique for assessment and visualization of stenotic flows. Magn Reson Med. 2015;73(3):939–50.

Chemical Shift Artifacts Produced by Center-out Radial Sampling: A Potential Pitfall in Clinical Diagnosis

18

Mark Bydder

Introduction

With Cartesian sampling of the k-space, chemical shift artifacts between water and fat manifest as a displacement of fat in the image relative to water [1]. Since the magnitude and polarity of the gradient used for frequency encoding are identical for all phase encoding lines, the chemical shift artifacts appear as a constant pixel shift of fat in the frequency encoding direction.

However, with radial and other types of non-Cartesian sampling of the k-space, where the frequency encoding gradient changes in sign, direction, and/or magnitude, the appearance of chemical shift artifacts between fat and water is less well known. This can be a potential problem since non-Cartesian techniques are being used more often in clinical practice and the artifacts that arise from them are unfamiliar to radiologists and may be mistaken for pathology [2].

Ultrashort echo time (UTE) imaging is one example of non-Cartesian imaging used in musculoskeletal, lung, and neurological imaging [3, 4], which employs center-out radial sampling of the k-space (Fig. 18.1a).

A concept that is useful in imaging systems for illustrating imperfections in the encoding and/or reconstruction is the point spread function (PSF). Essentially, the PSF is the image that would be obtained by encoding and reconstructing an infinitely narrow point object. Ideally, the result should be a single bright pixel in the image; however, practical limitations mean that the image and the object always differ. Typically, the finite resolution of the measuring apparatus causes the infinitely narrow point to have a finite width in the image (i.e., the point is spread out). The width is a property of the measurement process.

PSFs can be measured empirically or calculated numerically based on a model of the measurement system. Blurring can result not only from finite sampling since the resolution is obviously dependent on practical choices such as the matrix size and field of view but also from inherent properties of the object, including its T_2. As shown in Rahmer et al. [6], the rapid loss of signal from short-T_2 species means that there is only a short window of time available to spatially encode the object, and this broadens the PSF in a manner dependent on T_2 (also known as T_2 blurring).

In addition to blurring, other artifacts such as chemical shift and aliasing may be characterized in terms of the PSF. Of primary interest in this chapter is chemical shift artifact. With Cartesian sampling, the PSF is a displacement of the point from its true location, which is consistent with its well known appearance on clinical images. In the case of center-out radial sampling, PSFs are shown in Fig. 18.1b and c for the case of on-resonance and off-resonance points, respectively. These illustrate the effect of finite resolution (Fig. 18.1b) and the effect of the chemical shift (Fig. 18.1c).

A chemical shift effect with radial sampling of k-space is sometimes described as blurring or producing a horseshoe artifact, but this does not fully capture the range of artifacts that may be seen with this type of sampling. Although it is known that the off-resonance effect in center-out radial sampling of the k-space creates a ring-shaped PSF (Fig. 18.1c) [7, 8], there is a practical need to show how this manifests in clinical images.

UTE imaging is used to obtain signals from short- (1–10 ms) and ultrashort-T_2 tissues (0.1–1 ms) such as cortical bone, periosteum, entheses, the calcified and deep radial layers of the articular cartilage, and the cartilaginous endplates (CEPs) of intervertebral discs. Chemical shift artifacts arising from fat may be displaced into regions that have zero signal and be mistaken for real tissues, since it may not be obvious whether this signal has a normal appearance or is an artifact. Many short- and ultrashort-T_2 tissues are adjacent to fat, so image interpretation at these boundaries may be particularly problematic.

M. Bydder (✉)
Department of Radiological Sciences, David Geffen School of Medicine, University of California Los Angeles, Los Angeles, CA, USA

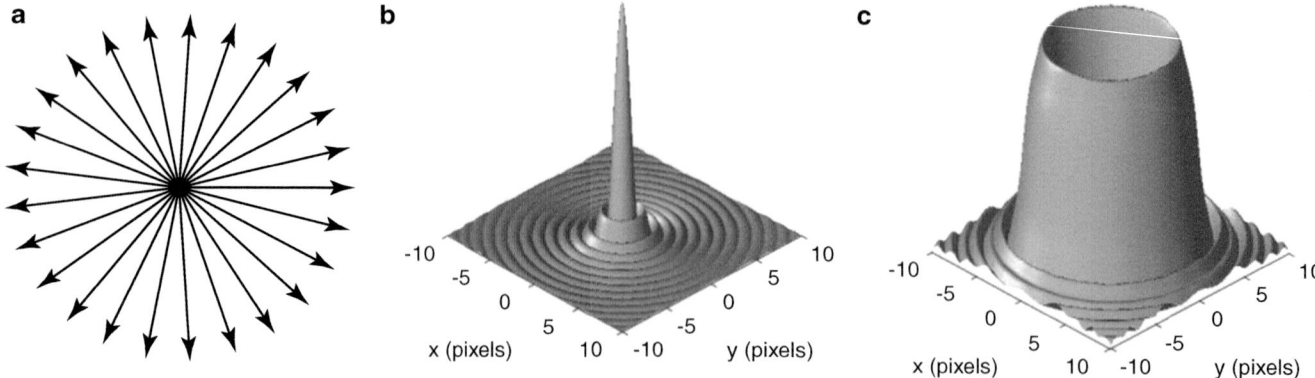

Fig. 18.1 A schematic of (**a**) center-out radial sampling of *k*-space. The gradient directions are indicated by arrows. (**b**) The point spread function (PSF) for this sampling with on-resonance spins (water). (**c**) The PSF for the same acquisition with the addition of off-resonance effects due to a chemical shift (fat). Panel (**b**) shows a sharp central peak surrounded by circular rings (Gibbs ringing). Panel (**c**) shows no central peak but complete displacement of the signal away from the center and formation of a ring shape. (Reproduced with permission from Bydder et al. [5])

The purpose of this chapter is to unequivocally demonstrate chemical shift artifacts in radial center-out sampling of the *k*-space in phantoms, show their appearance in normal human images, and describe their potential for misdiagnosis.

Phantom Studies

Two phantoms were constructed using vegetable oil (to simulate in vivo triglyceride) and water doped with gadopentetate dimeglumine (MultiHance, Bracco Diagnostics, NJ, USA). The first phantom was made with a syringe containing oil placed inside a water-filled beaker to illustrate a "point" source of signal. The second phantom was made using three beakers of different sizes in a "Russian-doll" arrangement, with a large beaker containing a medium-sized beaker containing a small beaker. The largest and smallest beakers contained water, and the medium-sized beaker contained vegetable oil. The purpose of this phantom was to show artifacts arising from structures with a thin layer of fat surrounded by a water-containing tissue on either side.

Figure 18.2 shows the results from the first phantom containing oil centrally within a syringe. This reveals a radially symmetric signal from the off-resonance oil, which is mid-gray in Fig. 18.2a. It is surrounded by a dark ring where the syringe material produces no detectable signal. As the bandwidth is decreased (Fig. 18.2b–d), a less central, mid-gray signal is seen, and the water surrounding it increases in signal as the signal from the oil is progressively displaced outward into it. At 4 kHz (Fig. 18.2e), no signal remains from the oil in the syringe at its correct location.

Figure 18.3 shows the results from the second phantom, which had an oil annulus surrounded by water in the two beakers internal and external to it. In Fig. 18.3a, there is a central ring of signal from the oil, which appears mid-gray. It is surrounded by narrow inner and outer dark rings from the material of the beakers. As the bandwidth decreases in Fig. 18.3b–e, the central mid-gray ring becomes thinner and less obvious until it is no longer seen in Fig. 18.3e. There is an increase in signal in the surrounding internal and external water, which becomes more extensive from Fig. 18.3b–e. There are slight asymmetries to the artifact, which are most evident at the lowest bandwidth, which reflect the susceptibility-induced off-resonance effects at the interfaces between the oil and water layers.

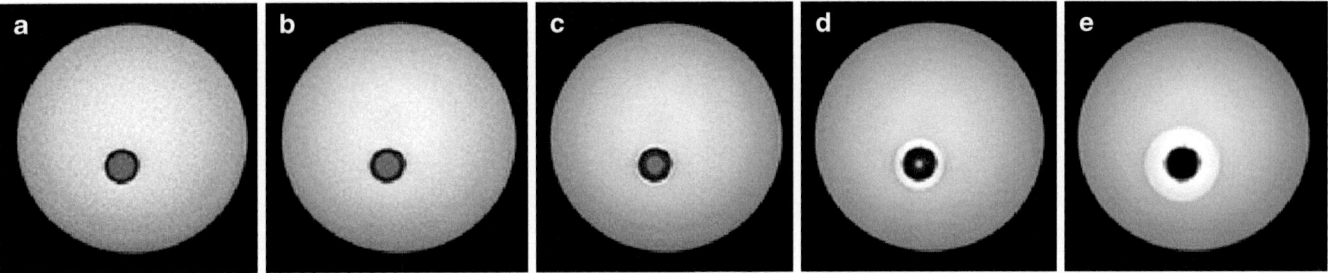

Fig. 18.2 An oil sample in a syringe surrounded by water imaged at different bandwidths: (**a**) 62.5, (**b**) 31, (**c**) 15, (**d**) 8, and (**e**) 4 kHz. (Reproduced with permission from Bydder et al. [5])

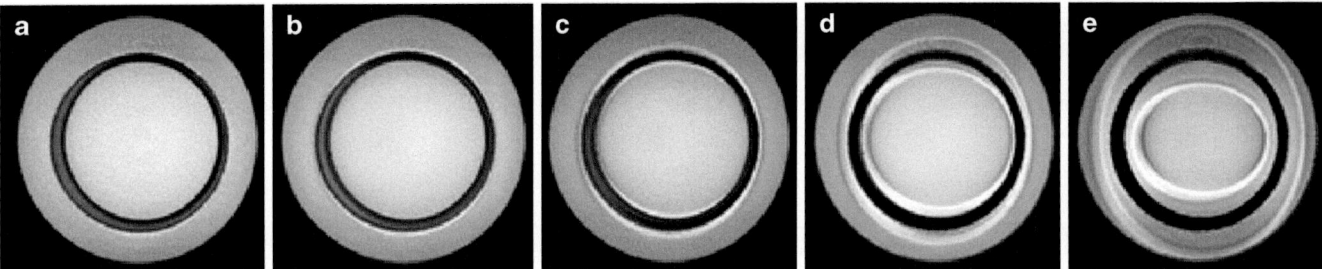

Fig. 18.3 An oil annulus situated between the outer and inner beakers, which contain water, imaged at bandwidths: (**a**) 62.5, (**b**) 31, (**c**) 15, (**d**) 8, and (**e**) 4 kHz. (Reproduced with permission from Bydder et al. [5])

Human Volunteer Studies

A human volunteer (male, age: 65 years) was scanned using the same imaging sequence and range of bandwidths as for the phantoms. Representative examples of images of the head, pelvis, and spine are shown.

Figure 18.4a shows a transverse image of the brain of the 65-year-old volunteer using a 62.5-kHz bandwidth, and Fig. 18.4b is the same slice imaged at a 4-kHz bandwidth. The latter figure shows the brain with areas of increased signal adjacent to it inside the skull. These areas (arrows) simulate the appearance of subdural hematomas. In addition, in Fig. 18.4b, an increased number of layers is seen in the surrounding scalp. The signal from fat in the red bone marrow (approximately 50%) between the inner and outer tables of the skull is centrally displaced inside the skull around the brain and peripherally outside the skull into the scalp. Unlike Cartesian chemical shift artifacts, which are seen in one direction only and have a single displacement polarity, radial center-out artifacts are seen in different directions and have two displacement polarities (i.e., both central and peripheral displacements of the signal).

Figure 18.5a shows a transverse image of the pelvis of the volunteer at 62.5 kHz. Figure 18.5b shows the same slice at a 4-kHz bandwidth. In this image, additional high signal is seen between the urine in the bladder and the surrounding pelvic tissues (arrows), giving the appearance of bladder wall thickening. This simulates a bladder tumor. The artifacts are seen in different directions and result from central displacement of the signal from more peripheral perivesical fat.

Figure 18.6a is a sagittal image of the lumbar spine of the volunteer obtained with a bandwidth of 62.5 kHz. Figure 18.6b is the same slice imaged with a bandwidth of 4 kHz. In the latter image, a high signal is seen at the upper and lower margins of the intervertebral discs (arrows) between the vertebral bodies. The appearances simulate those of CEPs seen with UTE subtraction imaging. The CEP has a zero signal with conventional long-TE imaging but shows a low signal with UTE imaging. When a short TE zero signal image is subtracted from the low signal UTE image, a relatively higher signal is seen in the CEPs. This genuine finding is simulated by the chemical shift artifacts shown in Fig. 18.6b. Unlike Cartesian chemical shift artifacts using sagittal frequency encoding, in which increased

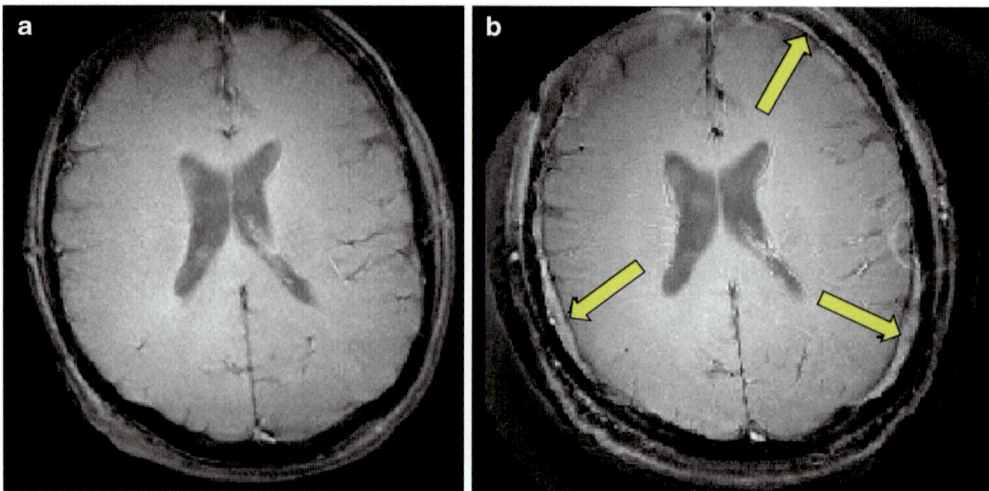

Fig. 18.4 (**a**) A transverse image of the brain of a 65-year-old volunteer using a bandwidth of 62.5 kHz. (**b**) The same slice imaged at a 4-kHz bandwidth. (Reproduced with permission from Bydder et al. [5])

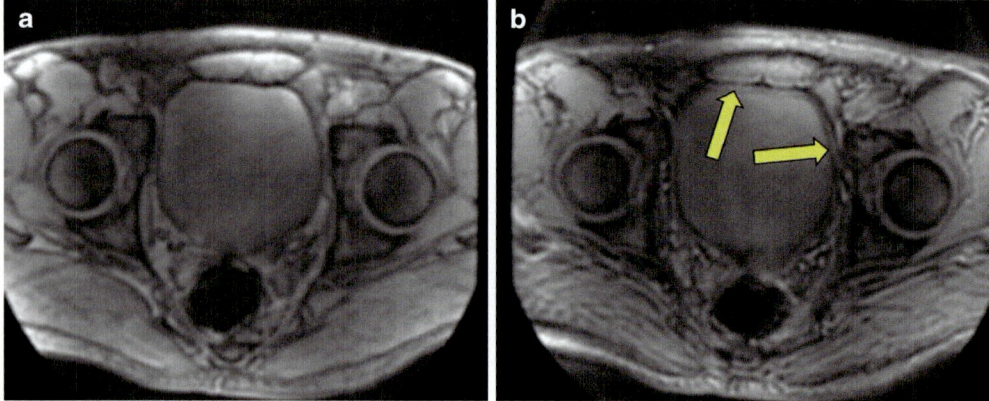

Fig. 18.5 (**a**) A transverse image of the pelvis using a bandwidth of 62.5 kHz. (**b**) The same slice at a 4-kHz bandwidth. (Reproduced with permission from Bydder et al. [5])

signal is only seen in the region of one CEP, with radial center-out sampling, increased signal is seen in the regions of both the upper and lower CEPs of the intervertebral discs.

In addition to the in-plane chemical shift shown thus far, the two-dimensional (2D) UTE sequence is vulnerable to through-slice off-resonance effects owing to the use of half pulses, which employ opposite polarity slice-selective gradients [9]. The degree of off-resonance required to produce a visible artifact is rather large, since the amplitude of the

slice-selective gradient is typically high compared to that of the readout gradient and is not manipulable by end users. Moreover, the artifacts do not mimic pathology in a potentially dangerous way like the in-plane artifacts shown in Figs. 18.4, 18.5, and 18.6. An example of off-resonance through-slice artifact is shown in Fig. 18, which compares a full RF pulse excitation (Fig. 18.7a) to the sum of two half pulses (Fig. 18.7b). These were acquired with a perturbation of 2 kHz to the scanner frequency. The image in panel (b) is significantly degraded.

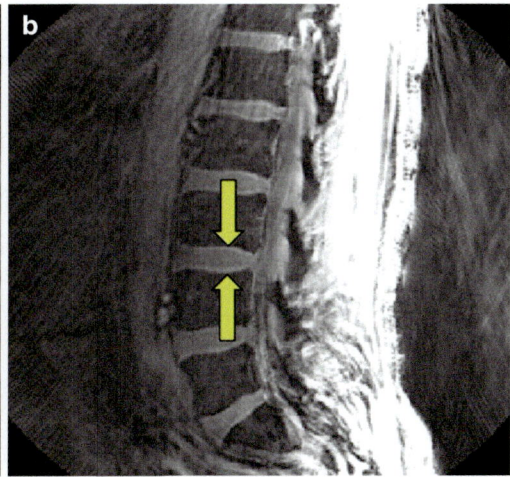

Fig. 18.6 Images of the lumbar spine of the volunteer. (**a**) A sagittal image obtained with a bandwidth of 62.5 kHz. (**b**) The same slice imaged with a bandwidth of 4 kHz. High signal artifacts are seen in the region of the CEPs (yellow arrows). (Reproduced with permission from Bydder et al. [5])

Fig. 18.7 A sagittal image of the brain acquired with a 2 kHz perturbation of the frequency using (**a**) full RF pulse excitation and (**b**) two half-pulse excitations. Artifacts are seen in panel (**b**). The artifacts degrade the image in a way that is unlikely to be mistaken for anatomy. It should be noted that this level of off-resonance was introduced for demonstration purposes and is unlikely to be seen in a scanner that is correctly operated

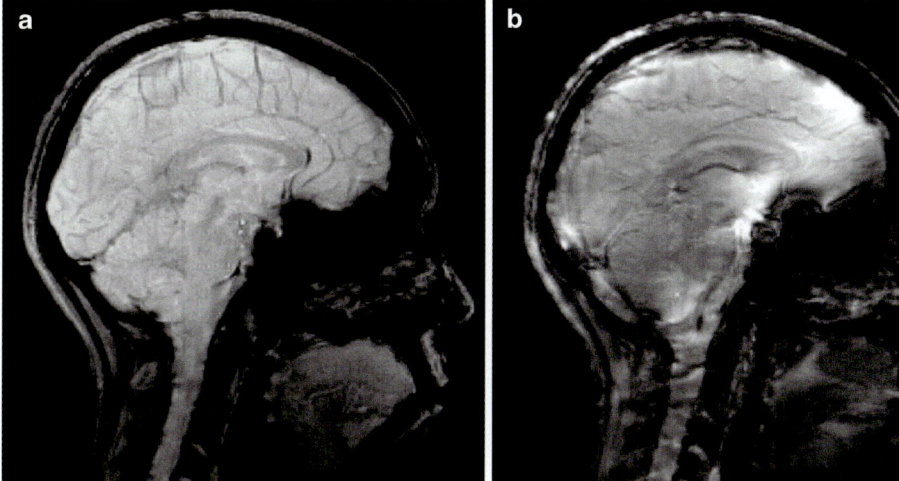

Conclusions

This chapter aims to develop an understanding of chemical shift artifacts seen with center-out radial UTE imaging and to demonstrate that these artifacts can simulate normal structures and disease. Chemical shift between water and fat may result in partial or complete loss of signal from its original location and increases in the central and peripheral signal around the original site of the fatty tissue. This can produce a reduction in the apparent size of the fatty tissue and additional signals that can extend beyond the original fatty tissue in different directions. At a low bandwidth, the artifact can take the form of discrete, well-defined signals displaced away from the original site of the fat, and these may mimic normal anatomy and/or disease. As with Cartesian scanning, the artifacts become more pronounced at low receiver bandwidths and high field strengths.

References

1. Hood MN, Ho VB, Smirniotopoulos JG, Szumowski J. Chemical shift: the artifact and clinical tool revisited. Radiographics. 1999;19(2):357–71.

2. Weiger M, Pruessman KP. Short-T_2 MRI: principles and recent advances. Prog Nucl Magn Reson Spectrosc. 2019;114–115:237–70.

3. Bergin CJ, Pauly JM, Macovski A. Lung parenchyma: projection reconstruction MR imaging. Radiology. 1991;179(3):771–81.

4. Robson MD, Gatehouse PD, Bydder M, Bydder GM. Magnetic resonance: an introduction to ultrashort TE imaging. J Comput Assist Tomogr. 2003;27(6):825–46.

5. Bydder M, Carl M, Bydder GM, Du J. MRI chemical shift artifact produced by center-out radial sampling of k-space: a potential pitfall in clinical diagnosis. Quant Imaging Med Surg. 2021;11(8):3677–83.

6. Rahmer J, Bornert P, Bos C. Three-dimensional radial ultrashort echo-time imaging with T_2 adapted sampling. Magn Reson Med. 2006;55(5):1075–82.

7. Mentrup D, Eggers H. Signal decay correction in 2D ultra-short echo time imaging. MAGMA. 2006;19(2):62–70.

8. Haake EM, Brown RW, Thompson MR, Venkatesan R. Magnetic resonance imaging: physical principles and sequence design. New York: Wiley; 1999. p. 327–8.

9. Pauly JM. Selective excitation for ultrashort echo time imaging. In: Bydder GM, Fullerton GD, Young IR, editors. MRI of tissues with short T_2 s or T_2*s. New York: Wiley; 2012. p. 69–78.

Pulse Sequences as Tissue Property Filters and the Central Contrast Theorem: A Way of Understanding the Signal, Contrast, and Weighting of Magnetic Resonance Images

19

Paul Condron, Samantha J. Holdsworth,
Graeme M. Bydder, and Daniel M. Cornfeld

Introduction

The most important advantage of magnetic resonance imaging (MRI) over X-ray computed tomography (CT) is its higher soft tissue contrast. This was first demonstrated in 1981 in 10 cases of multiple sclerosis (MS) in which 19 lesions were seen with CT and 112 lesions were seen with MRI [1]. This was a major clinical advance in an important disease of the central nervous system (CNS), where imaging previously had little to contribute. The lesion contrast was produced by an increase in T_1 in abnormal areas in the white matter of the brain and by the use of a highly T_1-sensitive inversion recovery (IR) pulse sequence.

In the following year, high soft tissue contrast was also demonstrated as a consequence of increased T_2 in lesions, and the use of long echo time (TE) spin echo (SE) pulse sequences. This was not only in MS but in many other diseases of the brain as well [2, 3].

The most common change in disease seen with MRI is concurrent increases in T_1 and T_2 relative to normal. With SE sequences, an increase in T_1 leads to negative contrast (i.e., a lower signal in the lesion relative to normal) and an increase in T_2 leads to positive contrast (i.e., a higher signal in the lesion). These two effects can can cancel each other out, leading to little or no lesion contrast. To avoid this problem, SE sequences are usually designed to maximize T_1 contrast and minimize opposed T_2 contrast (repetition time, TR about the T_1 of the lesion and a short TE) or to maximize T_2 contrast and minimize opposed T_1 contrast (long TR and TE about the T_2 of the lesion). This gives two principal types of SE images, i.e., T_1-weighted and T_2-weighted, with the names describing the single tissue property (TP), i.e., either T_1 or T_2, that is the dominant source of contrast.

There are difficulties with just designating a single TP as a source of contrast because a single image can be T_1-weighted for one tissue and T_2-weighted for another tissue shown in the same image, and this can lead to incorrect image interpretation. In 1986, this problem led to the American College of Radiology (ACR) Subcommittee on Nomenclature and Phantoms refusing to list the terms "T_1-weighted" and "T_2-weighted" in their Glossary of Terms and recommending that the terms be abandoned [4]. However, the ACR subcommittee did not provide an alternative, and the terms "T_1-weighted" and "T_2-weighted" have continued to be used in clinical practice to the present day.

The difficulties with the concept of weighting have been compounded by the use of additional TPs such as diffusion and susceptibility as well as newer pulse sequences, including the pulsed gradient spin echo (PGSE) sequence and the T_2-fluid-attenuated inversion recovery (T_2-FLAIR) sequence.

This has led to a new approach to understanding contrast that accommodates contrast arising from more than one TP, provides a basis for understanding more complex sequences, and facilitates using TPs synergistically to improve lesion contrast [5–8]. The approach uses the Bloch and Torrey equations with mathematical definitions of contrast and weighting as well as differential calculus to link changes in TPs to changes in signal (or contrast) and forms the subject of this chapter.

P. Condron · S. J. Holdsworth · D. M. Cornfeld
Mātai Medical Research Institute, Tairāwhiti Gisborne, New Zealand

Department of Anatomy and Medical Imaging and Centre for Brain Research, Faculty of Medical and Health Sciences, University of Auckland, Auckland, New Zealand
e-mail: p.condron@matai.org.nz; s.holdsworth@matai.org.nz; d.cornfeld@matai.org.nz

G. M. Bydder (✉)
Mātai Medical Research Institute, Tairāwhiti Gisborne, New Zealand

Department of Radiology, University of California, San Diego, La Jolla, CA, USA
e-mail: gbydder@health.ucsd.edu

J. Du, G. M. Bydder (eds.), *MRI of Short- and Ultrashort-T2 Tissues*, https://doi.org/10.1007/978-3-031-35197-6_19

Normal Tissue Properties (TPs), Changes of TPs in Disease, and the Effects of Contrast Agents

There are 20 or more TPs that affect MR images, and a critical part of MRI is relating differences or changes in TPs in disease to contrast seen on MR images. This is described as the central contrast problem in MRI. It requires a knowledge of pulse sequences and their pulse sequence parameters to link differences or changes in TPs to differences or changes in signal, i.e., contrast (Table 19.1).

It is useful to display the full extent of the values of TPs encountered in clinical practice along X-axes. Differences or changes in a TP can then be represented as horizontal green arrows (Fig. 19.1). Subsequent understanding of image signal and contrast includes all tissues and fluids visualized in the images. The TP X-axis can be either linear or logarithmic. The domain can be chosen to include particular tissues and fluids of clinical interest when, for example, with susceptibility, the values for metal are far outside those of the tissues. (In the subsequent text, the term "tissues" is assumed to include fluids unless otherwise stated.)

In many diseases (e.g., inflammation, demyelination, tumors, etc.) T_1 and T_2 are increased, but, in other conditions, including, for example, hemorrhage and iron deposition, T_1, T_2, and T_2^* are often decreased. Diffusion is frequently decreased in acute diseases of the brain (infarction, infection) and in some tumors but is increased in other tumors and many chronic diseases.

Gadolinium-based contrast agents (GBCAs) can decrease the T_1, T_2, and T_2^* of tissues and can thus create image contrast when appropriate sequences are used. However, the decrease in T_1, T_2, and T_2^* is opposite to the increase in T_1,

Table 19.1 The central contrast problem. Tissue properties (TPs) and their differences or changes (ΔTP, $\frac{\varnothing TP}{TP}$); pulse sequences and their pulse sequence parameters; signal (S) and phase (θ), signal contrast (absolute contrast $C_{ab} = \Delta S$, fractional contrast $C_{fr} = \frac{\varnothing S}{S}$), and phase contrast ($\Delta\theta$ = absolute phase contrast). The central contrast problem is to relate differences or changes in TPs (left column) to differences or changes in signal and phase, i.e. contrast (right column) through knowledge of the pulse sequences and their pulse sequence parameters (central column). Conventionally, this is performed using the concept of qualitative weighting and designates a sequence by the single TP considered to be most responsible for the contrast. Frequently, more than one TP is responsible for contrast between the different tissues imaged, and pulse sequences have different sensitivities to different TPs. This complexity leads to inconsistencies when using qualitative weighting with a single TP to interpret MR images

Tissue properties (TPs)	Pulse sequences and their pulse sequence parameters	Signal (S), phase (θ)
$\Delta TP \quad \dfrac{\varnothing TP}{TP}$		$C_{ab} = \Delta S \quad C_{fr} = \dfrac{\varnothing S}{S}$ $\Delta\theta$
$\Delta\rho_m \quad \dfrac{\Delta\rho_m}{\rho_m}$ $\Delta T_1 \quad \dfrac{\varnothing T_1}{T_1}$ $\Delta T_2 \quad \dfrac{\varnothing T_2}{T_2}$ $\Delta D^* \quad \dfrac{\Delta D^*}{D^*}$	Spin echo (SE) (TR, TE, etc.) Inversion recovery (IR) (TR, TI, TE, etc.) Pulsed gradient spin echo (PGSE) (TR, TE, b, etc.)	$C_{ab} = \Delta S \quad C_{fr} = \dfrac{\varnothing S}{S}$ $\Delta\theta$ = absolute phase contrast
$\Delta\chi$ susceptibility	Spoiled gradient echo (SGE) (TR, TE, α, etc.)	
$\Delta\delta$ chemical shift		
$\varnothing\dfrac{T_2}{T_1} \quad \dfrac{\varnothing\frac{T_2}{T_1}}{\frac{T_2}{T_1}}$	Balanced steady-state free precession (TR, TE, α, etc.)	
Δ ultrashort $T_2 \quad \dfrac{\varnothing \text{Ultrashort} T_2}{T_2}$	Ultrashort TE (UTE) (TR, TE, α, etc.)	
Δ flow, Δv	PGSE (TR, TE, δ, Δ, etc.)	
Δ GBCA concentration c, Δc	SE, IR, SGE, UTE, etc.	

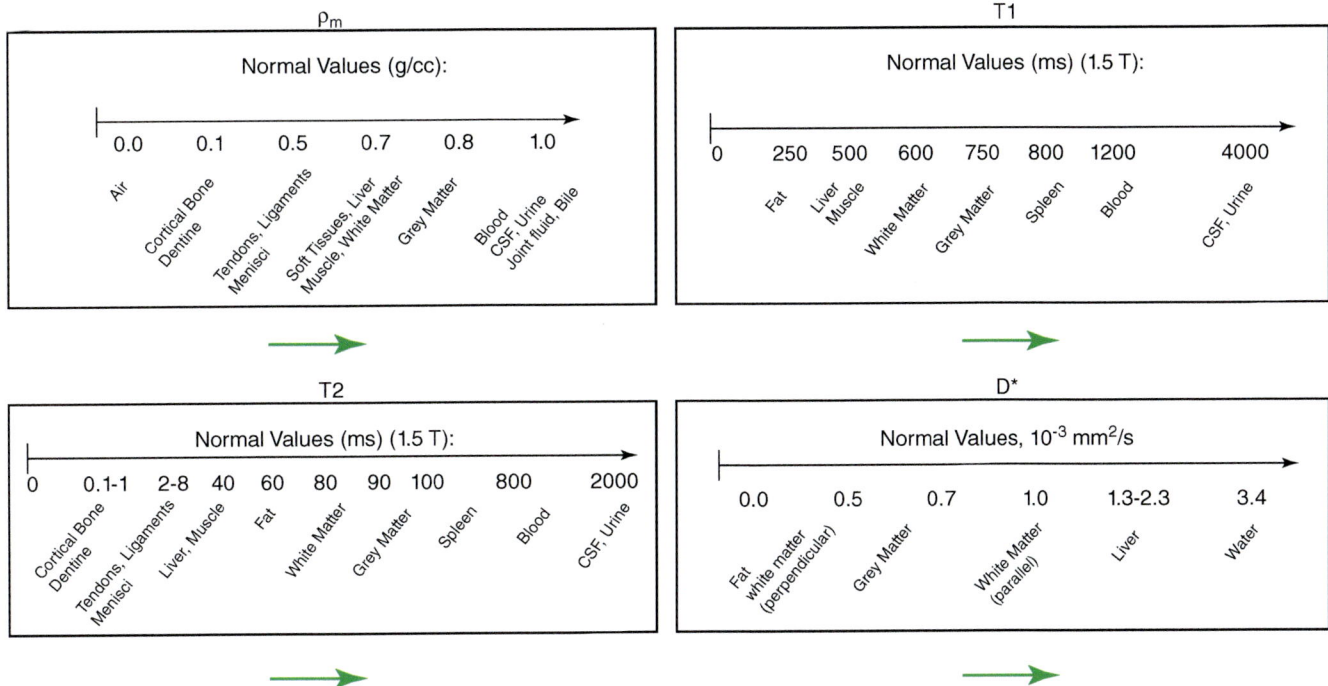

Fig. 19.1 Normal tissue properties (TPs) of ρ_m, T_1, T_2, and D^* ordered from zero to their maximum values along the X-axis using a linear X scale. Differences or changes in TPs are shown as green arrows along the horizontal X-axis

T_2, and T_2^* produced by a disease, and there is a risk that the two opposite effects may cancel each other out.

The signs and magnitudes of the changes in TPs as shown in Fig. 19.1 are also important for synergistic contrast MRI (scMRI). If concurrent changes in different TPs are present (which is usually the case), then there is an opportunity to use appropriate sequences and image processing to make each of the changes in TP synergistically contribute to the overall contrast of the images, irrespective of the sign of those changes.

Fluid properties are important in imaging the brain, for example, and often establish the upper or lower points of the image display dynamic range. Partial volume effects between extremely long T_1 and T_2 cerebrospinal fluid (CSF) and normal tissues may simulate increases in T_1 and T_2 in the tissue and thus in lesions. For this reason, it is often useful to selectively reduce CSF signals when heavily T_2-weighted sequences are used. This can be performed with techniques such as CSF nulling (T_2-FLAIR sequence). Ideally, these techniques should not reduce contrast between the tissues of primary clinical interest.

The Central Contrast Problem

The central contrast problem in clinical MRI is to relate differences or changes in TPs such as $\Delta\rho_m$, ΔT_1, and ΔT_2 (or fractional changes in these TPs, such as $\frac{\Delta\rho_m}{\rho_m}$, $\frac{\varnothing T_1}{T_1}$, and $\frac{\varnothing T_2}{T_2}$, respectively) (Table 19.1, left column) to differences or changes in the signal S, i.e., contrast $C_{ab} = \Delta S$ (or fractional contrast $C_{fr} = \frac{\varnothing S}{S}$) as well as phase θ and differences in phase ($\Delta\theta$) (Table 19.1, right column). This is performed via knowledge of the relevant pulse sequences and their pulse sequence parameters (Table 19.1, central column). Although the Bloch equations describing MRI relate TPs to S, the primary interest in clinical practice is actually to relate differences or changes in TPs to differences or changes in S (i.e., contrast).

The conventional way of doing this is to use qualitative weighting. This designates a single TP as the one believed to

Normal Brain   Abnormal Achilles Tendon

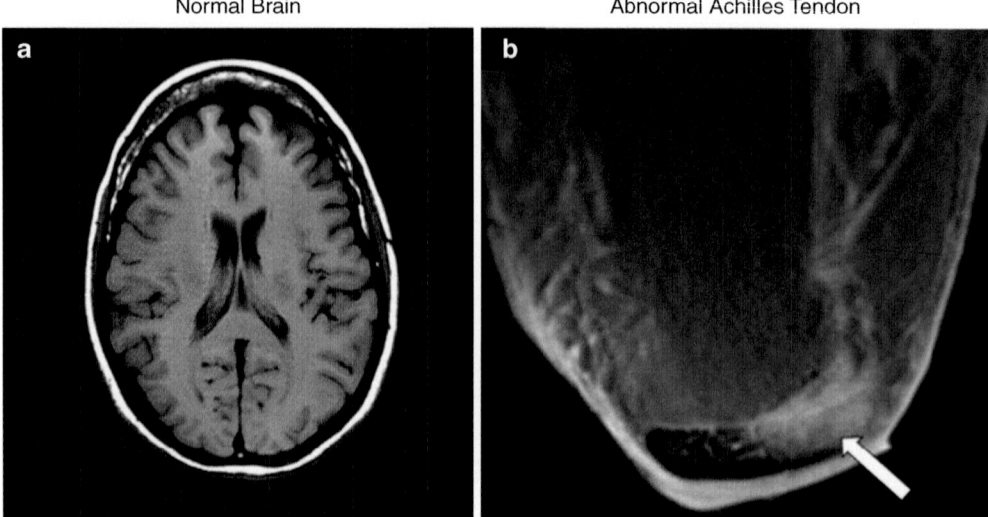

Fig. 19.2 A normal brain showing white and gray matter (**a**), and Achilles tendon showing normal and abnormal (white arrow) areas (**b**) examined with the same T_1-weighted SE (T_1-wSE) sequence. The sequence is T_1-weighted for white and gray matter in panel (**a**) where the increase in T_1 from normal white matter (white color) to normal gray matter (gray color) results in negative contrast. However, the same "T_1-wSE" sequence is T_2-weighted for the Achilles tendon in panel (**b**). The increase in T_2 from normal (black, low signal) to abnormal tissues (white, high signal) in the tendon results in high positive contrast (white arrow) (**b**). If the sequence is regarded as T_1-weighted in the Achilles tendon, then the high signal abnormality could be attributed to a decrease in T_1 and therefore be due to hemorrhage, fat, and/or GBCA enhancement. In fact, the abnormality is due to an increase in T_2 and is likely to be due to completely different pathology, e.g., degeneration, trauma, and/or edema

be most responsible for the contrast of interest and describes sequences and images accordingly as, for example, "T_1-weighted", "T_2-weighted," and "diffusion-weighted." However, contrast is often dependent on differences or changes in more than one of the ten TPs shown in Table 19.1. In addition, there are also at least six classes of pulse sequences, and these display varying sensitivities to differences or changes in TPs. There are also differences within pulse sequence classes, which depend on sequence parameters. This complexity leads to inconsistencies with qualitative weighting where only a single TP is used to describe the relationship between differences or changes in several TPs and the contrast they produce.

Problems with Qualitative Weighting

Examples of the problems encountered with the use of qualitative weighting include the following:

(a) A sequence that is T_1-weighted in one application, for example, showing contrast between the white and gray matter in the brain, can be T_2-weighted in other applications (such as showing contrast between the normal and diseased tissue in the Achilles tendon) even though the sequence is still usually described as T_1-weighted (Fig. 19.2).

(b) T_2-FLAIR sequences are highly T_2-weighted for the brain but are simultaneously highly T_1-weighted for CSF.

(c) "Diffusion-weighted" sequences may be more T_2-weighted than diffusion-weighted.

(d) Although reducing TE is said to reduce T_2-weighting, subtracted ultrashort TE (UTE) sequences with ultrashort TEs (e.g., 8 µs) can be highly T_2-weighted.

(e) "Fluid-sensitive" sequences used in the musculoskeletal system are insensitive to fluids such as pore water and matrix-bound water in cortical bone. On the other hand, subtracted UTE sequences that are sensitive to pore and matrix-bound water are insensitive to joint and bursal fluid.

These and other inconsistencies complicate the use of qualitative weighting for image interpretation and limit its usefulness for understanding more complex sequences as well as developing new applications of these sequences in clinical MRI.

In order to resolve these problems, it is necessary to recognize the fact that several different TPs often determine contrast with most pulse sequences and provide specific relationships between differences or changes in TPs and differences or changes in signal (i.e., contrast) with these sequences. This is outlined in the next sections.

Pulse Sequences as Tissue Property (TP) Filters

The Spin Echo (SE) Sequence (Univariate Model)

The usual explanation of image signal and contrast with the SE sequence utilizes the Bloch equations. First, it follows longitudinal magnetization (M_Z) over time TR, and, second, it follows transverse magnetization (M_{XY}) after the application of a 90° pulse (Fig. 19.3) for a further time TE. Contrast between two tissues, such as P with a shorter T_1 and T_2 and Q with a longer T_1 and T_2, is shown by the difference in M_{XY} at the time of data collection (dc) at TE, as shown in Fig. 19.3.

The voxel signal S for an SE sequence is derived from the simplified Bloch equations so that

$$S = K\rho_m \left(1 - e^{-t'/T_1}\right) e^{-t''/T_2} \qquad (19.1)$$

where K is a scaling function, ρ_m is the mobile proton density, and t' as well as t'' are variable times. T_1 and T_2 are time constants. Equation 19.1 describes ρ_m in the first segment, recovery of longitudinal magnetization (M_Z) over time t' in the second segment (which is in parentheses), and decay of transverse magnetization (M_{XY}) over time in the third segment. The equations in the second and third segments are of the forms $y = 1 - e^{-x}$ and $y = e^{-x}$, respectively.

It is useful to replace the variables t' and t'' in Eq. 19.1 by the constant times of the SE sequence TR and TE and to treat the two time constants T_1 and T_2 in Eq. 19.1 as variables. This changes Eq. 19.1 to

$$S = K\rho_m \left(1 - e^{-TR/T_1}\right) e^{-TE/T_2} \qquad (19.2)$$

or

$$S = KS\rho_m S_{T_1} S_{T_2} \qquad (19.3)$$

where the signals for the three segments $S\rho_m$, S_{T1}, and S_{T2} are given by

$$S\rho_m = \rho_m, \quad S_{T_1} = 1 - e^{-TR/T_1}, \quad S_{T_2} = e^{-TE/T_2} \qquad (19.4)$$

The second and third segments in Eq. 19.2 are of the forms $y = 1 - e^{-1/x}$ and $y = e^{-1/x}$, respectively, since T_1 and T_2 are now variables. These forms are quite different from the forms $y = 1 - e^{-x}$ and $y = e^{-x}$ shown in the second and third segments of the Bloch equations, respectively, in Eq. 19.1.

The three segments of Eqs. 19.2–19.4 have the features of a linear or exponential filter for ρ_m (depending on whether the X-axis is linear or natural logarithmic (ln)), a low-pass filter for T_1, and a high-pass filter for T_2 (Figs. 19.4, 19.5, and 19.6).

The signal levels on images are given by Eqs. 19.2–19.4 for ρ_m, S_{T1}, and S_{T2} and correspond to the signal or brightness of tissues seen on images.

Equations 19.2–19.4 can be plotted using linear or logarithmic X-axes. When using a linear axis, changes in x (i.e., changes in ρ_m, T_1, or T_2) represent the absolute differences in TPs. When using a logarithmic X-axis as in Figs. 19.4, 19.5, and 19.6, small changes in x (i.e., $\Delta\ln \rho_m$, $\Delta\ln T_1$, and $\Delta\ln T_2$) represent the fractional changes in TPs because of small differences $\Delta\ln x = \Delta x/x$.

In Fig. 19.4, which shows a ρ_m-filter, the absolute contrast C_{ab} (vertical blue arrow) is produced by an increase in ρ_m (horizontal green arrow) multiplied by the positive slope of the ρ_m-filter (red line). The difference in signal $\Delta S\rho_m$ equals C_{ab} (vertical blue arrow).

The absolute contrast (C_{ab}) or difference in signal ΔS_{T1} produced by the positive increase $\Delta\ln T_1$ $\left(= \dfrac{\emptyset T_1}{T_1}\right)$ between the T_1s of two tissues P and Q is shown in Fig. 19.5 using a ln X-axis. The positive change from P to Q of $\Delta\ln T_1$ along the X-axis (horizontal green arrow) produces a negative change from P to Q along the Y-axis (vertical blue arrow) or a negative change in signal ΔS_{T1}, i.e., negative contrast $C_{ab} = \Delta S_{T1}$.

The equation for C_{ab} for small changes in ΔT_1 and ΔS_{T1} using a linear X-axis is

$$C_{ab} = \Delta S_{T_1} = \frac{\partial S_{T_1}}{\partial T_1} \times \Delta T_1 \qquad (19.5)$$

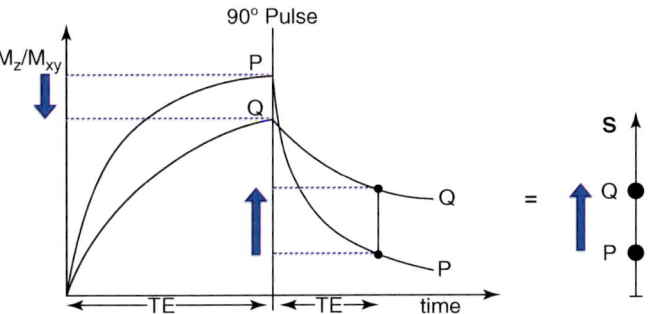

Fig. 19.3 A plot of M_Z/M_{XY} vs. times TR and TE for the SE sequence for two tissues, P (with a shorter T_1 and T_2) and Q (with a longer T_1 and T_2). T_1-dependent contrast (the first negative blue arrow on the left) and the overall T_1 and T_2 contrast (the second and third positive blue arrows in the center and on the right, respectively) are shown

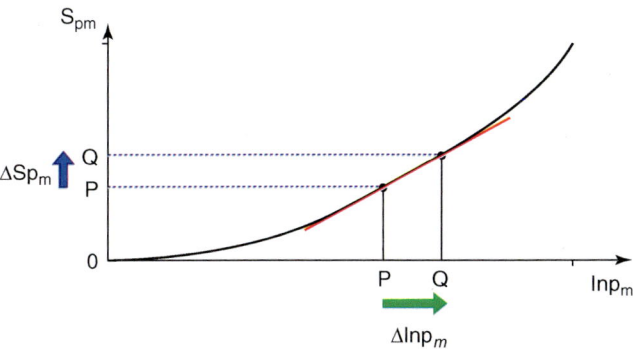

Fig. 19.4 An SE sequence. A ρ_m-filter with a ln ρ_m X-axis. The positive increase in ρ_m from P to Q $\Delta\ln \rho_m$ (positive horizontal green arrow) is multiplied by the positive slope of the filter (red line) to produce positive contrast (positive vertical blue arrow) $\Delta S\rho_m = C_{ab}$

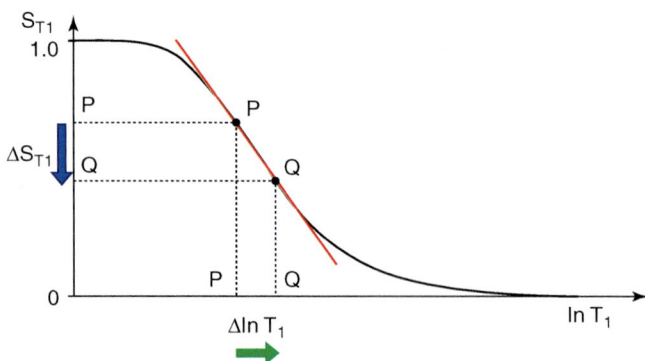

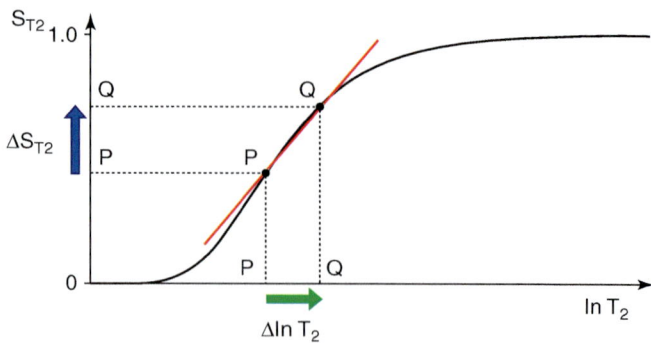

Fig. 19.5 An SE sequence. The T_1-filter with a ln T_1 X-axis. The positive increase in T_1 from P to Q Δln T_1 (positive horizontal green arrow) is multiplied by the negative slope of the filter (red line) to produce negative contrast (negative vertical blue arrow) $\Delta S_{T1} = C_{ab}$. ΔS_{T1} may be positive or negative. Δln T_1 may also be positive or negative

Fig. 19.6 An SE sequence. The T_2-filter with a ln T_2 X-axis. The positive increase in T_2 from P to Q Δln T_2 (positive horizontal green arrow) is multiplied by the positive slope of the filter (red line) to produce positive contrast (positive vertical blue arrow) $\Delta S_{T2} = C_{ab}$

where $\dfrac{\partial S_{T_1}}{\partial T_1}$ is the first partial derivative of the T_1-filter with respect to T_1, or the slope of the T_1-filter, x = multiplied, and ΔT_1 is the change in T_1 using a linear X-axis.

Using a ln X-axis, noting that Δln $T_1 = \dfrac{\varnothing T_1}{T_1}$ for small changes in T_1, and that $\dfrac{dy}{d(\ln x)} = x\,\dfrac{dy}{dx}$, where x is a variable, Eq. 19.5 becomes

$$C_{ab} = \Delta S_{T_1} = \frac{\partial S_{T_1}}{\partial \ln T_1} \times \frac{\Delta T_1}{T_1} \qquad (19.6)$$

where $\dfrac{\partial S_{T_1}}{\partial \ln T_1}$ is the slope of the filter, or the first partial derivative with respect to ln T_1 (when using a ln X-axis), x = multiplied in this and subsequence equations, and $\dfrac{\varnothing T_1}{T_1}$ is the fractional change in T_1, as shown in Fig. 19.5. For the T_1-filter, a positive change from P to Q along the X-axis results in a negative change from P to Q along the Y-axis, i.e., negative contrast C_{ab}. The slope of the curve (red line), which is the sequence weighting for the T_1 segment, is negative.

For the T_2-filter (Fig. 19.6), the positive change Δln $T_2 = \dfrac{\varnothing T_2}{T_2}$ from P to Q along the X-axis results in positive change $\Delta S_{T2} = C_{ab}$ from P to Q along the Y-axis, i.e., positive contrast. The slope of the T_2-filter (red line), which is the sequence weighting for the T_2 segment, is positive.

Putting the second derivative of the TP-filter to zero yields the TP value where the slope of the TP-filter, and therefore the contrast, is the highest. For the T_1 and T_2-filters, the slope is at TR = T_1 and TE = T_2, when using a ln X-axis, and at TR = 2 T_1 and TE = 2 T_2, when using a linear X-axis.

For the fractional contrast $C_{fr} = \Delta S/S$ (rather than $C_{ab} = \Delta S$), Eqs. 19.5 and 19.6 are divided by S_{T1} and S_{T2} for the nonzero values of S_{T1} and S_{T2}, respectively.

So, for T_1 using a ln X-axis,

$$C_{fr} = \frac{1}{S_{T_1}} \frac{\partial S_{T_1}}{\partial \ln T_1} \times \frac{\Delta T_1}{T_1} \qquad (19.7)$$

and for T_2 using a ln X-axis,

$$C_{fr} = \frac{1}{S_{T_2}} \frac{\partial S_{T_2}}{\partial \ln T_2} \times \frac{\Delta T_2}{T_2} \qquad (19.8)$$

The Spin Echo (SE) Sequence (Multivariate Model) and the Central Contrast Theorem (CCT)

The TP-filters can be either considered separately (i.e., a univariate model for each TP alone, as above) or combined in a multivariate model. This shows the contributions of the sequence weightings and changes in each TP to the overall contrast for each of ρ_m, T_1, and T_2 in the SE sequence and is illustrated in Fig. 19.7.

From Eqs. 19.3 and 19.4, for a small change in $\Delta\rho_m$, ΔT_1, and ΔT_2, and using a ln X-axis, the product rule from differential calculus gives

$$\Delta S = \frac{\partial S_{\rho_m}}{\partial \ln \rho_m} S_{T_1} S_{T_2} \times \frac{\Delta \rho_m}{\rho_m} + S_{\rho_m} \frac{\partial S_{T_1}}{\partial \ln T_1} S_{T_2} \times \frac{\Delta T_1}{T_1} + S_{\rho_m} S_{T_1} \frac{\partial S_{T_2}}{\partial \ln T_2} \times \frac{\Delta T_2}{T_2} \qquad (19.9)$$

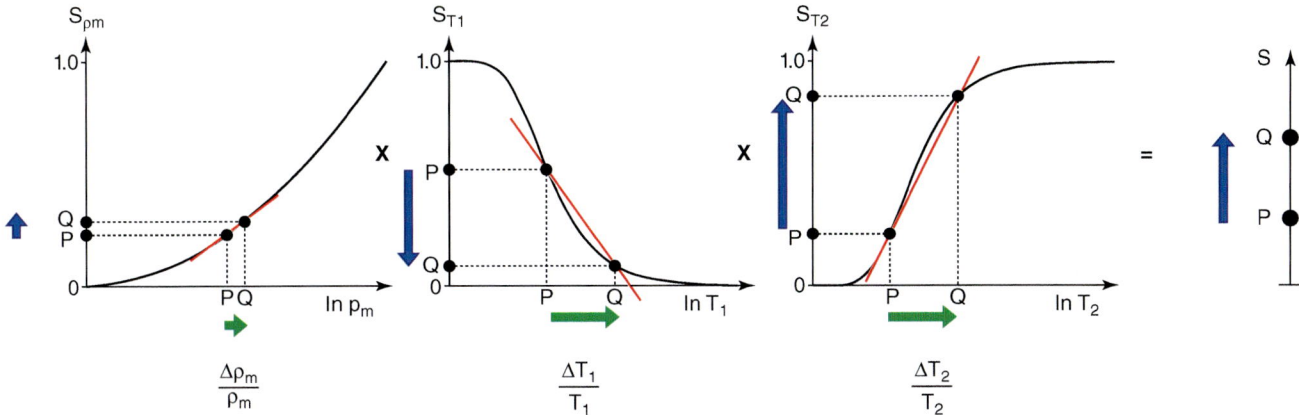

Fig. 19.7 An SE sequence with combination of ρ_m, T_1, and T_2-filters. Increases in $\Delta\rho_m/\rho_m$, $\Delta T_1/T_1$, and $\Delta T_2/T_2$ (positive horizontal green arrows) are multiplied by the slopes of their respective TP-filters (red lines) to produce positive, negative, and positive ρ_m, T_1, and T_2 contrasts with their respective TP-filters (vertical blue arrows with each TP-filter). The overall positive contrast (positive blue arrow on the right) is the algebraic sum of the TP contrasts produced by each of the three TP-filters (blue arrows with each TP-filter)

With linear X-axis, i.e. TP

$$C_{fr} = \sum_{TP}^{n} \frac{1}{S_{TP}} \frac{S_{TP}}{TP} \cdot \Delta TP$$

With logarithmic X-axis, i.e. lnTP

$$C_{fr} = \sum_{TP}^{n} \frac{1}{S_{TP}} \frac{S_{TP}}{TP} \cdot \frac{\Delta TP}{TP}$$

C_{fr}	=	$\Delta S/S$, fractional contrast
TP	=	ρ_m, T_1, T_2, T_2^*, D^*, T_2/T_1....
S_{TP}	=	TP-filter for each pulse sequence SE, IR, PGSE, SGE, bSSFP...
$\dfrac{S_{TP}}{TP}$	=	first partial derivative of S_{TP} with respect ot TP for linear X-axis; is sequence weighting and slope of filter
$\dfrac{S_{TP}}{lnTP}$	=	first partial derivative of S_{TP} with respect ot TP for logarithmic X-axis; is sequence weighting and slope of filter
ΔTP	=	difference or change in TP
$\dfrac{\Delta TP}{TP}$	=	fractional difference or change in TP

Fig. 19.8 The central contrast theorem (CCT) for MRI and a corollary. The signal equations for C_{fr} are shown with a linear X-axis (TP) (upper) and with a logarithmic X-axis (ln TP) (lower). The theorem relates the fractional contrast C_{fr} to differences or changes in TPs and provides solutions to the central contrast problem outlined in Table 19.1, i.e., the relationship between the differences or changes in TPs shown in the first column in Table 19.1 and the differences or changes in signal or contrast shown in the third column of Table 19.1

Normalizing Eq. 19.9 by dividing it by S and using Eq. 19.3 for the nonzero values of S, $S_{\rho m}$, S_{T1}, and S_{T2}, C_{fr} is given by

$$C_{fr} = \frac{\Delta S}{S} = \frac{1}{S_{\rho_m}} \frac{\partial S_{\rho_m}}{\partial \ln \rho_m} \times \frac{\Delta \rho_m}{\rho_m} + \frac{1}{S_{T_1}} \frac{\partial S_{T_1}}{\partial \ln T_1} \times \frac{\Delta T_1}{T_1} + \frac{1}{S_{T_2}} \frac{\partial S_{T_2}}{\partial \ln T_2} \times \frac{\Delta T_2}{T_2} \tag{19.10}$$

Thus, the contributions of the TPs to the overall contrast C_{fr} are, for each TP, its sequence weighting multiplied by the fractional change in the TP. The relative contributions of each TP to sequence and image weighting can be calculated and expressed as ratios.

From Eq. 19.10, the overall fractional contrast C_{fr} using a ln X-axis is given by

$$C_{fr} = \sum_{TP} \frac{1}{S_{TP}} \frac{\partial S_{TP}}{\partial \ln TP} \times \frac{\Delta TP}{TP} \tag{19.11}$$

where $1/S_{TP}$ $S_{TP}/\partial \ln$ TP is the sequence weighting for the tissue property and $\Delta TP/TP$ is the fractional change in the TP. This is one form of the central contrast theorem (CCT) for MRI and its corollaries, which are shown in Fig. 19.8. Using a ln X-axis, the contrast for each TP is the normalized first partial derivative with respect to ln TP multiplied by the fractional change in TP. The total fractional contrast C_{fr} is the algebraic sum of the contributions to contrast from each TP. For T_1 and T_2, if both fractional contrasts are positive or, if both are negative, then a synergistic contribution to overall

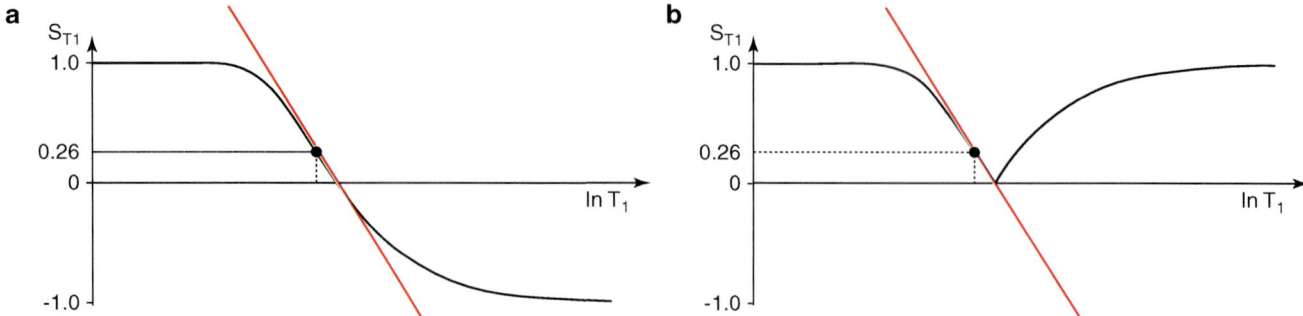

Fig. 19.9 IR T_1-filters with phase-sensitive (ps) (**a**) and magnitude (m) reconstruction (**b**) using ln T_1 X-axes. Panel (**a**) shows both positive and negative values for S_{T1}, whereas in panel (**b**), negative values are "reflected" across the X-axis and become positive. The maximum slopes of the T_1-filters are shown as red lines and are negative in both cases

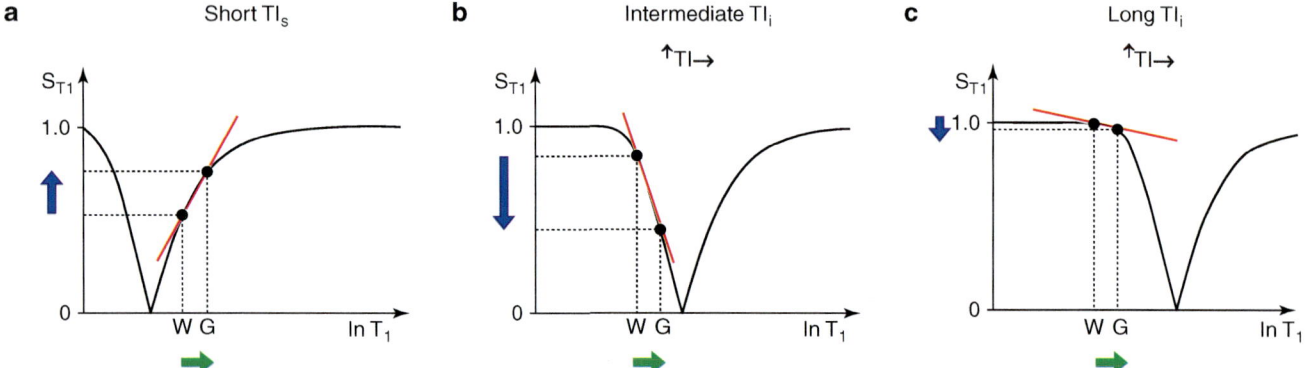

Fig. 19.10 The long-TR IR sequence. T_1-filters for short TI_s (**a**, left), intermediate TI_i (**b**, center), and long-TI_l (**c**, right) values. The positions of the white (W) and gray (G) matter are the same for each of the three TIs. TI is increased from TI_s (left) to TI_i (center) and then further to TI_l (right). The increase in T_1 from W to G along the X axis (green arrows) is multiplied by the relevant slopes of the T_1-filters (red lines) and produces strongly positive, strongly negative, and mildly negative contrast, respectively (blue arrows), as TI is increased from left to right

C_{fr} results. If one TP contrast is negative and the other is positive, then there is a reduction in the overall C_{fr} results. Thus, to achieve synergistic contrast, contributions to contrast of the same sign are sought from each of the relevant TPs to make their effects complementary.

The Inversion Recovery (IR) Sequence

The IR sequence has an additional T_1 filter (segment) to those of the SE sequence, which is shown in Fig. 19.12, where

$$S_{T_1} = \left(1 - 2e^{-TI/T_1}\right) \qquad (19.12)$$

This T_1-filter is shown in the phase-sensitive (ps) reconstructed form in Fig. 19.9a and in magnitude (m) reconstructed form in Fig. 19.9b.

When the inversion time (TI) is increased, the T_1-filter shifts to the right as shown for the m form in Fig. 19.10.

Figure 19.10a (left) shows the IR T_1-filter with a short TI_s (e.g., the short TI IR or STIR sequence) for the brain where gray matter (G) has a higher signal than white matter (W). The slope of the filter between W and G is strongly positive. When TI is increased to an intermediate TI_i as in Fig. 19.10b (center) with W and G fixed in the same position on the ln X-axis, W has a higher signal than G. The slope of the T_1-filter between them is strongly negative. When TI_i is increased further to a long TI_i as in Fig. 19.10c (right), W has a slightly higher signal than does G and the slope of the T_1-filter between them is negative but of smaller size than in Fig. 19.10b. The sequence T_1-weighting, which is the slope or first partial derivative of the T_1-filter, is highly positive in panel (a), highly negative in panel (b), and slightly negative in panel (c) using a short TI_s (a), an intermediate TI_i (b), and a long TI_l (c), respectively.

When the IR sequence repetition time (TR) is much greater than T_1, the other T_1-filter $(1 - e^{-TR/T1})$ becomes ~1, and the main determinant of contrast is the $(1 - 2e^{-TI/T1})$ T_1-filter.

Fig. 19.11 PGSE sequence T_2 and D^*-filters. Increases in both T_2 and D^* from P to Q (positive horizontal green arrows) result in positive and negative T_2 and D^* contrast, respectively, and low opposite negative overall contrast (negative short vertical blue arrow, right)

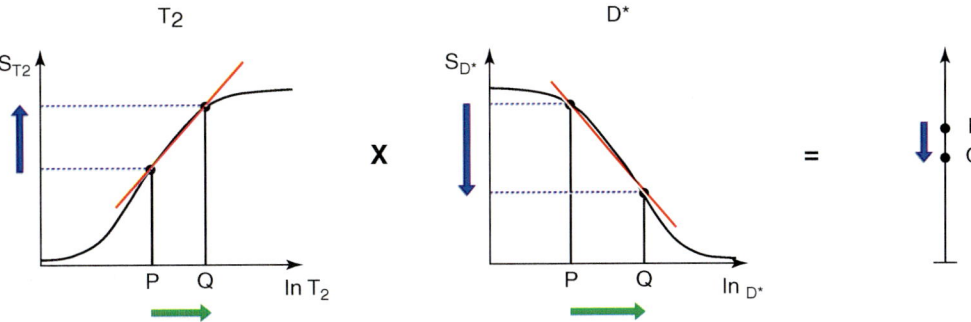

Fig. 19.12 PGSE sequence T_2 and D^*-filters. Increase in T_2 and decrease in D^* from P to Q (positive and negative horizontal green arrows, respectively) both produce positive contrast and, as a consequence, high positive overall synergistic contrast (positive long vertical blue arrow, right)

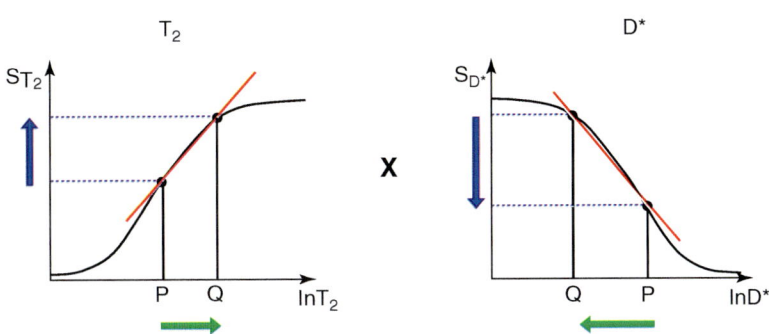

The Pulsed Gradient Spin Echo (PGSE) Sequence

For diffusion using the PGSE sequence, an additional segment is added to those shown in Fig. 19.7 for the SE sequence and is illustrated in Fig. 19.11 under the D^* heading. The extra segment is the D^* filter, which has the form of an exponential decay with its signal S_{D^*} given by

$$S_{D^*} = e^{-bD^*} \qquad (19.13)$$

b is the diffusion sensitivity parameter and D^* is the apparent diffusion coefficient. Significant D^*-weighting requires a long TE with the PGSE sequence using present-day clinical scanners. This is to provide time for the two pulsed diffusion gradients to be applied before and after the inversion pulse of the SE sequence. The long TE necessary for this creates T_2-weighting, and, so, the sequence simultaneously has both positive T_2-weighting (i.e. the positive slope of the T_2-filter shown in Fig. 19.11 under the T_2 heading) and negative D^*-weighting (i.e. the negative slope of the D^*-filter shown in Fig. 19.11 under the D^* heading). The positive change ΔT_2 from P to Q along the X-axis (horizontal green arrow) produces positive T_2 contrast (the positive vertical blue arrow). The positive change ΔD^* from P to Q along the X-axis produces negative D^* contrast (negative vertical blue arrow). The overall result of the opposed T_2 and D^* contrasts produced in this way is low negative contrast (negative short vertical blue arrow on the right in Fig. 19.11). This is the case in many tissues where disease

causes an increase in both T_2 and D^* and the resulting opposite diffusion and T_2 contrasts produce low overall contrast.

Figure 19.12 shows a situation in which T_2 is increased from P to Q under the heading T_2 and D^* is *decreased* from P to Q under the heading D^* (rather than increased as in Fig. 19.11). The changes in T_2 and D^* both result in positive contrast (blue arrows), and the algebraic sum of these is synergistic and produces high positive contrast (vertical long blue arrow on the right). In this situation, the PGSE T_2 and diffusion weightings work together with the changes in T_2 and D^* to produce synergistic contrast.

The Spoiled Gradient Echo (SGE) Sequence

(a) The SGE sequence has a T_1-filter, which is affected by two pulse sequence parameters TR and the flip angle α (Eq. 19.14). The T_1-filter, appears the same as the T_1-filter SE sequence for flip angle $\alpha = 90°$, but, as α is reduced, the curve flattens and there is less T_1 sequence weighting for a given value of TR (Fig. 19.13).

$$S = \frac{\sin \alpha}{1 - \cos \alpha e^{-\frac{TR}{T_1}}} \left(1 - e^{-\frac{TR}{T_1}} \right) \qquad (19.14)$$

S is the signal, α is the flip angle, and TR is the repetition time. The flip angle to maximize the signal α_S is determined by setting the first derivative of Eq. 19.14 to zero. The flip

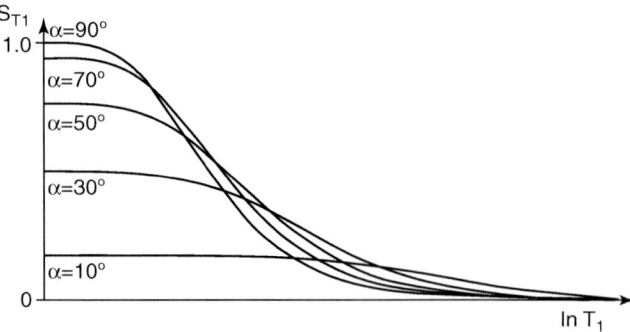

Fig. 19.13 An SGE sequence T_1-filter. For a given TR as α is decreased from 90° to 10°, the negative slope of the curve (which is its T_1 sequence weighting) generally decreases in size

angle to maximize the contrast α_C is determined by setting the second derivative of Eq. 19.14 to zero.

With the SGE sequence, the T_2-filter of the SE sequence becomes a $T_2{}^*$-filter and includes additional susceptibility effects, which make $T_2{}^*$-less than T_2. Chemical shift effects are modeled by including phase differences for water and fat and taking the vector sum and difference of these as with the Dixon technique.

Ultrashort Echo Time (UTE) and Zero Echo Time (ZTE) Sequences

The UTE and ZTE sequences are the subjects of much of this book. They both decrease the effective TE of acquisitions so that it is possible to detect signals from tissues with short and ultrashort T_2s. Their general behavior parallels that of the SGE sequence with a T_1-dependent segment in which both the signal and contrast depend on TR and α as well as a T_2-dependent segment in which contrast depends on $T_2{}^*$ and TE.

Use of an inversion pulse as preparation introduces an additional T_2-filter for tissues with T_2s comparable to, or less than, the duration of the inversion pulse. This pulse is typically used with a TI chosen to null the long-T_2 components, which are fully inverted. Short- and ultrashort-T_2 components are typically not fully inverted and are instead partially or fully saturated.

These two effects have the result of producing low-pass T_2 and T_1-filters in which short- and ultrashort-T_2 signals are detectable (with a UTE or ZTE acquisition), but long-T_2 and long-T_1 tissues and fluids are not detectable.

Lesions that increase T_2 in the short- and ultrashort-T_2 domains produce a reduction in signal with nulled inversion pulse preparations (negative contrast) and thus are synergistic with negative T_2 contrast produced by echo subtraction (ES), as explained in previous chapters.

Features of TP-Filters

Features of the TP-filter approach include the following:

(a) Placement of TPs along the X-axis, and the use of both linear and ln scales along this axis.
(b) Placement of signal S along the Y-axis and the use of both linear and logarithmic scales for this.
(c) Use of both the absolute contrast C_{ab} and the fractional contrast C_{fr}.
(d) Designation of the slope or first derivative of the TP-filter (or normalized slope of the TP-filter) as sequence weighting and calculation of this slope both for linear and ln X-axes.
(e) The use of the second derivatives of the TP-filter and points of inflection to calculate the values of sequence parameters (e.g., TR = T_1, TE = T_2 with ln X-axes) to maximize C_{ab}.
(f) Allocation of signs (positive or negative) to each of signal, contrast, image weighting, sequence weighting, and TP differences or changes. This helps make it possible to understand contrast and weighting in both semiquantitative and quantitative terms.
(g) Separation of sequence and image weighting and calculation of sequence and image weighting ratios to determine the relative contributions of different TPs to sequence weighting and image weighting.
(h) Ability to deal with the situation in which a single TP (e.g., T_1) is affected by two pulse sequence parameters (TR and α) or a single pulse sequence parameter (e.g., TE) has effects on two TPs (e.g., T_2 and D^*).
(i) TP values cover the full extent experienced in clinical practice so the graphics provide a complete representation of the contrast and weighting of images.
(j) The same approach can be used for sequence preparations and complete pulse sequences.
(k) Although developed here primarily for ρ_m, T_1, T_2, D^*, and $T_2{}^*$, the TP-filter approach is also applicable to other TPs.

Features of the Central Contrast Theorem (CCT) and Its Corollaries

Unlike conventional qualitative weighting, which only utilizes a single TP to explain contrast, the CCT makes it possible to deal with two or more TPs and to understand both their separate and combined contributions to contrast. As a result, use of the CCT resolves many of the inconsistencies associated with the use of conventional qualitative weighting. Resolution of one of these inconsistencies is shown in Fig. 19.14, which explains the fact that an SE sequence that is T_1-weighted for the brain can be T_2-weighted for disease in

Brain normal white matter (W) and gray matter (G): T_1-wSE sequence (upper)

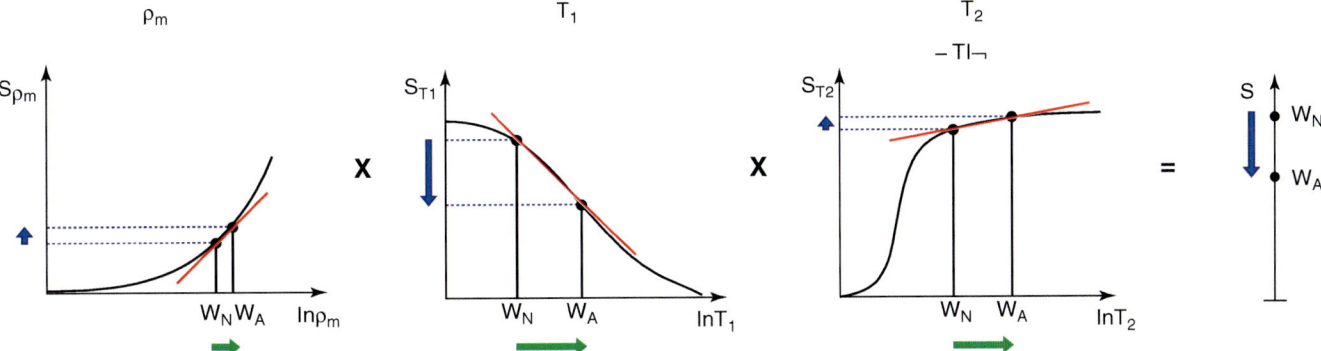

Achilles tendon normal (T_N) and abnormal (T_A): "T_1-wSE" sequence (lower)

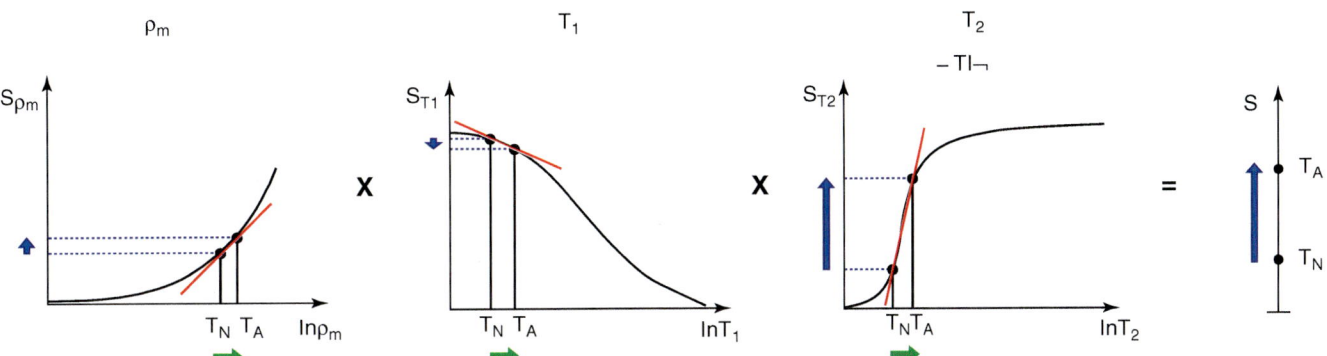

Fig. 19.14 Normal white matter (W) and gray matter (G) in the brain (upper) as well as normal (T_N) and abnormal (T_A) Achilles tendon (lower) imaged with the same T_1-wSE sequence. The T_1-wSE sequence ρ_m, T_1, and T_2-filters are the same in the upper and lower figures. In the upper figure, ρ_m, T_1, and T_2 are increased from W to G. The TP sequence weightings are the slopes of the TP-filters (red lines), which are positive for ρ_m, negative for T_1, and positive for T_2. The contrast produced by each filter is the increase in each TP (positive horizontal green arrows) multiplied by the slope of the relevant TP-filter (red lines), and these are shown as vertical blue arrows for each TP-filter. They are slightly positive for ρ_m, markedly negative for T_1, and slightly positive for T_2 (upper). The overall fractional contrast is the algebraic sum of the fractional contrasts for each TP. This is shown as the negative vertical blue arrow (on the upper right side). In the lower part of the figure, the normal T_1 of the Achilles tendon is shorter than that of W (upper) and corresponds to a flatter negative part of the T_1-filter (lower). The normal T_2 of the Achilles tendon (lower) is shorter than that of W (upper) and corresponds with a steeply positive sloping part of the T_2-filter (lower). The abnormality in the Achilles tendon shows an increase in ρ_m, T_1, and T_2 (positive green arrows) (lower). These changes are multiplied by the

positive ρ_m, slightly negative T_1, and highly positive slopes of the ρ_m, T_1, and T_2 filters, respectively (red lines). These produce positive, slightly negative, and strongly positive TP contrasts, respectively (vertical blue arrows for each TP-filter). The overall fractional contrast, which is the algebraic sum of the fractional TP contrasts, is highly positive (blue vertical arrow) (lower right side). Because of the shorter T_1 and T_2 of the Achilles tendon relative to the T_1 and T_2 of W and G, there is a shift from the dominant negative T_1-weighting and contrast for W relative to G (i.e., steeper T_1 and flatter T_2 in the corresponding parts of the T_1 and T_2-filters) (upper), to the dominant positive T_2-weighting and contrast for the change from normal (T_N) to abnormal (T_A) in the Achilles tendon (flatter T_1 and steeper T_2 in the corresponding parts of the T_1 and T_2-filters) (lower). The designation "T_1-weighted" is usually applied to the "T_1-wSE" sequence when it is used for the Achilles tendon even though the sequence and contrast are both actually T_2-weighted. This may be because there is already a long TR, long TE T_2-weighted SE sequence in regular use in the musculoskeletal system, and redesignating the "T_1-wSE" sequence as T_2-weighted as well could cause a different type of confusion

the Achilles tendon, as illustrated in Fig. 19.2. It also makes it possible to understand how T_2 and D^* contrast behave individually and how they interact with each other with the PGSE sequence (Figs. 19.11 and 19.12).

The CCT formalizes the relationship between differences/changes in TPs and the fractional contrast C_{fr} (Fig. 19.8). It is in two parts. First, for each TP, the fractional contrast generated is the normalized product of sequence weighting (the partial derivative of the TP-filter either with respect to the TP or ln TP) multiplied by the change in TP or the fractional change in TP. The second part is the algebraic sum of the fractional contrasts generated by each TP, which is the overall fractional contrast C_{fr}. For signal S, the CCT and its corol-laries are derived from the Bloch equations for ρ_m, T_1 and T_2, and the Torrey equations, which add diffusion D^*. The CCT is used in graphical form in this chapter.

The CCT can be used in qualitative form to determine which single TP among several is the most responsible for contrast for given changes in the TPs and a specific pulse sequence. It is the TP with the largest C_{fr}. It can also be used in semiquantitative or graphical form where the sign of differences or changes in TP and their relative magnitudes are considered. It can also be used in quantitative form where sequence and image weighting ratios are expressed in percentages with the relative contributions of each TP to sequence weighting and to image weighting using the equations:

$$sW^r\left(\rho_m : T_1 : T_2\right) = \left(\frac{1}{S_{\rho_m}}\frac{\partial S_{\rho_m}}{\partial \ln \rho_m} : \frac{1}{S_{T_1}}\frac{\partial S_{T_1}}{\partial \ln T_1} : \frac{1}{S_{T_2}}\frac{\partial S_{T_2}}{\partial \ln T_2}\right) \quad (19.15)$$

$$iW^r\left(\rho_m : T_1 : T_2\right) = \left(\frac{1}{S_{\rho_m}}\frac{\partial S_{\rho_m}}{\partial \ln \rho_m}\cdot\frac{\Delta\rho_m}{\rho_m} : \frac{1}{S_{T_1}}\frac{\partial S_{T_1}}{\partial \ln T_1}\cdot\frac{\Delta T_1}{T_1} : \frac{1}{S_{T_2}}\frac{\partial S_{T_2}}{\partial \ln T_2}\cdot\frac{\Delta T_2}{T_2}\right) \quad (19.16)$$

The sequence weighting ratio sW^r describes the relative weighting of the TPs within a sequence. The image weighting ratio (iW^r) uses the sequence weighting ratio and combines it with differences/changes in each TP to describe their relative effects on the contrast of the image. This is an important difference. The sequence T_1-filter may be steeper than the T_2-filter, meaning that it is more T_1-weighted than it is T_2-weighted for particular values of T_1 and T_2. However, if disease results in a larger change in T_2 than in T_1, contrast on the image can be dominated by the T_2 change and not the T_1 change so that the image has a dominant T_2-weighting in spite of the fact that the sequence has a dominant T_1-weighting.

The CCT and its corollaries employ the small change approximation of differential calculus. This is applicable, in particular, to the detection of effects due to small changes in TPs, which is appropriate for demonstration of subtle disease. When larger changes are present, the small change approximation may lead to larger errors, but this is a known issue and is usually not a problem in clinical practice since larger changes are usually easy to detect.

The use of fractional contrast involves normalization by the TP-filter signals S_{TP} and the overall signal S. If one or more of these is zero, or close to zero, when the image noise is taken into account, then the values may take the form 1/0 and be uninterpretable. It means that fractional contrast is only valid between certain limits.

It is also not obvious which of the absolute contrast C_{ab} or the fractional contrast C_{fr} best represents what is visually perceived by human observers and therefore provides the more appropriate model for understanding contrast. In this chapter, consideration is given to both forms of contrast.

The signal and contrast produced by sequences are subject to changes in window width and level performed by the observer. This has an effect on the perception of contrast and also needs consideration.

Conclusions

The use of TP-filters and the CCT resolves many of the problems associated with the use of conventional quantitative weighting to describe MR image contrast. They also provide a basis for understanding more complex sequences and for using synergistic contrast. Their use is somewhat counterintuitive. Instead of the basic diagrams used to explain T_1 and T_2 contrast being exponential recoveries and decays respectively, they are low and high-pass filters with slopes opposite to those commonly used. Sequence and image weighting are distinguished, and each of the quantities, namely, signal, contrast, sequence and image weighting, and TP changes, have positive or negative signs associated with them.

A particularly helpful way to understand and integrate the concepts is through the use of interactive applications (apps) for each segment of a pulse sequence as well as for the pulse sequence as a whole. This shows the dependence of contrast on TP changes of different types and the effects of varying pulse sequence parameters such as TR, TE, and TI.

The focus on TP-filters and CCT is on sequence preparations with smaller but important contributions from the acquisition, basic image processing, and quantitation.

The use of UTE and ZTE acquisitions allows signals to be obtained from tissues and/or tissue components that provide little or no signal with conventional SE, SGE, and other acquisitions. Basic image processing using multiplication, addition, subtraction, and/or division of sequences makes it possible to produce synergistic contrast and to amplify contrast. In addition, long inversion pulses may act as T_2 and T_1-filters for ultrashort- and short-T_2 tissues and produce additional contrast which can also be used synergistically.

References

1. Young IR, Hall AS, Pallis CA, Legg NJ, Bydder GM, Steiner RE. Nuclear magnetic resonance imaging of the brain in multiple sclerosis. Lancet. 1981;2(8255):1063–6.

2. Bailes DR, Young IR, Thomas D, Straughan K, Bydder GM, Steiner RE. NMR imaging of the brain using spin-echo sequences. Clin Radiol. 1982;33(4):395–414.

3. Bydder GM, Steiner RE, Young IR, Hall AS, Thomas D, Marshall J, Pallis CA, Legg NJ. Clinical NMR imaging of the brain: 140 cases. AJR Am J Roentgenol. 1982;139(2):215–36.

4. Axel L. Revised glossary of MR terms. Radiology. 1987;162(3):874.

5. Young IR, Szeverenyi NM, Du J, Bydder GM. Pulse sequences as tissue property filters (TP-filters): a way of understanding the signal, contrast and weighting of magnetic resonance images. Quant Imaging Med Surg. 2020;10(5):1080–120.

6. Ma Y-J, Fan S, Shao H, Du J, Szeverenyi NM, Young IR, Bydder GM. Clinical use of multiplied, added, subtracted and/or fiTted inversion recovery (MASTIR) pulse sequences. Quant Imaging Med Surg. 2020;10(6):1334–69.

7. Ma Y-J, Shao H, Fan S, Lu X, Du J, Young IR, Bydder GM. New options for increasing the sensitivity, specificity and scope of synergistic contrast magnetic resonance imaging (scMRI) using multiplied, added, subtracted and/or FiTted (MASTIR) pulse sequences. Quant Imaging Med Surg. 2020;10(10):2030–65.

8. Ma Y-J, Moazamian D, Cornfeld DM, Condron P, Holdsworth SJ, Bydder M, Du J, Bydder GM. Improving the understanding and performance of clinical MRI using tissue property filters and the central contrast theorem. MASDIR pulse sequences and synergistic contrast MRI. Quant Imaging Med Surg. 2022;12(9):4658–90.

MASDIR (Multiplied, Added, Subtracted, and/or Divided Inversion Recovery) Pulse Sequences and Synergistic Contrast MRI (scMRI)

20

Nivedita Agarwal, Letizia Losa, Denis Peruzzo, John D. Port, and Graeme M. Bydder

Introduction

This book is divided into four parts: (1) acquisition, (2) contrast mechanisms, (3) quantitation, and (4) applications. In the first part, acquisitions are broadly divided into two categories, namely, those using ultrashort echo time (UTE) approaches, in which the radiofrequency (RF) pulse is applied initially after which gradients are activated and data are collected, and those using zero echo time (ZTE) approaches, in which the gradients are initially activated, after which the RF pulses are applied and data are collected.

The second part of this book on contrast mechanisms describes sequence preparations such as inversion pulses, which are applied prior to data acquisition, different data acquisitions, and basic image processing processes, such as subtraction of images with different echo times (TEs). These techniques are used to increase image contrast and/or specificity.

In the preceding chapter of this book, it was explained that the conventional approach to understanding image contrast using qualitative weighting leads to contradictions and inconsistencies. The conventional approach is also poorly suited to understanding more complex sequences. To deal with this problem, an alternative approach using tissue property (TP) filters and the central contrast theorem (CCT) was described and illustrated for commonly used pulse sequences.

This chapter employs this alternative approach to understand combinations of inversion recovery (IR) sequences in which two or more IR sequences are multiplied, added, subtracted, and/or divided, i.e., MASDIR sequences. These provide more options for manipulating contrast than single IR sequences.

In particular, they provide options to develop synergistic contrast in which a single tissue property (TP) is used twice or more in the same sequence to increase contrast and/or two or more different TPs are used in the same sequence for the same purpose. The synergistic contrast developed by the TPs may be supplemented by suppression of unwanted high signals or use of opposed contrast for the same purpose. Synergistic contrast can be used to increase sensitivity and/or specificity.

This chapter describes MASDIR sequences and synergistic contrast MRI (scMRI) in more detail, including their uses with short- and ultrashort-T_2 tissues.

Development of MASDIR Sequences

The first combination of two IR sequences to form a single sequence was described in 1985 [1]. This was the use of two inversion pulses to suppress the signal from both fluid and fat. It was applied in the brain and body as a double IR (DIR) sequence, which is a multiplied IR (MIR) sequence. In 1994, its use was extended to suppress either white or gray matter signals as well as cerebrospinal fluid (CSF) [2]. Subtracted IR (SIR) sequences were used to show effects due to contrast enhancement [3], inhalation of O_2 [4], and to selectively show short- or ultrashort-T_2 components [5]. In 2010, the MP2RAGE (magnetization-prepared 2 rapid acquisition gradient echo) sequence was described [6]. It multiplies two IR sequences together and normalizes them. This was extended in the form of magnetization-prepared n rapid acquisition

N. Agarwal · L. Losa · D. Peruzzo
Istituto di Ricovero e Cura a Carattere Scientifico (IRCCS),
Eugenio Medea Bosisio Parini, Lecco, Italy
e-mail: nivedita.agarwal@lanostrafamiglia.it;
letizia.losa@lanostrafamiglia.it; denis.peruzzo@lanostrafamiglia.it

J. D. Port
Department of Radiology, Mayo Clinic, Rochester, MN, USA
e-mail: Port.John@mayo.edu

G. M. Bydder (✉)
Department of Radiology, University of California, San Diego,
La Jolla, CA, USA

Mātai Medical Research Institute, Tairāwhiti Gisborne,
New Zealand
e-mail: gbydder@health.ucsd.edu

gradient echo (MPnRAGE) [7]. The fluid and white matter suppression (FLAWS) sequence was initially described to produce separate images: one with fluid (i.e., CSF) suppression and the other with white matter suppression using IR sequences, but variants have been developed in which these two acquired images are multiplied, added, subtracted, and divided as the FLAWSdiv, FLAWShc, and FLAWShco (where div = divided, hc = high contrast, and hco = high contrast opposite) sequences [8, 9]. The MASTIR (multiplied, added, subtracted, and/or fitted IR (FIR)) group of sequences was described in 2020 [10] with the inclusion of division in 2022 to produce MASDIR sequences [11].

Classification of MASDIR Sequences

The classification of MASDIR sequences is shown in Table 20.1. They are divided into: (1) multiplied, (2) added, (3) subtracted, and (4) divided. Fitted IR sequences [7, 12–14] are treated as a separate category. Subsequent sections describe some of these sequences in more detail.

1. Multiplied IR (MIR) Sequences

    MIR sequences include DIR and MP2RAGE as mentioned above.
2. Added IR (AIR and A^{1}IR) Sequences

    One group of added IR (AIR) sequences adds two magnitude (m) reconstructed sequences with different inversion times (TIs) and is used with subtraction and division (see below). Another group of sequences (A^{1}IR) uses a single TI with images reconstructed in phase-sensitive (ps) and magnitude (m) forms. Addition of these two sequences shows shorter-T_1 tissues and suppresses the signal from longer-T_1 tissues and fluids. The A^{1}IRES sequence supplements this by echo subtraction (ES; see later) and so adds a T_2-filter, thus reducing the signal from longer-T_2 tissues and fluids to provide a combined T_1 and short T_2-filter. The subtracted AIR (S^{1}AIR) sequence subtracts a longer-TI image from a shorter one to selectively show a specific range of short-T_1 tissues.
3. Subtracted IR (SIR) Sequences

    Eight subgroups of SIR sequences are included in Table 20.1. The first five groups use subtraction of a longer TI image from a shorter TI one (or vice versa as the reversed or r form). They start with the basic sequence (SIR), add T_2-weighting to it as the subtracted IR echo subtraction (SIRES) sequence, and then add D*-weighting to this as the subtracted IR echo diffusion subtraction (SIREDS) sequence. The spin echo (SE) segment of the SIRES sequence is substituted by a gradient echo to produce the subtraction IR gradient echo subtraction (SIRGES) sequence. This can have added to it diffusion weighting as the subtraction IR diffusion and gradient echo subtraction (SIRDGES) sequence.

Table 20.1 MASDIR sequences

Groups of MASDIR sequences	Expansion of MASDIR sequence acronyms
MIR	Multiplied IR
DIR	Double IR (mTI$_l$ × mTI$_{s/l}$)
MP2RAGE	Magnetization-prepared 2 rapid acquisition gradient echo (psTI$_l$ × psTI$_i$) (also normalized)
AIR	Added IR
AIR	Added IR (mTI$_{s/i/l}$ + mTI$_{s/i/l}$)
A^{1}IR	Added IR (psTI$_{s/i/l}$ + mTI$_{s/i/l}$)
A^{1}IRES	AIR added IR echo subtraction
S^{1}AIR	Subtracted, added IR
SIR	Subtracted IR
SIR, rSIR	Subtracted IR (mTI$_{s/i/l}$ − mTI$_{s/i/l}$), reverse SIR
SIRES, rSIRES	Subtracted IR echo subtraction, reverse SIRES
SIREDS, rSIREDS	Subtracted IR echo diffusion subtraction, reverse SIREDS
SIRGES, rSIRGES	Subtraction IR gradient echo subtraction, reverse SIRGES
SIRDGES, rSIRDGES	Subtraction IR diffusion and gradient echo subtraction, reverse SIRDGES
DESIRE, STAIRES[a]	Double echo sliding IR, short TR adiabatic pulse prepared IR (TR × mTI$_{i/s}$) echo subtraction
shMOLLI[a]	Shortened modified Look–Locker inversion recovery
S^{1}IR	Subtracted IR (psTI$_{s/i/l}$ − mTI$_{s/i/l}$)
S^{2}IR	Subtracted SIR
IRES	IR echo subtraction
STIRES	Short TI IR echo subtraction
dIR	Divided IR
dSIR, drSIR	Divided SIR, divided reverse SIR
dSIRES, drSIRES	Divided SIRES, divided reverse SIRES
dSIREDS, drSIREDS	Divided SIREDS, divided reverse SIREDS
dSIRGES, drSIRGES	Divided SIRGES, divided reverse SIRGES
dSIRDGES, drSIRDGES	Divided SIRDGES, divided reverse SIRDGES
FIR	Fitted IR (multiple TIs)
MPnRAGE	Magnetization-prepared rapid acquisition gradient echo
shMOLLI[a]	Shortened modified Look–Locker inversion recovery
DESIRE[a]	Double echo sliding IR

[a]Included in both the subtracted and fitted categories

The sixth group includes the shortened modified Look–Locker IR (shMOLLI) [12] sequence, the DESIRE (double echo sliding IR) [13, 14] sequence, which uses a sliding TI window to obtain many IR images with different TIs followed by a UTE data collection (dc) and ES, and the STAIRES (short repetition time (TR) adiabatic IR echo subtraction) [15, 16] sequence. This sequence multiplies an extremely short TR segment by a short TI$_s$ segment to reduce to zero, or nearly zero, long-T_1 and long-T_2

signals from tissues, with a wide range of T_1s above a certain minimum. It is used with UTE data collection (dc) to provide selective imaging of ultrashort-T_2 tissues. This is followed by ES to reduce to zero the signal from any long-T_2 tissues, which are not completely nulled. Both the DESIRE and STAIRES sequences can be selectively used to image myelin and other ultrashort-T_2 tissues.

The seventh group uses the same TI and subtracts a ps image from an m image once (S^1IR), or twice (S^2IR) with different TIs, for example, to selectively show fluid or tissue.

The eighth group of subtracted IR sequences is a basic IR echo subtraction (IRES), and the STIRES (short TI IR echo subtraction; STIR and ES) sequence, which nulls the shorter-T_1 white adipose tissue (WAT) and uses Dixon subtraction of out-of-phase images from in-phase images to selectively show lipids present in brown adipose tissue (BAT) as a result of its longer T_1 compared to the T_1 of lipids in WAT.

4. Divided IR (dIR) Sequences

A central issue with division of IR sequences is the behavior of the TP-filter if, or when, the denominator takes a value of zero. This potentially leads to infinite values of the TP-filter. Even if zero values are avoided, there are values when the denominator approaches zero and division becomes unreliable as a result of noise and artifacts.

This problem can be largely avoided with two IR images by making the denominator the addition of the signals in the two images. The TP-filters have different TIs and, using magnitude reconstruction, the sum of them in the denominator is nonzero. If the numerator is two subtracted IR images, then division normalizes the sequence so that the effects of ρ_m and T_2 are reduced or eliminated, as are those due to receiver coil inhomogeneity.

5. Fitted IR (FIR) Sequences

These obtain multiple IR images primarily for quantification of T_1, e.g., MPnRAGE [7] and shMOLLI [12]. The DESIRE sequence can be used in this way but can also be used for selecting the best TI to null long-T_2 components in tissue or tissues with different T_1s. The DESIRE sequence is included in both the subtraction and fitted categories.

AIR, SIR, and dSIR Sequences

Two IR filters with different TIs are shown in Fig. 20.1a. The signal in a voxel is plotted against T_1 for each T_1-filter. They are subtracted to yield the SIR T_1-filter in Fig. 20.1b. This T_1-filter is steep in the X-axis region between the T_1s corresponding to the nulling TIs, i.e., in the middle domain (mD). The two sequences in Fig. 20.1a can also be added as the added IR (AIR) sequence, which is shown in Fig. 20.1c, in

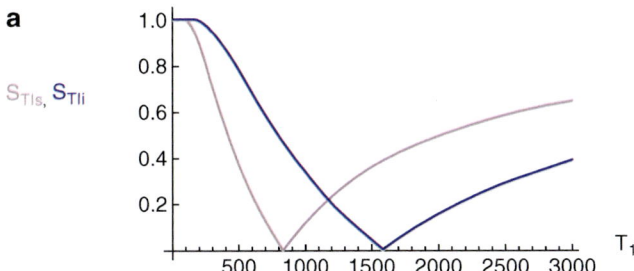

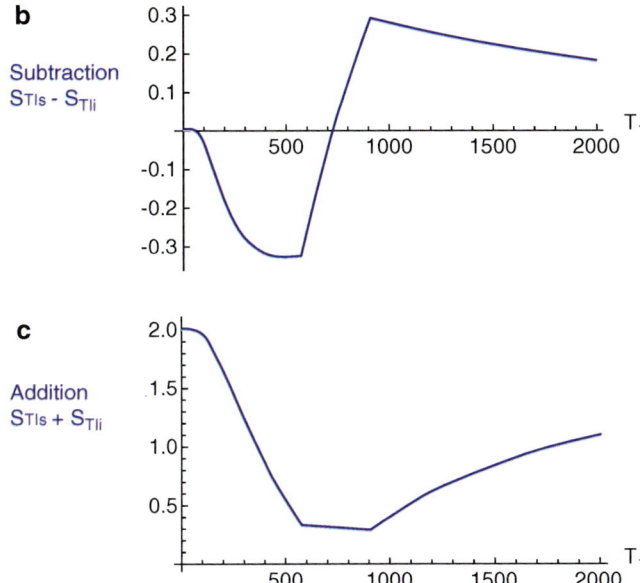

Fig. 20.1 SIR and AIR T_1-filters. Voxel signal S is shown along the Y-axis for S_{TIs} and S_{TIi}, and T_1 is shown along the X-axis. (**a**) The TI_s T_1-filter (pink) and the TI_i T_1-filter (blue). (**b**) The subtraction ($S_{TIs} - S_{TIi}$) IR or SIR T_1-filter. (**c**) The addition ($S_{TIs} + S_{TIi}$) IR or AIR T_1-filter. In panel (**b**), the slope of the curve in the mD is nearly double that of the S_{TIs} T_1-filter (pink in panel (**a**)). In panel (**c**), the signal at $T_1 = 0$ is doubled to 2.0, and the signal in the mD is reduced to about 0.35–0.33 in the nearly linear, slightly downward sloping central part of the AIR filter (i.e., the middle domain, mD)

which there are higher signal and higher slope regions outside of the mD. The mD in Fig. 20.1c has a low signal with a nearly linear, slightly downward, sloping curve.

Figure 20.2a shows the T_1-bipolar filter for the divided subtracted IR (dSIR) sequence in which the SIR T_1-filter in Fig. 20.1b is divided by the AIR T_1-filter in Fig. 20.1c. The dSIR T_1-bipolar filter shows a very highly sloping, positive mD.

Figure 20.2b compares the contrast from the short TI T_1-filter, S_{TIs} (pink), which is that of a conventional intermediate TI_i IR sequence such as MP-RAGE (magnetization-prepared rapid acquisition gradient echo), to that from the SIR T_1-filter (blue). The vertical pink and blue arrows on the right show that the contrast produced by the SIR T_1-filter (blue) is about double that produced by the S_{TIs} T_1-filter (pink) for the same change in T_1 across the mD (horizontal positive green arrow).

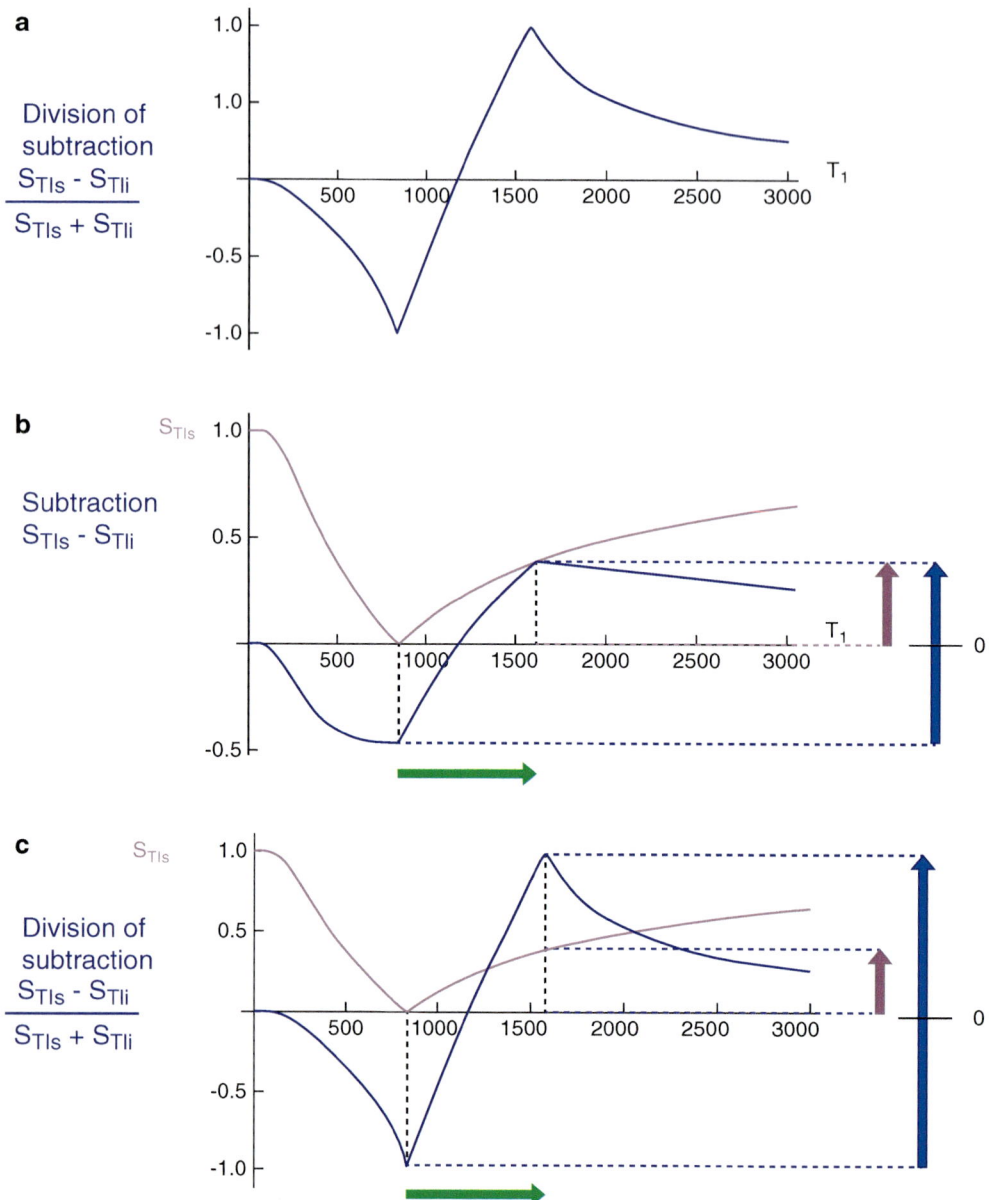

Fig. 20.2 A dSIR T_1-bipolar filter (**a**) and comparisons of the S_{TIs} T_1-filter with the SIR T_1-filter (**b**) and of the S_{TIs} T_1-filter with the dSIR T_1-bipolar filter (**c**) for an increase in T_1 in the mD. Voxel signals $S_{TIs} - S_{TIi}/S_{TIs} + S_{TIi}$ and $S_{TIs} - S_{TIi}$ are shown along the Y-axis. T_1 is shown along the X-axis. Panel (**a**) shows division (d) of the subtraction ($S_{TIs} - S_{TIi}$) T_1-filter by the addition ($S_{TIs} + S_{TIi}$) T_1-filter to produce ($S_{TIs} - S_{TIi})/(S_{TIs} + S_{TIi}$) or SIR/AIR = the dSIR T_1-bipolar filter. Panel (**b**) shows a comparison of the S_{TIs} T_1-filter (pink) and the subtraction SIR T_1-filter (blue). Panel (**c**) is a comparison of the S_{TIs} T_1-filter (pink) with the dSIR T_1-bipolar filter (blue). The dSIR T_1-bipolar filter in panels (**a**) and (**c**) has maximum and minimum values of 1 and −1, respectively, and is steeply sloping. In panel (**b**), the increase in signal (i.e., contrast) for the increase in T_1 extending from one end of the mD to the other, for example, from white to gray matter (horizontal green arrow), is about 0.35 for the S_{TIs} T_1-filter and about 0.75 for the subtraction (SIR) T_1-filter. This represents an increase in contrast for the SIR T_1-filter compared to the S_{TIs} T_1-filter of about two (right vertical arrows). In panel (**c**), for the same change in T_1 (horizontal green arrow), the change in the S_{TIs} T_1-filter is about 0.35, as shown also in panel (**b**), and that in the dSIR T_1-bipolar filter is 2.0, representing an increase in contrast of about five times (right vertical arrows)

Figure 20.2c compares the contrast produced by the short TI T_1-filter, S_{TIs} (pink), to that from the dSIR T_1-bipolar filter (blue). For the same change in T_1 (positive horizontal green arrow across the mD), the dSIR T_1-bipolar filter generates about five times the contrast (vertical blue arrow) produced by the S_{TIs} T_1-filter (vertical pink arrow). As the second TI is moved closer to the first TI, the slope of the T_1-bipolar filter in the mD becomes steeper, and, so, the T_1-dependent contrast in the mD increases. This is documented in Table 20.2. In this table, as the difference in TI (ΔTI) decreases from 90 to 13%, the ratio of the contrast produced by the dSIR T_1-bipolar filter to that produced by the conventional IR T_1-filter

Table 20.2 TI_s, TI_i, ΔTI, and S_{TIs} contrast at TI_i, S_{dSIR} contrast at TI_i, and ratio of S_{dSIR}/S_{TIs} contrast. As TI_i is reduced, the mD narrows, ΔTI decreases, and the signal for TI_s at TI_i (S_{TIs}) decreases. The ratio of the dSIR contrast to the S_{TIs} contrast increases from 5 to 20, as ΔTI decreases from 90% to 13% when the mD is narrowed

| TI_s (ms) | TI_i (ms) | ΔTI | | S_{TIs} contrast | S_{dSIR} contrast | Ratio of S_{dSIR}/S_{TIs} contrast |
		(ms)	%			
580	1100	520	90	0.40	2.0	5
580	840	260	45	0.25	2.0	8
580	710	130	22	0.15	2.0	13
580	655	75	13	0.10	2.0	20

increases from 5 to 20. The trade-off for this amplified contrast is a decreased width of the mD, which is the region where sequence T_1-weighting and the contrast ratio are high. The mathematical basis for this is described in the Appendix.

Synergistic Contrast MRI (scMRI)

Synergistic contrast arises in two main ways:

1. A single TP can be used twice or more in a sequence to increase contrast. For example, T_1 can be used in the T_1-dependent TR segment of an IR sequence and in the T_1-dependent TI segment. T_1 is also used twice in DIR sequences when two T_1-dependent segments are multiplied together and in the SIR sequence when using the subtraction: the short TI_s segment minus the intermediate TI_i segment. The synergistic T_1 contrast from the SIR sequence can be further increased using T_1 three or four times in the form of divided SIR (dSIR) and divided reverse SIR (drSIR) sequences.

   Synergistic contrast may arise from repeated use of T_2 when imaging ultrashort-T_2 tissues with an IR sequence when using a long adiabatic inversion pulse to invert and null long-T_2 signals while ultrashort-T_2 tissues that are saturated by the inversion pulse recover. This is followed by the 90° excitation pulse and ES. The two effects, first from the inversion pulse and nulling and second from the decay in transverse magnetization, produce synergistic negative T_2 contrast when there is an increase in T_2 in ultrashort-T_2 tissues.

2. Two or more different TPs can also be used to produce synergistic contrast as was first described with the short TI IR (STIR) sequence in 1985 [1]. Clinical pulse sequences have a basic structure consisting of ρ_m, T_1, and T_2 filters as seen in SE sequences. There are additional options, which can be added, such as those for T_1-dependent inversion pulses and D^* sensitization. In many circumstances, ρ_m is a minor determinant of contrast and T_1, T_2, and D^* are the major determinants. The most common change in TPs in disease is concurrent increases in ρ_m, T_1, T_2. In this situation with the SE sequence, the contrast developed by an increase in T_1 is negative, whereas

that developed by an increase in T_2 is positive so that simultaneous increases in T_1 and T_2 produce opposed contrast and the net, or overall, contrast is reduced. To avoid this problem, T_1-weighted sequences use a short TE to minimize the opposite T_2 contrast and T_2-weighted sequences use a long TR to minimize the opposed T_1 contrast. The dominant source of contrast in the resulting sequences is then a single TP, i.e., T_1 or T_2, and the sequences are described as T_1-weighted or T_2-weighted, respectively. They are not synergistic for T_1 and T_2 contrast but are opposed.

In particular circumstances, such as certain forms of the STIR and the DIR sequences, the T_1 contrast produced by an increase in T_1 is positive and so is the T_2 contrast produced by an increase in T_2. The effects of the concurrent increases in T_1 and T_2 are therefore synergistic and typically result in high positive lesion contrast.

The contrast produced above from (i) a single TP and/or (ii) two or more different TPs can be supplemented by increasing or decreasing signals from normal tissues and/or fluids. There may be little contrast between high signal lesions and high signal fat, long-T_2 tissues, or fluids. Reduction in the normal signal from these latter tissues or fluids (using the same or different TPs as those used to create the original synergistic contrast in (i) and/or (ii)) can increase the contrast between the high signal lesions and the zero or low signal-suppressed tissues and/or fluids. It may also result in a more appropriate dynamic range for the image.

In tissues with a mixture of ultrashort- and long-T_2 tissues, low abundance ultrashort-T_2 tissues may only become apparent if the more abundant signals from the long-T_2 tissues are reduced or suppressed. This also applies to edema in yellow bone marrow, where suppression of the more abundant fat signal may be necessary to show lower concentration edema. Signals can also be increased for the same purpose.

The synergistic contrast produced in (i) and/or (ii) can also be supplemented by opposed contrast outside the region of interest.

Thus, one or both of mechanisms (i) and (ii) described above may be used in any one synergistic contrast sequence with, or without, supplementary synergistic contrast from suppression or increase of signals from normal tissues as well as the use of opposed contrast. Achievement of synergistic contrast requires a knowledge of the sign of sequence weighting of the TP-filters involved as well as the sign of the change in each TP.

Image Processing to Achieve Synergistic Contrast

There are three situations within sequences in which the ability to reverse the sign of the weighting of a TP-filter of the sequence is important for achieving synergistic contrast. These are first the reversal of the sign of the T_1 contrast produced by a change in T_1 with IR sequences using different TIs (together with m reconstruction). The second is the reversal of the sign of T_2 contrast produced by a change in T_2 with an SE T_2-filter by the subtraction: shorter TE filter minus longer TE T_2-filter, i.e., ES. The third is the reversal of the sign of diffusion contrast produced by the pulsed gradient spin echo (PGSE) D^*-filter using the subtraction: low b-value (e.g., 0–20 s/mm²) filter minus high b-value (e.g., 500–1500 s/mm²) filter, i.e., diffusion subtraction (DS). This ability to change the sign of the sequence TP-filter and the resulting contrast for T_1, T_2, and D^* is crucial for creating synergistic contrast from either positive or negative changes in each of T_1, T_2, and D^* in disease.

In addition to changing the sign of the sequence weighting of a TP-filter within a sequence as above, it is also possible to reverse the order of subtraction of two sequences and so reverse the contrast produced by the sequences. This is reverse (r) subtraction.

Using the same change in a TP twice or more in the same sequence may result in higher synergistic contrast than just using it once. Using changes in different TPs may also be effective in increasing the overall contrast. This is because T_1, T_2, and D^* often change concurrently in disease, and using synergistic contrast developed by each of these TPs may result in higher overall contrast than using just a single TP. These are approaches targeted at increasing sequence sensitivity.

Image processing also includes late (extremely long TE) echo acquisition of signal from long-T_2 fluids such as CSF. This can be helpful when CSF is at the top or bottom of the display dynamic range and white or gray matter would be preferred in this location. It is also of value in avoiding problems with partial volume effects simulating lesions.

It is also possible to specifically include image acquisitions for their use in image processing. This includes, for example, short TE sequences for subtraction from them of longer TE sequences.

Synergistic contrast can also be used to improve sequence specificity, for example, using the reductions in both T_1 and T_2^* produced by organic iron to provide high-contrast visualization of its effects.

The Subtracted IR Echo Subtraction (SIRES) Sequence

As explained above, in order to create sequences with synergistic contrast, it is sometimes necessary to reverse the weighting of a conventional TP-filter. ES is used to reverse the T_2-weighting of the T_2-filter. This is accomplished by the subtraction: short TE T_2-filter minus long-TE T_2-filter, as shown in Fig. 20.3. Increases in T_2 in the chosen sloping region of the T_2-filter result in increased signal (Fig. 20.3a and b). For the ES filter, increase in T_2 results in a decreased signal in the sloping region shown in Fig. 20.3c. Thus, the T_2-filter weighting has changed from positive in Fig. 20.3a and b to negative in Fig. 20.3c.

Row I of Fig. 20.4 describes a TP-filter with a short TI and a long TE, resulting in positive contrast from the T_1 and T_2-filters (middle and right columns in Fig. 20.4b and c, respectively). Row II of Fig. 20.4 shows an intermediate TI T_1-filter with negative contrast from both the T_1 and T_2-filters in Fig. 20.4b and c respectively. Row II includes in the right column (Fig. 20.4c) the subtraction: intermediate TI_i short TE sequence minus intermediate TI_i long-TE sequence. Thus, ES reverses the sign of the conventional T_2-filter and produces synergistic contrast with T_1. In row III, the SIRES filter is created by the subtraction: row I minus row II, which produces the overall synergistic positive T_1 and T_2 contrast. Row IV shows the reverse SIRES (rSIRES), which produces overall negative contrast. Row

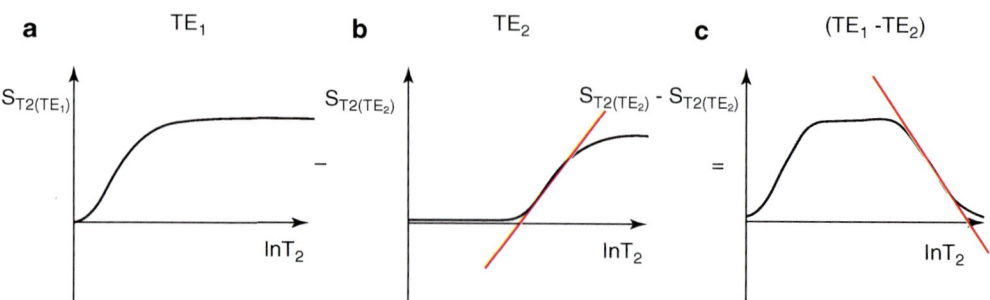

Fig. 20.3 Echo subtraction (ES). Short TE_1 (**a**), long TE_2 (**b**), and subtracted ($TE_1 − TE_2$) T_2-filters (**c**). The positive slope of the TE_2 T_2-filter (red line) becomes negative with the ($TE_1 − TE_2$) T_2-filter (red line)

Fig. 20.4 The SIRES sequence. Row I shows that increases in ρ_m, T_1, and T_2 (green arrows) produce synergistic positive contrast (blue arrows). Row II (which includes ES) shows that increases in T_1 and T_2 produce synergistic negative contrast. In row III, the subtraction (row I minus row II) results in synergistic positive contrast. In row IV, the reverse subtraction rSIRES produces negative synergistic contrast. Row V shows the divided forms of the sequences dSIRES and rdSIRES, which have increased positive and negative T_1 contrast, respectively

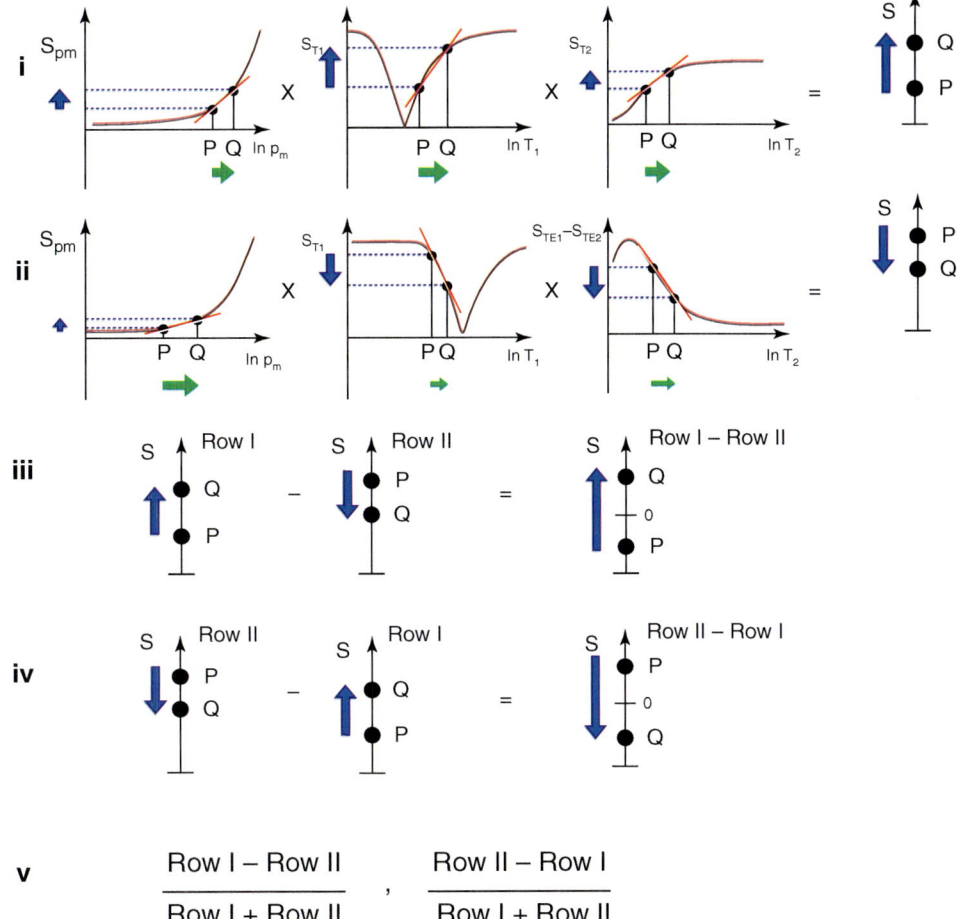

V shows the divided SIRES (dSIRES) and divided reverse SIRES (drSIRES) TP-filters, which result in further increases in positive and negative T_1 contrast, respectively.

The Subtracted IR Echo and Diffusion Subtracted (SIREDS) Sequence

Diffusion subtraction (DS) is used to reverse the weighting of the D^*-filter. This is accomplished by the subtraction: D^*-filter with b = "0" minus D^*-filter with a high b-value as shown in Fig. 20.5. For the short TE and b = "0" filter in Fig. 20.5a, an increase in D^* results in no change. For the diffusion D^*-filter in Fig. 20.5b, an increase in D^* results in negative contrast. For the subtracted D^*-filter, an increase in D^* produces positive contrast.

A SIREDS TP-filter that adds D^* to the SIRES TP-filter and includes DS to create synergistic T_1, T_2, and D^* contrast is shown in Fig. 20.6. Row I is a TP-filter with a short TI, a long TE, and a high b-value, resulting in positive synergistic contrast for increases in T_1 and T_2 and a decrease in D^* as seen in some acute diseases and many tumors. This results in positive synergistic D^* contrast. Row II is a TP-filter with negative synergistic contrast for increases in T_1 and T_2 and a decrease in D^*. Row II includes the subtraction: intermediate TI_i, short TE, b = "0" D^*-filter minus intermediate TI_i, short TE, high b-value (i.e., ES and diffusion subtraction (EDS)). Row III shows the subtraction: row I minus row II to yield the SIREDS TP-filter. Row IV shows the reverse SIREDS (rSIREDS) TP-filter. The divided SIREDS (dSIREDS) and divided reverse SIREDS (drSIREDS) TP-filters are shown in row V and increase the positive and negative T_1 weighting.

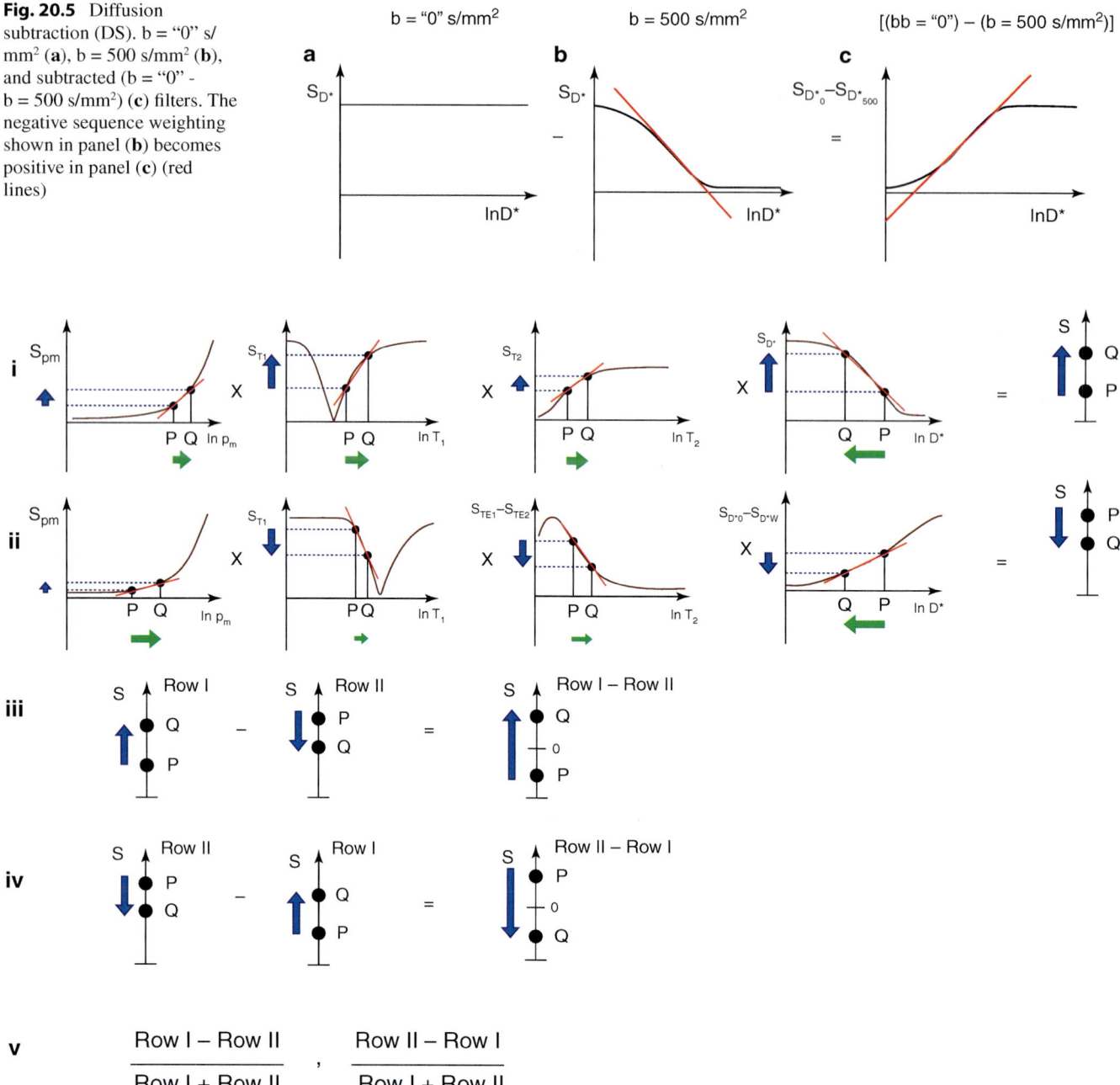

Fig. 20.5 Diffusion subtraction (DS). b = "0" s/mm² (**a**), b = 500 s/mm² (**b**), and subtracted (b = "0" - b = 500 s/mm²) (**c**) filters. The negative sequence weighting shown in panel (**b**) becomes positive in panel (**c**) (red lines)

Fig. 20.6 A SIREDS filter. The ρ_m, T_1 and T_2, and D^* contrasts are synergistic and positive in row I and the T_1, T_2, and D^* contrasts are synergistic and negative in row II. In row III, the subtraction (row I minus row II) results in overall synergistic positive contrast. Row IV shows the reverse subtraction. Row V shows the divided forms of the filters, dSIREDS, and drSIREDS, which have increased T_1 contrast

Contrast at Tissue Boundaries

In the previous sections of this chapter, contrast between two voxels was considered, but there was no reference to the location of voxels or contrast at the boundaries between two voxels.

In general terms, contrast detectability at boundaries between two voxels with different values of S can be related to $C_{ab} = \Delta S$ or $C_{fr} = \Delta S/S$ divided by the distance Δx between the voxels. Boundaries are more detectable when contrast is high and Δx is low, rather than in the opposite situation in which contrast is low and Δx is high.

At a boundary between two pure tissues P and Q, it is useful to define the tissue fraction f, which is the proportion of the second tissue Q in a voxel containing a mixture of both tissues. The proportion of the other tissue P is then $(1 - f)$.

The T_1 of the mixture of the two tissues (P and Q) can be expressed as a function.

$$T_{1P,Q} = \Gamma\left(T_{1P}, T_{1Q}, f\right) \qquad (20.1)$$

where $T_{1P,Q}$ is the T_1 of the mixture, T_{1P} is the T_1 of P, and T_{1Q} is the T_1 of Q.

It is also useful to consider $\dfrac{\partial f}{\partial x}$, the change in tissue fraction with distance x. This may be gradual, corresponding to a low value of $\dfrac{\partial f}{\partial x}$, or more abrupt, in parts corresponding to higher values of $\dfrac{\partial f}{\partial x}$.

Using the chain rule from differential calculus, for T_1

$$\frac{1}{S_{T_1}} \cdot \frac{\Delta S}{\Delta x} \approx \frac{1}{S_{T_1}} \cdot \frac{dS}{dx} = \frac{1}{S_{T_1}} \cdot \frac{\partial S_{T_1}}{\partial T_1} \cdot \frac{\partial T_1}{\partial f} \cdot \frac{\partial f}{\partial x} \qquad (20.2)$$

where $\dfrac{1}{S_{T1}} \cdot \dfrac{\partial S}{\partial x}$ is the change in the fractional contrast with distance x, S_{T1} is the T_1-filter signal, $\dfrac{dS}{dx}$ is a measure of the detectable contrast, $\dfrac{\partial S_{T1}}{\partial T_1}$ is the first partial derivative of S_{T1} with respect to T_1, i.e., the sequence T_1-weighting, $\dfrac{\partial T_1}{\partial f}$ is the change in T_1 with tissue fraction f, and $\dfrac{\partial f}{\partial x}$ is the change in f with distance x.

If the sequence weighting is high as within the mD of a dSIR sequence, then $\dfrac{\partial S_{T1}}{\partial T_1}$ is high (Fig. 20.7). In the brain, $\dfrac{\partial T_1}{\partial f}$ is increased from white–gray matter to gray matter–CSF to white matter–CSF at boundaries between tissue fluids. $\dfrac{\partial f}{\partial x}$ increases as the transition from one tissue changes from gradual to abrupt.

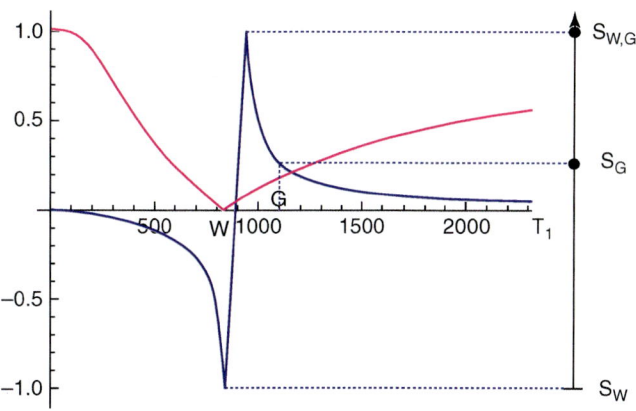

Fig. 20.7 A dSIR T_1-filter with a narrow mD extending from white matter (W) to a $T_{1W,G}$ between the TIs of white matter (W) and gray matter (G) (blue) and a W-nulled T_1-filter, e.g., MP-RAGE (pink). The peak signal ($S_{W,G}$) appears between W and G along the X-axis where there are partial volume effects producing a $T_{1W,G}$ between W and G, which corresponds to the peak signal $S_{W,G}$, i.e., the high signal peak $S_{W,G}$ is at a T_1 between those of W and G matter and is higher than the signals for W and G, i.e., S_W and S_G. This high signal boundary is shown in Fig. 20.8 for narrow and wider mD dSIR T_1-bipolar filter

At a boundary between two tissues, the actual T_1 of the voxels with mixtures of tissues within them spans the range of T_1 values between the two tissues. This is shown in Fig. 20.7. If the T_1-filter is such that a T_1 value between those of the two tissues results in a high value of S, then a high signal line results at the boundary between the two tissues, as seen in Fig. 20.8. The width and location of the line is dependent on the slope of the T_1-filter and the gradient of T_1 with f as well as the gradient of f with x. The high signal narrow boundary at the white–gray matter boundary inside the brain in Fig. 20.8a was obtained using a narrow mD and the wider boundary high signal was obtained with a wider mD (Fig. 20.8b). Thus, the width of the boundary can be changed by the choice of mD, which alters the slope of the T_1-filter. The location of the high signal boundary can also be shifted to between cortical gray matter and CSF by use of an even wider mD. High signal boundaries provide a useful basis for locating lesions and segmenting tissues.

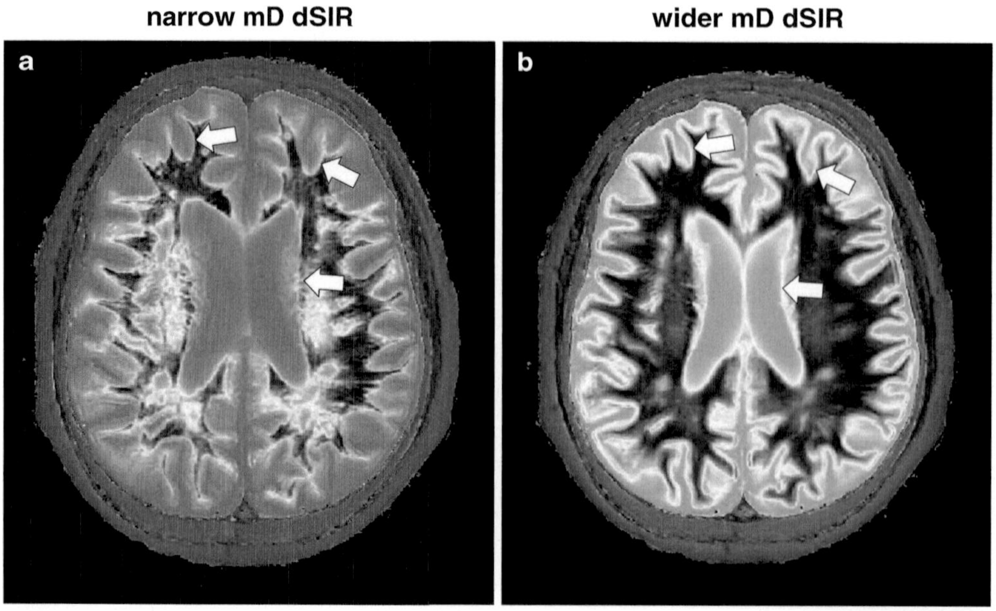

narrow mD dSIR   **wider mD dSIR**

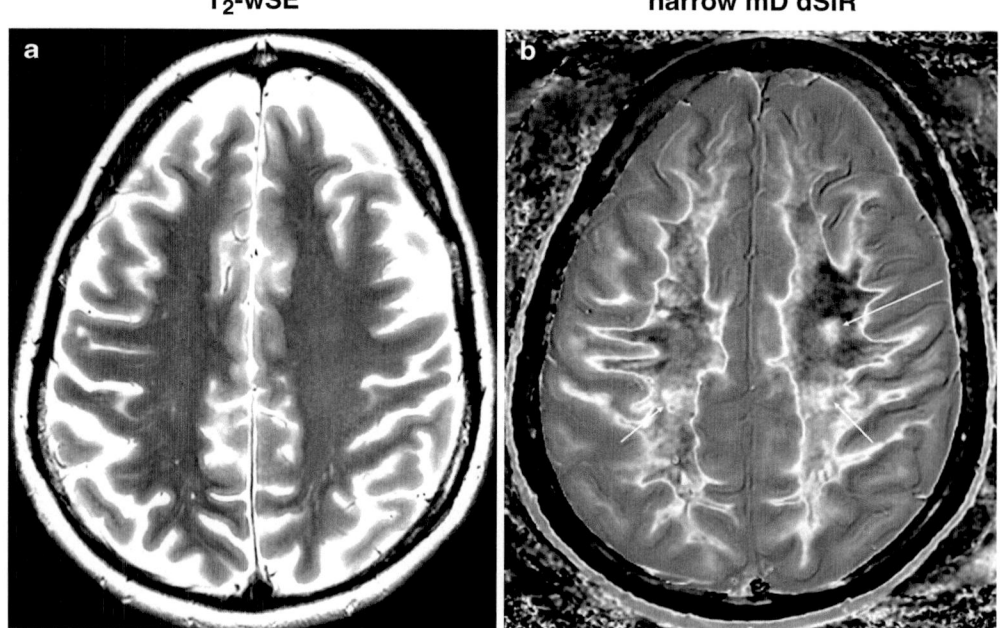

Fig. 20.8 A patient with small vessel disease of white matter with a narrow mD dSIR image (TI$_s$ = 540 ms and TI$_i$ = 640 ms, ΔTI = 18% at 3 T) (**a**) and an intermediate mD dSIR image (TI$_s$ = 540 ms and TI$_i$ = 840 ms, ΔTI = 56%) (**b**). In panel (**a**), where the slope of the T$_1$-filter is high, the high signal boundary between white and gray matter is narrow (arrows). In panel (**b**), where the slope of the T$_1$-filter is lower, the high signal boundary between white and gray matter is broader (corresponding paired white arrows in panels (**a**) and (**b**)). The same pattern is seen at white matter–CSF boundaries around the lateral ventricles (corresponding paired white arrows in panels (**a**) and (**b**))

Fig. 20.9 Case of MS. Comparison of T$_2$-wSE (**a**) and narrow mD dSIR (**b**) images. The T$_2$-wSE image appears normal. A focal lesion not seen on the T$_2$-wSE image is shown on the dSIR image (long arrow) and other abnormalities are seen in the corticospinal tracts (short arrows) as well as elsewhere in the white matter on the dSIR image. The normal white matter is black, and about 80% of the white matter on the dSIR image shows a higher signal and is abnormal. High signal boundaries are seen between white matter and cortical gray matter. These are not seen on the T$_2$-wSE image (**a**)

T$_2$-wSE   **narrow mD dSIR**

Examples

Application of these principles can be seen in a case of multiple sclerosis (MS) (Fig. 20.9).

In the figure, T$_2$-weighted SE (T$_2$-wSE) images are compared with dSIR images. No abnormality is seen on the T$_2$-wSE image (Fig. 20.9a), but a focal lesion is seen on the dSIR image (long arrow) (Fig. 20.9b). The corticospinal tracts are also seen (short arrows). There are areas of increased signal in much of the white matter (normal white matter appears black). High-signal, high-contrast boundaries are seen between white and gray matter.

In a case of small vessel disease, abnormalities are seen on the T$_2$-wSE image (Fig. 20.10a), but more extensive change is seen with the dSIR image (Fig. 20.10b).

A comparison of a T$_2$-fluid attenuated inversion recovery (T$_2$-FLAIR) image (Fig. 20.11a) and a DESIRE image (Fig. 20.11b) is shown in a case of MS. The lesions that exhibit a high signal due to their increase in T$_2$ in Fig. 20.11a show low signal due to myelin loss in Fig. 20.11b.

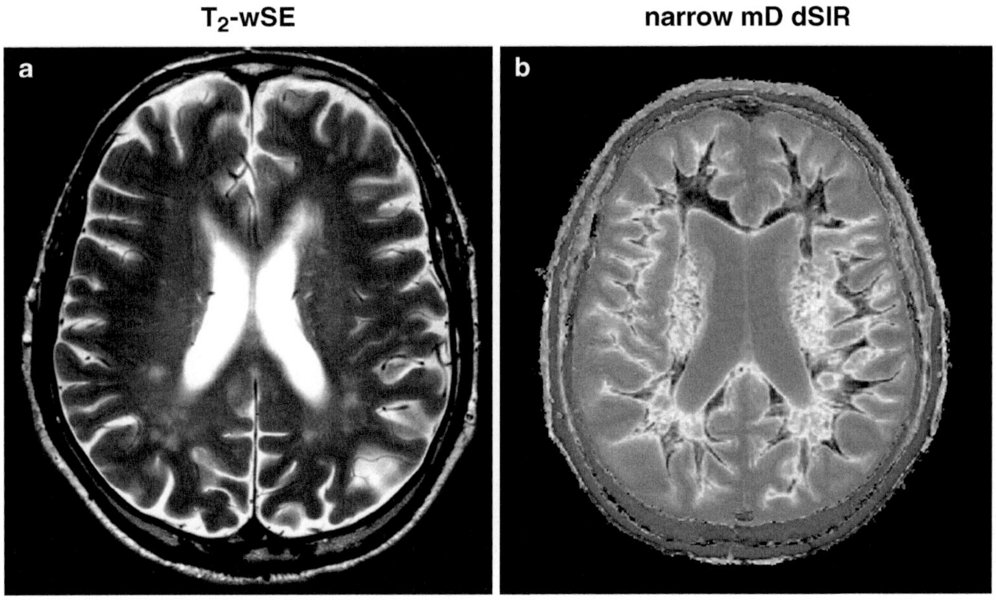

T₂-wSE   **narrow mD dSIR**

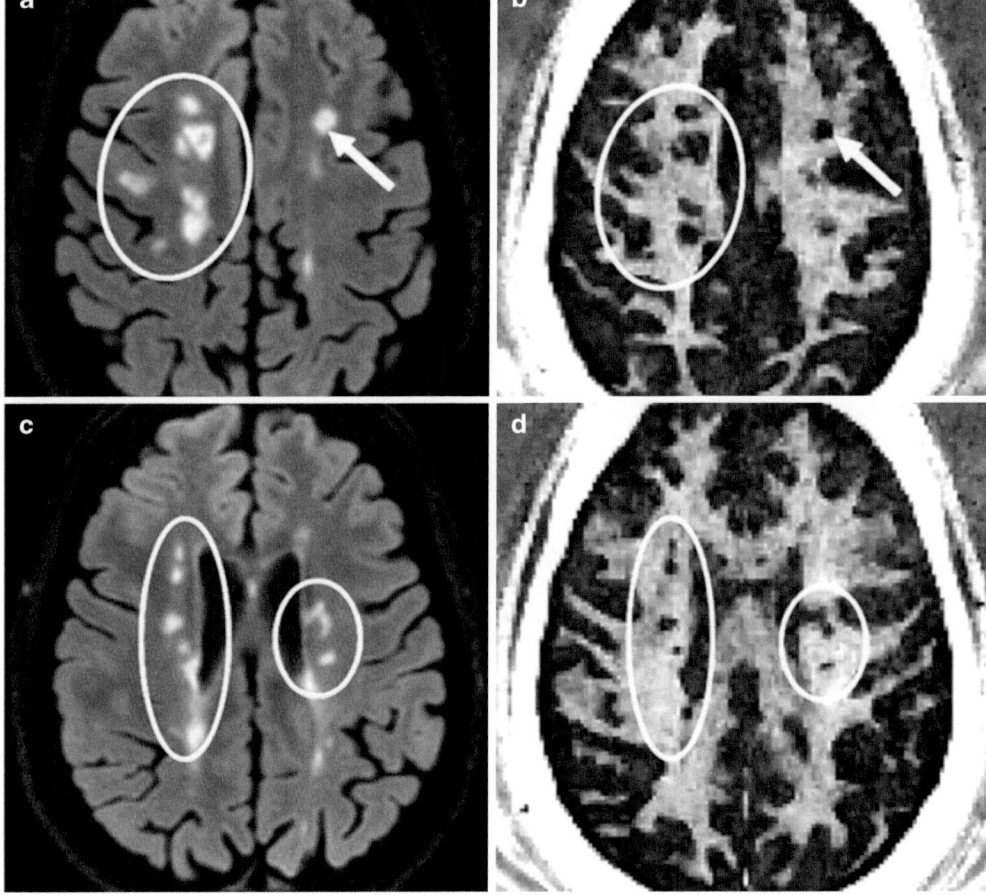

Fig. 20.10 A patient with small vessel disease of white matter T₂-wSE (**a**) and narrow mD dSIR (TIs 540 ms and 640 ms with ΔTI = 18% at 3 T) (**b**) images. The dSIR image shows much more abnormality than the T₂-wSE image. On the dSIR image (**b**), normal white matter is black (the lowest gray-scale value) and abnormal white matter with an increased T₁ is higher signal up to the highest, gray-scale display value. Normal gray matter and CSF show intermediate signal. There is a high signal boundary between normal white and gray matter as well as between white matter and CSF. Abnormal white matter, which has T₁ increased beyond that corresponding to the second nulled TI shows a high signal boundary at the maximum signal and an intermediate signal center. This appearance is seen in some lesions in the occipital white matter

Fig. 20.11 T₂-FLAIR (**a**, **c**) and corresponding DESIRE (**b**, **d**) images in a case of MS. The lesions have high signals due to increased T₂ on the T₂-FLAIR images (**a**, **c**) and show low signals due to loss of myelin on the DESIRE images (**b**, **d**). (Reproduced with permission from Ma et al. [13])

Conclusions

This chapter describes the concepts underlying MASDIR sequences and scMRI and explains how they can be applied. It is somewhat counterintuitive that successively nulling the signals from normal and abnormal tissues can lead to high contrast T_1-weighted images and that this contrast may be many times that produced by a single IR sequence. Likewise, the production of high signal, high contrast boundaries between white and gray matter with dSIR sequences is difficult to explain without the use of T_1-bipolar filters.

The work has a mathematical basis and uses differential calculus to understand TP-filters and the CCT as well as contrast at boundaries. The basic operations of arithmetic, namely, multiplication, addition, subtraction, and division are used to combine IR sequences. The graphics used to understand contrast are accessible using a basic level mathematical app such as Wolfram Alpha.

There are also many other options with MASDIR sequences, including perfusion, use of magnetization transfer, phase imaging, and fat and bone marrow imaging, in which synergistic contrast may be particularly useful.

Appendix: Features of the dSIR and drSIR Sequences, Including Their Use As T_1 Maps

The signals S_s and S_i for two long TR IR T_1-filters with short and intermediate TIs: TI_s and TI_i, respectively, are given by

$$S_s = 1 - 2e\left(-TI_s / T_1\right) \tag{20.3}$$

and

$$S_i = 1 - 2e\left(-TI_i / T_1\right) \tag{20.4}$$

Performing the subtraction: magnitude of the IR signal $|S_s|$ in Eq. 20.3 minus magnitude of the IR signal $|S_i|$ in Eq. 20.4 yields the signal of the SIR T_1-filter S_{SIR}, which is equal to $-S_s - S_i$, i.e.,

$$S_{SIR} = 2e\left(-TI_s / T_1\right) + 2e\left(-TI_i / T_1\right) - 2 \tag{20.5}$$

Addition of the magnitudes of the two IR signals $|S_s|$ and $|S_i|$ in Eqs. 20.3 and 20.4 S_{AIR} is equal to $-S_s + S_i$, i.e.,

$$S_{AIR} = 2e\left(-TI_s / T_1\right) - 2e\left(-TI_i / T_1\right) \tag{20.6}$$

Division of the signal of the subtraction T_1-filter S_{SIR} in Eq. 20.5 by the signal of the addition T_1-filter S_{AIR} in Eq. 20.6 yields the signal of the S_{dSIR} T_1-filter:

$$S_{dSIR} = \frac{e\left(-TI_s / T_1\right) + e\left(-TI_i / T_1\right) - 1}{e\left(-TI_s / T_1\right) - e\left(-TI_i / T_1\right)} \tag{20.7}$$

Although this expression is accurate, it does not provide an easy insight into the properties of the S_{dSIR} T_1-filter. To do this, a linear equation of the form $y = mx + c$ between the end points of the mD can be produced by fitting a straight line to the first and last points of the mD (i.e., first point at $x = TI_s/\ln 2$ and $y = 1$ and last point at $x = TI_i/\ln 2$ and $y = -1$). This can be used as an approximation for the S_{dSIR} T_1-filter so that

$$S_{dSIR} \approx \frac{\ln 4}{\Delta TI} T_1 - \frac{\Sigma TI}{\Delta TI} \tag{20.8}$$

where $\Delta TI = TI_i - TI_s$ and $\Sigma TI = TI_s + TI_i$.

The expression in Eq. 20.8 demonstrates four key features of the dSIR T_1-filter: first, it shows a linear change of signal with T_1 in the mD as an approximation to the T_1-filter, second, it has a slope equal to $\ln 4/\Delta TI$, third, it shows high sensitivity to small changes in T_1 when ΔTI is small, and, fourth, the equation can be used to map T_1 values directly from S_{dSIR} since

$$T_1 \approx \frac{\Delta TI}{\ln 4} S_{dSIR} + \frac{\Sigma TI}{\ln 4} \tag{20.9}$$

Thus, the dSIR image is also a T_1 map. The S_{dSIR} image/T_1 map shows high contrast and high spatial resolution as for the two source images since they are linear voxel rescaling of these images (e.g., Fig. 20.12) with the three caveats: (i) it only applies to T_1s in the mD; (ii) the reasoning applies to long TR IR images. If the TR is not long enough, then correction of the T_1 values is needed and (iii) accurate nulling is required.

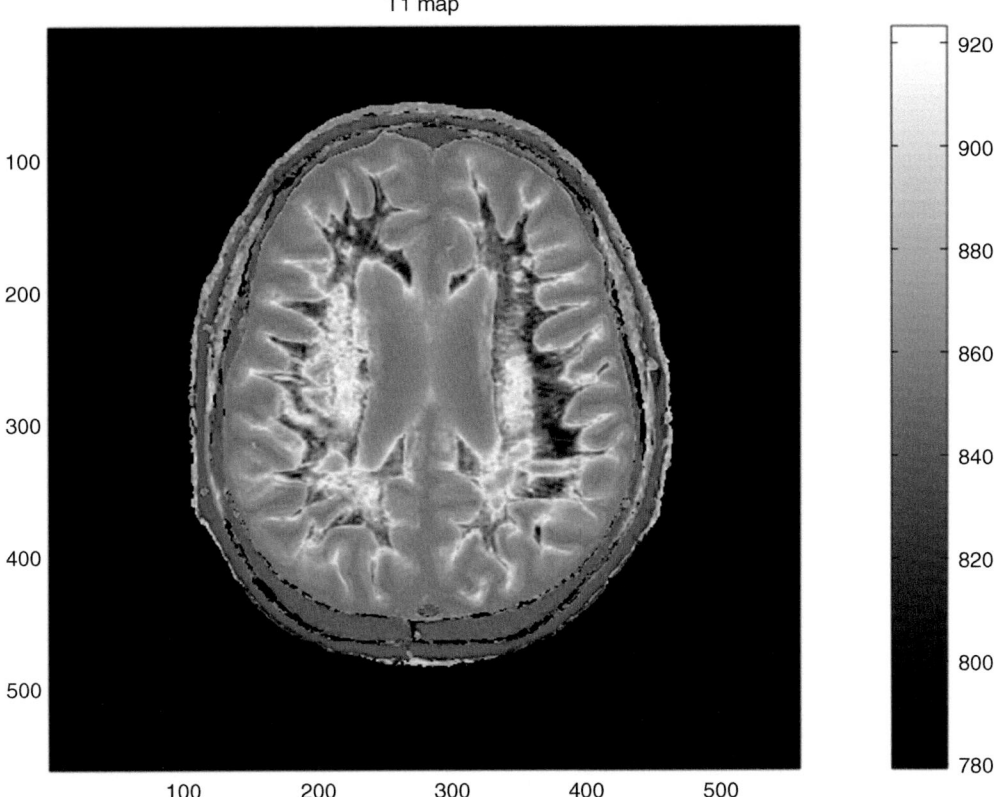

Fig. 20.12 A narrow mD dSIR image/T_1 map ($TI_s = 540$ ms and $TI_i = 640$ ms, TR $= 6000$ ms) in a patient with small vessel disease showing T_1 values within the mD on the gray scale on the right. The figure relates dSIR signal to the T_1 gray scale, which covers the mD that is within the white matter. The gray scale shows T_1 values over a range of 144 ms with the dark, low signal representing shorter, normal T_1 values in the white matter of 780 ms (i.e., 540/ln 2 ms) and above, and the higher signal representing abnormal increased T_1 values in the white matter up to the maximum of 924 ms (i.e., 640/ln 2 ms). Lesions with T_1 values greater than the maximum in the mD (i.e., greater than 924 ms) "overshoot" and appear mid-gray in their centers (where their T_1 values are not included) and are surrounded by high signal boundaries. The T_1 maps are only valid in the mD. They are obtained using long TR IR images as in this case. If the TR is short, then the T_1 values may be low and need correction

References

1. Bydder GM, Young IR. Clinical use of the inversion recovery sequence. J Comput Assist Tomogr. 1985;9(4):659–75.
2. Redpath TW, Smith FW. Technical note: use of a double inversion recovery pulse sequence to image selectively gray or white brain matter. Br J Radiol. 1994;67(804):1258–63.
3. McKinney A, Palmer C, Short J, Lucato L, Truwit C. Utility of fat-suppressed FLAIR and subtraction imaging in detecting meningeal abnormalities. Neuroradiology. 2006;48(12):881–5.
4. Edelman RR, Hatabu H, Tadamura E, Li W, Prasad PV. Noninvasive assessment of regional ventilation in the human lung using oxygen-enhanced magnetic resonance imaging. Nat Med. 1996;2(11):1236–9.
5. Robson M, Gatehouse PD, Bydder M, Bydder GM. Magnetic resonance: an introduction to ultrashort TE (UTE) imaging. J Comput Assist Tomogr. 2003;27(6):825–46.
6. Marques JP, Kober T, Krueger G, van der Zwaag W, Van de Moortele P-F, Gruetter R. MP2RAGE, a self bias-field corrected sequence for improved segmentation and T_1-mapping at high field. Neuroimage. 2010;49(2):1271–81.
7. Kecskemeti S, Samsonov A. MPnRAGE: a technique to simultaneously acquire hundreds of differently contrasted MP-RAGE images with applications to quantitative T_1 mapping. Magn Reson Med. 2016;75(3):1040–53.
8. Beaumont J, Saint-Jalmes H, Acosta O, Kober T, Tanner M, Ferré JC, Salvado O, Fripp J, Gambarota G. Multi T_1-weighted contrast MRI with fluid and white matter suppression at 1.5T. Magn Reson Imaging. 2019;63:217–25.
9. Beaumont J, Gambarota G, Saint-Jalmes H, Acosta O, Ferré J-C, Raniga P, Fripp J. High-resolution multi-T_1-weighted contrast and T_1 mapping with low B_1 sensitivity using the fluid and white matter suppression (FLAWS) sequence at 7T. Magn Reson Med. 2021;85(3):1364–78.
10. Ma Y-J, Fan S, Shao H, Du J, Szeverenyi NM, Young IR, Bydder GM. Use of multiplied, added, subtracted and/or fiTted inversion recovery (MASTIR) pulse sequences. Quant Imaging Med Surg. 2020;10(6):1334–69.
11. Ma Y-J, Moazamian D, Cornfeld DM, Condron P, Holdsworth SJ, Bydder M, Du J, Bydder GM. Improving the understanding and performance of clinical MRI using tissue property filters and the central contrast theorem, MASDIR pulse sequences and synergistic contrast MRI. Quant Imaging Med Surg. 2022;12(9):4658–90.
12. Mozes FE, Tunnicliffe EM, Moolla A, Marjot T, Levick CK, Pavlides M, Robson MD. Mapping tissue water T_1 in the liver using

the MOLLI T_1 method in the presence of fat, iron and B_0 inhomogeneity. NMR Biomed. 2019;32(2):e4030.

13. Ma Y-J, Searleman AC, Jang H, Wong J, Chang EY, Corey-Bloom J, Bydder GM, Du J. Whole-brain myelin imaging using 3D double-echo sliding inversion recovery ultrashort echo time (DESIRE UTE) MRI. Radiology. 2020;294(2):362–74.

14. Port JD. Why we DESIRE to directly image brain myelin using MRI. Radiology. 2020;294(2):375–6.

15. Ma Y-J, Jang H, Wei Z, Cai Z, Xue Y, Chang EY, Bydder GM, Corey-Bloom J, Du J. Myelin imaging in human brain using a short TR adiabatic inversion recovery prepared ultrashort echo time (STAIR-UTE) MRI sequence in multiple sclerosis. Radiology. 2020;297(2):392–404.

16. Messina SA, Port JD. On the STAIR-way to imaging myelin with clinical MRI. Radiology. 2020;297(2):405–6.

Quantitative Ultrashort Echo Time Magnetic Resonance Imaging: T_1

Yajun Ma, Xing Lu, Saeed Jerban, Hyungseok Jang, Jiang Du, and Graeme M. Bydder

Introduction

T_1 relaxation is a fundamental MR property of tissue, and quantitative T_1 measurement offers a better understanding of the imaging contrast mechanisms [1, 2]. Measured T_1s may be used as biomarkers of diseases such as degeneration of cartilage and tendon [3, 4] since they have an advantage over T_2 or T_2^* measurement because of their insensitivity to the magic angle effect [5]. In addition, other quantitative measures, such as $T_{1\rho}$ [6, 7], magnetization transfer modeling [8], and perfusion [9], are highly dependent on the accuracy of T_1 measurements. As a result, accurate T_1 quantification is essential in many MR imaging studies.

Many T_1 measurement techniques have been combined with ultrashort echo time (UTE) acquisitions to provide accurate T_1 measurements of short-T_2 species, such as saturation recovery (SR) [10–14] and inversion recovery (IR) [15–19], as well as gradient echo-based variable flip angle (VFA) [11, 20–26] and variable repetition time (VTR) [16, 27–29] methods. These techniques have been applied to T_1 measurement in many short-T_2 tissues, such as cortical bone, tendons, ligaments, the osteochondral junction, and myelin.

This chapter describes these quantitative UTE T_1 measurement techniques and discusses their advantages and disadvantages.

Saturation Recovery UTE (SR-UTE)

Figure 21.1 shows a diagram of the SR-UTE measurement sequence with different saturation recovery times (TSRs). A 90° nonselective pulse is utilized to saturate short-T_2 tissue magnetization, and UTE data acquisition starts after TSR. With a series of SR-UTE scans with different TSRs, T_1 can be estimated using the following equation [16, 30]:

$$S(\text{TSR}) = S_0\left(1-(1-k)\right)e^{-\frac{\text{TSR}}{T_1}} + C \qquad (21.1)$$

where $S(\text{TSR})$ is the acquired UTE signal and S_0 is the UTE signal with full longitudinal recovery. k accounts for the residual fraction of the longitudinal magnetization after application of the saturation pulse. C is the constant accounting for background noise and image artifacts. k can be estimated from the Bloch equations for a known tissue T_2. If the saturation module consists of several short 90° pulses, then the tissue magnetization is completely saturated, and Eq. 21.1 is simplified since $k = 0$. In this case, the T_1 measurement is more accurate because of the simplicity of the equation and the insensitivity of it to B_1 inhomogeneity.

Filho et al. applied the SR-UTE sequence to the measurement of T_1 in the Achilles tendon [10]. The signal intensities of the tendon increase with longer TSRs. The estimated T_1 of this tendon is around 611 ms. The SR-UTE sequence was also utilized for T_1 measurement in tibial cortical bone (Fig. 21.2), in which images were acquired with TSRs from 10 to 800 ms [14]. Excellent fitting was achieved with an estimated T_1 value of around 231 ms for this cortical bone. While the Achilles tendon shows a low signal at short TSRs, cortical bone shows a high signal on SR-UTE images even

Y. Ma (✉) · X. Lu · S. Jerban · H. Jang
Department of Radiology, University of California, San Diego, La Jolla, CA, USA
e-mail: yam013@ucsd.edu; xil135@health.ucsd.edu; sjerban@health.ucsd.edu; h4jang@health.ucsd.edu

J. Du
Department of Radiology, University of California, San Diego, La Jolla, CA, USA

Department of Bioengineering, University of California, San Diego, La Jolla, CA, USA

VA San Diego Healthcare System, San Diego, CA, USA
e-mail: jiangdu@health.ucsd.edu

G. M. Bydder
Department of Radiology, University of California, San Diego, La Jolla, CA, USA

Mātai Medical Research Institute, Tairāwhiti Gisborne, New Zealand
e-mail: gbydder@health.ucsd.edu

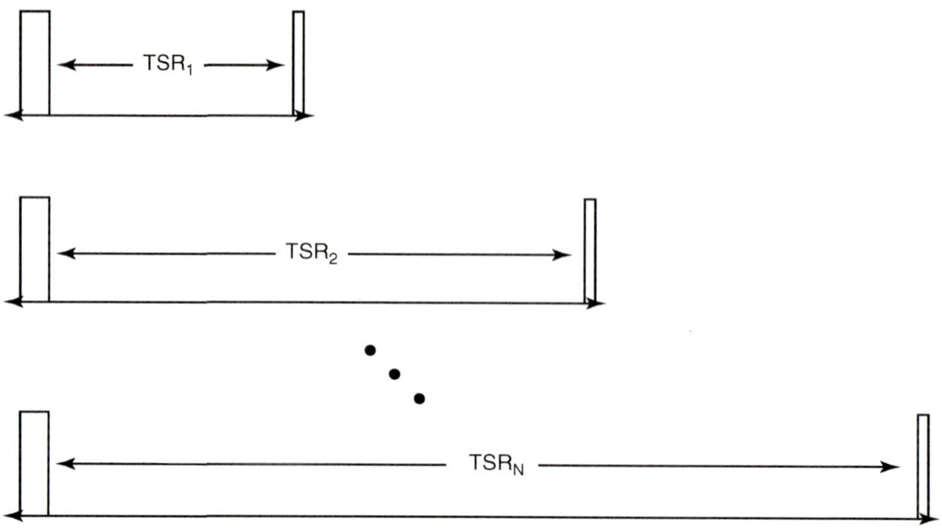

Fig. 21.1 A sequence diagram of the SR-UTE sequence. A saturation pulse, typically a 90° nonselective pulse, is used to saturate tissue magnetizations, followed by a UTE acquisition. A series of SR-UTE scans with different saturation recovery times (TSRs) are performed for T_1 quantification

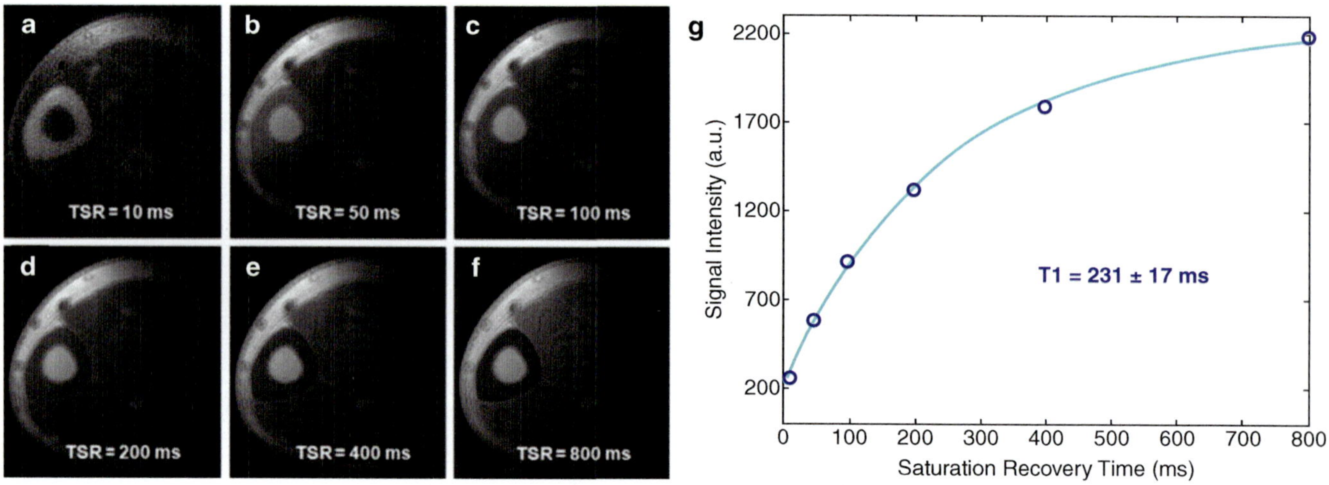

Saturation pulse   UTE excitation pulse

TSR_1

TSR_2

TSR_N

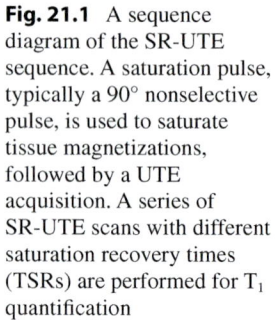

a   TSR = 10 ms

b   TSR = 50 ms

c   TSR = 100 ms

d   TSR = 200 ms

e   TSR = 400 ms

f   TSR = 800 ms

g

$T1 = 231 \pm 17$ ms

Signal Intensity (a.u.)

Saturation Recovery Time (ms)

Fig. 21.2 Representative normal tibial cortical bone SR-UTE images with TSRs of 10, 50, 100, 200, 400, and 800 ms (**a**) and the corresponding fitting (**b**). The signal intensities of the SR-UTE images increase with longer TSRs, and the estimated T_1 value of the tibial cortex is 231 ms. (Reproduced with permission from Du et al. [14])

with the shortest TSR of 10 ms. This is due to inefficient saturation of the extremely short-T_2 magnetization of cortical bone (i.e., a relatively high k value) and the fast signal recovery during TSR due to the short T_1 of cortical bone. To achieve a more reliable T_1 measurement using the SR-UTE technique, the TSR should be long enough to obtain a broader signal dynamic range and provide more reliable curve fitting.

Zhang et al. proposed using a three-dimensional (3D) SR-SWIFT (sweep imaging with Fourier transformation) Look–Locker sequence for T_1 measurement of extremely short-T_2 high-concentration iron oxide nanoparticle (IONP) suspensions [12]. Figure 21.3a shows the

sequence diagram. In this sequence, an adiabatic half-passage (AHP) pulse was utilized for signal saturation, and multiple datasets were acquired with different TSRs in a single TR. Fast T_1 measurement was achieved with this Look–Locker scheme. A phantom was constructed from six 5-mm nuclear magnetic resonance (NMR) tubes containing Ferrotec EMG 308 iron oxide nanoparticles (IONPs) of concentrations ranging from 0.0 to 53.6 mM of Fe (equivalent to 0.0–3.0 mg Fe/mL) in 1% agar solution. Figure 21.3b shows excellent linear correlations between measured R_1s and Fe concentrations, demonstrating the feasibility of obtaining T_1 measurements of high-concentration IONP suspensions.

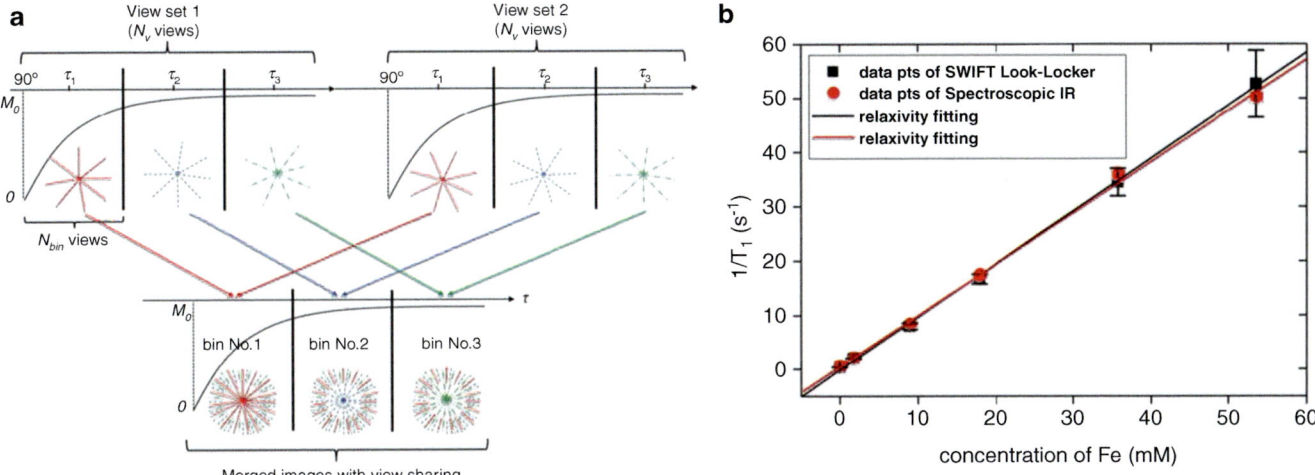

Fig. 21.3 An acquisition scheme for a 3D SWIFT Look–Locker sequence for T_1 measurement (**a**) and a correlation curve between the measured R_1s (by both the proposed method and a reference spectroscopic IR method) and concentration of Fe (**b**). N_v spokes are acquired at each TR, and these N_v views are equally divided into N_v/N_{bin} groups. N_{bin} is the total number of views in one group. The data acquired within groups with the same TSRs are combined and reconstructed into one image. A total of (N_v/N_{bin}) images are produced with different TSRs using this sequence. R_1s measured by both this method and a reference spectroscopic IR method have an excellent correlation with the concentration of Fe. (Reproduced with permission from Zhang et al.[12])

UTE with Variable TR (UTE-VTR)

Although the SR-UTE technique can accurately measure T_1 values for short-T_2 tissues, the scan time is quite long, especially when TSR is greater than 1000 ms. This long scan time makes the current SR-UTE sequence unsuitable for clinical use. A faster T_1 measurement technique using the variable TR (VTR) method has therefore been proposed [16].

For UTE-VTR T_1 measurement, the regular steady-state UTE sequence with radiofrequency (RF) spoiling and a gradient crusher is used for data acquisition. The steady-state signal S(TR) is provided in Ma et al. [24, 28]:

$$S(TR) = M_0 f_{xy}(\alpha, \tau, T_2) \frac{1-E}{1-E f_z(\alpha, \tau, T_2)} \quad (21.2)$$

where M_0 is the equilibrium magnetization and $E = \exp\left(-\dfrac{TR}{T_1}\right)$.

$f_{xy}(\alpha, \tau, T_2)$ and $f_z(\alpha, \tau, T_2)$ are the respective transverse and longitudinal magnetization mapping functions generated by the RF pulse, with $f_{xy}(\alpha, \tau, T_2) = M_{xy}^+ / M_z^-$ and $f_z(\alpha, \tau, T_2) = M_z^+ / M_z^-$. M_z^- is the longitudinal magnetization before RF excitation. M_{xy}^+ and M_z^+ are the transverse and longitudinal magnetizations after the RF excitation, respectively. α is the flip angle, and τ is the duration of the rectangular excitation pulse. Details of $f_{xy}(\alpha, \tau, T_2)$ and $f_z(\alpha, \tau, T_2)$ are as follows [24, 28]:

$$f_{xy}(\alpha, \tau, T_2) = e^{-\frac{\tau}{2T_2}} \alpha \, sinc\left(\sqrt{\alpha^2 - \left(\frac{\tau}{2T_2}\right)^2}\right) \quad (21.3)$$

$$f_z(\alpha, \tau, T_2) = e^{-\frac{\tau}{2T_2}} \left(\cos\left(\sqrt{\alpha^2 - \left(\frac{\tau}{2T_2}\right)^2}\right) + \frac{\tau}{2T_2} sinc\left(\sqrt{\alpha^2 - \left(\frac{\tau}{2T_2}\right)^2}\right) \right) \quad (21.4)$$

Since the RF pulse duration is much shorter than the tissue T_1, T_1 relaxation during the excitation can be neglected in the mapping functions. For short-T_2 tissues with T_2 values of the same order as the RF duration τ, both $f_{xy}(\alpha, \tau, T_2)$ and $f_z(\alpha, \tau, T_2)$ are determined not only by the flip angle α but also by τ and the tissue T_2. For relatively long-T_2 tissues with T_2s $\gg \tau$, both $f_{xy}(\alpha, \tau, T_2)$ and $f_z(\alpha, \tau, T_2)$ simplify to $\sin(\alpha)$ and $\cos(\alpha)$, respectively, so that Eq. 21.2 becomes

$$S(TR) = M_0 \sin(\alpha) \frac{1-E}{1-E\cos(\alpha)} \quad (21.5)$$

The UTE-VTR method acquires a series of UTE data with different TRs for T_1 fitting. The UTE-VTR method uses a fixed and relatively low flip angle for excitation (20°, for example). This low flip angle excitation allows using a pulse duration τ that is significantly shorter than the T_1 and T_2 of bone water so that the simplified Eq. 21.5 can be utilized for

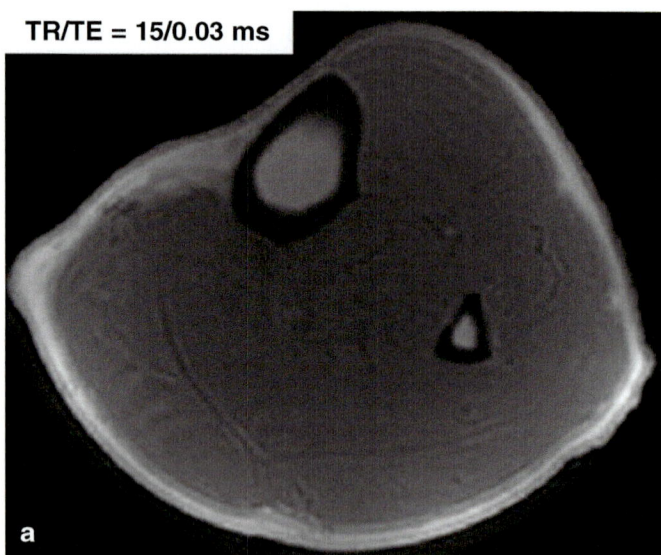

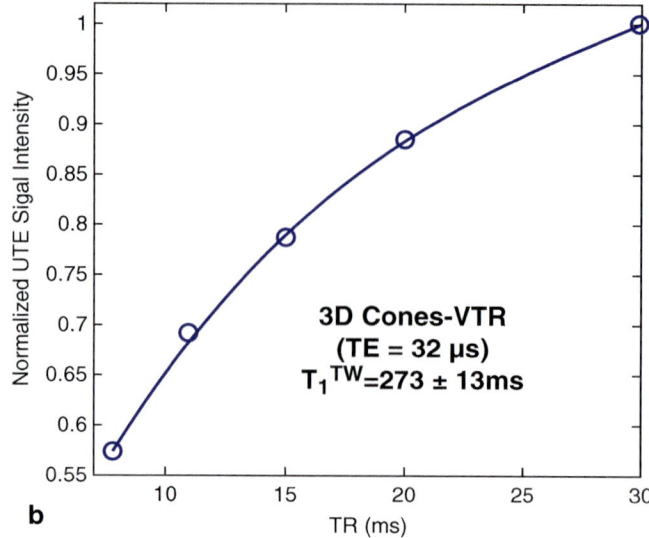

Fig. 21.4 A representative tibial UTE-VTR image from a healthy volunteer with a TR of 15 ms (**a**) and the corresponding fitting of the tibial cortical bone (**b**). Excellent fitting is achieved with the UTE-VTR T_1 fitting. The low flip angle excitation also allows fast longitudinal magnetization recovery for accurate T_1 measurement. The more time-efficient UTE-VTR scan benefits from this fast recovery (i.e., with use of a shorter TR). With the reduced TR, volumetric T_1 measurement is possible using a 3D UTE-VTR method. This is unlike SR-UTE T_1 measurement, which is typically a two-dimensional (2D) method due to its long scan time.

Chen et al. applied the 3D UTE-VTR technique to cortical bone volumetric T_1 measurement [16]. The representative 3D UTE-VTR image and a fitting curve of these authors are shown in Fig. 21.4. The steady-state UTE signal increases with longer TRs. The measured T_1 of cortical bone using the UTE-VTR method is around 273 ms, which is very similar to the value measured with the SR-UTE method shown in Fig. 21.2. The UTE-VTR sequence with a relatively long TE (e.g., 2.5 ms) was applied to pore water T_1 measurement. In this case, pure pore water signals were received and quantified after the bound water signals had decayed to zero, which was before the UTE-VTR data acquisition at a TE of 2.5 ms.

UTE Actual Flip Angle Imaging (UTE-AFI)

The UTE-VTR T_1 measurement method is sensitive to B_1 inhomogeneity. The B_1 distribution is more inhomogeneous when imaged with a higher magnetic field scanner, such as 3 T and 7 T. As a result, B_1 correction for accurate UTE-VTR T_1 measurement is critical on clinical 3T scanners.

The AFI method has been widely used for 3D B_1 mapping [31], which is a perfect fit with 3D T_1 measurement using

method, and the estimated T_1 value of the bone is 273 ± 13 ms. (Reproduced with permission from Chen et al. [16])

UTE sequences. Using the combination of UTE and AFI techniques, it is possible to measure B_1 maps for short-T_2 tissues. Recently, Ma et al. have combined the UTE-VTR and UTE-AFI methods to provide accurate T_1 measurement of short-T_2 tissues with B_1 correction [28]. The UTE-AFI sequence is shown in Fig. 21.4a, which uses a pair of interleaved TRs to produce accurate B_1 mapping.

The steady-state signals S_1 and S_2 acquired in TR_1 and TR_2 of the 3D UTE-AFI sequence are expressed as follows [24, 28]:

$$S_1 = M_0 f_{xy}\left(\alpha,\tau,T_2\right)\frac{1-E_2+\left(1-E_1\right)E_2 f_z\left(\alpha,\tau,T_2\right)}{1-E_1 E_2 f_z^2\left(\alpha,\tau,T_2\right)} \quad (21.6)$$

$$S_2 = M_0 f_{xy}\left(\alpha,\tau,T_2\right)\frac{1-E_1+\left(1-E_2\right)E_1 f_z\left(\alpha,\tau,T_2\right)}{1-E_1 E_2 f_z^2\left(\alpha,\tau,T_2\right)} \quad (21.7)$$

with

$$E_1 = \exp\left(-TR_1 / T_1\right)$$

$$E_2 = \exp\left(-TR_2 / T_1\right)$$

where M_0 is the equilibrium magnetization.

Two fundamental assumptions are necessary for accurate B_1 mapping with AFI: first is that complete spoiling of the transverse magnetization occurs during TR_1 and TR_2, and second is that TR_1s and TR_2s are short compared to T_1. For short-T_2 imaging, the first assumption is easily fulfilled due to the fast signal decay of the short-T_2 tissues. With TRs that are short relative to T_1, the signal ratio r of S_1 to S_2 can be simplified using a first-order approximation for the exponential terms [28, 31] so that

$$r = S_2 / S_1 \approx \frac{1 + n f_z(\alpha, \tau, T_2)}{n + f_z(\alpha, \tau, T_2)} \qquad (21.8)$$

where $n = TR_2/TR_1$. The ratio r can then be used as a T_1-independent measure of $f_z(\alpha, \tau, T_2)$:

$$f_z(\alpha, \tau, T_2) \approx \frac{rn - 1}{n - r} \qquad (21.9)$$

For long-T_2 tissues, $f_z(\alpha, \tau, T_2)$ becomes $\cos(\alpha)$. So, the actual flip angle α can be estimated with the following equation [28, 31]:

$$\alpha \approx \arccos\left(\frac{rn - 1}{n - r}\right) \qquad (21.10)$$

Then, the B_1 scaling factor (B_{1s}) is obtained by dividing the measured α by the nominal flip angle α_{nom}, which is expressed as follows:

$$B_{1s} = \alpha / \alpha_{nom} \qquad (21.11)$$

B_{1s} is used to quantify RF inhomogeneity. $B_{1s} = 1$ corresponds to a uniform RF field.

To achieve sufficient sensitivity for B_1 mapping, the AFI technique should use a relatively high flip angle (i.e., $\geq 40°$). However, with this high flip angle and the limited RF peak power of clinical scanners, the pulse duration τ (between 150 and 200 ms) is comparable to the T_2s of ultrashort-T_2 tissues such as cortical bone with a T_2 of ~0.3 ms [28]. The measurement of α or B_{1s} from Eq. 21.9 is complicated in this case. With known values of τ and tissue T_2, α can be calculated from the analytical expression of $f_z(\alpha, \tau, T_2)$ in Eq. 21.4 or through Bloch equation simulation. However, it is highly challenging to measure short-T_2 values accurately in practice.

To cope with these issues, Ma et al. proposed a new approach that avoids the calculation of α for B_1 mapping [28]. Instead, the value of $f_z(\alpha, \tau, T_2)$ in Eq. 21.9 is directly used as input for T_1 calculation using the UTE-VTR method (i.e., Eq. 21.2). To use this method, the RF pulse duration and flip angle need to be identical for both the UTE-VTR and UTE-AFI sequences (UTE-AFI-VTR). In this case, the longitudi-

nal function $f_z(\alpha, \tau, T_2)$ of the UTE-AFI sequence is identical to that of the UTE-VTR sequence. This way, $f_z(\alpha, \tau, T_2)$ maps, including information about both B_1 and excitation efficiency, are measured instead of the regular B_1 maps.

Once $f_z(\alpha, \tau, T_2)$ is known and substituted into Eq. 21.2, the regular UTE-VTR method is used for T_1 mapping of short-T_2 tissues. This framework also works for the T_1 measurement of long-T_2 tissues. Figure 21.5b and c shows representative UTE-AFI images of a bovine cortical bone sample with TRs of 20 and 100 ms. B_{1s} and f_z maps are calculated from these dual TR images, as shown in Fig. 21.5d and e, respectively. The B_{1s} map is calculated from Eqs. 21.10 and 21.11, which is inaccurate since the bone T_2 is not sufficiently long compared to the RF pulse duration. The opposite distribution in both B_{1s} and f_z maps is seen due to the B_1 inhomogeneity. Figure 21.5g and h shows T_1 maps obtained using the regular UTE-VTR and the newly developed UTE-AFI-VTR methods, respectively. The regular UTE-VTR method uses a short RF pulse of 60 μs and a flip angle of 20°. The B_1 distribution modulates the UTE-VTR T_1 map. The UTE-AFI-VTR T_1 map shows a much more homogeneous T_1 distribution. As shown in Fig. 21.6, much more uniform T_1 maps for in vivo tibial cortical bone were also achieved with the new UTE-AFI-VTR method compared to the B_1-uncorrected UTE-VTR method.

Furthermore, Zhao et al. proposed a faster version for short-T_2 tissue T_1 measurement, which only acquires dual-TR UTE-AFI data and UTE data with a single TR (UTE-STR) (UTE-AFI-STR) (a total of three datasets) [29]. In this approach, three equations, i.e., Eqs. 21.2, 21.6, and 21.7 are combined into a group for data fitting, with three unknown parameters in this group, i.e., $f_z(\alpha, \tau, T_2)$, $M_0 f_{xy}(\alpha, \tau, T_2)$, and T_1. Thus, the three acquired datasets are sufficient for fitting and parameter estimation. This new approach takes advantage of the identical M_0 and excitation parameters in both the UTE-AFI and UTE-STR sequences. Similar T_1 maps of cortical bone are achieved with both the faster UTE-AFI-STR and slower UTE-AFI-VTR methods.

Fig. 21.5 A UTE-AFI sequence diagram (**a**) and T_1 measurement results of an ex vivo bovine cortical bone (**b–g**). The UTE-AFI sequence acquires two datasets with two different interleaved TRs. Examples of two AFI images of cortical bone are shown in panels (**a**) and (**c**). Inhomogeneous distribution of B_1s (**d**) and f_z (**e**) maps can be seen in the cortical bone region. A much more uniform T_1 map is generated by the UTE-AFI-VTR method (**g**) compared to that generated by the regular UTE-VTR method (**f**). (Reproduced with permission from Ma et al. [28])

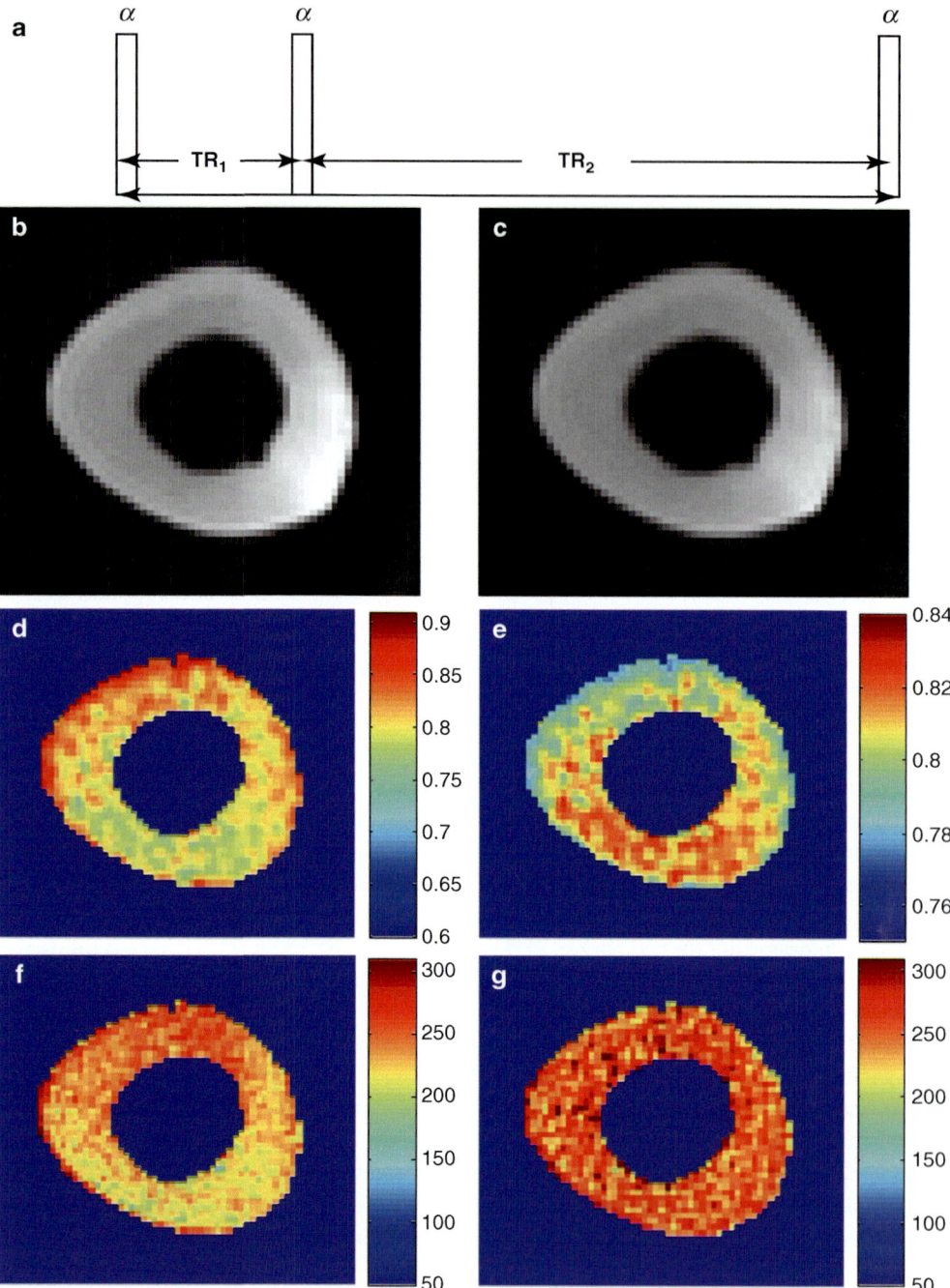

Fig. 21.6 Representative tibial cortical bone T_1 measurement with UTE-VTR and UTE-AFI-VTR for a healthy volunteer. Inhomogeneous distribution of B_1s (**a**) and f_z (**b**) maps can be seen in the cortical bone region. A much more uniform T_1 map is generated by the UTE-AFI-VTR method in panel (**d**) compared to that generated by the regular UTE-VTR method (**c**). (Reproduced with permission from Ma et al. [28])

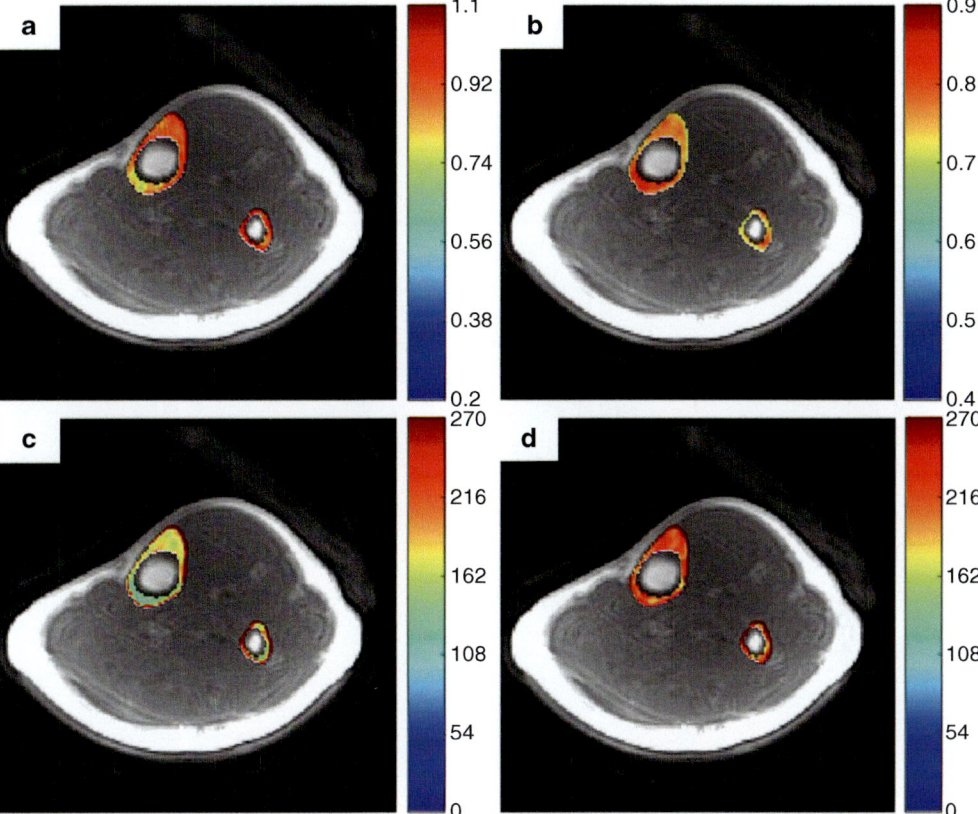

UTE with Variable FA (UTE-VFA)

The fast VFA technique has been widely used for T_1 measurement [31]. It has recently been combined with UTE acquisition for T_1 measurement of the whole knee joint [24, 26]. The UTE-VFA sequence has advantages in measuring tissues with a wide range of T_1s. However, as with the UTE-VTR method, the UTE-VFA method is susceptible to B_1 inhomogeneity.

The UTE-AFI sequence has been applied to measure B_1 maps for correction of UTE-VFA T_1 measurement (called UTE-AFI-VFA) [24, 26]. In this technique, the B_1 map is estimated from Eqs. 21.10 and 21.11, without consideration for the extremely short-T_2 tissues ($T_2 < 1$ ms), such as cortical bone [24]. Ma et al. performed a numerical simulation and found that the errors in T_1 estimation for tissues with a $T_2 > 1$ ms are less than 1% if a 150-μs RF pulse is utilized for signal excitation in the UTE-AFI-VFA acquisitions [24]. Apart from cortical bone, most tissues in the knee joint, such as cartilage, meniscus, ligaments, tendons, muscles, and fat, have T_2s longer than 1 ms. Thus, the UTE-AFI-VFA technique could provide a comprehensive T_1 measurement for all the soft tissues in the knee joint except cortical bone.

Figure 21.7 shows representative UTE images and estimated B_1 and T_1 maps in a healthy knee joint. In this study, an eight-channel transmit and receive (T/R) knee coil was utilized for RF excitation and signal reception [24]. Apparent B_1 variations can be found in estimated B_1 maps with this T/R knee coil. The B_1-corrected and B_1-uncorrected T_1 maps are shown in the second and third rows, respectively. More uniform T_1 values in the marrow fat and muscle regions can be seen in the B_1-corrected T_1 maps. This demonstrates the effectiveness of the B_1 correction using the UTE-AFI technique. Ma et al. also summarized the average T_1 values for principal tissues from 16 healthy knee joints. The UTE-AFI-VFA method showed a mean T_1 value and standard deviation (SD) of 833 ± 47 ms for the meniscus, 800 ± 66 ms for the quadriceps tendon, 656 ± 43 ms for the patellar tendon, 873 ± 38 ms for the anterior cruciate ligament (ACL), 832 ± 49 ms for the posterior cruciate ligament (PCL), 1098 ± 67 ms for the cartilage, 379 ± 18 ms for the marrow, and 1393 ± 46 ms for the muscle.

Maggioni et al. further optimized the spoiling scheme for faster UTE-AFI acquisitions with half the scan time [26]. The angle orientations of the gradient crushers in the x–y plane are randomized within different TRs. The phantom and in vivo knee joint experiments showed more stable T_1 esti-

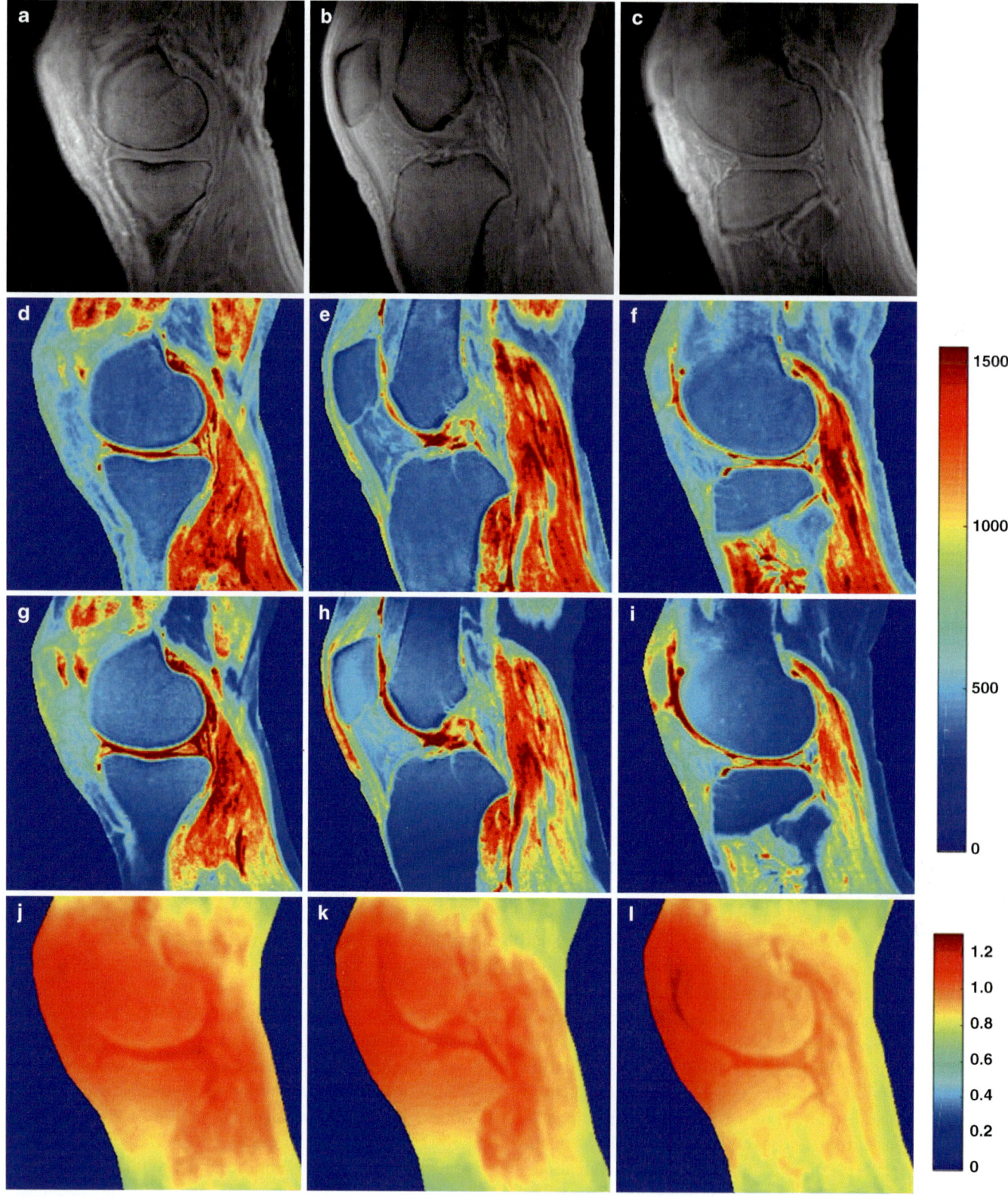

Fig. 21.7 Representative UTE images for three different slices (**a–c**) and the corresponding T$_1$ mapping results in a healthy knee joint. Much more uniform T$_1$ values in muscles and marrow fat regions are achieved using the B$_1$-corrected UTE-AFI-VFA method (**d–f**) compared to those generated by the B$_1$-uncorrected UTE-VFA method (**g–i**). The inhomogeneous distribution of the B$_1$ maps can be seen in the coil boundary region (**j–l**). (Reproduced with permission from Ma et al. [24])

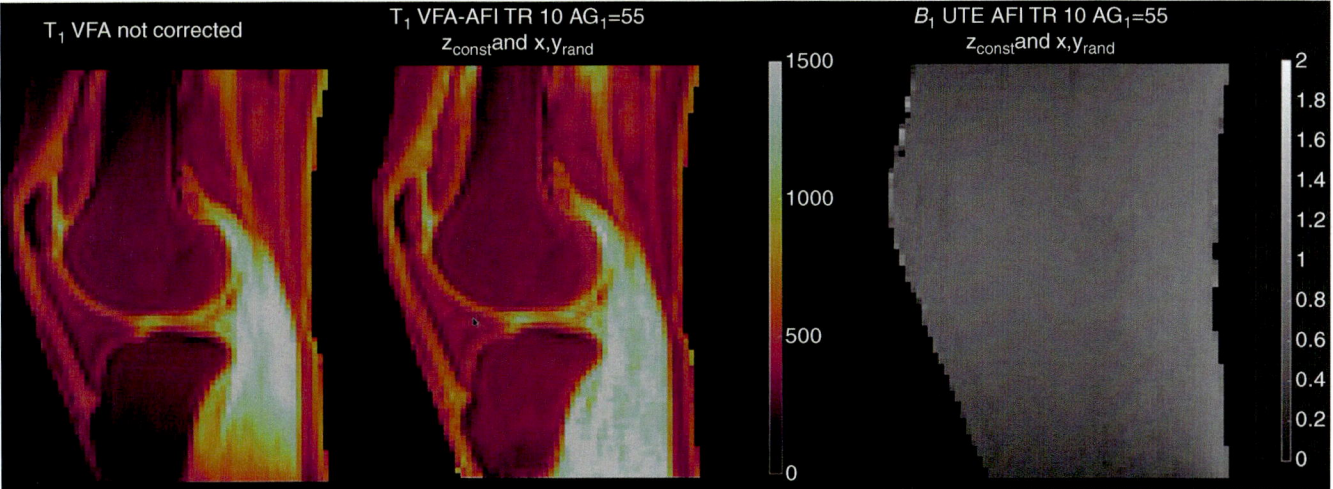

Fig. 21.8 Representative B_1 (last column) and T_1 mapping results from a healthy knee joint using the B_1-uncorrected UTE-VFA method (first column) and the optimized UTE-AFI-VFA method (second column). Much more uniform T_1 values are achieved in muscle and marrow fat regions using the B_1-corrected UTE-AFI-VFA method. (Reproduced with permission from Maggioni et al. [26])

mations using the optimized UTE-AFI sequence than the conventional AFI sequence. Figure 21.8 shows representative T_1 maps with and without B_1 correction for a healthy knee joint. With B_1 correction, T_1 maps in the muscle and marrow fat regions are spatially more uniform. The study also summarized T_1 values for different tissues in a healthy knee joint and showed a mean T_1 value and SD of 768 ± 38 ms for the quadriceps tendon, 640 ± 56 ms for the patellar tendon, 337 ± 8 ms for the bone marrow, and 1411 ± 156 ms for the muscle. These T_1 values are similar to the measurements in Ma et al.'s study, demonstrating the accuracy of the optimized protocol.

Inversion Recovery UTE (IR-UTE)

The IR sequence is the gold standard for T_1 measurement for long-T_2 tissues [32]. However, for the T_1 measurement of short-T_2 tissues, the relatively long IR pulse does not invert the longitudinal magnetizations efficiently [33, 34]. This makes the T_1 measurement of short-T_2 tissues more complicated.

Zhao et al. performed a phantom study to investigate the feasibility of T_1 measurement of short-T_2 tissues using an IR-UTE sequence [15]. This sequence uses an adiabatic full-passage (AFP) pulse for signal inversion, followed by a multispoke UTE acquisition. IR-UTE acquisitions with different inversion times (TIs) are acquired for curve fitting and T_1 estimation. To account for the imperfect inversion, an inversion efficiency factor Q is included in the signal equation. Q ranges from -1 (full inversion, for species with long

T_2s, e.g., $T_2 > 100$ ms) to 1 (no disturbance to the longitudinal magnetization, for species with extremely short T_2s, e.g., $T_2 < 1$ μs). Q is 0 when the magnetization is completely saturated (for tissues with ultrashort T_2s, e.g., $T_2 \sim 0.1$ ms). In this study, 12 5-mL tubes were filled with $MnCl_2$ aqueous solutions with concentrations ranging from 0 to 89.16 mM. The phantom T_2^* values ranged from 0.14 to 10.61 ms for the tubes with concentrations of 89.16–1.43 mM, which covers the T_2^* values for the major short-T_2 tissues in the body. Figure 21.9 shows the representative IR-UTE images with different TIs for two TRs of 50 and 400 ms, respectively. Different contrasts for the IR-UTE images were observed at different TIs. The R_1 values are well-correlated with the concentrations. The IR-UTE sequence with a longer TR (i.e., 400 ms) performs better for the T_1 measurement of longer-T_1 tissues. In comparison, the IR-UTE sequence with a shorter TR (i.e., 50 ms) performs better for the T_1 measurement of shorter-T_1 tissues. This study demonstrates the feasibility of T_1 measurement of short-T_2 tissues using the IR-UTE sequence.

Du et al. proposed an IR-UTE technique for T_1 measurement of short-T_2 components in the brain (i.e., myelin) [19] and cortical bone (i.e., bound water) [16, 17]. In this approach, long-T_2 components are suppressed by IR preparation, and UTE acquisitions detect only short-T_2 signals. Several IR-UTE scans are performed with different TRs, and TIs are carefully chosen at long-T_2 nulling points for each TR. Then, the acquired short-T_2 signals are fitted by the IR-UTE signal model for T_1 measurement. Figure 21.10 shows representative dual-echo

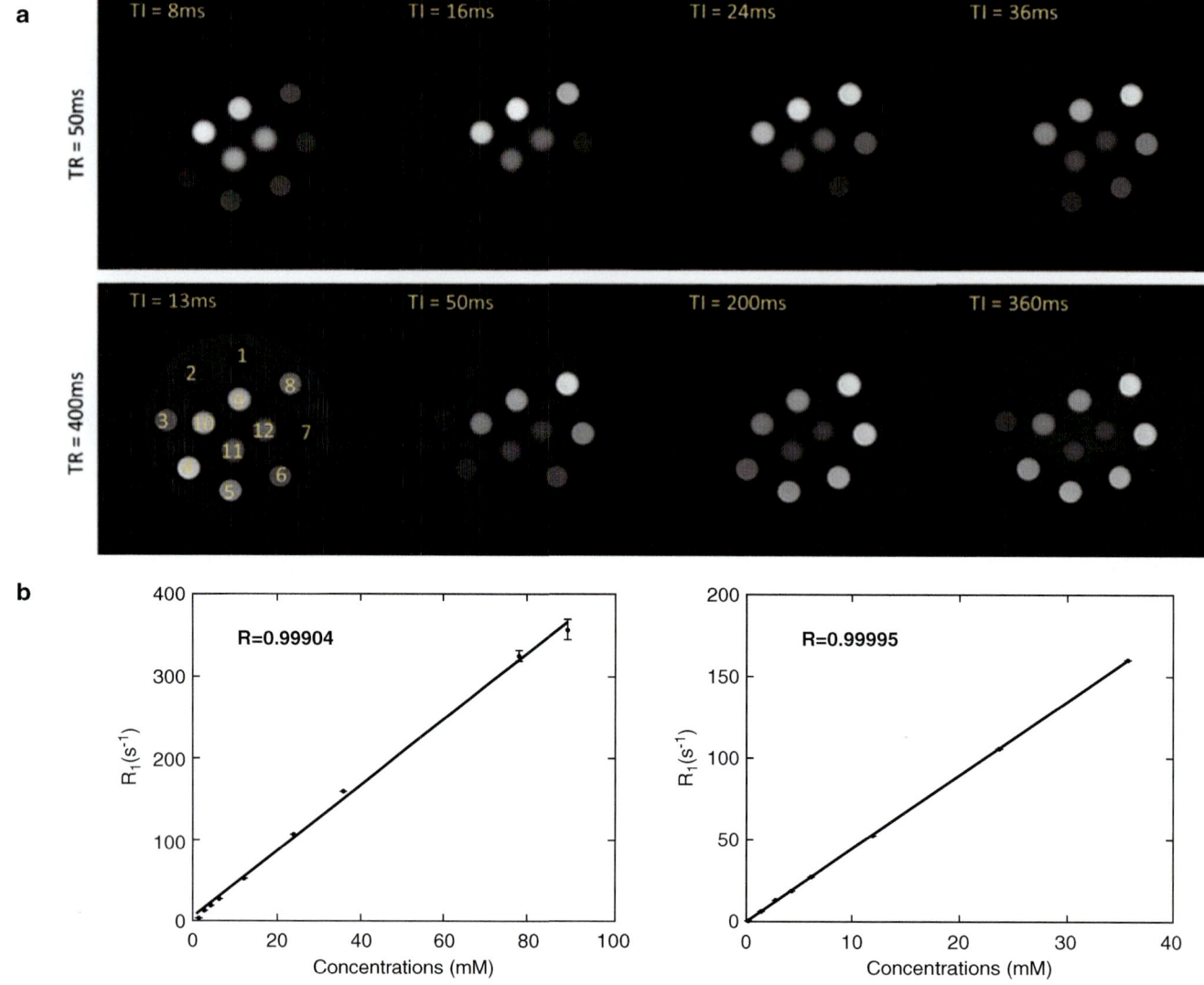

Fig. 21.9 Representative IR-UTE images with TRs of 50 and 400 ms (**a** and **b**, respectively) and the correlation curves between measured R_1s and MnCl$_2$ concentrations (**b**). Different image contrasts are observed on IR-UTE images with different TIs. Excellent correlations are achieved between R_1s and MnCl$_2$ concentrations for scans with TRs of 50 ms (the left column in panel (**b**), tubes 4–12) and 400 ms (the right column in panel (**b**), tubes 1–10). (Reproduced with permission from Wei et al. [15])

IR-UTE images and the corresponding fitting curves in a healthy brain [19]. The dual-echo subtracted images with different TRs offer high myelin contrast, and the myelin signal intensities increase with longer TRs. After fitting, the estimated T$_1$ of myelin is around 234 ms. The same technique has been applied to bound water T$_1$ measurement in cortical bone, and the estimated T$_1$ value of bound water is around 131 ms [16].

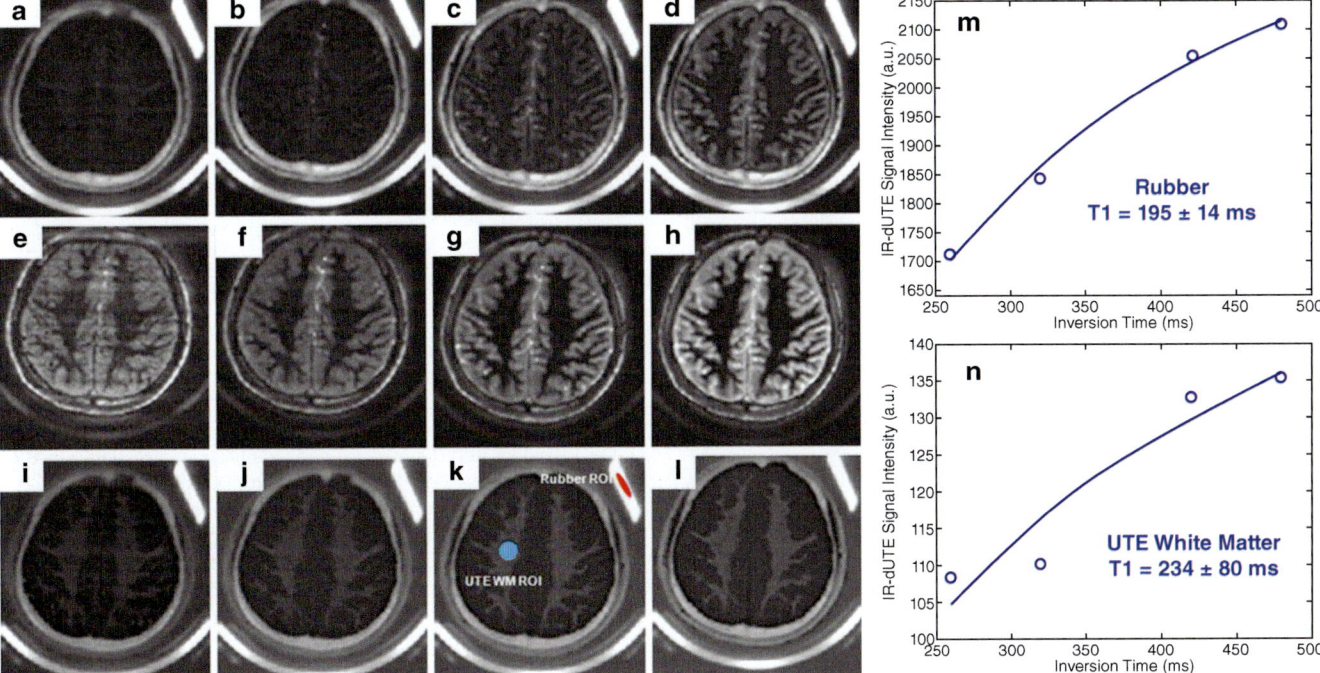

Fig. 21.10 Representative brain dual-echo IR-UTE images (**a–l**) and T_1 fitting curves (**m** and **n**) in a healthy volunteer. Pure myelin images (**i–l**) are achieved by echo subtraction between the first echo (**a–d**) and the second echo (**e–h**) images. The estimated T_1 values of rubber band and myelin in the brain are 195 ± 14 (**m**) and 234 ± 80 ms (**n**), respectively. (Reproduced with permission from Du et al. [19])

Conclusions

Current state-of-the-art UTE-T_1 measurement techniques are summarized in this chapter, including SR-UTE, IR-UTE, UTE-VTR, and UTE-VFA. The SR-UTE and IR-UTE techniques typically require long scan times. Utilizing the Look–Locker method could improve scan efficiency. The more time-efficient UTE-VTR and UTE-VFA methods are suitable for high-resolution volumetric T_1 mapping.

References

1. Bloch F. Nuclear induction. Phys Rev. 1946;70:460–74.
2. Goldman M. Formal theory of spin-lattice relaxation. J Magn Reson. 2001;149(2):160–87.
3. Burstein D, Velyvis J, Scott KT, et al. Protocol issues for delayed Gd (DTPA)(2-)- enhanced MRI (dGEMRIC) for clinical evaluation of articular cartilage. Magn Reson Med. 2001;45(1):36–41.
4. Tiderius CJ, Olsson LE, Leander P, Ekberg O, Dahlberg L. Delayed gadolinium-enhanced MRI of cartilage (dGEMRIC) in early knee osteoarthritis. Magn Reson Med. 2003;49(3):488–92.
5. Bydder M, Rahal A, Fullerton GD, Bydder GM. The magic angle effect: a source of artifact, determinant of image contrast, and technique for imaging. J Magn Reson Imaging. 2007;25(2):290–300.
6. Ma Y-J, Carl M, Shao H, Tadros AS, Chang EY, Du J. Three-dimensional ultrashort echo time cones $T_1\rho$ (3D UTE-cones-$T_1\rho$) imaging. NMR Biomed. 2017;30(6):10.1002/nbm.3709.
7. Ma Y, Carl M, Searleman A, Lu X, Chang EY, Du J. 3D adiabatic T1rho prepared ultrashort echo time cones (3D AdiabT1rho

8. UTE-cones) sequence for whole knee imaging. Magn Reson Med. 2018;80(4):1429–39.
8. Ma Y, Carl M, Chang EY, Du J. Quantitative magnetization transfer ultrashort echo time imaging using a time-efficient 3D multispoke cones sequence. Magn Reson Med. 2018;79(2):692–700.
9. de Bazelaire C, Rofsky NM, Duhamel G, et al. Combined T_2^* and T_1 measurements for improved perfusion and permeability studies in high field using dynamic contrast enhancement. Eur Radiol. 2006;16(9):2083–91.
10. Filho GH, Du J, Pak BC, et al. Quantitative characterization of the Achilles tendon in cadaveric specimens: T_1 and T_2^* measurements using ultrashort-TE MRI at 3 T. AJR Am J Roentgenol. 2009;192(3):W117–24.
11. Wright P, Jellus V, McGonagle D, Robson M, Ridgeway J, Hodgson R. Comparison of two ultrashort echo time sequences for the quantification of T_1 within phantom and human Achilles tendon at 3 T. Magn Reson Med. 2012;6(4):1279–84.
12. Zhang J, Chamberlain R, Etheridge M, et al. Quantifying iron-oxide nanoparticles at high concentration based on longitudinal relaxation using a three-dimensional SWIFT look-locker sequence. Magn Reson Med. 2014;71(6):1982–8.
13. Mahar R, Batool S, Badar F, Xia Y. Quantitative measurement of T_2, $T_1\rho$ and T_1 relaxation times in articular cartilage and cartilage-bone interface by SE and UTE imaging at microscopic resolution. J Magn Reson. 2018;297:76–85.
14. Du J, Carl M, Bydder M, Takahashi A, Chung CB, Bydder GM. Qualitative and quantitative ultrashort echo time (UTE) imaging of cortical bone. J Magn Reson. 2010;207(2):304–11.
15. Wei Z, Ma Y-J, Jang H, Yang W, Du J. To measure T1 of short T2 species using an inversion recovery prepared three-dimensional ultrashort echo time (3D IR-UTE) method: a phantom study. J Magn Reson. 2020;314:106725.
16. Chen J, Chang EY, Carl M, et al. Measurement of bound and pore water T1 relaxation times in cortical bone using three-dimen-

sional ultrashort echo time cones sequences. Magn Reson Med. 2017;77(6):2136–45.

17. Guo T, Ma Y, Jerban S, et al. T1 measurement of bound water in cortical bone using 3D adiabatic inversion recovery ultrashort echo time (3D IR-UTE) cones imaging. Magn Reson Med. 2020;84(2):634–45.

18. Zurek M, Johansson E, Risse F, Alamidi D, Olsson LE, Hockings PD. Accurate T_1 mapping for oxygen-enhanced MRI in the mouse lung using a segmented inversion-recovery ultrashort echo-time sequence. Magn Reson Med. 2014;71(6):2180–5.

19. Du J, Sheth V, He Q, Carl M, Chen J, Corey-Bloom J, Bydder GM. Measurement of T1 of the ultrashort T2* components in white matter of the brain at 3T. PLoS One. 2014;9(8):e103296.

20. Springer F, Steidle G, Martirosian P, Syha R, Claussen CD, Schick F. Rapid assessment of longitudinal relaxation time in materials and tissue with extremely fast signal decay using UTE sequences and the variable flip angle method. Investig Radiol. 2011;46(10):610–7.

21. Wang L, Corum CA, Idiyatullin D, Garwood M, Zhao Q. T1 estimation for aqueous iron oxide nanoparticle suspensions using a variable flip angle SWIFT sequence. Magn Reson Med. 2013;70(2):341–7.

22. Han M, Rieke V, Scott SJ, et al. Quantifying temperature-dependent T_1 changes in cortical bone using ultrashort echo-time MRI. Magn Reson Med. 2015;74(6):1548–55.

23. Alamidi DF, Smailagic A, Bidar AW, et al. Variable flip angle 3D ultrashort echo time (UTE) T1 mapping of mouse lung: a repeatability assessment. J Magn Reson Imaging. 2018;48(3):846–52.

24. Ma Y, Zhao W, Wan L, et al. Whole knee joint T1 values measured in vivo at 3T by combined 3D ultrashort echo time cones actual flip angle and variable flip angle methods. Magn Reson Med. 2019;81(3):1634–44.

25. Cai Z, Wei Z, Wu M, et al. Knee osteochondral junction imaging using a fast 3D T_1-weighted ultrashort echo time cones sequence at 3T. Magn Reson Imaging. 2020;73:76–83.

26. Maggioni MB, Krämer M, Reichenbach JR. Optimized gradient spoiling of UTE VFA-AFI sequences for robust T_1 estimation with B1-field correction. Magn Reson Imaging. 2021;82:1–8.

27. Akbari A, Abbasi-Rad S, Rad HS. T_1 correlates age: a short-TE MR relaxometry study in vivo on human cortical bone free water at 1.5 T. Bone. 2016;83:17–22.

28. Ma Y, Lu X, Carl M, et al. Accurate T_1 mapping of short T_2 tissues using a three-dimensional ultrashort echo time cones actual flip angle—variable TR (3D UTE-cones AFI-VTR) method. Magn Reson Med. 2018;80(2):598–608.

29. Wei Z, Jang H, Bydder GM, Yang W, Ma Y-J. Fast T_1 measurement of cortical bone using 3D UTE actual flip angle imaging and single-TR acquisition (3D UTE-AFI-STR). Magn Reson Med. 2021;85(6):3290–8.

30. Du J, Bydder GM. Qualitative and quantitative ultrashort-TE MRI of cortical bone. NMR Biomed. 2013;26(5):489–506.

31. Yarnykh VL. Actual flip-angle imaging in the pulsed steady state: a method for rapid three-dimensional mapping of the transmitted radiofrequency field. Magn Reson Med. 2007;57(1):192–200.

32. Stikov N, Boudreau M, Levesque IR, Tardif CL, Barral JK, Pike GB. On the accuracy of T_1 mapping: searching for common ground. Magn Reson Med. 2015;73(2):514–22.

33. Sussman MS, Pauly JM, Wright GA. Design of practical T_2-selective RF excitation (TELEX) pulses. Magn Reson Med. 1998;40(6):890–9.

34. Horch RA, Gochberg DF, Nyman JS, Does MD. Clinically compatible MRI strategies for discriminating bound and pore water in cortical bone. Magn Reson Med. 2012;68(6):1774–84.

Jiang Du, Arya Suprana, Xing Lu, Hyungseok Jang, Yajun Ma, and Saeed Jerban

Introduction

T_2^* relaxation, also called the apparent transverse relaxation, describes the exponential decay in M_{xy} following an initial radiofrequency (RF) excitation pulse as a function of time. T_2^* is an important tissue property that incorporates T_2 but is additionally affected by inhomogeneities in the main magnetic field B_0 and susceptibility-induced field distortions produced by tissue, with the latter usually dominant in short-T_2 tissues. Ultrashort echo time (UTE) sequences provide direct imaging of short-T_2 tissues and tissue components as well as quantitative assessment of their MR relaxation times and tissue properties. As a result, T_2^* measurements are commonly used to evaluate short-T_2 tissue degeneration [1–3], iron deposition [4–6], temperature [7], and soft tissue calcification [8, 9].

Biological tissues frequently contain different water compartments with distinct T_2 or T_2^* values [10–19]. Quantifying different water components may be problematic with clinical MR sequences, as conventional spin echo and gradient echo sequences usually have initial echo times (TEs) too long to detect the signal from shorter transverse relaxation time components. Signals from short- and ultrashort-T_2 water components in short-T_2 tissues, such as tendons and bone, can be detected using UTE-based sequences. Furthermore, multicomponent T_2^* analysis can evaluate different water components, including short-, ultrashort-, and long-T_2 compartments in biological tissues [20, 21].

Long-T_2 suppression pulses, such as adiabatic inversion recovery (IR)-based preparation pulses, may be of particular value in suppressing longer T_2/T_2^* components and providing selective imaging of short- and ultrashort-T_2^* components [22–27]. For example, adiabatic IR-based UTE (IR-UTE) imaging has been developed to image and quantify the T_2^* of bound water in cortical bone [24–26]. In addition, a short TR adiabatic inversion recovery UTE (STAIR-UTE) sequence has been developed to image and quantify the T_2^* of the trabecular bone as well as myelin in the white matter of the brain [28, 29]. Also, a dual adiabatic inversion UTE (dual-IR-UTE) sequence has been used to image the osteochondral junction selectively and quantify its T_2^*. This sequence minimizes partial volume effects by suppressing the signal from surrounding long-T_2 components [30–32].

UTE T₂* Single-Component Analysis

The T_2^* values of short-T_2 species can be quantified using single-component exponential fitting of UTE images acquired with different TEs. Figure 22.1 shows an example of a rubber band with a conventional clinical gradient echo sequence (a) and a basic UTE sequence (b) using ten different TEs of 8 µs, 0.1, 0.2, 0.3, 0.5, 0.8, 1.2, 1.6, 2.0, and 2.5 ms. The conventional clinical gradient echo sequence only detects noise following RF excitation. This is because the transverse magnetization of the rubber band decays to zero before the receive mode of the sequence is enabled. In contrast, the UTE sequence (b) shows a high signal from the rubber band due to its ultrashort nominal TE of 8 µs. Defects in the rubber band are depicted with a high spatial resolution and contrast. Excellent single-component exponential curve

J. Du (✉)
Department of Radiology, University of California, San Diego, La Jolla, CA, USA

Department of Bioengineering, University of California, San Diego, La Jolla, CA, USA

VA San Diego Healthcare System, San Diego, CA, USA
e-mail: jiangdu@health.ucsd.edu

A. Suprana
Department of Bioengineering, University of California, San Diego, La Jolla, CA, USA
e-mail: asuprana@eng.ucsd.edu

X. Lu · H. Jang · Y. Ma · S. Jerban
Department of Radiology, University of California, San Diego, La Jolla, CA, USA
e-mail: xil135@health.ucsd.edu; h4jang@health.ucsd.edu; yam013@ucsd.edu; sjerban@health.ucsd.edu

Fig. 22.1 MR image of a rubber band. This shows near-zero signal with a conventional gradient echo sequence (**a**) but high signal with a UTE sequence (arrow) (**b**). This allows excellent single-component exponential curve fitting of the UTE signal decay, which demonstrates an ultrashort-T_2* of 322 ± 4 μs (**c**)

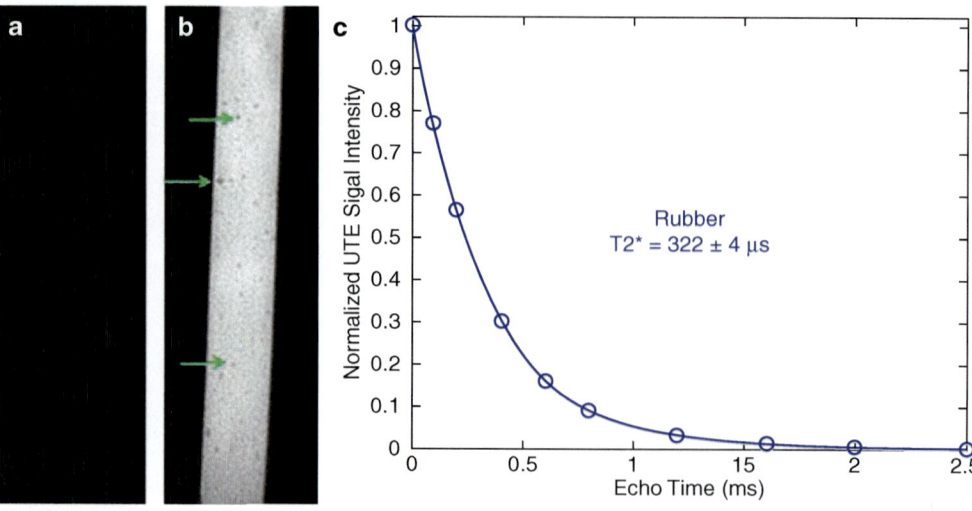

fitting of the signal decay can be achieved, demonstrating an ultrashort-T_2* of 322 ± 4 μs. Clinical gradient echo sequences cannot be used to quantify the T_2* of the rubber band due to the lack of detectable signal. The UTE technique may be directly applied to map T_2* of musculoskeletal tissues and regions such as the osteochondral junction, menisci, ligaments, tendons, and cortical bone [1–3]. Short-T_2 tissues usually have a highly organized extracellular matrix structure. An early sign of short-T_2 tissue degeneration is the disorganization of this matrix structure, leading to an increase in T_2* [1, 2]. UTE T_2* measurements have been used to evaluate outcomes after exercise therapy in patellar tendinopathy (PT) and have shown a statistically significant decrease in T_2* values in degenerative tissue compartments after treatment. The reduction in T_2* was associated with an improvement in symptom severity assessed by the Victorian Institute of Sports Assessment (VISA-P) score [3]. UTE T_2* can also quantify iron deposition in the liver, where higher iron concentration leads to greater susceptibility and, thus, a shorter T_2* [4, 5]. UTE-based R_2* ($1/T_2$*) quantification in patients with a massive iron overload correlates highly with biopsy-confirmed hepatic iron content [4]. UTE T_2* may also be used to assess hemosiderin in the knee joint of hemophilia patients [6] and map temperature during cryotherapy [7]. Furthermore, UTE T_2* measurement allows the characterization of calcified carotid plaques and shows a high correlation with CT-measured mineral density [8, 9].

UTE T_2* Bicomponent Analysis

Biological tissues usually contain distinct water compartments, which typically have quite different T_2*s [10–19]. For example, cortical bone comprises not only pore water residing in macroscopic pores but bound water, which is loosely or tightly bound to collagen and mineral [10]. The T_2* of collagen-bound water is about ten times shorter than that of pore water [11]. This absolute difference allows bound and pore water to be separated using bicomponent modeling of UTE T_2* signal decay, which provides information about the fractions of ultrashort- and long-T_2* components and their relaxation times [11–13]. Bicomponent analysis can be performed using UTE images and a series of gradient echoes with longer TEs (e.g., from 8 μs to 8 ms). Figure 22.2 shows UTE imaging of the cortex of a cadaveric human tibial sample, which was subject to single- and bicomponent fitting analyses. The single-component model provides poor fitting of the UTE signal decay, suggesting that more than one water component exists within cortical bone.

In contrast, the bicomponent model provides excellent fitting and shows two distinct water compartments in cortical bone: one with a short-T_2* of 0.34 ms, representing water bound to the organic matrix (or bound water) occupying 75.4% of the detected volume, and the other with a longer T_2* of 2.92 ms, representing water, which resides in the microscopic pores (or pore water) and occupies 24.6% of the detected volume.

Bicomponent exponential T_2* fitting has been investigated to quantify matrix density and porosity. Significant correlations have been reported between pore water fractions acquired from bicomponent T_2* analysis and microcomputed tomography (μCT)-derived cortical porosity in human cortical bone samples [12]. Additionally, moderate correlations have been observed between bicomponent T_2* results and the mechanical properties of human cortical bone strips. Recently, UTE bicomponent T_2* analysis and its efficacy were investigated through comparison with histomorphometry measures of bone porosity [13]. Bicomponent T_2* was found to be capable of detecting bone porosity, including pores that were undetectable using μCT [13]. Excellent

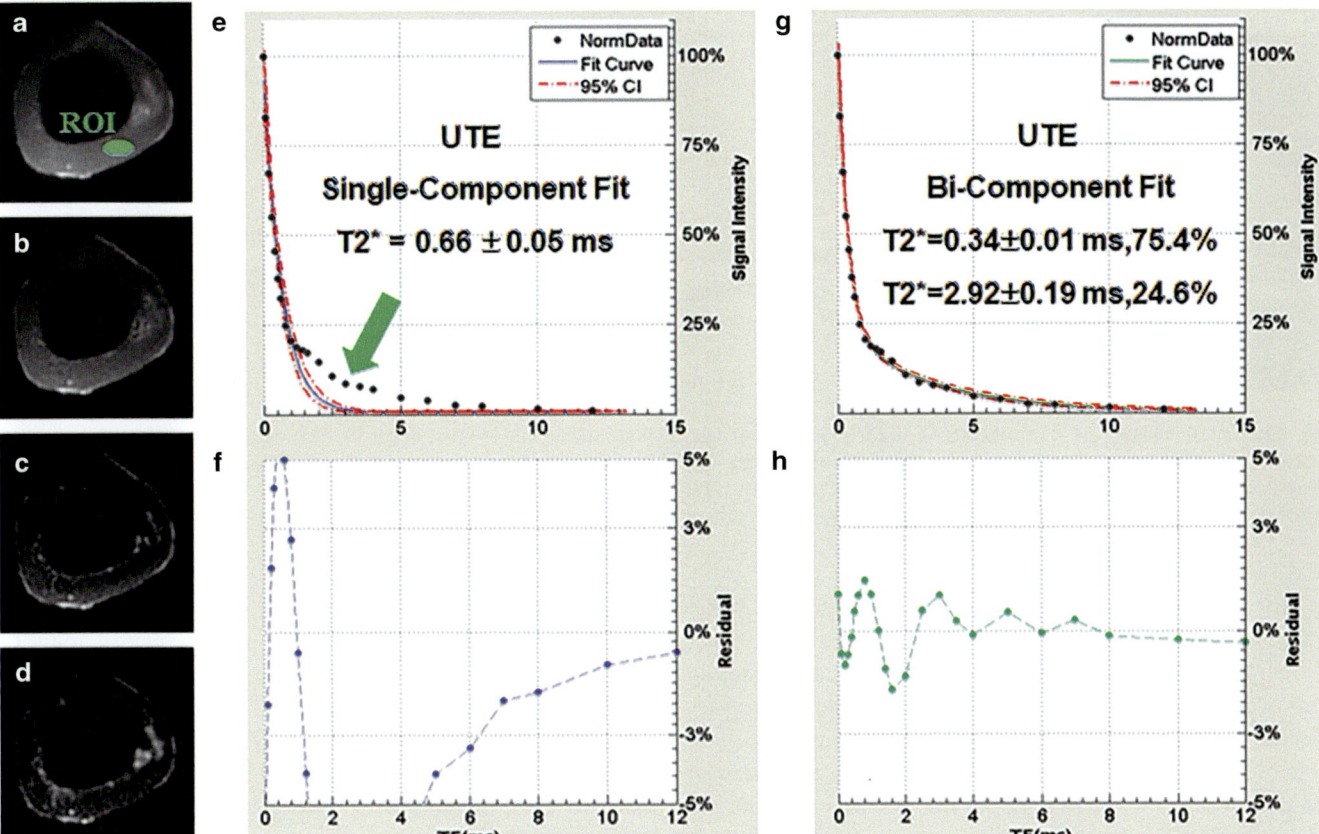

Fig. 22.2 Selected UTE images of the cortex of a cadaveric human tibial sample with TEs of 32 µs (**a**), 0.6 ms (**b**), 1.6 ms (**c**), and 4.0 ms (**d**), as well as a single-component fitting of UTE images (**e**) and residues (**f**), with bicomponent fitting (**g**) and its residues (**h**). The poor single-component fitting and excellent bicomponent fitting are consis-tent with the presence of two water components in cortical bone: colla-gen-bound water with an ultrashort-T_2^* of 0.34 ± 0.01 ms and a fraction of 75.4%, as well as pore water with a longer T_2^* of 2.92 ± 0.19 ms and a fraction of 24.6%

bicomponent T_2^* decay has been observed in other musculo-skeletal tissues such as the Achilles tendon [14, 15], patellar tendon [3, 16], menisci [14, 15], and articular cartilage [17–19].

UTE T_2^* Tri-Component Analysis

Biological tissues may contain not only different water com-ponents with distinct T_2^* relaxation times but micro- or mac-roscopic fat. For example, human cortical bone may have a considerable amount of fat [33, 34], particularly in the regions near the endosteum, where larger pores can be found. Fat in cortical bone pores probably has comparable proper-ties to the bone marrow fat within the endosteum. It is believed that adipocytes secrete cytokines and adipokines, which stimulate or inhibit osteoblastic activity in nearby bone [34]. This raises the possibility that increased forma-tion of fat cells could cause a decrease in the rate of bone

remodeling. Bone fat is low in neonates and accumulates steadily over a lifetime [34]. Lu et al. recently proposed tri-component fitting incorporating a model fat spectrum [20] that improved estimation of bound and pore water in cortical bone. This tri-component T_2^* fit model was applied to the entire cross sections of tibial cortex samples. Estimated water fractions using tri-component T_2^* fitting demonstrated improved correlations with the µCT-based porosity com-pared to bicomponent analyses [20]. Figure 22.3 compares µCT images of a cortical bone sample and the corresponding UTE bi- and tri-component fitting results. The bone sample was harvested from a 57-year-old female with a µCT poros-ity of 33%. The sample shows a significant oscillating signal at a TE of around 2 ms due to the chemical shift between fat and water. The signal oscillations are very well fitted using the tri-component model, whereas the bicomponent model lacks accuracy. The bound water fraction is significantly lower when applying the tri-component fitting model. The tri-component model results in substantially lower T_2^* val-

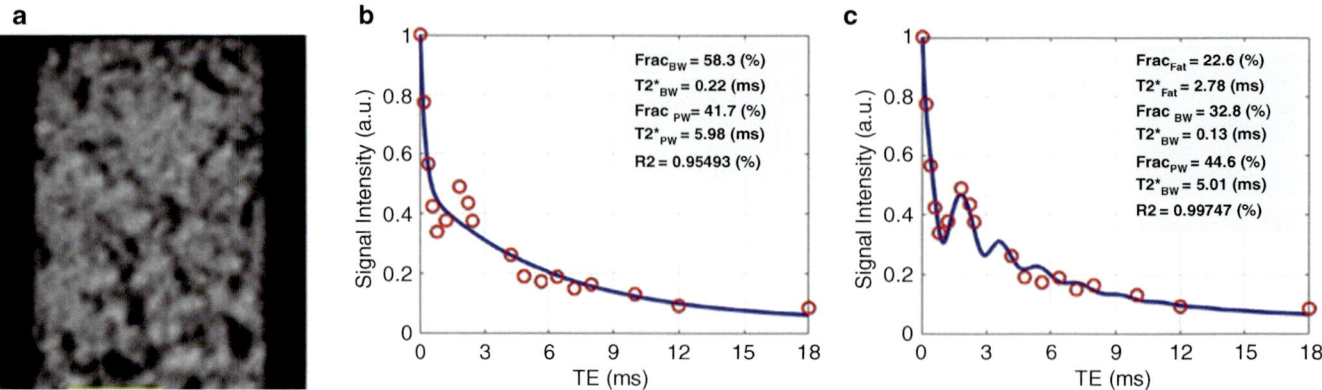

Fig. 22.3 μCT imaging of a representative cortical bone strip harvested from a 57-year-old female donor with a porosity of 33% (**a**). The corresponding bicomponent (**b**) and tri-component (**c**) fittings of UTE signal decay are presented. The oscillating signal decay in the cortical bone specimens is fitted better by including the signal contribution of fat in the tri-component model (**c**). (Reproduced with permission from Ref. [21])

ues for both bound and pore water and a lower pore water fraction.

Including the fat contribution in signal decay modeling improves the estimation of water fractions, which helps predict the microstructural and mechanical properties of cortical bone with higher accuracy [21]. Specifically, summation of the pore water fraction and the fat fraction derived from the tri-component model shows the strongest correlation with bone porosity. Pore sizes show only moderate correlations with bone biomechanics [21]. In the bicomponent fitting model, fat and pore water are regarded as one component (i.e., parts of a single longer T_2^* component). Bound water is regarded as the other component (i.e., the shorter T_2^* component). In this approach, fat and pore water oscillation leads to signal cancellation and, thus, to a reduced long-T_2^* fraction (thereby underestimating the contributions from pore water and fat) as well as an increased short-T_2^* fraction (thereby overestimating the organic matrix content and density).

IR-UTE T_2^* Measurement

Adiabatic IR preparation has been used to provide efficient long-T_2 signal suppression and help create high contrast for short-T_2 tissues in IR-UTE imaging [22–27]. The adiabatic inversion pulse can also selectively suppress signals from longer T_2^* components in ultrashort-T_2 tissues (e.g., cortical bone), therefore providing selective imaging of ultrashort-T_2^* components such as collagen-bound water [24, 25]. The fundamental physics behind IR-UTE imaging shows that the adiabatic inversion pulse can efficiently invert only long-T_2 components. Ultrashort-T_2 components are only partially inverted and are saturated as their T_2s are far shorter than the duration of the long adiabatic inversion pulse. This is due to

transverse magnetization relaxation during the long adiabatic inversion process [22–25]. The efficiency of long-T_2 signal suppression depends highly on the choice of the inversion time (TI), which is related to the T_1 of the long-T_2 components and the repetition time (TR). Figure 22.4 shows magnitude and phase images from a human tibia sample using IR-UTE imaging with a TR of 300 ms and a short TI of 20 ms. The IR-UTE images show a positive phase with TEs less than 0.4 ms (e.g., 0.27 for TE = 8 μs and 0.74 for TE = 0.4 ms), suggesting that the un-inverted bound water magnetization dominates the IR-UTE signal. In contrast, IR-UTE images with TEs longer than 0.6 ms show a negative phase (e.g., −2.47 for TE = 0.6 ms and −2.03 for TE = 1.4 ms), suggesting that the inverted pore water magnetization dominates the IR-UTE signal [35]. This signal decay behavior could be explained by the fact that the bound water fraction is significantly higher than the pore water fraction in cortical bone, leading to a faster decay of the bound water signal compared to pore water and eventually leaving the negative pore water signal dominating the IR-UTE signal at longer TEs [35].

When an appropriate TI is chosen, the pore water component can be nulled entirely so that bound water can be imaged selectively using IR-UTE imaging. Figure 22.5 shows an example of the IR-UTE sequence applied to the same cadaveric human tibial cortex shown in Fig. 22.2. The IR-UTE images show a single component with a T_2^* of 0.31 ms, which is close to the T_2^* value of 0.34 ms derived from the UTE T_2^* bicomponent analysis. The short-T_2^* fraction was increased from 24.6% with UTE imaging to 100% with IR-UTE imaging, consistent with the longer T_2^* pore water component being selectively inverted and nulled by the adiabatic inversion pulse so that only bound water is detected with IR-UTE imaging. Subtraction of bound water (derived

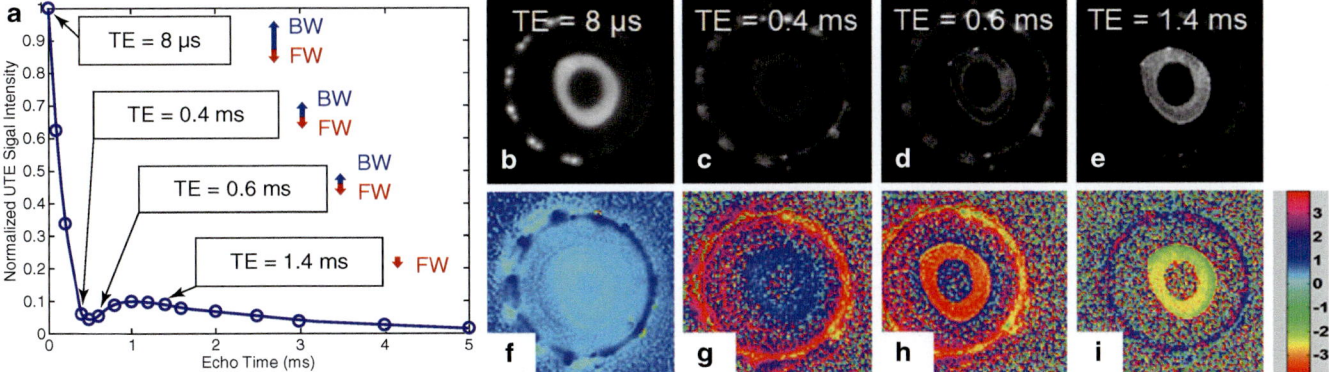

Fig. 22.4 Normalized magnitude signal decay for IR-UTE images of a human tibial bone sample with a TR of 300 ms and a TI of 20 ms using a series of TEs ranging from 8 μs to 5 ms (**a**), and the corresponding magnitude images at selected TEs of 8 μs (**b**), 0.4 ms (**c**), 0.6 ms (**d**), and 1.4 ms (**e**), as well as the corresponding phase images (**f–i**). Schematic longitudinal magnetizations of bound water (BW) and free water (FW) (i.e., pore water) at different TEs are also shown in (**a**), where the positive signal from BW dominates the IR-UTE signal at short TEs (e.g., TE < 0.4 ms). In contrast, the negative signal from FW dominates at longer TEs (e.g., TE > 0.6 ms). (**f**)–(**i**) Show the signals at opposite phases before and after a TE of 0.5 ms (i.e., 0.27 at TE = 8 μs, 0.74 at TE = 0.4 ms, −2.47 at TE = 0.6 ms, and −2.03 at TE = 1.4 ms), which is consistent with a transition from positive to negative net magnetization at TE ~0.5 ms. (Reproduced with permission from Ref. [35])

from IR-UTE imaging) from total water (derived from UTE imaging) provides a fast and reliable measurement of pore water [24]. This technique is promising, as pore water mapping accurately assesses cortical porosity [10–12]. This is challenging or impossible with other imaging techniques, such as DEXA or CT, as they do not have sufficient resolution to resolve small pore sizes in cortical bone. UTE and IR-UTE techniques successfully solve this technical challenge by comprehensively mapping bound water (organic matrix density) and pore water (cortical porosity) and doing this without ionizing radiation.

Quantitative mapping (e.g., T$_2$*, T$_1$, T$_2$, T$_{1\rho}$) of short-T$_2$ tissues or tissue components frequently requires robust suppression of associated long-T$_2$ signals within the tissues or tissue components. An example is T$_2$* quantification of short-T$_2$ components in white matter of the brain, which has ultrashort-T$_2$ values of less than 1 ms. These components are "invisible" with conventional clinical MRI sequences [36–38]. UTE sequences with minimum nominal TEs of ~8 μs, which are ~100 times shorter than the TEs of conventional clinical sequences, are potentially able to directly detect signals from myelin using a whole-body clinical MRI scanner [39–45]. The major challenge is the concurrent detection of signals from long-T$_2$ water components, which may show far higher signal intensities than the short-T$_2$ components [45]. An adiabatic IR preparation can selectively null the long-T$_2$ water components allowing selective imaging of the short-T$_2$ components. Figure 22.6 shows IR-UTE images of a brain specimen using a clinical 3T scanner (MR750, GE Healthcare, Milwaukee, WI, USA). The longitudinal magnetization of long-T$_2$ water components is inverted and nulled, as evidenced by the near-zero signal at a TE of 0.6 ms (Fig. 22.6e). Subtraction of the TE = 0.6 ms image (Fig. 22.6e) from the TE = 10 μs image (Fig. 22.6a) provides selective detection of ultrashort-T$_2$ components in the white matter (h), which have T$_2$*s of ~0.21 ms (i) [42].

Fig. 22.5 Selected IR-UTE images of the tibial cortex of a cadaveric human bone sample with TEs of 32 μs (**a**), 0.6 ms (**b**), 1.6 ms (**c**), and 4.0 ms (**d**), as well as the corresponding single-component fitting of IR-UTE images (**e**) and their residues (**f**). IR-UTE images show only one component with a short-T_2^* of 0.38 ± 0.01 ms, consistent with the selective imaging of bound water. Longer T_2^* component pore water is nulled by the adiabatic inversion pulse

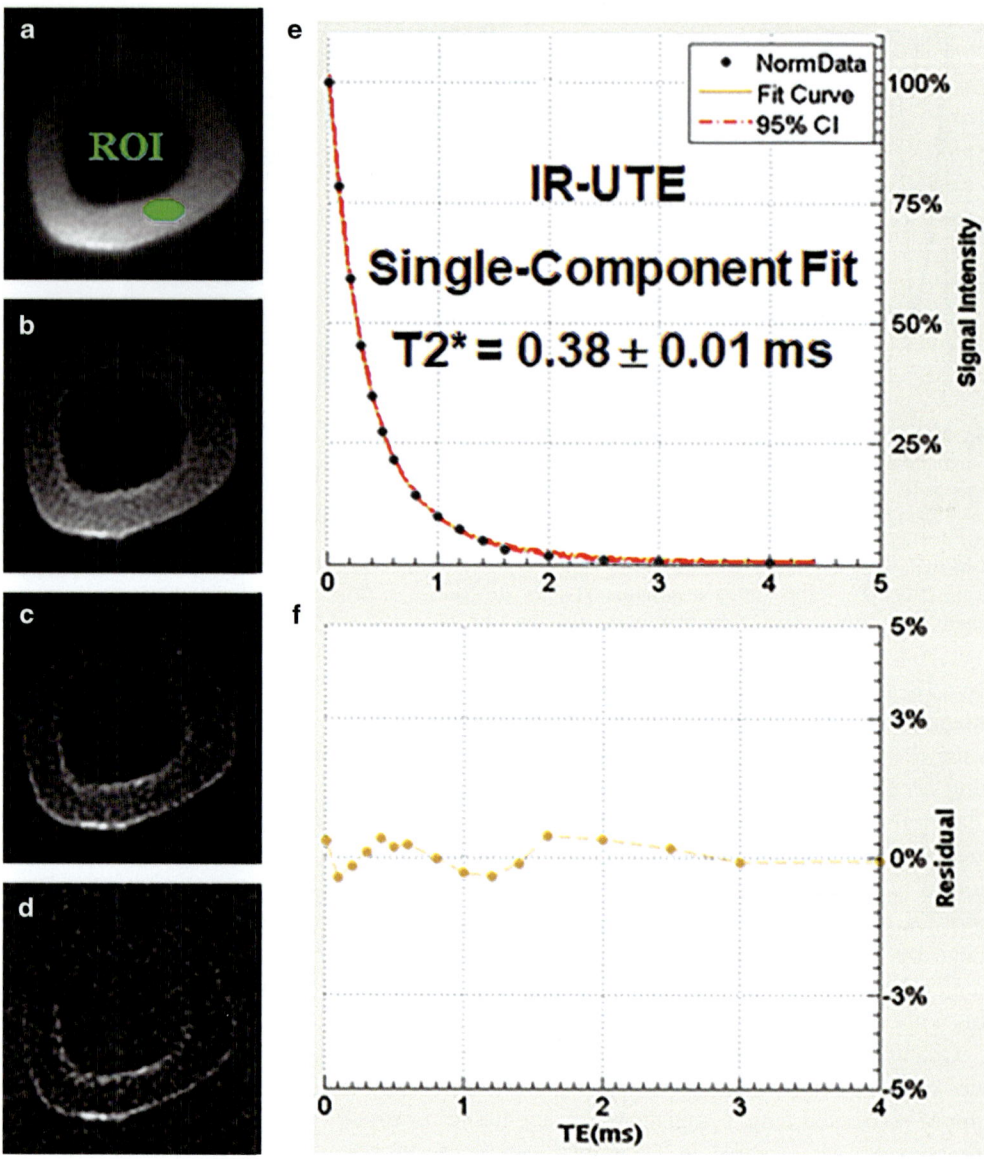

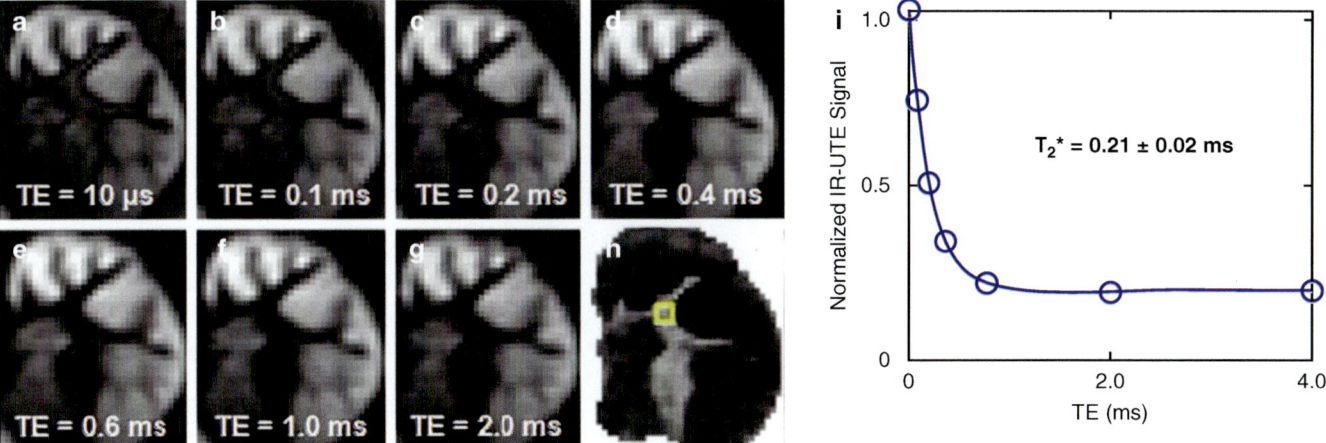

Fig. 22.6 IR-UTE imaging of a brain specimen with TEs of 10 μs (**a**), 0.1 ms (**b**), 0.2 ms (**c**), 0.4 ms (**d**), 0.6 ms (**e**), 1.0 ms (**f**), and 2.0 ms (**g**), as well as the subtraction image (TE 10 μs–TE 0.6 ms) (**h**). Single-component exponential fitting of the region of interest in white matter (yellow box in **h**) shows a short-T_2^* of 0.21 ± 0.02 ms (**i**). (Reproduced with permission from Ref. [42])

STAIR-UTE T₂* Measurement

Short-T_2^* mapping can be much more challenging in body regions with large amounts of fat, such as trabecular bone. Trabecular bone has an extremely low proton density and an ultrashort-T_2^*, which lead to a very low signal even when using UTE imaging. Trabecular bone is mixed with a large amount of fat in both yellow and red marrow. Fat has a high proton density and a short T_1. Fat-related off-resonance artifacts result in blurring with UTE imaging due to the ring-shaped point spread function of fat. This is quite different from the linear chemical shift artifacts seen with Cartesian sampling of k-space [46]. The strong fat signal and associated chemical shift artifacts may significantly affect T_2^* relaxation time mapping. Therefore, efficient fat suppression is critical for robust T_2^* mapping of trabecular bone.

The STAIR-UTE sequence was developed to address this problem. It is based on a regular IR-UTE data acquisition, but uses a very short TR and high flip angle (FA) and is operated within specific absorption rate limits for clinical imaging [28, 29]. The combination of a very short TR and TI provides robust suppression of signals from long-T_2 tissues, which may have T_1s above a particular value. The STAIR-UTE sequence is insensitive to B_1 and B_0 inhomogeneities when using Silver-Hoult adiabatic full-passage pulses with a relatively wide spectral bandwidth. The 3D STAIR-UTE sequence provides high contrast imaging of cortical and trabecular bone in the lumbar spine, with excellent suppression

of signals from long-T_2 fat and water-containing tissues [29]. Figure 22.7a–e shows STAIR-UTE images of the lumbar spine of a 36-year-old male volunteer. Long-T_2 signals from the surrounding muscle, spinal cord, CSF, and bone marrow are all efficiently suppressed. Only ultrashort-T_2^* components from trabecular bone are visualized, as evidenced by an excellent single-component curve fitting with a T_2^* of 0.31 ± 0.01 ms, which is close to the T_2^* of cortical bone [10–15].

Other contrast mechanisms, such as a dual-echo acquisition with echo subtraction [47], long-T_2 saturation [48], adiabatic IR (AIR) [25], or spectral presaturation with IR (SPIR) [49], may not be able to suppress signals from bone marrow fat efficiently so that the residual fat signal can be higher than that from trabecular bone. Figure 22.7f–j shows SPIR-UTE images of the fingers [49]. The measured T_2^* for the capitate is 2.42 ± 0.56 ms at 3 T, which is much longer than the T_2^* value of 0.31 ± 0.01 ms for trabecular bone of the spine measured with STAIR-UTE at the same field strength [29], or the T_2^* value of ~0.3 ms for cortical bone measured with various IR-based UTE techniques [11–15]. The much longer T_2^* value suggests that SPIR-UTE imaging of trabecular bone is subject to significant fat signal contamination. In comparison, STAIR-UTE-measured T_2^* values for trabecular bone are remarkably close to those measured on IR-UTE imaging for cortical bone. This suggests that bone marrow fat is completely suppressed, leaving signals from trabeculae selectively detected with STAIR-UTE imaging [29].

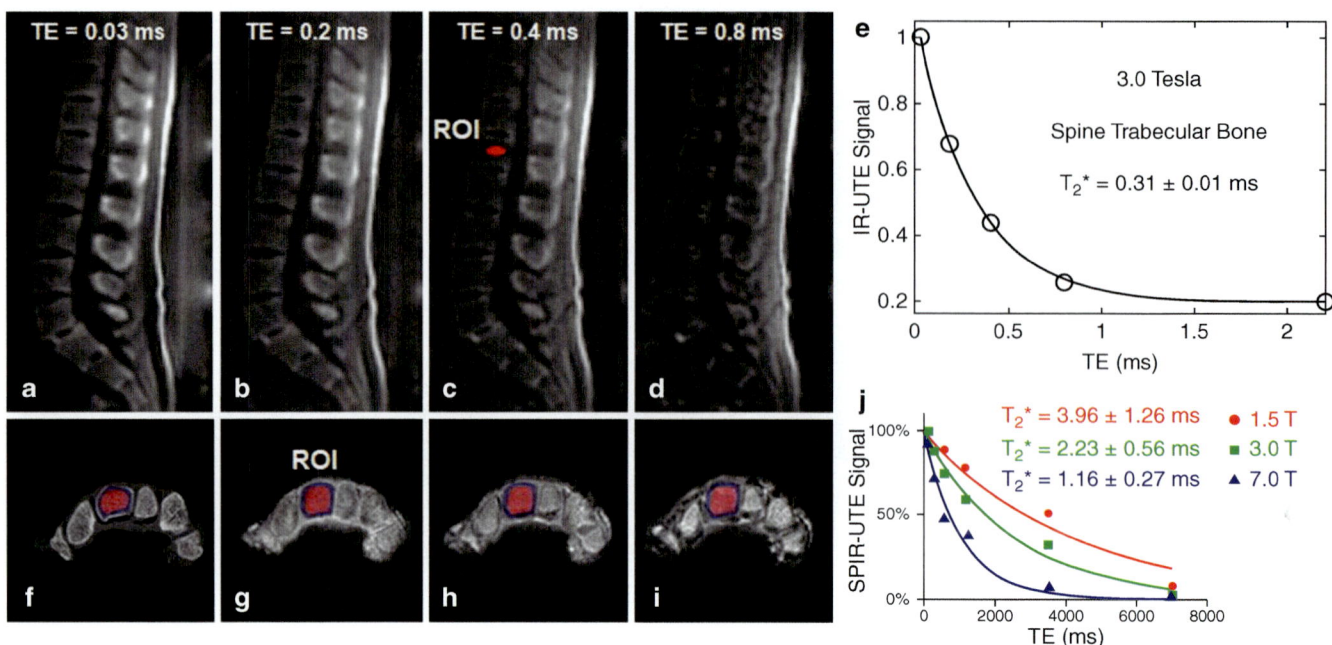

Fig. 22.7 Selected STAIR-UTE images of the spine of a 36-year-old male volunteer with TEs of 0.03 ms (**a**), 0.2 ms (**b**), 0.4 ms (**c**), 0.8 ms (**d**), and the single-component T_2^* fitting curve (**e**). μCT (**f**) and SPIR-UTE imaging of the fingers at 1.5 T (**g**), 3.0 T (**h**), 7.0 T (**i**), and the corresponding single-component T_2^* fitting curves (**j**) are shown. Trabecular bone of the spine shows a short-T_2^* of 0.31 ± 0.01 ms using the STAIR-UTE sequence, while trabecular bone in the fingers shows short-T_2^* values of 1.16 ± 0.27 ms at 1.5 T, 2.23 ± 0.56 ms at 3.0 T, and 3.96 ± 1.26 ms at 7.0 T, respectively, using the SPIR-UTE sequence. (Reproduced with permission from Refs. [29, 49])

Dual-IR-UTE T_2^* Measurement

As mentioned previously, long-T_2 signal contamination is one of the major challenges in accurate mapping of short-T_2^* tissues or tissue components. Long-T_2 tissues typically have higher proton densities and show higher signal intensities. This is especially the case for T_2^* mapping of thin structures such as those at the osteochondral junction and cartilaginous endplate. The osteochondral junction has a very thin and curved structure with a thickness of 0.1–0.2 mm [50]. While its T_2^* can be measured using regular UTE data acquisitions with variable TEs [51], the fitted T_2^* values are likely to be subject to significant errors due to partial volume effects with other tissues. The same holds for the cartilaginous endplate, which ranges in thickness from 0.5 to 1.0 mm [52]. The cartilaginous endplate anchors the disc to the vertebral body and modulates nutrient transportation and waste product elimination. Accurate T_2^* mapping may help evaluate the status of this critical structure in spine function [53–55]. Efficient

long-T_2 signal suppression is essential for precise quantification of its T_2^* and other relaxation times, as well as the proton density of the cartilaginous endplate, the osteochondral junction, and other short-T_2 tissues. The dual adiabatic IR UTE (dual-IR-UTE) technique employs two long Silver-Hoult adiabatic inversion pulses to separately invert the longitudinal magnetization of long-T_2 water and fat [30–32]. An appropriate combination of TI and TR allows robust and efficient simultaneous suppression of long-T_2 water and fat signals without sensitivity to chemical shift effects. Figure 22.8 shows conventional clinical proton density-weighted fast spin echo (PD-FSE), T_1-FSE, gradient recalled echo (GRE), basic UTE, and dual-IR-UTE images at different TEs in a cadaveric human patella sample [32]. The dual-IR-UTE sequence provides high-contrast images of the osteochondral junction, which appears as a linear, well-defined area of high signal (arrows). This layer shows an excellent single-component exponential signal decay and demonstrates a short-T_2^* of 1.79 ± 0.20 ms.

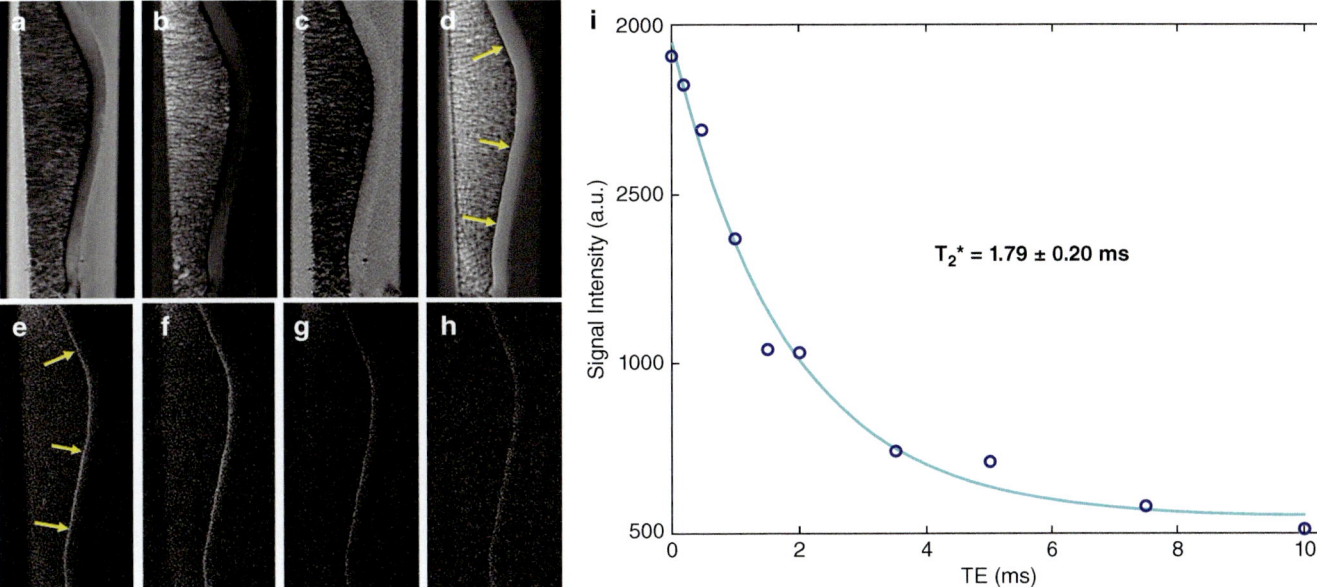

Fig. 22.8 A cadaveric human patellar sample imaged with clinical PD-FSE (**a**), T_1-FSE (**b**), GRE (**c**), basic UTE (**d**), and dual-IR-UTE sequences at different TEs of 8 µs (**e**), 0.2 ms (**f**), 1 ms (**g**), and 2 ms (**h**), as well as single-component exponential curve fitting, which demonstrates a short-T_2^* of 1.79 ± 0.20 ms for the osteochondral junction (**i**). (Reproduced with permission from Ref. [32])

Conclusion

T_2^* mapping of short-T_2 tissues or tissue components, such as the osteochondral junction, the cartilaginous endplate, menisci, ligaments, and tendons, as well as cortical and trabecular bone, can be quantified using UTE-type sequences. Single-, bi-, and tri-component fitting models have been employed to evaluate different water components and fat. Significant confounders are contamination from signals coming from long-T_2 water as well as from fat due to chemical shift artifacts compounded by susceptibility effects. Adiabatic IR preparations can selectively invert and null longer T_2^* components and allow reliable assessment of the shorter T_2^* components. Efficient long-T_2 suppression using STAIR-UTE, dual-IR-UTE, and other contrast mechanisms is of critical importance for accurate T_2^* mapping of short-T_2 tissues or tissue components, such as trabecular bone, the osteochondral junction, and the cartilaginous endplate. UTE T_2^* mapping can also be used to diagnose short-T_2 tissue degeneration and monitor therapeutic effects [1–7, 56].

References

1. Williams A, Qian Y, Golla S, Chu CR. UTE-T_2^* mapping detects subclinical meniscus injury after anterior cruciate ligament tear. Osteoarthr Cartil. 2012;20(6):486–94.
2. Chu CR, Williams AA, West RV, Qian Y, Fu FH, Do BH, Bruno S. Quantitative magnetic resonance imaging UTE-T_2^* mapping of cartilage and meniscus healing after anatomic anterior cruciate ligament reconstruction. Am J Sports Med. 2014;42(8):1847–56.
3. Breda SJ, de Vos RJ, Poot DHJ, Krestin GP, Hernandez-Tamames JA, Oei EHG. Association between T_2^* relaxation times derived from ultrashort echo time MRI and symptoms during exercise therapy for patellar tendinopathy: a large prospective study. J Magn Reson Imaging. 2021;54(5):1596–605.
4. Krafft AJ, Loeffler RB, Song R, Tipirneni-Sajja A, McCarville MB, Robson MD, Hankins JS, Hillenbrand CM. Quantitative ultrashort echo time imaging for assessment of massive iron overload at 1.5 and 3 Tesla. Magn Reson Med. 2017;78(5):1839–51.
5. Doyle EK, Toy K, Valdez B, Chia JM, Coates T, Wood JC. Ultrashort echo time images quantify high liver iron. Magn Reson Med. 2018;79(3):1579–85.
6. Jang H, von Drygalski A, Wong J, et al. Ultrashort echo time quantitative susceptibility mapping (UTE-QSM) for detection of hemosiderin deposition in hemophilic arthropathy: a feasibility study. Magn Reson Med. 2020;84(6):3246–55.
7. Wansapura JP, Daniel BL, Pauly J, Butts K. Temperature mapping of frozen tissues using eddy current compensated half excitation RF pulses. Magn Reson Med. 2001;46(5):985–92.
8. Du J, Peterson M, Kansal N, Bydder GM, Kahn A. Mineralization in calcified plaque is like that of cortical bone—further evidence from ultrashort echo time (UTE) magnetic resonance imaging of carotid plaque calcification and cortical bone. Med Phys. 2013;40(10):102301.
9. Du J, Corbeil J, Znamirowski R, Angle N, Peterson M, Bydder GM, Kahn A. Direct imaging and quantification of carotid plaque calcification. Magn Reson Med. 2011;65(4):1013–20.
10. Nyman JS, Ni Q, Nicolella DP, Wang X. Measurements of mobile and bound water by nuclear magnetic resonance correlate with mechanical properties of bone. Bone. 2008;42(1):193–9.
11. Biswas R, Bae W, Diaz E, et al. Ultrashort echo time (UTE) imaging with bi-component analysis: bound and free water evaluation of bovine cortical bone subject to sequential drying. Bone. 2012;50(3):749–55.

12. Bae WC, Chen PC, Chung CB, Masuda K, Lima D, Du J. Quantitative ultrashort echo time (UTE) MRI of human cortical bone: correlation with porosity and biomechanical properties. J Bone Miner Res. 2012;27(4):848–57.

13. Jerban S, Ma Y, Wong JH, et al. Ultrashort echo time magnetic resonance imaging (UTE-MRI) of cortical bone correlates well with histomorphometric assessment of bone microstructure. Bone. 2019;123:8–17.

14. Diaz E, Chung CB, Bae WC, et al. Ultrashort echo time spectroscopic imaging (UTESI): an efficient method for quantifying bound and free water. NMR Biomed. 2012;25(1):161–8.

15. Du J, Diaz E, Carl M, Bae W, Chung C, Bydder GM. Ultrashort echo time imaging with bicomponent analysis. Magn Reson Med. 2012;67(3):645–9.

16. Kijowski R, Wilson JJ, Liu F. Bicomponent ultrashort echo time T2* analysis for assessment of patients with patellar tendinopathy. J Magn Reson Imaging. 2017;46(5):1441–7.

17. Qian Y, Williams A, Chu CR, Boada FE. Multi-component T2* mapping of knee cartilage: technical feasibility ex vivo. Magn Reson Med. 2010;64(5):1426–31.

18. Pauli C, Bae WC, Lee M, et al. Ultrashort-echo time MR imaging of the patella with bicomponent analysis: correlation with histopathologic and polarized light microscopic findings. Radiology. 2012;264(2):484–93.

19. Shao H, Chang EY, Zanganeh S, et al. UTE bi-component analysis of T_2* relaxation in articular cartilage. Osteoarthr Cartil. 2016;24(2):364–73.

20. Lu X, Jerban S, Wan L, et al. Three dimensional ultrashort echo time imaging with tri-component analysis for human cortical bone. Magn Reson Med. 2019;82(1):348–55.

21. Jerban S, Lu X, Dorthe EW, Alenezi S, Ma Y, Kakos L, Jang H, Sah RL, Chang EY, D'Lima D, Du J. Correlation of cortical bone microstructural and mechanical properties with water proton fractions obtained from ultrashort echo time (UTE) MRI tricomponent T_2* model. NMR Biomed. 2020;33(3):e4233.

22. Reichert ILH, Robson MD, Gatehouse PD, He T, Chappell KE, Holmes J, Girgis S, Bydder GM. Magnetic resonance imaging of cortical bone with ultrashort TE pulse sequences. Magn Reson Imaging. 2005;23(5):611–8.

23. Larson PE, Conolly SM, Pauly JM, Nishimura DG. Using adiabatic inversion pulses for long-T_2 suppression in ultrashort echo time (UTE) imaging. Magn Reson Med. 2007;58(5):952–61.

24. Du J, Carl M, Bydder M, Takahashi A, Chung CB, Bydder GM. Qualitative and quantitative ultrashort echo time (UTE) imaging of cortical bone. J Magn Reson. 2010;207(2):304–11.

25. Horch R, Gochberg D, Nyman J, Does M. Clinically-compatible MRI strategies for discriminating bound and pore water in cortical bone. Magn Reson Med. 2012;68(6):1774–84.

26. Ma Y, Jerban S, Jang H, Chang D, Chang EY, Du J. Quantitative ultrashort echo time (UTE) magnetic resonance imaging of bone: an update. Front Endocrinol (Lausanne). 2020;11:567417.

27. Masoud-Afsahi A, Ma Y, Jang H, Jerban S, Chung C, Chang EY, Du J. Ultrashort echo time (UTE) MRI techniques: met and unmet needs in musculoskeletal imaging. J Magn Reson Imaging. 2022;55(6):1597–612.

28. Ma Y, Jang H, Wei Z, Cai Z, Xue Y, Chang EY, Corey-Bloom J, Du J. Myelin imaging in human brain using a short repetition time adiabatic inversion recovery prepared ultrashort echo time (STAIR-UTE) MRI sequence in multiple sclerosis. Radiology. 2020;297(2):392–404.

29. Ma Y, Chen Y, Li L, Cai Z, Zhao W, Jerban S, Jang H, Chang EY, Du J. Trabecular bone imaging using a 3D adiabatic inversion recovery prepared ultrashort echo time cones sequence at 3T. Magn Reson Med. 2020;83(5):1640–51.

30. Du J, Takahashi A, Bae WC, Chung CB, Bydder GM. Dual inversion recovery, ultrashort echo time (DIR UTE) imaging: creating high contrast for short-T_2 species. Magn Reson Med. 2010;63(2):447–55.

31. Bae W, Dwek JR, Znamirowski R, Statum S, Hermida JC, D'Lima DD, Sah RL, Du J, Chung CB. Ultrashort echo time MR imaging of osteochondral junction of the knee at 3 T: identification of anatomic structures contributing to signal intensity. Radiology. 2010;254(3):837–45.

32. Du J, Carl M, Bae WC, Statum S, Chang EY, Bydder GM, Chung CB. Dual inversion recovery ultrashort echo time (DIR-UTE) imaging and quantification of the zone of calcified cartilage (ZCC). Osteoarthr Cartil. 2013;21(1):77–85.

33. Sundh D, Rudäng R, Zoulakis M, Nilsson AG, Darelid A, Lorentzon M. A high amount of local adipose tissue is associated with high cortical porosity and low bone material strength in older women. J Bone Miner Res. 2016;31(4):749–57.

34. Devlin MJ, Rosen CJ. The bone-fat interface: basic and clinical implications of marrow adiposity. Lancet Diabetes Endocrinol. 2015;3(2):141–7.

35. Li S, Ma L, Chang EY, Shao H, Chen J, Chung CB, Bydder GM, Du J. Effects of inversion time on inversion recovery prepared ultrashort echo time (IR-UTE) imaging of free and bound water in cortical bone. NMR Biomed. 2015;28(1):70–8.

36. Waldman A, Rees JH, Brock CS, Robson MD, Gatehouse PD, Bydder GM. MRI of the brain with ultra-short echo time pulse sequences. Neuroradiology. 2003;45(12):887–92.

37. Horch RA, Gore JC, Does MD. Origins of the ultrashort T_2 1H NMR signals in myelinated nerve: a direct measure of myelin content? Magn Reson Med. 2011;66(1):24–31.

38. Wilhelm MJ, Ong HH, Wehrli SL, Li C, Tsai PH, Hackney DB, Wehrli FW. Direct magnetic resonance detection of myelin and prospects for quantitative imaging of myelin density. Proc Natl Acad Sci U S A. 2012;109(24):9605–10.

39. Du J, Ma G, Li S, Carl M, Szeverenyi N, VandenBerg S, Corey-Bloom J, Bydder GM. Ultrashort TE echo time (UTE) magnetic resonance imaging of the short T_2 components in white matter of the brain using a clinical 3T scanner. NeuroImage. 2013;87:32–41.

40. Du J, Sheth V, He Q, Carl M, Chen J, Corey-Bloom J, Bydder GM, Du J. Measurement of T_1 of the ultrashort T_2* components in white matter of the brain at 3T. PLoS One. 2014;9(8):e103296.

41. Sheth V, Shao H, Chen J, VandenBerg S, Corey-Bloom J, Bydder GM, Du J. Magnetic resonance imaging of myelin using ultrashort echo time (UTE) pulse sequence: phantom, specimen, volunteers and multiple sclerosis patient studies. NeuroImage. 2016;136:37–44.

42. Fan S, Ma Y, Chang EY, Bydder GM, Du J. Inversion recovery ultrashort echo time imaging of ultrashort T_2 tissue components in ovine brain at 3T: a sequential D_2O exchange study. NMR Biomed. 2017;30(10): https://doi.org/10.1002/nbm.3767.

43. Fan S, Ma Y, Searleman A, Zhu Y, Bydder GM, Du J. Yet more evidence that myelin protons can be directly imaged with ultrashort echo time (UTE) sequences on a clinical 3T scanner: bi-component T_2* analysis of native and deuterated ovine brain specimens. Magn Reson Med. 2018;80(2):538–47.

44. Ma Y, Jang H, Chang EY, Hiniker A, Head BP, Lee RR, Corey-Bloom J, Bydder GM, Du J. Ultrashort echo time (UTE) magnetic resonance imaging of myelin: technical developments and challenges. Quant Imaging Med Surg. 2020;10(6):1186–203.

45. Ma Y, Searleman AC, Jang H, Fan SJ, Wong J, Xue Y, Cai Z, Chang EY, Corey-Bloom J, Du J. Volumetric imaging of myelin in vivo using 3D inversion-recovery ultrashort echo time cones magnetic resonance imaging. NMR Biomed. 2020;33(10):e4326.

46. Bydder M, Carl M, Bydder GM, Du J. MRI chemical shift artifact produced by center-out radial sampling of k-space: a potential pitfall in clinical diagnosis. Quant Imaging Med Surg. 2021;11:3677–83.

47. Du J, Bydder M, Takahashi AM, Carl M, Chung CB, Bydder GM. Short T_2 contrast with three-dimensional ultrashort echo time imaging. Magn Reson Imaging. 2011;29(4):470–82.

48. Larson PE, Gurney PT, Nayak K, Gold GE, Pauly JM, Nishimura DG. Designing long-T2 suppression pulses for ultrashort echo time imaging. Magn Reson Med. 2006;56(1):94–103.

49. Wurnig MC, Calcagni M, Kenkel D, Vich M, Weiger M, Andreisek G, Wehrli FW, Boss A. Characterization of trabecular bone density with ultra-short echo-time MRI at 1.5, 3.0, and 7.0 T—comparison with micro-computed tomography. NMR Biomed. 2014;27(10):1159–66.

50. Lane LB, Bullough PG. Age-related changes in the thickness of the calcified zone and the number of tidemarks in adult human articular cartilage. J Bone Joint Surg Br. 1980;62(3):372–5.

51. Foreman SC, Ashmeik W, Baal JD, Han M, Bahroos E, von Schacky CE, Carl M, Krug R, Joseph GB, Link TM. Patients with type 2 diabetes exhibit a more mineralized deep cartilage layer compared with nondiabetic controls: a pilot study. Cartilage. 2021;13(1_Suppl):428S–36S.

52. Berg-Johansen B, Han M, Fields AJ, et al. Cartilage endplate thickness variation measured by ultrashort echo-time MRI is associated with adjacent disc degeneration. Spine. 2018;43(10):E592–E600.

53. Bae WC, Statum S, Zhang Z, Yamaguchi T, Wolfson T, Gamst AC, Du J, Bydder GM, Masuda K, Chung CB. Morphology of the cartilaginous endplates in human intervertebral disks with ultrashort echo time MR imaging. Radiology. 2013;266(2):564–74.

54. Wei Z, Lombardi A, Lee R, Wallace M, Koichi M, Chang EY, Du J, Bydder GM, Yang W, Ma Y. Comprehensive assessment of in vivo lumbar spine intervertebral discs using a 3D adiabatic $T_{1}\rho$ prepared ultrashort echo time (UTE-Adiab-$T_1\rho$) pulse sequence. Quant Imaging Med Surg. 2022;12(1):269–80.

55. Lombardi A, Wei Z, Wong J, Carl M, Lee R, Wallace M, Koichi M, Chang EY, Du J, Ma Y. High contrast cartilaginous endplate imaging using a 3D adiabatic inversion-recovery-prepared fat-saturated ultrashort echo time (3D IR-FS-UTE) sequence. NMR Biomed. 2021;34(10):e4579.

56. Kaggie JD, Markides H, Graves MJ, et al. Ultra short echo time MRI of iron-labelled mesenchymal stem cells in an ovine osteochondral defect model. Sci Rep. 2020;10(1):8451.

Jiang Du, Soo Hyun Shin, Michael Carl, Hyungseok Jang, Eric Y. Chang, and Yajun Ma

Introduction

$T_{1\rho}$ relaxation refers to spin-lattice relaxation which occurs in the rotating frame in the presence of an external radiofrequency (RF) pulse or spin-lock pulse [1]. $T_{1\rho}$ is sensitive to molecular processes with a frequency close to that of the precession of the spin-lock pulse, which typically ranges from a few hundred Hz up to a kHz on clinical whole-body MRI scanners [2]. $T_{1\rho}$ provides information about relatively low-frequency molecular processes such as proton exchange and slow dipolar interactions. That is a significant difference from spin-lattice relaxation (or T_1 relaxation), which is maximal for spins moving at the Larmor frequency determined by the main magnetic field strength (e.g., 128 MHz at 3 T). While imaging T_1 is challenging to characterize low-frequency motion atoms and molecules, $T_{1\rho}$ reflects slow interactions between motion-restricted water molecules and their local macromolecular environment [1–3]. Recent studies suggest that $T_{1\rho}$ has a high sensitivity to proteoglycan (PG) loss in cartilage samples as well as to osteoarthritis (OA) in patients [4–6]. $T_{1\rho}$ values increase with decreasing PG content and progression of OA. It has been shown that $T_{1\rho}$ provides more sensitive detection of PG loss at the initial stages of cartilage degeneration than T_2 [3]. $T_{1\rho}$ has also been shown to be sensitive to changes in collagen content, fiber orientation, and hydration [7, 8]. Furthermore, $T_{1\rho}$ has been proposed as a probe of other biochemical changes such as fibrosis in the liver [9] and annulus fibrosis degeneration in intervertebral discs [10], as well as amyloid and tau protein accumulation in the brain [11, 12].

$T_{1\rho}$ relaxation depends on the power of the spin-lock pulse. Without a spin-lock pulse, the magnetization undergoes transverse relaxation with a T_2 or T_2^* decay. The spin-lock pulse forces spins to process along its direction and slows the transverse magnetization relaxation process. As a consequence, $T_{1\rho}$ is always longer than T_2 or T_2^* but is shorter than T_1. A stronger spin-lock pulse tends to "lock" the transverse magnetization more efficiently along its direction, leading to longer values of $T_{1\rho}$. The dependence of $T_{1\rho}$ on spin-lock field strength is called $T_{1\rho}$ dispersion. The self-diffusion effect dominates at low spin-lock powers (i.e., $\omega_1 < 100$ Hz). At higher spin-lock powers (ω_1 = several hundred or thousand Hz), the chemical exchange effect between the fast exchangeable solute protons and water protons makes a significant contribution [13, 14]. $T_{1\rho}$ approaches T_1 at high spin-lock power.

With conventional $T_{1\rho}$ imaging, the spin-lock pulse is applied to magnetization processing in the transverse plane. Two-dimensional (2D) or 3D MRI data are acquired with a series of spin-lock pulse durations or spin-lock times (TSLs). $T_{1\rho}$ can be estimated by fitting the MRI data using the following equation:

$$S(\text{TSL}) = S(0) \times e^{-\text{TSL}/\text{T1}\rho} + \text{constant} \qquad (23.1)$$

where $S(\text{TSL})$ is the signal of a pixel or region of interest (ROI) in the corresponding $T_{1\rho}$ image acquired with a pre-

J. Du (✉)
Department of Radiology, University of California, San Diego, La Jolla, CA, USA

Department of Bioengineering, University of California, San Diego, La Jolla, CA, USA

VA San Diego Healthcare System, San Diego, CA, USA
e-mail: jiangdu@health.ucsd.edu

S. H. Shin
Department of Bioengineering, University of California, San Diego, La Jolla, CA, USA
e-mail: shs033@health.ucsd.edu

M. Carl
GE Healthcare, San Diego, CA, USA
e-mail: Michael.Carl@ge.com

H. Jang · Y. Ma
Department of Radiology, University of California, San Diego, La Jolla, CA, USA
e-mail: h4jang@health.ucsd.edu; yam013@health.ucsd.edu

E. Y. Chang
Department of Radiology, University of California, San Diego, La Jolla, CA, USA

VA San Diego Healthcare System, San Diego, CA, USA
e-mail: e8chang@health.ucsd.edu

© The Author(s), under exclusive license to Springer Nature Switzerland AG 2023
J. Du, G. M. Bydder (eds.), *MRI of Short- and Ultrashort-T$_2$ Tissues*, https://doi.org/10.1007/978-3-031-35197-6_23

defined TSL. A constant term is introduced to account for background noise and artifacts associated with data acquisition and image reconstruction. Mono-exponential fitting of the signal decay provides accurate estimation of $T_{1\rho}$ on the condition that there is enough signal, or in other words, $S(TSL)$ is significantly above the noise floor. This assumption typically holds for long-T_2 tissues but may fail with short-T_2 tissues due to significant signal decay before the MR receiving mode is enabled when conventional spin echo or gradient echo data acquisitions are used.

$T_{1\rho}$ imaging techniques have been applied to many biological tissues and organs with relatively long T_2s, such as articular cartilage [4–8], muscle [15], liver [9], spine [10], and brain [11, 12]. However, their application to short-T_2 tissues has been limited because short-T_2 tissues show little or no signal with conventional MRI sequences when echo times (TEs) are of the same order or shorter than the T_2s of interest. The osteochondral junction, menisci, ligaments, tendons, rotator cuff, and cartilaginous endplate have short T_2s and are essentially "invisible" with conventional clinical MR sequences [16]. As a result, $T_{1\rho}$ cannot be accurately measured due to the limited signal detected with relatively long TEs. Ultrashort echo time (UTE) sequences allow direct imaging of short-T_2 tissues and tissue components by reducing the nominal TEs of sequences to 0.1 ms or less [16–18]. Combining a spin-lock preparation pulse with UTE data acquisition allows imaging and quantification of $T_{1\rho}$ and $T_{1\rho}$ dispersion in both short- and long-T_2 tissues of the body [17–21]. This information may help evaluate changes in PGs and collagen in healthy and degenerate tissues.

UTE $T_{1\rho}$ Imaging

UTE combined with continuous wave (CW) spin-lock (SL) $T_{1\rho}$ (UTE-$T_{1\rho}$) has been developed to evaluate PG depletion in short-T_2 tissues (Fig. 23.1a) [19–21]. The initial spin-lock pulse cluster consists of a short rectangular 90° pulse followed by a spin-lock pulse and another short rectangular −90° pulse. The first 90° pulse is applied along the X-axis to flip the longitudinal magnetization into the transverse plane along the Y-axis. A composite pulse is then applied along the Y-axis to spin-lock the transverse magnetization. The second 90° pulse flips this spin-locked magnetization back along the Z-axis. Finally, any residual transverse magnetization is dephased with a crusher gradient. The magnetization stored along the Z-axis is subsequently detected by 2D or 3D UTE data acquisition. Figure 23.1b–e shows a comparison between 3D magnetization-prepared angle-modulated partitioned k-space spoiled gradient echo snapshots (MAPSS) imaging and 2D UTE-$T_{1\rho}$ imaging of the Achilles tendon and meniscus in a young, healthy volunteer [19, 22]. The 3D MAPSS sequence provides little or no signal for the meniscus and Achilles tendon, which have significantly decayed transverse magnetizations when the receiving mode is enabled with conventional gradient echo imaging. In contrast, the UTE-$T_{1\rho}$ sequence provides a much higher signal for both the meniscus and Achilles tendon. The receiving mode is enabled shortly after the RF excitation, thus allowing detection of the free induction decay (FID) from short-T_2 tissues such as the meniscus and Achilles tendon before significant loss of signal.

The high signal from UTE-$T_{1\rho}$ imaging allows robust quantification of $T_{1\rho}$ values for both long-T_2 tissues such as the articular cartilage and muscle, and short-T_2 tissues such as the Achilles tendon and meniscus. For example, Fig. 23.2 shows 2D gradient recalled echo (GRE)-based $T_{1\rho}$ (GRE-$T_{1\rho}$) and 3D UTE-$T_{1\rho}$ imaging of the Achilles tendon in a young, healthy volunteer [21]. The GRE-$T_{1\rho}$ sequence provides near-zero signal for the Achilles tendon precluding quantitative $T_{1\rho}$ measurement. In distinction, the UTE-$T_{1\rho}$ sequence shows a much higher signal in the Achilles tendon and demonstrates a short $T_{1\rho} \sim 3.0$ ms. While the conventional GRE-$T_{1\rho}$ sequences provide a very low signal for the Achilles tendon and cannot reliably quantify its $T_{1\rho}$, sequences of this type have been applied to tissues with longer but still relatively short T_2s, such as the meniscus [23–25].

Significant differences have been reported between healthy subjects, mild osteoarthritis (OA) patients, and severe OA patients, with mean GRE-$T_{1\rho}$ values of 14.7 ± 5.5, 16.1 ± 6.6, and 19.3 ± 7.6 ms, respectively. Meniscal $T_{1\rho}$ values correlated with clinical findings of OA, suggesting the potential of GRE-$T_{1\rho}$ for differentiating healthy subjects from patients with mild or severe OA [23]. In another study, significantly elevated GRE-$T_{1\rho}$ values were found in the lateral meniscus in patients with acute anterior cruciate ligament (ACL) injuries compared with healthy controls ($P < 0.01$) [24]. In addition, a significant correlation ($R^2 = 0.47$, $P = 0.007$) was found between GRE-$T_{1\rho}$ values of the posterior horn of lateral meniscus and GRE-$T_{1\rho}$ values of the posterior sub-compartment of the lateral tibial cartilage in ACL patients. This study demonstrated a strong injury-related relationship between the meniscus and cartilage biochemical changes [24]. Entire meniscus GRE-$T_{1\rho}$ values in healthy controls (28 ± 4 ms) were also reported to be significantly lower than those of both Kellgren and Lawrence KL1–2 (33 ± 6 ms) and KL3–4 OA subjects (34 ± 6 ms), respectively, suggesting GRE-$T_{1\rho}$ mapping might be sensitive to meniscus degeneration [25]. In addition, the longer T_2 components in the meniscus contribute significantly to the detected signal with GRE-$T_{1\rho}$ imaging. UTE-type sequences with much shorter TEs are expected to provide a better depiction and more robust characterization of the meniscus, especially short-T_2 tissues such as the Achilles tendon.

Fig. 23.1 The UTE-T$_{1\rho}$ sequence. This employs a spin-lock (SL) preparation pulse followed by a UTE FID data acquisition (**a**). The preparation pulse consists of a hard 90° pulse followed by a composite spin-lock pulse and another −90° hard pulse. The phase of the second half of the composite spin-lock pulse is shifted 180° from the first half to reduce artifacts caused by B_1 inhomogeneity. 2D UTE-T$_{1\rho}$ imaging of a healthy volunteer shows signal in both the Achilles tendon (**b**) and meniscus (**d**). 3D MAPSS imaging of the same volunteer shows very little signal from the Achilles tendon (**c**) and mostly low signal from the meniscus (**e**). (Reproduced with permission from Ref. [19])

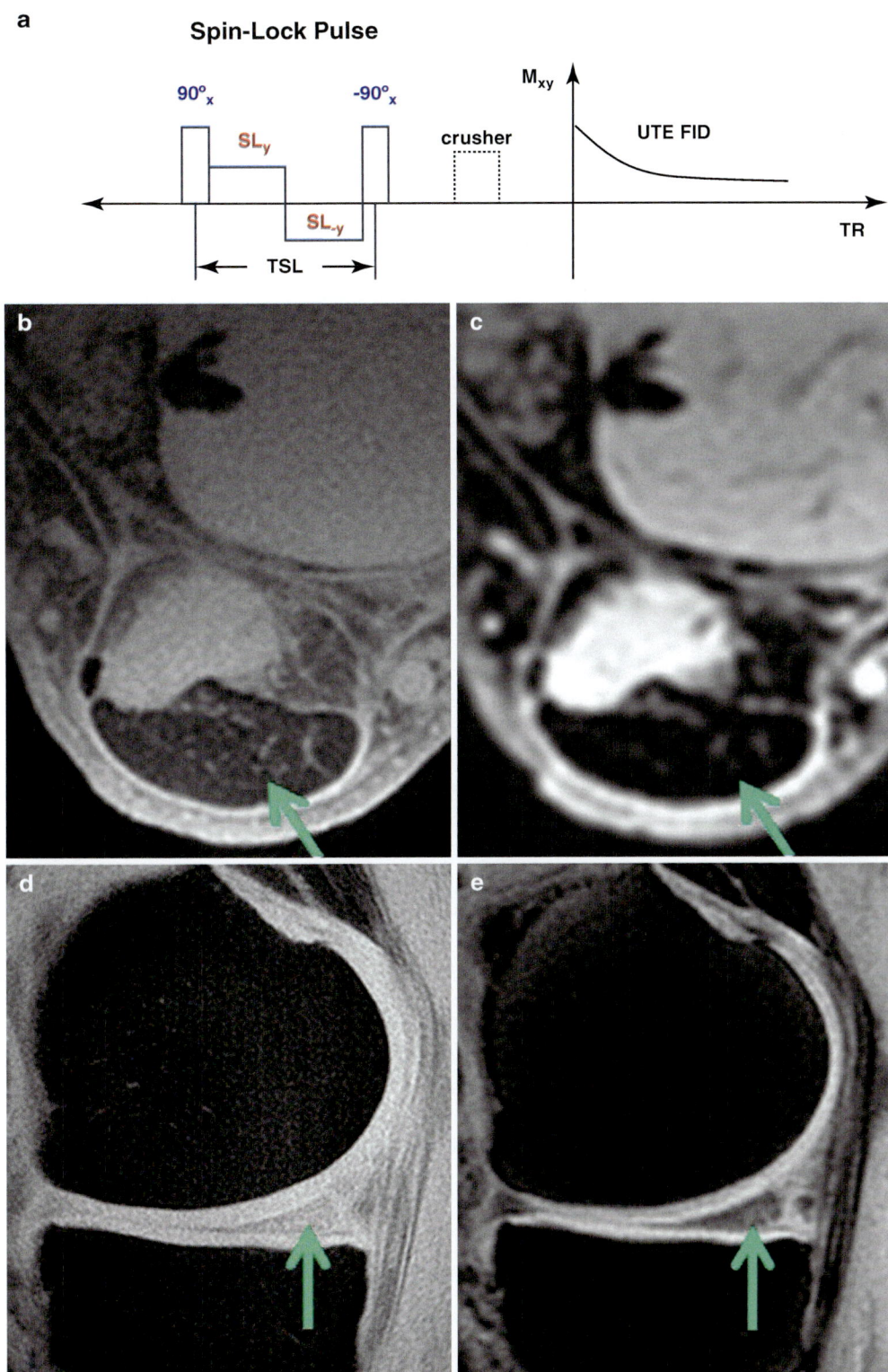

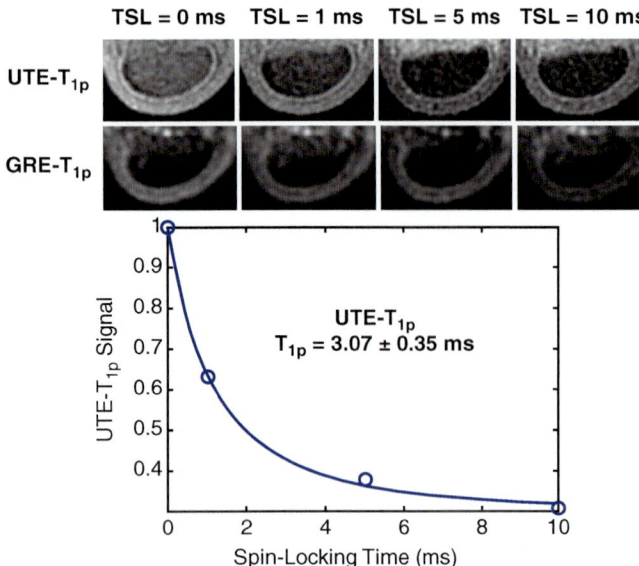

Fig. 23.2 3D UTE-$T_{1\rho}$ (**first row**) and 2D GRE-based spiral $T_{1\rho}$ (**second row**) imaging of the Achilles tendon of the same volunteer with four spin-lock times of 0, 1, 5, and 10 ms. 2D GRE-based $T_{1\rho}$ imaging shows near-zero signal in the Achilles tendon (**second row**), which is shown with much higher signal when using 3D UTE-$T_{1\rho}$ imaging (**first row**). Excellent exponential curve fitting demonstrates a short $T_{1\rho}$ of 3.07 ± 0.35 ms (**third row**). (Reproduced with permission from Ref. [21])

UTE-$T_{1\rho}$ Dispersion

UTE-$T_{1\rho}$ dispersion can be investigated by repeating UTE-$T_{1\rho}$ measurements with different spin-lock pulse powers. In a recent study, 2D UTE-$T_{1\rho}$ dispersion was investigated in the Achilles tendon and meniscus of cadavers and healthy volunteers. Ankle and knee joints were scanned with four to six TSLs ranging from 0.2 to 10 ms using three spin-lock field strengths of 250, 500, and 1000 Hz, respectively [19]. The range of spin-lock pulse powers was limited to 1000 Hz because of the limited maximal RF power available on clinical MR scanners. UTE-T_2^* was also measured for comparison using similar data acquisition parameters. Figure 23.3 shows UTE-$T_{1\rho}$ imaging of the Achilles tendon of a cadaveric ankle specimen. The Achilles tendon was depicted with high signal, contrast, and spatial resolution. Also, excellent single-component exponential curve fitting was achieved for UTE-$T_{1\rho}$ imaging of the Achilles tendon at all three spin-lock field strengths. As shown in Fig. 23.3e–p, significant UTE-$T_{1\rho}$ dispersion was observed in the Achilles tendon, with $T_{1\rho}$ increasing from 2.19 ± 0.12 ms with a spin-lock field of 250 Hz to 4.95 ± 0.23 ms with a spin-lock field of 500 Hz and 7.43 ± 0.56 ms with a spin-lock field of 1000 Hz, corresponding to an overall increase of 239% [19]. In comparison, a very short T_2^* of 0.78 ± 0.07 ms was observed in the Achilles tendon of this ankle specimen. In addition, UTE-$T_{1\rho}$ dispersion has been observed in the meniscus of healthy volunteers, with UTE-$T_{1\rho}$ values of 6.93 ± 0.44, 8.24 ± 0.49, and 12.96 ± 0.54 ms with spin-lock fields of 250, 500, and 1000 Hz, respectively [19].

$T_{1\rho}$ is sensitive to molecular motions and interactions on the time scale of the frequency-locking B_1 field. Variation or dispersion of $T_{1\rho}$ with locking field strength provides information on relatively slow molecular motions and chemical exchange [26, 27]. Cross-relaxation in the rotating frame allows exchanging protons to be affected by non-exchanging protons in macromolecules through dipolar coupling with dispersion reflecting motions on the time scale of γB_1 [28]. $T_{1\rho}$ dispersion can be fitted to a model described by Chopra et al. for estimating exchange rates [29]. According to the Cobb study, the calculated exchange values increased by a factor of four as pH increased in low-stiffness gels, consistent with chemical exchange being the dominant contributor to $T_{1\rho}$ dispersion [28]. These authors also observed increased chemical exchange rates with stiffness and attributed this to modified side-chain exchange kinetics. UTE-$T_{1\rho}$ dispersion can potentially be used to estimate chemical exchange in the menisci, ligaments, tendons, and other short-T_2 tissues and provides another tool to evaluate musculoskeletal tissue degeneration in OA.

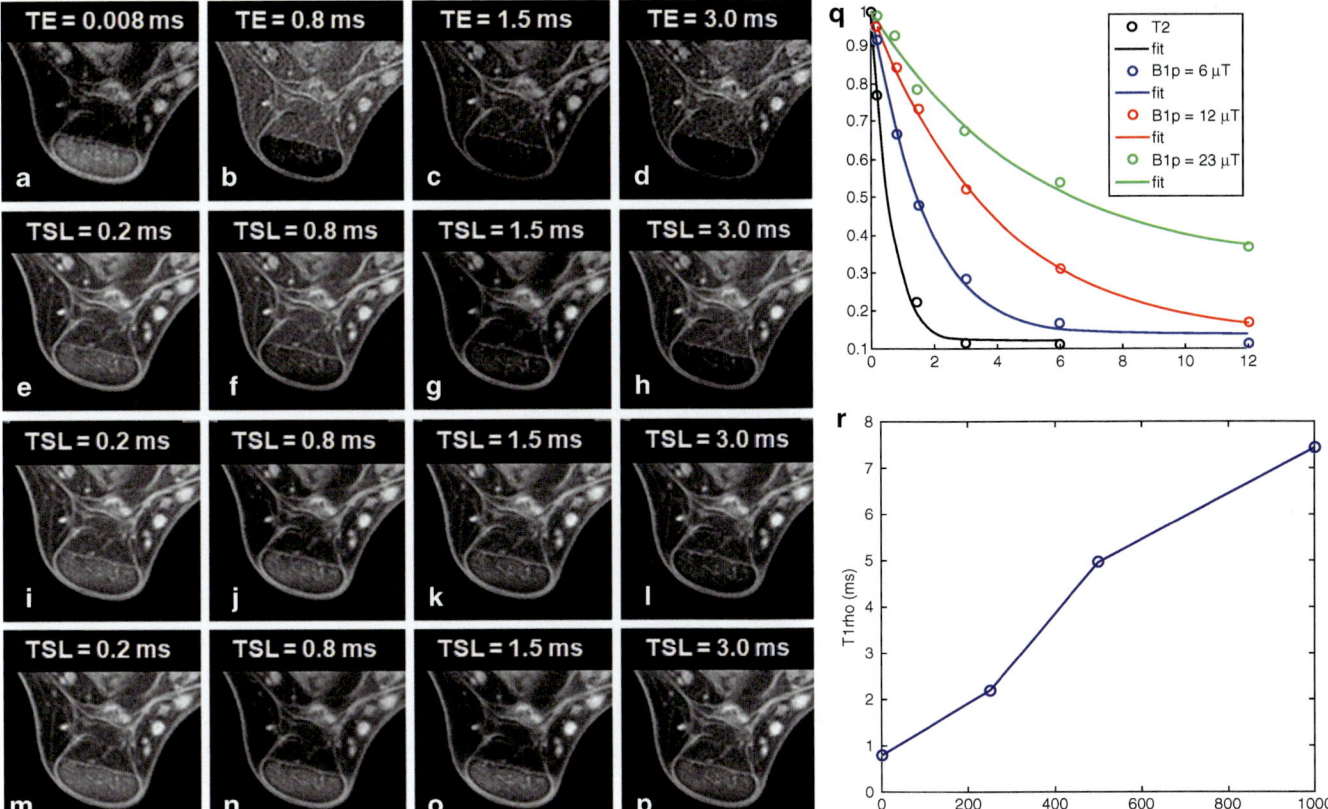

Fig. 23.3 The Achilles tendon of an ankle specimen. This was subject to UTE-T_2^* imaging with four TEs of 8 μs (**a**), 0.8 (**b**), 1.5 (**c**), and 3.0 ms (**d**), and UTE-$T_{1\rho}$ imaging with three spin-lock powers of 250 (**e–h**), 500 (**i–l**), and 1000 Hz (**m–p**), using four spin-lock times of 0.2, 0.8, 1.5, and 3.0 ms, respectively. Excellent single-component fitting was achieved and provided robust quantification of T_2^* and $T_{1\rho}$ (**q**). Significant $T_{1\rho}$ dispersion was observed in the Achilles tendon (**r**). (Reproduced with permission from Ref. [19])

Dual Adiabatic Inversion Recovery UTE $T_{1\rho}$ Imaging

Short-T_2 tissues or tissue components such as the osteochondral junction may have much lower signal intensities than long-T_2 tissues, primarily due to the following two factors. First, short-T_2 tissues and tissue components may experience significant signal loss during MR data acquisition because of their fast signal decay. Second, short-T_2 tissues and tissue components typically have higher macromolecular contents and lower mobile proton densities, leading to significantly lower signal levels than long-T_2 tissues. As a result of the low signal from short-T_2 tissues, long-T_2 signal contamination is a major challenge in accurately quantifying short-T_2 tissues, including their T_1s, T_2s, T_2^*s, $T_{1\rho}$s, and proton densities. Long-T_2 signal contamination is especially prominent in thin structures such as the osteochondral junction, which is a curved, very thin structure with a thickness of 0.1–0.2 mm [30, 31]. Another case is the cartilaginous endplate (CEP) which anchors the intervertebral disc to the vertebral body and modulates nutrient transportation and waste product elimination [32, 33]. Both of these structures are adjacent to long-T_2 fat and water-containing bone marrow and are also subject to significant susceptibility effects. Efficient long-T_2 suppression from these tissues is critical for accurate $T_{1\rho}$ quantification. The dual adiabatic inversion recovery UTE (dual-IR-UTE) technique employs two long adiabatic inversion pulses (Silver–Hoult pulses) to separately invert the longitudinal magnetizations of long-T_2 water and fat, respectively [34–37]. An appropriate combination of inversion time (TI) and repetition time (TR) allows simultaneous robust and efficient suppression of long-T_2 water and fat signals as a function of both of their T_1s (and not the chemical shift of fat in the presence of susceptibility differences). Figure 23.4 shows conventional clinical GRE, proton density-weighted fast spin echo (PD-FSE), T_1-weighted FSE (T_1-FSE), 2D UTE, and dual-IR-UTE-$T_{1\rho}$ imaging of a cadaveric human patellar sample [36]. The dual-IR-UTE-$T_{1\rho}$ sequence shows high contrast imaging of the osteochondral junction, which appears as a linear, well-defined area of high signal (arrows). Excellent single-component exponential signal decay was observed in this layer, which demonstrated a short UTE-$T_{1\rho}$ of 4.61 ± 0.07 ms. This is too short to be accurately quantified with conventional $T_{1\rho}$ sequences. It is

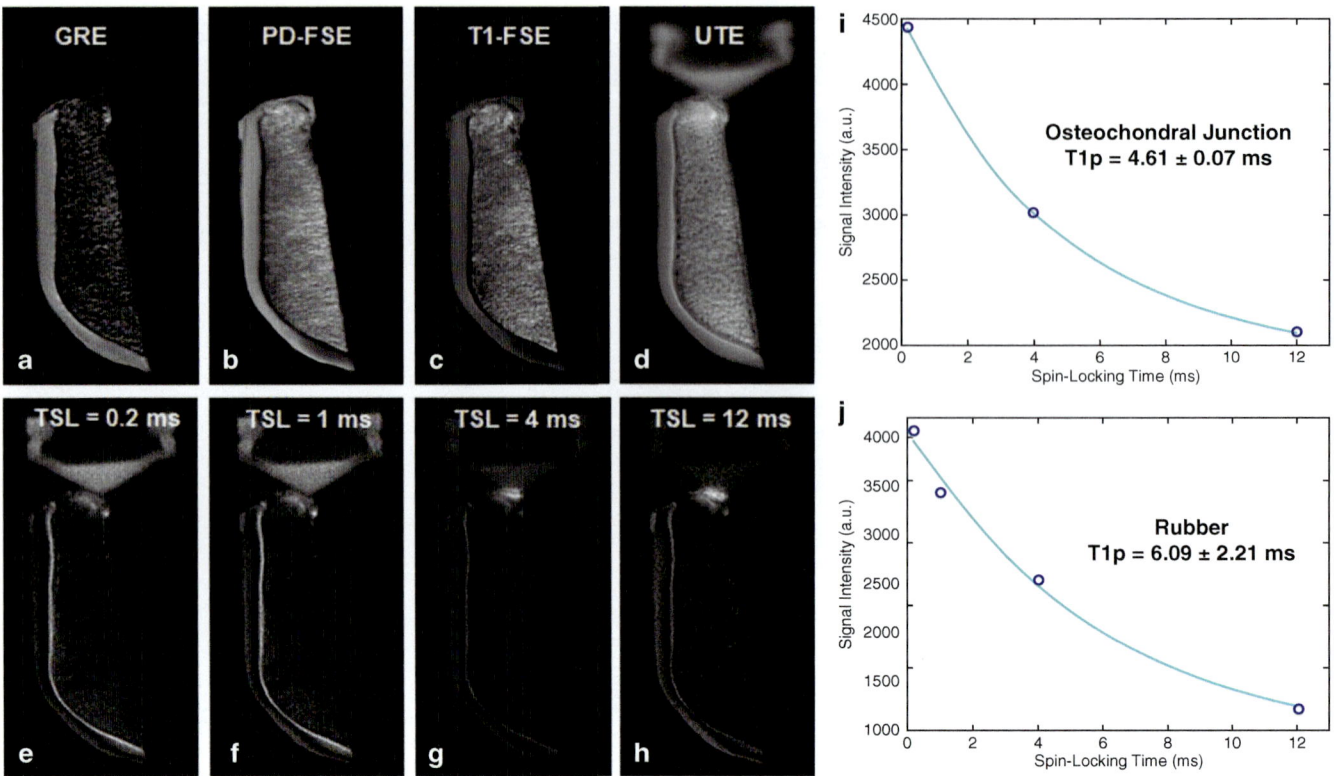

Fig. 23.4 Axial imaging of a cadaveric human patellar sample with clinical GRE (**a**), PD-FSE (**b**), T_1-FSE (**c**), 2D UTE (**d**), and dual-IR-UTE-$T_{1\rho}$ sequences with TSLs of 0.2 (**e**), 1.0 (**f**), 4 (**g**), and 12 ms (**h**), as well as mono-exponential fitting of the osteochondral junction signal which shows a short UTE-$T_{1\rho}$ of 4.61 ± 0.07 ms (**i**), and for the rubber stopper in the syringe which shows a UTE-$T_{1\rho}$ of 6.09 ± 2.21 ms (**j**). The dual IR preparation allows efficient suppression of signals from the superficial layers of cartilage and marrow fat and shows high contrast imaging of the osteochondral junction. This may improve the quantification of UTE-$T_{1\rho}$ values. (Reproduced with permission from Ref. [36])

also challenging with regular UTE sequences due to the high signals from surrounding superficial layers of articular cartilage and marrow fat–water and the partial volume effects with these tissues. The dual-IR-UTE sequence is expected to provide more accurate T_2* mapping of this thin layer than regular UTE sequences without long-T_2 signal suppression. It is interesting to note that the $T_{1\rho}$ value for the osteochondral junction of this patellar sample was 41% longer than its UTE-T_2* value of 3.26 ± 0.23 ms. In comparison, the rubber stopper in the syringe had a UTE-$T_{1\rho}$ of 6.09 ± 2.21 ms, which was 16 times longer than its short UTE-T_2* of 0.38 ± 0.01 ms. The quite different behaviors of UTE-T_2*, UTE-$T_{1\rho}$, and UTE-$T_{1\rho}$ dispersion (not shown) may be related to the biochemical differences between the osteochondral junction and rubber.

Magic Angle Effects with $T_{1\rho}$ and UTE-$T_{1\rho}$ Imaging

Recent studies suggest that $T_{1\rho}$, like T_2, is sensitive to the magic angle effect because of the contribution of dipole–dipole interactions to $T_{1\rho}$ relaxation [38]. Water protons in highly ordered collagen fibers are subject to dipolar interactions which are modulated by the term $(3\cos^2\theta - 1)$, where θ is the angle between the fiber orientation and the static magnetic field B_0. These interactions are minimized when the fibers are oriented at 55° or 125° (the magic angles) relative to B_0 when $3\cos^2\theta - 1$ approximates zero. This relationship between angle-dependent dipolar interactions and $T_{1\rho}$ relaxation is a significant confounding factor when using $T_{1\rho}$ as a biomarker of biochemical changes in biological tissues. Studies show that $T_{1\rho}$ values can increase by more than 200% in the middle and deep zones of articular cartilage when θ is oriented from 0° to 54° [38]. $T_{1\rho}$ changes due to the magic angle effect can be significantly higher than changes caused by degeneration (typically of the order of 10–30%) [39], which complicates the evaluation of tissue degeneration.

The magic angle effect is generally greater in short-T_2 tissues than in long-T_2 tissues, as their collagen fibers tend to be more ordered than in long-T_2 tissues. The UTE-$T_{1\rho}$ sequence has been used to measure the $T_{1\rho}$ of ligament and tendon specimens at a series of angular orientations to investigate the contribution of dipole–dipole interaction to $T_{1\rho}$ relaxation [20]. Figure 23.5 shows UTE-$T_{1\rho}$ images of a goat ACL at 0° and 55° relative to the B_0 field. The UTE-$T_{1\rho}$

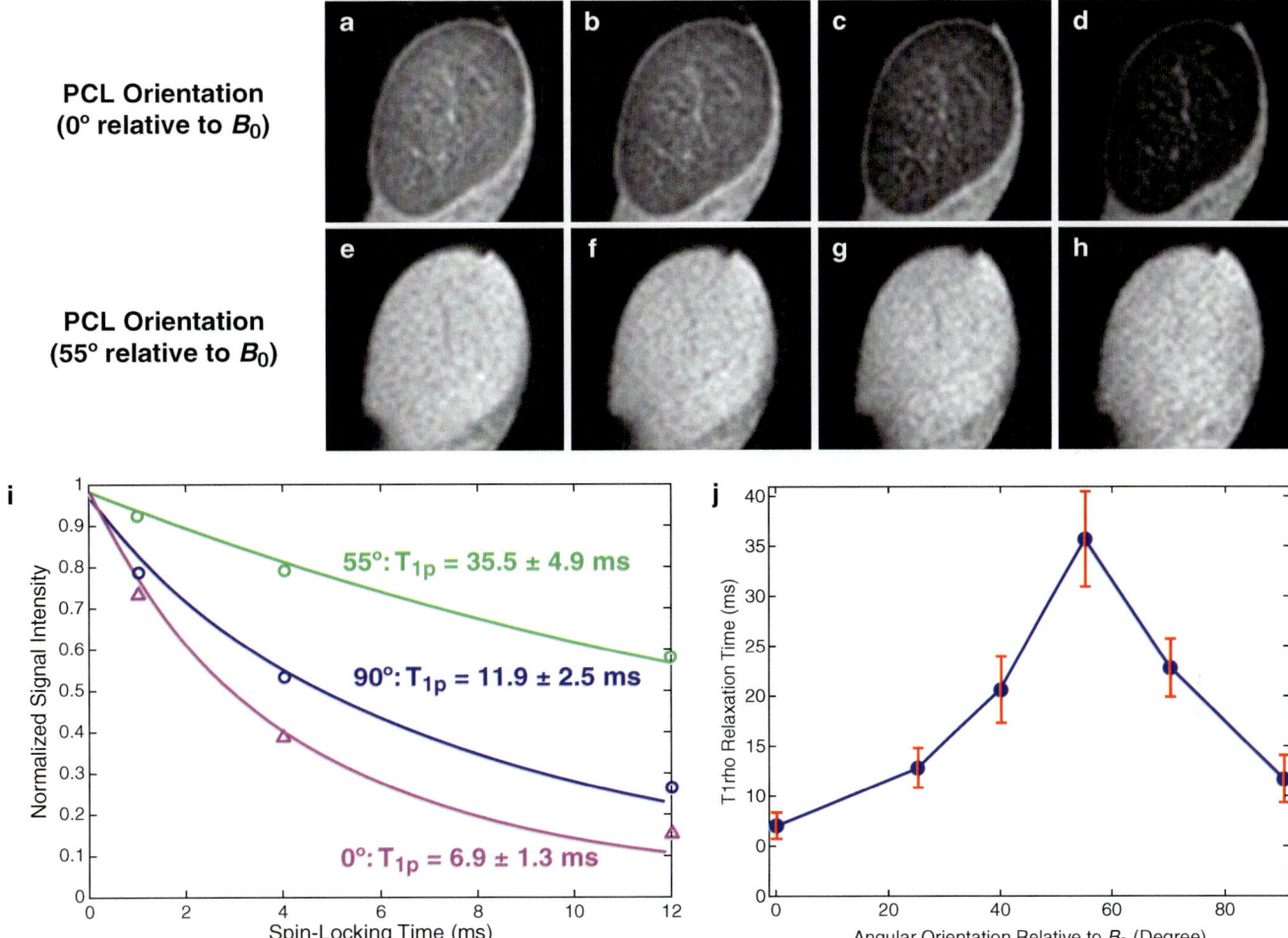

Fig. 23.5 UTE-T$_{1\rho}$ images of a goat PCL specimen at 0° (**a–d**) and 55° (**e–h**) relative to the B_0 field at TSLs of 8 μs (**a, e**), 1 ms (**b, f**), 4 ms (**c, g**), and 12 ms (**d, h**), respectively. The PCL signal decays much more slowly at 55°, consistent with a longer T$_{1\rho}$. An ROI drawn in the central portion of the goal ACL was used for subsequent T$_{1\rho}$ fitting. Exponential fitting of UTE-T$_{1\rho}$ images shows T$_{1\rho}$ values of 6.9 ± 1.3 ms at 0°, 35.5 ± 4.9 ms at 55°, and 11.9 ± 2.5 ms at 90°, respectively (**i**). Measurement of T$_{1\rho}$ as a function of the angular orientation relative to the B_0 field shows a strong magic angle effect, with the UTE-T$_{1\rho}$ value peaking at 55° relative to the B_0 field (**j**). (Reproduced with permission from Ref. [20])

images show a low signal in the bulk of the tendon and clearly depict the longer T$_2$ fascicular pattern at 0°, consistent with a short T$_{1\rho}$. In distinction, there is a higher signal in the bulk of the tendon at 55° with near-complete disappearance of the fascicular pattern. Figure 23.5i shows the selected T$_{1\rho}$ curve fitting for an ROI drawn in the central portion of the goat ACL. There is a marked change in the UTE-T$_{1\rho}$ value, which increases from 6.9 ± 1.3 ms at 0° to 36 ± 5 ms at 55° and then decreases to 12 ± 3 ms at 90°. The UTE-T$_{1\rho}$ magic angle behavior is depicted in Fig. 23.5j, where mean T$_{1\rho}$ values and standard deviations at six angles of 0°, 25°, 40°, 55°, 70°, and 90° relative to the B_0 field are displayed. The UTE-T$_{1\rho}$ value is increased by more than five-fold at 55°.

UTE Adiabatic T$_{1\rho}$

As explained above, T$_{1\rho}$ imaging is subject to magic angle effects [38]. More recently, trains of adiabatic inversion pulses have been employed to generate contrast that differs from conventional CW spin-lock-based T$_{1\rho}$ relaxation [40–42]. This adiabatic T$_{1\rho}$ relaxation is less sensitive to the magic angle effect than both T$_{1\rho}$ and T$_2$ relaxations [43]. Adiabatic T$_{1\rho}$ shows a higher sensitivity to the trypsin-induced changes in bovine patellar cartilage than the commonly used T$_2$ and magnetization transfer approaches [40]. In a rabbit model of anterior cruciate ligament transection (ACLT), early superficial cartilage degeneration was observed, including significant loss of PGs in both medial

Fig. 23.6 3D UTE-AdiabT$_{1\rho}$ imaging. A train of adiabatic inversion pulses is employed to generate T$_{1\rho}$ contrast. This is followed by multispoke sampling to speed up data acquisition (**a**). Selected UTE-AdiabT$_{1\rho}$ images of the knee in a 23-year-old normal volunteer with regions of interest (red circles or triangles) drawn in the quadriceps tendon (**b**), PCL (**c**), and meniscus (**d**), as well as the corresponding exponential curve fitting which demonstrates UTE-AdiabT$_{1\rho}$ values of 13.7 ± 1.0 ms (**e**), 22.5 ± 1.2 ms (**f**), and 21.5 ± 1.1 ms (**g**), respectively. (Reproduced with permission from Ref. [44])

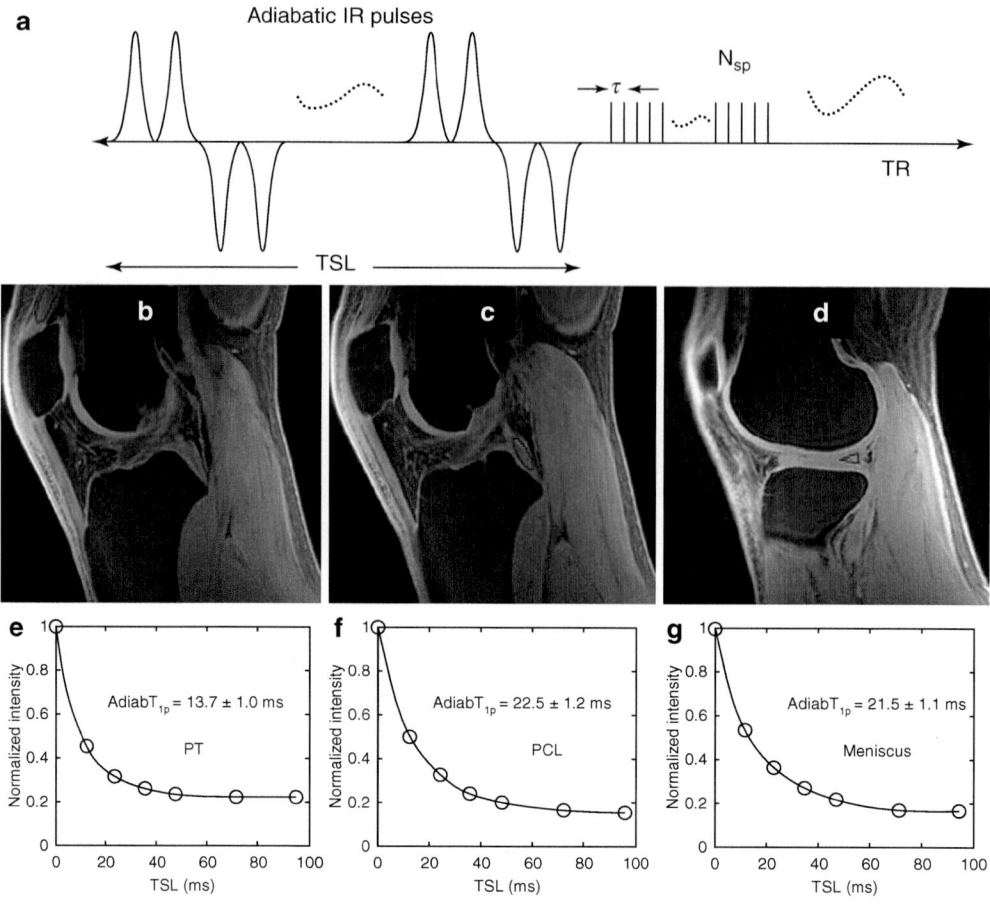

and lateral compartments as confirmed by digital densitometry, increased collagen fibril anisotropy in the lateral condyle as confirmed by polarized light microscopy and decreased biomechanical properties in both medial and lateral compartments as confirmed by indentation testing [41]. However, conventional T$_{1\rho}$ was prolonged only in the lateral compartment of ACLT joints. T$_2$ and magnetization transfer (MT) did not show a statistically significant difference between the ACLT and control groups.

In distinction, adiabatic T$_{1\rho}$ detected degenerative changes in both lateral and medial condyles ($P < 0.05$) [41]. However, due to the lack of detectable signals, AdiabT$_{1\rho}$ imaging based on conventional clinical pulse sequences is of limited value for detecting PG depletion in short-T$_2$ tissues or tissue components. Combining the 3D UTE sequence with an AdiabT$_{1\rho}$ preparation (UTE-AdiabT$_{1\rho}$) provides magic angle-insensitive imaging of both short- and long-T$_2$ tissues in the knee joint [44–46]. The UTE-AdiabT$_{1\rho}$ sequence is described in Fig. 23.6a, where a train of adiabatic inversion pulses is followed by a 3D UTE data acquisition to generate T$_{1\rho}$ contrast.

Figure 23.6b–g shows representative 3D UTE-AdiabT$_{1\rho}$ images of the knee joint in a 23-year-old male volunteer, with high signal and contrast achieved in all the primary knee joint tissues [44]. Excellent single-component fitting shows UTE-AdiabT$_{1\rho}$ values of 13.7 ± 1.0 ms for the quadriceps tendon, 22.5 ± 1.2 ms for the PCL, and 21.5 ± 1.1 ms for the meniscus. Conventional T$_{1\rho}$, adiabatic T$_{1\rho}$, T$_2$, and other quantitative MRI measurements are unavailable for these knee joint tissues due to their fast signal decay and low or zero signal intensity when imaged with conventional pulse sequences.

The UTE-AdiabT$_{1\rho}$ sequence has also been applied to the nucleus pulposus (NP) and annulus fibrosis (AF) of intervertebral discs (IVDs). Figure 23.7 shows a UTE-AdiabT$_{1\rho}$ map with adiabatic T$_1\rho$ values corresponding with values for glycosaminoglycan (GAG) content in the anterior and posterior NP regions. This result demonstrates the potential of the UTE-AdiabT$_{1\rho}$ for the diagnosis of degenerative disc changes at the biochemical level, compared to clinical images that only provide morphological evaluation.

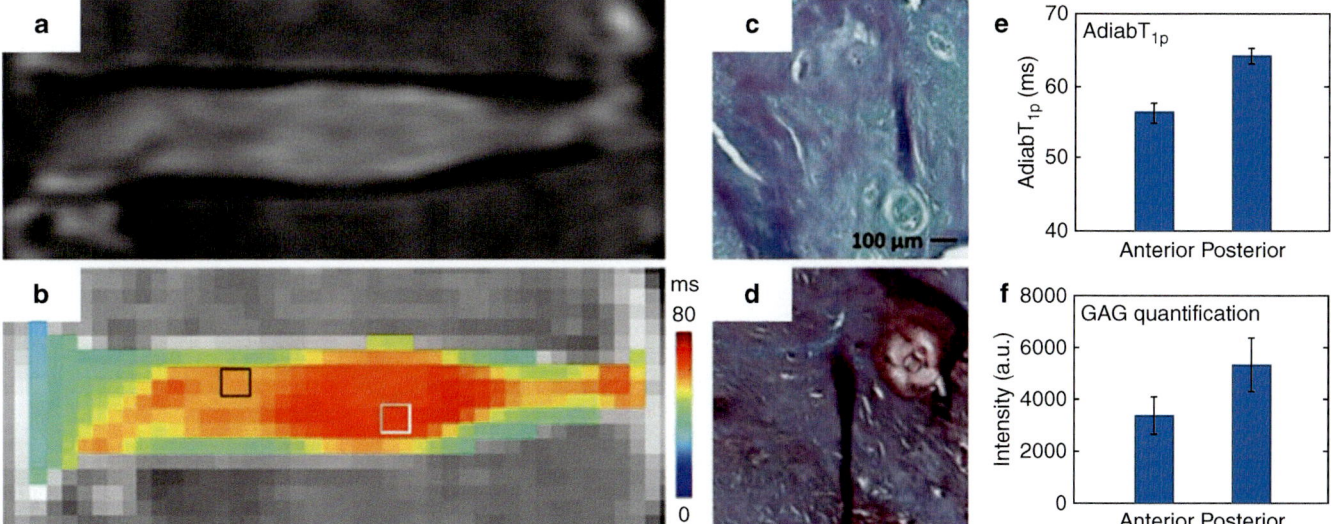

Fig. 23.7 Clinical T_2-FSE image (**a**) and UTE-AdiabT$_{1\rho}$ map (**c**) in a lumbar L2–L3 intervertebral disc. The Safranin O-stained images (**b, d**) correspond to the regions within the left (anterior) and right (posterior) boxes in (**c**), respectively. The UTE-AdiabT$_{1\rho}$ and GAG content for the left and right regions are shown in (**e**) and (**f**), respectively. There is a close correspondence between the AdiabT$_{1\rho}$ values and GAG content

Magic Angle Effect in UTE-AdiabT$_{1\rho}$

Prior studies suggest that AdiabT$_{1\rho}$ is much less sensitive to magic angle effects than conventional $T_{1\rho}$ and T_2 [43]. The magic angle effect in 3D UTE-AdiabT$_{1\rho}$ imaging was also investigated by repeating the sequence on cadaveric human patellar samples at different orientations ranging from 0° to 90° relative to the B_0 field [46]. UTE-AdiabT$_{1\rho}$ values increased from the radial layer to the superficial layer at all angular orientations. The superficial layer showed the least angular dependence (around 4.4%), while the radial layer showed the strongest angular dependence (around 34.4%). UTE-AdiabT$_{1\rho}$ values showed a much reduced magic angle effect compared to UTE-$T_{1\rho}$ and UTE-T_2* values in all examined layers and the global ROI. Figure 23.8 shows the angular dependence of 3D UTE-AdiabT$_{1\rho}$, UTE-$T_{1\rho}$, and UTE-T_2* sequences for the superficial, transitional, and deep radial layers and global ROIs covering all three layers of the patellar sample. The 3D UTE-AdiabT$_{1\rho}$ values show much-reduced magic angle effects compared to the regular 3D UTE-$T_{1\rho}$ and UTE-T_2* values for all examined layers and the global ROI. On average, over eight patellae, UTE-AdiabT$_{1\rho}$ values increased by 27.2% (4.4% for superficial, 23.8% for transitional, and 34.4% for radial layers), UTE-$T_{1\rho}$ values increased by 76.9% (11.3% for superficial, 59.1% for transitional, and 117.8% for radial layers), and UTE-T_2* values increased by 237.5% (87.9% for superficial, 262.9% for transitional, and 327.3% for radial layers) near the magic angle.

It is still unclear why the AdiabT$_{1\rho}$ and UTE-AdiabT$_{1\rho}$ sequences are less sensitive to magic angle effects [43, 45, 46]. One explanation is that the adiabatic spin-lock pulse has a relatively high power, which helps reduce the angular dependence of the magnetization exchange. Conventional $T_{1\rho}$ imaging studies have demonstrated that the angular dependence is highly related to the power of the spin-lock pulse and that a higher power leads to a reduced magic angle effect [43]. This could partly explain the reduced magic angle sensitivity associated with the AdiabT$_{1\rho}$ and UTE-AdiabT$_{1\rho}$ sequences. Another explanation is that the pairs of adiabatic spin-lock pulses have a relatively broad spectral bandwidth, much broader than CW spin-lock pulses. One of the main advantages of using trains of adiabatic fast passage pulses for spin-locking is their insensitivity to B_1 inhomogeneity, which is a significant limitation of conventional spin-lock pulses [47]. More research is needed to explain the reduced magic angle sensitivity of the 3D UTE-AdiabT$_{1\rho}$ sequence compared with 3D UTE-$T_{1\rho}$ sequence and conventional $T_{1\rho}$ sequences.

UTE-AdiabT$_{1\rho}$ Imaging in Knee Joint Degeneration

The feasibility and efficacy of 3D UTE-AdiabT$_{1\rho}$ imaging have been investigated for in vivo assessment of whole knee cartilage in healthy volunteers and patients with varying degrees of OA [48]. Subregional and global UTE-AdiabT$_{1\rho}$ values of articular cartilage were correlated with clinical evaluation of OA patients measured by KL grade and Whole-Organ Magnetic Resonance Imaging Score (WORMS). All subjects were classified into normal controls (KL = 0), doubtful-minimal OA (KL ≤ 2), and moderate-

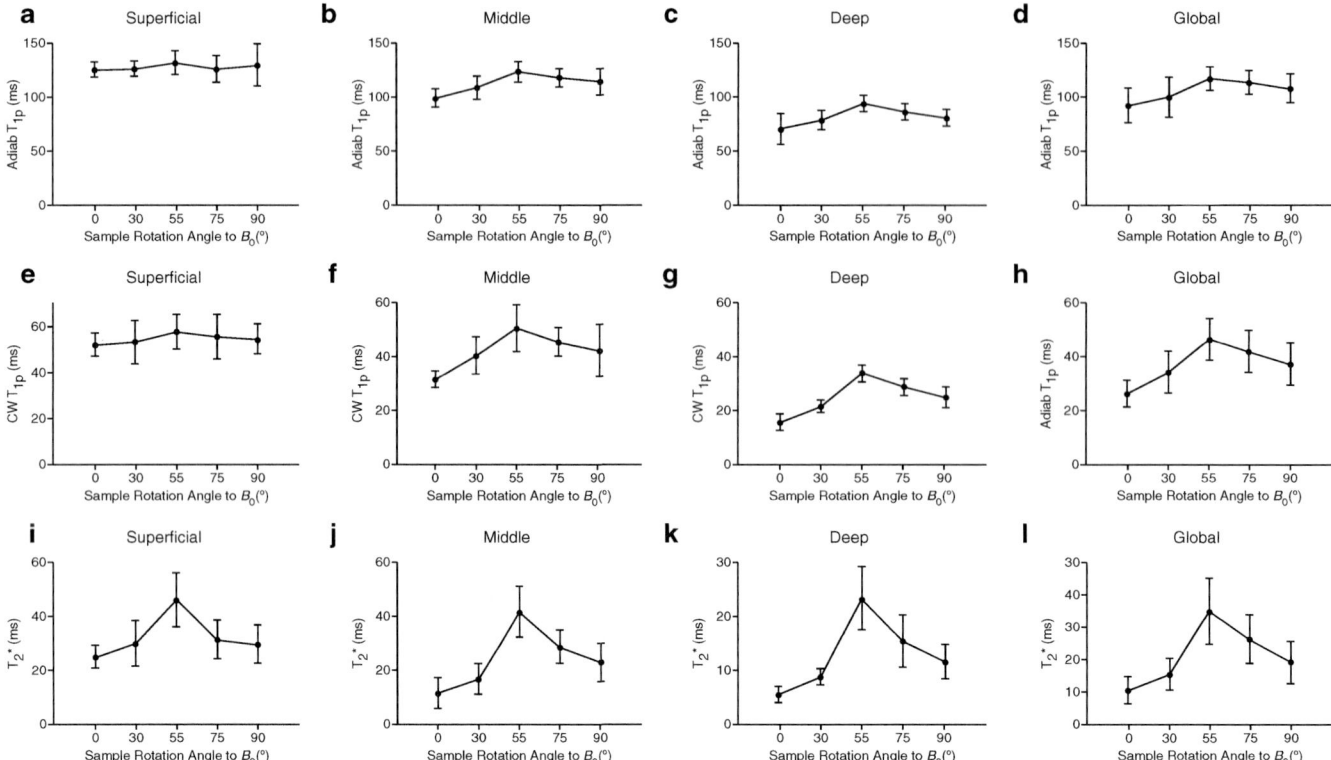

Fig. 23.8 The angular dependence of 3D UTE-AdiabT$_{1\rho}$ (**a–d**), CW T$_{1\rho}$ (**e–h**), and UTE-T$_2$* (**i–l**) values for the superficial (**a, e, i**), middle (**b, f, j**), and deep layers (**c, g, k**), as well as a global ROI (**d, h, l**) of a cadaveric human patellar sample. The superficial layers show a reduced magic angle effect compared to the middle and deep radial layers of articular cartilage. The UTE-AdiabT$_{1\rho}$ values show a much reduced magic angle effect compared to the regular CW T$_{1\rho}$ and T$_2$*. (Reproduced with permission from Ref. [46])

severe OA (KL ≥ 3) according to KL grade. The whole knee articular cartilage was divided into 13 subregions, which were further divided into two respective subcategories according to the extent and depth of cartilage lesions [48]. The extent groups included controls (WORMS = 0), regional lesions (WORMS = 1, 2, and 2.5), and diffuse lesions (WORMS = 3, 4, and 5). The depth groups included controls (WORMS = 0), partial-thickness lesions (WORMS = 1, 2, 3, and 4), and full-thickness lesions (WORMS = 2.5 and 5). Figure 23.9 shows representative UTE-AdiabT$_{1\rho}$ fitting in the femoral condyle of two human subjects, including a 36-year-old healthy volunteer and a 43-year-old patient with doubtful-minimal OA. Excellent single-component exponential fitting was achieved for both ROIs drawn in the femoral condyle, demonstrating UTE-AdiabT$_{1\rho}$ values of 32.3 ± 3.7 ms for the healthy volunteer and 40.8 ± 5.6 ms for the doubtful-minimal OA patient, respectively. Similar exponential fitting was achieved for all the 3D UTE-AdiabT$_{1\rho}$ data for a total of 713 cartilage subregions from 66 human subjects. Excellent interobserver agreement measured by interclass correlation coefficient (ICC = 0.938–0.966, $P < 0.05$) was achieved between two radiologists for KL grading, WORMS grading, and quantitative analyses. Figure 23.9e, f shows the boxplot of 3D UTE-AdiabT$_{1\rho}$ val-

ues in different WORMS groups. Statistically significant differences were observed in UTE-AdiabT$_{1\rho}$ values between the WORMS extent and depth groups. The mean UTE-AdiabT$_{1\rho}$ values of cartilage were 37.3 ± 5.45 ms for normal controls, 39.1 ± 6.46 ms for doubtful-minimal OA, and 39.0 ± 6.42 ms for moderate-severe OA. Higher UTE-AdiabT$_{1\rho}$ values were observed in more extensive and deeper lesions, with 44.1 ± 5.6 ms for cartilage with diffuse lesions and 46.8 ± 6.5 ms for cartilage with full-thickness lesions compared to 35.5 ± 4.9 ms for normal cartilage. The diagnostic threshold value of UTE-AdiabT$_{1\rho}$ for doubtful-minimal OA was 38.5 ms with 64.5% sensitivity and 54.5% specificity, and the diagnostic threshold value of UTE-AdiabT$_{1\rho}$ for mild cartilage degeneration was 39.4 ms with higher sensitivity (80.8%) and specificity (63.5%) [48]. The 3D UTE-AdiabT$_{1\rho}$ sequence may significantly improve the robustness of quantitative evaluation of articular cartilage degeneration. A systematic evaluation of UTE-AdiabT$_{1\rho}$ values for all the principal components in the knee joint, including the menisci, ligaments, tendons, muscles, and bones, remains to be conducted. No current grading systems involve morphological and quantitative imaging of all primary knee joint tissues, especially tissues with short T$_2$ relaxation times. Further research is needed in this area.

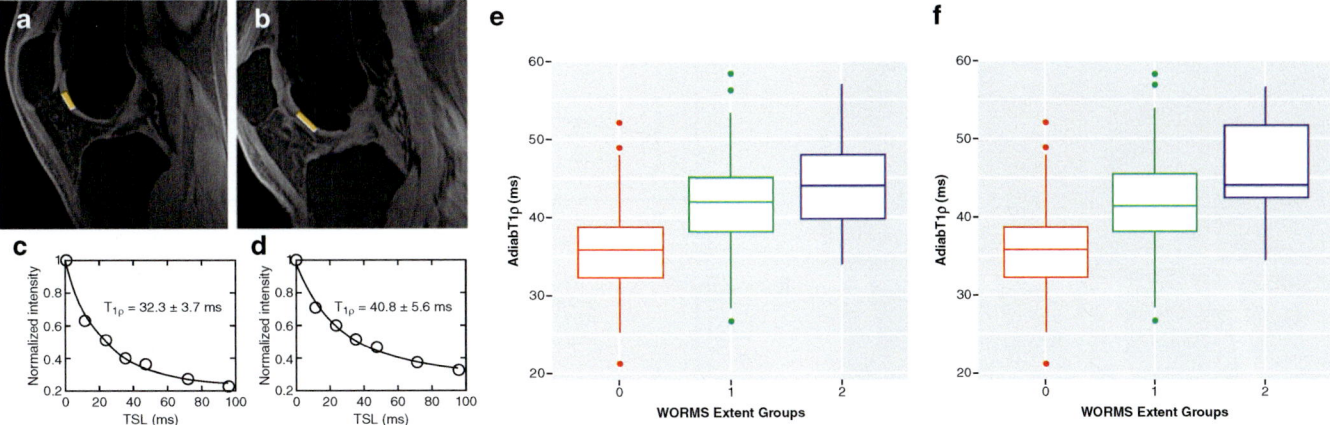

Fig. 23.9 Excellent single-component exponential UTE-AdiabT$_{1\rho}$ fitting was achieved for normal cartilage (**a, c**) (T$_{1\rho}$ = 32.3 ± 3.7 ms) in a 36-year-old healthy volunteer, and abnormal cartilage (**b, d**) (WORMS = 2, T$_{1\rho}$ = 40.8 ± 5.6 ms) in a 43-year-old patient with doubt-ful-minimal OA. Boxplot of UTE-AdiabT$_{1\rho}$ values in different WORMS extent groups (**e**) and WORMS depth groups (**f**) for a total of 713 cartilage subregions from 66 human subjects with varying degrees of knee joint degeneration. (Reproduced with permission from Ref. [48])

UTE-AdiabT$_{1\rho}$ Imaging in Spine Degeneration

Past studies have demonstrated that quantitative T$_{1\rho}$ mapping is a promising technique for detecting biochemical changes in IVDs during the process of degeneration [3, 10]. Research on T$_{1\rho}$ measurement in IVDs has focused on changes in the NP [49] and the AF [10]. The cartilaginous endplate (CEP) may be degraded and affect nutrient availability and cell metabolism in the rest of the IVD and, thus, contribute to the degeneration of the NP and AF [50]. Recently, Wei et al. conducted a feasibility study on 17 human subjects (nine women and eight men) with a mean age of 43 ± 16 years and a range of 25–71 years [51]. Each subject underwent 3D UTE-AdiabT$_{1\rho}$ and T$_2$-FSE imaging of the lumbar spine. Each lumbar IVD was manually segmented into seven subregions, including outer anterior AF, inner anterior AF, outer posterior AF, inner posterior AF, superior CEP, inferior CEP, and NP. The UTE-AdiabT$_{1\rho}$ values of these subregions were correlated with modified Pfirrmann grades and subjects' ages. In addition, UTE-AdiabT$_{1\rho}$ values were compared in subjects with and without low back pain (LBP). Correlations of UTE-AdiabT$_{1\rho}$ values of the outer posterior AF, superior CEP, inferior CEP, and NP with modified Pfirrmann grades were significant ($P < 0.05$) with R values of 0.51, 0.36, 0.38, and −0.94, respectively. Correlations of UTE-AdiabT$_{1\rho}$ values of the outer anterior AF, outer posterior AF, and NP with

ages were significant, with R values of 0.52, 0.71, and −0.76, respectively. UTE-AdiabT$_{1\rho}$ differences in the outer posterior AF, inferior CEP, and NP between the subjects with and without LBP were significant ($P = 0.005$, 0.020, and 0.000, respectively). Figure 23.10 shows UTE-AdiabT$_{1\rho}$ maps (first row) and corresponding T$_2$-FSE images (second row) from four subjects [51]. The modified Pfirrmann grading is a widely used method of determining the degree of disc degeneration through qualitative assessment of disc morphology and the signal intensity of the NP and AF using clinical T$_2$-FSE images [52]. More degraded discs with higher modified Pfirrmann grades showed lower UTE-AdiabT$_{1\rho}$ values in the NP. Figure 23.10 also shows scatter plots of UTE-AdiabT$_{1\rho}$ values for the outer anterior AF, superior CEP, inferior CEP, and NP as a function of the modified Pfirrmann grade for all 17 subjects. Spearman's analysis showed that the correlations were all statistically significant ($P < 0.05$). UTE-AdiabT$_{1\rho}$ values of the outer posterior AF, superior CEP, and inferior CEP showed moderate positive correlations with Pfirrmann grades with R values of 0.51, 0.36, and 0.38, respectively. Conversely, UTE-AdiabT$_{1\rho}$ values of the NP were inversely correlated with Pfirrmann grades with an R of −0.94, which is consistent with reported trends for the NP [49]. The UTE-AdiabT$_{1\rho}$ sequence can quantify the T$_{1\rho}$ of whole IVDs, including CEPs. This is a technical advance and of value for a comprehensive assessment of IVD degeneration.

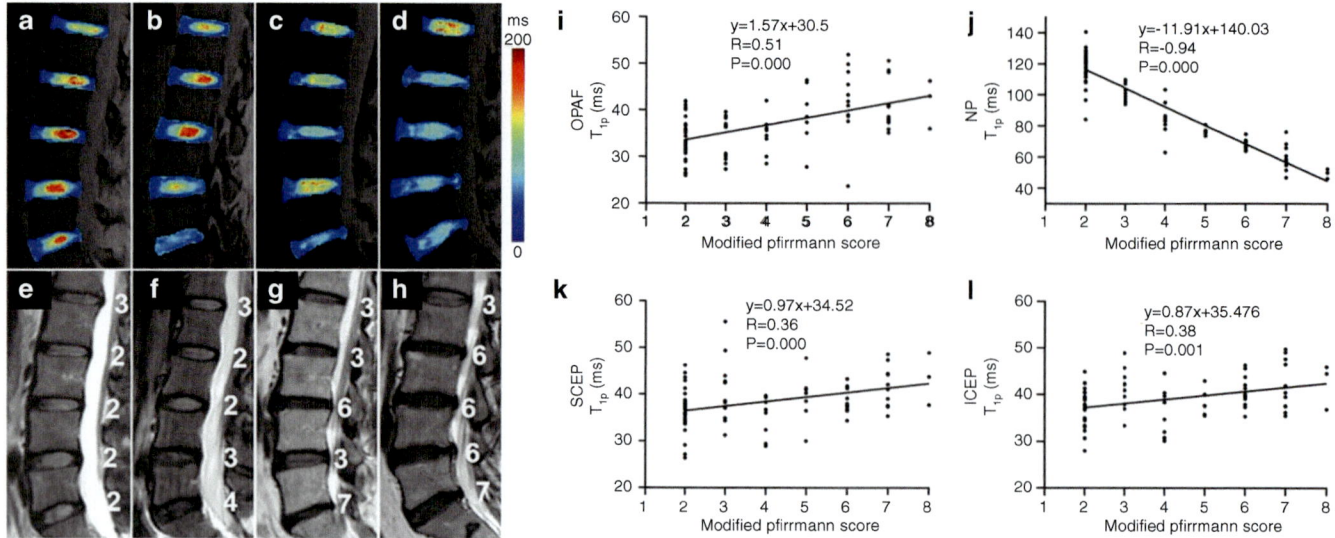

Fig. 23.10 UTE-AdiabT$_{1\rho}$ maps (**a–d**) and corresponding T$_2$-FSE images (**e–h**) from four subjects (first column, 29-year-old female; second column, 32-year-old female; third column, 60-year-old female; fourth column, 55-year-old male). The modified Pfirrmann grades for each disc are shown on the T$_2$-FSE images. Spearman's correlation coefficients between modified Pfirrmann grades and T$_{1\rho}$ values of outer posterior AF (**i**), superior CEP (**j**), inferior CEP (**k**), and NP (**l**) from 17 in vivo subjects (aged from 25 to 71 years old, nine female, five discs each) are shown. A strong negative correlation is seen for the NP, and moderate positive correlations are observed for the outer posterior AF, superior CEP, and inferior CEP. (Reproduced with permission from Ref. [51])

Conclusion

The UTE-T$_{1\rho}$ sequence provides reliable T$_{1\rho}$ mapping of short-T$_2$ tissues and tissue components, such as the menisci, ligaments, and tendons. It can be combined with long-T$_2$ signal suppression pulses to produce selective T$_{1\rho}$ mapping of short-T$_2$ tissue components such as the osteochondral junction. However, the UTE-T$_{1\rho}$ sequence is subject to magic angle effects, which can be alleviated using UTE-AdiabT$_{1\rho}$ imaging. This sequence is relatively insensitive to magic angle effects and allows more robust mapping of T$_{1\rho}$ for both short- and long-T$_2$ tissues. Preliminary studies have demonstrated the efficacy of the sequence in detecting early changes in the knee joint, including early changes in articular cartilage and menisci. Future research will include UTE-T$_{1\rho}$ dispersion and modeling of chemical exchange rates and pH levels in both short-T$_2$ musculoskeletal tissues such as the menisci, ligaments, tendons, and long-T$_2$ tissues such as articular cartilage, muscle, and synovium.

References

1. Redfield AG. Nuclear magnetic resonance saturation and rotary saturation in solids. Phys Rev. 1955;98:1787–809.
2. Sepponen RE, Pohjonen JA, Sipponen JT, Tanttu JI. A method for T$_1$ rho imaging. J Comput Assist Tomogr. 1985;9:1007–11.
3. Wang YX, Zhang Q, Li X, Chen W, Ahuja A, Yuan J. T$_1$rho magnetic resonance: basic physics principals and applications in knee and intervertebral disc imaging. Quant Imaging Med Surg. 2015;5:858–85.
4. Duvvuri U, Reddy R, Patel SD, Kaufman JH, Kneeland JB, Leigh JS. T$_1$rho-relaxation in articular cartilage: effects of enzymatic degradation. Magn Reson Med. 1997;38:863–7.
5. Keenan KE, Besier TF, Pauly JM, Rosenberg J, Smith RL, Delp SL, Beaupre GS, Gold GE. Prediction of glycosaminoglycan content in human cartilage by age, T$_{1\rho}$ and T$_2$ MRI. Osteoarthr Cartil. 2011;19:171–9.
6. Li X, Benjamin Ma C, Link TM, et al. In vivo T$_1$rho and T$_2$ mapping of articular cartilage in osteoarthritis of the knee using 3T MRI. Osteoarthr Cartil. 2007;15:789–97.
7. Menezes NM, Gray ML, Hartke JR, Burstein D. T$_2$ and T$_1$rho MRI in articular cartilage systems. Magn Reson Med. 2004;51:503–9.
8. Mlynarik V, Trattnig S, Huber M, Zembsch A, Imhof H. The role of relaxation times in monitoring proteoglycan depletion in articular cartilage. J Magn Reson Imaging. 1999;10:497–502.
9. Allkemper T, Sagmeister F, Cincinnati V, Beckebaum S, Kooijman H, Kanthak C, Stehling C, Heindel W. Evaluation of fibrotic liver disease with whole-liver T$_{1\rho}$ MR imaging: a feasibility study at 1.5 T. Radiology. 2014;271:408–15.
10. Wang YX, Zhao F, Griffith JF, Mok GS, Leung JC, Ahuja AT, Yuan J. T$_1$rho and T$_2$ relaxation times for lumbar disc degeneration: an in vivo comparative study at 3.0-Tesla MRI. Eur Radiol. 2013;23:228–34.
11. Borthakur A, Gur T, Wheaton AJ, et al. In vivo measurement of plaque burden in a mouse model of Alzheimer's disease. J Magn Reson Imaging. 2006;24:1011–7.
12. Nestrasil I, Michaeli S, Liimatainen T, Rydeen CE, Kotz CM, Nixon JP, Hanson T, Tuite PJ. T$_1$rho and T$_2$rho MRI in the evaluation of Parkinson's disease. J Neurol. 2010;257:964–8.
13. Knispel RR, Thompson RT, Pintar MM. Dispersion of proton spin-lattice relaxation in tissues. J Magn Reson. 1974;14:44–51.
14. Zu ZL, Afzal A, Li H, Xie JP, Gore JC. Spin-lock imaging of early tissue pH changes in ischemic rat brain. NMR Biomed. 2018;31:e3893.

15. Virta A, Komu M, Lundbom N, Kormano M. T_1 rho MR imaging characteristics of human anterior tibial and gastrocnemius muscles. Acad Radiol. 1998;5:104–10.

16. Robson MD, Gatehouse PD, Bydder M, Bydder GM. Magnetic resonance: an introduction to ultrashort TE (UTE) imaging. J Comput Assist Tomogr. 2003;27:825–46.

17. Chang E, Du J, Chung C. UTE imaging in the musculoskeletal system. J Magn Reson Imaging. 2015;41:870–83.

18. Afsahi AM, Ma Y, Jang H, et al. Ultrashort echo time magnetic resonance imaging techniques: met and unmet needs in musculoskeletal imaging. J Magn Reson Imaging. 2022;55:1591–612.

19. Du J, Carl M, Diaz E, et al. Ultrashort TE T_1rho (UTE T_1rho) imaging of the Achilles tendon and meniscus. Magn Reson Med. 2010;64:834–42.

20. Du J, Statum S, Znamirowski R, Bydder GM, Chung CB. Ultrashort TE T_1rho magic angle imaging. Magn Reson Med. 2013;69:682–7.

21. Ma YJ, Carl M, Shao H, Tadros AS, Chang EY, Du J. Three-dimensional ultrashort echo time cones T_1rho (3D UTE-cones-T1rho) imaging. NMR Biomed. 2017;30:3709.

22. Li X, Han ET, Ma B, Busse RF, Majumdar S. In vivo $T_{1\rho}$ mapping in cartilage using 3D magnetization-prepared angle-modulated partitioned k-space spoiled gradient echo snapshots (3D MAPSS). Magn Reson Med. 2008;59:298–307.

23. Rauscher I, Stahl R, Cheng J, Li X, Huber MB, Luke A, Majumdar S, Link TM. Meniscal measurements of T_1rho and T_2 at MR imaging in healthy subjects and patients with osteoarthritis. Radiology. 2008;249(2):591–600.

24. Bolbos RI, Link TM, Ma CB, Majumdar S, Li X. T1rho relaxation time of the meniscus and its relationship with T_1rho of adjacent cartilage in knees with acute ACL injuries at 3 T. Osteoarthr Cartil. 2009;17(1):12–8.

25. Wang L, Chang G, Bencardino J, Babb JS, Krasnokutsky S, Abramson S, Regatte RR. T_1rho MRI of menisci in patients with osteoarthritis at 3 Tesla: a preliminary study. J Magn Reson Imaging. 2014;40(3):588–95.

26. Hills BP. The proton-exchange cross-relaxation model of water relaxation in biopolymer systems. 2. The sol and gel states of gelatin. Mol Phys. 1992;76:509–23.

27. Duvvuri U, Goldberg AD, Kranz JK, Hoang L, Reddy R, Wehrli FW, Wand AJ, Englander SW, Leigh JS. Water magnetic relaxation dispersion in biological systems: the contribution of proton exchange and implications for the noninvasive detection of cartilage degradation. Proc Natl Acad Sci U S A. 2001;98:12479–84.

28. Cobb JG, Xie J, Gore JC. Contributions of chemical exchange to T$_{1\rho}$ dispersion in a tissue model. Magn Reson Med. 2011;66:1563–71.

29. Chopra S, Mcclung RED, Jordan RB. Rotating-frame relaxation rates of solvent molecules in solutions of paramagnetic-ions undergoing solvent exchange. J Magn Reson. 1984;59:361–72.

30. Lane LB, Bullough PG. Age-related changes in the thickness of the calcified zone and the number of tidemarks in adult human articular cartilage. J Bone Joint Surg Br. 1980;62:372–5.

31. Foreman SC, Ashmeik W, Baal JD, Han M, Bahroos E, von Schacky CE, Carl M, Krug R, Joseph GB, Link TM. Patients with type 2 diabetes exhibit a more mineralized deep cartilage layer compared with nondiabetic controls: a pilot study. Cartilage. 2021;13(1_Suppl):428S–36S.

32. Berg-Johansen B, Han M, Fields AJ, et al. Cartilage endplate thickness variation measured by ultrashort echo-time MRI is associated with adjacent disc degeneration. Spine. 2018;43:592–600.

33. Kim YJ, Cha JG, Shin YS, Chaudhari AS, Suh YJ, Yoon SH, Gold GE. 3D ultrashort TE MRI for evaluation of cartilaginous endplate of cervical disk in vivo: feasibility and correction with disk degeneration in T_2-weighted spin-echo sequence. AJR Am J Roentgenol. 2018;210:1131–40.

34. Du J, Takahashi A, Bae WC, Chung CB, Bydder GM. Dual inversion recovery, ultrashort echo time (DIR UTE) imaging: creating high contrast for short-T_2 species. Magn Reson Med. 2010;63:447–55.

35. Bae W, Dwek JR, Znamirowski R, Statum S, Hermida JC, D'Lima DD, Sah RL, Du J, Chung CB. Ultrashort echo time MR imaging of osteochondral junction of the knee at 3 T: identification of anatomic structures contributing to signal intensity. Radiology. 2009;254:837–45.

36. Du J, Carl M, Bae WC, Statum S, Chang EY, Bydder GM, Chung CB. Dual inversion recovery ultrashort echo time (DIR-UTE) imaging and quantification of the zone of calcified cartilage (ZCC). Osteoarthr Cartil. 2013;21:77–85.

37. Ma YJ, Zhu Y, Lu X, Carl M, Chang EY, Du J. Short T_2 imaging using a 3D double adiabatic inversion recovery prepared ultrashort echo time cones (3D DIR-UTE-Cones) sequence. Magn Reson Med. 2018;79:2555–63.

38. Shao H, Pauli C, Li S, Ma Y, Tadros AS, Kavanaugh A, et al. Magic angle effect plays a major role in both T_1rho and T_2 relaxation in articular cartilage. Osteoarthr Cartil. 2017;25:2022–30.

39. Mosher TJ, Zhang Z, Reddy R, Boudhar S, Milestone BN, Morrison WB, et al. Knee articular cartilage damage in osteoarthritis: analysis of MR image biomarker reproducibility in ACRIN-PA 4001 multi-center trial. Radiology. 2011;258:832–42.

40. Ellermann J, Ling W, Nissi MJ, Arendt E, Carlson CS, Garwood M, Michaeli S, Mangia S. MRI rotating frame relaxation measurements for articular cartilage assessment. Magn Reson Imaging. 2013;31:1537–43.

41. Rautiainen J, Nissi MJ, Liimatainen T, Herzog W, Korhonen RK, Nieminen MT. Adiabatic rotating frame relaxation of MRI reveals early cartilage degeneration in a rabbit model of anterior cruciate ligament transection. Osteoarthr Cartil. 2014;22:1444–52.

42. Casula V, Nissi MJ, Podlipska J, et al. Elevated adiabatic $T_{1\rho}$ and T2ρ in articular cartilage are associated with cartilage and bone lesions in early osteoarthritis: a preliminary study. J Magn Reson Imaging. 2017;46:678–89.

43. Hänninen N, Rautiainen J, Rieppo L, Saarakkala S, Nissi MJ. Orientation anisotropy of quantitative MRI relaxation parameters in ordered tissue. Sci Rep. 2017;7:9606.

44. Ma Y, Carl M, Searleman A, Lu X, Chang EY, Du J. Three dimensional adiabatic $T_{1\rho}$ prepared ultrashort echo time cones (3D AdiabT1ρ UTE-cones) sequence for whole knee imaging. Magn Reson Med. 2018;80:1429–39.

45. Wu M, Ma Y, Wan L, et al. Magic angle effect on adiabatic $T_{1\rho}$ imaging of the Achilles tendon using 3D ultrashort echo time cones trajectory. NMR Biomed. 2020;33:e4322.

46. Wu M, Ma Y, Kasibhatla A, et al. Convincing evidence for magic angle less-sensitive quantitative $T_{1\rho}$ imaging of articular cartilage using the 3D ultrashort echo time cones adiabatic $T_{1\rho}$ (3D UTE cones-AdiabT1ρ) sequence. Magn Reson Med. 2020;84:2551–60.

47. Garwood M, DelaBarre L. The return of the frequency sweep: designing adiabatic pulses for contemporary NMR. J Magn Reson. 2001;153:155–77.

48. Wu M, Ma YJ, Liu M, Xue Y, Gong L, Wei Z, Jerban S, Jang H, Chang DG, Chang EY, Ma L, Du J. Quantitative assessment of articular cartilage degeneration using 3D ultrashort echo time cones adiabatic T1ρ (3D UTE-cones-AdiabT$_{1\rho}$) imaging. Eur Radiol. 2022;32:6178–86.

49. Adams MA, Roughley PJ. What is intervertebral disc degeneration, and what causes it? Spine. 2006;31:2151–61.

50. Wei Z, Lombardi AF, Lee RR, Wallace M, Masuda K, Chang EY, Du J, Bydder GM, Yang W, Ma Y. Comprehensive assessment of in vivo lumbar spine intervertebral discs using a 3D adiabatic $T_{1\rho}$ prepared ultrashort echo time (UTE-Adiab-$T_{1\rho}$) pulse sequence. Quant Imaging Med Surg. 2022;12:269–80.

51. Griffith JF, Wang YX, Antonio GE, Choi KC, Yu A, Ahuja AT, Leung PC. Modified Pfirrmann grading system for lumbar intervertebral disc degeneration. Spine. 2007;32:708–12.

Quantitative Ultrashort Echo Time Magnetic Resonance Imaging: Proton Density

Yajun Ma, Saeed Jerban, Hyungseok Jang, Eric Y. Chang, and Jiang Du

Introduction

Proton density (PD) is a fundamental MR property of tissue, and PD-weighted imaging has been widely used for clinical diagnosis [1]. Measured tissue PD has also been recognized as a useful biomarker for evaluating tissue changes in disease [2–6]. Since protons in semisolid tissues (e.g., collagen and protein) are usually undetectable with conventional MRI sequences due to their very short T_2s (~10 μs) [6, 7], most PD measurement studies have been focused on the quantification of water content in tissues. For example, water content or PD in cortical bone provides information about bone quality [4]. The free water in cortical bone resides in the microscopic pores of the Haversian and the Lacunocanalicular systems and is described as pore water. Its density and other MR properties are related to bone porosity and poroelasticity. The bound water in cortical bone is tightly bound to the collagen matrix or embedded in the crystals of bone minerals and affects bone viscoelastic properties. Changes in bone water PD are also correlated with age [8, 9]. The development of accurate water PD quantification techniques is of central importance in understanding changes with age and in disease in cortical bone and other tissues.

Y. Ma (✉) · S. Jerban · H. Jang
Department of Radiology, University of California, San Diego, La Jolla, CA, USA
e-mail: yam013@ucsd.edu; sjerban@health.ucsd.edu; h4jang@health.ucsd.edu

E. Y. Chang
Department of Radiology, University of California, San Diego, La Jolla, CA, USA

VA San Diego Healthcare System, San Diego, CA, USA
e-mail: e8chang@health.ucsd.edu

J. Du
Department of Radiology, University of California, San Diego, La Jolla, CA, USA

VA San Diego Healthcare System, San Diego, CA, USA

Department of Bioengineering, University of California, San Diego, La Jolla, CA, USA
e-mail: jiangdu@health.ucsd.edu

Ultrashort echo time (UTE) sequences with echo times (TEs) shorter than 100 μs can detect signals from both short- and long-T_2 components in tissue, thus allowing quantitative PD mapping of these separate tissue compartments and more comprehensive assessment of tissue changes [10]. Several UTE PD mapping techniques have been developed and successfully used to evaluate PD changes in cortical bone, trabecular bone, and brain myelin [4–6]. This chapter describes these quantitative UTE PD measurement techniques and their applications.

Total Bone Water PD Mapping in Cortical Bone

There are two distinct water compartments in cortical bone: bound water and pore water. The bound water component contributes most to the total water content in cortical bone (i.e., ~70%) [11]. However, the bound water has a very short T_2 relaxation time of ~300 μs, and clinical gradient echo (GRE) and fast spin echo (FSE) sequences cannot detect the fast-decaying signals from bound water. Thus, UTE sequences and their variants (e.g., ZTE, WASPI, and PETRA) with TEs less than 100 μs are currently the only options available to image both bound water and pore water signals in cortical bone. Techawiboonwong et al. have proposed a simple method to quantify total bone water content in cortical bone [4]. The cortical bone is scanned with a reference phantom with known MR properties using a regular UTE sequence. The steady-state signal of this UTE sequence, $S(\text{TE})$, is expressed as follows:

$$S(\text{TE}) = C\rho_0 f_{xy} \frac{1 - e^{-\frac{\text{TR}}{T_1}}}{1 - f_z e^{-\frac{\text{TR}}{T_1}}} e^{-\frac{\text{TE}}{T_2^*}} \qquad (24.1)$$

$$= C\rho_0 f_{xy} e^{-\frac{\text{TE}}{T_2^*}}$$

Where ρ_0 is the PD of cortical bone. C is a constant that includes information on receiver gain and coil sensitivities. f_{xy} and f_z are functions of the excitation flip angle α and pulse duration τ, as well as tissue T_2^*, which are described as follows:

$$f_{xy} = e^{-\frac{\tau}{2T_2^*}} \alpha \, sinc\left(\sqrt{\alpha^2 - \left(\frac{\tau}{2T_2^*}\right)^2}\right) \qquad (24.2)$$

$$f_z = e^{-\frac{\tau}{2T_2^*}} \left(\cos\left(\sqrt{\alpha^2 - \left(\frac{\tau}{2T_2^*}\right)^2}\right) + \frac{\tau}{2T_2^*} sinc\left(\sqrt{\alpha^2 - \left(\frac{\tau}{2T_2^*}\right)^2}\right) \right) \qquad (24.3)$$

When the pulse duration τ is much shorter than the tissue T_2^*, f_{xy} and f_z revert to $\sin(\alpha)$ and $\cos(\alpha)$, respectively.

The PD of cortical bone ρ_{bone} can be estimated using the following equation:

$$\rho_{bone} = \rho_{ref} \frac{I_{bone} F_{ref}}{I_{ref} F_{bone}} e^{-\frac{TE}{T_{2,ref}^*} + \frac{TE}{T_{2,bone}^*}} \qquad (24.4)$$

where I_{ref} and I_{bone} are the UTE signal intensities of reference phantom and cortical bone, respectively. The MR properties of the reference phantom, including ρ_{ref} and $T_{2,ref}^*$, are known. The T_1 of bone is measured with the saturation recovery prepared UTE (SR-UTE) sequence [12].

The reference phantom (10% H_2O in D_2O doped with 27 mmol/L $MnCl_2$) has a similar T_2^* to cortical bone (i.e., ~300 μs). As can be seen in Figs. 24.1b, d, f, the phantom was placed close to the cortical bone during MR imaging [4]. Signals from both the phantom and cortical bone were detected in the UTE images shown in Figs. 24.1b, d, f, while no signals were detected with the GRE sequence in the phantom or cortical bone (Figs. 24.1a, c, e). Three groups of female subjects were recruited in this study, including two healthy cohorts with respective age ranges of 20–40 years (premenopausal) and 60–80 years (postmenopausal), as well as one patient group (age range of 40–60 years) with renal osteodystrophy (ROD). Figure 24.1g, h shows the scatterplots of bone water PD and bone mineral density (BMD) measurements from these three groups. The bone water PD of the postmenopausal group is much higher than that of the premenopausal group. Moreover, the ROD patient group showed significantly higher bone water PDs than the pre-

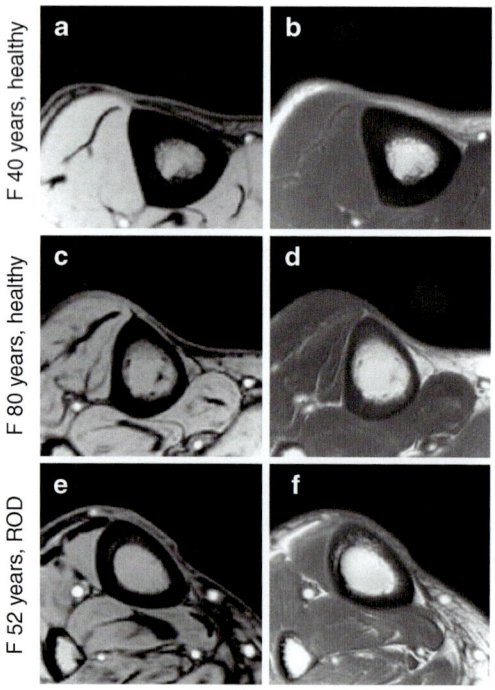

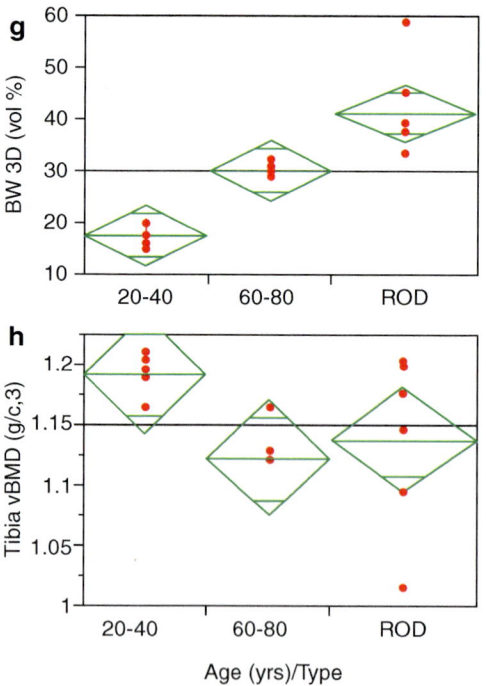

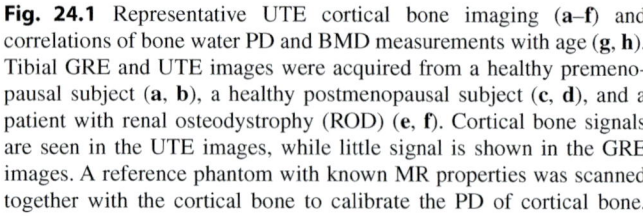

Fig. 24.1 Representative UTE cortical bone imaging (**a–f**) and correlations of bone water PD and BMD measurements with age (**g**, **h**). Tibial GRE and UTE images were acquired from a healthy premenopausal subject (**a**, **b**), a healthy postmenopausal subject (**c**, **d**), and a patient with renal osteodystrophy (ROD) (**e**, **f**). Cortical bone signals are seen in the UTE images, while little signal is shown in the GRE images. A reference phantom with known MR properties was scanned together with the cortical bone to calibrate the PD of cortical bone.

Cortical bone PD increases from the premenopausal group to the postmenopausal group and further increases in the ROD patient group (**g**). BMD decreased from the premenopausal group to the postmenopausal group and to the ROD patient group, while no significant difference was found between the postmenopausal group and ROD patient group (**h**). (Reproduced with permission from Ref. [4])

Fig. 24.2 Flow diagram of image post-processing and bone water PD quantification for in vivo human cortical bone. (Reproduced with permission from Ref. [13])

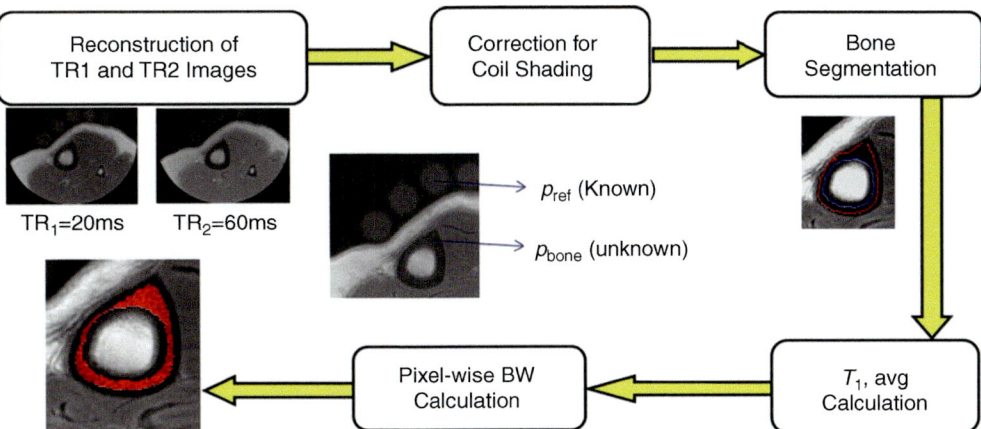

menopausal and postmenopausal groups. However, the areal BMD measured by dual X-ray absorptiometry (DXA) did not show significant differences between the ROD patient group and the postmenopausal group. Though the BMD measurements showed substantial differences between the premenopausal and postmenopausal groups, the changes were much lower (i.e., 38%) than those with bone water PD measurements (i.e., 135%). These results demonstrate the advantage of the UTE bone water PD mapping technique, which has great potential for better clinical evaluation of disease.

T_1 is an important input for accurate bone water PD measurement. However, the SR-UTE T_1 measurement sequence is slow and thus not generally suitable for clinical 3D imaging. Later, the same group as in reference [4] employed a faster 3D T_1 measurement technique that utilized UTE data with two different TRs for T_1 quantification [13]. In each subject, the estimated average T_1 value for bone water PD quantification was used. The data processing procedure is shown in Fig. 24.2. Variation in RF coil sensitivity was corrected for by dividing the 3D UTE signal from bone or the reference phantom by the 3D UTE signal obtained from a separate scan of a homogenous water phantom. This phantom was large enough to cover both the cortical bone and reference phantom regions. The UTE data with a shorter TR (i.e., 20 ms) was utilized for PD quantification using Eqs. (24.1) to (24.4). The cortical bone regions were manually segmented for T_1 averaging and pixel-wise bone water PD mapping.

Bound Water, Pore Water, and Total Water PD Mapping in Cortical Bone

Since the bound water and pore water compartments contribute in different ways to cortical bone biomechanical properties, it is likely to be useful to map both of them.

Bae et al. combined the total water PD measurement (described above) and bicomponent analysis to quantify the PDs of bound water and pore water [14]. Bound water and pore water fractions were estimated by biexponential T_2^* fitting using multi-TE UTE data [11]. Given known total water PDs and the estimated fractions of both water compartments, the PDs of bound water and pore water can be easily calculated. Bone water PDs measured from 44 rectangular bone sample slabs were correlated with μCT porosity and biomechanical properties. As can be seen in Fig. 24.3, total and pore water PDs significantly correlated positively with porosity [14]. Total water PD correlated negatively with failure energy ($R^2 = 0.1$, $p < 0.05$) and ultimate stress ($R^2 = 0.25$, $p < 0.001$). Free water PD correlated negatively with failure strain ($R^2 = 0.14$, $p < 0.05$) and bound water PD correlated negatively with ultimate stress ($R^2 = 0.22$, $p < 0.01$). These results suggest that UTE PD measures for both water compartments are sensitive to the structural and failure properties of cortical bone and may provide a unique way of evaluating cortical bone quality.

Horch et al. proposed another technique to quantify bound water and pore water PDs using adiabatic inversion recovery (AIR), and double adiabatic full-passage (DAFP) prepared UTE sequences [15]. The sequence diagrams are shown in Fig. 24.4a, b. For AIR-UTE imaging, the pore water signal is suppressed using an appropriate inversion time (TI) with the AIR preparation. The bound water signal is then selectively acquired at the pore water nulling time during UTE readout. The bound water signal S_{AIR} is expressed as follows:

$$S_{AIR} \approx$$
$$S_0^{bw} \sin(\theta) \frac{1 - \left(1 - \alpha^{bw}\right) e^{-R_1^{bw} TI} - \alpha^{bw} e^{-R_1^{bw} TR}}{1 - \alpha^{bw} e^{-R_1^{bw} TR} \cos(\theta)} e^{-R_2^{*bw} TE} \quad (24.5)$$

where S_0^{bw} is the bound water PD and θ is the excitation flip angle. R_1^{bw} and R_2^{*bw} are the T_1 and T_2^* ratios of bound

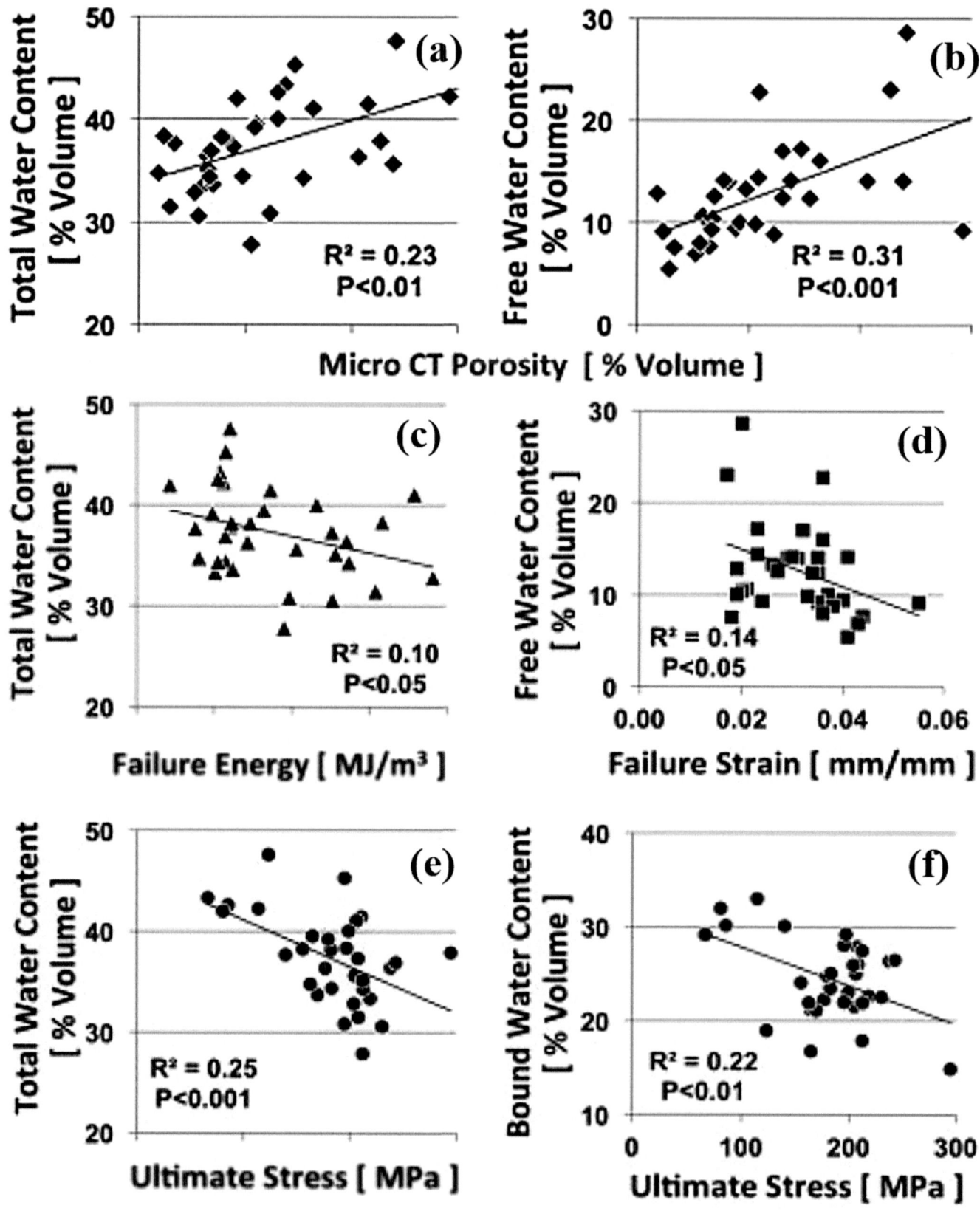

Fig. 24.3 Correlations. Correlations between total water content and μCT porosity (**a**), free water content and μCT porosity (**b**), total water content and failure energy (**c**), free water content and failure strain (**d**), total water content and ultimate stress (**e**), and bound water content and ultimate stress (**f**). (Reproduced with permission from Ref. [14])

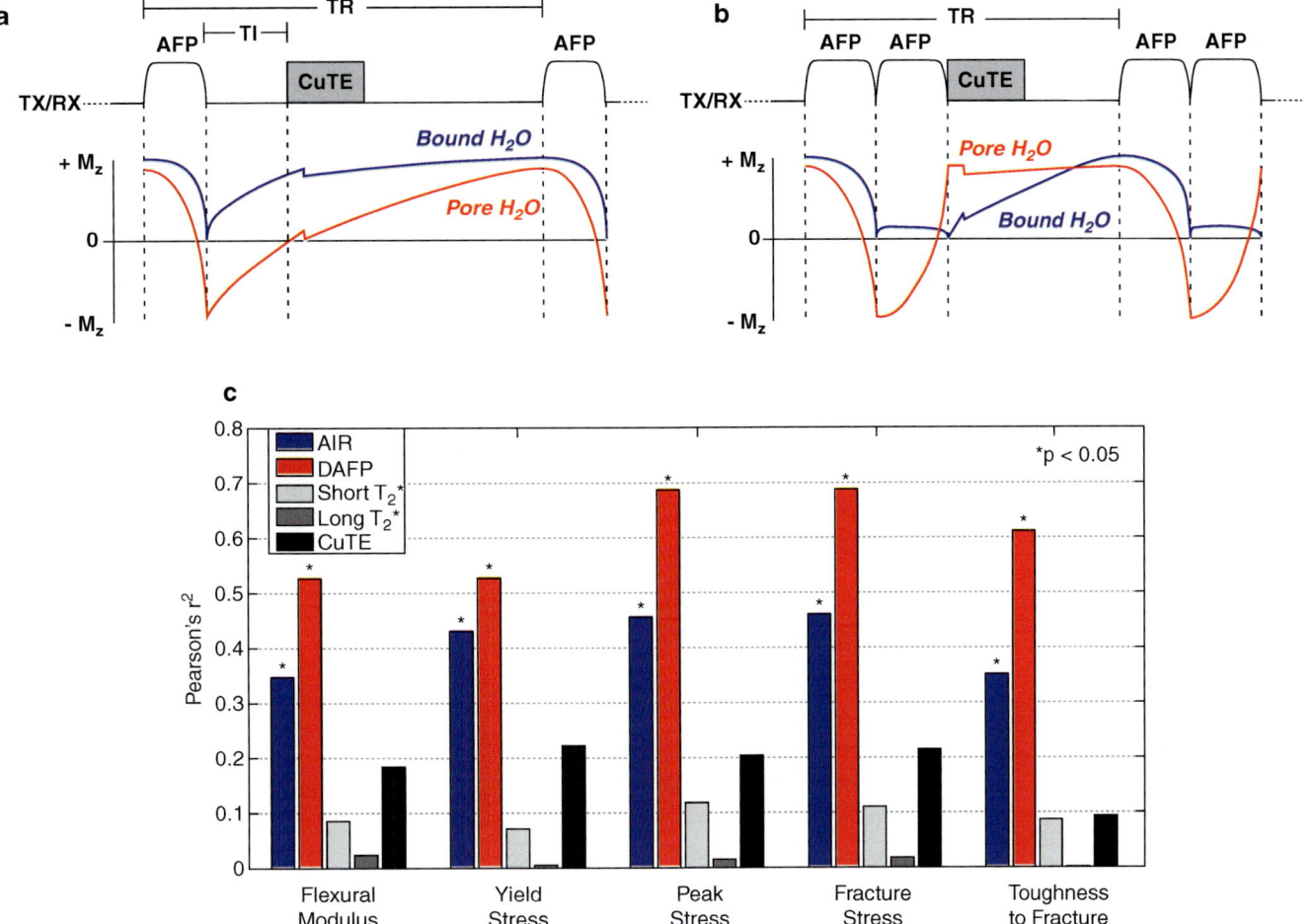

Fig. 24.4 AIR- and DAFP-UTE sequence diagrams (**a, b**) and Pearson correlation coefficients between UTE measurements and biomechanical properties (i.e., flexural modulus, yield stress, peak stress, fracture stress, and toughness to fracture) (**c**). The AIR- and DAFP-UTE measured PDs show significantly higher correlations with all the mechanical properties than either T_2^* measured by bicomponent analysis, or total water PD measured by regular UTE imaging (**c**). (Reproduced with permission from Ref. [15])

water, respectively. α^{bw} is the inversion efficiency representing the change in longitudinal magnetization of bound water caused by the AFP pulse.

According to the numerical simulations, the bound water signals can be efficiently suppressed with DAFP preparation while pore water signals are largely preserved. The pore water signals are acquired immediately after the DAFP preparation. The pore water signal S_{DAFP} is expressed as follows:

$$S_{DAFP} \approx S_0^{pw} \sin(\theta) \frac{\left(\alpha^{bw}\right)^2 e^{-R_1^{pw} TR}}{1 - \left(\alpha^{bw}\right)^2 e^{-R_1^{pw} TR} \cos(\theta)} e^{-R_2^{*pw} TE} \quad (24.6)$$

where S_0^{pw} is the pore water PD, and θ is the excitation flip angle. R_1^{pw} and R_2^{*pw} are the pore water T_1 and T_2^* relaxation rates.

To quantify PDs for both bound water and pore water, a reference phantom with known MR properties is scanned together with the cortical bone. Then the PDs of bound and

pore water components are estimated using a signal ratio similar to Eq. (24.4). Figure 24.4c shows the Pearson correlation coefficients between bone water measures and bone biomechanical properties [15]. The bound water and pore water PDs measured by the AIR- and DAFP-UTE sequences have higher correlations with bone biomechanical properties, including flexural modulus, yield stress, peak stress, fracture stress, and toughness to fracture, than T_2^*s measured by bicomponent analysis and total water PD measured by regular UTE sequence. Only the correlations of the AIR- and DAFP-UTE measurements had statistical significance ($p < 0.05$). These results demonstrate the clinical value of the bound water and pore water PDs measured by the AIR- and DAFP-UTE sequences.

Manhard et al. further investigated the feasibility of translating AIR- and DAFP-UTE-based bone water PD measurements techniques in vivo studies on a clinical 3T scanner [16]. The lower leg and wrist of five healthy volunteers were scanned three times. Figure 24.5a shows representative

Fig. 24.5 Representative cortical bone PD measurements for the tibia and radius (**a**), and PD measurement comparisons for 2D and 3D UTE sequences (**b**). Pore water (upper three rows in **a**) and bound water (lower three rows in **a**) PD maps show excellent consistency in three repeated studies. Similar contrast can be seen in 2D and 3D AIR- and DAFP-UTE images (upper two rows in **b**), and consistent PD measurements are achieved for 2D and 3D UTE techniques (lower two rows in **b**). (Reproduced with permission from Ref. [16])

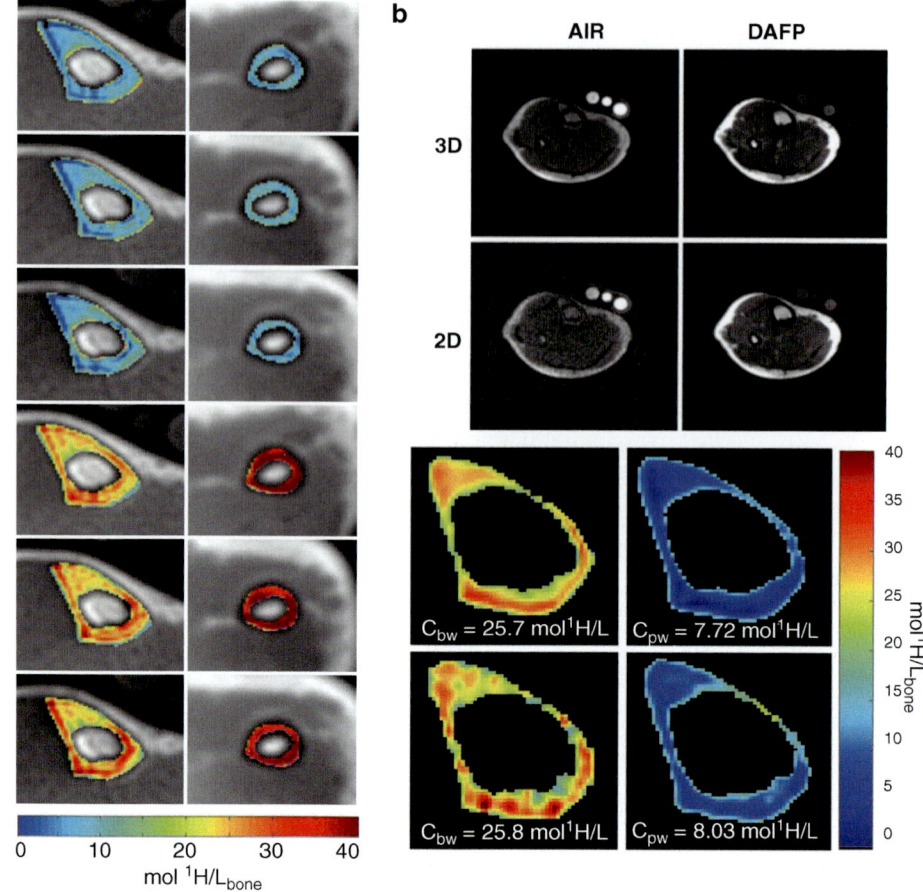

bound and pore water PD maps for the tibia and radius. Similar PD measures can be seen for the three repeated studies, demonstrating excellent sequence reproducibility for both the AIR- and the DAFP-UTE sequences. The same group also developed a fast 2D imaging protocol for bound water and pore water PD measurements on a 3T clinical scanner [17]. The 30s 2D scans show results comparable with the 3D scans which took a much longer scan time of ~14 min. Figure 24.5b shows similar contrast between 2D and 3D scans for both the AIR- and the DAFP-UTE sequences, though the 2D UTE images show a slightly lower signal-to-noise ratio. Minor PD measurement differences were found between the 2D and 3D techniques (bound water PD: 25.7 vs. 25.8 mol/L and pore water PD: 7.72 vs. 8.03 mol/L). These results demonstrate the potential of 2D fast bone water PD quantification for clinical use.

Water and Collagen PD Mapping in Cortical Bone

UTE sequences can detect bound and pore water signals in bone [11], but they cannot be utilized for collagen imaging due to the relatively long effective TE of current UTE

sequences compared to the super short-T_2 of collagen protons ($\approx 10\,\mu s$) [7]. The collagen matrix, one of the essential components of bone, provides tensile strength and elasticity and thus contributes significantly to the mechanical properties of bone [18]. Quantifying collagen matrix may, therefore, provide valuable information about bone quality.

Recently, Ma et al. have developed a UTE-based two-pool magnetization transfer (MT) modeling technique to quantify macromolecular fraction (MMF) in cortical bone [19, 20]. With this technique, the collagen matrix can be accessed indirectly. Saeed et al. further combined UTE-MT modeling and water mapping techniques to quantify cortical bone collagen and water PDs [18, 21]. This technique provides a biomarker panel for the evaluation of bone quality, including mapping of bound water, pore water, total water, and collagen PDs [18]. Similar to previous water PD imaging studies, a reference phantom with known MR properties is scanned together with the cortical bone. The bound water PD is quantified with the AIR-UTE technique [15], and total water PD is quantified with a regular UTE imaging technique [4]. A series of UTE-MT datasets with different MT powers and frequency offsets are acquired for UTE-MT modeling to estimate MMF values in cortical bone [18]. With known

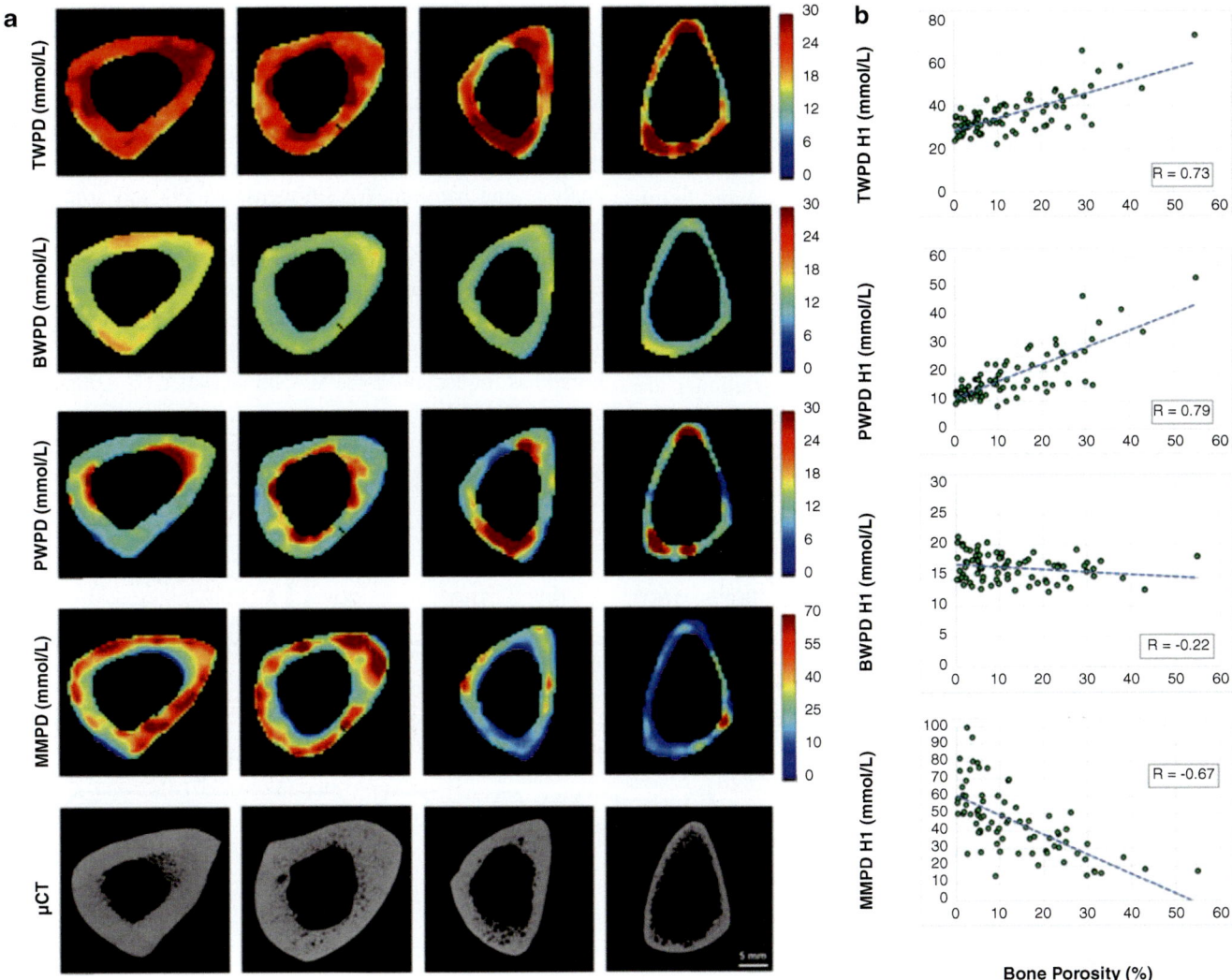

Fig. 24.6 Representative PD maps for total water, bound water, pore water, and macromolecular PD (MMPD) from four cortical bone samples (**a**) and correlation curves between PD values and bone porosity (**b**). Total water, pore water, and macromolecular proton PDs show strong correlations with bone porosity with Rs not less than 0.65. (Reproduced with permission from Ref. [18])

bound water, total water PDs, and MMF, the pore water PD and macromolecular PD (MMPD) can easily be calculated. Figure 24.6a shows representative PD maps for four human bone samples from donors of different ages and the corresponding μCT images for comparison. The total water and pore water PDs show positive correlations with μCT-measured BMD, while bound water PD and MMPD show negative correlations with BMD (Fig. 24.6b). All correlations were statistically significant, but total water and pore water PDs and MMPF have much higher correlations than bound water PD. As expected, pore water showed the highest correlation with bone porosity. Conversely, BWPD and

MMPD were lower for the old group compared with the young group in the ex vivo study. In vivo imaging was also performed in this study, and excellent reproducibility was found with this protocol. This study demonstrated the feasibility of clinical translation for the comprehensive UTE PD mapping protocol. Moreover, ten young and five elderly healthy subjects were scanned for bone PD mapping [18]. On average, total and pore water PDs and MMPF showed significant differences between the two cohorts. The PDs of all the major proton pools in the cortical bone were quantified with this protocol. Future patient studies will be necessary to establish the clinical value of this technique.

Water- and Fat-Suppressed Proton Projection MRI (WASPI)

Wu et al. proposed a special version of the UTE sequence to selectively image short-T_2 components in the bone while suppressing signals from both free water and fat [22–24]. As can be seen in Fig. 24.7a, low-power chemical-selective pulses are utilized for free water and fat signal suppression [22]. These pulses are relatively long and do not saturate short-T_2 components in bone. After the long-T_2 signal saturation module, short-T_2 signals are acquired with a zero echo time (ZTE)-type acquisition scheme. In this ZTE acquisition, readout gradients are turned on before signal excitation, so the gradient encoding can begin simultaneously with signal excitation to minimize TE.

Three pellet phantoms were made with polymer densities of 0.56, 0.80, and 1.17 g/cm^3, respectively, to calibrate the WASPI signals. The PD of short-T_2 components in bone is estimated by signal calibration according to the correlation curve between WASPI signal and polymer pellet density. Figure 24.7b shows the correlations between WASPI-measured PD and gravimetric analysis and between WASPI-measured PD and amino acid analysis for three pieces of cortical bone, eight pieces of trabecular bone, and five bone/glass mixture specimens [23]. Excellent correlations were found between WASPI-measured PDs and both analysis results which demonstrated the accuracy of short-T_2 PD quantification by WASPI. Furthermore, the same group has implemented the WASPI sequence on a clinical 3T scanner. WASPI efficiently suppresses both long-T_2 water and marrow fat signals, and excellent bone contrast can be seen on WASPI images.

Fig. 24.7 Diagram of the WASPI sequence (**a**) and correlations between PDs measured by WASPI and bone matrix density measured by gravimetric (**b**) and amino acid (**c**). Chemical-selective long RF pulses suppress free water and fat signals in WASPI, and this is followed by ZTE-type acquisitions. Excellent correlations are shown between WASPI-measured PDs and gravimetric and amino acid-measured bone matrix density with R^2s ≥ 0.95. (Reproduced with permission from Ref. [22])

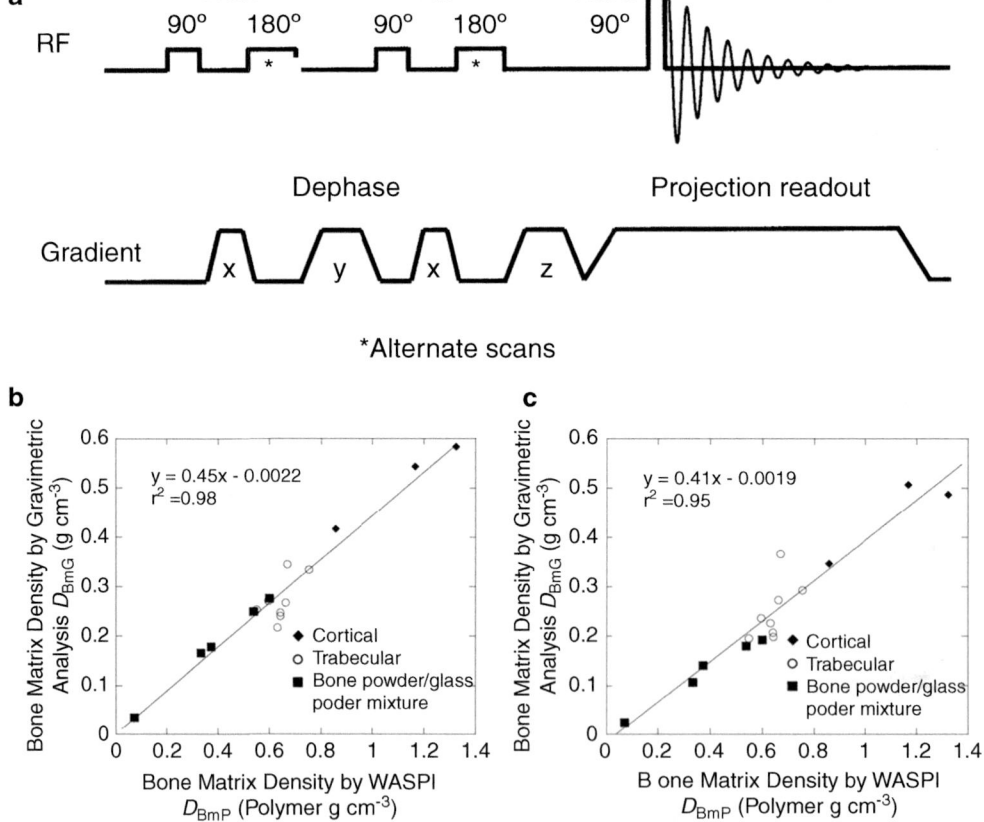

Bound Water PD Mapping in Trabecular Bone

Bone collagen matrix can be accessed by quantifying bound water content in bone. However, bound water imaging in trabecular bone is very challenging because trabecular bone has a much lower PD than cortical bone. A high concentration of long-T_2 components, including marrow fat and free water in trabecular bone, also makes efficient long-T_2 signal suppression more difficult. Ma et al. have recently proposed a short TR adiabatic inversion recovery prepared UTE (STAIR-UTE) sequence for high contrast bound water imaging of trabecular bone with excellent suppression of all long-T_2 components [6]. Then, bound water PD is quantified using a method similar to AIR-UTE described above [15].

The major difference between the STAIR-UTE and AIR-UTE sequences is that the TR of the STAIR-UTE sequence is much shorter. Numerical simulations suggested that the shorter TR used in STAIR-UTE, the better the long-T_2 signal suppression that is achieved [6]. The shortest TR in STAIR-UTE is typically limited by the maximum allowed RF heating (i.e., a SAR issue). For spine and hip imaging, a TR of 150 ms was used in the STAIR-UTE protocol. The T_2^* of a vertebra was measured by the single exponential fitting of multi-TE STAIR-UTE data. The estimated T_2^* was around 0.3 ms, close to the bound water T_2^* in cortical bone. This demonstrates that long-T_2 components around trabecular bone are well suppressed.

Figure 24.8 shows representative STAIR-UTE images of the lumbar spine in a healthy volunteer. Compared to the clinical T_2-weighted FSE image, the soft tissue signals in the spine are largely suppressed in the STAIR-UTE images. Due to the inhomogeneous coil sensitivity distribution of the spine array coil, the STAIR-UTE image with no coil sensitivity correction suffers from spatial signal variations. To generate a coil sensitivity profile for the spine coil, two sets of data are acquired with a fast regular UTE sequence using spine and body coils for the reception. The coil sensitivity profile is estimated from the STAIR-UTE signal ratio between the spine coil image and the body coil image. After coil sensitivity correction, the STAIR-UTE images are more uniform. A rubber band with known MR properties was placed under the back of the volunteer and scanned together with the volunteer during the MR imaging. The bound water PD in the vertebra was calculated from the signal ratio between trabecular bone and rubber band. Liu et al. further applied this STAIR-UTE PD mapping technique to evaluate osteoporosis [25]. As can be seen in Fig. 24.9, the STAIR-UTE measured PDs in vertebra decrease with lower BMDs measured by quantitative CT and DXA. Excellent correlations were found between measured PDs and BMDs. This demonstrates that the STAIR-UTE-measured PDs may be a good surrogate for CT and not require the use of ionizing radiation.

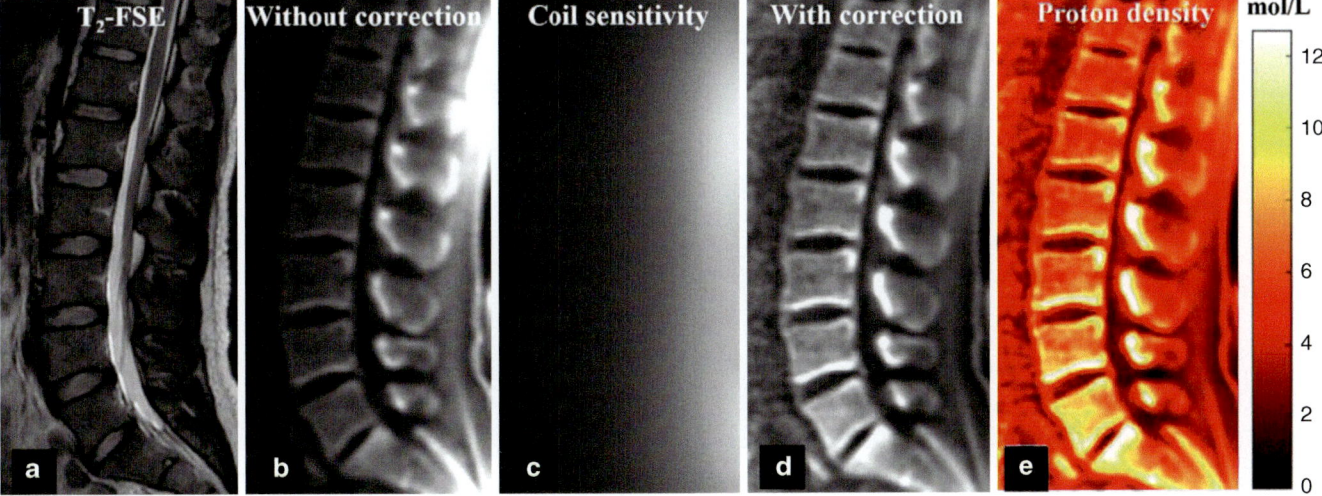

Fig. 24.8 Representative STAIR-UTE imaging of the lumbar spine in a healthy volunteer. Soft tissue signals are well suppressed in the STAIR-UTE image (**b**) compared to the clinical T_2-FSE image (**a**). Coil sensitivity profile (**c**) is utilized to correct the signal variations in trabecular bone, and the trabecular bone signal is more uniform after coil sensitivity correction (**d**). With a rubber band as a reference phantom, the trabecular bone PD map is calculated using a similar method as proposed in the AIR-UTE study (**e**). (Reproduced with permission from Ref. [6])

Fig. 24.9 Representative quantitative CT-measured BMD (first column), DXA measured T score (second column), and STAIR-UTE measured PD (last column) maps of the lumbar spine in three subjects with normal bone mass (50-year-old male) (**a**), osteopenia (54-year-old female) (**b**), and osteoporosis (66-year-old male) (**c**), respectively. As can be seen, BMD, T score, and PD values all decrease from subject (**a**) to (**c**). (Reproduced with permission from Ref. [25])

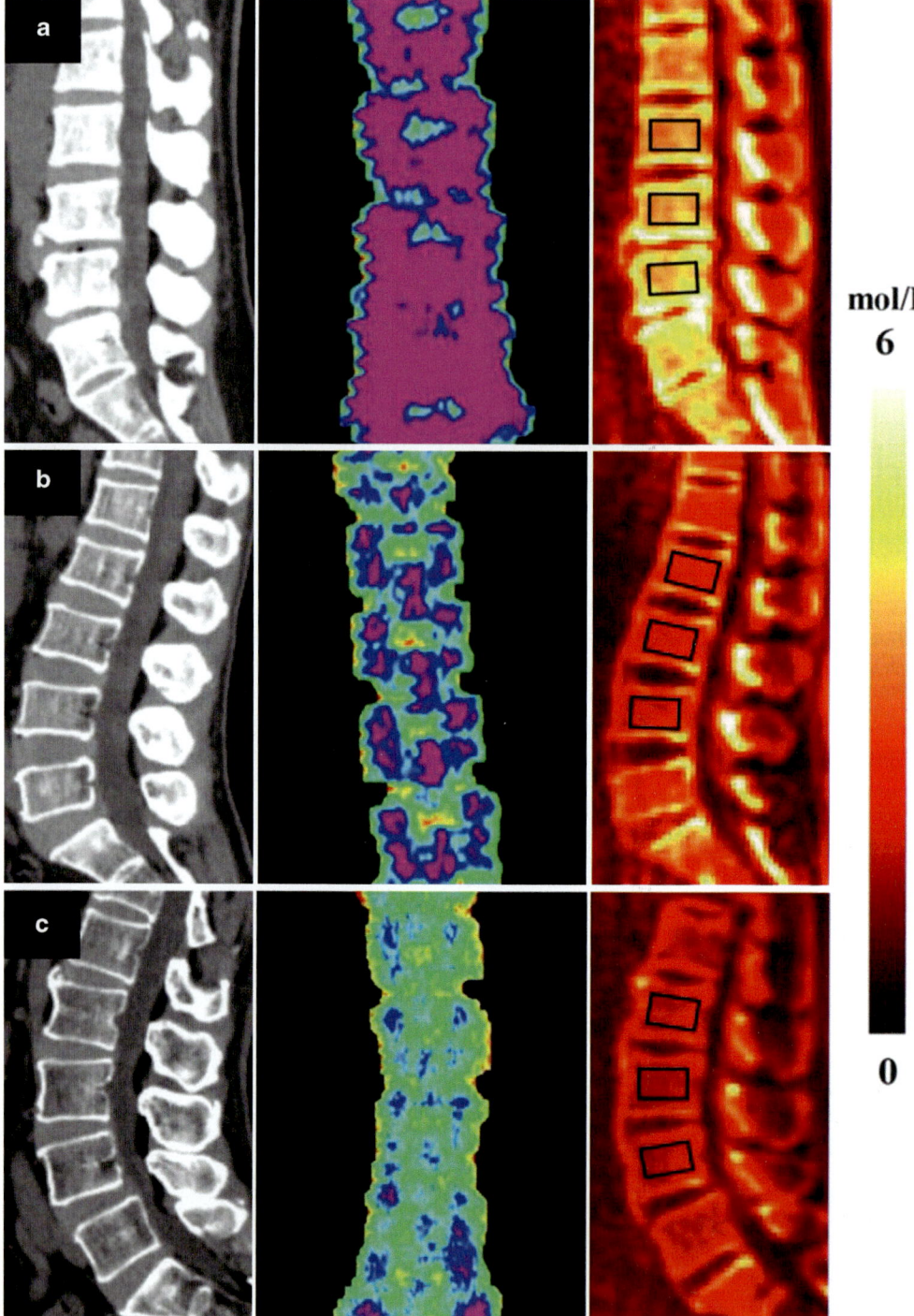

Myelin PD Mapping in Brain

In addition to PD mapping in cortical or trabecular bone, UTE PD mapping can also be applied to ultrashort-T_2 myelin quantification in the brain to evaluate demyelination in multiple sclerosis (MS) [5, 26, 27]. Like bone-bound water imaging, an IR-UTE sequence is utilized to suppress the long-T_2 water components in the brain and selectively image ultrashort-T_2 myelin.

To investigate whether the UTE sequence can capture short-T_2 signals from the semisolid myelin lipids and proteins, purified bovine myelin extracts of different concentrations were suspended in D_2O and were imaged using an IR-UTE sequence (Fig. 24.10a) [27]. An excellent linear correlation was found between the myelin density and IR-UTE signals. This demonstrates that the IR-UTE sequence can capture ultrashort-T_2 signals from myelin. Seifert et al. have applied the IR-UTE sequence for PD mapping of the ovine

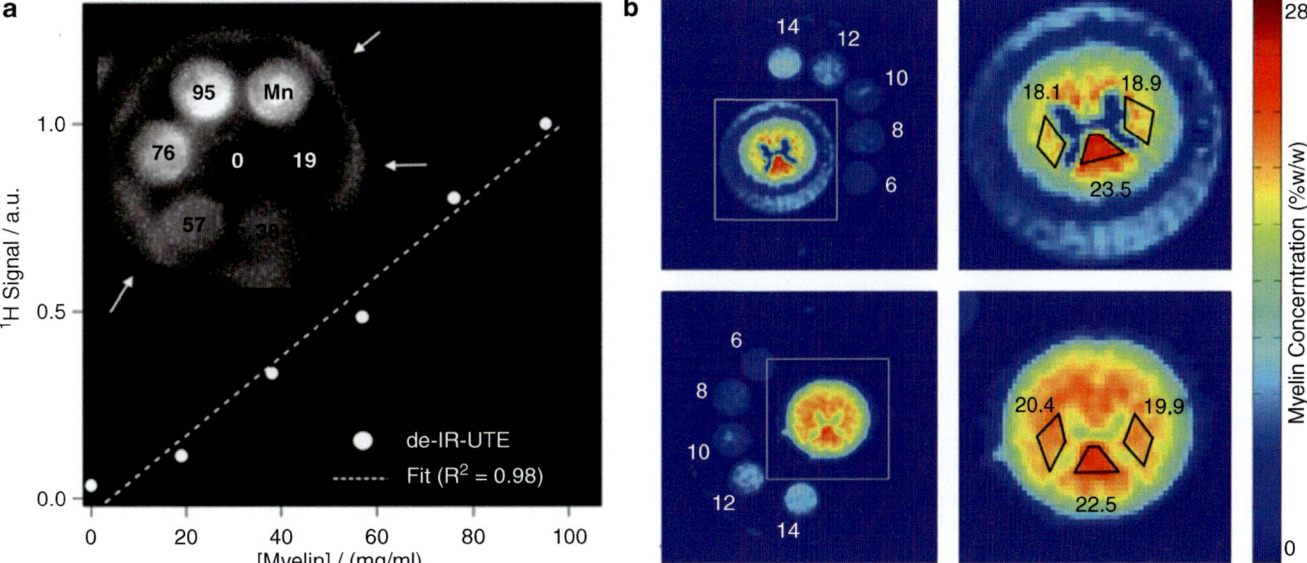

Fig. 24.10 Linear correlation between IR-UTE signals and myelin densities (**a**) and PD measurements for spinal cord with and without D_2O exchange (**b**). Myelin phantoms are made from purified bovine myelin extracts suspended in D_2O at six different concentrations. A strong linear correlation was found between IR-UTE signals and myelin densities with $R^2 = 0.98$. Comparable myelin PD maps are found between the spinal cord samples with and without D_2O exchange. (Reproduced with permission from Ref. [27])

spinal cord before and after D_2O exchange [28]. The PDs of spinal cords were determined by the calibration curves between the known concentration of myelin phantoms and the corresponding IR-UTE signals (Fig. 24.10b). The D_2O exchanged spinal cord has a very low water concentration and thus provides a good reference standard to validate whether IR preparation suppresses the water content effectively in the fresh cord samples. The PDs measured for the two samples were comparable, demonstrating the feasibility of PD mapping of myelin in translational studies.

Ma et al. further applied the STAIR-UTE sequence to whole-brain myelin mapping [5]. As mentioned in the trabecular bone imaging section, the STAIR-UTE sequence can suppress tissue signals with a wide range of T_1s. This allows robust water signal suppression in the whole brain and, thus, selective myelin imaging. The shortest TR that could be applied in STAIR-UTE acquisition for in vivo brain myelin imaging was 140 ms. The study recruited and scanned ten healthy volunteers and patients with MS. Significantly lower myelin PDs were found in both MS lesions and normal-appearing white matter regions in MS patients compared to normal white matter regions in healthy brains. This study demonstrated the clinical potential of quantitative PD mapping of myelin to evaluate MS and other demyelinating diseases.

Conclusion

This chapter has summarized the UTE PD mapping techniques applied to cortical bone, trabecular bone, and brain myelin imaging. The cortical bone studies have shown that the measured PDs for different proton pools correlate well with porosity and bone biomechanical properties. The trabecular bone study has demonstrated that bound water PD is a promising surrogate for BMD measured with quantitative CT or DXA for clinically evaluating osteoporosis. Current UTE myelin PD mapping techniques have shown clinical potential, though further studies will be needed to establish their clinical value.

References

1. Nitz WR, Reimer P. Contrast mechanisms in MR imaging. Eur Radiol. 1999;9(6):1032–46.
2. Abbas Z, Gras V, Möllenhoff K, Keil F, Oros-Peusquens A-M, Shah NJ. Analysis of proton-density bias corrections based on T_1 measurement for robust quantification of water content in the brain at 3 Tesla. Magn Reson Med. 2014;72(6):1735–45.
3. Mezer A, Rokem A, Berman S, Hastie T, Wandell BA. Evaluating quantitative proton-density-mapping methods. Hum Brain Mapp. 2016;37(10):3623–35.

4. Techawiboonwong A, Song HK, Leonard MB, Wehrli FW. Cortical bone water: in vivo quantification with ultrashort echo-time MR imaging. Radiology. 2008;248(3):824–33.

5. Ma Y-J, Jang H, Wei Z, et al. Myelin imaging in human brain using a short repetition time adiabatic inversion recovery prepared ultrashort echo time (STAIR-UTE) MRI sequence in multiple sclerosis. Radiology. 2020;297(2):392–404.

6. Ma Y-J, Chen Y, Li L, et al. Trabecular bone imaging using a 3D adiabatic inversion recovery prepared ultrashort TE cones sequence at 3T. Magn Reson Med. 2020;83(5):1640–51.

7. Ma Y-J, Chang EY, Bydder GM, Du J. Can ultrashort-TE (UTE) MRI sequences on a 3-T clinical scanner detect signal directly from collagen protons: freeze-dry and D_2O exchange studies of cortical bone and Achilles tendon specimens. NMR Biomed. 2016;29(7):912–7.

8. Li C, Seifert AC, Rad HS, et al. Cortical bone water concentration: dependence of MR imaging measures on age and pore volume fraction. Radiology. 2014;272(3):796–806.

9. Abbasi-Rad S, Saligheh RH. Quantification of human cortical bone bound and free water in vivo with ultrashort echo time MR imaging: a model-based approach. Radiology. 2017;283(3):862–72.

10. Afsahi AM, Ma Y, Jang H, et al. Ultrashort echo time magnetic resonance imaging techniques: met and unmet needs in musculoskeletal imaging. J Magn Reson Imaging. 2022;55(6):1597–612.

11. Du J, Diaz E, Carl M, Bae W, Chung CB, Bydder GM. Ultrashort echo time imaging with bicomponent analysis. Magn Reson Med. 2012;67(3):645–9.

12. Zhao X, Song HK, Wehrli FW. In vivo bone ^{31}P relaxation times and their implications on mineral quantification. Magn Reson Med. 2018;80(6):2514–24.

13. Rad HS, Lam SCB, Magland JF, et al. Quantifying cortical bone water in vivo by three-dimensional ultra-short echo-time MRI. NMR Biomed. 2011;24(7):855–64.

14. Bae WC, Chen PC, Chung CB, Masuda K, D'Lima D, Du J. Quantitative ultrashort echo time (UTE) MRI of human cortical bone: correlation with porosity and biomechanical properties. J Bone Miner Res. 2012;27(4):848–57.

15. Horch RA, Gochberg DF, Nyman JS, Does MD. Clinically compatible MRI strategies for discriminating bound and pore water in cortical bone. Magn Reson Med. 2012;68(6):1774–84.

16. Manhard MK, Horch RA, Gochberg DF, Nyman JS, Does MD. In vivo quantitative MR imaging of bound and pore water in cortical bone. Radiology. 2015;277(1):221–9.

17. Manhard MK, Harkins KD, Gochberg DF, Nyman JS, Does MD. 30-Second bound and pore water concentration mapping of cortical bone using 2D UTE with optimized half-pulses. Magn Reson Med. 2017;77(3):945–50.

18. Jerban S, Ma Y, Li L, et al. Volumetric mapping of bound and pore water as well as collagen protons in cortical bone using 3D ultrashort echo time cones MR imaging techniques. Bone. 2019;127:120–8.

19. Ma Y-J, Tadros A, Du J, Chang EY. Quantitative two-dimensional ultrashort echo time magnetization transfer (2D UTE-MT) imaging of cortical bone. Magn Reson Med. 2018;79(4):1941–9.

20. Ma Y, Carl M, Chang EY, Du J. Quantitative magnetization transfer ultrashort echo time imaging using a time-efficient 3D multispoke cones sequence. Magn Reson Med. 2018;79(2):692–700.

21. Jerban S, Ma Y, Nazaran A, et al. Detecting stress injury (fatigue fracture) in fibular cortical bone using quantitative ultrashort echo time-magnetization transfer (UTE-MT): an ex vivo study. NMR Biomed. 2018;31(11):e3994.

22. Wu Y, Ackerman JL, Chesler DA, Graham L, Wang Y, Glimcher MJ. Density of organic matrix of native mineralized bone measured by water- and fat-suppressed proton projection MRI. Magn Reson Med. 2003;50(1):59–68.

23. Cao H, Ackerman JL, Hrovat MI, Graham L, Glimcher MJ, Wu Y. Quantitative bone matrix density measurement by water-and fat-suppressed proton projection MRI (WASPI) with polymer calibration phantoms. Magn Reson Med. 2008;60(6):1433–43.

24. Wu Y, Hrovat MI, Ackerman JL, et al. Bone matrix imaged in vivo by water-and fat-suppressed proton projection MRI (WASPI) of animal and human subjects. J Magn Reson Imaging. 2010;31(4):954–63.

25. Liu J, Liao J-W, Li W, et al. Assessment of osteoporosis in lumbar spine: in vivo quantitative MR imaging of collagen bound water in trabecular bone. Front Endocrinol (Lausanne). 2022;13:801930.

26. Ma YJ, Searleman AC, Jang H, et al. Whole-brain myelin imaging using 3D double-echo sliding inversion recovery ultrashort echo time (DESIRE-UTE) MRI. Radiology. 2020;294(2):362–74.

27. Wilhelm MJ, Ong HH, Wehrli SL, et al. Direct magnetic resonance detection of myelin and prospects for quantitative imaging of myelin density. Proc Natl Acad Sci U S A. 2012;109(24):9605–10.

28. Seifert AC, Li C, Wilhelm MJ, Wehrli SL, Wehrli FW. Towards quantification of myelin by solid-state MRI of the lipid matrix protons. NeuroImage. 2017;163:358–67.

Yajun Ma, Saeed Jerban, Hyungseok Jang, Xing Lu,
Eric Y. Chang, and Jiang Du

Introduction

Magnetization transfer (MT) in MRI describes the exchange of magnetization between different proton pools, such as between free water and macromolecular proton pools [1]. Like tissue relaxation times, the MT effect is an important phenomenon in MRI which produces specific image contrast related to macromolecular density and integrity [1, 2].

Proton MRI typically detects signals from only those protons that are mobile, such as water protons. The motion of semisolid protons is more restricted, leading to a much broader spectrum than that of mobile protons [3]. The transverse magnetizations of semisolid protons dephase too quickly (with T_2s around ten μs) to be detected by typical MR scanners [1, 4]; however, MT sequences can evaluate semisolid tissues indirectly by taking advantage of the magnetization exchange between mobile and less mobile protons.

An overwhelming concentration of water protons in macromolecular abundant tissues, such as cartilage, meniscus, tendon, ligament, and cortical bone, is tightly bound to collagen fibers [5–7], creating bound water pools which have shorter T_2s than free water pools. Ultrashort echo time (UTE) sequences with nominal echo times (TEs) less than 100 μs have been developed to efficiently detect signals from water pools (including both free and bound water) [5–7]. Building on this foundation, sequences combining ultrashort TE (UTE) and MT (i.e., UTE-MT) techniques provide a unique way to access the semisolid proton information from macromolecular abundant tissues [2].

Recently, quantitative UTE-MT imaging techniques, including UTE-MT ratio (UTE-MTR) and UTE-MT modeling, have been developed and applied to imaging tissues in the musculoskeletal and nervous systems [6, 8–10]. In this chapter, we introduce the basic mechanisms underlying the most commonly utilized quantitative UTE-MT techniques in the field and briefly review their applications.

UTE-Magnetization Transfer Ratio (UTE-MTR)

As seen in Fig. 25.1a, many tissues can be regarded as two-pool models: one water pool and one macromolecular pool [1]. Both pools have intrinsic proton densities and relaxation times (i.e., T_1 and T_2) and constantly interact with each other through magnetization exchange. The macromolecular proton pool has a much broader spectrum than the more mobile water proton pool (Fig. 25.1b) [3]. To create MT contrast, an off-resonance radiofrequency (RF) pulse (also called an "MT pulse") is applied to the macromolecular proton pool only. The magnetizations of the macromolecular proton pool experience strong saturation due to their fast signal decay, and these saturated magnetizations exchange with the unsaturated magnetizations present in the water pools. As a result, part of the water magnetization becomes saturated, leading to reduction in the detectable water signal.

A simple way to quantify the MT effect is to measure the signal reduction ratio using the following equation for the MT ratio (MTR):

Y. Ma (✉) · S. Jerban · H. Jang · X. Lu
Department of Radiology, University of California, San Diego, La Jolla, CA, USA
e-mail: yam013@ucsd.edu; sjerban@health.ucsd.edu; h4jang@health.ucsd.edu; xil135@health.ucsd.edu

E. Y. Chang
Department of Radiology, University of California, San Diego, La Jolla, CA, USA

VA San Diego Healthcare System, San Diego, CA, USA
e-mail: e8chang@health.ucsd.edu

J. Du
Department of Radiology, University of California, San Diego, La Jolla, CA, USA

VA San Diego Healthcare System, San Diego, CA, USA

Department of Bioengineering, University of California, San Diego, La Jolla, CA, USA
e-mail: jiangdu@health.ucsd.edu

J. Du, G. M. Bydder (eds.), *MRI of Short- and Ultrashort-T₂ Tissues*, https://doi.org/10.1007/978-3-031-35197-6_25

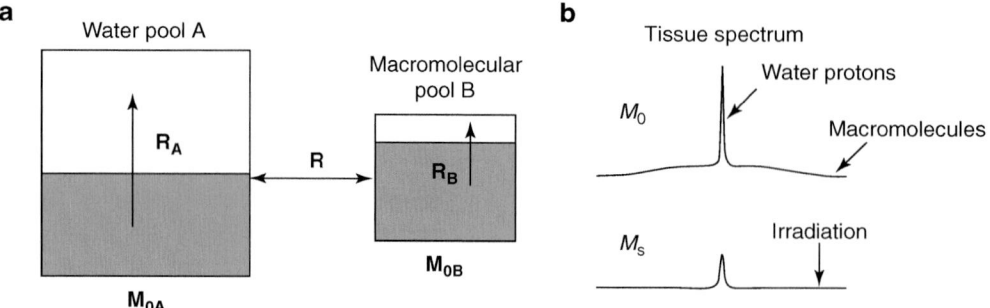

Fig. 25.1 A diagram of the two-pool MT model (**a**) consisting of water and macromolecular pools. Each pool has its intrinsic proton density and relaxation times, and the respective magnetizations of the two pools are in constant exchange. The linewidth of the macromolecular pool is much broader than that of the water pool (**b**). When an off-resonance RF pulse is applied to the macromolecular pool, the water pool signal decreases due to the MT effect. (Reproduced with permission from Refs. [1, 3])

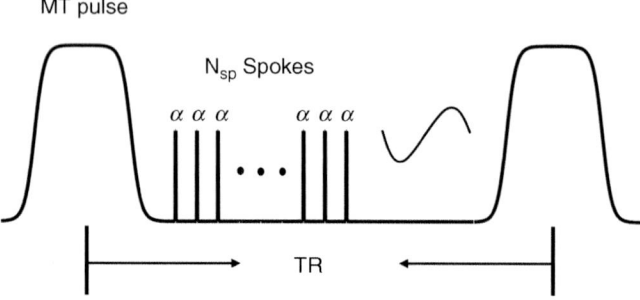

Fig. 25.2 Sequence diagram for the UTE-MT sequence. An off-resonance RF pulse, or "MT pulse," is applied to saturate the magnetizations of the macromolecular pool, followed by N_{sp} UTE spokes for fast data acquisition. (Reproduced with permission from Ref. [11])

$$MTR = \frac{MT_{off} - MT_{on}}{MT_{off}} \qquad (25.1)$$

where MT_{on} and MT_{off} are the signals obtained from images acquired with and without the applied MT pulse. The MTR value is affected by both the flip angle and the off-resonance frequency of the MT pulse. UTE-MT imaging with a higher power (or flip angle) and/or a lower off-resonance frequency for the MT pulse creates stronger MT contrast and, in turn, a higher MTR value.

The sequence diagram for a typical UTE-MT pulse sequence is shown in Fig. 25.2 [11]. During each TR prior to data acquisition, an MT pulse with a Gaussian or Fermi shape is applied to create MT contrast, and this is followed by a series of UTE acquisition spokes. The number of spokes per TR (N_{sp}) for 2D UTE-MT imaging is typically set to one, whereas for 3D UTE-MT imaging, N_{sp} is generally set to five or greater to reduce scan time. In this latter case, the TR should not be too long (ideally less than 150 ms) because the MT contrast is also determined by the average mean power per second of the MT pulse [12].

In one of the very first UTE-MT imaging studies performed, Springer et al. investigated the technical feasibility of UTE-MTR measurement in bovine and human cortical bone using a clinical 3T scanner [8]. Figure 25.3a shows a representative UTE-MTR map of tibial cortical bone from a healthy volunteer. The UTE-MTR values of cortical bone are much higher than those of surrounding soft tissues such as muscle. An in vivo study of three healthy subjects showed an average MTR value of 0.30 ± 0.08 for cortical bone. Chang et al. further investigated the correlations of UTE-MTR with μCT porosity and biomechanical properties in human cortical bone samples (Fig. 25.3b) [13]. A moderate correlation was found between UTE-MTR and μCT porosity with an R^2 value of 0.51, suggesting that collagen content may be related to bone porosity. In pathologic bone, an increase in cortical porosity (and, therefore, pore water) is typically accompanied by a decrease in the organic matrix density. Weak but significant correlations were found between UTE-MTR and Young's modulus ($R^2 = 0.12$) and between UTE-MTR and yield stress ($R^2 = 0.30$), suggesting that UTE-MTR may be a surrogate marker for biomechanical properties of cortical bone.

The UTE-MT technique has also been used to evaluate the biochemical changes in the Achilles tendon of athletes after long-distance running [14]. The UTE-MTR values of the Achilles tendon were measured 1 week pre-marathon race, 2 days post-race, and 4 weeks post-race. Representative UTE-MTR maps at these three time points in a runner are shown in Fig. 25.4a. In most tendon regions, the UTE-MTR values decreased significantly 2 days post-race, then increased significantly after 4 weeks post-race back toward their pre-race value (Fig. 25.4b). Additionally, this study showed excellent sequence reproducibility for UTE-MTR measurement with intraclass correlation coefficients (ICCs) measuring ≥0.896. The authors concluded that UTE-MTR is a promising biomarker for detecting dynamic changes in the Achilles tendon before and after long-distance running.

A recent study also showed that UTE-MTR (TE = 0.076 ms) might be a better biomarker for the presence of demyelination than short TE-based MTR (STE-MTR,

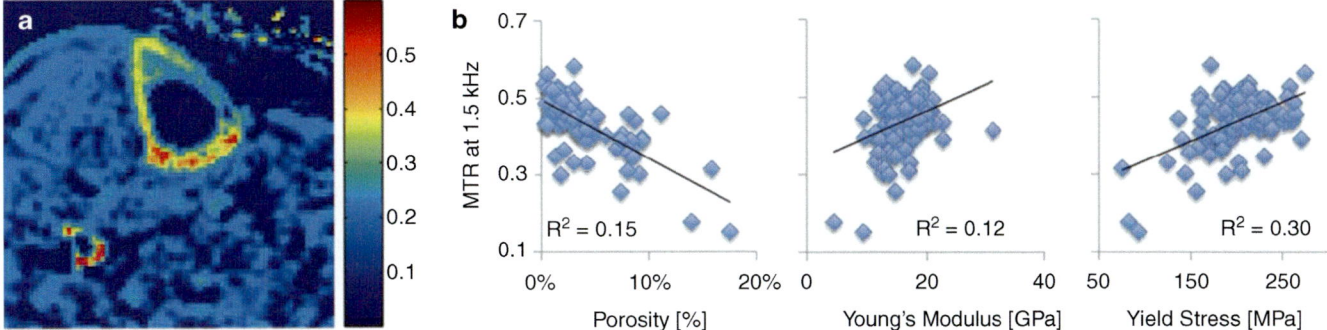

Fig. 25.3 Representative UTE-MTR map of tibial cortical bone from a healthy volunteer (**a**) and correlations between UTE-MTR and bone porosity as well as mechanical properties (**b**). UTE-MTR shows a negative correlation with bone porosity ($R^2 = 0.51$) and positive correlations with Young's Modulus ($R^2 = 0.12$) and yields stress ($R^2 = 0.30$). (Reproduced with permission from Refs. [8, 13])

Fig. 25.4 Representative UTE-MTR maps measured at three time points (i.e., 1 week pre-marathon race (first column), 2 days post-race (second column), and 4 weeks post-race (third column)) for a 43-year-old runner (**a**), and summary plots at these time points for the muscle–tendon junction (MTJ), middle part (MID), and bulk regions of the Achilles tendon (**b**). The UTE-MTR first decreases 2 days post-race, then increases back toward the pre-race value, after 4 weeks rest. (Reproduced with permission from Ref. [14])

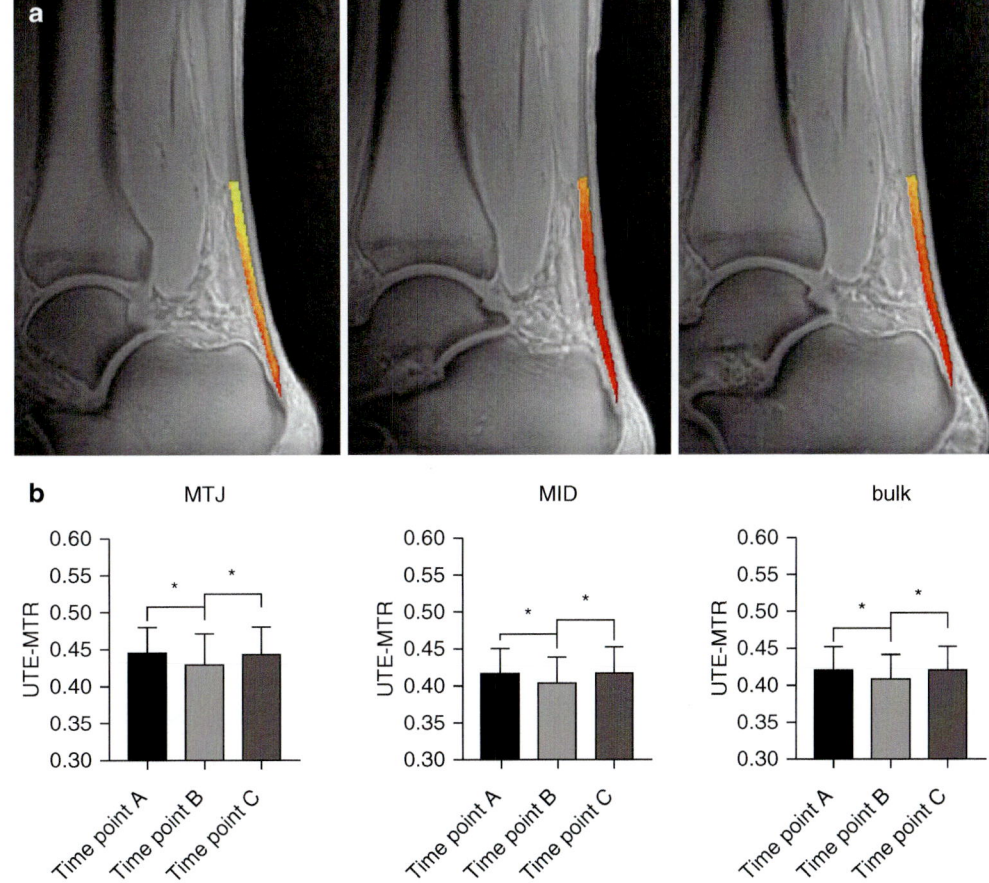

TE = 3 ms) [10]. Representative UTE-MTR and STE-MTR maps obtained from a control mouse brain are shown in Fig. 25.5a. The white matter regions were visible as bright, hyperintense MR signals on the UTE-MTR and STE-MTR maps, but the UTE-MTR map showed higher white matter contrast. A stronger positive correlation was also found between UTE-MTR and myelin basic protein (MBP) content ($R^2 = 0.76$) compared to that between STE-MTR and MBP content ($R^2 = 0.46$) (Fig. 25.5b). In addition, the study found that UTE-MTR allowed detection of cuprizone-induced alterations in multiple white and grey matter regions, including the cerebral cortex, a capability that STE-MTR lacked, suggesting that UTE-MTR may be more sensitive to MT saturation of the myelin and other brain tissues than STE-MTR.

Another interesting brain study utilized the UTE-MT technique for high contrast phase imaging [15]. With UTE acquisition (TE = 0.106 ms), the phase difference between the images with and without MT pulse showed much higher contrast than that with non-UTE acquisitions (TEs = 5 and

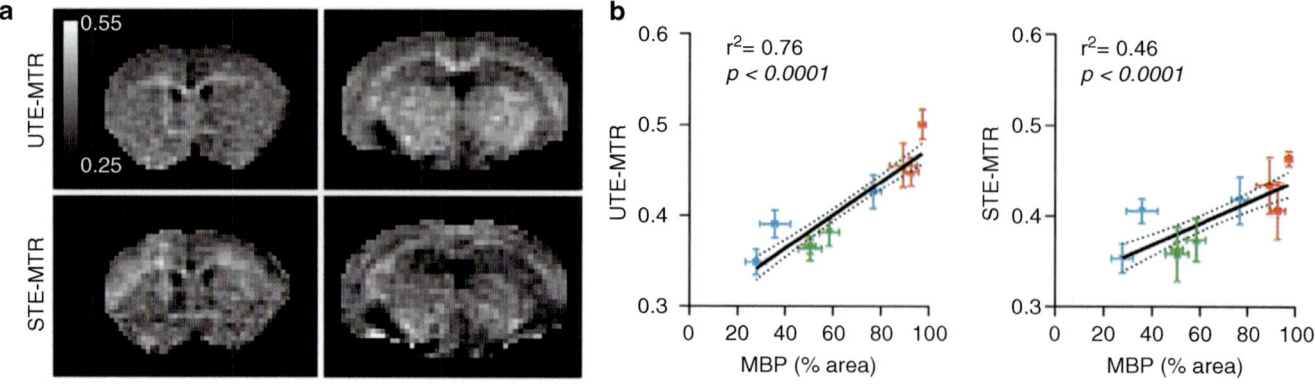

Fig. 25.5 Representative UTE-MTR (first row) and STE-MTR (second row) maps for a control mouse brain (**a**) and correlations between UTE-MTR and MBP (first column) and between STE-MTR and MBP (second column) (**b**). The UTE-MTR maps show better image contrast between white and gray matter and correlate better with MBP content than STE-MTR maps. (Reproduced with permission from Ref. [10])

15 ms). This high phase contrast is probably related to direct and indirect saturation (i.e., an MT effect) of the off-resonance myelin proton pool.

2D UTE-Magnetization Transfer (UTE-MT) Modeling

Although UTE-MTR measurement is a technically simple approach with rapid data acquisition, MTR measurements are inherently semiquantitative and reflect a complex combination of biological parameters (such as T_1 relaxation) and experimental parameters (such as flip angle) [16, 17].

To describe tissue properties more precisely and quantitatively, several quantitative MT models have been proposed since the 1990s [1]. The two-pool model is the most widely used one for quantitative MT analysis. This approach divides the spins within a biological tissue into two pools: (1) a water proton pool (A) and (2) a macromolecular proton pool (B) [4, 12, 18, 19], with each pool having its own longitudinal and transverse relaxation times. Magnetization exchange between the two pools is modeled using a first-order rate constant (R). Henkelman et al. were among the first to incorporate modified Bloch equations into the mathematical description of the MT phenomenon by using non-Lorentzian lineshapes for the macromolecular pool, shown as follows [4]:

$$\frac{dM_z^A}{dt} = R_{1A}\left(M_{0A} - M_z^A\right) - RM_{0B}M_z^A + RM_{0A}M_z^B + w_1 M_y^A \quad (25.2)$$

$$\frac{dM_z^B}{dt} = R_{1B}\left(M_{0B} - M_z^B\right) - RM_{0A}M_z^B + RM_{0B}M_z^A - R_{RFB}\left(w_1, \Delta f\right) M_y^B \quad (25.3)$$

$$\frac{dM_x^A}{dt} = -\frac{M_x^A}{T_{2A}} - 2\pi \Delta f M_y^A \quad (25.4)$$

$$\frac{dM_y^A}{dt} = -\frac{M_y^A}{T_{2A}} + 2\pi \Delta f M_x^A - w_1 M_z^A \quad (25.5)$$

where $M_{0A, 0B}$ are the magnetizations of water (A) and macromolecular (B) proton pools in the equilibrium state, respectively; $M_{x,y,z}^{A,B}$ are the x, y, and z components of the magnetization of water and macromolecular proton pools, respectively; w_1 is the angular frequency of precession induced by the off-resonance MT pulse; Δf is the frequency offset of the MT pulse in Hz; $R_{1A, 1B}$ are the longitudinal rate constants; $T_{2A, 2B}$ are the transverse relaxation times; and R_{RFB} (radiofrequency (RF)) is the rate of loss of longitudinal magnetization of the macromolecular proton pool (B) due to the direct saturation of the MT pulse. This is related to the absorption lineshape $G(2\pi\Delta f)$ of the spins in the macromolecular proton pool and is given by:

$$R_{RFB} = \pi w_1^2 G\left(2\pi \Delta f\right) \quad (25.6)$$

Because the protons in the macromolecular proton pool do not experience the same motional narrowing as the protons in the water proton pool, their spectrum cannot be characterized by a Lorentzian lineshape function and instead have been characterized by alternatives such as Gaussian and super-Lorentzian lineshapes, which have been reported to provide good representations of this proton pool [4, 18]. The Gaussian and super-Lorentzian lineshapes are expressed as $G_G(2\pi\Delta f)$ and $G_{sL}(2\pi\Delta f)$, respectively, where:

$$G_G\left(2\pi \Delta f\right) = \frac{T_{2B}}{\sqrt{2\pi}} \exp\left(-\frac{\left[2\pi \Delta f T_{2B}\right]^2}{2}\right) \quad (25.7)$$

$$G_{sL}\left(2\pi\,\Delta f\right)=\int\limits_{0}^{\pi/2}d\theta\sin\theta\sqrt{\frac{2}{\pi}}\frac{T_{2B}}{\left|3\cos^2\theta-1\right|}$$
$$\exp(-2\left[\frac{2\pi\,\Delta f\,T_{2B}}{\left|3\cos^2\theta-1\right|}\right]^2) \qquad (25.8)$$

where θ is the angle between the B_0 and the axis of molecular orientation.

Henkelman et al. employed a single, long (~5 s), constant amplitude RF pulse to drive the longitudinal magnetization of the system to a steady state and built a continuous wave (CW) power model to solve the Bloch equations [4]. However, due to scan time limitations and concerns regarding specific absorption rate (SAR), the long CW pulse is usually replaced by short Gaussian or Fermi pulses that are distributed throughout the imaging sequence. Ramani et al. modified Henkelman et al.'s CW model by converting the shaped pulse to a rectangular CW pulse with the same mean saturating power in each TR, the so-called "CW power equivalent (CWPE) approximation" [12]. With a known tis-

sue's apparent T_1 (extra measurement) and a fixed T_{1B} (=1), there are a total of five unknown parameters in the CWPE model, including R_{1A}, T_{2A}, T_{2B}, RM_{0A}, and MMF. RM_{0A} is the exchange rate from the macromolecular pool to the water pool, and MMF is the macromolecular proton fraction defined as $M_{0B}/(M_{0A} + M_{0B})$. This means that at least five sets of images with different MT contrasts—either with different flip angles or frequency offsets for the MT pulse—need to be acquired for parameter estimation. The CWPE method has been applied in exploratory and clinical investigations and was initially utilized in brain studies [12, 20].

Recently, Ramani et al.'s CWPE model was successfully applied to 2D UTE-MT imaging and modeling for the assessment of compositional changes in the Achilles tendon and cortical bone [9, 21]. For Achilles tendon imaging, 2D UTE-MT images with four different MT powers and five different frequency offsets were acquired for two-pool MT modeling [9]. As seen in Fig. 25.6a, images with higher MT powers or lower frequency offsets suffer greater signal attenuation in the Achilles tendon. After parameter fitting, a sig-

Fig. 25.6 Representative UTE-MT images of the Achilles tendon in a healthy volunteer with zero MT power (**a**), an MT power of 1400° and a frequency offset of 10 kHz (**b**), and an MT power of 1400° and a frequency offset of 2 kHz (**c**), as well as a scatterplot of MMF measurements vs. age for eight healthy volunteers and a psoriatic arthritis patient (**d**). A significantly lower MMF value was found in the patient compared to the healthy volunteers. (Reproduced with permission from Ref. [9])

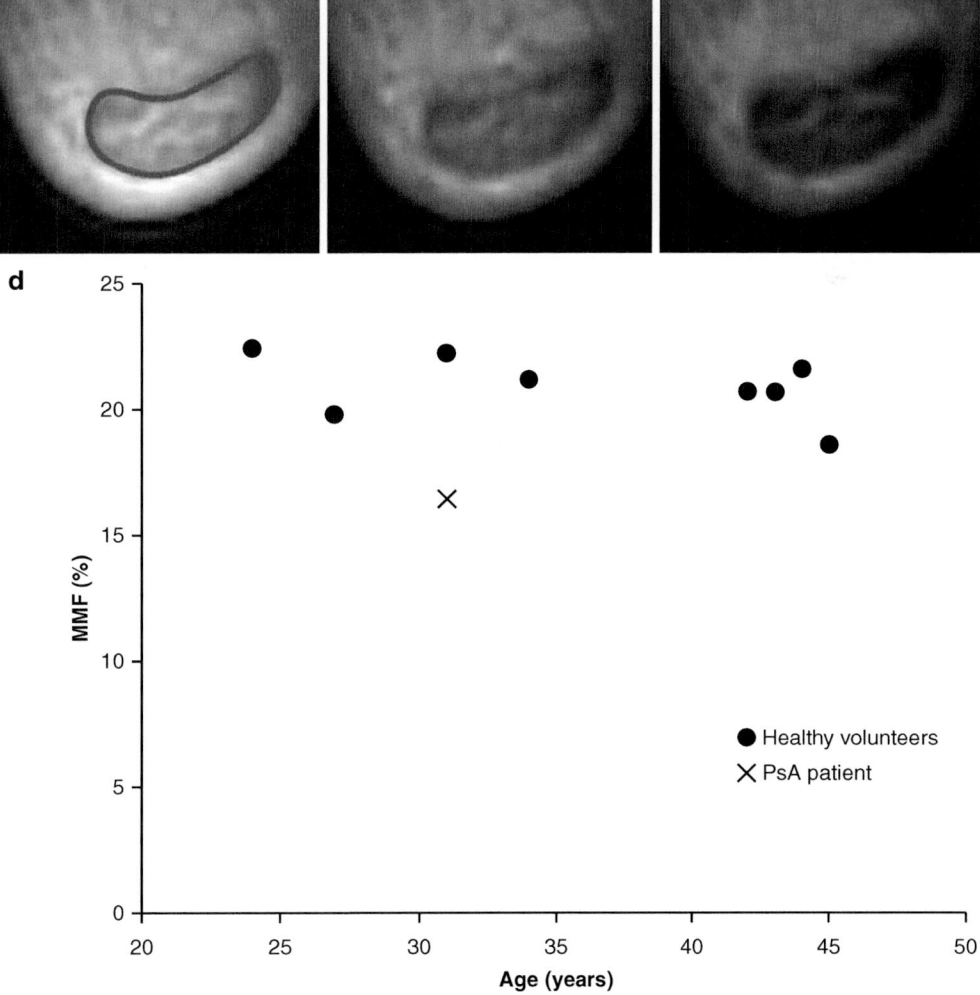

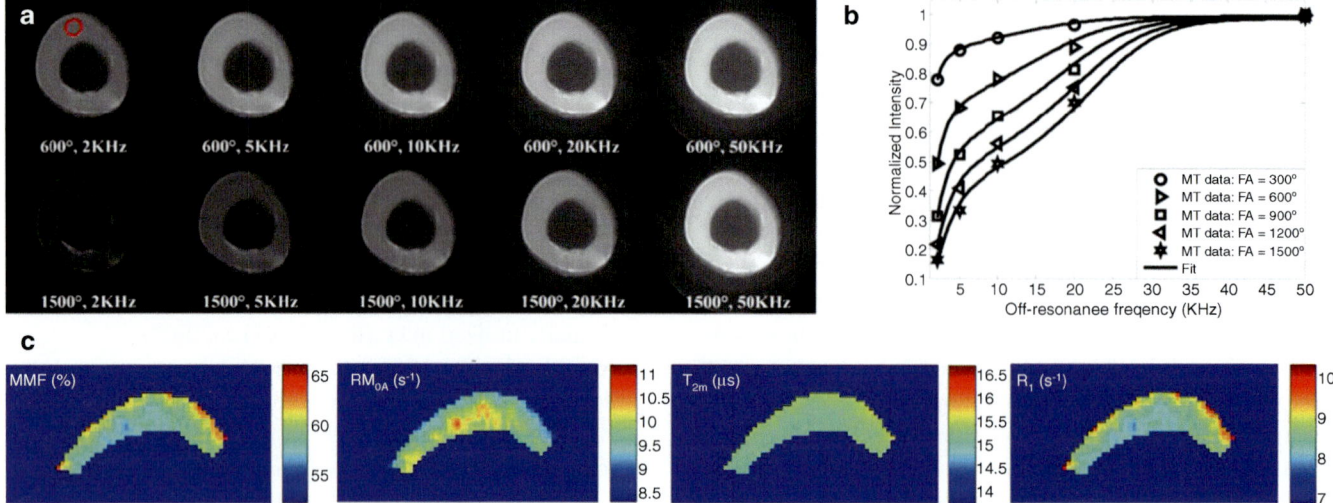

Fig. 25.7 2D UTE-MT imaging signal intensities in an ex vivo bovine cortical bone sample. These decrease as MT powers increase from 600° to 1500°, and increase as the frequency offsets increase from 2 to 50 kHz (**a**). Excellent fitting curves for the bone region (red circle in **a**) (**b**) and the representative parameter maps of MMF, RM_{0A}, T_{2B}, and R_1 are also shown (**c**). (Reproduced with permission from Ref. [21])

nificantly lower MMF was found in the Achilles tendon of a patient with psoriatic arthritis (i.e., 16.4%) compared to healthy volunteers (i.e., 21.0%) (Fig. 25.6b). This study demonstrates the clinical feasibility of 2D UTE-MT modeling and may be useful for assessing the collagen and water changes that occur in Achilles tendinopathy.

Figure 25.7a shows representative bovine cortical bone images acquired with a 2D UTE-MT sequence. Similar to the tendon study shown in Fig. 25.6, UTE-MT imaging with higher MT powers and lower frequency offsets produces greater signal attenuation [21]. Excellent curve fitting is achieved with MT modeling using the CWPE model (Fig. 25.7b). A Gaussian lineshape was used to represent the spectrum distribution of the macromolecular proton pool in cortical bone, while a super-Lorentzian lineshape was used in the previous tendon study. This is because collagen structure in cortical bone is more highly organized than in softer tissues such as tendon. Figure 25.7c shows the parameter maps of cortical bone for MMF, RM_{0A}, T_{2B}, and R_1.

3D UTE-Magnetization Transfer (UTE-MT) Modeling

2D UTE-MT imaging has demonstrated the feasibility of ex vivo and in vivo studies. However, the earlier developed conventional 2D UTE sequence is a single-slice technique, and this does not offer sufficient coverage for many anatomical structures such as the knee joint. As a result, 3D UTE sequences have been developed for morphological and quantitative UTE imaging [22].

Recently, Ma et al. described a 3D UTE-MT sequence for volumetric MT modeling [11]. This uses a multispoke acquisition strategy to speed up the 3D data acquisition to a clinically realistic time (Fig. 25.2). Furthermore, a modified rectangular pulse (RP) approximation MT model (based on Sled and Pike's original RP model for two-pool MT modeling [18, 23]) was developed to improve the accuracy of parameter estimation. Two separate comparison studies have demonstrated that the RP model is more accurate than the CWPE model for parameter estimation [24, 25]. In the original RP model, the effect of the shaped MT pulse on the macromolecular pool was modeled as a rectangular pulse (i.e., RP approximation) whose width is equal to the full width at half the maximum of the curve obtained by squaring the MT pulse throughout its duration. The RP pulse has an average equivalent power to the original MT pulse. On the other hand, the effect of the MT pulse on the water pool is modeled as an instantaneous fractional saturation of the longitudinal magnetization. Such instantaneous saturation is obtained by numerically solving Eqs. (25.2), (25.4), and (25.5) when R and R_{1A} are set to zero. For the modified RP model, the instantaneous saturation of the water component induced by the excitation pulses is $\cos^{N_{sp}}(\alpha)$, where α is the excitation flip angle and N_{sp} is the number of spokes or excitations after each MT pulse preparation. Deviations of the modified model from the original RP model are described in Ref. [11].

Both numerical simulations and small sample studies were performed to investigate whether the modified RP model provides a reasonable approximation for modeling multispoke UTE-MT acquisitions [11]. Simulation results demonstrated that the RP model is more accurate than the

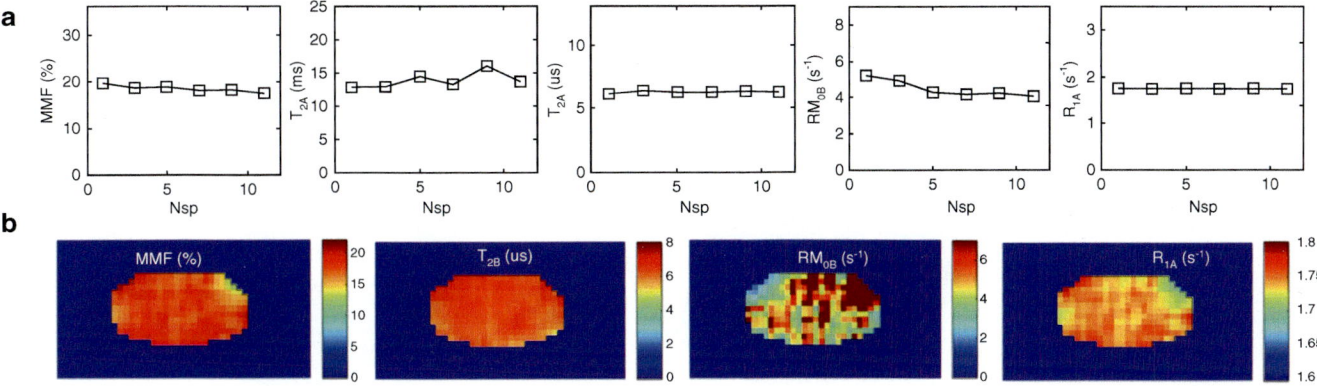

Fig. 25.8 3D UTE-MT modeling parameters vs. N_{sp} for an Achilles tendon sample (**a**) and representative parameters maps of MMF, T_{2B}, RM_{0B}, and R_{1A} when $N_{sp} = 9$ (**b**). (Reproduced with permission from Ref. [11])

CWPE model when N_{sp} gets larger. The parameters of MMF, RM_{0B}, R_{1A}, and T_{2B} are also consistent across different N_{sp} values. As can be seen in Fig. 25.8a for the tendon sample study, most of the parameters estimated only experience very minor changes when the value of N_{sp} is increased, especially MMF, RM_{0B}, and T_{2B}. This demonstrates the accuracy of the modified RP model for 3D UTE-MT modeling with multi-spoke acquisitions. Figure 25.8b shows parameter maps when $N_{sp} = 9$.

Jerban et al. applied this 3D UTE-MT modeling technique to assess bone stress injury (BSI) [26]. Fourteen human fibular samples were subjected to cyclic loading on a four-point bending setup. MMF maps were produced before and after loading, as shown in a representative cortical bone sample in Fig. 25.9a. Obvious MMF decreases were seen after loading. On average, MMF demonstrated a significant decrease ($12\% \pm 20\%$, $p = 0.02$) which may be related to rupture of the collagenous matrix or collagen softening due to loading. This study indicates that the UTE-MT modeling may be a useful technique for detecting early fatigue fractures in cortical bone.

The same group also investigated the relationship between MMF and bone mechanical properties in a study in which 156 rectangular human cortical bone strips were harvested from the tibial and femoral midshafts of 43 donors [27]. As seen in Fig. 25.9b, MMF showed significant correlations with cortical bone porosity ($R = -0.72$, $p < 0.01$), bone mineral density (BMD) ($R = 0.71$, $p < 0.01$), Young's modulus ($R = 0.61$, $p < 0.01$), yield stress ($R = 0.60$, $p < 0.01$), ultimate stress ($R = 0.60$, $p < 0.01$), and failure energy ($R = 0.45$, $p < 0.01$). These results suggest that the UTE-MT model which focuses on the organic matrix of bone can potentially serve as a novel tool to detect variations in intracortical porosity and bone mechanical properties.

The 3D UTE-MT modeling technique has also been used in a cadaveric knee joint loading study [28]. Fourteen knee joints were scanned under loads of 300 and 500 N and com-

pared with the unloaded state. Figure 25.10a shows the UTE-MT fitting curves and corresponding estimated parameters for the posterior meniscus region, where MMF values increased with a greater load. Representative MMF maps for a knee joint including cartilage and meniscus regions are shown in Fig. 25.10b. Noticeable MMF increases were found in both cartilage and meniscus. Another study found significantly lower MMF values in an elderly cohort (75 ± 8 years old, 22 subjects) compared with a younger cohort (29 ± 6 years old, 26 subjects) for both the anterior tibialis tendon (ATT) (decreased by 16.8%, $p = 0.03$) and the posterior tibialis tendon (PTT) (decreased by 23.0%, $p < 0.01$) [29]. Representative MMF maps for four of the subjects and bar plots are shown in Fig. 25.11. This study demonstrated that MMF may be a valuable biomarker for assessing the impact of aging on human tendons.

The 3D UTE-MT modeling technique was also utilized to evaluate in vivo knee cartilage and meniscus degeneration [30, 31]. Figure 25.12a shows representative MT fitting curves and the corresponding MMF maps for articular cartilage from three knee joints with different osteoarthritis grades (i.e., Kellgren–Lawrence (KL) and Whole-Organ Magnetic Resonance Imaging Score (WORMS)). MMF values decreased significantly with higher KL ($R = -0.53$, $p < 0.05$) and WORMS scores (different extent groups: $R = -0.48$, $p < 0.05$; different depth groups: $R = -0.47$, $p < 0.05$) (Fig. 25.12b) [30]. Similarly, the knee meniscus also showed that MMF values decreased with higher WORMS scores [31]. Representative MMF maps for three different knee joints are shown in Fig. 25.13a–l, with MMF showing a higher correlation with WORMS scores ($R = -0.769$, $p < 0.01$) than MTR values did ($R = -0.320$, $p < 0.01$) (Fig. 25.13m, n). The cartilage and meniscus studies demonstrate that UTE-MT modeling techniques can detect compositional changes in important tissue components of the knee. These may be valuable in clinical diagnosis.

Fig. 25.9 MMF maps of an ex vivo tibial cortical bone sample pre- and post-loading (**a**) and correlations between MMF and μCT-measured bone porosity and BMD (first row), and between MMF and Young's modulus and yield stress (second row), as well as ultimate stress and failure energy (third row) (**b**). (Reproduced with permission from Ref. [27])

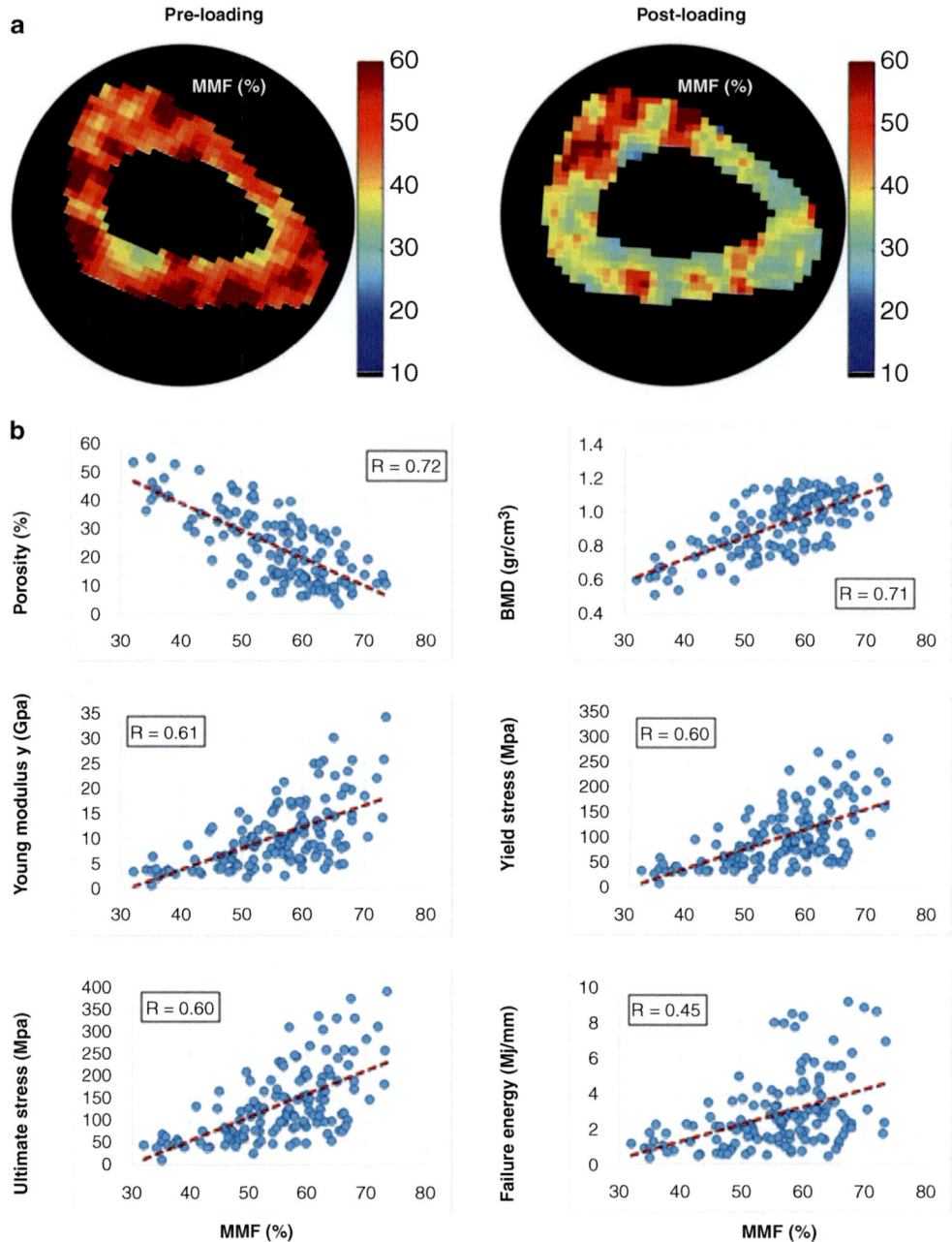

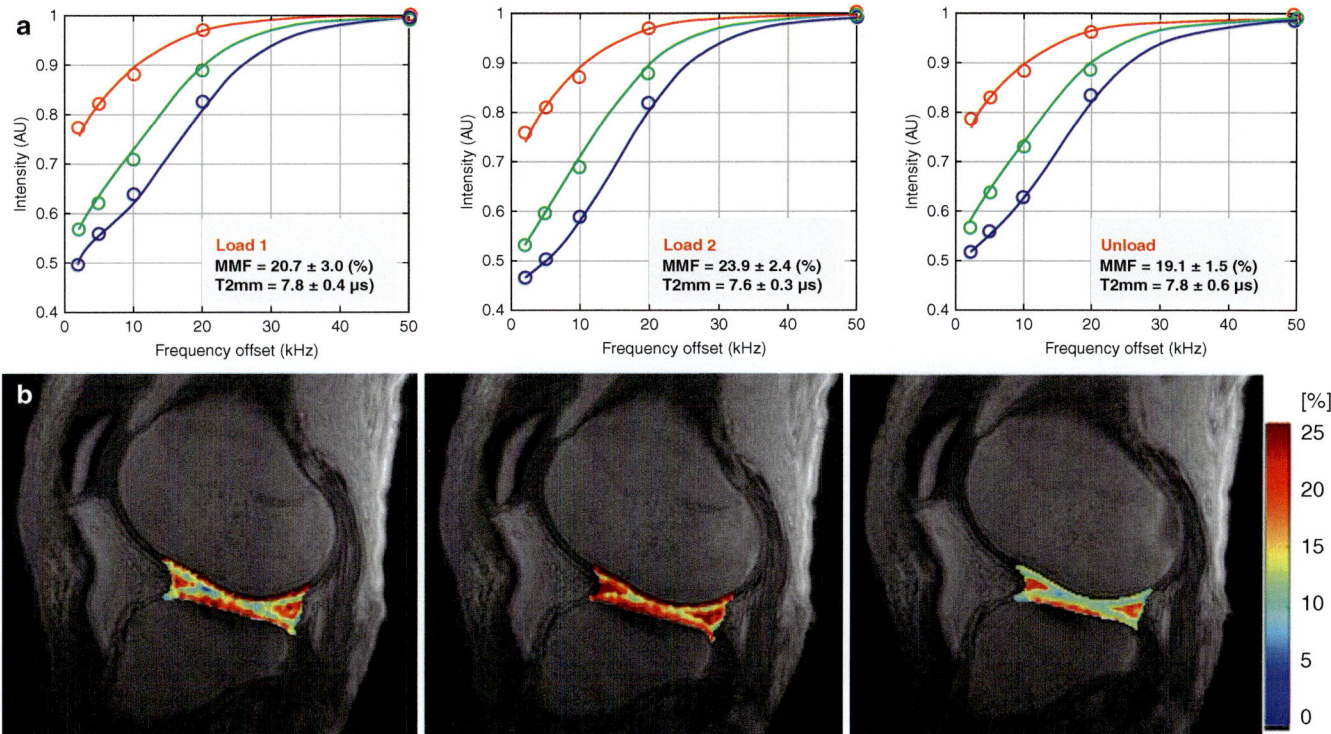

Fig. 25.10 Representative 3D UTE-MT fitting curves for the meniscus in an ex vivo knee joint at load 1 (300 N), load 2 (500 N), and no load (0 N) (**a**), and representative MMF maps for cartilage and meniscus for the three loading conditions (**b**). MMF values of both cartilage and meniscus increase with higher loads. (Reproduced with permission from Ref. [28])

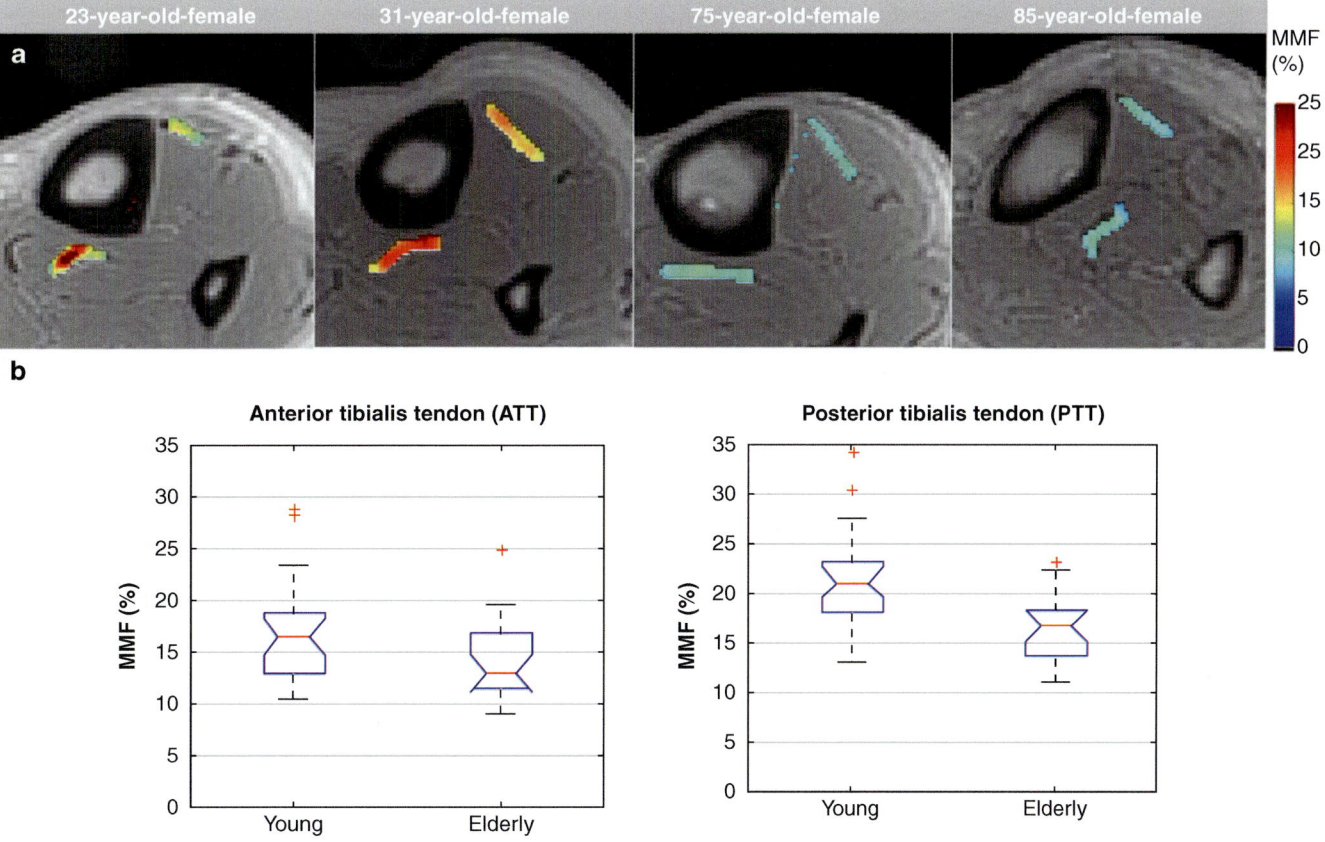

Fig. 25.11 Representative MMF maps for the ATT and the PTT in two young, healthy volunteers (first two columns) and two elderly, healthy volunteers (second two columns) (**a**), and summary plots of MMF values for 26 young and 22 elderly subjects (**b**). A significant decrease in MMF was found in the ATT and the PTT in elderly subjects compared to young subjects. (Reproduced with permission from Ref. [29])

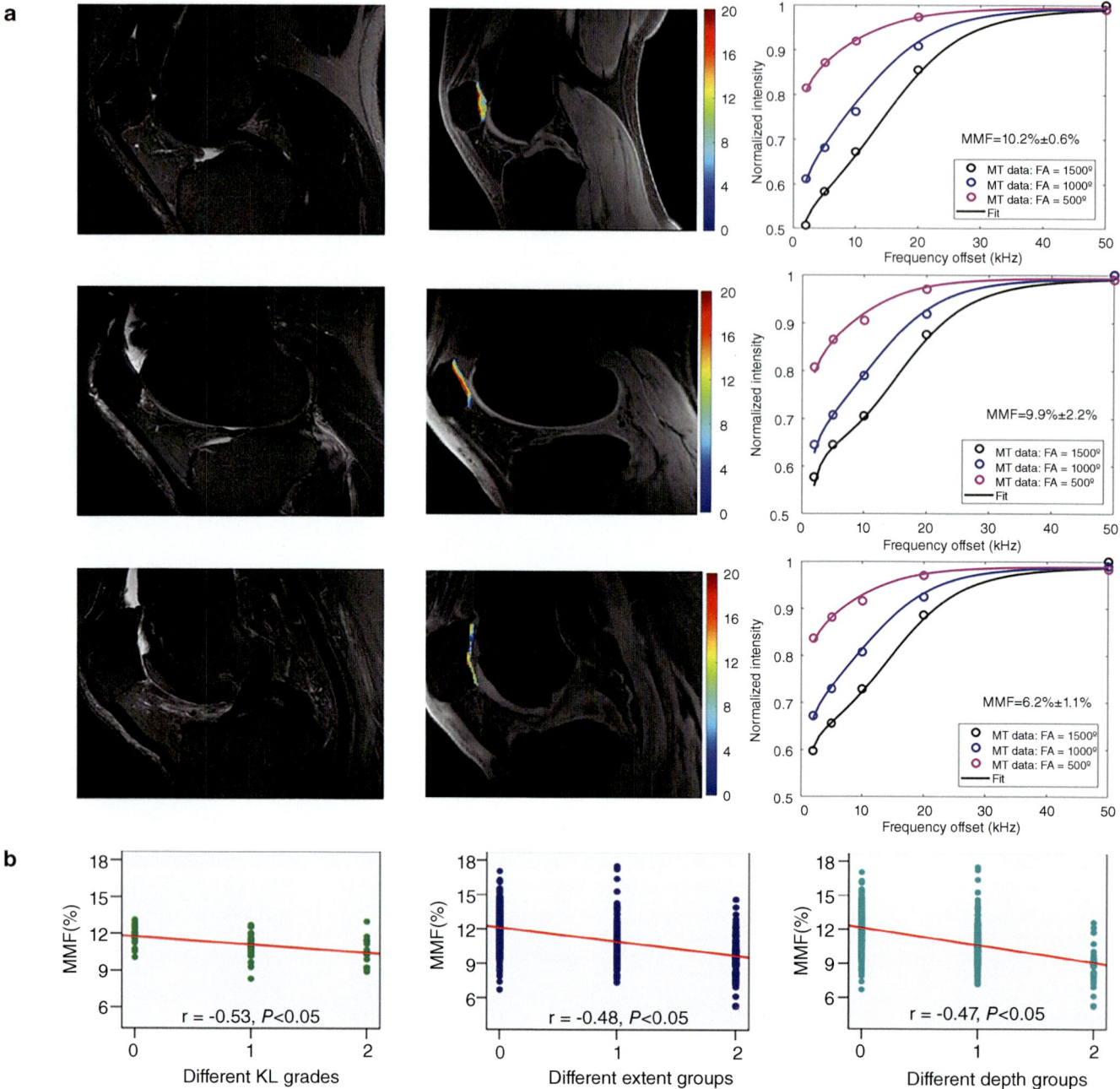

Fig. 25.12 Representative clinical T_2-weighted fast spin echo (FSE) images (first column), MMF maps (second column), and the corresponding MT fittings (third column) for three subjects with different KL and WORMS grades (first row: KL = 0 and WORMS = 0, second row: KL = 1 and WORMS = 2, and third row: KL = 3 and WORMS = 4) (**a**), and correlations between MMF and KL grades, and between MMF and two WORMS groups (i.e., different extent groups and different depth groups) (**b**). MMF values decrease significantly with both higher KL grades and higher WORMS scores. (Reproduced with permission from Ref. [30])

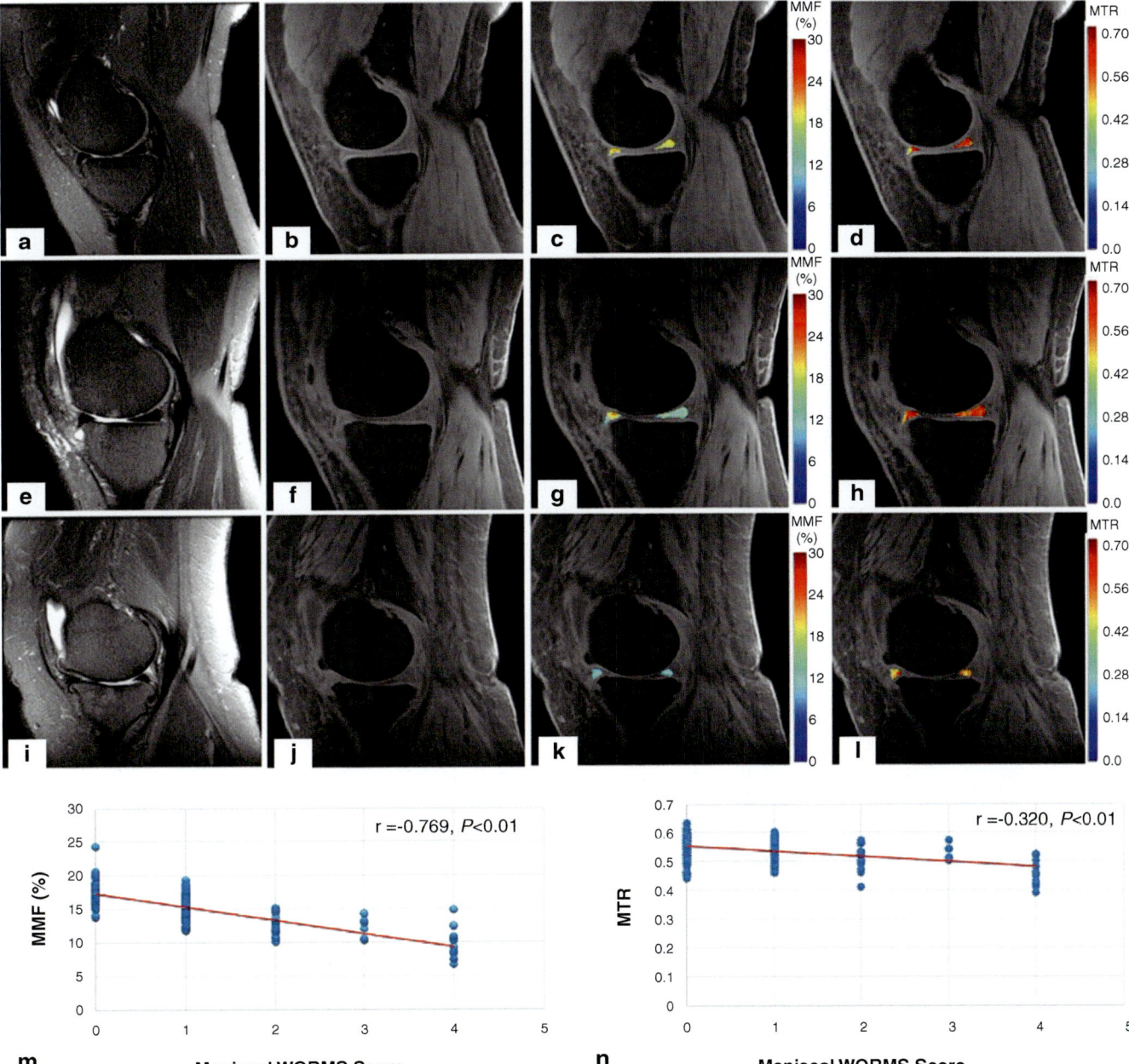

Fig. 25.13 Representative clinical T_2-weighted fast spin echo (FSE) images (first column), UTE images (second column), MMF maps (third column), and MTR maps (fourth column) for a healthy volunteer (first row), a patient with mild OA (second row), and a patient with advanced OA (third row) (**a**), and correlations between MMF and meniscal WORMS scores, and between MTR and WORMS scores (**b**). (**c–n**) MMF shows a higher correlation with WORMS scores ($R = -0.769$, $p < 0.01$) than MTR values ($R = -0.320$, $p < 0.01$). (Reproduced with permission from Ref. [31])

Magic Angle Effect Sensitivity

Ma et al. investigated the sensitivity of UTE-MT modeling to the magic angle effect [32]. Four Achilles tendon samples were scanned at five orientations to the main B_0 field ranging from 0° to 90°. The coefficient of variation (CV) values of MMF measurements for the five angle orientations were less than 3.1%, which is much lower than those for T_2^* measurements where the CV was 54.8% or higher. Figure 25.14a shows graphs of T_2^* and MMF values with five orientations: the T_2^* values first increased and reached a maximum value close to the magic angle of 55°, then decreased with higher orientations. In comparison, the MMF values were consistent across the different orientations.

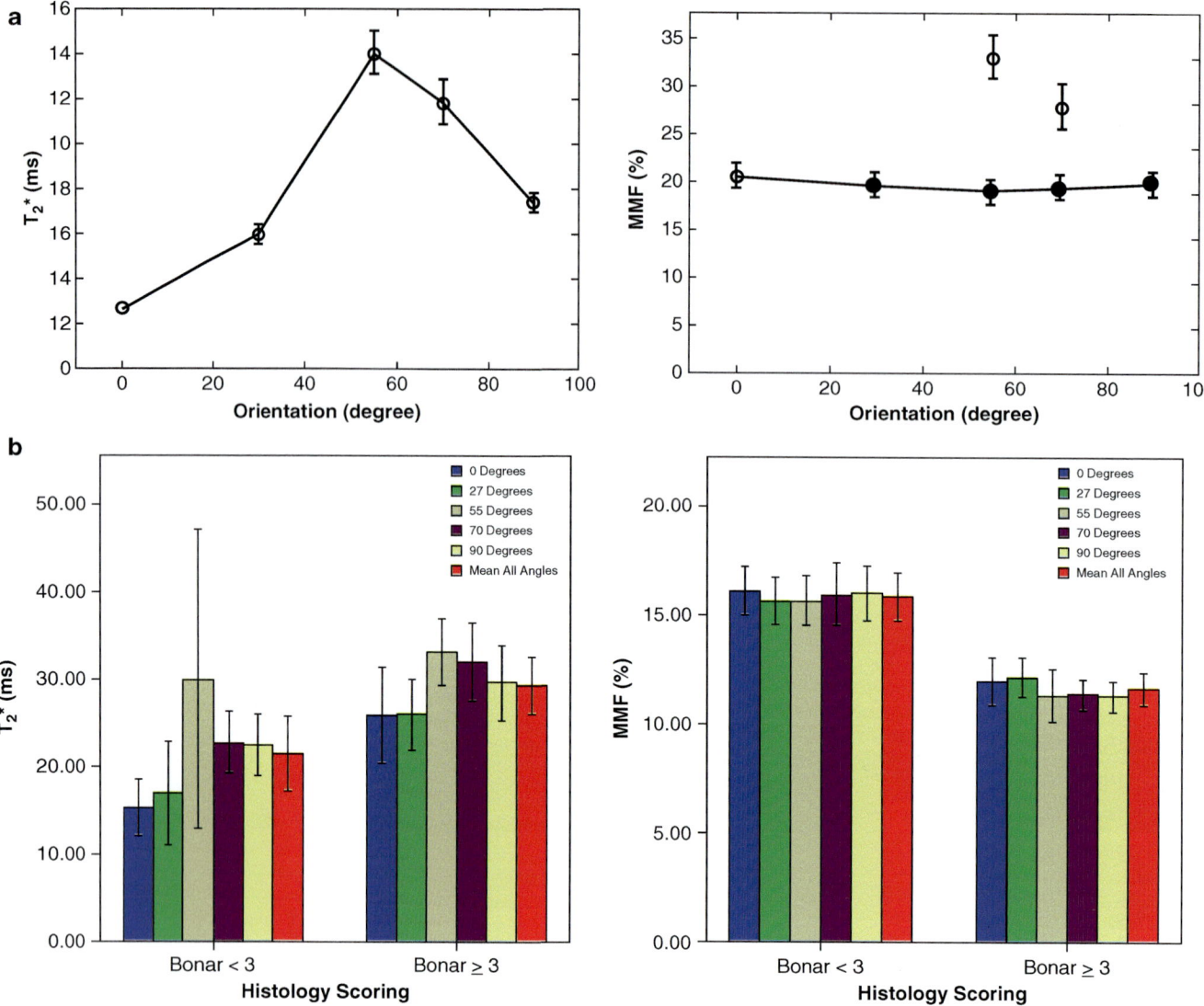

Fig. 25.14 T_2^* and MMF values vs. angular orientations relative to the B_0 direction for an ex vivo Achilles tendon study (**a**) and bar graphs of T_2 and MMF values for mild and severe tendinopathy groups in an ex vivo rotator cuff study (**b**). The T_2^* and T_2 values change significantly with different angular orientations. In contrast, MMF values remain consistent across different angular orientations, demonstrating that MMF is much less sensitive to the magic angle effect than T_2 and T_2^*. MMF values decrease significantly with more advanced rotator cuff tendon degeneration. (Reproduced with permission from Refs [32, 33])

Zhu et al. investigated the magic angle effect sensitivity of MMF and T_2 measurements in normal and abnormal rotator cuff tendon samples [33]. The abnormality of each sample was characterized through histology (Fig. 25.14b). Significant overlap in T_2 values was observed between normal and abnormal samples as all rotator cuff tendon samples were subject to a strong magic angle effect. In comparison, almost no changes were observed in MMF values among the five different angular orientations for any rotator cuff tendon sample. The abnormal samples all showed significantly reduced MMF values compared to the normal ones.

Both studies demonstrated that MMF derived from the UTE-MT modeling technique is almost insensitive to the magic angle effect. Biochemical changes probably caused the changes in MMF values that were observed rather than the magic angle effect. This is a significant advantage for the UTE-MT technique compared to T_2 and T_1rho, which are both sensitive to magic angle effects [34].

Conclusion

The UTE-MT imaging technique provides reliable mapping of short- and long-T_2 tissues, such as cortical bone, Achilles tendon, cartilage, and menisci. Quantitative UTE-MT imaging biomarkers such as MMF are insensitive to the magic angle effect, which allows robust evaluation of tissue degeneration. Both ex vivo and in vivo studies have demonstrated the efficacy of this technique in detecting changes in cortical bone, tendons, articular cartilage, and menisci, as well as myelin in the mouse brain. More investigations, including longitudinal studies, need to be performed to validate the clinical use of UTE-MT imaging and quantification.

References

1. Henkelman RM, Stanisz GJ, Graham SJ. Magnetization transfer in MRI: a review. NMR Biomed. 2001;14(2):57–64.
2. Tyler DJ, Robson MD, Henkelman RM, Young IR, Bydder GM. Magnetic resonance imaging with ultrashort TE (UTE) pulse sequences: technical considerations. J Magn Reson Imaging. 2007;25(2):279–89.
3. Balaban RS. Magnetization transfer between water and macromolecules in proton MRI. eMagRes. 2007
4. Henkelman RM, Huang X, Xiang Q-S, Stanisz GJ, Swanson SD, Bronskill MJ. Quantitative interpretation of magnetization transfer. Magn Reson Med. 1993;29(6):759–66.
5. Chang EY, Du J, Chung CB. UTE imaging in the musculoskeletal system. J Magn Reson Imaging. 2015;41(4):870–83.
6. Afsahi AM, Ma Y, Jang H, et al. Ultrashort echo time magnetic resonance imaging techniques: met and unmet needs in musculoskeletal imaging. J Magn Reson Imaging. 2022;55(6):1597–612.
7. Afsahi AM, Sedaghat S, Moazamian D, et al. Articular cartilage assessment using ultrashort echo time MRI: a review. Front Endocrinol (Lausanne). 2022;13:892961.
8. Springer F, Martirosian P, Machann J, Schwenzer NF, Claussen CD, Schick F. Magnetization transfer contrast imaging in bovine and human cortical bone applying an ultrashort echo time sequence at 3 Tesla. Magn Reson Med. 2009;61(5):1040–8.
9. Hodgson RJ, Evans R, Wright P, et al. Quantitative magnetization transfer ultrashort echo time imaging of the Achilles tendon. Magn Reson Med. 2011;65(5):1372–6.
10. Guglielmetti C, Boucneau T, Cao P, Van der Linden A, Larson PE, Chaumeil MM. Longitudinal evaluation of demyelinated lesions in a multiple sclerosis model using ultrashort echo time magnetization transfer (UTE-MT) imaging. NeuroImage. 2020;208:116415.
11. Ma Y, Carl M, Chang EY, Du J. Quantitative magnetization transfer ultrashort echo time imaging using a time-efficient 3D multispoke cones sequence. Magn Reson Med. 2018;79(2):692–700.
12. Ramani A, Dalton C, Miller DH, Tofts PS, Barker GJ. Precise estimate of fundamental in-vivo MT parameters in human brain in clinically feasible times. Magn Reson Imaging. 2002;20(10):721–31.
13. Chang EY, Bae WC, Shao H, et al. Ultrashort echo time magnetization transfer (UTE-MT) imaging of cortical bone. NMR Biomed. 2015;28(7):873–80.
14. Fang Y, Zhu D, Wu W, Yu W, Li S, Ma Y-J. Assessment of Achilles tendon changes after long-distance running using ultrashort echo time magnetization transfer MR imaging. J Magn Reson Imaging. 2022;56(3):814–23.
15. Wei H, Cao P, Bischof A, Henry RG, Larson PE, Liu C. MRI gradient-echo phase contrast of the brain at ultra-short TE with off-resonance saturation. NeuroImage. 2018;175:1–11.
16. Berry I, Barker GJ, Barkhof F, et al. A multicenter measurement of magnetization transfer ratio in normal white matter. J Magn Reson Imaging. 1999;9(3):441–6.
17. Helms G, Dathe H, Kallenberg K, Dechent P. High-resolution maps of magnetization transfer with inherent correction for RF inhomogeneity and T_1 relaxation obtained from 3D FLASH MRI. Magn Reson Med. 2008;60(6):1396–407.
18. Sled JG, Pike GB. Quantitative interpretation of magnetization transfer in spoiled gradient echo MRI sequences. J Magn Reson. 2000;145(1):24–36.
19. Gochberg DF, Kennan RP, Gore JC. Quantitative studies of magnetization transfer by selective excitation and T_1 recovery. Magn Reson Med. 1997;38(2):224–31.
20. Tozer D, Ramani A, Barker GJ, Davies GR, Miller DH, Tofts PS. Quantitative magnetization transfer mapping of bound protons in multiple sclerosis. Magn Reson Med. 2003;50(1):83–91.
21. Ma Y-J, Tadros A, Du J, Chang EY. Quantitative two-dimensional ultrashort echo time magnetization transfer (2D UTE-MT) imaging of cortical bone. Magn Reson Med. 2018;79(4):1941–9.
22. Carl M, Bydder GM, Du J. UTE imaging with simultaneous water and fat signal suppression using a time-efficient multi-spoke inversion recovery pulse sequence. Magn Reson Med. 2016;76(2):577–82.
23. Sled JG, Pike GB. Quantitative imaging of magnetization transfer exchange and relaxation properties in vivo using MRI. Magn Reson Med. 2001;46(5):923–31.
24. Cercignani M, Barker GJ. A comparison between equations describing in vivo MT: the effects of noise and sequence parameters. J Magn Reson. 2008;191(2):171–83.
25. Portnoy S, Stanisz GJ. Modeling pulsed magnetization transfer. Magn Reson Med. 2007;58(1):144–55.
26. Jerban S, Ma Y, Nazaran A, et al. Detecting stress injury (fatigue fracture) in fibular cortical bone using quantitative ultrashort echo time-magnetization transfer (UTE-MT): an ex vivo study. NMR Biomed. 2018;31(11):e3994.
27. Jerban S, Ma Y, Dorthe EW, et al. Assessing cortical bone mechanical properties using collagen proton fraction from ultrashort echo time magnetization transfer (UTE-MT) MRI modeling. Bone Rep. 2019;11:100220.
28. Jerban S, Kasibhatla A, Ma Y, et al. Detecting articular cartilage and meniscus deformation effects using magnetization transfer ultrashort echo time (MT-UTE) modeling during mechanical load application: ex vivo feasibility study. Cartilage. 2021;13(1_Suppl):665S–73S.
29. Jerban S, Ma Y, Namiranian B, et al. Age-related decrease in collagen proton fraction in tibial tendons estimated by magnetization transfer modeling of ultrashort echo time magnetic resonance imaging (UTE-MRI). Sci Rep. 2019;9(1):1–7.
30. Xue Y-P, Ma Y-J, Wu M, et al. Quantitative 3D ultrashort echo time magnetization transfer imaging for evaluation of knee cartilage degeneration in vivo. J Magn Reson Imaging. 2021;54(4):1294–302.
31. Zhang X, Ma Y-J, Wei Z, et al. Macromolecular fraction (MMF) from 3D ultrashort echo time cones magnetization transfer (3D UTE-Cones-MT) imaging predicts meniscal degeneration and knee osteoarthritis. Osteoarthr Cartil. 2021;29(8):1173–80.
32. Ma Y-J, Shao H, Du J, Chang EY. Ultrashort echo time magnetization transfer (UTE-MT) imaging and modeling: magic angle independent biomarkers of tissue properties. NMR Biomed. 2016;29(11):1546–52.
33. Zhu Y, Cheng X, Ma Y, et al. Rotator cuff tendon assessment using magic-angle insensitive 3D ultrashort echo time cones magnetization transfer (UTE-Cones-MT) imaging and modeling with histological correlation. J Magn Reson Imaging. 2018;48(1):160–8.
34. Shao H, Pauli C, Li S, et al. Magic angle effect plays a major role in both T1rho and T2 relaxation in articular cartilage. Osteoarthr Cartil. 2017;25(12):2022–30.

Hyungseok Jang, Saeed Jerban, Xing Lu, Yajun Ma,
Sam Sedaghat, Eric Y. Chang, and Jiang Du

Introduction

Magnetic susceptibility is one of the fundamental physical properties of materials. In biological systems, tissues create their own local magnetic field called a dipole field in response to an external magnetic field. The strength of the local dipole field is proportional to the tissue's magnetic susceptibility and is generated in a parallel or antiparallel direction to the external magnetic field. Negative magnetic susceptibility is referred to as diamagnetism, meaning that the created local dipole field is in the direction opposite to that of the external magnetic field. Positive magnetic susceptibility, which includes paramagnetism, superparamagnetism, and ferromagnetism, creates dipole fields in the same direction as the external magnetic field. In the human body, most tissues are diamagnetic including bone mineral and dystrophic calcification. Paramagnetic tissues include ferritin, hemosiderin, and deoxyhemoglobin.

In an MRI system, any tissue in the B_0 field creates a dipole field that distorts the applied B_0 field which is already inhomogeneous. The additional field inhomogeneity plays a critical role in MRI. Tissues with strong magnetic susceptibilities may degrade MR image quality due to perturbation of the B_0 field. This can result in signal dropout due to rapid signal dephasing and/or spatial distortion, particularly in the presence of strong field inhomogeneities and larger off-resonance frequency shifts. To address these issues in MR systems, B_0 shimming is utilized in which additional static linear or higher-order gradient fields are superimposed on B_0 to mitigate field distortions. On the other hand, susceptibility-induced phenomena are actively used to create image contrast specific to the susceptibility of tissues in the form of susceptibility-weighted sequences which are widely used in clinical studies. Susceptibility-weighted imaging (SWI) [1, 2] and blood oxygenation level-dependent (BOLD) imaging [3, 4] are two imaging techniques that utilize MR signal changes induced by susceptibility to create contrast. SWI is widely used for cardiovascular imaging as well as neuroimaging. In SWI, strong T_2*-weighting is utilized to create susceptibility-weighted contrast in which both magnitude and phase information are combined to increase contrast and discriminate between paramagnetic and diamagnetic tissues. SWI is effective for the identification of hemorrhage, hemosiderin, and calcification. BOLD imaging is a standard technique that is used to assess brain activity in functional MRI based on changes in blood oxygenation in the brain. BOLD signal change is associated with the relative level of deoxygenated hemoglobin which is paramagnetic and can be detected with heavily T_2*-weighted imaging. However, these methods only provide susceptibility weighting in qualitative or semiquantitative form. They are not genuine quantitative measurements of tissue susceptibility.

Quantitative susceptibility mapping (QSM) has been actively developed to estimate susceptibility and provide a diagnostic tool to characterize the microenvironment of targeted tissues [5–9]. QSM has been used in a variety of applications, such as neuroimaging [7, 10, 11], body imaging [12–14], and cardiovascular imaging [15, 16]. However, QSM of the musculoskeletal (MSK) system is still at an early stage of development for many MSK tissues due to the

H. Jang (✉) · S. Jerban · X. Lu · Y. Ma · S. Sedaghat
Department of Radiology, University of California, San Diego,
La Jolla, CA, USA
e-mail: h4jang@health.ucsd.edu; sjerban@health.ucsd.edu;
xil135@health.ucsd.edu; yam013@health.ucsd.edu; ssedaghat@
health.ucsd.edu

E. Y. Chang
Department of Radiology, University of California, San Diego,
La Jolla, CA, USA

VA San Diego Healthcare System, San Diego, CA, USA
e-mail: e8chang@health.ucsd.edu

J. Du
Department of Radiology, University of California, San Diego,
La Jolla, CA, USA

VA San Diego Healthcare System, San Diego, CA, USA

Department of Bioengineering, University of California, San
Diego, La Jolla, CA, USA
e-mail: jiangdu@health.ucsd.edu

J. Du, G. M. Bydder (eds.), *MRI of Short- and Ultrashort-T2 Tissues*, https://doi.org/10.1007/978-3-031-35197-6_26

limitations and challenges caused by the short-T_2s of tissues such as bone, tendon, ligament, and meniscus. Problems with adipose tissue, which has a large chemical shift, also complicate accurate estimation of susceptibility [17–20]. Recently, ultrashort echo time (UTE) based QSM (UTE-QSM) has been developed to enable QSM of short- and ultrashort-T_2 tissues [19, 21–23]. In this chapter, the theory and practice underpinning UTE-QSM are explained.

Quantitative Susceptibility Mapping (QSM)

QSM displays tissue susceptibility using measurements of B_0 field distortions. In MRI, the total field distortion is assessed by measuring the phase evolution after RF excitation using gradient recalled echo (GRE)-based sequences. Multiple gradient echo images are acquired and their phase evolution is fitted linearly to estimate the total field map (including effects due to B_0 and tissue inhomogeneities). The time course of phase evolution needs to be unwrapped since phase only has values between $-\pi$ to $+\pi$, and phase accrual beyond this range is wrapped. To address this issue, region-growing, graph-cut, and Laplacian-based phase unwrapping approaches are utilized in QSM [24, 25].

The B_0 field distortion has contributions from B_0 inhomogeneity due to MR system imperfections (i.e., background field) and tissue susceptibility (i.e., local field effects). For QSM that maps tissue susceptibility, the local field effects need to be separated from background field imperfections. Two commonly used methods to remove background field effects are high-pass filtering (HPF) [26] and projection onto dipole fields (PDF) [27]. The HPF method is based on traditional image processing techniques where the background field is estimated by low-pass filtering of acquired complex images. The PDF method is based on the projection theorem in Hilbert space in which background and local fields are decomposed by projecting the measured field map onto subspace spanned by the dipole fields. Figure 26.1 shows simulated results using these two methods. PDF offers significantly reduced error (3.21%) compared with HPF (23.51%) in this simulation.

Once the local field map is obtained, tissue susceptibility can be estimated. This step assumes that the local field map is the net sum of dipole fields generated by individual particles in tissues. In signal or image processing, this is often modeled using a convolution operation, described by the following equation [28].

$$b = d * \chi \tag{26.1}$$

where b is the measured local field map, d is the dipole kernel, * indicates the convolution operator, and χ is the tissue susceptibility map.

The dipole kernel d can be modeled using

$$d = \frac{3\cos^2\left(\theta_{r-r'}\right)-1}{4\pi\left|r'-r\right|^3} \tag{26.2}$$

where r and r' indicate locations of dipoles with respect to the susceptibility source and θ_r represents the azimuthal angle in the spherical coordinate system. The most straightforward approach to deconvolve χ from b is utilizing Fourier transformation (FT), which is commonly done in signal processing. In the FT domain (i.e., k-space), the equation becomes

$$B = DX \tag{26.3}$$

where B, D, and X are, respectively, the local field map, dipole kernel, and susceptibility map in k-space. Thinking simplistically, X could be estimated by dividing B by D. Unfortunately, direct deconvolution in this way is not feasible due to zero values of D.

Figure 26.2 demonstrates a dipole kernel in the spatial (Fig. 26.2a, b) and k-space domains (Fig. 26.2c). Due to the zero values on the conic surfaces at the magic angle (~54.7° from the direction of B_0) in (Fig. 26.2c), the deconvolution problem to solve for susceptibility is ill-posed. Hence, no deterministic solution exists for this dipole inversion problem. Thus, the inverse approach is not effective in QSM. To find the optimal solution, a forward approach is implemented, using iterative non-linear optimization in which the solution (i.e., the susceptibility map) is repeatedly updated with successive iterations designed to minimize L1 or L2 norm, the distance between measured data and forward-modeled data (i.e., the field map estimated based on susceptibility map), combined with appropriate regularization terms such as a smoothness promoting operator. The optimization is typically done using a gradient descent algorithm (i.e., Newton's method) or a conjugate gradient descent method. Unfortunately, these approaches are still affected by the zero conic surfaces in the dipole field, which produce streaking artifacts across the estimated susceptibility map. To overcome this problem, several approaches have been proposed.

The calculation of susceptibility through multiple orientation sampling (COSMOS) method was introduced by Liu et al. [29]. The key idea of COSMOS is to reduce the impact of the zero conic surfaces by compensating for them using multiple acquisitions at different angles to B_0 (Fig. 26.3). COSMOS allows accurate production of susceptibility maps without significant streaking artifacts. Unfortunately, the clinical feasibility of COSMOS is relatively low because the imaged object needs to be placed at three different optimal angles (0°, 60°, and 120°) within the MRI system bore, and this is not practical for adult human subjects due to the limited bore size. In addition, COSMOS is affected by other factors such as rotational angles, image registration, and anisotropic susceptibility.

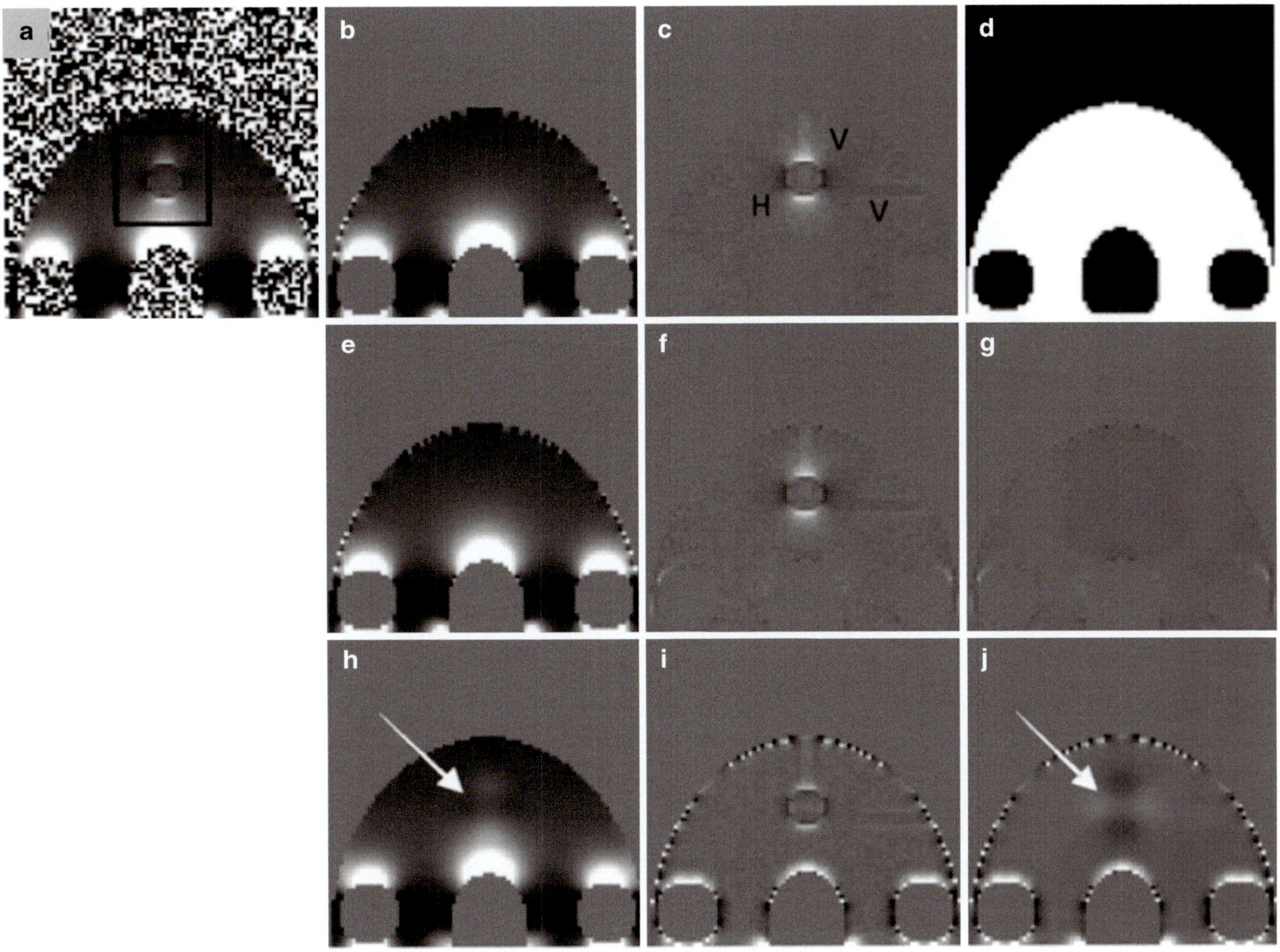

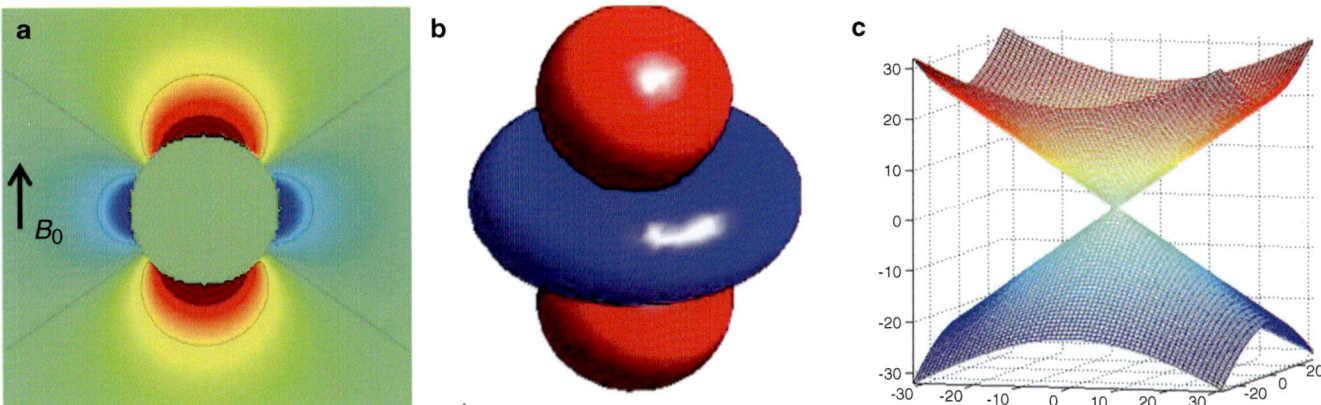

Fig. 26.1 Background field removal. (**a**) Simulated total field map, (**b**) the ground truth background field map, (**c**) the ground truth local field with simulated hemorrhage (annotated with H) and veins (annotated with V), (**d**) object mask, (**e**) the background field map estimated with projection onto dipole fields (PDF), (**f**) the local field map estimated with PDF, (**g**) error in local field map with PDF, (**h**) the background field map estimated with high-pass filtering (HPF), (**i**) the local field map estimated with HPF, and (**j**) error in local field map with HPF. The local field estimated with PDF (**f**) shows much less error (**g**) near the strong susceptibility sources (H and Vs in (**c**)) than HPF (**i**) and (**j**). (Adapted with permission from Ref. [27])

Fig. 26.2 Dipole field in the spatial domain (**a**), its surface rendering (**b**), and zero surfaces of the dipole kernel in k-space (**c**). The zero surfaces in the dipole kernel in k-space make the dipole inversion problem ill-posed. (Adapted with permission from Ref. [5])

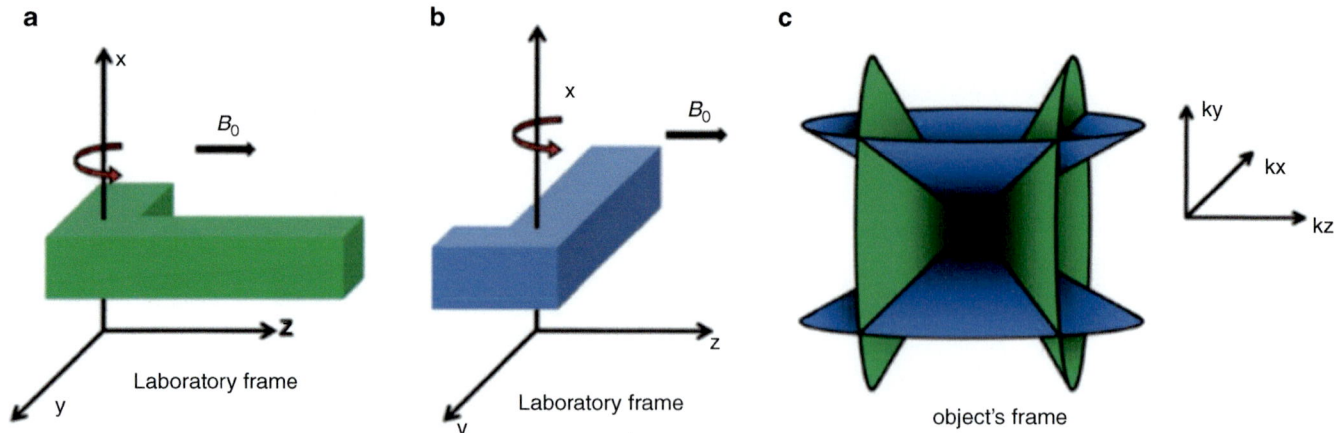

Fig. 26.3 Calculation of susceptibility through multiple orientation sampling (COSMOS). The scan is performed with the first original orientation (**a**). The scan is then repeated with the object rotated about the x-axis (**b**). In k-space in the object's frame, this results in the two dipole kernels being placed at different angles which removes zero surfaces (**c**). However, lines of zero values remain where the two kernels inter- cept. A third acquisition with proper rotation can remove these zero values, and only leave the origin of the k-space with a zero value. The zero value only affects the DC offset of the estimated susceptibility, and this can be corrected by using an appropriate reference standard. (Adapted with permission from Ref. [29])

Another approach to reducing streaking artifacts has been proposed by Liu et al. This utilizes morphological information and is called morphology-enabled dipole inversion (MEDI) [30]. MEDI uses magnitude information to weight the objective function so that the optimization process becomes less affected by signals with low signal-to-noise ratios (SNRs) which are often the source of streaking artifacts. Wei et al. have proposed another technique called streaking artifact reduction for quantitative susceptibility mapping (STAR-QSM), which is based on a two-level reconstruction in which strong susceptibility sources are estimated separately [31] (Fig. 26.4). More recently, deep learning-based QSM methods have been investigated and have shown robust dipole inversion with reduced streaking artifacts [32, 33].

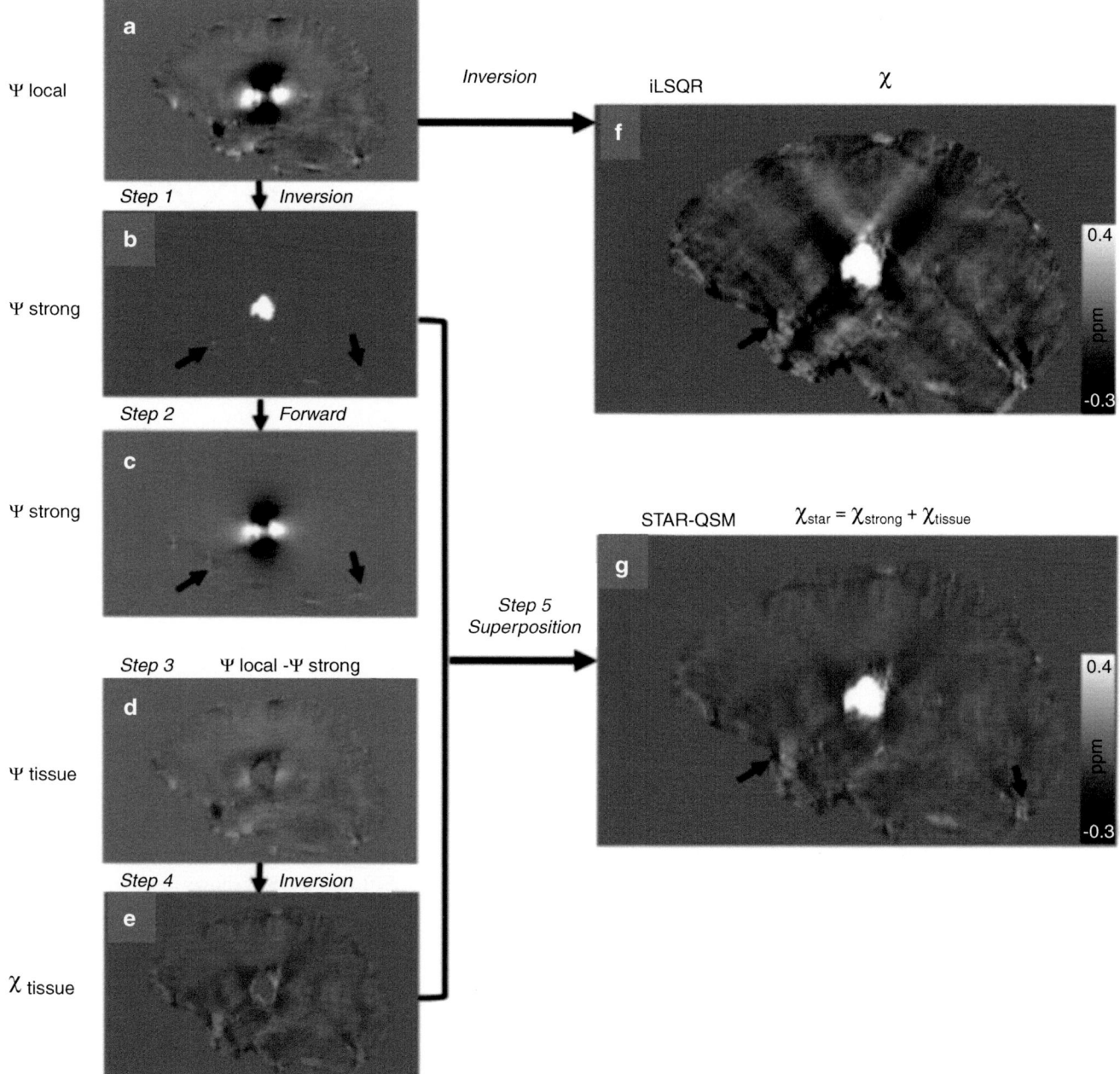

Fig. 26.4 Streaking artifact reduction for quantitative susceptibility mapping (STAR-QSM) utilizing two-level reconstruction. (**a**) Local field map, (**b**) estimation of strong susceptibility source, (**c**) dipole field generated based on the strong susceptibility source, (**d**) residual local dipole field without strong susceptibility, (**e**) resultant susceptibility without strong susceptibility, (**f**) QSM result without two-level recon-struction using the improved sparse linear equation and least squares (iLSQR) algorithm, and (**g**) the final susceptibility map based on super-position of two susceptibility maps (with and without strong suscepti-bility, i.e., (**c**) and (**e**)). (Adapted with permission from Ref. [31])

UTE-QSM

Despite its promise, the utilization of QSM on short-T_2 tis-sues, such as bone, tendon, meniscus, and ligament, is still at an early stage. Conventional QSM is typically based on GRE imaging which is used to acquire phase evolution from the acquired free induction decay (FID). However, TEs used in GRE imaging (i.e., of the order of a few ms) are much longer than T_2s of ultrashort-T_2^* tissues, resulting in insufficient signal to map phase evolutions. QSM based on UTE resolves this problem by allowing acquisition of signals using much shorter TEs (<1 ms).

Fig. 26.5 Interleaved UTE imaging for UTE-QSM. Pulse sequences with (**a**) 3D radial trajectory and (**b**) 3D cones trajectory. Because of the limited performance of MRI gradient systems, echo spacing is inherently limited. Interleaved UTE imaging is typically utilized in UTE-QSM to acquire images with echo spacings less than the allowed hardware values for single acquisitions. The 3D cones trajectory allows more efficient encoding of 3D k-space with reduced scan times

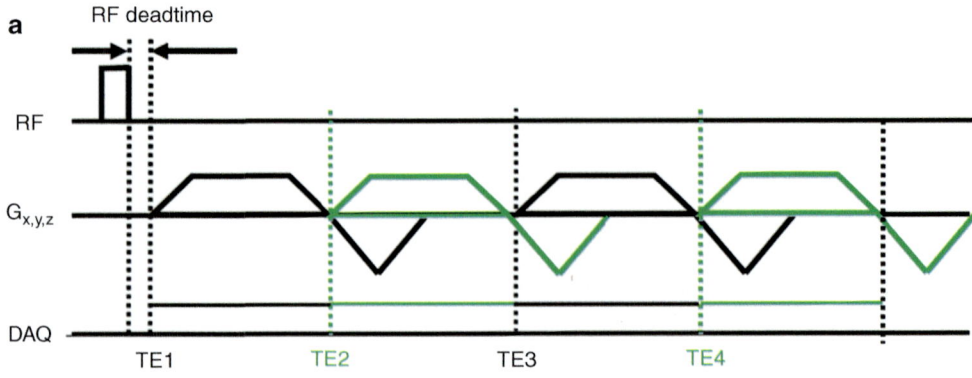

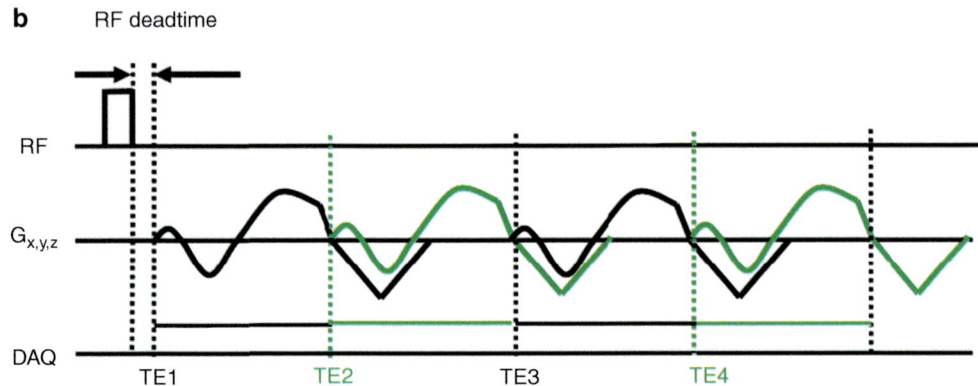

Figure 26.5a shows the pulse sequence diagram used for UTE-based QSM (UTE-QSM), utilizing a center-out 3D radial acquisition [34]. A GRE scheme is used to acquire multiple images at different TEs. Since the minimum attainable echo spacing of the gradient echo train is limited by the performance of the gradient system (i.e., maximum slew rate and amplitude), multiple interleaved acquisitions are utilized. With this approach, the gradients are delayed by different times, allowing flexible echo spacings which are much shorter than the duration of readout and rewinding gradients for single acquisitions (green lines in Fig. 26.5). This enables acquisition of images at many desired TEs from UTE (near-zero ms) to later TEs (few ms) at the expense of the longer times required for the different scans. The 3D cones trajectory (Fig. 26.5b) allows more efficient sampling with a smaller number of spokes to cover 3D spherical k-space, and so significantly reduces scan time (>2× acceleration) [35]. UTE-QSM also benefits from the use of 3D cones trajectories. An alternative is continuous single-point imaging (CSPI) which was developed by Jang et al. [20]. In this method, a 3D pure phase encoding scheme is used to capture true phase information with near-zero readout duration.

Continuous sampling is performed at one k-space coordinate to allow efficient encoding and yield various images. Autocalibration-based parallel imaging is applied to shorten the scan time [36]. CSPI-based QSM shows more robust estimation of susceptibility with reduced ringing artifacts around strong susceptibility sources.

UTE-QSM with different sampling strategies was investigated by Lu et al. [22]. In their study, 3D CSPI, 3D radial sampling, and 3D cones trajectories with various stretch factors (i.e., lengthened readout duration in a 3D spiral arm) were tested using a phantom with six different concentrations of iron nanoparticles (2, 6, 10, 14, 18, and 22 mM). All three UTE techniques achieved highly linear correlations between estimated susceptibility and iron concentration (Pearson's correlation >0.98). In the experiment with UTE-QSM using cones trajectories with different stretching factors, no significant differences were observed.

After data acquisition and reconstruction of UTE images, the same standard QSM processing pipelines can be applied to UTE-QSM, which has a series of data processing steps that include phase unwrapping, total field map estimation, background field removal, and dipole inversion.

Chemical Shift in UTE-QSM

One major challenge with UTE-QSM is how to minimize chemical shift effects, which are a major cause of streaking artifacts [37]. The off-resonant fat signal causes strong phase evolution over different TEs and complicates the estimation of true field maps. In conventional QSM, TEs can be selected near the time delay at which fat and water signals are in phase (i.e., the phase of the fat signal becomes 2π) to minimize chemical shift-induced phase errors, leaving only B_0 inhomogeneity-induced phase evolution. However, this strategy may not be effective with UTE-QSM, when several images before the in-phase echo need to be acquired to characterize the short-T_2 signal. A potential alternative is to use a fat saturation pulse and suppress fat signals as demonstrated in work by Wei et al. [18]. However, with this approach, the fat saturation pulse attenuates signal from short-T_2 tissues that have broad spectra which include the frequency of the principal fat resonance peak that is saturated [38, 39].

Another approach is to use comprehensive signal modeling and take the fat signal into account in the estimation of field inhomogeneity (i.e., a total field map). This approach has been used for fat and water signal separation and is referred to as m-point Dixon [40] or iterative decomposition of water and fat with echo asymmetry and least square estimation (IDEAL) [41]. In this approach, multiple off-resonant peaks in the fat spectrum are included to allow more accurate signal modeling, as in the following equation.

$$s(t) = \left(\rho_w e^{-R_{2w}^* t} + \rho_f \sum_n \alpha_n e^{-i2\pi f_n t} \right) e^{-i2\pi f_s t} \quad (26.4)$$

where α_n and f_n are the relative amplitude and chemical shift of the nth spectral peak of fat, respectively; f_s is a field inhomogeneity; ρ_w and ρ_f are amplitude of water and fat at zero TE; and R_{2w}^* indicates R_2^* of the water component. Using the above equation, T_2^* of water signal and the field map, as well as water and fat signals, are simultaneously estimated using the signal modeling. Multiple input images are required to achieve accurate signal modeling because of the need to fit Eq. (26.4) with multiple free parameters. Once the field map, f_s, is acquired, it is processed using the QSM pipeline with conventional non-UTE QSM.

In the literature, Dimov et al. [19], Jerban et al. [21], and Jang et al. [23] have demonstrated the feasibility of UTE-QSM based on fat–water signal modeling. The potential downsides are that the complexity of the signal modeling is high, multiple images are required, and the signal fitting is prone to errors caused by noise and artifacts.

UTE-QSM for Quantitative Imaging of Bone Mineral Density

Measurement of bone mineral density (BMD) is a standard diagnostic tool for evaluating osteoporosis (OP) and osteopenia. Modern noninvasive imaging tools to diagnose OP in the clinic are dual-energy X-ray absorptiometry (DEXA) and quantitative computed tomography (qCT). DEXA has limited specificity due to its 2D nature and low spatial resolution. qCT provides high-resolution, volumetric and quantitative measures of BMD, but imposes a potential risk due to exposure to ionizing radiation. MRI is an alternative that allows 3D imaging with high spatial resolution and is free from ionizing radiation. Unfortunately, due to the ultrashort-T_2 of bone, it is impossible to image bone with conventional MRI techniques. Recently, quantitative UTE MRI has emerged as a promising technique to provide a comprehensive evaluation of bone, including its pore water, collagenous organic matrix, and mineral components.

UTE-QSM has been used to provide a quantitative evaluation of BMD. Biomaterials containing calcium, such as bone, are diamagnetic and QSM can be effective in characterizing bone organic matrix. However, due to the ultrashort-T_2s of water bound to hydroxyapatite calcium phosphate crystals and the collagenous matrix of bone ($T_2^* \sim 300$ μs), it is virtually impossible to perform QSM with conventional GRE-based sequences. To work around this issue, De Rochefort et al. proposed an approach for indirect estimation of field distortion based on a piecewise constant susceptibility model [42]. They used a gradient echo sequence to estimate bone susceptibility in vivo and reported that the susceptibility of bone was −2.20 ppm. However, this method is based on indirect estimation of field distortion inside the bone utilizing tissue segmentation and the assumption of constant susceptibility which may be unreliable in subjects with complex anatomical structures.

As an alternative, UTE-QSM has been investigated for quantification of BMD in bone, using a signal model that includes fat. Dimov et al. performed UTE-QSM on a porcine hoof and healthy volunteers [19]. They utilized an interleaved 3D radial UTE sequence implemented on a 3T MRI scanner with images acquired at TEs of 0.04, 0.24, 3.0, and 4.0 ms in two scans. The background field was estimated using a fat signal model with peaks at −3.82, −3.46, −2.74, −1.86, −0.5, and 0.5 ppm. A graph-cut algorithm was used for phase unwrapping during the field map estimation. The background field removal was performed using the PDF method, and dipole inversion was performed using MEDI. The estimated susceptibility in the porcine hoof bone (Fig. 26.6a) showed a high linear correlation ($R^2 = 0.77$) with

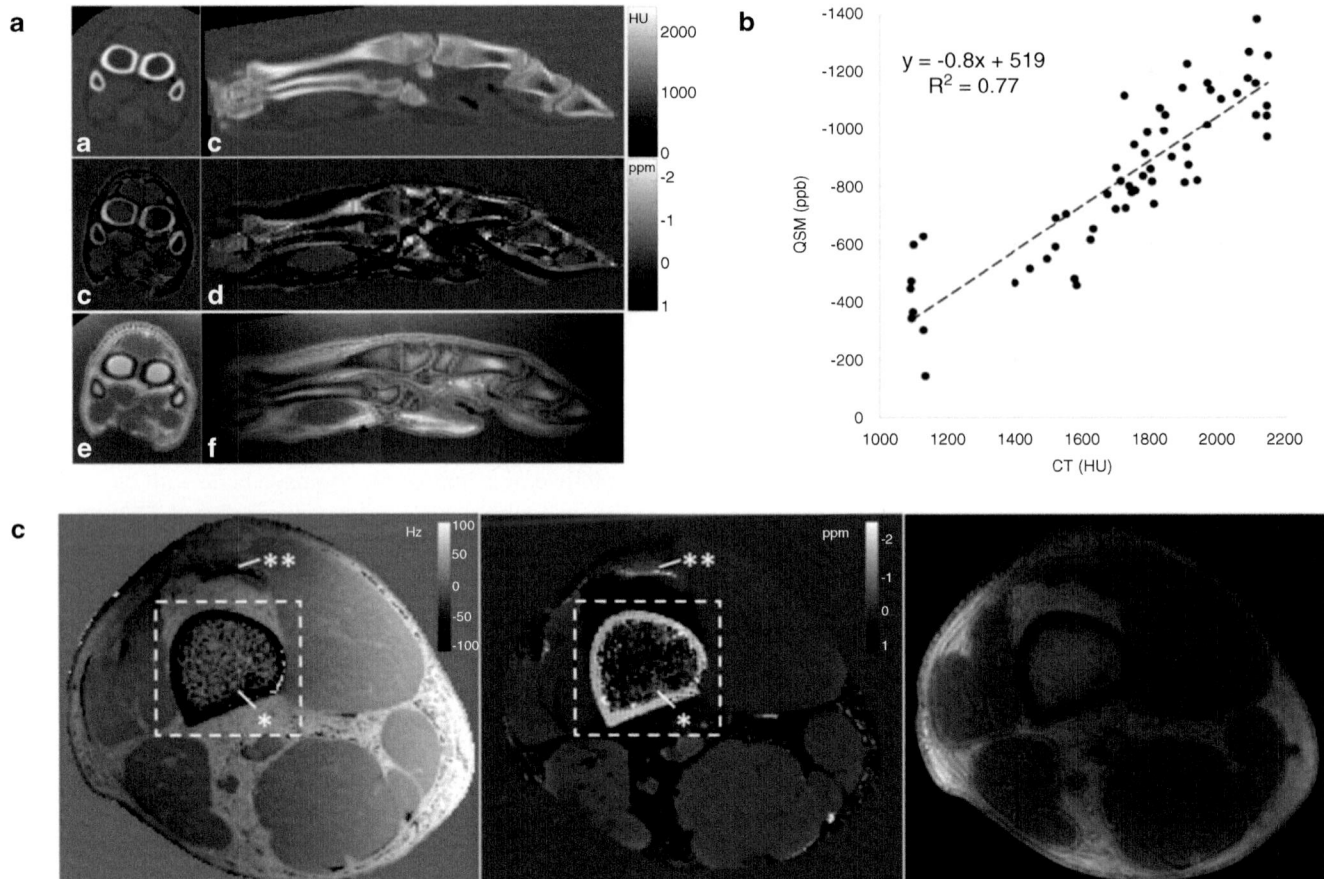

Fig. 26.6 Bone UTE-QSM. (**a**) CT image (upper) compared with a susceptibility map obtained from UTE-QSM (middle) and magnitude UTE imaging (lower). (**b**) Linear regression of mean susceptibility values from UTE-QSM and CT in multiple ROIs from a porcine hoof.

(**c**) In vivo results show the estimated field map (left), susceptibility map (center), and the magnitude UTE image (right) from the femur of a healthy volunteer. (Adapted with permission from Ref. [19])

radiodensity measured in Hounsfield Units (HUs) derived from CT imaging (Fig. 26.6b). In the in vivo experiment, the estimated susceptibility of cortical bone in a femoral midshaft ranged from −2.3 to −1.8 ppm showing strong diamagnetism (Fig. 26.6c). Jang et al. also demonstrated UTE-QSM in bone using the CSPI technique, and the estimated bone susceptibility ranged from −2.1 to −1.6 ppm [20], which corresponded well with results from Dimov's study.

Jerban et al. investigated the correlation between bone density estimated by μCT and susceptibility estimated by UTE-QSM [21]. They studied nine cadaveric cortical bone specimens from the tibial midshaft on a clinical 3T MRI scanner using a 3D UTE cones sequence. A total of six images at TEs of 0.032, 0.2, 0.4, 1.2, 1.8, and 2.4 ms were acquired using three interleaved scans. UTE-QSM was performed using a similar method to Dimov's PDF and MEDI study. Nine ROIs were drawn in different zones in the cortical bone samples, yielding 81 data points to compare UTE-QSM and μCT. Figure 26.7a shows the resultant susceptibility map from UTE-QSM (upper left), μCT (upper right), μCT-based porosity (lower left), and μCT-based BMD (lower right). This study showed significant linear correlations of −0.70 between susceptibility and BMD and 0.68 between susceptibility and porosity (Fig. 26.7b).

Fig. 26.7 Correlation between UTE-QSM and μCT. (**a**) Cadaveric tibial midshaft cortical bone (45-year-old female) and (**b**) scatter plot and linear regressions of average quantitative susceptibility mapping (QSM) of the nine studied bone specimens with bone mineral density (BMD) (left) and bone porosity (right). (Adapted with permission from Ref. [21])

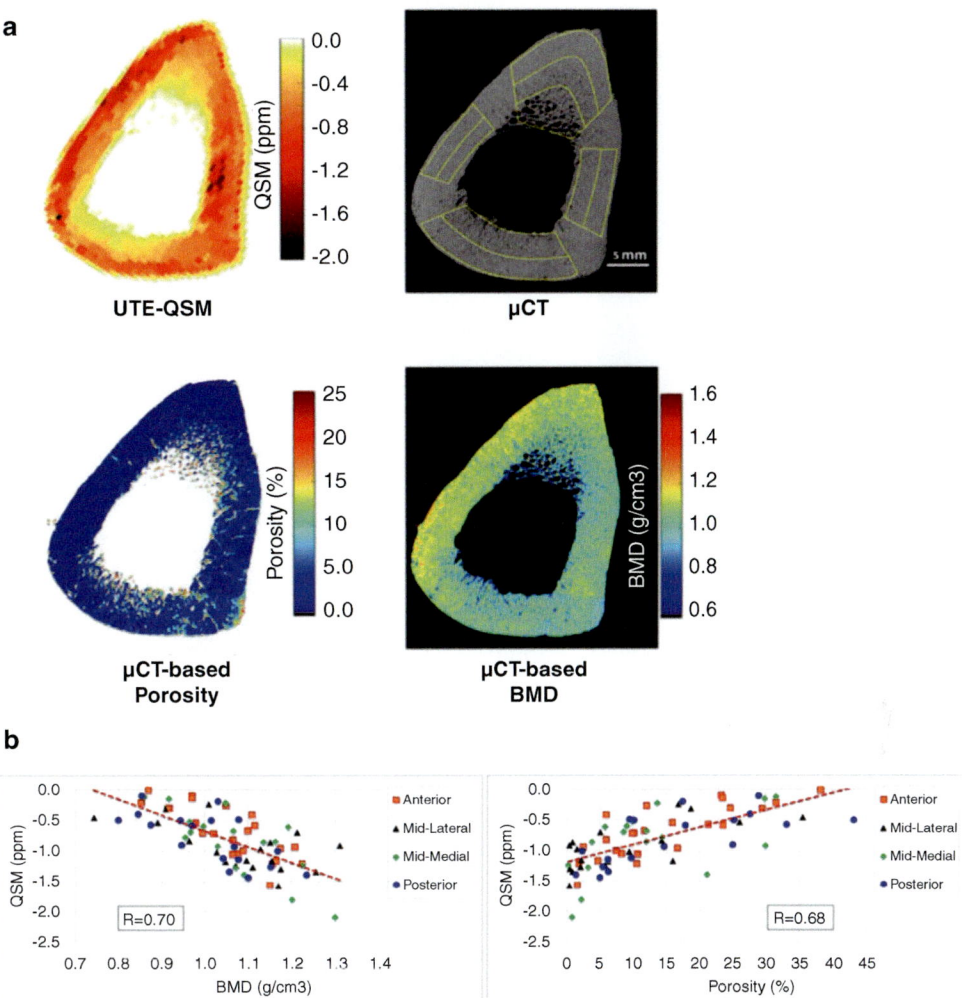

UTE-QSM for Detection of Iron Overload

Organic iron is usually paramagnetic and of fundamental importance in the human body. However, excessive iron deposition is seen in diseases and may be toxic. Iron content is an important biomarker for diagnosing dysfunctionality of organs such as the liver, pancreas, heart, and brain [43]. Gradient echo-based MRI has been effective for quantifying iron content. However, highly concentrated iron has a short-T_2 and T_2^* and shows little or no signal with conventional GRE acquisition. UTE-based R_2^* (i.e., $1/T_2^*$) quantification has been an effective method for quantifying iron over a wide range of concentrations [44]. UTE-QSM has also been investigated to quantify high iron concentrations. Lu et al. demonstrated simultaneous susceptibility and R_2^* mapping using UTE imaging. As a proof of concept, they performed a experiment using a phantom with various concentrations of iron oxide nanoparticles (IONPs) [45]. This was repeated with different first echo times (TE₁s) to investigate the effect

of the first TE. Figure 26.8 shows the phantom (left), the resultant R_2^* values from UTE-QSM (middle), and the susceptibility values from UTE-QSM (right). R_2^* and susceptibility showed higher values with increased iron concentrations, exhibiting high linearity. The linearity was impaired with longer values of TE₁ (i.e., non-UTE sequences) due to mis-estimation of R_2^* and susceptibility at higher iron concentrations. This shows that UTE imaging is necessary to estimate iron content with QSM accurately, and demonstrates the value of UTE-QSM.

Jang et al. have recently demonstrated the feasibility of another application using UTE-QSM which is in hemophilia [23]. In hemophilic patients, spontaneous bleeding in joints can cause hemophilic arthropathy. Recurrent bleeding causes accumulation of hemosiderin in the synovium and other joint tissues and results in a high level of tissue iron deposition which creates a toxic environment. Jang et al. have shown that the hemosiderin in knee and ankle joints can be quantified using the UTE-QSM technique.

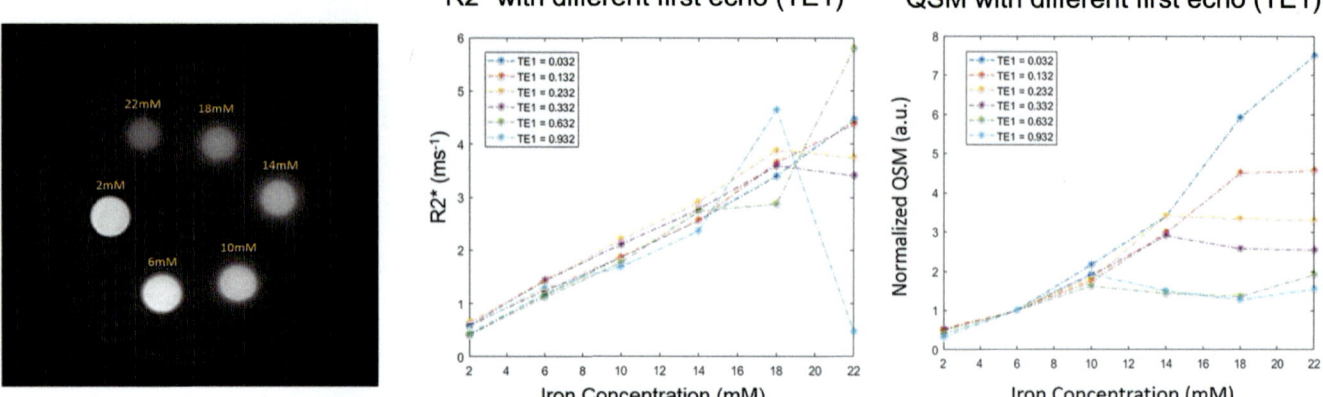

Fig. 26.8 R_2^* and QSM with different first echoes TEs (TE$_1$). The result shows that the shortest TE$_1$ is most desirable for accurately estimating R_2^* and QSM for materials with high susceptibility (i.e., highly concentrated iron in this study). (Adapted with permission from Ref. [45])

UTE-QSM for Stem Cell Tracking

Stem cell therapies have emerged as a promising treatment for various conditions such as Parkinson's disease and multiple sclerosis [46]. With the increasing number of clinical trials with stem cell therapies, there has been interest in the development of imaging techniques to noninvasively monitor the delivery of cells. With the development of various IONP-based stem cell labeling techniques, it has become possible to utilize MRI to track injected stem cells [47–49]. In MRI, the T$_1$ and T$_2$ of stem cells decrease with increasing IONP concentration, which creates a contrast with T$_1$-weighted or T$_2$-weighted MRI [50, 51]. However, highly concentrated IONPs typically cause strong susceptibility artifacts (i.e., blooming artifacts) using conventional MRI, preventing the scans from accurately localizing labeled stem cells.

As an alternative, Athertya et al. have recently reported the use of UTE techniques to provide quantitative evaluation of labeled stem cells [52]. Figure 26.9 shows results in a stem cell phantom scanned using quantitative UTE imaging techniques, including UTE-QSM, UTE-T$_1$, UTE-T$_2^*$, and spin echo-based T$_2$ with the Carr–Purcell–Meiboom–Gill (CPMG) sequence. The susceptibility values estimated with UTE-QSM showed highly linear fitting to the density of labeled stem cells. In contrast, CPMG-T$_2$ showed impaired estimation, presumably due to the rapid T$_2$ decay in signal from highly concentrated IONPs, resulting in a significantly decreased SNR. They also showed an ex vivo study with a post-mortem mouse that was injected with labeled stem cells. In the experiment, T$_2^*$ and UTE-QSM showed the best detection of the injected stem cells, while T$_1$ and CPMG-T$_2$ did not detect injected stem cells. In a comparison between T$_2^*$ and UTE-QSM, UTE-QSM exhibited better performance with clearly detected injection points. In contrast, the injection points on the T$_2^*$ map tended to be obscured by the surrounding tissues which were highly inhomogeneous. In vivo experiments are yet to be performed.

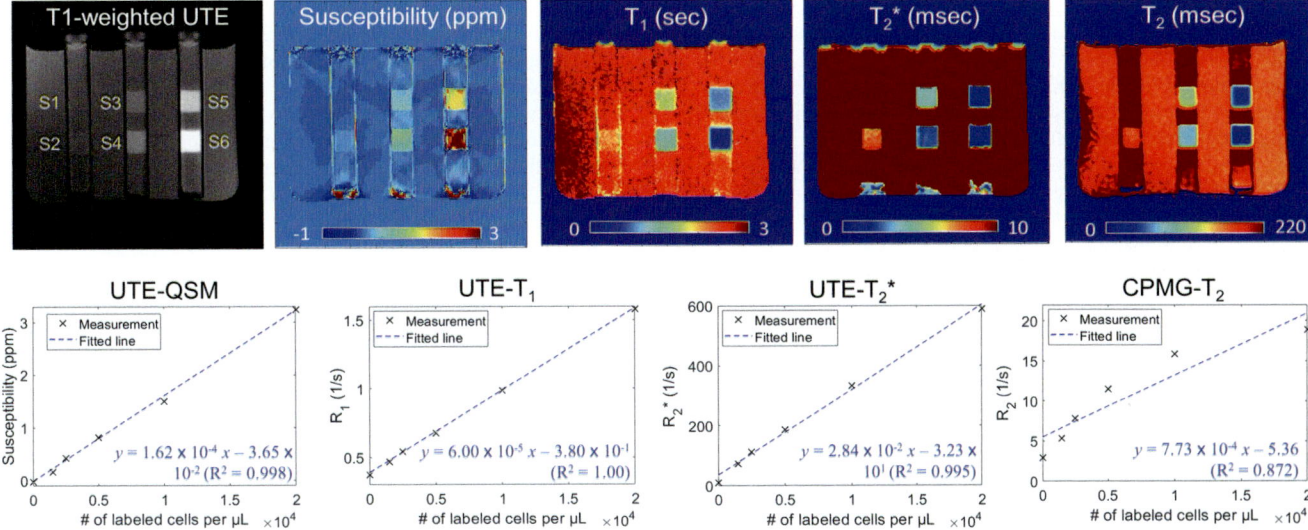

Fig. 26.9 Detection of stem cells labeled with IONPs. Phantom experiment. All qUTE parameters showed a highly linear relationship with the number of labeled cells ($R^2 > 0.99$), while clinical CPMG-based T_2 mapping showed poor linearity ($R^2 \sim 0.87$). (Adapted with permission from Ref. [52])

Conclusion

In this chapter, we have reviewed the status of UTE-QSM and its applications. UTE-QSM remains an active research topic with the development of UTE-QSM still at an early stage. The most promising area of application is MSK disorders. UTE-QSM has shown its efficacy in bone imaging targeting OP. UTE-QSM can also provide a meaningful biomarker for osteoarthritis by assessing tissue susceptibility in cartilage, tendons, ligaments, and menisci. However, UTE-QSM has not yet been investigated in patients with MSK pathologies due to technical challenges associated with current UTE-QSM implementations, such as limited spatial resolution, low SNR due to fast signal decay, and phase errors caused by eddy currents and chemical shift. Besides MSK applications, UTE-QSM has shown promising results in iron detection, which can provide quantitative assessment of iron and hemosiderin overload in tissues and labeled cell tracking. UTE-QSM for brain imaging can also be effective in detecting iron overload and hemorrhage [53].

In UTE-QSM, the chemical shift of fat is a significant source of error and causes strong streaking artifacts if not compensated for. Despite recent advances in UTE-QSM techniques which account for the fat signal model with multiple off-resonant peaks, residual errors in the signal fitting may be seen and these can cause artifacts that can affect estimated QSM values. Another source of error is motion between scans. Since interleaved scans are necessary to acquire multiple UTE images with a short echo spacing, inter-scan motion cannot be avoided. The motion causes misregistration between pixels and yields erroneous field mapping and dipole inversion. To avoid this, appropriate motion registration should be incorporated with in vivo scans [54, 55]. Another concern related to the interleaved scans is frequency shifting. As UTE sequences use strong gradients with a high-duty cycle, the temperature in the MRI bore of permanent magnets can increase over time, which results in varying B_0 field strength. Although prescan processing in modern MRI systems can address the resonant frequency (or center frequency) shift to some degree, there may still be remaining errors that can add different phase offsets in different scans, causing inaccurate field maps. Further studies are needed to address these issues.

In conclusion, UTE-QSM has a considerable potential to provide an additional layer of information that could be valuable for diagnosing pathologies associated with tissue degeneration and alterations in the tissue microenvironment. The technique still needs further development to explore more applications and establish its diagnostic value in clinical practice.

References

1. Barbosa JHO, Santos AC, Salmon CEG. Susceptibility weighted imaging: differentiating between calcification and hemosiderin. Radiol Bras. 2015;48(2):93–100.
2. Hodel J, Blanc R, Rodallec M, et al. Susceptibility-weighted angiography for the detection of high-flow intracranial vascular lesions: preliminary study. Eur Radiol. 2013;23(4):1122–30.
3. Le Bihan D. Diffusion, confusion and functional MRI. NeuroImage. 2012;62(2):1131–6.
4. Chen JJ, Pike GB. Human whole blood T_2 relaxometry at 3 tesla. Magn Reson Med. 2009;61(2):249–54.

5. Wang Y, Liu T. Quantitative susceptibility mapping (QSM): decoding MRI data for a tissue magnetic biomarker. Magn Reson Med. 2015;73(1):82–101.

6. Langkammer C, Liu T, Khalil M, Enzinger C, Jehna M, Fuchs S, Fazekas F, Wang Y, Ropele S. Quantitative susceptibility mapping in multiple sclerosis. Radiology. 2013;267(2):551–9.

7. Acosta-Cabronero J, Betts MJ, Cardenas-Blanco A, Yang S, Nestor PJ. In vivo MRI mapping of brain iron deposition across the adult lifespan. J Neurosci. 2016;36(2):364–74.

8. Deistung A, Schweser F, Wiestler B, et al. Quantitative susceptibility mapping differentiates between blood depositions and calcifications in patients with glioblastoma. PLoS One. 2013;8(3):e57924.

9. Liu S, Wang C, Zhang X, Zuo P, Hu J, Haacke EM, Ni H. Quantification of liver iron concentration using the apparent susceptibility of hepatic vessels. Quant Imaging Med Surg. 2018;8(2):123–34.

10. Barbosa JHO, Santos AC, Tumas V, Liu M, Zheng W, Haacke EM, Salmon CEG. Quantifying brain iron deposition in patients with Parkinson's disease using quantitative susceptibility mapping, R_2 and R_2*. Magn Reson Imaging. 2015;33(5):559–65.

11. Wisnieff C, Ramanan S, Olesik J, Gauthier S, Wang Y, Pitt D. Quantitative susceptibility mapping (QSM) of white matter multiple sclerosis lesions: interpreting positive susceptibility and the presence of iron. Magn Reson Med. 2015;74(2):564–70.

12. Xie L, Dibb R, Cofer GP, Li W, Nicholls PJ, Johnson GA, Liu C. Susceptibility tensor imaging of the kidney and its microstructural underpinnings. Magn Reson Med. 2015;73(3):1270–81.

13. Jafari R, Sheth S, Spincemaille P, et al. Rapid automated liver quantitative susceptibility mapping. J Magn Reson Imaging. 2019;50(3):725–32.

14. Bechler E, Stabinska J, Thiel T, et al. Feasibility of quantitative susceptibility mapping (QSM) of the human kidney. MAGMA. 2021;34(3):389–97.

15. Dibb R, Qi Y, Liu C. Magnetic susceptibility anisotropy of myocardium imaged by cardiovascular magnetic resonance reflects the anisotropy of myocardial filament α-helix polypeptide bonds. J Cardiovasc Magn Reson. 2015;17(1):60.

16. Wen Y, Nguyen TD, Liu Z, et al. Cardiac quantitative susceptibility mapping (QSM) for heart chamber oxygenation. Magn Reson Med. 2018;79(3):1545–52.

17. Wang L, Nissi MJ, Toth F, Johnson CP, Garwood M, Carlson CS, Ellermann J. Quantitative susceptibility mapping detects abnormalities in cartilage canals in a goat model of preclinical osteochondritis dissecans. Magn Reson Med. 2017;77(3):1276–83.

18. Wei H, Dibb R, Decker K, Wang N, Zhang Y, Zong X, Lin W, Nissman DB, Liu C. Investigating magnetic susceptibility of human knee joint at 7 tesla. Magn Reson Med. 2017;78(5):1933–43.

19. Dimov AV, Liu Z, Spincemaille P, Prince MR, Du J, Wang Y. Bone quantitative susceptibility mapping using a chemical species-specific R_2* signal model with ultrashort and conventional echo data. Magn Reson Med. 2018;7(1):121–8.

20. Jang H, Lu X, Carl M, Searleman AC, Jerban S, Ma Y, von Drygalski A, Chang EY, Du J. True phase quantitative susceptibility mapping using continuous single-point imaging: a feasibility study. Magn Reson Med. 2019;81(3):1907–14.

21. Jerban S, Lu X, Jang H, Ma Y, Namiranian B, Le N, Li Y, Chang EY, Du J. Significant correlations between human cortical bone mineral density and quantitative susceptibility mapping (QSM) obtained with 3D cones ultrashort echo time magnetic resonance imaging (UTE-MRI). Magn Reson Imaging. 2019;62:104–10.

22. Lu X, Jang H, Ma Y, Jerban S, Chang E, Du J. Ultrashort echo time quantitative susceptibility mapping (UTE-QSM) of highly concentrated magnetic nanoparticles: a comparison study about different sampling strategies. Molecules. 2019;24(6):1143.

23. Jang H, Drygalski A, Wong J, et al. Ultrashort echo time quantitative susceptibility mapping (UTE-QSM) for detection of hemosiderin deposition in hemophilic arthropathy: a feasibility study. Magn Reson Med. 2020;84(6):3246–55.

24. Li W, Avram AV, Wu B, Xiao X, Liu C. Integrated laplacian-based phase unwrapping and background phase removal for quantitative susceptibility mapping. NMR Biomed. 2014;27(2):219–27.

25. Bechler E, Stabinska J, Wittsack H. Analysis of different phase unwrapping methods to optimize quantitative susceptibility mapping in the abdomen. Magn Reson Med. 2019;82(6):2077–89.

26. Al-Radaideh AM, Wharton SJ, Lim SY, Tench CR, Morgan PS, Bowtell RW, Constantinescu CS, Gowland PA. Increased iron accumulation occurs in the earliest stages of demyelinating disease: an ultra-high field susceptibility mapping study in clinically isolated syndrome. Mult Scler J. 2013;19(7):896–903.

27. Liu T, Khalidov I, de Rochefort L, Spincemaille P, Liu J, Tsiouris AJ, Wang Y. A novel background field removal method for MRI using projection onto dipole fields (PDF). NMR Biomed. 2011;24(9):1129–36.

28. de Rochefort L, Nguyen T, Brown R, Spincemaille P, Choi G, Weinsaft J, Prince MR, Wang Y. In vivo quantification of contrast agent concentration using the induced magnetic field for time-resolved arterial input function measurement with MRI. Med Phys. 2008;35(12):5328–39.

29. Liu T, Spincemaille P, de Rochefort L, Kressler B, Wang Y. Calculation of susceptibility through multiple orientation sampling (COSMOS): a method for conditioning the inverse problem from measured magnetic field map to susceptibility source image in MRI. Magn Reson Med. 2009;61(1):196–204.

30. Liu J, Liu T, De Rochefort L, et al. Morphology enabled dipole inversion for quantitative susceptibility mapping using structural consistency between the magnitude image and the susceptibility map. NeuroImage. 2012;59(3):2560–8.

31. Wei H, Dibb R, Zhou Y, Sun Y, Xu J, Wang N, Liu C. Streaking artifact reduction for quantitative susceptibility mapping of sources with large dynamic range. NMR Biomed. 2015;28(10):1294–303.

32. Feng R, Zhao J, Wang H, et al. MoDL-QSM: model-based deep learning for quantitative susceptibility mapping. NeuroImage. 2021;240:118376.

33. Yoon J, Gong E, Chatnuntawech I, et al. Quantitative susceptibility mapping using deep neural network: QSMnet. NeuroImage. 2018;179:199–206.

34. Rahmer J, Börnert P, Groen J, Bos C. Three-dimensional radial ultrashort echo-time imaging with T_2 adapted sampling. Magn Reson Med. 2006;55(5):1075–82.

35. Wan L, Zhao W, Ma Y, Jerban S, Searleman AC, Carl M, Chang EY, Tang G, Du J. Fast quantitative 3D ultrashort echo time MRI of cortical bone using extended cones sampling. Magn Reson Med. 2019;82(1):225–36.

36. Wiens CN, Artz NS, Jang H, McMillan AB, Reeder SB. Externally calibrated parallel imaging for 3D multispectral imaging near metallic implants using broadband ultrashort echo time imaging. Magn Reson Med. 2017;77(6):2303–9.

37. Dimov AV, Liu T, Spincemaille P, Ecanow JS, Tan H, Edelman RR, Wang Y. Joint estimation of chemical shift and quantitative susceptibility mapping (chemical QSM). Magn Reson Med. 2015;73(6):2100–10.

38. Carl M, Nazaran A, Bydder GM, Du J. Effects of fat saturation on short T_2 quantification. Magn Reson Imaging. 2017;43:6–9.

39. Jang H, Carl M, Ma Y, Jerban S, Guo T, Zhao W, Chang EY, Du J. Fat suppression for ultrashort echo time imaging using a single-point Dixon method. NMR Biomed. 2019;32(5):e4069.

40. Glover G. Multipoint Dixon technique for water and fat proton and susceptibiltiy imaging. J Magn Reson Imaging. 1991;1(5):521–30.

41. Reeder SB, Pineda AR, Wen Z, Shimakawa A, Yu H, Brittain JH, Gold GE, Beaulieu CH, Pelc NJ. Iterative decomposition of water and fat with echo asymmetry and least-squares estimation (IDEAL): application with fast spin-echo imaging. Magn Reson Med. 2005;54(3):636–44.

42. De Rochefort L, Brown R, Prince MR, Wang Y. Quantitative MR susceptibility mapping using piece-wise constant regularized inversion of the magnetic field. Magn Reson Med. 2008;60(4):1003–9.

43. Wood JC. Guidelines for quantifying iron overload. Hematology Am Soc Hematol Educ Program. 2014;2014(1):210–5.

44. Hong W, He Q, Fan S, Carl M, Shao H, Chen J, Chang EY, Du J. Imaging and quantification of iron-oxide nanoparticles (IONP) using MP-RAGE and UTE based sequences. Magn Reson Med. 2017;78(1):226–32.

45. Lu X, Ma Y, Chang EY, He Q, Searleman A, von Drygalski A, Du J. Simultaneous quantitative susceptibility mapping (QSM) and R_2^* for high iron concentration quantification with 3D ultrashort echo time sequences: an echo dependence study. Magn Reson Med. 2018;79(4):2315–22.

46. Lindvall O, Kokaia Z. Stem cells for the treatment of neurological disorders. Nature. 2006;441(7097):1094–6.

47. Nedopil A, Klenk C, Kim C, Liu S, Wendland M, Golovko D, Schuster T, Sennino B, McDonald M, Heike D, Daldrup-Link E. MR signal characteristics of viable and apoptotic human mesenchymal stem cells in MASI for treatment of asteoarthritis. Investig Radiol. 2010;45(10):634–40.

48. Henning TD, Boddington S, Daldrup-Link HE. Labeling hESCs and hMSCs with iron oxide nanoparticles for non-invasive in vivo tracking with MR imaging. J Vis Exp. 2008;13:685.

49. Simon GH, Von Vopelius-Feldt J, Fu Y, Schlegel J, Pinotek G, Wendland MF, Chen MH, Daldrup-Link HE. Ultrasmall supraparamagnetic iron oxide-enhanced magnetic resonance imaging of antigen-induced arthritis: a comparative study between SHU 555 C, ferumoxtran-10, and ferumoxytol. Investig Radiol. 2006;41(1):45–51.

50. Gutova M, Frank JA, D'Apuzzo M, et al. Magnetic resonance imaging tracking of ferumoxytol-labeled human neural stem cells: studies leading to clinical use. Stem Cells Transl Med. 2013;2(10):766–75.

51. Khurana A, Nejadnik H, Chapelin F, et al. Ferumoxytol: a new, clinically applicable label for stem-cell tracking in arthritic joints with MRI. Nanomedicine. 2013;8(12):1–23.

52. Athertya JS, Akers J, Sedaghat S, Wei Z, Moazamian D, Dwek S, Thu M, Jang H. Detection of iron oxide nanoparticle (IONP)-labeled stem cells using quantitative ultrashort echo time imaging: a feasibility study. Quant Imaging Med Surg. 2023;13:585.

53. Jang H, Sedaghat S, Athertya JS, Moazamian D, Carl M, Ma Y, Lu X, Ji A, Chang EY, Du J. Feasibility of ultrashort echo time quantitative susceptibility mapping with a 3D cones trajectory in the human brain. Front Neurosci. 2022;16:1033801.

54. Wu M, Zhao W, Wan L, Kakos L, Li L, Jerban S, Jang H, Chang EY, Du J, Ma Y. Quantitative three-dimensional ultrashort echo time cones imaging of the knee joint with motion correction. NMR Biomed. 2020;33(1):1–11.

55. Klein S, Staring M, Murphy K, Viergever MA, Pluim JPW. Elastix: a toolbox for intensity-based medical image registration. IEEE Trans Med Imaging. 2010;29(1):196–205.

Chun Zeng, Jiang Du, Jiyo Athertya, and Graeme M. Bydder

Introduction

Dynamic contrast-enhanced magnetic resonance imaging (DCE-MRI) has been used to study perfusion in various tissues and organs in the body, such as the liver, breast, spine, brain, muscle, and bone marrow [1–3]. The technique typically employs fast repeated T_1-weighted images to capture signal changes induced by exogenous intravascular non-diffusible contrast agents, such as Gadolinium-Based Contrast Agents (GBCAs), in tissues or organs as a function of time. To generate a bolus, the paramagnetic contrast agent is injected intravenously, typically through the forearm. DCE-MRI involves the acquisition of baseline images without contrast enhancement and contrast-enhanced images after the arrival of the contrast agent in the tissue or organ of interest [2]. The basic principle of DCE-MRI imaging is relatively simple. As the paramagnetic contrast agent particle enters and is dispersed within the tissue, it changes the local T_1, T_2, or T_2^* (depending on the local concentration of the contrast agent), leading to change in the MR signal. A series of images can be used to analyze the temporal pattern of enhancement within the target tissue and allow assessment not only of perfusion but other microvascular parameters such as vessel permeability and fluid volume fractions [2].

However, it is challenging to study perfusion in solid tissues such as bone and many connective tissues, including menisci, ligaments, tendons, and periosteum, as well as the falx and meninges around the brain [4–6]. These tissues show rapid transverse magnetization relaxation and show little or no signal with conventional clinical pulse sequences. It is of considerable interest to study perfusion in these tissues. For example, it is clinically significant to differentiate the vascular red zone from the avascular white zone of the meniscus of the knee using noninvasive MRI. The white zone occupies the central ~70% of the meniscus, while the red zone occupies the more peripheral ~30% of the meniscus. As tears in the vascular portion are more likely to heal than those in the avascular region, meniscus-preserving surgical techniques are more effective for tears in the red zone, while debridement is more appropriate for those in the white zone [7].

Another example is bone which is highly vascularized [8]. There is a strong association between bone perfusion, bone remodeling, and fracture repair [9]. Increased cortical bone turnover and inflammation are associated with increased blood flow [10]. There is also a strong correlation between bone perfusion and bone mineral density [11]. However, the nature of bone makes it difficult to investigate its perfusion using conventional DCE-MRI techniques due to its extremely fast signal decay [12]. The same applies to many soft tissues with short- or ultrashort-T_2s, which are difficult or impossible to study with conventional techniques, including menisci, ligaments, and tendons, as well as the falx and meninges.

Ultrashort echo time (UTE) MRI sequences allow direct imaging of short- and ultrashort-T_2 tissues such as cortical bone, menisci, ligaments, and tendons. The nominal echo

C. Zeng
Department of Radiology, The First Affiliated Hospital of Chongqing Medical University, Chongqing, China

Department of Radiology, University of California, San Diego, La Jolla, CA, USA
e-mail: c3zeng@health.ucsd.edu

J. Du (✉)
Department of Radiology, University of California, San Diego, La Jolla, CA, USA

Department of Bioengineering, University of California, San Diego, La Jolla, CA, USA

VA San Diego Healthcare System, San Diego, CA, USA
e-mail: jiangdu@health.ucsd.edu

J. Athertya
Department of Radiology, University of California, San Diego, La Jolla, CA, USA
e-mail: jathertya@health.ucsd.edu

G. M. Bydder
Department of Radiology, University of California, San Diego, La Jolla, CA, USA

Mātai Medical Research Institute, Tairāwhiti Gisborne, New Zealand
e-mail: gbydder@health.ucsd.edu

J. Du, G. M. Bydder (eds.), *MRI of Short- and Ultrashort-T₂ Tissues*, https://doi.org/10.1007/978-3-031-35197-6_27

time (TE) can be reduced to less than 0.1 ms, which is shorter than the T_2^* of most tissues in the body. UTE sequences typically employ a short TR, which, together with the ultrashort TE, provides T_1-weighted imaging. This is helpful for GBCA-enhanced DCE-MRI of short- and ultrashort-T_2 tissues in the body.

Contrast-Enhanced MRI of Menisci

The knee menisci are C-shaped structures that span and cushion the space between the femur and the tibia in the knee joint. They play a vital protective role in the knee's long-term health by facilitating shock absorption and load distribution [13]. The menisci consist of highly organized collagen fibers, which lead to strong dipole–dipole interactions and a short T_2 [14]. As a result, the meniscus is only partially "visible" with conventional clinical sequences [15], and the red and white zones cannot be distinguished with MRI following contrast administration [16]. When UTE-type sequences with TEs of less than 0.1 ms are used, the menisci show moderate or high signals [17]. Their short-T_2 signal is detected before it decays to the very low level seen with conventional clinical pulse sequences with much longer TEs. Figure 27.1 shows the normal red zone of the meniscus using UTE subtraction images before and after contrast enhancement. In the pre-enhancement image, the meniscus appears isointense to articular cartilage and perimeniscal tissue at TE = 0.08 ms and has a generally lower signal at TE = 5.95 ms. Echo subtraction of the longer TE image from the UTE image shows the meniscus as moderate signal intensity with a low signal in the perimeniscal tissue (Fig. 27.1a). After contrast administration, the red zone of the meniscus is highlighted while the white zone remains unchanged (Fig. 27.2b) [5].

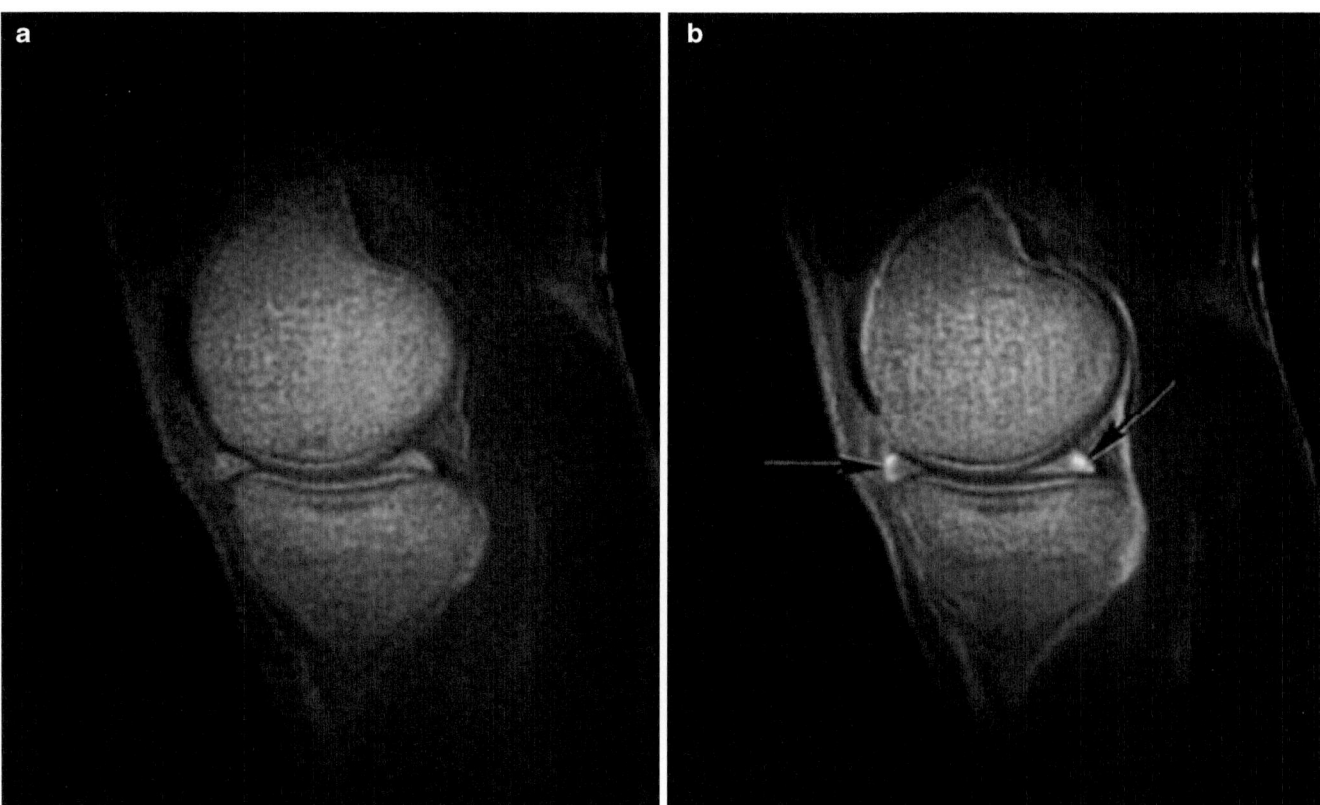

Fig. 27.1 Contrast enhancement of the red zone of the meniscus in a healthy volunteer. Sagittal UTE subtraction images with a TE of 0.08 ms minus a TE of 5.95 ms before (**a**) and after (**b**) enhancement. The red zone of the meniscus is highlighted on the contrast-enhanced image (**b**) (arrows). (Reproduced with permission from Ref. [5])

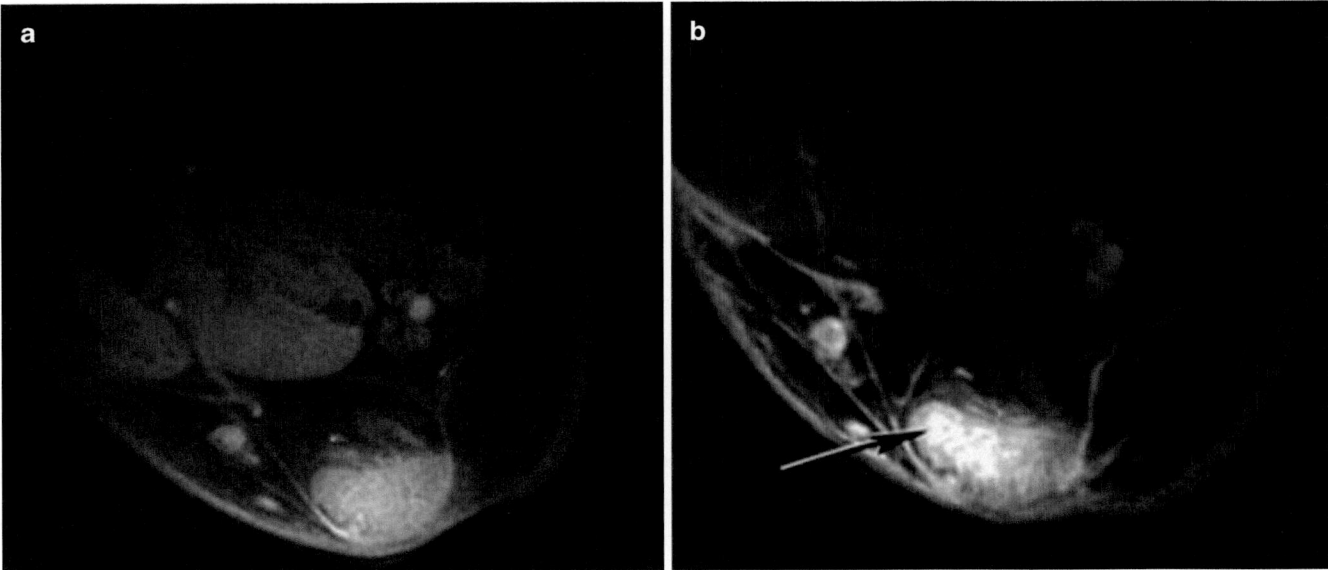

Fig. 27.2 Fat-saturated UTE imaging of Achilles tendinopathy before (**a**) and after (**b**) contrast enhancement using a TR of 500 ms and a TE of 0.08 ms. There is more significant enhancement on the right (arrow). (Reproduced with permission from Ref. [5])

Contrast-Enhanced MRI of Tendons

Tendons are dense fibrous connective tissues that attach muscle to bone. A tendon is primarily composed of collagenous fibers which contain bunches of collagen fibrils. The tendon shows a generally uniform parallel alignment of collagen molecules along the long axis, which provides the tensile strength necessary for mechanical motion of the body [18]. Tendons are poorly vascularized and rely heavily on synovial fluid to provide nutrition [19]. There is also a requirement for cell infiltration from blood to provide the necessary reparative factors for tissue healing during tendon injury from spontaneous rupture to chronic tendinitis or tendinosis. Contrast-enhanced MRI of the tendons can be used to study perfusion and potentially the response of the vasculature to tendon damage, including how and when revascularization or neovascularization occurs. Other potential applications include the study of the revascularization of the tendon during its use as a tendon graft in both ligament reconstruction and tendon–tendon grafting. However, stiff collagen molecules are immobile, leading to strong dipole–dipole coupling. As a result, tendons typically show a signal void with conventional clinical MR sequences when their fibers are aligned parallel to the B_0 field. UTE sequences can directly detect signals from tendons, allowing their perfusion to be studied using contrast-enhanced UTE MRI. Figure 27.2 shows contrast enhancement in abnormal Achilles tendons [5]. Distinct differences are observed with much higher signal enhancement on the right, the more abnormal Achilles tendon, consistent with increased vascularity in Achilles tendinopathy.

Contrast-Enhanced MRI of Bone

Bone is a composite material that is made up of hard and brittle calcium, containing mineral hydroxyapatite, soft and flexible protein collagen, and water. It has at least six significant functions, including support, movement, protection, production of blood cells, storage of ions, and endocrine regulation. Bone is divided into trabecular and cortical components, with the latter accounting for 80% of the skeleton. The highly vascularized trabecular bone and the inner two-thirds of cortical bone receive blood supply via the marrow cavity. In contrast, the outer third of cortical bone receives perfusion from the periosteum [20]. Perfusion plays a critical role in the growth and development of bone as well as in disease and healing. Bone perfusion can be assessed with nuclear medicine-based techniques, such as 18F-Fluoride positron emission tomography (PET), which is expensive, has a low spatial resolution, and subjects patients to ionizing radiation [21]. MRI can provide much higher spatial resolution without ionizing radiation and has advantages for studying bone perfusion. However, most MRI studies have focused on perfusion in the bone marrow [20], partly because cortical and trabecular bone show extremely fast signal decay and are invisible with conventional MRI sequences [22]. UTE sequences with nominal TEs less than 0.1 ms allow direct imaging of cortical bone. Figure 27.3 shows representative 2D UTE images of the tibial midshaft of a 38-year-old healthy volunteer pre-injection and at the enhancement peak after intravenous GBCA injection, as well as contrast-enhanced curves and signal modeling [6]. The corresponding kinetic analysis demon-

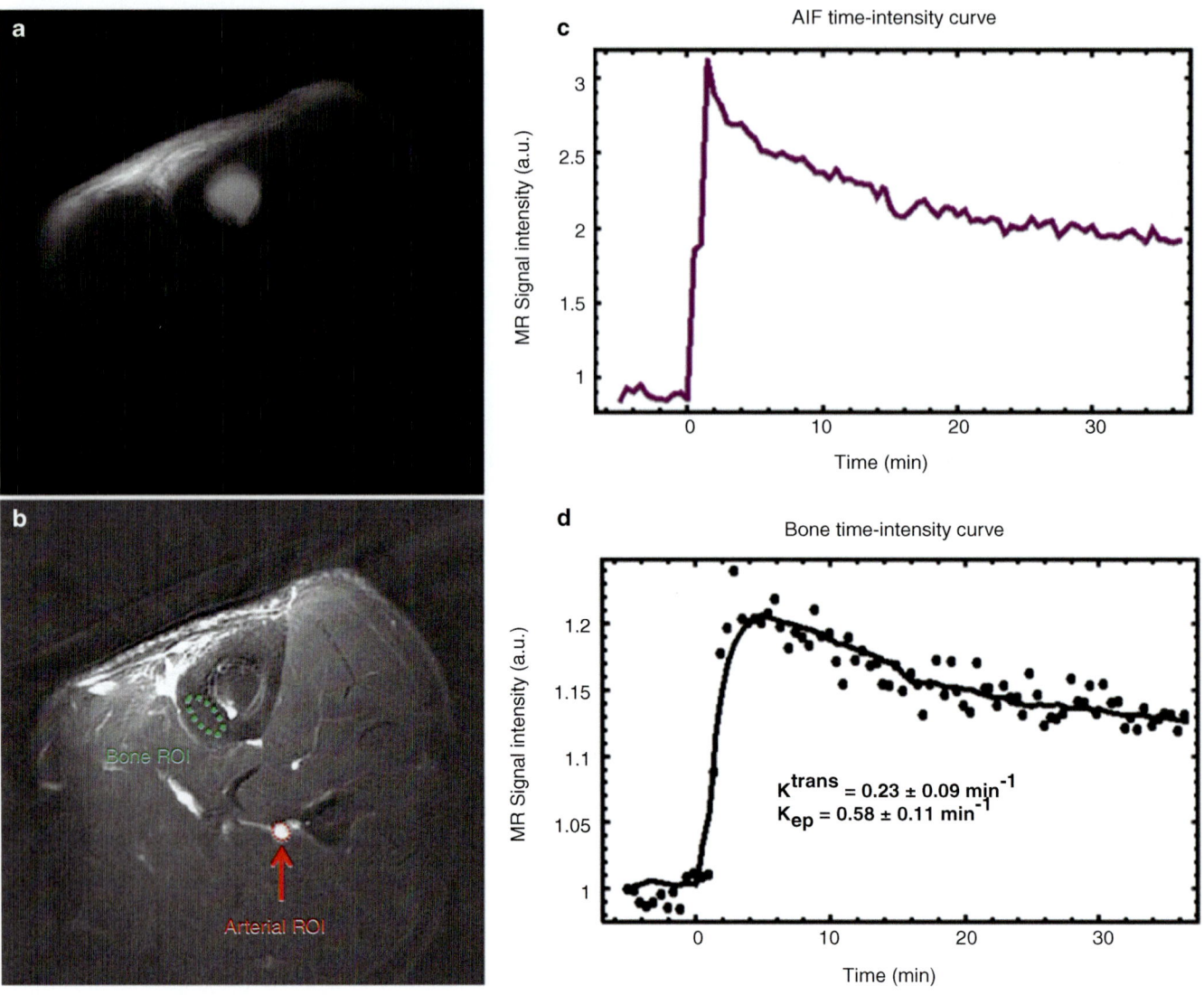

Fig. 27.3 UTE-based DCE-MRI of the tibial midshaft of a 38-year-old healthy volunteer: baseline image (**a**), subtraction of the peak enhancement from baseline image (**b**), a dynamic curve for an arterial region of interest (ROI) (**c**), and bone ROI (**d**). Kinetic analysis showed a K^{tran} of 0.23 ± 0.09 min^{-1} and K_{ep} of 0.58 ± 0.11 min^{-1} for the tibial midshaft. (Reproduced with permission from Ref. [6])

strated a K^{tran} of 0.23 ± 0.09 min^{-1} and K_{ep} of 0.58 ± 0.11 min^{-1} for the tibial midshaft.

The UTE bone signal comes from water in the vascular space (also called pore water) and water bound to the organic matrix (also called bound water), accounting for most of the total signal [23]. Bound water concentration is an indirect measure of organic matrix density, while pore water concentration is an indirect measure of cortical porosity. Adiabatic inversion recovery prepared UTE (IR-UTE) imaging has been developed to selectively image bound water in bone. UTE bone signal shows a bicomponent T_2^* decay with a longer T_2^* of a few ms and a shorter T_2^* of ~0.3 ms, while IR-UTE signal shows a mono-component T_2^* decay with a T_2^* of ~0.3 ms, consistent with selective suppression of the

longer T_2^* component or pore water and selective detection of the bound water component [24]. The IR-UTE sequence can be used for dynamic imaging organic matrix enhancement in cortical bone [6]. Figure 27.4 shows representative 2D IR-UTE imaging of the tibial midshaft of two human volunteers aged 68 and 40 years, respectively, at three specific time points (pre-contrast, peak, and post-contrast), as well as the corresponding bone perfusion curves. The 2D IR-UTE sequence shows excellent contrast for cortical bone before contrast enhancement and some increase in signal after contrast injection. Different contrast enhancement patterns were observed for the 68-year-old subject, where the curve shows an early peak, a rapid decline, and then a plateau. For the 40-year-old subject, a less peaked curve is shown [6].

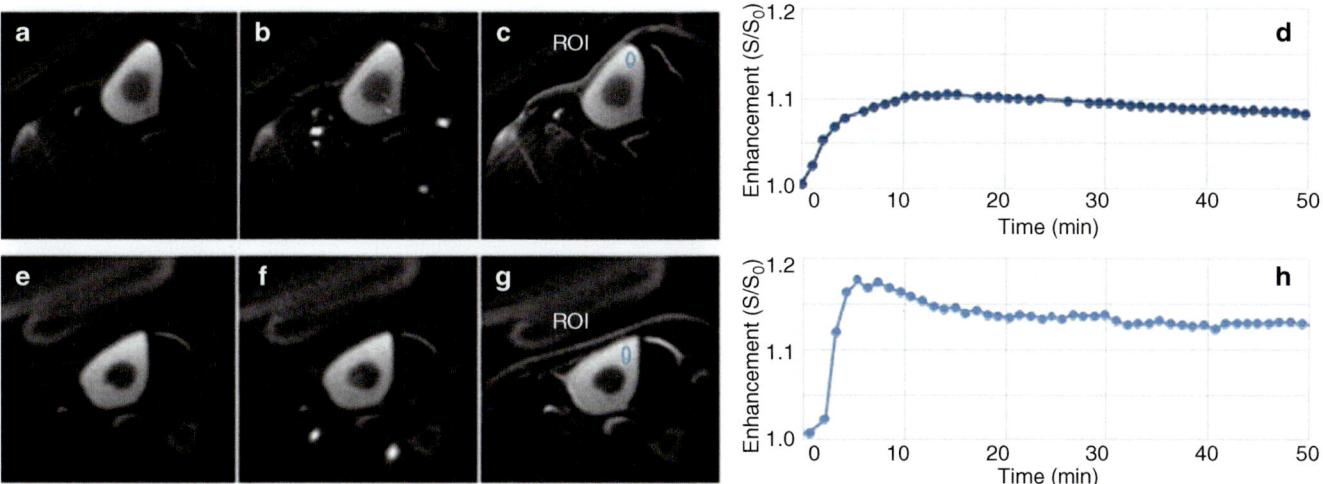

Fig. 27.4 IR-UTE imaging of two volunteers aged 68 and 40 years, respectively, at pre-contrast (**a, e**), peak enhancement (**b, f**), and post-contrast (**c, g**), and the corresponding bone perfusion curves (**d, h**) derived from two small ROIs shown in (**c, g**). Distinct contrast enhancement patterns are observed in the two volunteers. (Reproduced with permission from Ref. [6])

Maximum enhancement and enhancement slope can be used for further evaluation of cortical bone perfusion using the technique described by Griffith et al. [25]. Maximum enhancement can be calculated as the signal difference between maximal and minimal bone signal divided by the baseline signal. Enhancement slope can be calculated as the difference between maximal signal and baseline signal divided by the baseline signal and further separated by the time interval between the two time points at which the minimal and maximal signal intensities of interest were reached (10% and 90% of the maximum signal intensity, respectively) [6]. Both parameters can be derived from the first-pass phase of contrast enhancement and reflect the arrival of the contrast agent into the arteries and capillaries of cortical bone as well as its diffusion into the extracellular space and subsequent departure [6, 25]. Figure 27.5 shows perfusion curves using global regions of interest (ROIs) for cortical bone and the arterial input function, contrast enhancement, and enhancement slope, respectively. The younger volunteer shows higher enhancement with a higher enhancement slope [6]. IR-UTE-based DCE-MRI can potentially be used to study bone remodeling, which involves bone resorption by osteoclasts and the formation of new bone by osteoblasts. If an osteoclast or osteoblast-specific molecular agent is combined with gadolinium or iron, the IR-UTE sequence can potentially detect osteoclast or osteoblast activity.

Contrast-enhanced DCE-MRI has also been used to study perfusion in many other short-T_2 tissues of the body. For example, contrast enhancement can be observed in the normal periosteum and ligamentum flavum and anterior and posterior longitudinal ligaments of the lumbar spine. The contrast enhancement seen in disc disease is more obvious with DCE-MRI based on UTE sequences than with conven-

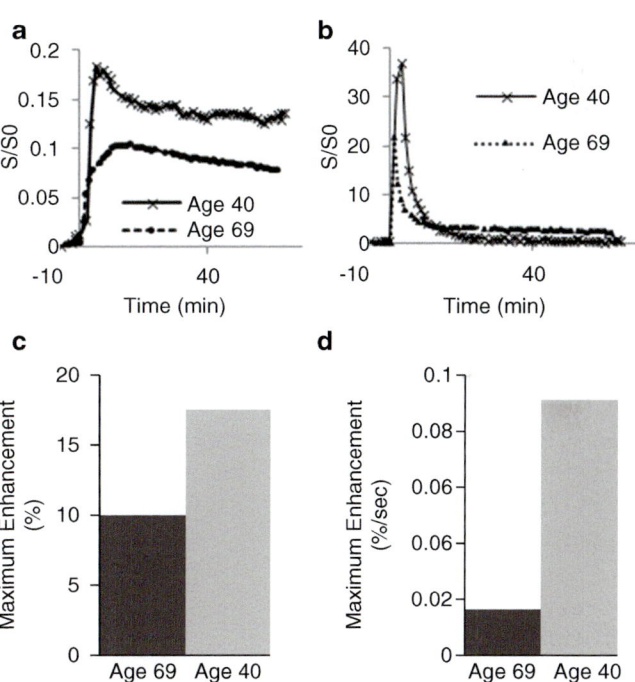

Fig. 27.5 Global contrast enhancement curves for tibial midshaft (**a**), AIF (**b**), maximum enhancement (**c**), and enhancement slope (**d**) of the 69-year-old and 40-year-old volunteers, respectively, based on 2D IR-UTE imaging. The 40-year-old volunteer shows an early peak with a rapid decline and then a plateau, with a higher maximum enhancement and enhancement slope than the 69-year-old volunteer, who shows a flatter contrast enhancement curve. (Reproduced with permission from Ref. [6])

tional clinical sequences. UTE-based sagittal post-enhancement images of the lumbar spine can depict disc prolapse, which is otherwise invisible with clinical T_1-weighted imaging [5]. Contrast-enhanced fat-suppressed

UTE imaging can be used to evaluate injury to the posterior cruciate ligament where scar tissue shows more obvious enhancement [5]. In fat-suppressed UTE, there is an extensive enhancement in blood vessels due to fracture of the tibial plateau 2 days after injury, with specific enhancement of the periosteum distinguished from that of blood vessels [5]. Contrast-enhanced UTE MRI can also highlight the falx and meninges, which are low signal with conventional clinical MRI sequences [5].

Conclusion

UTE-based dynamic MRI can detect contrast enhancement in short-T_2 tissues in which signal changes are poorly demonstrated or not seen with conventional pulse sequences. For the first time, contrast enhancement can be observed in the knee menisci, tendons, ligaments, bone, meninges, falx, dura, and many other short-T_2 tissues of the body. The red zone of the meniscus can be selectively highlighted and separated from the white zone of the meniscus, facilitating the diagnosis and treatment of tears and other diseases of the meniscus. Abnormal tendons in tendinopathy can be depicted with high contrast in the UTE perfusion study of the tendons. Perfusion in the cortical bone can be studied with MRI with much higher spatial resolution without ionization than with PET, which is the standard functional imaging technique to visualize and quantify regional bone metabolism and blood flow. IR-UTE-based DCE-MRI can be used to study perfusion in the organic matrix of bone and potentially the osteoclast and/or osteoblast activity. UTE- and IR-UTE-based dynamic MRI paves the way for perfusion and molecular imaging in hard tissues and many connective tissues that are otherwise "invisible" with conventional clinical MRI techniques. The clinical significance of this technique remains to be established.

References

1. Tofts PS, Kermode AG. Measurement of the blood-brain barrier permeability and leakage space using dynamic MR imaging. 1. Fundamental concepts. Magn Reson Med. 1991;17(2):357–67.
2. Sourbron S. Technical aspects of MR perfusion. Eur J Radiol. 2010;76(3):304–13.
3. Cha S. Perfusion MR imaging: basic principles and clinical applications. Magn Reson Imaging Clin N Am. 2003;11(3):403–13.
4. Gatehouse PD, He T, Puri BK, Thomas RD, Resnick D, Bydder GM. Contrast-enhanced MRI of the menisci of the knee using ultrashort echo time (UTE) pulse sequences: imaging of the red and white zones. Br J Radiol. 2004;77(920):641–7.
5. Robson MD, Gatehouse PD, So PW, Bell JD, Bydder GM. Contrast enhancement of short T_2 tissues using ultrashort TE (UTE) pulse sequences. Clin Radiol. 2004;59(8):720–6.
6. Wan L, Wu M, Sheth V, Shao H, Jang H, Bydder G, et al. Evaluation of cortical bone perfusion using dynamic contrast enhanced ultrashort echo time imaging: a feasibility study. Quant Imaging Med Surg. 2019;9(8):1383–93.
7. Newman AP, Daniels AU, Burks RT. Principles and decision making in meniscal surgery. Arthroscopy. 1993;9(1):33–51.
8. Sider KL, Song J, Davies JE. A new bone vascular perfusion compound for the simultaneous analysis of bone and vasculature. Microsc Res Tech. 2010;73(7):665–72.
9. McFarlane SI, Muniyappa R, Shin JJ, Bahtiyar G, Sowers JR. Osteoporosis and cardiovascular disease: brittle bones and boned arteries, is there a link? Endocrine. 2004;23(1):1–10.
10. McCarthy I. The physiology of bone blood flow: a review. J Bone Joint Surg Am. 2006;88(Suppl 3):4–9.
11. Wang YX, Griffith JF, Kwok AW, Leung JC, Yeung DK, Ahuja AT, et al. Reduced bone perfusion in proximal femur of subjects with decreased bone mineral density preferentially affects the femoral neck. Bone. 2009;45(4):711–5.
12. Du J, Carl M, Bydder M, Takahashi A, Chung CB, Bydder GM. Qualitative and quantitative ultrashort echo time (UTE) imaging of cortical bone. J Magn Reson. 2010;207(2):304–11.
13. Englund M. The role of the meniscus in osteoarthritis genesis. Rheum Dis Clin N Am. 2008;34(3):573–9.
14. Szeverenyi NM, Bydder GM. Dipolar anisotropy fiber imaging in a goat knee meniscus. Magn Reson Med. 2011;65(2):463–70.
15. McWalter EJ, Gold GE. UTE T_2* mapping detects sub-clinical meniscus degeneration. Osteoarthr Cartil. 2012;20(6):471–2.
16. Hauger O, Frank LR, Boutin RD, Lektrakul N, Chung CB, Haghighi P, et al. Characterization of the "red zone" of knee meniscus: MR imaging and histologic correlation. Radiology. 2000;217(1):193–200.
17. Gold GE, Pauly JM, Macovski A, Herfkens RJ. MR spectroscopic imaging of collagen: tendons and knee menisci. Magn Reson Med. 1995;34(5):647–54.
18. Fullerton GD, Rahal A. Collagen structure: the molecular source of the tendon magic angle effect. J Magn Reson Imaging. 2007;25(2):345–61.
19. Fenwick SA, Hazleman BL, Riley GP. The vasculature and its role in the damaged and healing tendon. Arthritis Res. 2002;4(4):252–60.
20. Ma HT, Griffith JF, Zhao X, Lv H, Yeung DK, Leung PC. Relationship between marrow perfusion and bone mineral density: a pharmacokinetic study of DCE-MRI. In: Annu Int Conf IEEE Eng Med Biol Soc, vol. 2012; 2012. p. 377–9.
21. Dyke JP, Aaron RK. Noninvasive methods of measuring bone blood perfusion. Ann N Y Acad Sci. 2010;1192:95–102.
22. Tyler DJ, Robson MD, Henkelman RM, Young IR, Bydder GM. Magnetic resonance imaging with ultrashort TE (UTE) PULSE sequences: technical considerations. J Magn Reson Imaging. 2007;25(2):279–89.
23. Biswas R, Bae W, Diaz E, Masuda K, Chung CB, Bydder GM, et al. Ultrashort echo time (UTE) imaging with bi-component analysis: bound and free water evaluation of bovine cortical bone subject to sequential drying. Bone. 2012;50(3):749–55.
24. Afsahi AM, Ma Y, Jang H, Jerban S, Chung CB, Chang EY, et al. Ultrashort echo time magnetic resonance imaging techniques: met and unmet needs in musculoskeletal imaging. J Magn Reson Imaging. 2022;55(6):1597–612.
25. Griffith JF, Yeung DK, Antonio GE, Lee FK, Hong AW, Wong SY, et al. Vertebral bone mineral density, marrow perfusion, and fat content in healthy men and men with osteoporosis: dynamic contrast-enhanced MR imaging and MR spectroscopy. Radiology. 2005;236(3):945–51.

UTE Diffusion-Weighted Imaging (UTE-DWI)

Hyungseok Jang, Soo Hyun Shin, Michael Carl, Yajun Ma, and Jiang Du

Introduction

Diffusion refers to the net movement or flow of energy or particles, such as atoms, molecules, and ions, in a physical system. A molecule in a free space undergoes random thermal motion called random walk or Brownian motion. The resultant random displacements typically follow a Gaussian distribution. In MRI, diffusion of protons (or spins) can be an unwanted adverse effect that limits spatial resolution. Conversely, diffusion effects can be utilized to create diffusion dependent image contrast and estimate apparent diffusivity. A pair of motion-sensitizing gradients are usually used to capture diffusion information. In this technique, the first gradient is applied to spins. After a certain time (i.e., T_{mix}), the second gradient is applied to rephase the spins. If there is no motion of the spins, they will be completely rephased, and there will be no residual phase modulation. If there is motion, the spins undergo different degrees of dephasing and rephasing, resulting in overall dephasing which reduces the signal from the spins. This approach, which is based on pulsed gradients, was first proposed by Stejskal and Tanner [1]. The signal reduction due to molecular water diffusion is as follows:

H. Jang (✉) · S. H. Shin · Y. Ma
Department of Radiology, University of California, San Diego, La Jolla, CA, USA
e-mail: h4jang@health.ucsd.edu; shs033@health.ucsd.edu; yam013@health.ucsd.edu

M. Carl
GE Healthcare, San Diego, CA, USA
e-mail: Michael.Carl@ge.com

J. Du
Department of Radiology, University of California, San Diego, La Jolla, CA, USA

Department of Bioengineering, University of California, San Diego, La Jolla, CA, USA

VA San Diego Healthcare System, San Diego, CA, USA
e-mail: jiangdu@health.ucsd.edu

$$\frac{S}{S_0} = \exp\left[-\gamma^2 G^2 \delta^2 \left(\Delta - \frac{\delta}{3} \right) D \right] \qquad (28.1)$$

where S_0 is the initial signal intensity without diffusion weighting, S is the diffusion-weighted signal, γ is the gyromagnetic ratio, G is the amplitude of diffusion-weighting gradient, δ is the duration of the gradient waveform, and Δ is the timing between two diffusion-weighting gradients also called T_{mix}. D is the diffusivity in the unit of mm²/s, also known as the apparent diffusion coefficient (ADC) [2]. This equation is often simplified by defining $b = \gamma^2 G^2 \delta^2 \left(\Delta - \frac{\delta}{3} \right)$, which yields the following equation:

$$S(b) = S_0 \exp(-bD) \qquad (28.2)$$

where b is the diffusion-weighting sensitivity factor in the unit of s/mm². To estimate D, diffusion-weighted imaging (DWI) is repeated multiple times with different b-values, and the signal decay is fitted using the above equations. Several approaches have been proposed to achieve signal preparation with diffusion weighting, such as spin echo- (SE), gradient echo-, and stimulated echo-based sequences. For data readout, echo planar imaging (EPI) is often used in clinical DWI to provide fast data acquisition [3].

As molecular diffusivity is closely related to the cellular microenvironment in living systems, diffusion-weighted MRI has been actively investigated and has become essential in clinical MRI examinations of the nervous system [4–6], body [7–9], cardiovascular system [10, 11], and musculoskeletal system [12–14]. However, DWI of short-T_2 tissues remains relatively unexplored. To achieve DWI for short-T_2 tissues, ultrashort echo time (UTE)-type sequences are necessary to enable the MR system receiving mode before short-T_2 signals decay to the noise level. However, a significant challenge for UTE-based diffusion imaging is that the minimum echo time (TE) is limited by the need for diffusion preparation. Transverse magnetization decays when diffusion encoding gradients are applied, and if these are of moderately long duration (of the order of a few ms), the signal from short-T_2 tissues ($T_2^* < 1$ ms) may have decayed to near zero, or zero, before the completion of the diffusion-weighting preparation and application of the spatial encoding gradients. As an alternative, stimulated echo-based UTE-DWI and double echo steady state (DESS)-based UTE-DWI techniques have been implemented. In this chapter, we review these two approaches.

Challenges with UTE Diffusion-Weighted Imaging (UTE-DWI)

As mentioned above, there are two conflicting factors: first, the requirement for a short enough TE to detect signal from short-T_2 tissues and second, a sufficiently high b-value to achieve useful diffusion sensitization. The transverse magnetization undergoes T_2^* decay during the diffusion gradient and T_2 decay during T_{mix}. Therefore, the resultant image has both T_2-weighting and diffusion weighting, which is not desirable for UTE-DWI. The duration of the gradient can be decreased by using a fast-ramping high-amplitude gradient waveform, but this is limited by hardware performance in the gradient system and FDA regulations for gradient slew rates [15].

Stimulated Echo Acquisition Mode (STEAM)-UTE-DWI

As an alternative, STEAM-based diffusion-weighted (DW) [16, 17] UTE (STEAM-DW-UTE) has been investigated [18]. Figure 28.1 shows the pulse sequence diagram. In this approach, diffusion weighting is achieved by using the preceding preparation module. In this module, a 90° tip-down

pulse is first applied, and this is followed by a diffusion gradient. As soon as the gradient is completed, the transverse magnetization is sent back to the longitudinal plane using a tip-up pulse with a −90° flip angle. A subsequent spoiler removes the remaining transverse magnetization. After that, another set of 90° tip-down RF pulse, diffusion encoding gradient, and a tip-up RF pulse is applied, followed by a UTE readout. This approach removes the T_2 decay during T_{mix} since the magnetization is stored in the longitudinal plane where the spins undergo T_1 recovery. However, T_2^* decay during the RF pulses and diffusion gradients cannot be avoided. Therefore, higher b-values cause higher T_2^*-weighting in the signal, which is not desirable with STEAM-UTE-DWI. b-values that are too low with STEAM-UTE-DWI can induce artifacts due to the banding effect that is generated when the phase labeling cycle is larger than the pixel dimension. The wavelength of the banding artifact is given by $\lambda = 2\pi/(\gamma\delta G)$. The diffusion gradient moment needs to be large enough so that λ is smaller than the pixel dimension in the corresponding axis. Figure 28.2 shows two phantom images with different diffusion gradient moments applied on the X-axis (left to right). The lower gradient moment results in a smaller λ.

Carl et al. showed the feasibility of STEAM-UTE-DWI using a cones trajectory [18]. In this approach, a STEAM-based diffusion-weighted preparation is followed by a 3D UTE cones data readout, with multiple spokes acquired per preparation. The multispoke imaging reduces the total imaging time, but the signal variation between spokes due to T_1 recovery can cause artifacts that contaminate the diffusion weighting produced by the diffusion preparation module. T_1 contamination is minimized by using an RF cycling scheme, in which the last tip-up pulse in the STEAM module alternates between +90° and −90°, and the average signal is taken. The MRI experiment was performed on a 3T clinical MR scanner

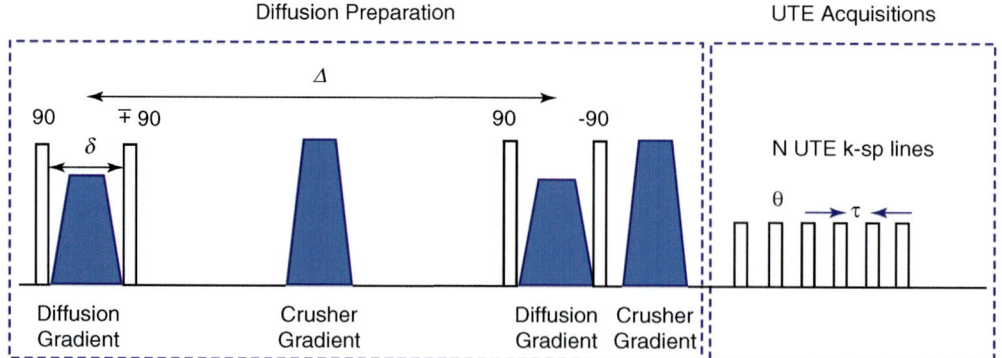

Fig. 28.1 STEAM-UTE-DWI. The first RF pulse (tip-down) flips the magnetization onto the transverse plane where the first diffusion gradient dephases the transverse magnetization, and the second RF pulse (tip-up) places it back into the longitudinal plane. After mixing time, Δ (or T_{mix}), another set of RF pulses and gradient is applied, and this rephases magnetization. Moving spins undergo dephasing during the

application of gradients which results in diffusion weighting. In the RF cycling scheme, the acquisition of data is repeated twice with the alternated polarity of the second or the fourth RF pulses (tip-up pulses), and the signal is averaged to reduce the effect of T_1 recovery. (Adapted with permission from Ref. [18])

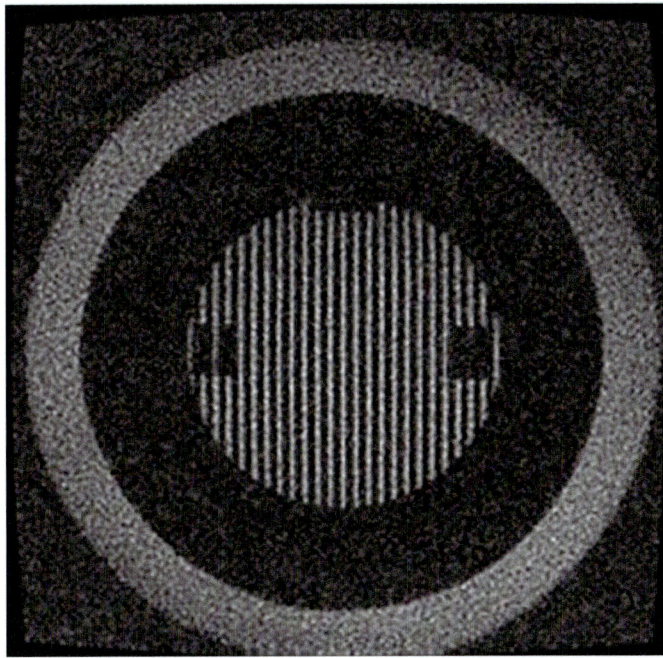 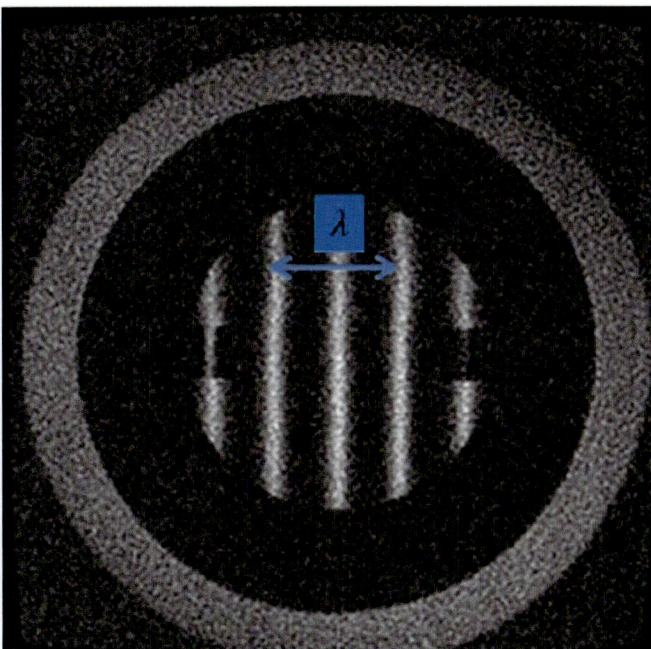

Fig. 28.2 Banding artifact with STEAM-UTE-DWI with small diffusion gradient moments. A higher diffusion-weighted gradient moment yields narrower banding with $\lambda = 9$ mm (left), whereas a lower diffusion gradient moment yields wider banding with $\lambda = 46$ mm (right). Use of a large diffusion gradient can remove the banding artifact because the wavelength of the banding becomes smaller than the pixel resolution. (Adapted with permission from Ref. [18])

(HDXt, GE Healthcare) using a T/R head coil with a doped water phantom with $T_1 = 100$ ms and $T_2 = 65$ ms. Figure 28.3 shows simulated STEAM-UTE-DWI data with different combinations of RF pulses: 90°, −90°, 90°, and −90° (Fig. 28.3a), 90°, 90°, 90°, and −90° (Fig. 28.3b), and RF cycled (Fig. 28.3c). Without RF cycling, the signal shows over- or underestimation due to the T_1 recovery effect. With RF cycling, the simulated signal is close to the expected signal decay. In an MRI experiment with the phantom, RF cycled STEAM-UTE-DWI showed an improved signal decay curve, reducing signal bias due to the T_1 effect, which was close to diffusion-weighted SE-based EPI (DW-SE-EPI) (Fig. 28.3d).

To investigate the influence of T_1, T_2, and TR on the accuracy of ADC estimated with STEAM-UTE-DWI, a phantom experiment was performed by Baron et al. using six tubes filled with 2% agarose gel and different concentrations of $MnCl_2$ (from 10 to 80 mg/L) [19]. The phantom was imaged using a STEAM-UTE-DWI sequence with $T_{mix} = 120$ ms and b-values = 14, 57, 127, and 227 s/mm², respectively. The experiment was repeated with different TRs of 200, 300, and 500 ms. As reference values, T_1, T_2, and ADC were measured using clinical inversion recovery (IR)-prepared spin echo (SE), SE, and DW-SE-EPI sequences, respectively. The measured mean T_1s with the IR-SE sequence were 238.0, 388.2, 387.3, 698.0, 924.1, and 1312.5 ms for tubes 1–6 (Fig. 28.4a). The measured mean T_2s with the SE sequence were 17.0,

24.9, 28.3, 35.2, 48.5, and 44.2 ms for tubes 1–6 (Fig. 28.4b). The measured mean ADC with the DW-SE-EPI sequence was 2.15×10^{-3} mm²/s in all tubes. Figure 28.4c–e shows the estimated ADC map from UTE-DWI with three different TRs. With a shorter TR, UTE-DWI tends to overestimate the ADC, presumably due to the residual signal that builds a coherent pathway. With TR = 200 ms, the ADC was overestimated up to 40% compared to the ADC estimated by DW-SE-EPI. Figure 28.4f shows the ADC map corrected by a Bloch simulation that simulated random diffusion weighting to spoil the coherent signal buildup. This dramatically reduced errors. This study shows that imaging parameters such as TR should be carefully selected for accurate ADC estimation when using STEAM-UTE-DWI.

Carl et al. have demonstrated the feasibility of in vivo STEAM-UTE-DWI of the human knee joint [20]. In their study, diffusion weighting was performed on the Z-axis (i.e., in the slice direction) to reduce the banding artifacts shown in Fig. 28.2, where b-values from 0 to 250 s/mm² were used. In addition, a conventional DW-SE-EPI sequence was used as a comparison. Figure 28.5a shows the resultant UTE images with $b = 1$, 136, and 240 s/mm². Figure 28.5b shows the mean signal in regions of interest (ROIs) in muscle, fat, posterior cruciate ligament (PCL) and the fitted lines. The measured ADC in the ROI of muscle was 1.3×10^{-3} mm²/s with DW-SE-EPI and 1.2×10^{-3} mm²/s with STEAM-UTE-

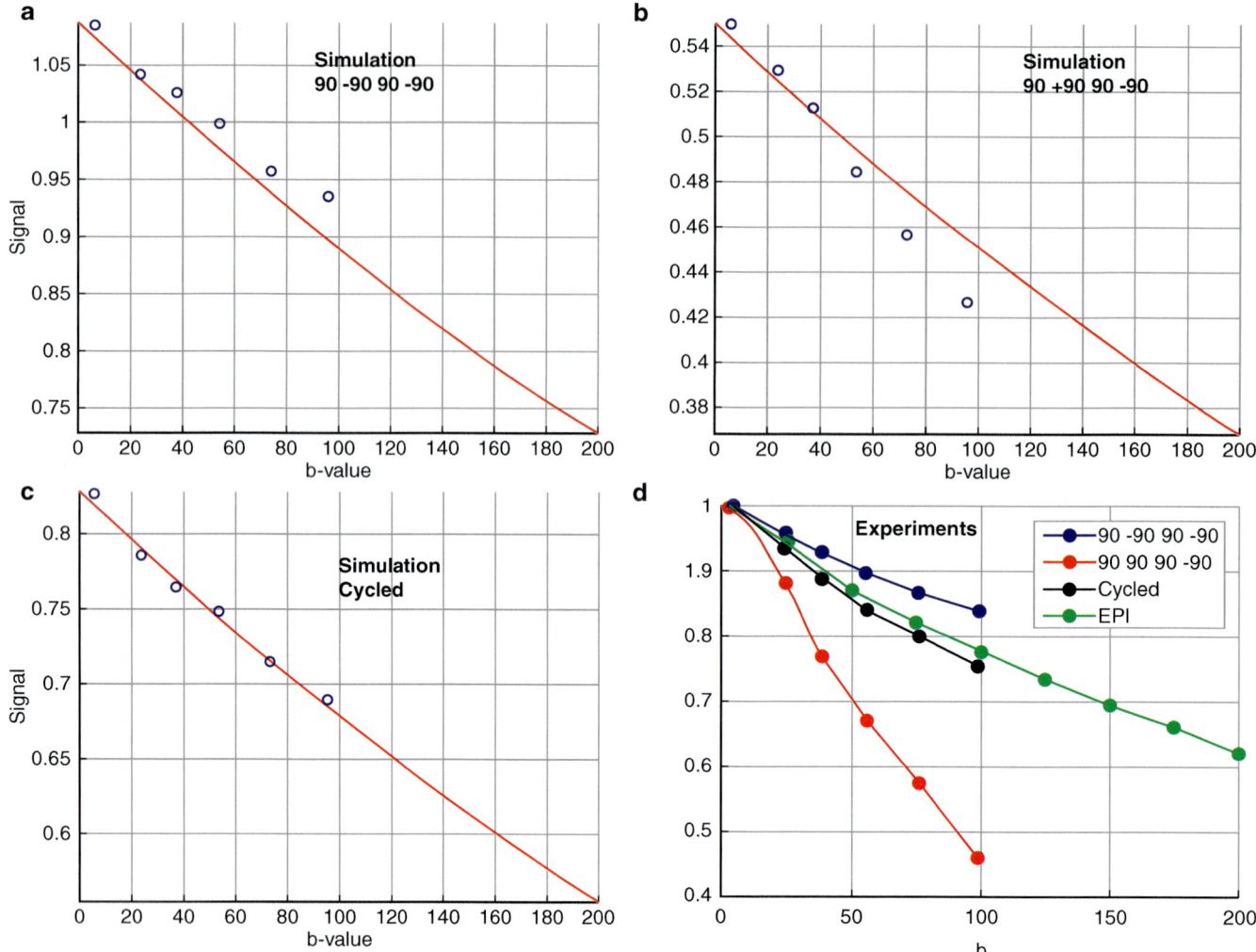

Fig. 28.3 RF cycling with STEAM-UTE-DWI. Bloch-simulated diffusion-weighted signal curves with a combination of RF pulses of (**a**) 90°, −90°, 90°, and −90°, (**b**) 90°, 90°, 90°, and −90°, (**c**) RF cycled, and (**d**) actual signal decay tested in a phantom. The simulation results show that RF cycled UTE-DWI reduces bias in the diffusion signal decay by reducing the T_1 recovery effect seen with multispoke imaging.

The result from an actual imaging experiment (**d**) demonstrates good agreement with the Bloch simulation and shows that RF cycling improves the diffusion-weighted signal curve with different *b*-values, yielding similar decay to that from DW-SE-EPI. (Adapted with permission from Ref. [18])

Fig. 28.4 Impact of T_1, T_2, and TR with STEAM-UTE-DWI. (**a**) T_1 map estimated from an IR-based SE (IR-SE) sequence, (**b**) T_2 map estimated from a SE sequence, and the measured ADC maps from STEAM-UTE-DWI with (**c**) TR = 500 ms, (**d**) TR = 200 ms, (**e**) TR = 300 ms, and (**f**) TR = 300 with signal correction based on the Bloch equations. The bias in the ADC map gets larger with shorter TRs due to the coherent buildup of the residual signal with successive RF excitations. (Adapted with permission from Ref. [19])

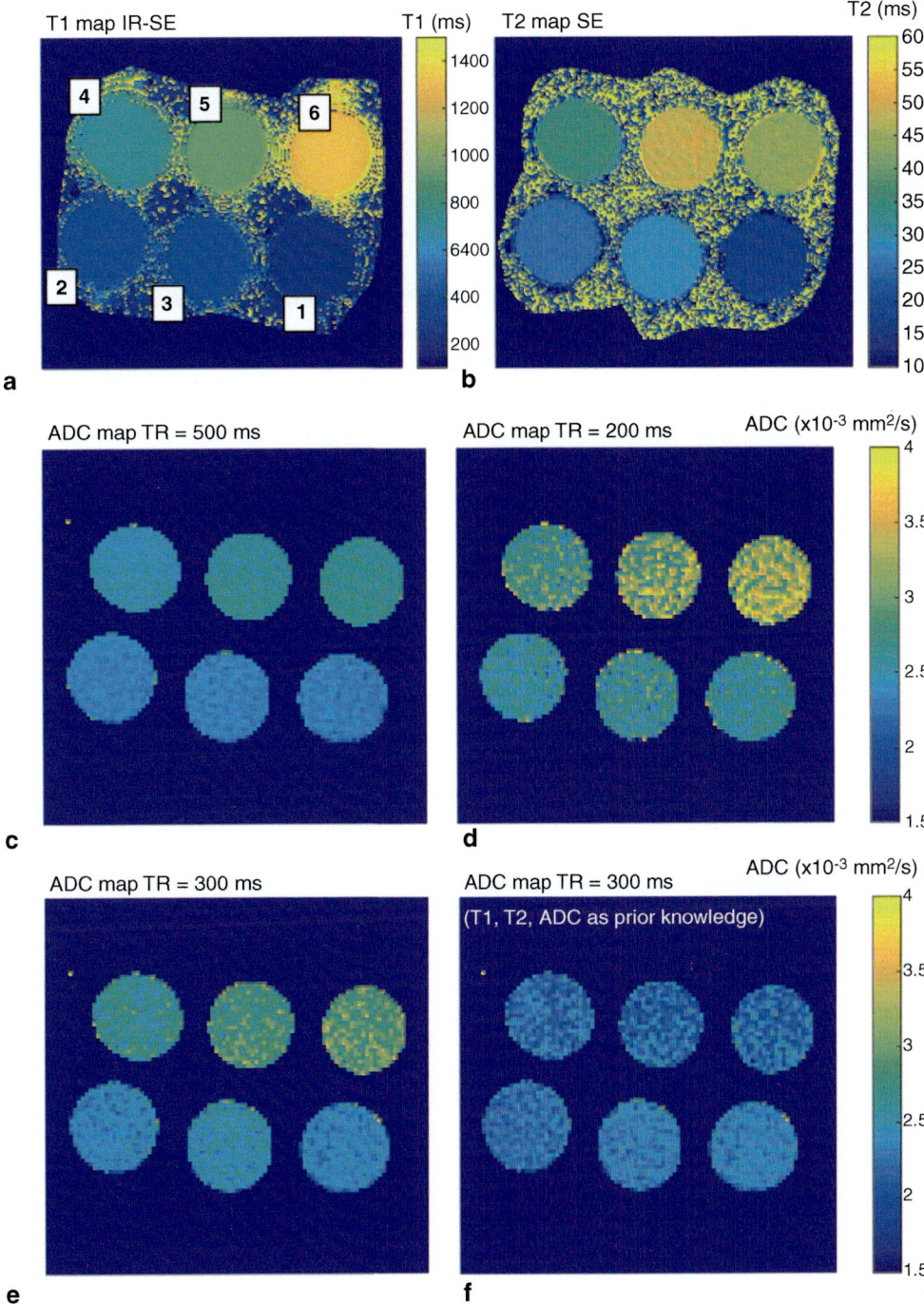

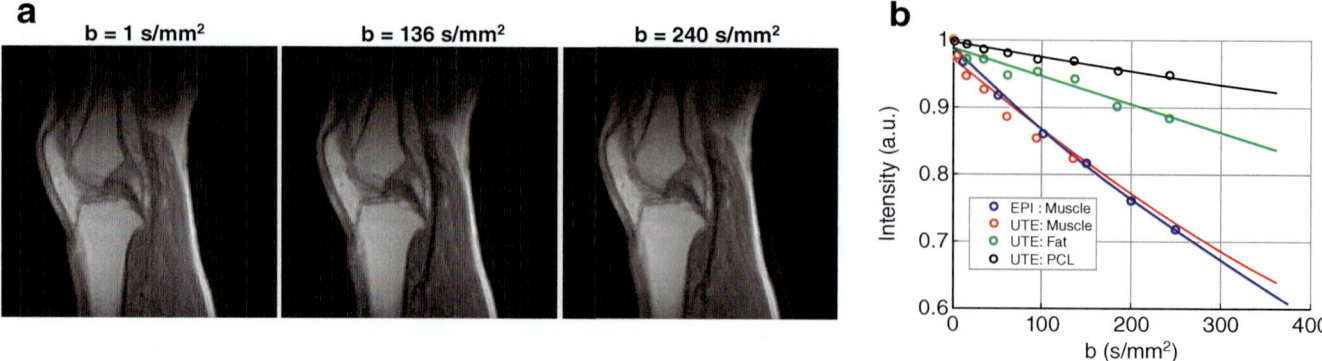

Fig. 28.5 STEAM-UTE-DWI in the PCL. (**a**) Diffusion-weighted UTE images and (**b**) the measured mean diffusion-weighted signal in ROIs in muscle, fat, and PCL with *b*-values from 0 to 250 s/mm². The measured signal with STEAM-UTE-DWI shows good agreement with that from DW-SE-EPI in muscle. (Adapted with permission from Ref. [20])

DWI. With STEAM-UTE-DWI, the measured ADCs for fat and PCL were 0.45×10^{-3} and 0.21×10^{-3} mm²/s, respectively.

diffusion weightings [37]. The parameter fitting was based on the SSFP signal model established by Freed et al. [38]. Staroswiecki et al. have also estimated ADC using the DESS signal model [39].

Quantitative UTE-Based Double Echo Steady State (qUTE-DESS)

Double Echo Steady State (DESS)

DESS imaging comes from the steady-state free precession (SSFP) [21] family of sequences. With SSFP, steady-state transverse magnetization is achieved by repeated RF pulses which create stimulated echoes and establish coherent signal pathways that contribute toward the steady state. DESS is a variant of balanced SSFP (bSSFP). Unlike bSSFP, where gradients are perfectly balanced, DESS utilizes an unbalanced gradient interleaved in the middle of the sequence to separate the signal into two echoes called S⁺ and S⁻. Both FID and stimulated echoes from previous signal pathways contribute to S⁺, while only stimulated echoes contribute to S⁻. S⁺ has more FID-like characteristics, while S⁻ is more spin echo or stimulated echo like. Due to the longer signal pathways contributing to the S⁻ signal, S⁻ is more T_2-weighted than S⁺. Both S⁺ and S⁻ signals are diffusion weighted due to the gradient interleaved in the middle of the sequence, but S⁻ typically shows more substantial diffusion weighting than S⁺.

DESS has been widely used in musculoskeletal imaging [22–29] and neuroimaging [30–35] due to its flexibility and versatility including controllable T_1, T_2, and diffusion weighting. The diffusion weighting of DESS has been useful in suppressing synovial fluid signal in cartilage imaging and blood signal in peripheral nerve imaging. Quantitative diffusion mapping has been investigated with DESS [23, 25, 35–37]. Bieri et al. investigated diffusion mapping with DESS in human knee cartilage using images acquired with different

UTE-Based Double Echo Steady State (UTE-DESS)

UTE-DESS was first introduced by Chaudhari et al. [40]. UTE-DESS is similar to DESS except for the readout scheme, which utilizes center-out radial acquisitions to shorten TE. Recently, Jang et al. demonstrated the feasibility of a UTE cones-based DESS (UTE-Cones-DESS) sequence that allows more flexible data encoding using 3D-spiral-cones trajectories [41]. Like DESS, UTE-DESS utilizes steady-state transverse magnetization established by repeated RF pulses. The SSFP signal is separated into S⁺ and S⁻ using a spoiling gradient interleaved between readout gradients. To allow UTE imaging of the S⁺ signal, a readout gradient is played out immediately after the RF dead-time to perform data encoding in a center-out *k*-space trajectory. The S⁻ signal is acquired using a gradient with a time-reversed shape and amplitude opposite in sign to that of the first readout gradient, so that data are acquired in the manner of a flyback. To encode 3D *k*-space for S⁺ and S⁻, the encoding gradients are rotated with successive TRs. In contrast, the interleaved spoiling gradient remains unchanged to allow coherent signal buildup in the steady state. The encoding gradient can be either trapezoidal (radial) or spiral (cones). Figure 28.6 shows a pulse sequence diagram for UTE-Cones-DESS. The projection radial (PR) mode can be realized by straightening the spiral arms. The spoiling gradient moment (GM) (i.e., the area under the gradient) is adjusted to achieve different degrees of diffusion weighting for qUTE-DESS.

Figure 28.7 shows S⁺ and S⁻ images acquired using the UTE-Cones-DESS sequence with different imaging parame-

Fig. 28.6 UTE-DESS with 3D-spiral-cones trajectory. (**a**) Pulse sequence diagram and (**b**) cones *k*-space trajectory. The spiral-cones trajectory allows more efficient encoding of the *k*-space with a much reduced number of spokes. For quantitative ADC mapping with UTE-DESS, the gradient moment of the spoiler is controlled by adjusting either the gradient amplitude, G_{max}, or the gradient pulse width (G_{pw}). (Adapted with permission from Ref. [42])

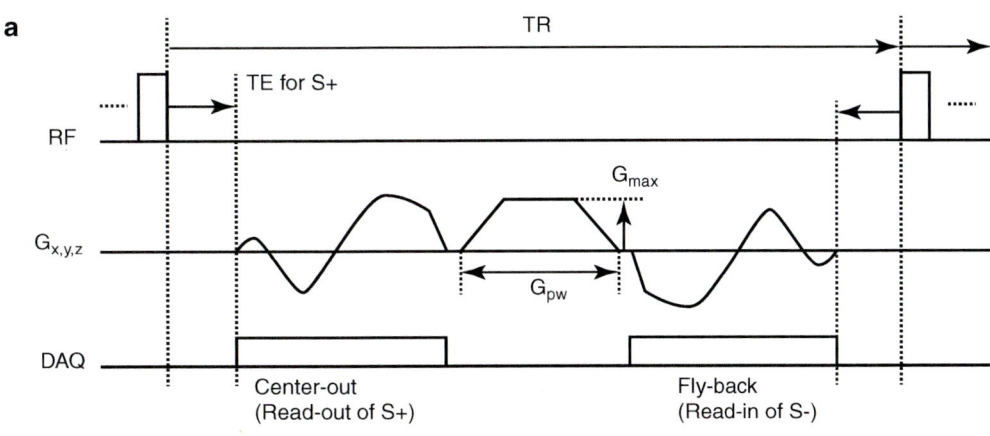

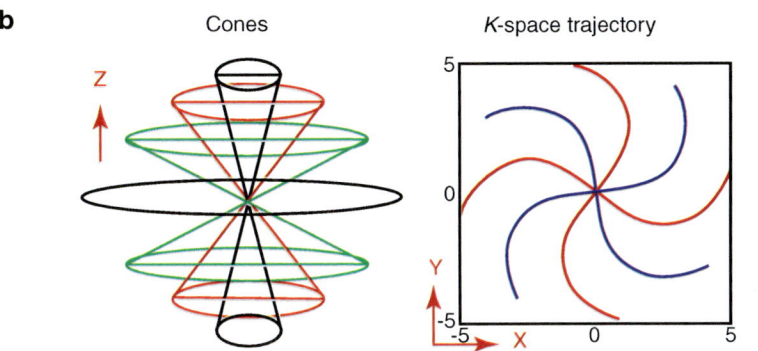

Fig. 28.7 Signal weighting with qUTE-DESS. T_2-weighting can be achieved between S^+ and S^- echoes. T_1-weighting is adjusted by use of different flip angles. Diffusion weighting is controlled by the spoiling gradient moments. (Adapted with permission from Ref. [42])

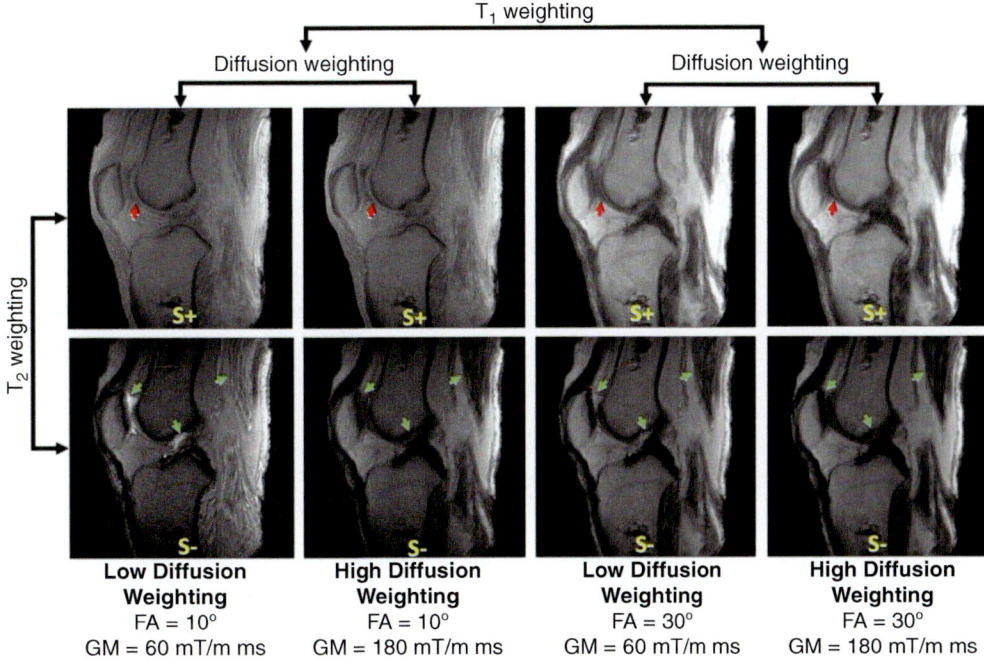

ters: FA = 10° or 30°, GM = 60, or 180 mT/m ms. In a comparison of images acquired with low and high GMs, the differences due to diffusion weighting are clearly observed in S^- (green arrows). In S^+, the different diffusion weighting is also seen in fluid which has high diffusivity (red arrows). Different

T_1-weighting is observed between the images acquired with different flip angles, while T_2-weighting differences are observed between S^+ and S^- images. Using the images with different signal weightings, quantitative T_1, T_2, and ADC values can be simultaneously estimated with qUTE-DESS [42].

Fat Suppression with UTE-DESS

Diffusion of lipid molecules is much slower than that of water diffusion. Without fat suppression, the ADC of water-containing tissues adjacent to fat can be underestimated with DWI due to the partial volume effects between water and fat. Unfortunately, conventional fat saturation techniques, including chemical shift selective (CHESS) imaging [43], IR-based fat suppression such as short tau IR (STIR) [44], spectral presaturation with IR (SPIR) [45], and spectral attenuated IR (SPAIR) [46, 47], cannot be used with DESS because they ruin the coherence signal pathway necessary to establish steady-state transverse magnetization. As an alternative, water excitation using composite RF pulses has been used with conventional DESS [24, 25, 27, 28, 32, 33]; however, it cannot be applied to UTE-DESS due to the long effective TE and T_2^* decay in the long binomial RF pulses used with this technique [48, 49]. Chaudhary et al. showed the feasibility of using a two-point Dixon approach to separate water and fat signals with UTE-DESS [40]. Despite the promising results from the two-point Dixon approach, it requires twice the scan time to acquire the additional images with different timings. Alternatively, Jang et al. proposed using a single-point Dixon approach adapted for UTE-DESS and this achieves direct fat and water separation without the need for an additional acquisition [41].

Eddy Current Correction for UTE-DESS

Eddy currents are generated within conductors in the magnet when magnetic fields are changed. Even with the good shielding of the modern MR systems, eddy currents cannot be completely avoided. Generated eddy currents create additional magnetic fields that vary in time and space, and are typically subdivided into different spatial orders [50]. Zero-order eddy currents generate a constant magnetic field in space and shift the net B_0 field. This is known as the B_0 eddy current. First-order eddy currents generate linear ramping magnetic fields in space, which mimic gradient fields, and are known as linear eddy currents. In general, linear eddy currents are more problematic with UTE sequences than with conventional Cartesian sequences due to the use of ramp sampling. They can result in imaging artifacts due to the distorted k-space trajectories [51, 52]. B_0 eddy currents are less problematic with regular UTE imaging. However, correcting for B_0 eddy current effects is more critical with UTE-DESS. In UTE-DESS, the S^+ image is acquired with a center-out gradient, while the S^- image is acquired with a flyback gradient. Due to the different gradient shapes with opposite polarities, S^+ and S^- signals are affected by various forms of eddy currents, but especially B_0 eddy currents which induce phase modulation in k-space of S^+ and S^- signals in opposite directions. This results in misregistration of S^+ and S^- images. The B_0 eddy current effect can be compensated for by demodulating the phase error from the acquired k-space data. The efficacy of B_0 eddy current correction in UTE-DESS has been demonstrated in the literature [53].

ADC Mapping with qUTE-DESS

As with STEAM-based UTE-DWI, qUTE-DESS suffers from the problem that diffusion weighting is limited by the rapid signal decay of short-T_2 tissues. With qUTE-DESS, higher diffusion sensitivity (i.e., higher diffusion weighting) requires higher gradient moments which need gradients with higher gradient amplitudes (G_{max}) and/or longer pulse widths (G_{pw}). However, higher GMs increase the minimum TR required to accommodate the longer G_{pw} and to keep the gradient duty cycle within safe limits. The attainable diffusion weighting is related to the steady-state coherent signal pathway, which is determined by imaging parameters such as flip angle, TR and GM, as well as tissue properties such as T_1, T_2, and ADC. It is essential to adjust imaging parameters for the targeted short-T_2 tissues. Figure 28.8 shows ex vivo knee imaging with a qUTE-DESS sequence tested using different imaging parameters. Figure 28.8a, b displays the resultant S^+ and S^- images, including various tissues of interest such as cartilage, menisci, and tendons. These images showed apparent diffusion weighting in cartilage and fluid with long T_2s, while the low signal intensity obscures diffusion-weighting effects in menisci and tendons with short T_2s. The results show that TR and GM are important imaging parameters for qUTE-DESS, which depend on the MR properties of the targeted tissues. A short TR provides higher sensitivity for short-T_2 tissues but can limit diffusion sensitivity and vice versa.

Figure 28.9 shows the T_1, T_2, and ADC mapping results from qUTE-DESS in two ex vivo cadaveric knee joints with a TR of 12.3 ms and maximum GM of 120 mT/m ms. Overall, qUTE-DESS shows reasonable values of T_1, T_2, and ADC for both long and short-T_2 tissues (red and gray arrows, respectively), while the clinical DW-SE-EPI sequence shows marked spatial distortion due to the B_0 inhomogeneities and eddy current effects.

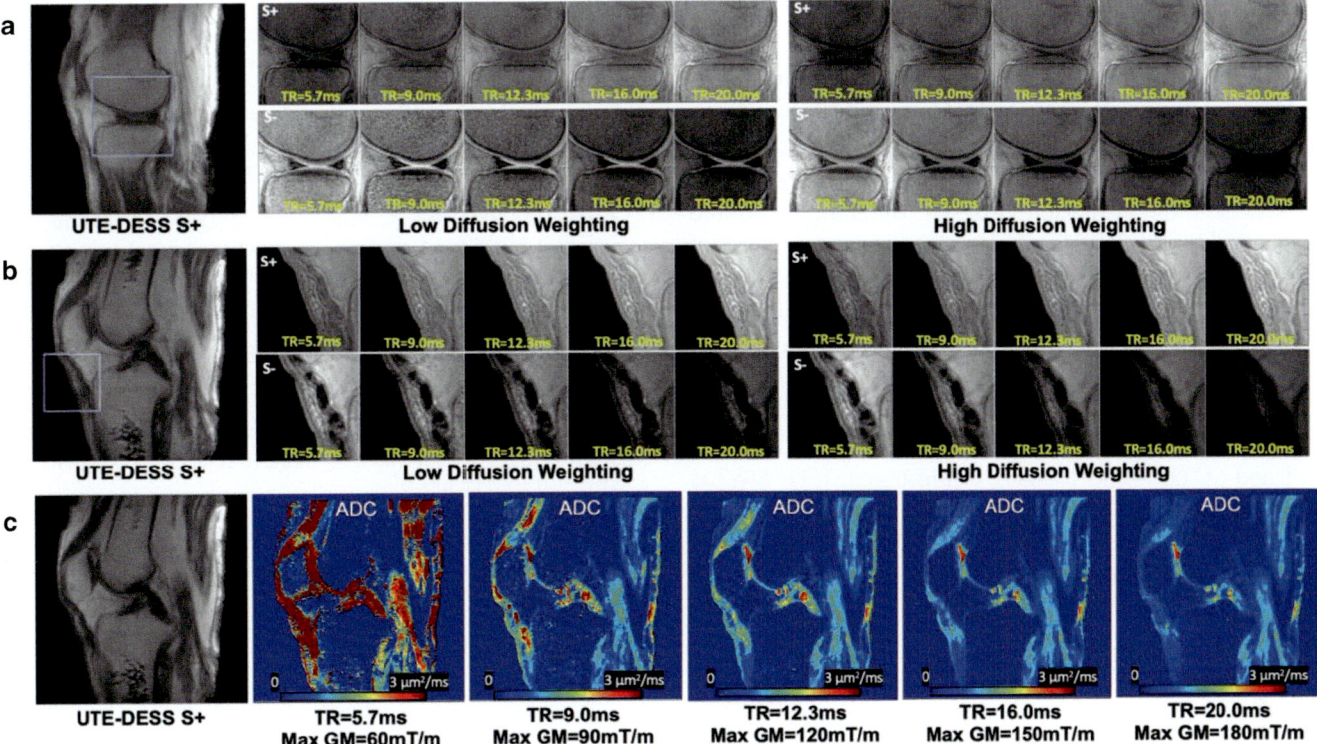

Fig. 28.8 Diffusion weighting and ADC mapping with qUTE-DESS using various gradient moments. S+ and S− images from two different slices (**a**, **b**) were acquired with varying gradient moments and TRs. (**c**) Shows the resultant ADC maps. (Adapted with permission from Ref. [42])

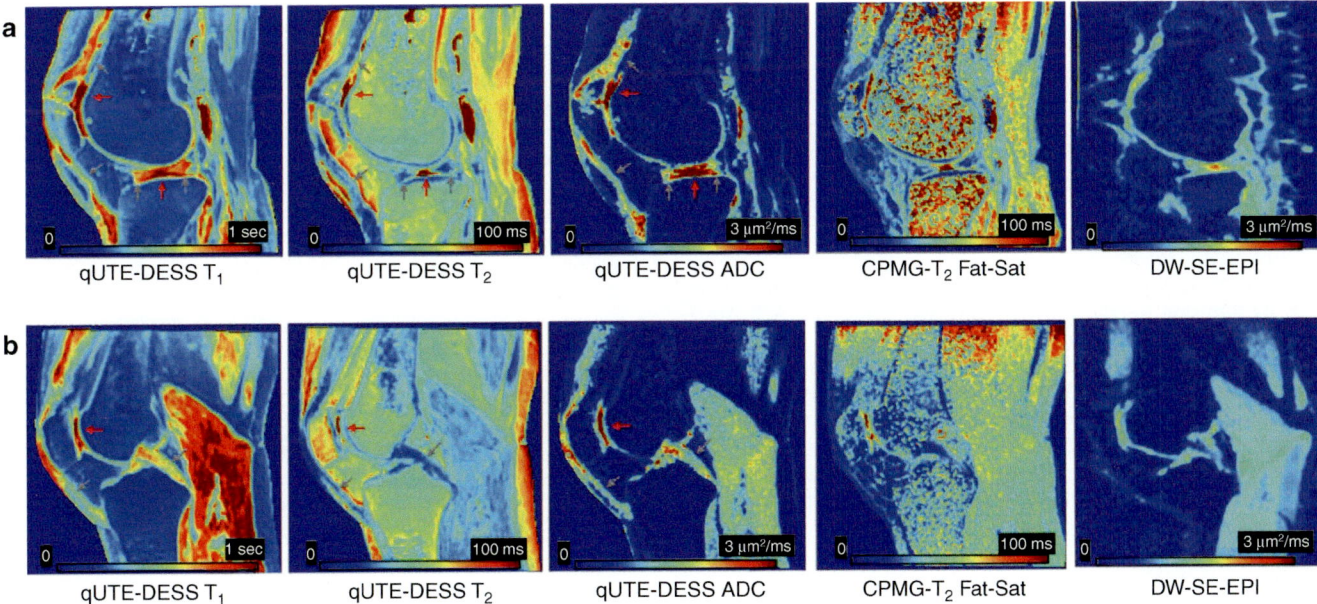

Fig. 28.9 Estimated T_1, T_2, and ADC from qUTE-DESS and T_2 calculated using CPMG and ADC evaluated by DW-SE-EPI. Ex vivo knee joints (**a**) 87-year-old donor and (**b**) 54-year-old donor. Compared to qUTE-DESS, the ADC map from DW-SE-EPI shows strong spatial distortion due to the EPI readout being sensitive to B_0 inhomogeneity and eddy currents. qUTE-DESS allows parameter estimation for both long (red arrows) and short (gray arrows) components. (Adapted with permission from Ref. [42])

Conclusion

Diffusion-weighted imaging of short-T_2 tissues is fundamentally limited by the short-T_2 signal decay and hardware performance, making it challenging to pursue both diffusion and short-T_2 sensitivity simultaneously. With current clinical MR scanners, the achievable diffusion weighting is limited for the short-T_2 tissues as a direct consequence of their T_2s. Clinical ADC mapping is not likely to be feasible for the tissues with ultrashort-T_2s, such as bone, due to the extremely rapid signal decay that does not allow effective diffusion encoding. However, UTE-DWI can be useful for tissues with moderately short-T_2s, such as tendons, ligaments, cartilage, and menisci. In this chapter, the feasibility of STEAM-UTE-DWI and qUTE-DESS imaging is illustrated. UTE-DWI is still at an early stage of development and needs further work. The potential applications of UTE-DWI include various musculoskeletal diseases involving cartilage, tendon, ligament, and meniscus.

References

1. Stejskal EO, Tanner JE. Spin diffusion measurements: spin echoes in the presence of a time-dependent field gradient. J Chem Phys. 1965;42(1):288–92.
2. Le Bihan D. Apparent diffusion coefficient and beyond: what diffusion MR imaging can tell us about tissue structure. Radiology. 2013;268(2):318–22.
3. Bammer R. Basic principles of diffusion-weighted imaging. Eur J Radiol. 2003;45(3):169–84.
4. Huisman TAGM. Diffusion-weighted and diffusion tensor imaging of the brain, made easy. Cancer Imaging. 2010;10(Spec no A(1A)):S163–71.
5. Wu EX, Cheung MM. MR diffusion kurtosis imaging for neural tissue characterization. NMR Biomed. 2010;23(7):836–48.
6. Baron CA, Beaulieu C. Oscillating gradient spin-echo (OGSE) diffusion tensor imaging of the human brain. Magn Reson Med. 2014;72(3):726–36.
7. Koh D-M, Collins DJ, Orton MR. Intravoxel incoherent motion in body diffusion-weighted MRI: reality and challenges. AJR Am J Roentgenol. 2011;196(6):1351–61.
8. Ichikawa S, Motosugi U, Ichikawa T, Sano K, Morisaka H, Araki T. Intravoxel incoherent motion imaging of the kidney: alterations in diffusion and perfusion in patients with renal dysfunction. Magn Reson Imaging. 2013;31(3):414–7.
9. Cercueil J-P, Petit J-M, Nougaret S, et al. Intravoxel incoherent motion diffusion-weighted imaging in the liver: comparison of mono-, bi- and tri-exponential modelling at 3.0-T. Eur Radiol. 2015;25(6):1541–50.
10. Yan X, Zhou M, Ying L, et al. Evaluation of optimized b-value sampling schemas for diffusion kurtosis imaging with an application to stroke patient data. Comput Med Imaging Graph. 2013;37(4):272–80.
11. Paschoal AM, Leoni RF, dos Santos AC, Paiva FF. Intravoxel incoherent motion MRI in neurological and cerebrovascular diseases. NeuroImage Clin. 2018;20:705–14.

12. Padhani AR, Van Ree K, Collins DJ, D'Sa S, Makris A. Assessing the relation between bone marrow signal intensity and apparent diffusion coefficient in diffusion-weighted MRI. AJR Am J Roentgenol. 2013;200(1):163–70.
13. Nguyen A, Ledoux J-B, Omoumi P, Becce F, Forget J, Federau C. Application of intravoxel incoherent motion perfusion imaging to shoulder muscles after a lift-off test of varying duration. NMR Biomed. 2016;29(1):66–73.
14. Koutoulidis V, Fontara S, Terpos E, et al. Quantitative diffusion-weighted imaging of the bone marrow: an adjunct tool for the diagnosis of a diffuse MR imaging pattern in patients with multiple myeloma. Radiology. 2017;282(2):484–93.
15. U.S. Food and Drug Administration. Testing and labeling medical devices for safety in the magnetic resonance (MR) environment: guidance for industry and Food and Drug Administration Staff. 2021. p. 1–26.
16. Zhang H, Sun A, Li H, Saiviroonporn P, Wu EX, Guo H. Stimulated echo diffusion weighted imaging of the liver at 3 tesla. Magn Reson Med. 2017;77(1):300–9.
17. Spinner GR, Stoeck CT, Mathez L, von Deuster C, Federau C, Kozerke S. On probing intravoxel incoherent motion in the heart-spin-echo versus stimulated-echo DWI. Magn Reson Med. 2019;82(3):1150–63.
18. Carl M, Ma Y, Brydder G, Du J. Diffusion weighted 3D UTE imaging using stimulated echoes: technical considerations. In: Proc Intl Soc Magn Reson Med; 2016:3021.
19. Baron P, Poot DHJ, Wielopolski PA, Oei EHG, Juan A. Accuracy of ADC measurements with an ultrashort echo time diffusion weighted stimulated echo 3D Cones sequence (DW-STEAM 3D Cones UTE). In: Proc Intl Soc Mag Reson Med; 2017. p. 3452.
20. Carl M, Ma Y, Bydder GM, Du J. Diffusion weighted 3D UTE in the posterior cruciate ligament. In: Proc Intl Soc Mag Reson Med; 2016. p. 4496.
21. Chavhan GB, Babyn PS, Jankharia BG, Cheng H-LM, Shroff MM. Steady-state MR imaging sequences: physics, classification, and clinical applications. Radiographics. 2008;28(4):1147–60.
22. Hardy PA, Recht MP, Piraino D, Thomasson D. Optimization of a dual echo in the steady state (DESS) free-precession sequence for imaging cartilage. J Magn Reson Imaging. 1996;6(2):329–35.
23. Welsch GH, Scheffler K, Mamisch TC, et al. Rapid estimation of cartilage T_2 based on double echo at steady state (DESS) with 3 Tesla. Magn Reson Med. 2009;62(2):544–9.
24. Moriya S, Miki Y, Yokobayashi T, Ishikawa M. Three-dimensional double-echo steady-state (3D-DESS) magnetic resonance imaging of the knee: contrast optimization by adjusting flip angle. Acta Radiol. 2009;50(5):507–11.
25. Friedrich KM, Reiter G, Kaiser B, et al. High-resolution cartilage imaging of the knee at 3T: basic evaluation of modern isotropic 3D MR-sequences. Eur J Radiol. 2011;78(3):398–405.
26. Siorpaes K, Wenger A, Bloecker K, Wirth W, Hudelmaier M, Eckstein F. Interobserver reproducibility of quantitative meniscus analysis using coronal multiplanar DESS and IWTSE MR imaging. Magn Reson Med. 2012;67(5):1419–26.
27. Moriya S, Miki Y, Matsuno Y, Okada M. Three-dimensional double-echo steady-state (3D-DESS) magnetic resonance imaging of the knee: establishment of flip angles for evaluation of cartilage at 1.5 T and 3.0 T. Acta Radiol. 2012;53(7):790–4.
28. Kohl S, Meier S, Ahmad SS, et al. Accuracy of cartilage-specific 3-Tesla 3D-DESS magnetic resonance imaging in the diagnosis of chondral lesions: comparison with knee arthroscopy. J Orthop Surg Res. 2015;10:191.
29. Chaudhari AS, Kogan F, Pedoia V, Majumdar S, Gold GE, Hargreaves BA. Rapid knee MRI acquisition and analysis tech-

niques for imaging osteoarthritis. J Magn Reson Imaging. 2020;52(5):1321–39.

30. Muhle C, Ahn JM, Biederer J, et al. MR imaging of the neural foramina of the cervical spine: comparison of 3D-DESS and 3D-FISP sequences. Acta Radiol. 2002;43(1):96–100.

31. Du R, Auguste KI, Chin CT, Engstrom JW, Weinstein PR. Magnetic resonance neurography for the evaluation of peripheral nerve, brachial plexus, and nerve root disorders. J Neurosurg. 2010;112(2):362–71.

32. Qin Y, Zhang J, Li P, Wang Y. 3D double-echo steady-state with water excitation MR imaging of the intraparotid facial nerve at 1.5T: a pilot study. AJNR Am J Neuroradiol. 2011;32(7):1167–72.

33. Fujii H, Fujita A, Yang A, et al. Visualization of the peripheral branches of the mandibular division of the trigeminal nerve on 3D double-echo steady-state with water excitation sequence. AJNR Am J Neuroradiol. 2015;36(7):1333–7.

34. Raval SB, Britton CA, Zhao T, et al. Ultra-high field upper extremity peripheral nerve and non-contrast enhanced vascular imaging. PLoS One. 2017;12(6):e0175629.

35. Burian E, Sollmann N, Ritschl LM, et al. High resolution MRI for quantitative assessment of inferior alveolar nerve impairment in course of mandible fractures: an imaging feasibility study. Sci Rep. 2020;10(1):11566.

36. Gras V, Farrher E, Grinberg F, Shah NJ. Diffusion-weighted DESS protocol optimization for simultaneous mapping of the mean diffusivity, proton density and relaxation times at 3 Tesla. Magn Reson Med. 2017;78(1):130–41.

37. Bieri O, Ganter C, Scheffler K. Quantitative in vivo diffusion imaging of cartilage using double echo steady-state free precession. Magn Reson Med. 2012;68(3):720–9.

38. Freed DE, Scheven UM, Zielinski LJ, Sen PN, Hürlimann MD. Steady-state free precession experiments and exact treatment of diffusion in a uniform gradient. J Chem Phys. 2001;115(9):4249–58.

39. Staroswiecki E, Granlund KL, Alley MT, Gold GE, Hargreaves BA. Simultaneous estimation of $T(2)$ and apparent diffusion coefficient in human articular cartilage in vivo with a modified three-dimensional double echo steady state (DESS) sequence at 3 T. Magn Reson Med. 2012;67(4):1086–96.

40. Chaudhari AS, Sveinsson B, Moran CJ, et al. Imaging and T2 relaxometry of short-T2 connective tissues in the knee using ultrashort echo-time double-echo steady-state (UTEDESS). Magn Reson Med. 2017;78(6):2136–48.

41. Jang H, Ma Y, Carl M, Jerban S, Chang EY, Du J. Ultrashort echo time cones double echo steady state (UTE-Cones-DESS) for rapid morphological imaging of short T_2 tissues. Magn Reson Med. 2021;86(2):881–92.

42. Jang H, Ma Y, Masoud-Afsahi A, et al. Quantitative UTE double echo steady state (qUTE-DESS) for simultaneous mapping of T_1, T_2, and diffusivity of short T_2 tissues—ex vivo study. In: Proc Intl Soc Mag Reson Med; 2022. p. 1411.

43. Haase A, Frahm J, Hanicke W, Matthaei D. 1H NMR chemical shift selective (CHESS) imaging. Phys Med Biol. 1985;30(4):341–4.

44. Krinsky G, Rofsky NM, Weinreb JC. Nonspecificity of short inversion time inversion recovery (STIR) as a technique of fat suppression: pitfalls in image interpretation. AJR Am J Roentgenol. 1996;166(3):523–6.

45. Kaldoudi E, Williams SCR, Barker GJ, Tofts PS. A chemical shift selective inversion recovery sequence for fat-suppressed MRI: theory and experimental validation. Magn Reson Imaging. 1993;11(3):341–55.

46. Tannús A, Garwood M. Adiabatic pulses. NMR Biomed. 1997;10(8):423–34.

47. Del Grande F, Santini F, Herzka DA, et al. Fat-suppression techniques for 3-T MR imaging of the musculoskeletal system. Radiographics. 2014;34(1):217–33.

48. Hardy PA, Recht MP, Piraino DW. Fat suppressed MRI of articular cartilage with a spatial-spectral excitation pulse. J Magn Reson Imaging. 1998;8(6):1279–87.

49. Schick F, Forster J, Machann J, Huppert P, Claussen CD. Highly selective water and fat imaging applying multislice sequences without sensitivity to B_1 field inhomogeneities. Magn Reson Med. 1997;38(2):269–74.

50. Vannesjo SJ, Haeberlin M, Kasper L, et al. Gradient system characterization by impulse response measurements with a dynamic field camera. Magn Reson Med. 2013;69(2):583–93.

51. Jang H, Wiens CN, McMillan AB. Ramped hybrid encoding for improved ultrashort echo time imaging. Magn Reson Med. 2016;76(3):814–25.

52. Jang H, McMillan AB. A rapid and robust gradient measurement technique using dynamic single-point imaging. Magn Reson Med. 2017;78(3):95–962.

53. Jang H, Athertya JS, Jerban S, et al. Correction of B0 and linear eddy currents: Impact on morphological and quantitative ultrashort echo time double echo steady state (UTE-DESS) imaging. NMR Biomed. 2023:e4939.

Deep Learning for Automated Segmentation and Quantitative Mapping with UTE MRI

Xing Lu, Hyungseok Jang, Yajun Ma, and Jiang Du

Introduction

Artificial intelligence (AI) technology, powered by advanced computing power, a large amount of data, and new algorithms, is becoming increasingly popular. With advances in computing power using graphics processing units and the availability of large data acquisitions, deep neural networks outperform human or other machine learning (ML) capabilities in computer vision and speech recognition tasks. The advances making this possible are also being applied to healthcare problems, including computer-aided detection/ diagnosis of disease, disease prediction, image segmentation, and image generation.

Deep learning is a type of machine learning and AI that imitates the way humans gain certain types of knowledge. The emergence of deep learning is driven by breakthroughs in convolution neural networks (CNNs) which are a set of techniques and algorithms that enable computers to discover complicated patterns in large data sets [1]. Feeding the breakthroughs is increased access to data ("big data"), user-friendly software frameworks, and an explosion of available computing power that enables the use of neural networks that are deeper than ever before. The typical compositions of CNNs are convolutional, pooling, and fully connected layers. The primary role of the convolutional layer is to identify patterns, lines, edges, and so on. Each hidden layer of a CNN consists of convolutional layers that convolve input arrays with weight-parameterized convolution kernels. The kernels generate multiple feature images and succeed in various vision tasks such as segmentation and classification.

Deep learning methods are increasingly used to improve clinical practice, and the list of examples of this is long and growing daily. Deep learning is assisting medical professionals and researchers in discovering hidden data opportunities and better-serving healthcare needs. Deep learning in healthcare provides doctors with accurate diagnosis of disease and helps improve treatment decisions. Specifically, in radiology, it may include early detection of cancer and other lesions, computer-assisted diagnosis (CAD), treatment planning, and survival analysis. MRI is a major medical imaging modality, in which deep learning has important applications, including image reconstruction, functional data analysis, segmentation, and quantification. In this chapter, we discuss essential aspects of these uses.

Deep Learning in MRI

Reconstruction

CNN and recurrent neural network (RNN)-based image reconstruction methods are gaining more attention. They were first proposed in 2016 by Yang et al. [2] and Wang et al. [3]. Later, various MRI reconstruction techniques with different CNN architectures were developed. In 2018, Qin et al. proposed the use of dynamic MR image reconstruction with convolutional RNNs [4], and reconstructing fast cardiac MR images from highly undersampled complex-valued k-space data by learning spatiotemporal dependencies with promising reconstructed image qualities. In the same year, a unified framework for image reconstruction [5], called automated transform by manifold approximation (AUTOMAP), was reported by Zhu et al. This consisted of a deep convolutional neural network (DCNN) with a convolutional autoencoder, which generated image reconstructions generically from MRI examinations such as those collected from the Human

X. Lu (✉) · H. Jang · Y. Ma
Department of Radiology, University of California, San Diego, La Jolla, CA, USA
e-mail: xil135@health.ucsd.edu; h4jang@health.ucsd.edu; yam013@health.ucsd.edu

J. Du
Department of Radiology, University of California, San Diego, La Jolla, CA, USA

Department of Bioengineering, University of California, San Diego, La Jolla, CA, USA

VA San Diego Healthcare System, San Diego, CA, USA
e-mail: jiangdu@health.ucsd.edu

J. Du, G. M. Bydder (eds.), *MRI of Short- and Ultrashort-T₂ Tissues*, https://doi.org/10.1007/978-3-031-35197-6_29

Connectome Project. The images were transformed from the k-space domain. Yang et al. proposed deep de-aliasing generative adversarial networks (DAGAN) for MRI reconstruction with deep Generative Adversarial Networks (GAN) [6]. In 2020, Yaman et al. reported the use of a self-supervised style of deep learning for MRI reconstruction with undersampled data. The acquired sub-sampled k-space data was divided into two sets; one was used to keep data consistency in the unrolled network, and the other was used for network training. Results demonstrated that the proposed method could reconstruct images from sub-sampled data, and had a similar performance to the supervised approach that was trained with fully sampled references [7].

Registration

Medical image registration is a fundamental part of various applications in medical image analysis. It is widely used to process data for downstream tasks such as lesion detection, organ segmentation, and classification, as well as quantification in parametric MRI. As a result, the performance of many tasks is heavily influenced by the quality of the image registration algorithm used to place the images in a common coordinate frame of fixed size and spatial resolution. Recently, deep learning-based algorithms have been applied to MRI registration to improve accuracy and speed. Some examples include elastic registration between 3D MRI and transrectal ultrasound for guiding targeted prostate biopsies [8], and deformable registration for brain MRI [9].

Segmentation

Image segmentation is one of the core functions of different types of quantitative image analysis and includes annotating images into multiple regions that share similar attributes including morphological designations. Initially, classical approaches were used for medical image segmentation and tissue classification [10–12]. Later, atlas-based and other complex segmentation methods and approaches were reported [13–15]. Deep learning-based techniques, mostly CNNs, are now penetrating the whole field of medical image segmentation with applications to the brain, liver, lung, knee, and spine [16–22].

Quantification

One important area that is gaining more and more attention in deep learning-based MRI is the estimation of quantitative tissue parameters with specific physical meanings from raw complex-valued data. Quantitative MRI (qMRI) provides unique opportunities for observing biological microstructural processes such as measuring tissue atrophy using morphological imaging. This allows more comprehensive characterization of tissue changes, including early effects on microstructural integrity and recognition of disease-specific changes. So far, qMRI techniques have been extensively investigated to quantify the specific tissue properties T_1, T_2, $T_{1\rho}$, susceptibility, magnetization transfer (MT), perfusion, and diffusion. Numerous studies suggest that qMRI of tissue properties will add valuable clinical information, including the detection of microstructural tissue damage in areas that appear normal on conventional MRI and unveiling microstructural correlates of clinical manifestations.

Although the application of deep learning in quantitative MRI are less explored compared to other techniques, a number of early studies have recently shown its great promise to improve the speed, efficiency, and quality of MR tissue property mapping. Rasmussen and coworkers used a U-Net-based convolutional neural network to perform field-to-source inversion to directly invert the magnetic dipole kernel convolution in quantitative susceptibility mapping (QSM), a technique called DeepQSM [23]. Magnetic resonance fingerprinting (MRF) uses a pseudo-randomized acquisition that causes the signals from different tissues to have a unique signal evolution ("fingerprint"). Mapping the signals back to known tissue parameters (T_1, T_2, and mobile proton density ρ_m) is a challenging inverse problem. Cohen et al. [24] have used voxel-wise MRI data acquired with MRF sequences (MRF-EPI, 25 frames in ~3 s; or MRF-FISP, 600 frames in ~7.5 s) with a four-layer neural network consisting of two hidden layers with 300×300 fully connected nodes and two nodes in the output layer, to produce T_1 and T_2 parametric maps. The MRF Deep RecOnstruction NEtwork (DRONE) was trained by an adaptive moment estimation stochastic gradient descent algorithm with a mean squared error loss function [25]. Liu et al. proposed a model-augmented neural network with incoherent k-space sampling (MANTIS) for efficient MR parameter mapping with physical models [26]. A major limitation of traditional qMRI is the long scan time required for reliable and repeatable measurements. Further development in deep learning-based qMRI is expected to significantly reduce the total scan time required for data acquisition, and thereby provide fast and robust maps of MR morphology and tissue properties.

Deep Learning in Knee Osteoarthritis with MRI

Knee osteoarthritis (OA) is a progressive disease that affects the entire knee joint and causes significant disability in patients worldwide. This disease is characterized by irreversible degeneration of the articular cartilage on the surfaces of the femur, tibia, and patella. Early detection of knee OA is crucial for therapy, such as weight reduction and exercises that have been found to be effective in halting disease progression and delaying the need for total knee replacement (TKR) [27].

Recent OA studies using fully automatic methods have mostly focused on MRI as it provides excellent soft tissue contrast and spatial resolution of the knee joint. MRI does not require ionizing radiation [28]. In addition, knee OA is a "whole-organ disease" that involves all the principal joint tissues and tissue components. Volumetric MRI can visualize the complex 3D structure of the knee joint while discriminating multiple tissue types and hence provide a better evaluation of OA than two-dimensional (2D) radiography [29, 30].

Most techniques used in deep learning studies in the OA field are based on CNNs. Most CNN segmentation studies utilize U-Net architecture which is a symmetrical network consisting of an encoder and a decoder. The network first learns to encode by convolution downsampling and then decode into a segmentation mask representing the object of interest in the image by upsampling the "deconvolutions" [30]. Several studies have adopted the 2D encoder–decoder U-Net model proposed by Ronneberger et al. [31] in knee compartment segmentation studies. Norman et al. utilized 2D U-Net to segment six subcompartments of the knee, including articular cartilages and menisci [32]. Liu et al. presented automated segmentation of knee bone and cartilage by combining 2D SegNet and 3D simplex deformable modeling. 3D deformable modeling allows the final segmentation of the output to produce the desired smooth surface and shape [33].

Though morphological changes in knee OA may be detected by conventional MRI sequences, such as dual-echo steady state (DESS), fast spin echo (FSE), and gradient recalled echo (GRE) [34], these changes typically occur during the late stages of OA when treatment is likely to be much less effective. Novel MRI techniques, such as ultrashort echo time (UTE), can potentially detect changes that occur in the early stages of OA [35–37]. With UTE MRI, short-T_2 tissues such as the osteochondral junction, menisci, ligaments, tendons, and bone, which are otherwise "invisible" with conventional MRI sequences, can be directly imaged and quantified, thereby providing a truly "whole-organ disease" approach for the diagnosis of OA. These morphological, and especially quantitative, UTE-based MRI techniques may allow more robust detection of early joint degeneration.

Deep learning-based methods have also been implemented with UTE MRI of short-T_2 tissues. This application of AI, especially deep learning, for automated segmentation and quantitative mapping with UTE MRI will be described in the following parts of this chapter. We will focus on UTE-based deep learning applications in knee OA, including knee compartment segmentation, quantitative parametric mapping, and an integrated deep learning framework for simultaneous segmentation and quantification.

Deep Learning in Knee Osteoarthritis with UTE MRI

Segmentation with UTE MRI

UTE MRI allows high-resolution morphological and quantitative imaging of both short- and long-T_2 tissues in the knee joint. A U-Net-based CNN has been developed for fully automated segmentation of short-T_2 tissues, such as the meniscus, and long-T_2 tissues, such as articular cartilage, including extraction of quantitative parameters such as UTE-based T_1, T_2*, $T_{1\rho}$, and macromolecular proton fraction (MPF).

Attention U-Net-Based Meniscus Segmentation

As a pilot study, Byra et al. developed an attention 2D U-Net CNN based on transfer learning and a relatively small set of UTE MR data [38]. In this study, a pre-trained model was used on a large set of nonmedical images. The deep learning approach was based on the U-Net architecture, as shown in Fig. 29.1. Gray colors indicate the convolutional blocks initiated with the weights extracted from the VGG19 network. For each block, the number of filters is indicated below the block type. Each convolutional block, except for the first and the last block, used a 3×3 convolutional filter and the rectifier linear unit (ReLu) as the activation function. The first block used a 1D 1×1 convolutional filter and no activation function. The last block used the sigmoid activation function suitable for binary classification. Attention layers (ALs) were applied to process the feature maps propagated through the skip connections to let the network focus more on particular regions in feature maps instead of analyzing the entire image representation.

Additionally, ALs to process the feature maps propagated through the skip connections were applied. ALs could help the network focus more on small regions instead of analyzing the entire field of view. This is done by filtering the encoder feature maps based on the output of the decoder convolution layers to incorporate information about initial menisci localization. Therefore, areas of feature maps far from the initial menisci localization are compressed and less noisy feature maps are propagated through the skip connections.

The transfer learning-based approach was also implied in the model development. The weights of this U-Net's first two convolutional blocks were initiated with the weights of the corresponding first two convolutional blocks of the VGG 19 model pre-trained on the ImageNet dataset. The first several layers of pre-trained CNNs, like the VGG 19, commonly

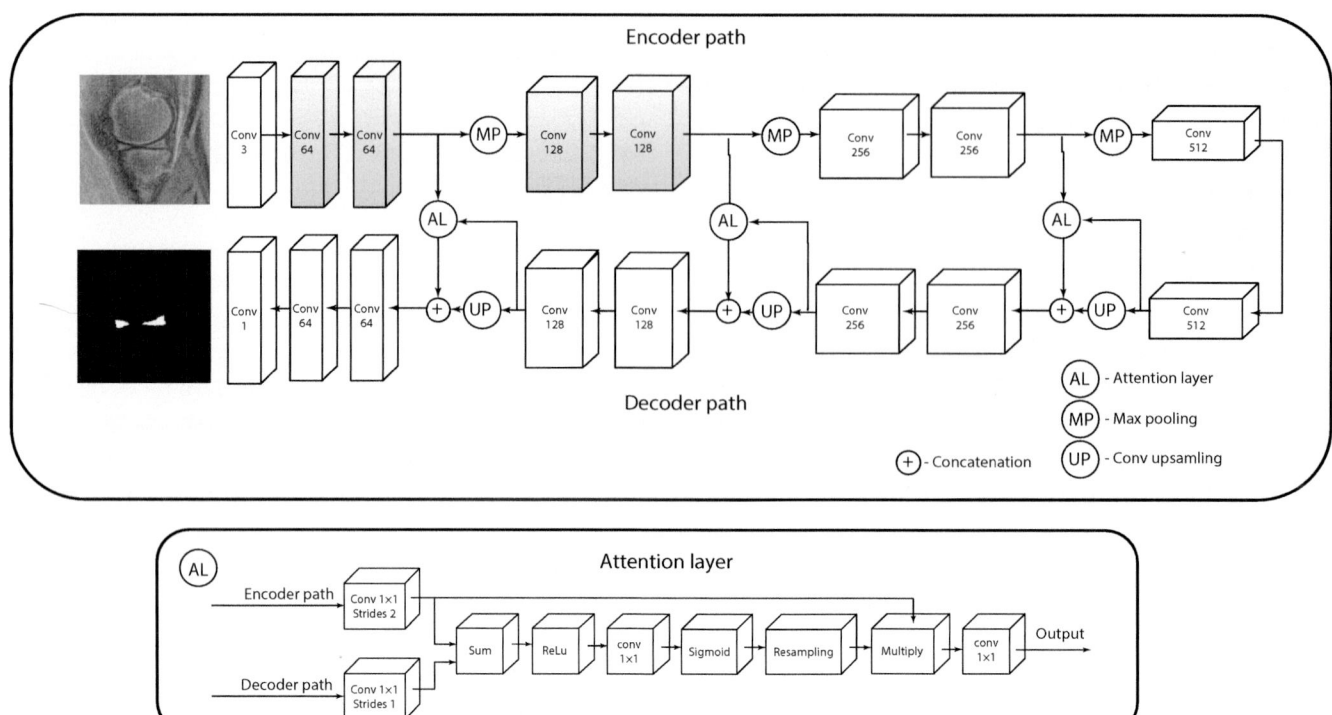

Fig. 29.1 The 2D attention U-Net CNN for the knee menisci segmentation. AL, attention layer; Conv, 2D convolutional block; Max pool, max pooling operator; Up, upsampling with a 2D transposed convolutional block (kernel size of 2 × 2, stride of 2 × 2). (Reproduced with permission from Ref. [38])

include blob and edge detectors, while the deeper layers extract features more related to the particular recognition problem. Transfer learning methods utilizing the VGG 19 CNN performed well for various medical image analysis problems across different medical imaging modalities.

The Dice score-based loss function is used for training the network. The Dice score (or coefficient) is defined in the following way:

$$\text{Dice score} = \frac{2|M \cap A|}{|M| + |A|} \tag{29.1}$$

where M is the manual segmentation region of interest (ROI), A is the automatic segmentation ROI predicted by the CNN, and $|\cdot|$ refers to set cardinality.

A total of 61 human subjects (aged 20–88 years, 30 males, 31 females) were recruited for this retrospective study, which included 23 healthy volunteers, 25 patients with mild OA, and 13 patients with moderate OA. Whole knee joint imaging was performed using a 3D UTE Cones sequences on a 3T MR750 scanner (GE Healthcare Technologies, Milwaukee, WI). UTE-based T_1, T_2^*, and $T_{1\rho}$ were measured for the whole knee joint. The Elastix motion registration based on the Insight Segmentation and Registration Toolkit was applied to the 3D UTE Cones data before quantification to account for possible motion during the relatively long data acquisitions. All UTE datasets were registered to the first set of UTE-T_2^* data. The Dice score was used for model selection during training. After the training, the best performing CNN model determined by the best Dice score on the validation dataset was employed to calculate the ROIs using the test dataset, which contained 191 2D images from 15 menisci. In the next step, the manual and automatic segmentations were used to calculate average UTE-T_1, UTE-$T_{1\rho}$, and UTE-T_2^*s for each 2D ROI. Figure 29.2 shows manual and automatic segmentations obtained from the test dataset in four cases. Figure 29.2a, b illustrates cases where a high level of agreement between radiologists and models was achieved. Figure 29.2c, d presents examples with a lower level of agreement between the radiologists and models.

Dice scores, Pearson's linear correlation coefficient, and Bland–Altman plots were implemented to evaluate the level of agreement between the CNNs and radiologists. Four cases were examined: Rad 1 vs. Rad 2, Rad 1 vs. CNN 1, Rad 2 vs. CNN 2, and CNN 1 vs. CNN 2. Figure 29.3 demonstrates the relationships and Bland–Altman plots for the average UTE-T_1 values calculated using the manual and automatic segmentations provided by the radiologists and the CNNs, respectively.

Attention U-Net-Based Cartilage Segmentation

As reported by Xue et al., a model architecture similar to that used for the meniscus was implemented for the study of

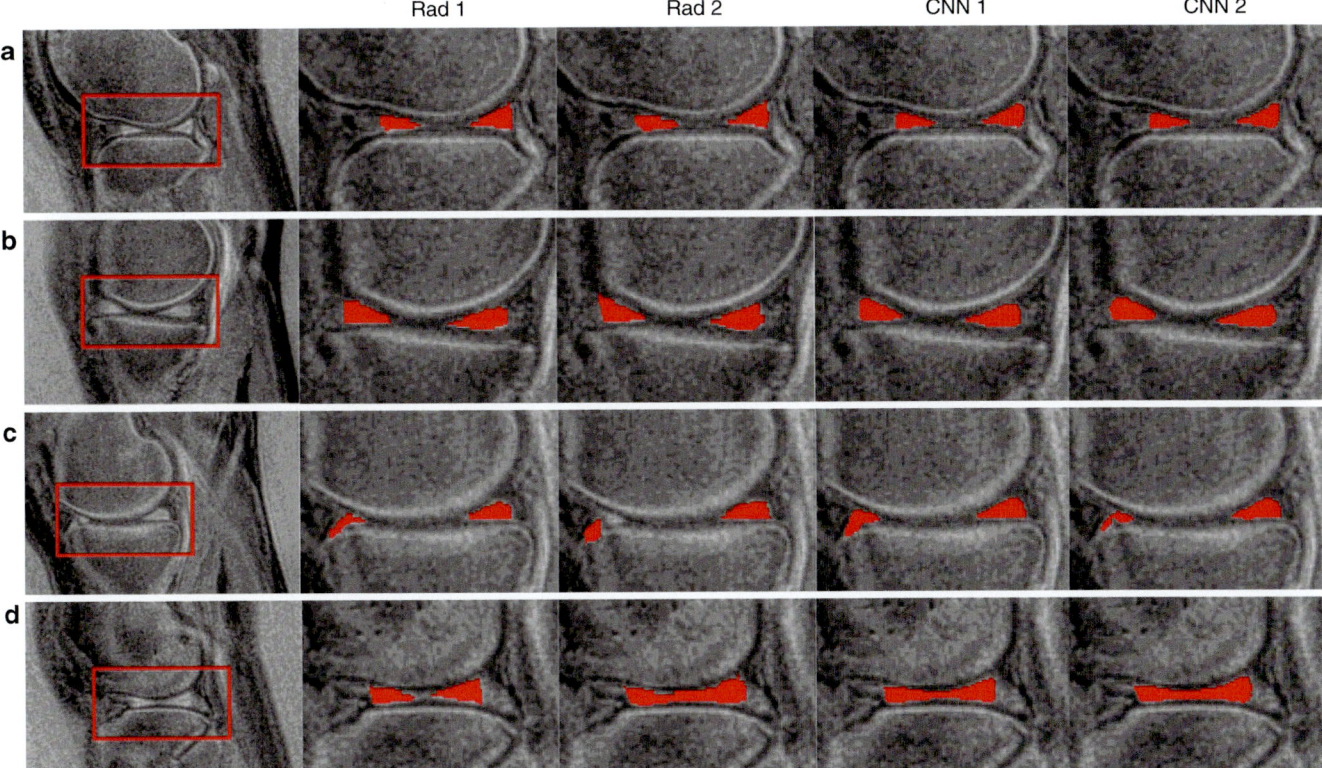

Fig. 29.2 Typical results of manual and automatic segmentations of the meniscus. (**a**) and (**b**) Show results with high-level agreement between radiologists (Rad 1 and Rad 2) and models (CNN 1 and CNN 2). Lesion levels of agreement are shown in (**c**) and (**d**). Both CNNs gave correct predictions, while there were some errors in the annotations by the radiologists. (Reproduced with permission from Ref. [38])

articular cartilage [39]. As shown in Fig. 29.4, the attention gates of this model account for the output of decoder convolutional blocks to determine the critical regions of the images and, consequently, to filter feature maps accordingly from the encoder path.

A total of 65 human subjects (33 females) were included in this study. The whole knee joint (29 left, 36 right) was scanned using a transmit/receive 8-channel knee coil on a 3T clinical MR system. The MRI protocol included a series of 3D UTE Cones sequences to measure T_1, $T_{1\rho}$, T_2^*, and MPF. Motion registration was applied to all quantitative 3D UTE Cones images using Elastix software [40], in which a rigid affine transform was followed by a nonrigid b-spline registration [41]. Fat-saturated adiabatic $T_{1\rho}$-weighted MR images provided the best cartilage contrast and were used for manual segmentation by two musculoskeletal radiologists (Rad 1 and Rad 2) with 18 and 13 years' experience, respectively. The manually segmented data was inputted to the CNN model as the ground truth. The same manual segmentation masks were applied to registered 3D UTE-based T_1, T_2^*, and MT data for subsequent quantitative processing. As shown in Fig. 29.5, the CNN models provided reliable cartilage segmentation similar to that provided by manual segmentation. Three representative subjects (a, 24-year-old

female, KL = 0; b, 43-year-old male, KL = 1; and c, 74-year-old female, KL = 3) were chosen to show the input 3D UTE Cones MR images, the corresponding manual labels drawn by Rad 1 and Rad 2, and the labels produced by CNN 1 and CNN 2, respectively. Strong interobserver agreement was shown between Rad 1 and CNN 1 and between Rad 2 and CNN 2. The morphology of labels produced by each CNN model showed high similarity with the labels produced by the corresponding radiologist.

Mean Dice scores were 0.81 ± 0.11 for Rad 1 vs. CNN 1 and 0.82 ± 0.08 for Rad 2 vs. CNN 2, respectively. The Dice score between labels produced by CNN 1 and CNN 2 was 0.87, which was higher than the Dice score between the two radiologists (0.83), indicating improved interobserver agreement in automatic segmentation compared with manual segmentation. The mean values of the volumetric overlap errors (VOEs) between manual and automatic segmentation were 28.43 ± 7.31%, 30.43 ± 13.03%, 29.28 ± 10.83%, and 22.15 ± 10.51% for Rad 1 vs. Rad 2, Rad 1 vs. CNN 1, Rad 2 vs. CNN 2, and CNN 1 vs. CNN 2, respectively.

Figure 29.6 shows scatter plots for UTE-T_1 between Rad 1 vs. CNN 1, Rad 2 vs. CNN 2, Rad 1 vs. Rad 2, and CNN 1 vs. CNN 2, with the corresponding Pearson correlation coefficients which ranged from 0.91 to 0.99, respectively. High

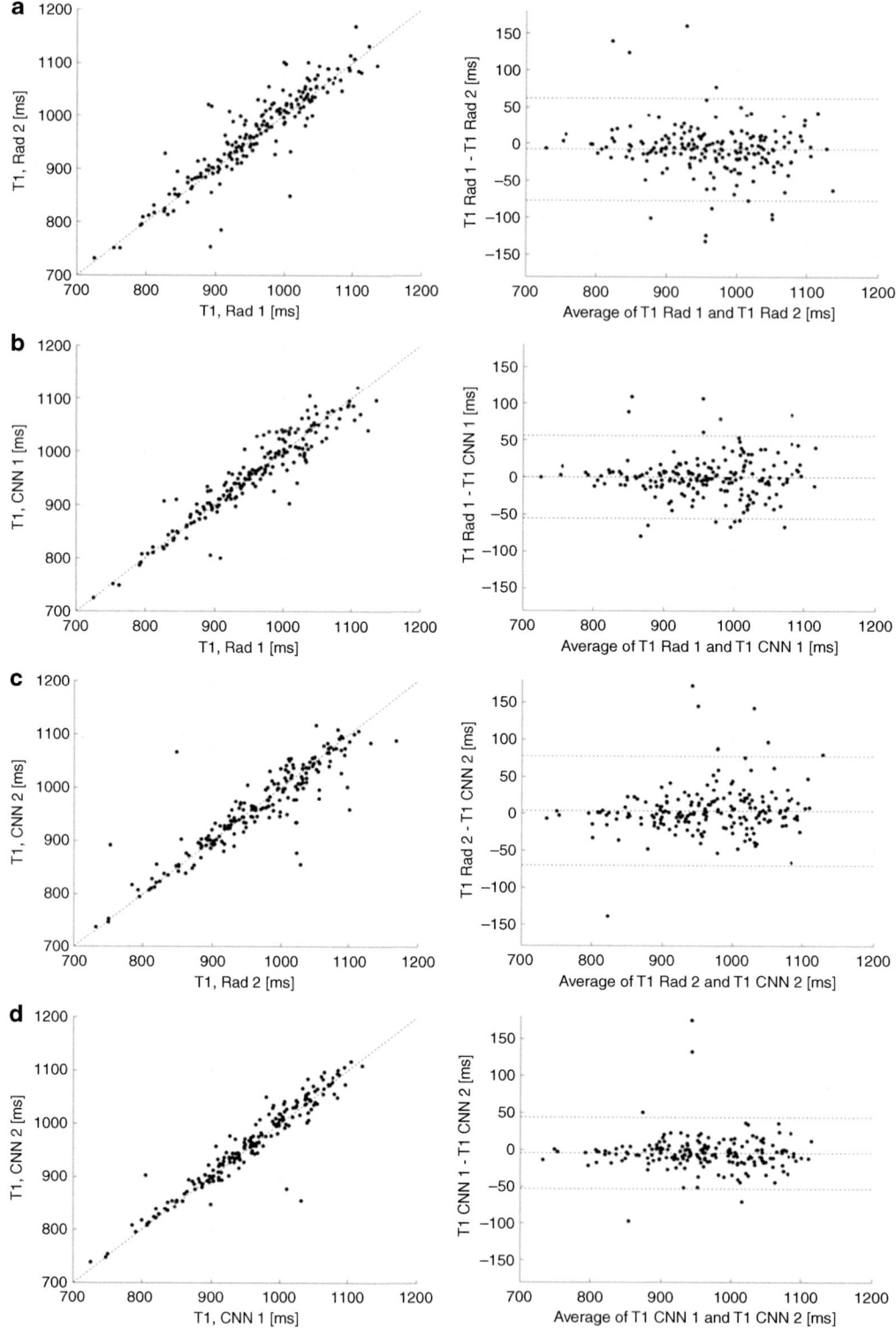

Fig. 29.3 Relationships and Bland–Altman plots for average UTE-T_1 values calculated using the segmentations provided by the radiologists and the CNNs, (**a**)–(**d**) demonstrate the relationships of UTE-T_1 values for Rad 1 vs. Rad 2 ($r = 0.91$), CNN 1 vs. Rad 1 ($r = 0.95$), CNN 2 vs. Rad 2 ($r = 0.94$), and CNN 1 vs. CNN 2 ($r = 0.9$). (Reproduced with permission from Ref. [38])

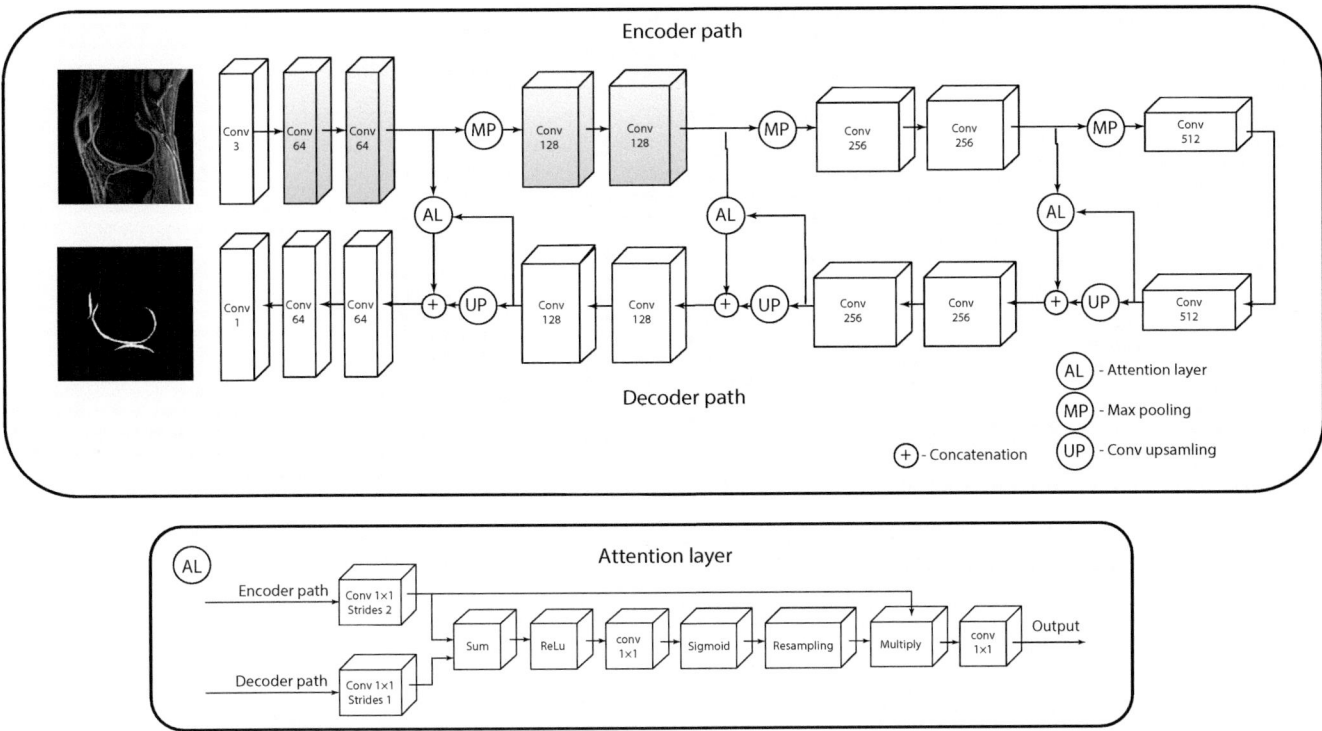

Fig. 29.4 The proposed 2D attention U-Net CNN for cartilage segmentation. (Reproduced with permission from Ref. [39])

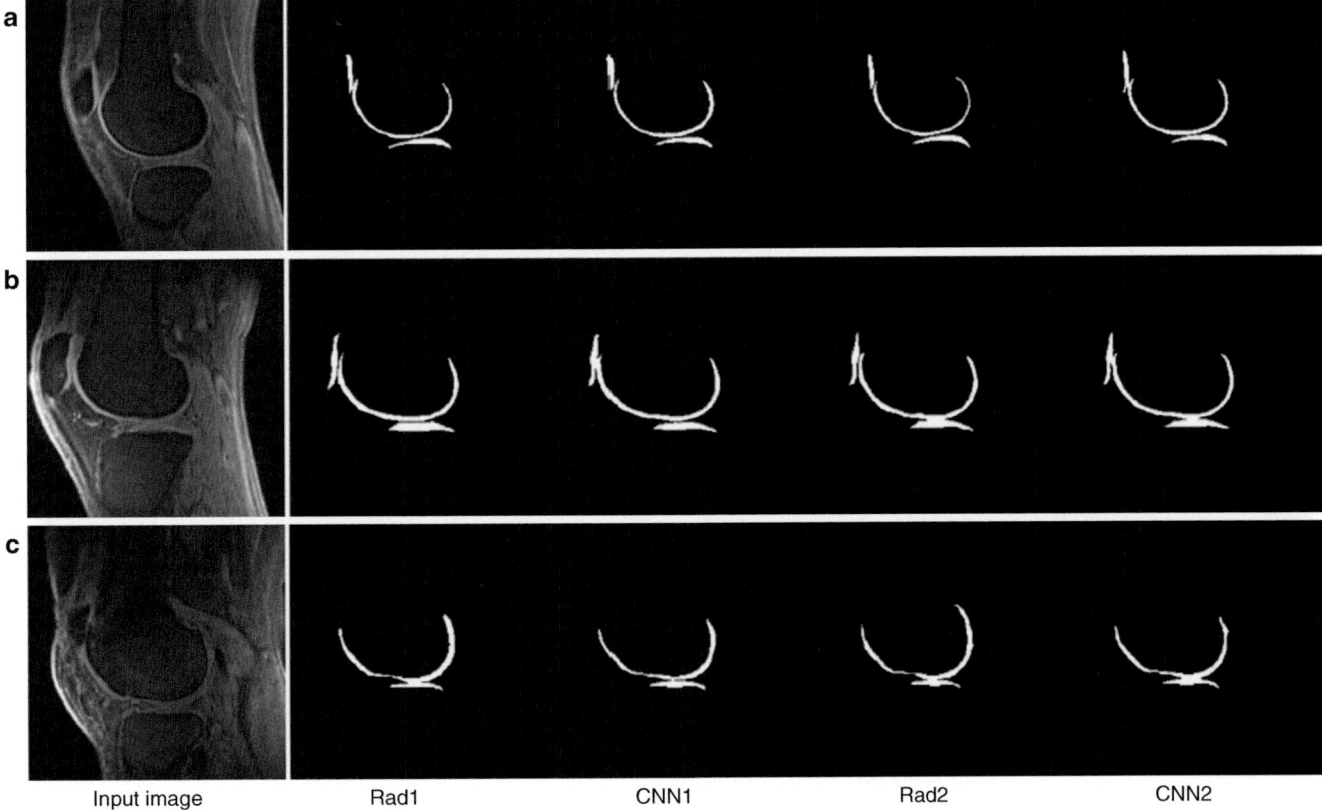

Fig. 29.5 The segmentation performance of the CNN model in three representative subjects (**a**–**c**). (Reproduced with permission from Ref. [39])

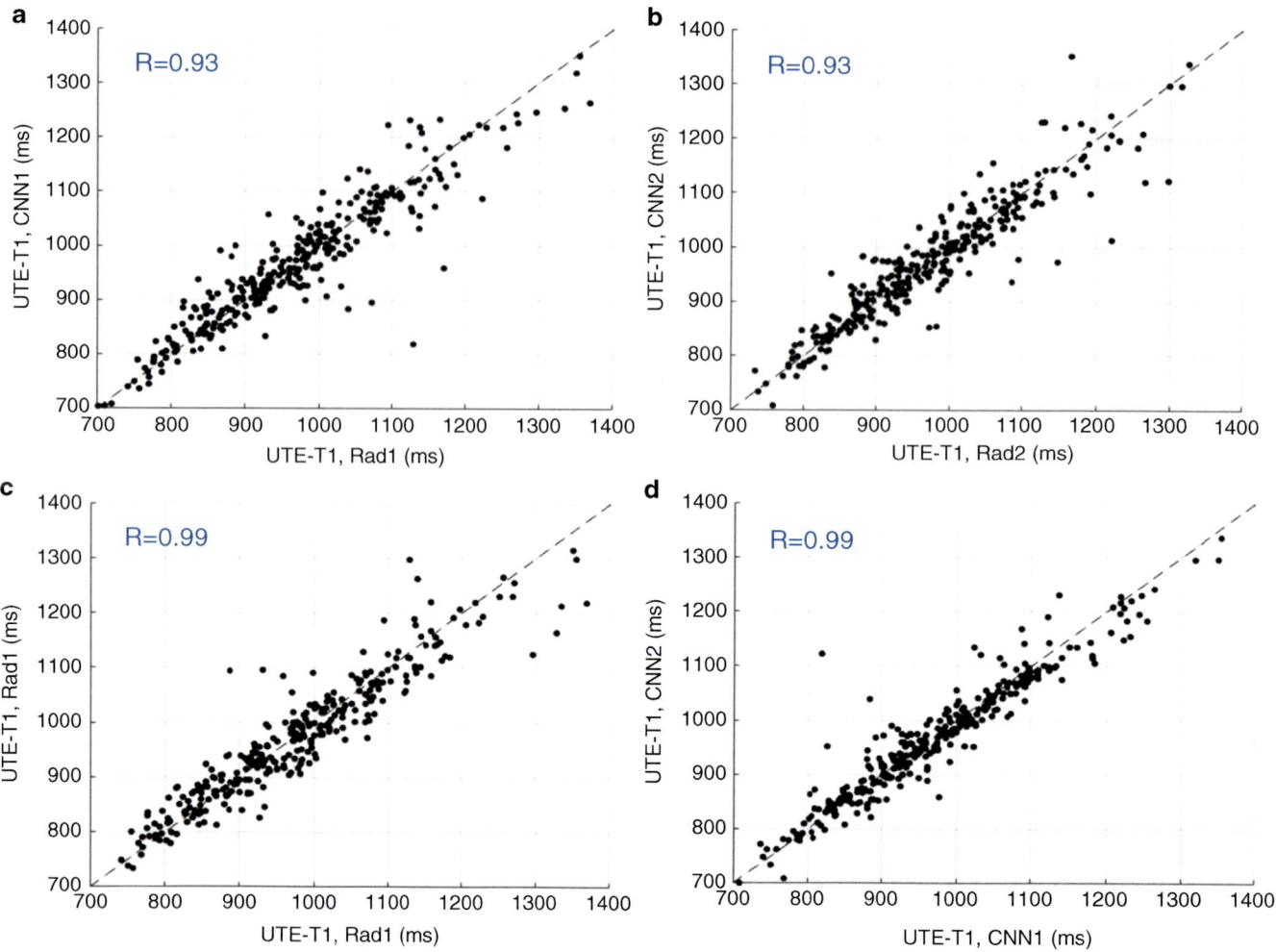

Fig. 29.6 Scatter plots for average UTE-T_1 values with manual and automatic segmentations obtained from the radiologists and the CNN models. (**a**)–(**d**) Show the relationships of UTE-T_1 values for Rad 1 vs. CNN 1, Rad 2 vs. CNN 2, Rad 1 vs. Rad 2, and CNN 1 vs. CNN 2. (Reproduced with permission from Ref. [39])

consistency was observed between the two radiologists and the CNN models. Significant increases in UTE-based T_1, $T_{1\rho}$, and T_2^* values ($P < 0.05$), as well as a decrease in MPF ($P < 0.001$), were observed in doubtful-minimal OA and/or moderate-severe OA compared with normal controls, suggesting that fully automated quantitative 3D UTE biomarkers may be useful in the evaluation of OA.

This study evaluated a transfer learning-based U-Net CNN model to automatically segment whole knee full-thickness cartilage and extract quantitative MR parameters using 3D UTE Cones MR imaging in vivo. Maps of UTE-based T_1, $T_{1\rho}$, and T_2^*s, as well as MPF, were automatically generated for whole knee cartilage. The robustness of this novel approach was validated by the high consistency in global mean values of T_1, $T_{1\rho}$, T_2^*, and MPF obtained from manually and automatically segmented cartilage.

Quantification with UTE MRI

Tissue properties such as T_1, $T_{1\rho}$, and T_2^* can be measured using qMRI techniques and can be used as potential biomarkers of disease [42]. Traditional qMRI parametric mapping is achieved by fitting a series of data with least square algorithms. The total scan time is significantly increased due to the need for data acquired with a series of repetition times (TRs) or flip angles (FAs) for T_1 mapping, spin-locking times (TSLs) for $T_{1\rho}$ mapping, or echo times (TEs) for T_2^* mapping [43–47]. As a result, the application of quantitative MRI in clinical practice is severely limited by the scan time that increases exponentially with data dimension. Deep learning-based quantification has been investigated to accelerate UTE parametric mapping.

Conventional method

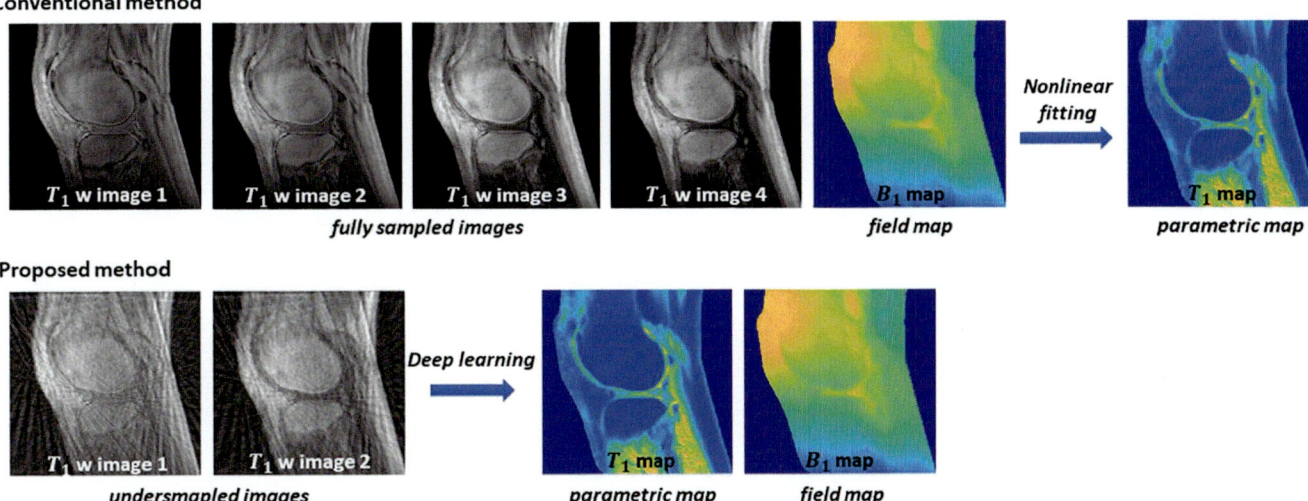

Fig. 29.7 Deep learning-based quantitative parametric mapping strategy compared to conventional nonlinear fitting methods. (Reproduced with permission from Ref. [48])

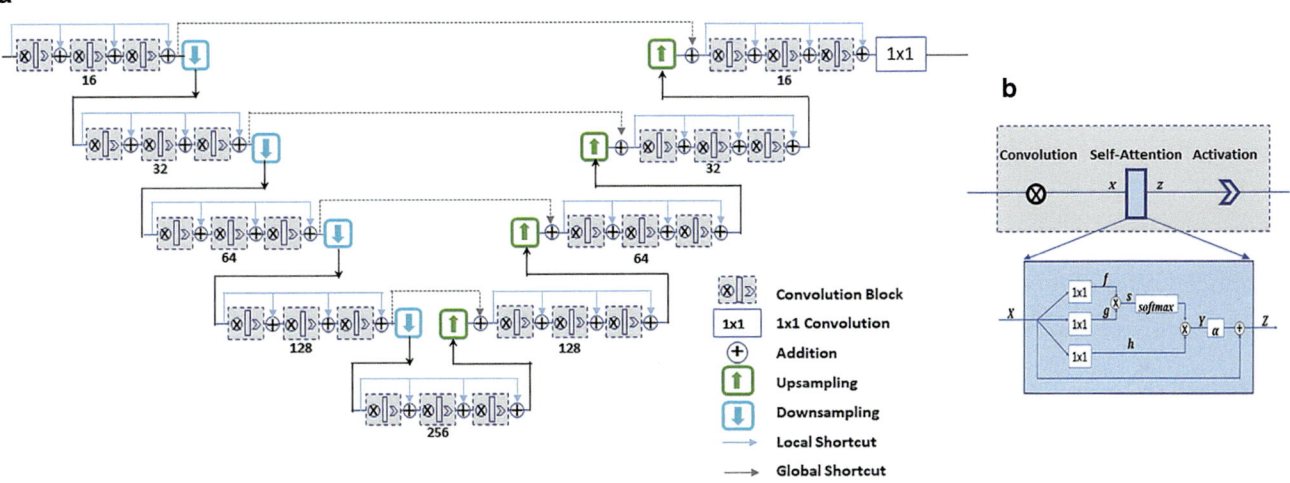

Fig. 29.8 Self-attention CNN. (**a**) The architecture of the self-attention CNN. (**b**) The composition of a convolutional block, where a novel self-attention layer is integrated. (Reproduced with permission from Ref. [48])

Wu et al. proposed a modified V-Net for shortening the UTE-T_1 mapping time [48]. Figure 29.7 shows conventional T_1 mapping derived from the least square fitting of UTE images acquired with different TRs and using RF field inhomogeneity corrected by B_1 mapping. T_1 and B_1 maps were predicted directly from two highly undersampled T_1-weighted images using deep learning.

A modified V-Net was used in this study, as shown in Fig. 29.8. It consists of an encoder and a decoder along which the resolution of feature maps first shrinks and then expands. Global shortcut connections were established between the corresponding levels of the two paths to compensate for details lost in downsampling. Local shortcut con-

nections were also established within the same level of a single path to facilitate residual learning.

Figure 29.9 demonstrates the feasibility of the modified V-Net for accelerated UTE-based T_1 and B_1 mapping. In Fig. 29.9d, the T_1 map predicted from two jointly reconstructed images (corresponding to 10° and 30° FAs) is highly consistent with the ground truth T_1 map (Fig. 29.9a) and is very similar to the T_1 map (Fig. 29.9e) predicted from four jointly reconstructed images (corresponding to 5°, 10°, 20°, and 30° FAs). This means that reducing the number of input images does not have a substantial impact on the fidelity of the predicted parametric map.

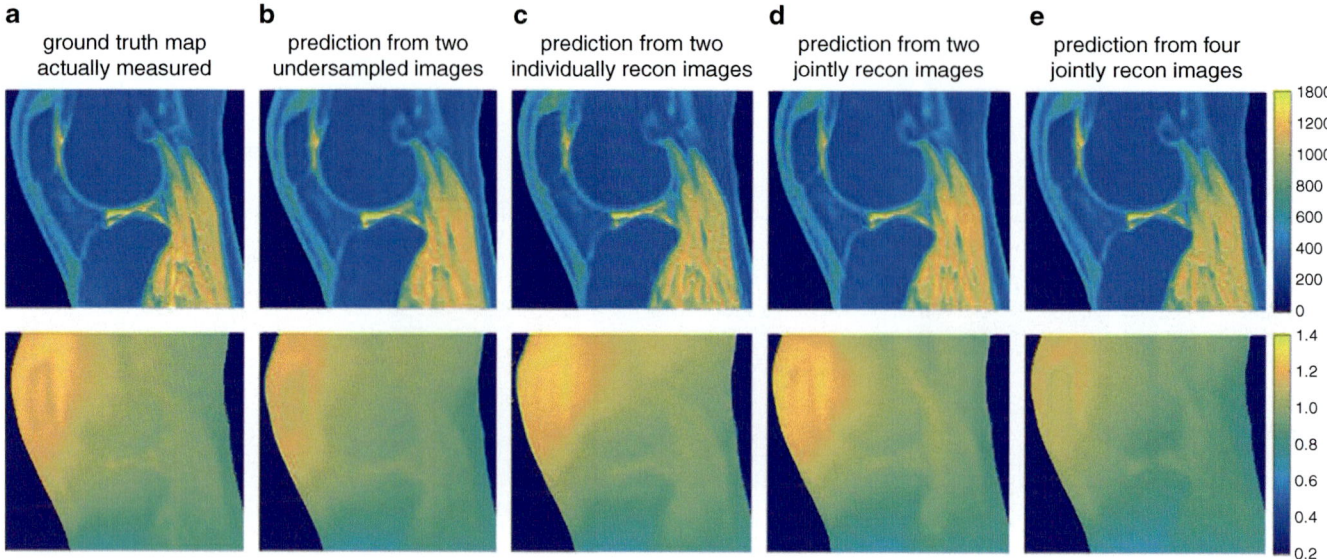

Fig. 29.9 T_1 and B_1 maps were predicted from various input images with an acceleration factor of four in every input image. (**a**) Ground truth of the T_1 and B_1 maps, (**b**) maps predicted from two undersampled images with $10°$ and $30°$ FAs, (**c**) maps derived from two individually reconstructed images with $10°$ and $30°$ FAs, (**d**) maps derived from two jointly reconstructed images with $10°$ and $30°$ FAs, and (**e**) maps derived from four jointly reconstructed images with $5°$, $10°$, $20°$, and $30°$ FAs. (Reproduced with permission from Ref. [48])

Using the proposed method, spatiotemporal correlation between images is exploited to allow undersampling and reduction in the number of different contrast images required. This greatly accelerates quantitative UTE parametric mapping without compromising its accuracy. In addition, acquisition of the B_1 map is no longer necessary, which further reduces the total scan time.

Simultaneous Segmentation and Quantification with UTE MRI

As OA is a "whole-organ" disease [49], it would be of great clinical value to simultaneously segment and quantify the principal joint tissues accurately and effectively. The feasibility of DCNNs with physical constraints for simultaneous segmentation and T_1 mapping of the whole knee joint tissues using UTE MRI has been shown. It would be highly desirable to develop similar techniques for automatic segmentation and mapping of a panel of UTE biomarkers, including T_1, $T_{1\rho}$, T_2, T_2^*, and MPF for all the primary tissues in the joint. A series of networks, including the Multi-Tissue Segmentation and Quantification Net (MSQ-Net), the Physical Constraint MSQ-Net (pcMSQ-Net), and the Multi-Tissue Segmentation Multi-Parameter Quantification Net (MSMQ-Net), are proposed to address these challenges [50, 51].

MSQ-Net and pcMSQ-Net

Deep learning models with multi-task or multi-head design, generally with one major task and other tasks as auxiliary with weaker constraints, have been widely used in deep learning architectures to achieve several tasks simultaneously. Also, limitations on the auxiliary task normally help improve the performance of the major task. The multi-task design strategy has been adopted for designing the MSQ-Net.

Although quantitative parametric mapping can be straightforwardly generated with U-Net style nets, as introduced in Sect. 29.3, each voxel on the quantification maps has physical meaning. As a result, physical constraints have been added to produce more meaningful quantification maps. Liu et al. proposed MANTIS, which added physics feedback to predict the MR parametric mapping [26]. Also, as introduced by Yang et al., multiple compartments are very important to simultaneously segment cartilage and so provide systematic evaluation of this tissue in OA [52]. A pcMSQ-Net including physics constraints and multi-tissue segmentation is therefore proposed (Fig. 29.10).

As shown in Fig. 29.10, the MSQ-Net network is based on a U-Net style DCNN but with two branches for outputs, named the Reg_branch and the Seg_branch. Along the encoder path, downsamplings are applied to enable subsequent feature extractions at coarser scales. Latent features are shared for both upsampling branches, and upsamplings are conducted to support subsequent feature extractions at finer scales. Between convolutional blocks, skip connections are established. For the Reg_branch, quantitative MRI parametric maps are generated according to voxel-fitting-based maps as the ground truth, with l1 loss ($loss_{map}$) as the constraint. For Seg_branch, the meniscus and cartilage masks

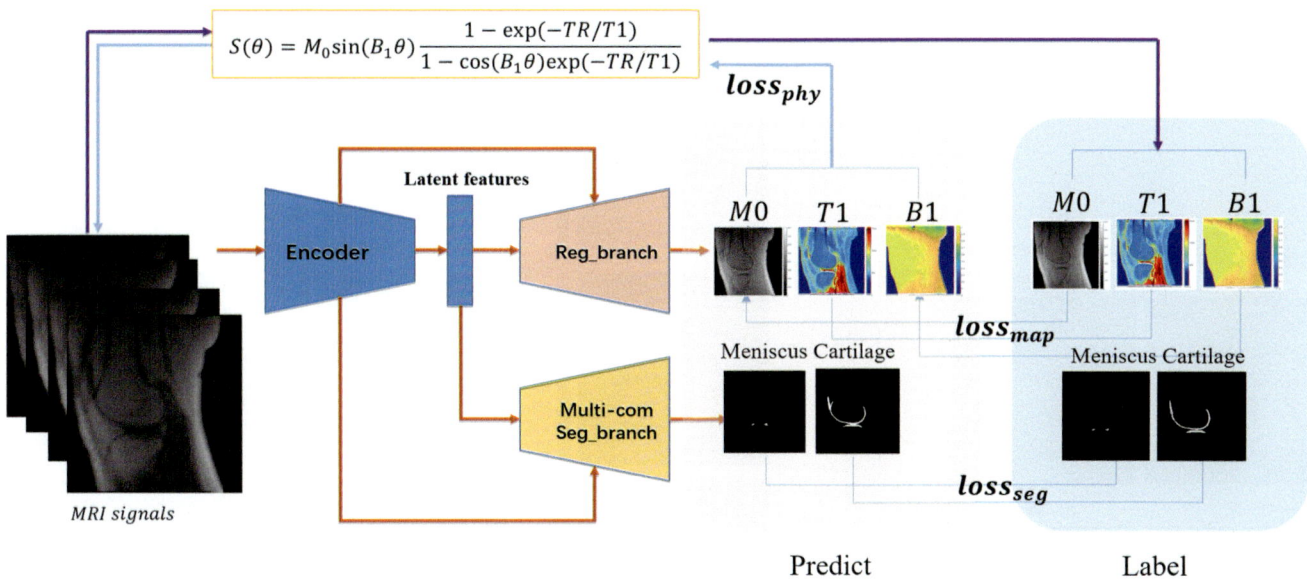

$$S(\theta) = M_0 \sin(B_1\theta) \frac{1 - \exp(-TR/T1)}{1 - \cos(B_1\theta)\exp(-TR/T1)}$$

Fig. 29.10 The network architecture of the MSQ-Net and pcMSQ-Net. The main difference between pcMSQ-Net and MSQ-Net is that the pcMSQ-Net has an additional loss for physical constraints. (Reproduced with permission from Ref. [50])

are generated with binary cross entropy loss and dice loss-based segmentation loss ($loss_{seg}$). For MSQ-net, the total loss ($loss_{MSQ}$) consists of $loss_{map}$ and $loss_{seg}$. A physical-constraint loss ($loss_{phy}$) is also applied to feed the predicted maps back to generate input MRI signals with different flip angles. MSQ-net with $loss_{phy}$ is the same as pcMSQ-net. The total loss for pcMSQ-net ($loss_{pcMSQ}$) consists of $loss_{map}$, $loss_{seg}$, and $loss_{phy}$. A structural similarity (ssim) score [53] is adopted to measure the performance of both MSQ-Net and pc-MSQ-Net.

A series of T_1-weighted images were acquired for each subject using a 3D UTE variable flip angle (UTE-VFA) technique. 3D spiral sampling was performed with conical view ordering using a very short TE of 32 μs, a TR of 20 ms, and four FAs of 5°, 10°, 20°, and 30°. Subsequently, image registration was performed to minimize inter-scan motion. M_0, T_1, and B_1 maps were derived via nonlinear fitting using the Levenberg-Marquardt algorithm.

Figure 29.11 shows typical results for the outputs of the MSQ-Net and pcMSQ-Net, demonstrating that both techniques can simultaneously generate reasonable parameter maps and segmentation masks. In this subject, the T_1 map of MSQ-Net had a ssim score of 0.806 relative to the GT, while pcMSQ-Net had a ssim score of 0.91. ROI analysis based on the T_1 maps and masks generated from both models was applied to all test datasets, as shown in Fig. 29.12, where the MSQ-Net and pcMSQ-Net results are comparable to the ground truth.

MSMQ-Net

The MSQ-Net and pcMSQ-Net have only been investigated for mapping of a single parameter: T_1. It is of great interest to study whether it is feasible to map several parameters simultaneously. The network architecture of the pcMSQ-Net was modified with more parameter regression to produce a new network, Multi-Tissue Segmentation with Multi-Parameter Quantification Net (MSMQ-Net), designed to predict both T_1 and $T_{1\rho}$ simultaneously on the quantification path [51], as shown in Fig. 29.13. The MSMQ-Net, similar to pcMSQ-Net, is based on a U-Net style DCNN with two output branches, Reg_branch and Seg_branch.

Along the encoder path, downsamplings are applied to enable subsequent feature extractions at coarser scales. Latent features are shared for both upsampling branches. Upsamplings are conducted to support subsequent feature extractions at finer scales. Between convolutional blocks, skip connections are established. $T_{1\rho}$ parameter quantification was added in the Reg_branch to test the extendibility of the previous pcMSQ-Net architecture. For $T_{1\rho}$ mapping, the scan parameters were TR = 500 ms, FA = 10°, with seven TSLs = 0, 12, 24, 36, 48, 72, and 96 ms. Subsequently, image registration was performed to minimize inter-scan motion. M_0, T_1, $T_{1\rho}$, and B_1 maps were derived via nonlinear fitting using the Levenberg–Marquardt algorithm. ROIs for the cartilage and meniscus area were labeled with homemade Matlab code by three experienced radiologists. A total of 1056 slice images from 44 subjects (including healthy volunteers and patients with different degrees of OA) were used for model training, and 144 images of six additional subjects were used for model validation. In order to evaluate the effect of reduced input images, two MSMQ-Net models were trained: one with total data inputs (4 FAs and 7 TSLs) and the other with partial data inputs (2 FAs = 5°, 10°, and 3 TSLs = 0, 12, 24 ms) with the same datasets and hyper-

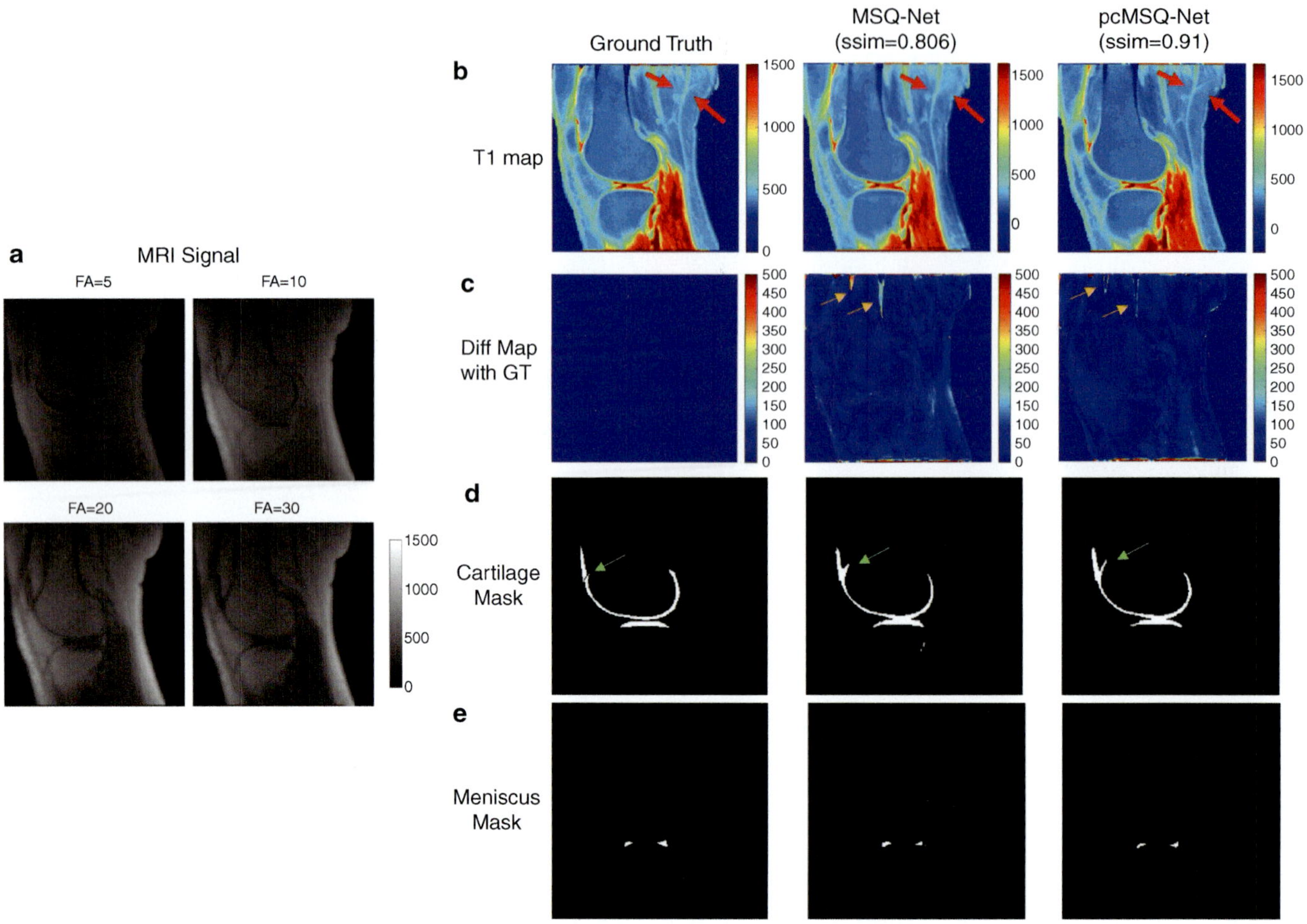

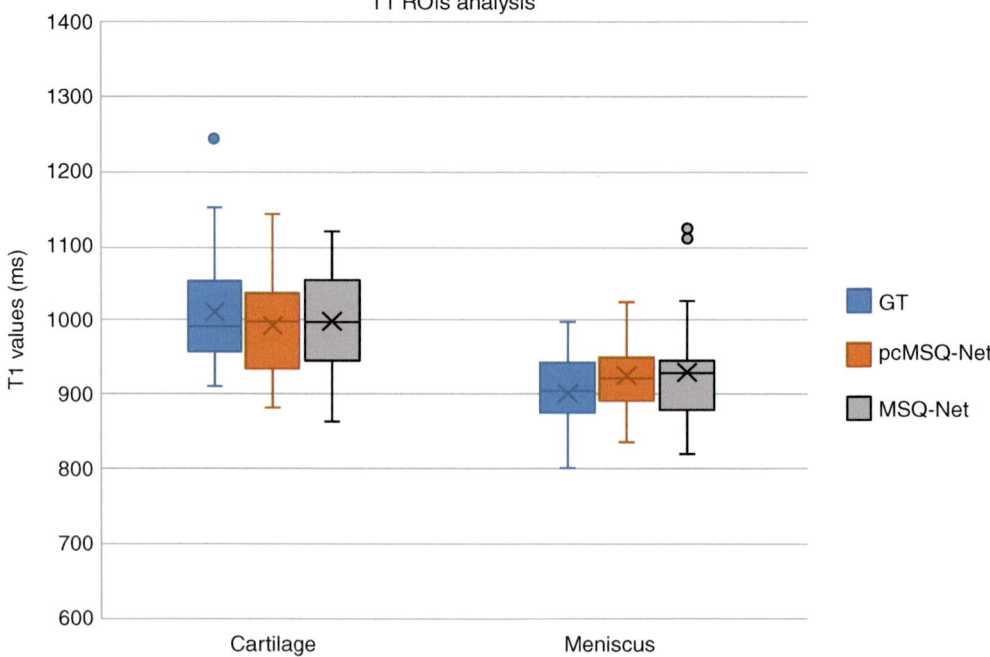

Fig. 29.11 Typical results of MSQ-Net and pcMSQ-Net. (**a**) MRI input signals with different FAs; (**b**) UTE-T_1 maps of ground truth (GT) and predictions by MSQ-Net and pcMSQ-Net; (**c**) the difference between predicted and ground truth T_1 maps, (**d**) and (**e**) show masks of cartilage and meniscus of ground truth and predicted masks with MSQ-Net and pcMSQ-Net. (Reproduced with permission from Ref. [50])

Fig. 29.12 T_1 ROI analysis for cartilage and meniscus with ground truth, MSQ-Net, and pcMSQ-Net. (Reproduced with permission from Ref. [50])

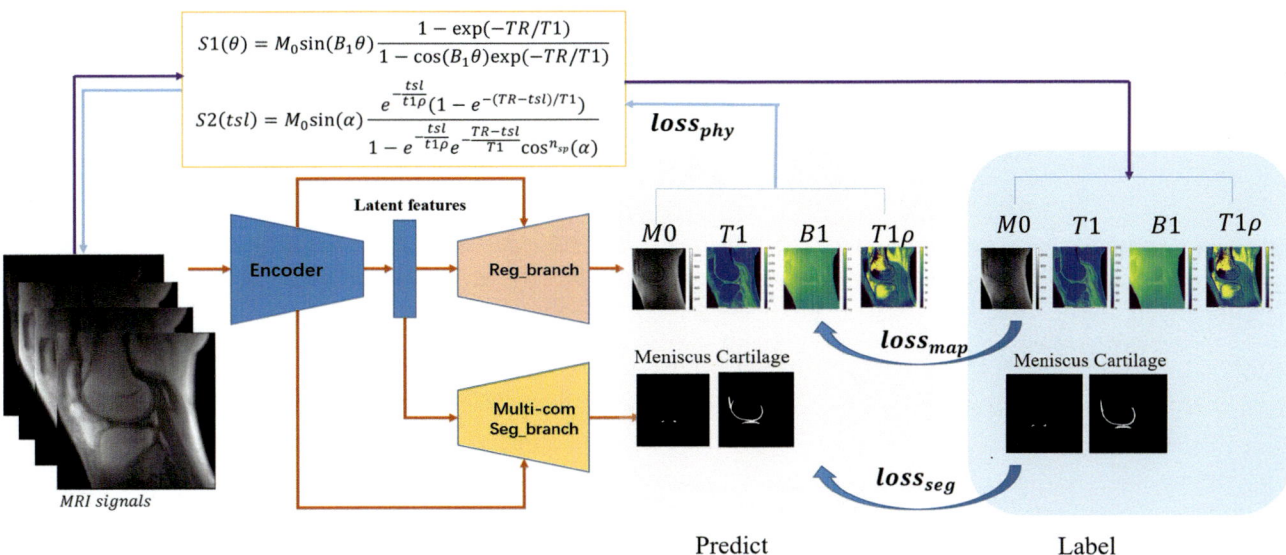

Fig. 29.13 The model architecture of MSMQ-Net, with modified physics constraints for multi-parameter quantification. (Reproduced with permission from Ref. [51])

parameters, including Adam optimizer, learning rate from 0.001 with a cosine-annealing strategy, and epochs of 300.

To compare the performance of the MSMQ-Net with full versus partial data for T_1 and $T_{1\rho}$ mapping, both violin distri-bution and Bland–Altman analysis were performed. Figure 29.14 shows the violin distributions of both T_1 and $T_{1\rho}$ values for the ROIs drawn in cartilage and meniscus from the full and partial data models, respectively.

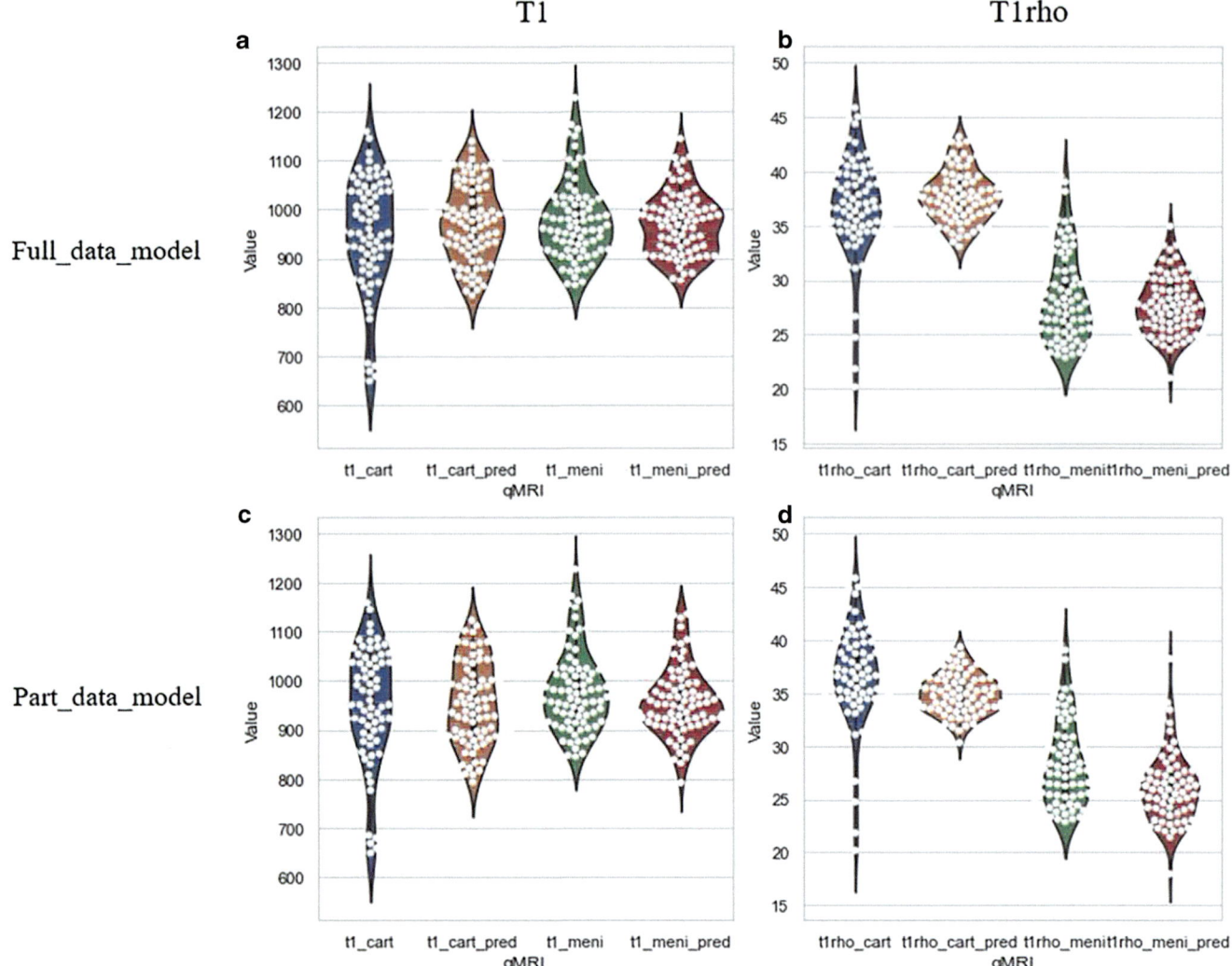

Fig. 29.14 Violin distribution of T_1 and $T_{1\rho}$ values of cartilage and meniscus predicted by MSMQ-Net with both the full_data and partial_data, which are also compared with the ground truth. In the x-axis of all subfigures, "_cart" and "_meni" represent the cartilage and meniscus, respectively, while "_pred" means prediction. -NetFor (**a**) and (**c**), the ground truth of the T_1 values of the cartilage and meniscus ROIs are shown in blue and green, respectively, while the T_1 values of the cartilage ROIs predicted by the MSMQ-Net-Net (including T_1 mapping and segmentation region). For (**b**) and (**d**), the same colors refer to corresponding $T_{1\rho}$ value distributions for cartilage and meniscus and different model outputs. (Reproduced with permission from Ref. [51])

Conclusion

CNN-based deep learning has been implemented in almost every aspect of the medical imaging arena. This chapter introduces several cutting-edge techniques for deep learning-based segmentation and quantification of UTE MRI. In moving toward a more automatic approach, it has been shown that the CNNs, especially U-Net architecture, can be used to provide highly accurate segmentation and/or quantification in the knee joint. For a more automatic and efficient protocol for "whole-organ" analysis of the OA, MSMQ-Net has been proposed and its feasibility has been demonstrated for simul-taneous segmentation of multiple tissues and quantification of multiple parameters. Several directions still need further development to achieve automatic analysis of OA with UTE MRI. First, advanced deep learning network architectures, such as transformers and GAN, will be adopted to further improve the segmentation and quantification performance. Second, the input of current models is still the image domain. We still need to include the reconstruction step from the raw MRI k-space data. In the next step, we may integrate the reconstruction into the whole network pipeline to make it more integrated. Third, 3D convolution-based DCNNs will be implemented with MRI volumes as input with the accumulation of the data. Fourth, direct assessment for the grading of OA based on the "whole-organ" information will be performed with a second-stage network or machine learning models. Information from different parts of the knee and different modalities will be fused to better predict the severity of OA.

References

1. LeCun Y, Bengio Y, Hinton G. Deep learning. Nature. 2015;521(7553):436–44.
2. Yang Y, Sun J, Li H, Xu Z. Deep ADMM-Net for compressive sensing MRI. In: Lee D, Sugiyama M, Luxburg U, Guyon I, Garnett R, editors. Advances in neural information processing systems, vol. 29. NeuralIPS; 2016. p. 10–8.
3. Wang S, Su Z, Ying L, Peng X, Zhu S, Liang F, et al. Accelerating magnetic resonance imaging via deep learning. In: Proc IEEE Int Symp Biomed Imaging. IEEE; 2016. p. 514–7.
4. Qin C, Hajnal JV, Rueckert D, Schlemper J, Caballero J, Price AN. Convolutional recurrent neural networks for dynamic MR image reconstruction. IEEE Trans Med Imaging. 2019;38(1):280–90.
5. Zhu B, Liu JZ, Cauley SF, Rosen BR, Rosen MS. Image reconstruction by domain-transform manifold learning. Nature. 2018;555(7697):487–92.
6. Yang G, Yu S, Dong H, et al. DAGAN: deep de-aliasing generative adversarial networks for fast compressed sensing MRI reconstruction. IEEE Tran Med Imaging. 2018;37(6):1310–21.
7. Yaman B, Hosseini SAH, Moeller S, Ellermann J, Uğurbil K, Akçakaya M. Self-supervised physics-based deep learning MRI reconstruction without fully-sampled data. In: Proc IEEE Int Symp Biomed Imaging. IEEE; 2020. p. 921–5.
8. Haskins G, Kruecker J, Kruger U, Xu S, Pinto PA, Wood BJ, Yan P. Learning deep similarity metric for 3D MR-TRUS image registration. Int J Comput Assist Radiol Surg. 2019;14(3):417–25.
9. Cao X, Yang J, Zhang J, Wang Q, Yap P-T, Shen D. Deformable image registration using a cue-aware deep regression network. IEEE Trans Biomed Eng. 2018;65(9):1900–11.
10. Zhu C, Ni J, Li Y, Gu G. General tendencies in segmentation of medical ultrasound images. In: Int Conf on ICICSE; 2009. p. 113–7.
11. Taxt T, Lundervold A, Fuglaas B, Lien H, Abeler V. Multispectral analysis of uterine corpus tumors in magnetic resonance imaging. Magn Reson Med. 1992;23(1):55–76.
12. Lundervold A, Storvik G. Segmentation of brain parenchyma and cerebrospinal fluid in multispectral magnetic resonance images. IEEE Trans Med Imaging. 1995;14(2):339–49.
13. Cabezas M, Oliver A, Lladó X, Freixenet J, Cuadra MB. A review of atlas-based segmentation for magnetic resonance brain images. Comput Methods Prog Biomed. 2011;104(3):e158–77.
14. Garciá-Lorenzo D, Francis S, Narayanan S, Arnold DL, Collins DL. Review of automatic segmentation methods of multiple sclerosis white matter lesions on conventional magnetic resonance imaging. Med Image Anal. 2013;17(1):1–18.
15. Dora L, Agrawal S, Panda R, Abraham A. State-of-the-art methods for brain tissue segmentation: a review. IEEE Rev Biomed Eng. 2017;10:235–49.
16. Litjens G, Kooi T, Bejnordi BE, et al. A survey on deep learning in medical image analysis. Med Image Anal. 2017;42:60–88.
17. Hesamian MH, Jia W, He X, Kennedy P. Deep learning techniques for medical image segmentation: achievements and challenges. J Digit Imaging. 2019;32(4):582–96.
18. Liu X, Song L, Liu S, Zhang Y. A review of deep-learning-based medical image segmentation methods. Sustainability. 2021;13(3):1224.
19. Gao X, Qian Y. Segmentation of brain lesions from CT images based on deep learning techniques. In: SPIE Medical Imaging; 2018. p. 105782L.
20. Hamidian S, Sahiner B, Petrick N, Pezeshk A. 3D convolutional neural network for automatic detection of lung nodules in chest CT. Proc SPIE Int Soc Opt Eng. 2017;10134:1013409.
21. Christ PF, Ettlinger F, Grün F, et al. Automatic liver and tumor segmentation of CT and MRI volumes using cascaded fully convolutional neural networks. 2017. https://arxiv.org/abs/1702.05970
22. Cai J, Lu L, Xing F, Yang L. Pancreas segmentation in CT and MRI images via domain specific network designing and recurrent neural contextual learning. 2018. https://arxiv.org/abs/1803.11303.
23. Bollmann S, Rasmussen KGB, Kristensen M, Blendal RG, Østergaard LR, Plocharski M, O'Brien K, Langkammer C, Janke A, Barth M. DeepQSM—using deep learning to solve the dipole inversion for quantitative susceptibility mapping. NeuroImage. 2019;195:373–83.
24. Ma D, Gulani V, Seiberlich N, Liu K, Sunshine JL, Duerk JL, Griswold MA. Magnetic resonance fingerprinting. Nature. 2013;495(7440):187–92.
25. Cohen O, Zhu B, Rosen MS. MR fingerprinting deep reconstruction network (DRONE). Magn Reson Med. 2018;80(3):885–94.
26. Liu F, Feng L, Kijowski R. MANTIS: model-augmented neural network with incoherent k-space sampling for efficient MR parameter mapping. Magn Reson Med. 2019;82(1):174–88.
27. Yeoh PSQ, Lai KW, Goh SL, Hasikin K, Hum YC, Tee YK, Dhanalakshmi S. Emergence of deep learning in knee asteoarthritis diagnosis. Comput Intell Neurosci. 2021;2021:4931437.
28. Morales Martinez A, Caliva F, Flament I, et al. Learning osteoarthritis imaging biomarkers from bone surface spherical encoding. Magn Reson Med. 2020;84(4):2190–203.
29. Nasser Y, Jennane R, Chetouani A, Lespessailles E, Hassouni ME. Discriminative regularized auto-encoder for early detection of knee osteoarthritis: data from the osteoarthritis initiative. IEEE Trans Med Imaging. 2020;39(9):2976–84.
30. Pedoia V, Norman B, Mehany SN, Bucknor MD, Link TM, Majumdar S. 3D convolutional neural networks for detection and severity staging of meniscus and PFJ cartilage morphological degenerative changes in osteoarthritis and anterior cruciate ligament subjects. J Magn Reson Imaging. 2019;49(2):400–10.
31. Ronneberger O, Fischer P, Brox T. U-Net: convolutional networks for biomedical image segmentation. In: MICCAI; 2015. p. 234–41.
32. Norman B, Pedoia V, Majumdar S. Use of 2D U-Net convolutional neural networks for automated cartilage and meniscus segmentation of knee MR imaging data to determine relaxometry and morphometry. Radiology. 2018;288(1):177–85.
33. Liu F, Zhou Z, Jang H, Samsonov A, Zhao G, Kijowski R. Deep convolutional neural network and 3D deformable approach for tissue segmentation in musculoskeletal magnetic resonance imaging. Magn Reson Med. 2018;79(4):2379–91.
34. Gan HS, Ramlee MH, Wahab AA, et al. From classical to deep learning: review on cartilage and bone segmentation techniques in knee osteoarthritis research. Artif Intell Rev. 2021;54:2445–94.
35. Chu CR, Williams AA, West RV, et al. Quantitative magnetic resonance imaging UTE-T_2^* mapping of cartilage and meniscus healing after anatomic anterior cruciate ligament reconstruction. Am J Sports Med. 2014;42(8):1847–56.
36. Williams A, Qian Y, Golla S, Chu CR. UTE-T_2^* mapping detects sub-clinical meniscus injury after anterior cruciate ligament tear. Osteoarthr Cartil. 2012;20(6):486–94.

37. Zhang X, Ma YJ, Wei Z, et al. Macromolecular fraction (MMF) from 3D ultrashort echo time cones magnetization transfer (3D UTE-Cones-MT) imaging predicts meniscal degeneration and knee osteoarthritis. Osteoarthr Cartil. 2021;29(8):1173–80.

38. Byra M, Wu M, Zhang X, Jang H, Ma YJ, Chang EY, Shah S, Du J. Knee menisci segmentation and relaxometry of 3D ultrashort echo time cones MR imaging using attention U-Net with transfer learning. Magn Reson Med. 2020;83(3):1109–22.

39. Xue YP, Jang H, Byra M, Cai ZY, Wu M, Chang EY, Ma YJ, Du J. Automated cartilage segmentation and quantification using 3D ultrashort echo time (UTE) cones MR imaging with deep convolutional neural networks. Eur Radiol. 2021;31(10):7653–63.

40. Klein S, Staring M, Murphy K, Viergever MA, Pluim JPW. Elastix: a toolbox for intensity-based medical image registration. IEEE Trans Med Imaging. 2010;29(1):196–205.

41. Wu M, Zhao W, Wan L, et al. Quantitative three-dimensional ultrashort echo time cones imaging of the knee joint with motion correction. NMR Biomed. 2020;33(1):e4214.

42. Chang EY, Du J, Chung CB. UTE imaging in the musculoskeletal system. J Magn Reson Imaging. 2015;41(4):870–83.

43. Lu X, Jerban S, Wan L, Ma Y, Jang H, Le N, Yang W, Chang EY, Du J. Three-dimensional ultrashort echo time imaging with tricomponent analysis for human cortical bone. Magn Reson Med. 2019;82(1):348–55.

44. Ma YJ, Carl M, Searleman A, Lu X, Chang EY, Du J. 3D adiabatic $T_{1\rho}$ prepared ultrashort echo time cones sequence for whole knee imaging. Magn Reson Med. 2018;80(4):1429–39.

45. Jerban S, Lu X, Jang H, Ma Y, Namiranian B, Le N, Li Y, Chang EY, Du J. Significant correlations between human cortical bone mineral density and quantitative susceptibility mapping (QSM) obtained with 3D Cones ultrashort echo time magnetic resonance imaging (UTE-MRI). Magn Reson Imaging. 2019;62:104–10.

46. Jerban S, Lu X, Dorthe EW, Alenezi S, Ma Y, Kakos L, Jang H, Sah RL, Chang EY, D'Lima D, Du J. Correlations of cortical bone microstructural and mechanical properties with water proton fractions obtained from ultrashort echo time (UTE) MRI tricomponent T_2^* model. NMR Biomed. 2020;33(3):e4233.

47. Lu X, Ma Y, Chang EY, He Q, Searleman A, von Drygalski A, Du J. Simultaneous quantitative susceptibility mapping (QSM) and R_2^* for high iron concentration quantification with 3D ultrashort echo time sequences: an echo dependence study. Magn Reson Med. 2018;79(4):2315–22.

48. Wu Y, Ma Y, Du J, Xing L. Accelerating quantitative MR imaging with the incorporation of B_1 compensation using deep learning. Magn Reson Imaging. 2020;72:78–86.

49. Brandt KD, Radin EL, Dieppe PA, Putte L. Yet more evidence that osteoarthritis is not a cartilage disease (Editorial). Ann Rheum Dis. 2006;65(10):1261–4.

50. Lu X, Ma YJ, Jerban S, et al. Deep CNNs with physical constraints for simultaneous multi-tissue segmentation and quantification (MSQ-Net) of knee from UTE MRIs. In: Proc Intl Soc Mag Reson Med; 2021:4051.

51. Lu X, Ma YJ, et al. Deep CNNs with physical constraints for simultaneous multi-tissue segmentation and multi-parameter quantification (MSMQ-Net) of knee. In: Proc Intl Soc Mag Reson Med; 2022:3462.

52. Yang M, Colak C, Chundru KK, Gaj S, Nanavati A, Jones MH, Winalski CS, Subhas N, Li X. Automated knee cartilage segmentation for heterogeneous clinical MRI using generative adversarial networks with transfer learning. Quant Imaging Med Surg. 2022;12(5):2620–33.

53. Wang Z, Bovik AC, Sheikh HR, Simoncelli EP. Image quality assessment: from error visibility to structural similarity. IEEE Trans Image Process. 2004;13(4):600–12.

Part IV

Applications

Fritz Schick

Introduction

Collagen is the most abundant protein in the human body. Because it forms mechanically stable macromolecular structures, collagen is an essential component of bones and connective tissues. It forms the matrix of cartilage, tendons, and ligaments and plays a major role in making the skin highly durable. Connective tissue structures containing collagen are also found in the extracellular matrix of most parenchymal organs and help maintain their structure. The connective tissues that transfer force from muscles such as aponeuroses and tendons largely consist of collagen.

Chemical Structure and Synthesis of Collagen

Chemically, collagen fibrils are helical chains of different amino acids [1, 2]. Compared to other proteins, glycine plays a special role in collagen, where it forms every third amino acid of the collagen primary chains. In other proteins, the glycine content is much lower. Since glycine produces a characteristic signal pattern with proton magnetic resonance spectroscopy (^{1}H-MRS), even when incorporated into a protein, it is important in spectrally resolved magnetic resonance (MR) investigations.

Collagen is mainly synthesized in fibroblasts but also in chondroblasts, osteoblasts, and other cell types. Figure 30.1 shows the main steps of collagen synthesis in fibroblasts: first, chains of amino acids (polypeptides) are assembled in the rough endoplasmic reticulum. Three of these chains are enzymatically linked to form a triple helix structure and packed as procollagen into special vesicles, which are transported through the cell and released into the intercellular

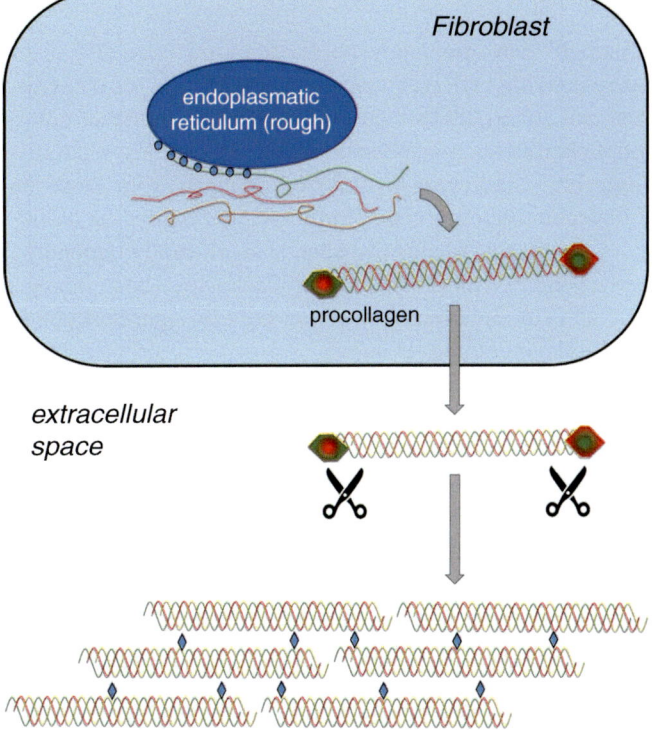

Fig. 30.1 Intracellular collagen biosynthesis in fibroblasts and extracellular cross-linking of fibrils to form solid collagen fibers. Polypeptide chains are produced by the rough endoplasmic reticulum. Three chains join together in a zipper-like manner to form a triple helix. The triple helixes are transported through the vesicles across the Golgi apparatus to the cell membrane and secreted into the extracellular space (ECS). In the extracellular space, cleavage of the procollagen end pieces triggers self-assembly of collagen fibrils and cross-linking. As a result, mechanically stable collagen fibers are formed

space. Outside the cell, the end pieces of the procollagen molecules are enzymatically separated and the collagen fibrils are connected with covalent cross-links between hydroxylysine and lysine residues of different fibrils. These cross-links and the tight winding are crucial for the high ten-

F. Schick (✉)
Department of Diagnostic and Interventional Radiology, Section of Experimental Radiology, University of Tübingen, Tübingen, Germany
e-mail: fritz.schick@med.uni-tuebingen.de

J. Du, G. M. Bydder (eds.), *MRI of Short- and Ultrashort-T₂ Tissues*, https://doi.org/10.1007/978-3-031-35197-6_30

sile strength of collagen fibers, which can be several thousand times their weight.

More than 25 different types of collagen are known. The most common of these in the body (types I–III) are unidirectional fibers as seen in tendons and aponeuroses. However, there are also collagen types that contribute to more net-like structures, which form direct connections between cells.

It should also be mentioned that extracellular collagen fiber formation is partially reversible, as fibroblasts are also able to degrade collagen with the help of enzymes (collagenases).

The MR Visibility of Collagen

Although there are many publications on magnetic resonance imaging (MRI) of tissues with large collagen contents, there are uncertainties regarding the MR visibility of collagen. In particular, misunderstandings can result from not distinguishing studies on hydrolyzed collagen from those on collagen in tissues in vivo. This is mainly because the mobility of amino acid chains can change significantly depending on the condition and pretreatment of collagen. These changes have an extremely large impact on the MR signals obtained from collagen-bound ^{1}H nuclei.

Organized collagen in fixed spatial structures, as present in bone, tendons, ligaments, and cartilage, shows extremely limited mobility in the vast majority of protein chains. This means that dipolar interactions are not compensated for and that the signals have extremely short cross-relaxation times. Therefore, ^{1}H spectroscopy of preparations of those tissues (e.g., the Achilles tendons of cows from a slaughterhouse) using whole-body MR systems do not reveal visible lines of collagen molecules in the spectrum, even when using pulse-acquire (or FID = free induction decay) sequences. The transverse relaxation times (T_2 and T_2^*) are so short that there is extreme line broadening, and no clear signal components of collagen-bound ^{1}H nuclei appear [3]. The signals visible in MR acquisitions with extremely short echo times (TEs) originate from bound or free water pools. These signals disappear after freeze-drying or deuterated water (D_2O)–water (H_2O) exchange. However, use of small-bore solid-state spectrometers [4] and the application of magic angle spinning (MAS) [5] during spectroscopy allow direct detection of ^{1}H signals from collagen, even in native (non-hydrolyzed) preparations of tendon tissue. Unfortunately, small-bore spectrometers and MAS are not suitable for in vivo studies.

Preparations of healthy tendons, which largely consist of organized collagen, do not produce clear signals from collagen molecules that can be directly detected with whole-body MR systems. This changes after mechanical crushing of tendons and addition of enzymes (e.g., trypsin or collagenase) that break down collagen molecules into smaller fragments. After this treatment, the same tendons show clear signals that can be assigned to the amino acids of collagen [6].

MR Studies of Collagen In Vitro

Various widely used products are made from collagen-containing components of animals. Two examples are described below and are suitable as samples for MRI and magnetic resonance spectroscopy (MRS) examinations. It should be noted that the organized collagen components in these products are present in a form that is chemically altered from that in tissues. They are the so-called hydrolysates of collagen, which consist of relatively short polypeptide chains that have high mobility. They provide a good representation of the signals from the ^{1}H nuclei that can be detected.

1. **Gelatine**: For the production of nutritional gelatine, components of the skin of pigs and cattle are mostly used, but their bones may also be used. In the production of gelatine, the collagen filaments are denatured by hydrolysis and split into smaller mobile peptide chains. These peptide chains partially cross-link again in the prepared gelatine, producing its firm consistency. However, the amino acid chains in the peptides remain at least partially mobile and so produce detectable signals even with the usual clinical MRI sequences, which have TEs of a few milliseconds.

2. **Collagen powder**: This is a food supplement. Hydrolyzed collagen (i.e., collagen broken down into smaller units) in powder form is marketed to counteract the breakdown of proteins in the body and thus improve joint function and the firmness of skin, hair, and nails. In general, the objective is to strengthen the connective tissue and prevent diseases involving collagen. While in the past, mostly pork and bovine ingredients were used, today, fish skins are commonly used for the production of food supplements. Collagen products made from fish are said to have good bioavailability. On the packages of collagen powders, it is often stated that they mainly contain collagen types I and III. The powders are highly soluble in water and are extremely suitable for the production of MR phantoms.

Tissue-derived collagen has been investigated using high-field nuclear magnetic resonance (NMR), with organized collagen being hydrolyzed with enzymes or acid/alkali treatments prior to investigation in order to be able to investigate the dissolved polypeptides derived from tissue collagen [7].

Some results of studies on aqueous solutions of commercially available collagen powder (i.e., collagen hydrolysate) are presented in Fig. 30.2a, which show a pulse-acquire

Collagen Hydrolysate, 10% in H₂O

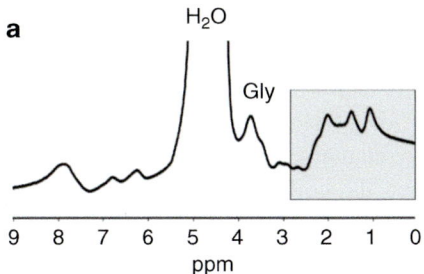

Collagen Hydrolysate, 10% in H₂O

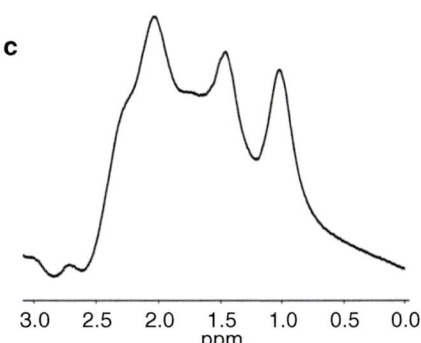

STEAM Spectra of
Collagen Hydrolysate, 10% in H₂O

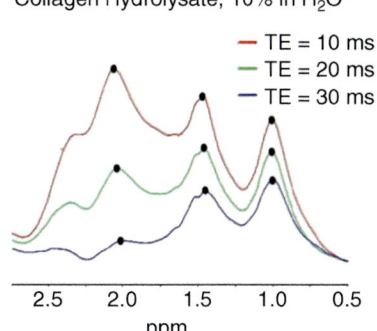

Collagen Hydrolysate, 10% in D₂O

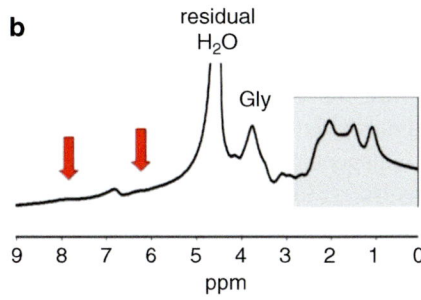

Amino Acids Spectra at 600 MHz

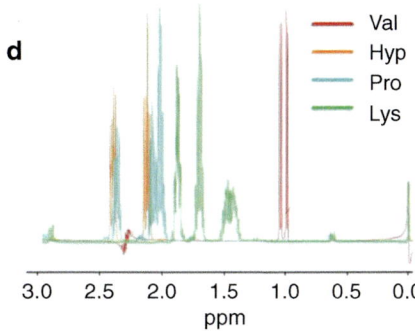

Fig. 30.2 ¹H spectroscopy of aqueous solution of collagen hydrolysate at 3 Tesla. (**a**) A pulse-acquire spectrum of collagen hydrolysate with H₂O as the solvent within a small glass sphere of 4-cm diameter used to obtain a homogeneous static field distribution after shimming. (**b**) A pulse-acquire spectrum of the collagen hydrolysate using D₂O as the solvent (in the glass sphere). The red arrows indicate vanishing signals due to exchanging ¹H/D atoms. (**c**) The signal pattern in the range from 0.0 to 3.0 ppm as indicated in panels (**a**) and (**b**), which show three main signal contributions. (**d**) The signal pattern of amino acids in high-field NMR spectra (600 MHz) of aqueous solutions is shown for comparison. The broad signals of the collagen hydrolysate correspond to common amino acids. (**e**) Nonlocalized stimulated echo acquisition mode (STEAM) spectra of collagen hydrolysate (10% in aqueous solution). These show signal decay from TE = 10 ms to TE = 30 ms

spectrum of a 10% aqueous solution of collagen placed in a glass sphere. With this arrangement, after shimming, a highly homogeneous B_0 field is achieved in the area of the solution. The (non-volume-localized) spectrum shows several frequency ranges with signals from the ¹H nuclei in the polypeptide chains of the collagen hydrolysate. The signal at 3.9 ppm (parts per million) is typical for the amino acid glycine, which is highly abundant in collagen. If the solvent H₂O is replaced by 99% deuterated water (D₂O), a reduction in the ¹H spectrum signal is seen in the two frequency ranges (Fig. 30.2b). The reduced intensities probably result from replacement of amide protons in peptides by the D (or ²H) nuclei through exchange with deuterated water. A closer examination of the spectral range between 0.0 and 3.0 ppm essentially shows three broad frequency ranges with signal contributions from the collagen hydrolysate (Fig. 30.2c). The ranges agree quite well with some signals from amino acids. The spectra of amino acids recorded at 600 MHz (14 Tesla) are shown in Fig. 30.2d for comparison. The decay of the signals in the range between 0.0 and 3.0 ppm due to

transverse relaxation was determined by means of a nonlocalized spin echo sequence with TEs = 10 ms, 20 ms, and 30 ms (Fig. 30.2e). Due to the superposition of several signal components and J-coupling effects, the mono-exponential behavior of the signal decay is not to be expected. It is obvious that the signals of collagen hydrolysate in an aqueous solution are easily detectable even with somewhat longer TEs > 10 ms.

Collagen-Related Signals in Tissues Without Long-T₂ Signal Components

Some tissues of the musculoskeletal system show almost no signal in MRI examinations with standard clinical sequences. These tissues include tendons, fibrocartilage (in the menisci), and compact bone. However, it is known that the ¹H nuclei are present in protein structures (especially with high concentrations of collagen) and in the numerous water molecules in healthy tendons and menisci (a water content of approximately 60% by weight is often quoted for these tissues). However, the signals of these water molecules have cross-relaxation times that are too short to be easily detectable with standard sequences. Only in the case of pathological changes in tendon areas (e.g., in achillodynia) or degenerative changes or tears in menisci are clear signals detectable when standard clinical sequences are used. These are visible in clinical MR images as high-signal areas. They are caused by the penetration of more mobile water molecules into the abnormal areas.

Healthy tendon tissue with its high degree of organization can, under certain circumstances, also show signals in measurements with standard sequences and longer TEs. This is the case if the fibers are positioned in relation to the magnetic field in such a way that the dipolar effects are balanced [8]. This is called the magic angle effect and can simulate pathologies [9].

While the aforementioned tissue classes only produce visible signals in the case of pathological changes, this is different in the case of articular cartilage due to the higher mobility of its water molecules; clear ^1H signals of hyaline articular cartilage can be seen with common clinical MR sequences and experimental sequences with longer TEs [10, 11]. The articular cartilage does have fibrous structures (collagen and proteoglycans) in the extracellular substance. However, these structures hardly affect the mobility of the predominant number of water molecules (water content 60–80%).

This chapter on collagen does not discuss in detail the different tissue types that produce clear signals only with ultrashort echo time (UTE) imaging—these tissue classes are covered in detail in separate chapters in this book. Some general comments on the effects of collagen on ^1H signal characteristics of these tissues will nevertheless be made:

Tendons: As already noted, the transverse relaxation times of healthy tendons are relatively short [12], and a significant detected signal can only be achieved using extremely short TEs with clinical MR scanners as demonstrated in Fig. 30.3. It may be assumed that the water molecules in the spaces between the collagen fiber bundles, but also some water in the sparse cells and blood vessels in tendons, are essentially responsible for the signals [13]. With increasing severity of degenerative changes, more mobile water penetrates the space between the collagen fiber bundles whose integrity has been disturbed, causing an increase in the water content and relatively long-T_2 values [14]. In later stages of the disease, the tendon ruptures (tears) with penetration by inflammatory and repair cells and replacement tissue can also be observed. In the case of pathological changes, but also after exercise, the interactions between the fibers and the MR-visible water result in measurable changes [15].

Fibrocartilage: The situation in fibrocartilage is similar to that in tendon, although there is no continuous unidirectional arrangement of collagen fibers but a multilayered, three-dimensional network. As with tendons, in fibrocartilage (e.g., menisci), signals from water with longer T_2s are increasingly observed in degenerative disease [17].

Bone: Compact bone has a rather complex structure with hard mineral components, collagen fibers, cellular components, and blood vessels. This gives rise to several water compartments, but these have short transverse relaxation times. Therefore, healthy compact bone appears practically signal free on the images using standard clinical sequences. With UTE sequences, distinct signals (probably almost exclusively from water molecules) can be detected, especially when signal components from the surrounding tissues are suppressed (see Fig. 30.4). It remains difficult to assess which compartments and to what extent different compartments (water-filled small "pores" in compact bone or water molecules associated with collagen) contribute to the signal in UTE studies [18–20]. Suitable MR methods are still being developed for this purpose.

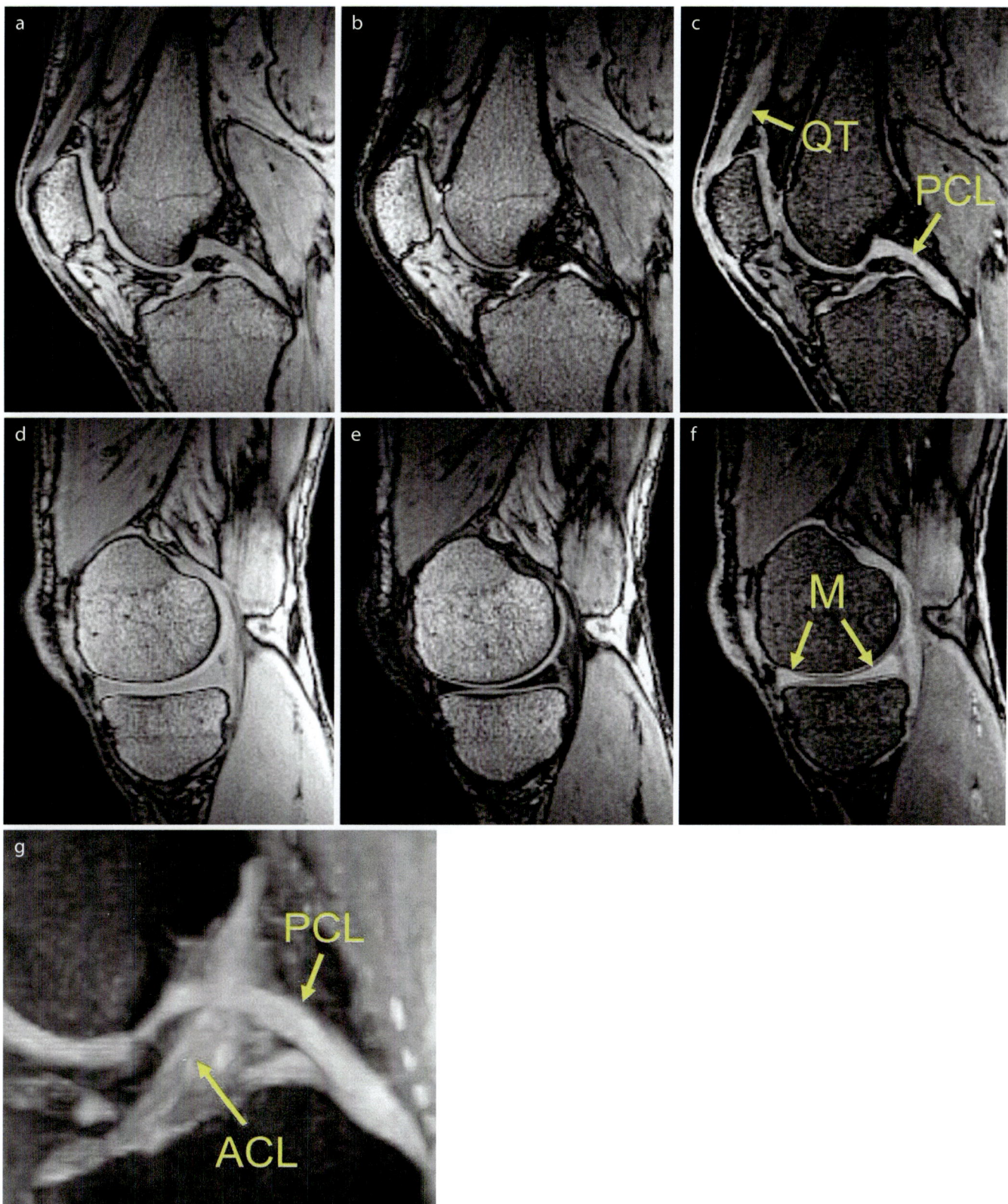

Fig. 30.3 Three-dimensional (3D) imaging of the knee joint of a healthy volunteer using a sub-DESS (double echo steady-state) sequence (sequence parameters: flip angle (FA) = 8°, repetition time (TR) = 6.14 ms, bandwidth (BW) = 575 Hz/pixel) at 3 T. The effective TE of the first echo (**a, d**) corresponds to TE = 1.2 ms, whereas the second echo (**b, e**) is clearly more T_2-weighted. (**c, f**) Subtraction images (first echo minus second echo) revealing tissues with short T_2s such as the quadriceps tendon (QT), anterior and posterior cruciate ligaments (ACL and PCL, respectively), and menisci (M) with positive contrast. (**g**) A maximum intensity projection (MIP) image of both cruciate ligaments. (Reproduced with permission from Martirosian et al. [16])

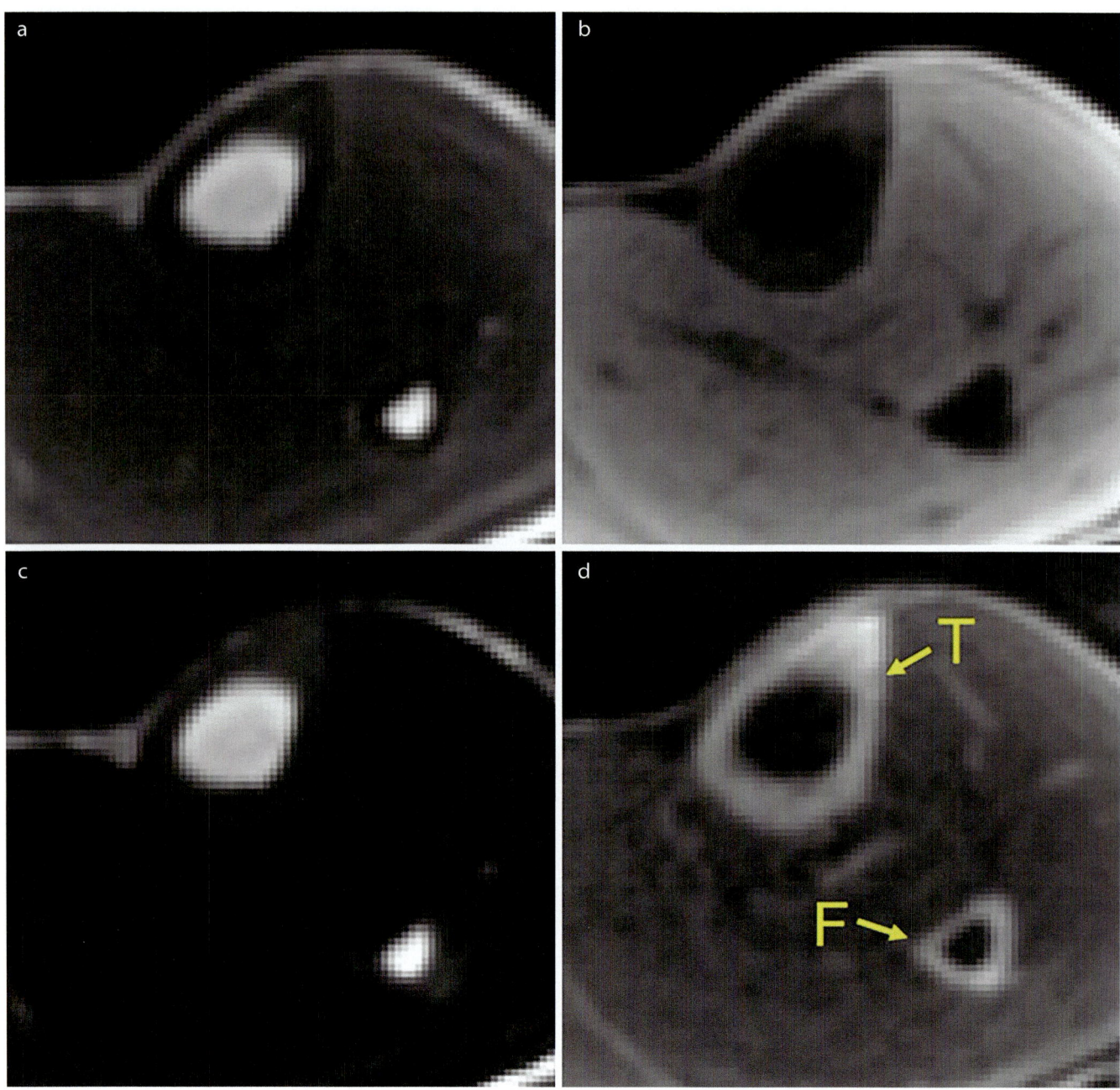

Fig. 30.4 Magnetization-prepared UTE imaging of cortical bone at 3 T. Images show a cross-sectional image of the lower leg of a healthy volunteer, including the tibia (T) and fibula (F). A radial 3D UTE sequence with a rectangular excitation pulse was applied (FA = 40°, TR = 34 ms, BW = 2370 Hz/pixel). (**a**) A UTE sequence without preparation of magnetization. (**b**) A UTE sequence with spectral fat saturation. (**c**) A UTE sequence with "long-T_2" signal suppression. (**d**) A UTE sequence with fat suppression and "long-T_2" signal suppression. This provides improved visualization of the cortical bone

MR Studies in Collagen in the Parenchymal Tissue and Organ Fibrosis

Collagen provides cohesion of cells and is contained in many organs as connective and supporting tissues, which take up mechanical loads and maintain the integrity of the organs. In muscles, the proportion of collagen is quite high, especially during the transition from muscle to tendon, as strong forces have to be transmitted through the tissues. However, other organs that are not subjected to particular mechanical stresses, such as the lungs or the liver, also contain collagen. The amount of connective tissue in parenchymatous organs is normally regulated to suit mechanical requirements. If the amount of connective tissue exceeds the necessary level, then this often results in a reduction of organ function and a harder organ consistency with reduced mobility and is described as organ fibrosis. The collagen fiber content of most organs naturally increases with age. Collagen fibers are also laid down when functioning organ cells die. In many diseases, cell damage (e.g., inflammatory processes and ischemia) leads to activation of fibroblasts, which often produce extremely large quantities of collagen fibers resulting in severe organ fibrosis.

Although acute inflammation (due to increased blood flow and prolongation of T_2) and ischemic conditions (due to reduced blood perfusion and, in stroke, changes in diffusion properties) can usually be successfully investigated with standard clinical MRI, determining the degree of fibrosis is more difficult. The most commonly used method to detect organ fibrosis is through the measurement of the mechanical properties (elastic modulus) by special ultrasound methods [21] or by MR elastography [22]. With these methods, advanced fibrosis can be detected, at least in some organs or systems such as the liver and musculature. Unfortunately, the elasticity and mechanical consistency of an organ only change significantly when microscopically extended and cross-linked fibrous networks are present. Often, at this stage, the fibrosis is advanced and is no longer reversible.

Due to the fact that parenchymal tissues always produce distinct ^{1}H signals from both cells and interstitium, selective determination of signals attributable to collagen fiber structures is difficult. As mentioned, organized collagen molecules hardly produce detectable ^{1}H signals with whole-body MRI systems, but water molecules associated with collagen with short T_2*s can be measurable. For this determination, the decrease in signal amplitude in UTE sequences with multiple echoes is usually determined and signal components with extremely short T_2*s are assigned to collagen water (i.e., water at least partially bound to collagen) [23].

Other approaches to determining tissue fibrosis are even more indirect: One can work with magnetization transfer pre-pulses and thus determine the interaction of mobile water molecules with macromolecules (direct proton exchange or exchange between the hydrated shell and the free state of the water molecules) [24]. Another approach is to measure the so-called $T_{1\rho}$ relaxation time [25], which also depends on the exchange of water molecules or the ^{1}H nuclei between different pools. In some organs, such as liver (and to some extent myocardium), the proton T_1 is longer in the interstitium (extracellular space) than in the intracellular space and the volume fraction of the extracellular space (ECS) can be estimated using the measured T_1 [26]. If the T_1 values are highly similar, then the use of an interstitial contrast agent offers a way of assessing the ECS [27]. Often, this approach equates the ECS with fiber content (since col-

lagen fibers are found in the extracellular space), but this may not always be the case.

In the following section, some UTE studies used to determine the fiber/fibrosis content in clinically interesting parenchymal tissues are briefly described:

The Skeletal Muscles

Multi-spin echo measurements using Carr–Purcell–Meiboom–Gill (CPMG) methods have shown that the water signal from skeletal muscle has several components that do not exchange rapidly, leading to multi-exponential signal decay [28, 29]. An interesting study on the determination of connective tissue components in healthy skeletal muscle using UTE sequences with multiple TEs was published in 2017 [30]. By fitting the signal dependence of TE (0.2–26.5 ms), the proportion of connective tissue could be estimated pixel by pixel. In the signal model used, two different water components (with short and long T_2*s) as well as the fat signal resonances of the triglyceride structure were characterized.

The Myocardium

Various quantitative methods have been used to examine the myocardium. Myocardial fibrosis is usually derived from an increase in the ECS (indirectly via T_1 determination with and without contrast media) [31]. However, there have also been experiments suggesting that myocardial fibrosis can be detected by determining fast transverse relaxing water components with UTE methods [32]. Studies with UTE in mice with myocardial infarction (replacement fibrosis) and diffuse fibrosis have shown corresponding results [33]. In 2011, it was demonstrated in patients that the replacement fibrous tissue in areas of myocardial infarction has a rapidly relaxing component [34]. This and other cardiac studies using UTE sequences for the diagnosis of fibrosis have been discussed in a recent review [35].

The Liver

The diagnosis of chronic nonalcoholic steatohepatitis (NASH) is another application of MRI. NASH is a chronic liver inflammatory disease that develops quite frequently in the presence of fatty liver and can lead to liver fibrosis/cirrhosis and hepatocellular carcinoma. Diagnosis of NASH is currently the subject of much scientific debate. Ultrasound and MRI are being further developed to be able to examine the condition of the liver in NASH noninvasively and thus avoid liver biopsy. While studies of the liver using the methods already mentioned (ultrasound elastography [21], MR elastography [22], T_1 determination for estimation of the ECS [26], mapping of $T_{1\rho}$ [25], magnetization transfer [24]) to determine the degree of fibrosis of the liver have been performed, few studies have been conducted on short-T_2 components in the liver. In 2003, healthy and diseased livers were examined in a study using UTE sequences [36]. It was shown that both the iron content and the degree of fibrosis influenced the signal behavior at short TEs. A more recent study from 2019 has integrated the fast-relaxing water signals into the signal model using the iterative decomposition of water and fat with echo asymmetry and the least squares estimation (IDEAL) method in order to characterize the short-T_2^* components associated with fibrosis, in addition to slow-relaxing water and fat components [37].

The Lungs

For MRI of the lungs, UTE sequences are often used because hardly any signal can be detected with standard sequences in healthy lung parenchyma. However, the reason for this is not that lung tissue consists only of tissue components (e.g., connective tissue) with extremely short T_2s but lies within the special microscopic structure of the lung. At higher magnetic field strengths, the many boundaries between air and tissue components (with their different magnetic susceptibilities) result in an extremely inhomogeneous microscopic magnetic field in the lung. This leads to rapid signal dephasing with not only gradient echo sequences but also with spin echo sequences, since diffusion of the water molecules in the magnetically inhomogeneous environment prevents rephasing.

Proliferation of the connective tissue (fibrosis) is frequently observed in lung disease. However, since both normal microscopic tissue structure and collagen fiber proliferation result in signal components with rapid signal decays, differentiation of these two tissues is difficult.

A number of studies have been conducted using UTE sequences for lung imaging, and these are addressed in more detail in Chapter 42 ("Lung Imaging with UTE MRI") of this book. A review of this topic is also provided in Torres et al. [38]. An interesting work on pulmonary fibrosis imaging was published in 2013 [39]: Bleomycin administration in mice caused an easily detectable histological increase in fiber content that correlated well with signal enhancement on UTE images. UTE applications in patients with cystic fibrosis (who show other changes besides fibrosis, such as hyperinflation and accumulation of secretions in the lungs) led to interesting results [40], which, however, must be interpreted extremely cautiously with regard to the increase in collagen fibers.

Challenges and New Methodological Approaches

In most cases, it is assumed that collagen in the extracellular space of tissues is largely present in an organized fibrous structure (collagen molecules with cross-links) and that the signals of the amino acid chains cannot be directly detected with whole-body MR tomography. Spectroscopic examinations of intact tissues with FID sequences do not show clear signals from collagen in the typical chemical shift regions, unlike the situation with MR examinations of relatively short amino acid chains of hydrolyzed collagen (collagen powder or gelatine) dissolved in water.

Whether or not there are pathological conditions (e.g., degenerate tendons, ligaments, or menisci with fraying of the collagen bundles), in which signals from collagen molecules become directly detectable at short TEs through increased mobility of some protein chains, is, in the author's opinion, not yet clear. The same applies to acute and chronic inflammatory stages of parenchymal organs such as the liver, musculature, and kidneys. It is clear that in the course of inflammation, fibroblasts in these organs can produce increased extracellular collagen. Furthermore, it is obvious that during the process of fibrosis, there must also be un-cross-linked precursors of collagen within cells and in the interstitium. Possibly, however, their proportion is so small that the signals are too low compared to the other signals and are therefore lost in the noise. In any case, metabolomic studies on fibroblasts show interesting differences between different fibroblast types, but only weak signals can be assigned to amino acids in procollagen [41].

The basis of in vivo investigations of collagen in tissues is the determination of the signal properties of the water in the vicinity of the collagen bundles. It has long been common practice in the clinic to detect degenerative changes in tendons or menisci by recording water signals, which are clearly visible even at longer TEs [17]. This is mainly attributed to mobile water that has penetrated the damaged fibrous structure. Only with extremely short TEs (<2 ms) can clear water signals also be recorded from healthy tendons, ligaments, and menisci [12]. The extremely short transverse relaxation times of the water molecules forming the hydration shell around collagen molecules in the solid collagen matrix can be explained by their limited mobility—in contrast to the more mobile water molecules in degenerate tissues.

It is clear that the signal strength and MR properties of water in different tissues with collagen fiber structures (i.e., bones, tendons, ligaments, cartilage, but also the extracellular space in healthy and especially fibrosed tissues) are influenced by the presence of collagen and partly by other macromolecules (e.g., glucosaminoglycans in cartilage). However, the indirect detection of collagen behavior through quantitative analysis of signals from water associated with the collagen is not easy. Whether, and to what extent, the effects are visible depends on the microscopic structure and also on the exchange of magnetization between collagen and water molecules as well as between different water compartments (H_2O in hydrate shells versus free water). In water-containing parenchymal tissues, the influence of collagen on the measured overall signal is small and often mainly limited to a (relatively small) water compartment with a short transverse relaxation time, which plays a marginal role in observation with standard MR images. Here, the determination of the signal decay at extremely short TEs, which can be performed with UTE sequences, can make the effects associated with collagen visible. However, it must be taken into account that in many tissue types (e.g., in the musculature through the contractile elements), there are also other macromolecules that can interact with water molecules.

As described earlier, many properties of water signals such as relaxation times T_1, $T_{1\rho}$, T_2, and T_2^* and the response to off-resonant radiofrequency (RF) excitation have already been investigated to characterize tissues containing collagen. However, there is also evidence that the resonance frequency of water signals depends on the geometric distribution of water in tissues with different magnetic susceptibilities [8]. These effects and their variation with TE are difficult to detect with the usual amplitude-only signals of UTE sequences.

The common methods for studying signals from tissues with short T_2s (i.e., both the signals of water present in the immediate surroundings of collagen and the signals of mobile peptide chains of collagen or its degradation products) are as follows:

1. Spectroscopic investigations with extremely short intervals between RF excitation and signal recording using pulse-acquire sequences (which are sometimes called FID = "free induction decay" sequences): This method is mostly used in vitro to examine aqueous solutions with collagen components. Its advantage is the option for spectral analysis of the signals. Its disadvantage is the lack of (or highly coarse) spatial selectivity and resolution so that targeted investigations of tissues in vivo are hardly possible.

2. Imaging with UTE sequences (with or without preparation of the magnetization): Imaging methods have been highly successful in imaging tissues such as bone, tendon, ligament, and menisci with high spatial resolution. However, since usually only signal amplitudes are determined as a function of TE, signal components with differing Larmor frequencies can often hardly be differentiated. In case of deviations from a mono-exponential signal decay with increasing TE, the presence of several water compartments is often assumed.

The first step toward phase-sensitive UTE imaging was made with the special UTE multi-echo sequences for quantitative susceptibility mapping (QSM) [42, 43]. This technique can be used to study the frequency shift of a single water component in tissues whose susceptibility is significantly different from that of water.

Recently, a three-dimensional (3D) multi-echo UTE sequence has been presented, in which signals detected with the UTE sequence were decomposed into their spectral components [44]. However, a relatively long measurement time has to be accepted with this technique, since TEs must be closely spaced in the time domain to enable Fourier transformation for spectral analysis. Furthermore, a rather arduous correction of the signal phases is necessary, since the intensive gradient switching in the UTE sequence with the recording of "stacked spirals" causes heating of the MR system and a distinct B_0 field drift during the measurement. Ultimately, however, this sequence allows both the recording of signals with the spatial resolution and sensitivity known from UTE imaging as well as spectral decomposition of the signal components of each picture element. This means that the signal components of mobile collagen peptides that are off-resonance, and possibly shifted water signal components, can be determined pixel by pixel (see Fig. 30.5).

Collagen-specific contrast agents represent another interesting recent development. Specific antibodies can be used to produce MR-visible contrast agents (e.g., by coupling the antibodies to iron oxide particles) that accumulate in the region of collagen [45]. This seems particularly interesting for detecting early (and still reversible) stages of fibrosis in inflamed tissues. The investigation of collagen or fibrosis in tissues is clinically of great importance and continues to offer interesting challenges in method development.

Fig. 30.5 Spectral UTE imaging with the UTE-FID sequence [44]. (**a**) Multi-echo UTE-FID imaging with echo shifting in successive scans in order to acquire signals from narrowly spaced points in the time domain. A dwell time of about 1 ms provides 1-kHz spectral width, which is suitable for ^1H signals. Phase correction of signals from the different scans is necessary to compensate for frequency shifts (due to B_0 field drift) during the measurement. In this scheme, 36 time points were recorded. Further points in the time domain can be extrapolated. This technique allows pixel-by-pixel reconstruction of the FID. (**b**) Imaging of a phantom with a central tube (diameter 2.5 cm) filled with 50% collagen hydrolysate in pure distilled water. (**c**) A true FID spectrum from a nonlocalized pulse-acquire sequence recorded from a sphere filled with aqueous collagen hydrolysate. (**d**) A spectrum derived from the reconstructed FID recorded by the UTE-FID sequence in a region of pure water (region of interest (ROI) 2 in panel **b**). (**e**) A spectrum derived from the FID recorded by the UTE-FID sequence in a region in the tube containing collagen hydrolysate (ROI 1 in panel **b**). The spectrum shows a highly similar pattern of signals from the ^1H nuclei of collagen as the true FID spectrum

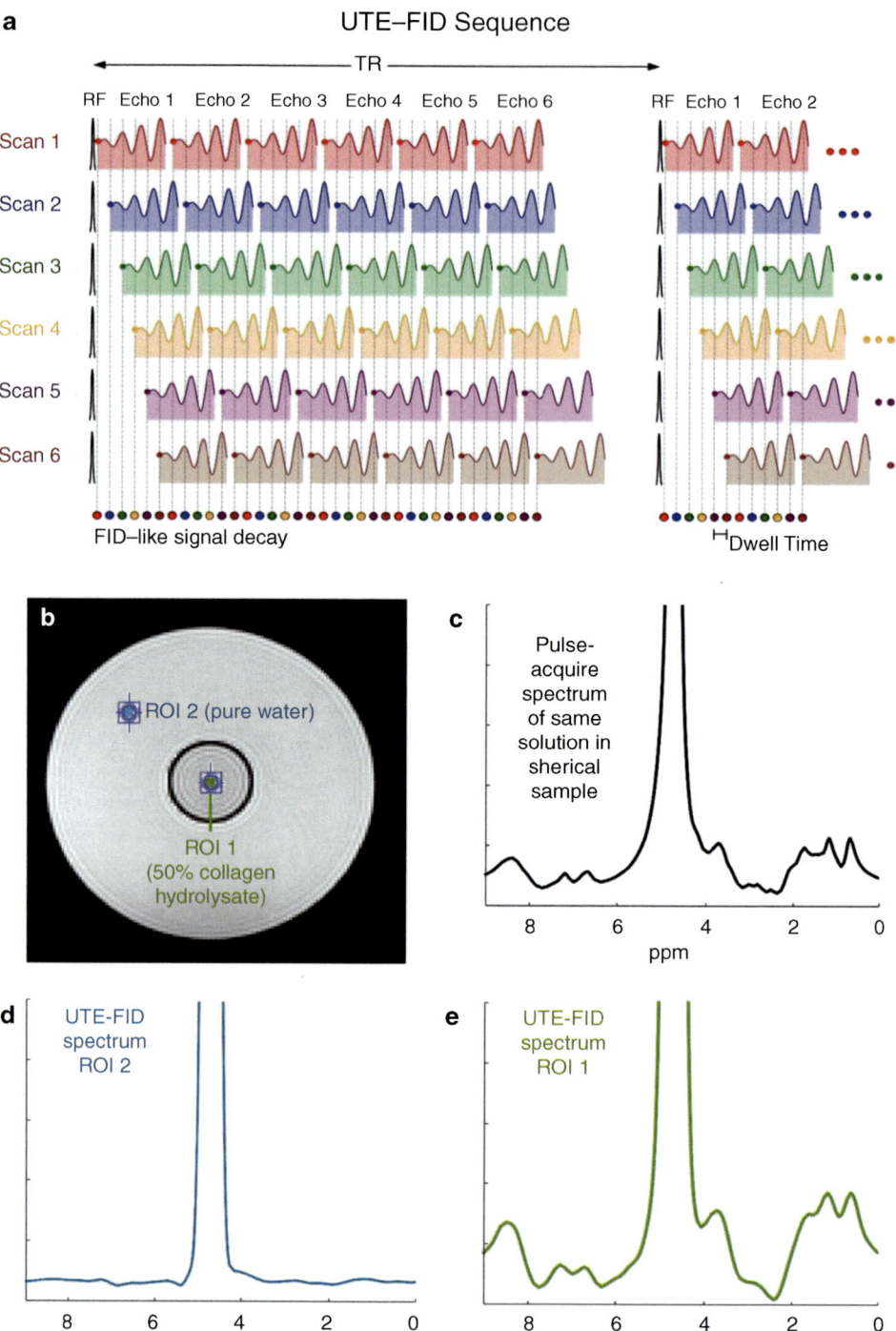

Acknowledgments The content of this chapter and the illustrations were supported by my working group, in particular Tobias Winkler, Tobias Lober, and Anja Fischer.

References

1. Onursal C, Dick E, Angelidis I, Schiller HB, Staab-Weijnitbz CA. Collagen biosynthesis, processing, and maturation in lung ageing. Front Med (Lausanne). 2021;8:593874.

2. Shoulders MD, Raines RT. Collagen structure and stability. Annu Rev Biochem. 2009;78(1):929–58.

3. Ma YJ, Chang EY, Bydder GM, Du J. Can ultrashort-TE (UTE) MRI sequences on a 3-T clinical scanner detect signal directly from collagen protons: freeze-dry and D_2O exchange studies of cortical bone and achilles tendon specimens. NMR Biomed. 2016;29(7):912–7.

4. Goldberga I, Li R, Duer MJ. Collagen structure-function relationships from solid-state NMR spectroscopy. Acc Chem Res. 2018;51(7):1621–9.

5. Singh C, Rai RK, Kayastha AM, Sinha N. Ultra fast magic angle spinning solid—state NMR spectroscopy of intact bone. Magn Reson Chem. 2016;54(2):132–5.

6. Riemer T, Nimptsch A, Nimptsch K, Schiller J. Determination of the glycosaminoglycan and collagen contents in tissue samples by high-resolution $_1H$ NMR spectroscopy after DCl-induced hydrolysis. Biomacromolecules. 2012;13(7):2110–7.

7. López-Morales CA, Vázquez-Leyva S, Vallejo-Castillo L, Carballo-Uicab G, Muñoz-García L, Herbert-Pucheta JE, et al. Determination of peptide profile consistency and safety of collagen hydrolysates as quality attributes. J Food Sci. 2019;84(3):430–9.

8. Krasnosselskaia LV, Fullerton GD, Dodd SJ, Cameron IL. Water in tendon: orientational analysis of the free induction decay. Magn Reson Med. 2005;54(2):280–8.

9. Erickson SJ, Cox IH, Hyde JS, Carrera GF, Strandt JA, Estkowski LD. Effect of tendon orientation on MR imaging signal intensity: a manifestation of the "magic angle" phenomenon. Radiology. 1991;181(2):389–92.

10. Gründer W. MRI assessment of cartilage ultrastructure. NMR Biomed. 2006;19(7):855–76.

11. Chalian M, Li X, Guermazi A, Obuchowski NA, Carrino JA, Oei EH, et al. The QIBA profile for MRI-based compositional imaging of knee cartilage. Radiology. 2021;301(2):423–32.

12. Krämer M, Maggioni MB, Brisson NM, Zachow S, Teichgräber U, Duda GN, et al. T_1 and T_2^* mapping of the human quadriceps and patellar tendons using ultra-short echo-time (UTE) imaging and bivariate relaxation parameter-based volumetric visualization. Magn Reson Imaging. 2019;63:29–36.

13. Du J, Diaz E, Carl M, Bae W, Chung CB, Bydder GM. Ultrashort echo time imaging with bicomponent analysis. Magn Reson Med. 2012;67(3):645–9.

14. Schick F, Dammann F, Lutz O, Claussen CD. Adapted techniques for clinical MR imaging of tendons. MAGMA. 1995;3(2):103–7.

15. Syha R, Springer F, Grözinger G, Würslin C, Ipach I, Ketelsen D, et al. Short-term exercise-induced changes in hydration state of healthy Achilles tendons can be visualized by effects of off-resonant radiofrequency saturation in a three-dimensional ultrashort echo time MRI sequence applied at 3 tesla. J Magn Reson Imaging. 2014;40(6):1400–7.

16. Martirosian P, Schraml C, Springer F, Schwenzer NF, Würslin C, Schick F, et al. Positive contrast MR imaging of tendons, ligaments, and menisci by subtraction of signals from a double echo steady state sequence (sub-DESS). Magn Reson Med. 2014;71(1):294–301.

17. Nebelung S, Tingart M, Pufe T, Kuhl C, Jahr H, Truhn D. Ex vivo quantitative multiparametric MRI mapping of human meniscus degeneration. Skelet Radiol. 2016;45(12):1649–60.

18. Biswas R, Bae W, Diaz E, Masuda K, Chung CB, Bydder GM, et al. Ultrashort echo time (UTE) imaging with bi-component analysis: bound and free water evaluation of bovine cortical bone subject to sequential drying. Bone. 2012;50(3):749–55.

19. Jerban S, Ma Y, Wan L, Searleman AC, Jang H, Sah RL, et al. Collagen proton fraction from ultrashort echo time magnetization transfer (UTE-MT) MRI modelling correlates significantly with cortical bone porosity measured with micro-computed tomography (μCT). NMR Biomed. 2019;32(2):e4045.

20. Jerban S, Ma Y, Namiranian B, Ashir A, Shirazian H, Wei Z, et al. Age-related decrease in collagen proton fraction in tibial tendons estimated by magnetization transfer modeling of ultrashort echo time magnetic resonance imaging (UTE-MRI). Sci Rep. 2019;9(1):17974.

21. Ozturk A, Grajo JR, Dhyani M, Anthony BW, Samir AE. Principles of ultrasound elastography. Abdom Radiol (NY). 2018;43(4):773–85.

22. Manduca A, Bayly PJ, Ehman RL, Kolipaka A, Royston TJ, Sack I, et al. MR elastography: principles, guidelines, and terminology. Magn Reson Med. 2021;85(5):2377–90.

23. Gatehouse PD, Bydder GM. Magnetic resonance imaging of short T_2 components in tissue. Clin Radiol. 2003;58(1):1–19.

24. Yarnykh VL, Tartaglione EV, Ioannou GN. Fast macromolecular proton fraction mapping of the human liver in vivo for quantitative assessment of hepatic fibrosis. NMR Biomed. 2015;28(12):1716–25.

25. Singh A, Reddy D, Haris M, Cai K, Rajender Reddy K, Hariharan H, et al. $T_{1\rho}$ MRI of healthy and fibrotic human livers at 1.5 T. J Transl Med. 2015;13:292.

26. Pavlides M, Banerjee R, Tunnicliffe EM, Kelly C, Collier J, Wang LM, et al. Multiparametric magnetic resonance imaging for the assessment of non-alcoholic fatty liver disease severity. Liver Int. 2017;37(7):1065–73.

27. Barison A, Grigoratos C, Todiere G, Aquaro GD. Myocardial interstitial remodelling in non-ischaemic dilated cardiomyopathy: insights from cardiovascular magnetic resonance. Heart Fail Rev. 2015;20(6):731–49.

28. Saab G, Thompson RT, Marsh GD. Multicomponent T_2 relaxation of in vivo skeletal muscle. Magn Reson Med. 1999;42(1):150–7.

29. Sharafi A, Chang G, Regatte RR. Bi-component $T_{1\rho}$ and T_2 relaxation mapping of skeletal muscle in-vivo. Sci Rep. 2017;7(1):14115.

30. Araujo ECA, Azzabou N, Vignaud A, Guillot G, Carlier PG. Quantitative ultrashort TE imaging of the short-T_2 components in skeletal muscle using an extended echo-subtraction method. Magn Reson Med. 2017;78(3):997–1008.

31. Everett RJ, Stirrat CG, Semple SI, Newby DE, Dweck MR, Mirsadraee S. Assessment of myocardial fibrosis with T_1 mapping MRI. Clin Radiol. 2016;71(8):768–78.

32. Schuijf JD, Ambale-Venkatesh B, Kassai Y, Kato Y, Kasuboski L, Ota H, et al. Cardiovascular ultrashort echo time to map fibrosis-promises and challenges. Br J Radiol. 2019;92(1103):20190465.

33. van Nierop BJ, Bax NA, Nelissen JL, Arslan F, Motaal AG, de Graaf L, et al. Assessment of myocardial fibrosis in mice using a T_2^*-weighted 3D radial magnetic resonance imaging sequence. PLoS One. 2015;10(6):e0129899.

34. de Jong S, Zwanenburg JJ, Visser F, der Nagel R, van Rijen HV, Vos MA, et al. Direct detection of myocardial fibrosis by MRI. J Mol Cell Cardiol. 2011;51(6):974–9.

35. Karamitsos TD, Arvanitaki A, Karvounis H, Neubauer S, Ferreira VM. Myocardial tissue characterization and fibrosis by imaging. JACC Cardiovasc Imaging. 2020;13(5):1221–34.

36. Chappell KE, Patel N, Gatehouse PD, Main J, Puri BK, Taylor-Robinson SD, et al. Magnetic resonance imaging of the liver with

ultrashort TE (UTE) pulse sequences. J Magn Reson Imaging. 2003;18(6):709–13.

37. Zhu A, Hernando D, Johnson KM, Reeder SB. Characterizing a short T(2)* signal component in the liver using ultrashort TE chemical shift-encoded MRI at 1.5T and 3.0T. Magn Reson Med. 2019;82(6):2032–45.

38. Torres L, Kammerman J, Hahn AD, Zha W, Nagle SK, Johnson K, et al. Structure-function imaging of lung disease using ultrashort echo time MRI. Acad Radiol. 2019;26(3):431–41.

39. Egger C, Cannet C, Gérard C, Jarman E, Jarai G, Feige A, et al. Administration of bleomycin via the oropharyngeal aspiration route leads to sustained lung fibrosis in mice and rats as quantified by UTE-MRI and histology. PLoS One. 2013;8(5):e63432.

40. Heidenreich JF, Weng AM, Metz C, Benkert T, Pfeuffer J, Hebestreit H, et al. Three-dimensional ultrashort echo time MRI for functional lung imaging in cystic fibrosis. Radiology. 2020;296(1):191–9.

41. Ban HY, Shin JW, Chun SI, Kang YG, Wu Y, Kim JE, et al. Distinguishing tendon and ligament fibroblasts based on ¹H nuclear magnetic resonance spectroscopy. Tissue Eng Regen Med. 2016;13(6):677–83.

42. Jerban S, Lu X, Jang H, Ma Y, Namiranian B, Le N, et al. Significant correlations between human cortical bone mineral density and quantitative susceptibility mapping (QSM) obtained with 3D cones ultrashort echo time magnetic resonance imaging (UTE-MRI). Magn Reson Imaging. 2019;62:104–10.

43. Jang H, von Drygalski A, Wong J, Zhou JY, Aguero P, Lu X, et al. Ultrashort echo time quantitative susceptibility mapping (UTE-QSM) for detection of hemosiderin deposition in hemophilic arthropathy: a feasibility study. Magn Reson Med. 2020;84(6):3246–55.

44. Fischer A, Martirosian P, Benkert T, Schick F. Spatially resolved free-induction decay spectroscopy using a 3D ultra-short echo time multi-echo imaging sequence with systematic echo shifting and compensation of B(0) field drifts. Magn Reson Med. 2022;87(5):2099–110.

45. Salarian M, Turaga RC, Xue S, Nezafati M, Hekmatyar K, Qiao J, et al. Early detection and staging of chronic liver diseases with a protein MRI contrast agent. Nat Commun. 2019;10(1):4777.

Quantitative Ultrashort Echo Time Magnetic Resonance Imaging of the Knee in Osteoarthritis

Mei Wu, Yajun Ma, Saeed Jerban, Dina Moazamian, Eric Y. Chang, Christine B. Chung, Susan V. Bukata, and Jiang Du

Introduction

Knee osteoarthritis (OA) is one of the most prevalent diseases in the world. It affects more than 50 million Americans and costs the United States more than $60 billion annually [1]. About 25% of individuals affected by knee OA are unable to perform activities of daily living, leading to significant public health issues, which will become even more critical as society ages. It is generally believed that it is necessary to develop techniques that improve the detection of OA at an early stage to allow timely intervention, since OA therapy is likely to be more effective early in the disease rather than later after irreversible damage and/or loss of tissue have occurred.

Knee OA is a heterogeneous and multifactorial disease that is associated with progressive loss of articular cartilage [2]. The most important early biochemical and microscopic signs of OA include loss of proteoglycans (PGs) as well as

M. Wu · Y. Ma · S. Jerban · D. Moazamian
Department of Radiology, University of California, San Diego, La Jolla, CA, USA
e-mail: mew140@health.ucsd.edu; yam013@health.ucsd.edu; sjerban@health.ucsd.edu; dmoazamian@health.ucsd.edu

E. Y. Chang · C. B. Chung
Department of Radiology, University of California, San Diego, La Jolla, CA, USA

VA San Diego Healthcare System, San Diego, CA, USA
e-mail: e8chang@health.ucsd.edu; cbchung@health.ucsd.edu

S. V. Bukata
Department of Orthopaedics, University of California, San Diego, La Jolla, CA, USA
e-mail: sbukata@health.ucsd.edu

J. Du (✉)
Department of Radiology, University of California, San Diego, La Jolla, CA, USA

VA San Diego Healthcare System, San Diego, CA, USA

Department of Bioengineering, University of California, San Diego, La Jolla, CA, USA
e-mail: jiangdu@health.ucsd.edu

changes in collagen microstructure and water content [3]. Current diagnostic approaches include arthroscopy, radiography, and magnetic resonance imaging (MRI). Arthroscopy is an invasive method with limited value for detecting early OA. Plain film radiography may only provide indirect signs of knee cartilage thinning (e.g., joint space narrowing) and is severely limited in its ability to visualize cartilage [2]. Magnetic resonance imaging (MRI) provides excellent soft tissue contrast at high spatial resolution, allowing accurate assessment of morphological changes in articular cartilage in OA [4]. However, conventional clinical MRI sequences perform poorly in detecting the initial stages of knee OA. There are three significant barriers to progress in this area:

First, human knee joints are composed of different tissues that allow joints to function interactively over a long period [5–7]. Disease of cartilage is generally considered a primary initiator of OA. However, not all cartilage degeneration leads to OA. Recent understanding of OA development has moved away from a cartilage-centric focus to the concept of a "whole-joint organ disease" [5–7]. Thus, it is believed that when one tissue begins to deteriorate, it is likely to affect others and contribute to failure of the joint as a whole. Unfortunately, clinical magnetic resonance (MR) sequences can only evaluate joint tissues or tissue components, such as the more superficial layers of articular cartilage, which have relatively long-T_2 values. Many joint tissues, including the osteochondral junction (OCJ), menisci, ligaments, tendons, and bone, have short- or ultrashort-T_2s and show little or no signal with conventional clinical sequences [8–10]. Thus, the short- or ultrashort-T_2^*s of relevant tissues present a significant problem in detecting abnormalities in the early stages of OA.

Second, there are two distinct groups of protons in most joint tissues, namely, water and macromolecular protons [11, 12]. Macromolecular changes such as PG depletion and collagen degradation are involved in the extremely early stages of OA [4]. Developing techniques to evaluate these changes in different joint tissues is essential. Conventional MRI sequences have difficulty assessing distinct proton groups,

J. Du, G. M. Bydder (eds.), *MRI of Short- and Ultrashort-T₂ Tissues*, https://doi.org/10.1007/978-3-031-35197-6_31

especially within the short- and ultrashort-T_2 tissues in the knee joint.

Third, over the past two decades, extensive research in knee OA has focused on two particular biomarkers, $T_{1\rho}$ and T_2. Most $T_{1\rho}$ and T_2 measurements have been performed on articular cartilage, with $T_{1\rho}$ being sensitive to PG depletion and T_2 showing sensitivity to collagen degradation [13–16]. However, the magic angle effect is a major confounding factor in $T_{1\rho}$ and T_2 measurements [17]. The effect may result in a several-fold increase in $T_{1\rho}$ and T_2 when collagen fibers are reoriented from 0 to 54° relative to the B_0 field. This change often far exceeds that produced by the disease (typically ~10–30% [14]) and may make interpretation of elevated $T_{1\rho}$s and T_2s highly challenging. This is a particular problem when employing clinical $T_{1\rho}$ and T_2 measurements of articular cartilage to detect early OA. Comprehensive evaluation of knee OA requires systematic imaging of water and macromolecular components of all the principal joint tissues without confounding problems caused by the magic angle effect.

Ultrashort echo time (UTE) sequences with echo times (TEs) of less than 0.1 ms allow direct imaging of both short- and long-T_2 tissues of the joints [8–10]. Combining UTE with a series of preparation schemes can demonstrate alterations in joint structure and quantify the biochemical integrity of joint tissues. For example, conventional UTE acquisitions with a series of TEs allow T_2^* mapping of primary joint tissues such as articular cartilage, menisci, ligaments, and tendons [18, 19]. UTE bicomponent analysis quantifies T_2^* and the relative fractions of bound and free water components in both short- and long-T_2 tissues of the joints [12, 20, 21]. This information may considerably help evaluate changes in collagen microstructure and water content of joint tissues. In addition, the spin-lock prepared UTE sequence provides imaging and quantification of $T_{1\rho}$ in human joint tissues. This information may help evaluate PG changes in healthy and degenerate tissues, regardless of their T_2 values [22, 23]. UTE sequence can also be combined with paired adiabatic inversion pulses for UTE-based adiabatic $T_{1\rho}$ (UTE-AdiabT$_{1\rho}$) imaging [24, 25] to minimize confounding magic angle effects. UTE, in combination with magnetization transfer (UTE-MT) imaging, allows indirect assessment of macromolecular protons in all major joint tissues [26]. As a consequence, UTE-based sequences may depict microstructural changes and other early alterations in OA, which are not visible with conventional clinical MRI sequences. UTE imaging can also be used to track super-

paramagnetic iron oxide (SPIO) nanoparticle-labeled multipotent mesenchymal stem cells (MSCs) after they have been injected into joints containing osteochondral defects, thereby providing a method for monitoring stem cell distribution in OA [27].

UTE Versus Conventional Clinical MRI in the Knee Joint

Conventional clinical sequences provide high-resolution imaging of musculoskeletal tissues with relatively long-T_2 values, such as the more superficial layers of articular cartilage, which have T_2 values of up to about 40 ms. Synovial fluid and muscle have even longer T_2s and are well depicted with clinical MRI sequences. However, many joint tissues have relatively short-T_2s. These tissues or tissue components include the OCJ, the medial and lateral menisci, the anterior cruciate ligament, the posterior cruciate ligament, and the collateral ligament (ACL, PCL, and CL, respectively), the quadriceps and popliteus tendons, as well as cortical and subchondral bone [8–10]. Their T_2s range from sub-milliseconds to several (<10) ms, which are often too short to be usefully depicted with conventional clinical sequences. UTE sequences with nominal TEs of 0.1 ms or shorter can robustly detect signals from short-T_2 tissues using clinical whole-body scanners. Figure 31.1 shows such an example. A cadaveric human knee joint was imaged using conventional clinical two-dimensional (2D) fast spin echo (FSE), three-dimensional (3D) gradient echo (GRE), and 3D UTE sequences. The menisci, the PCL, and the patellar tendon all show a high signal with the 3D UTE sequence but little or no signal with clinical sequences.

Quantitative imaging of musculoskeletal tissues has been limited to long-T_2 tissues or tissue components such as the more superficial layers of articular cartilage, muscles, and synovium. This also limits quantification since it usually requires direct detection of MR signals from the targeted tissue. However, with the introduction of UTE imaging, useful MR signals can be obtained from both long- and short-T_2 tissues. As a result, it is possible to quantitatively evaluate all the principal tissues of the knee joint, including their MR relaxation times such as T_1, T_2, T_2^*, and $T_{1\rho}$, as well as other tissue properties, including water content, macromolecular fraction, diffusion, perfusion, and susceptibility using UTE or UTE-type sequences.

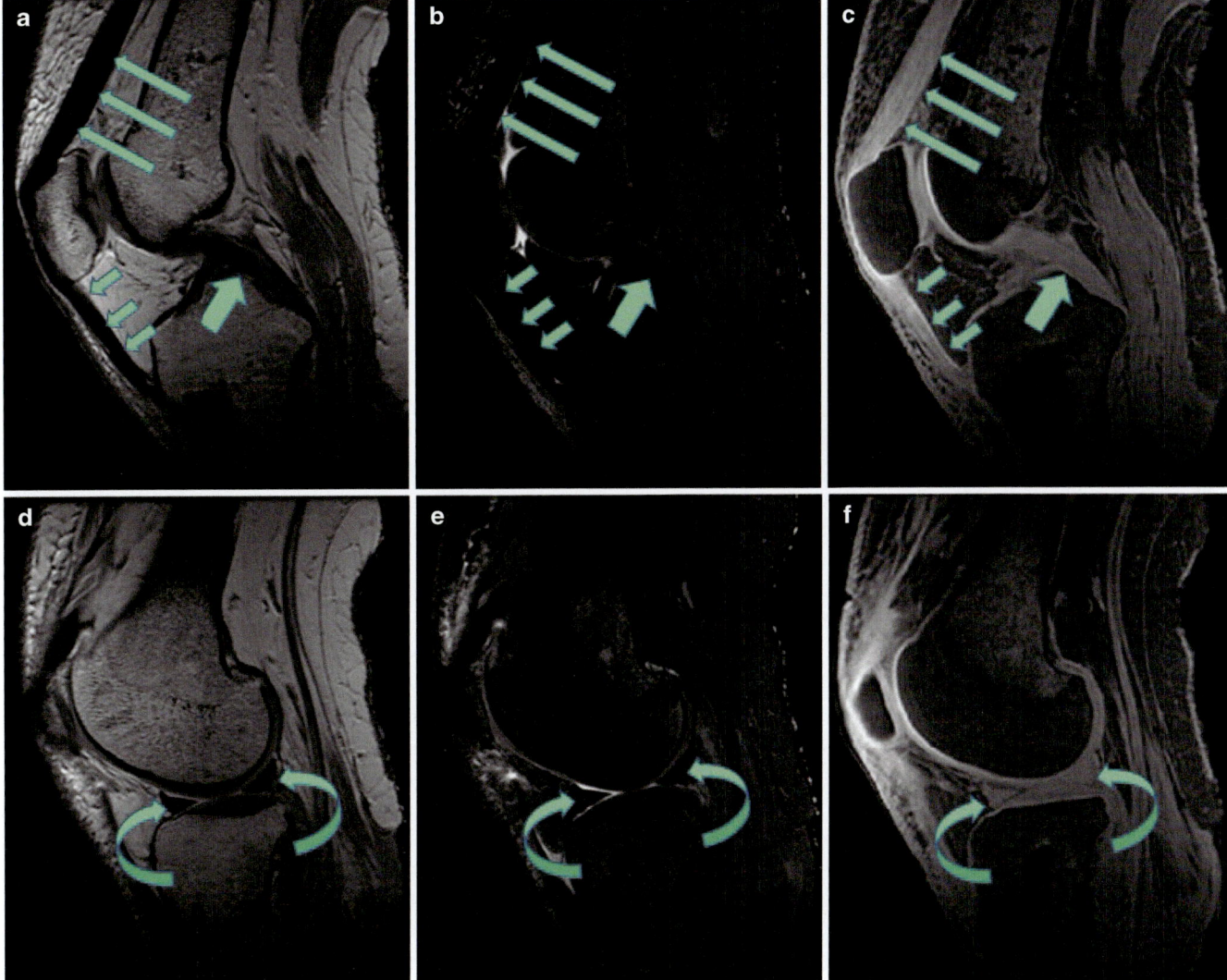

Fig. 31.1 Sagittal imaging of the PCL (thick arrows), the patellar tendon (short thin arrows), and the quadriceps tendon (long thin arrows) in a cadaveric human knee joint imaged with conventional clinical 2D proton density (PD)-FSE (**a**), fat-saturated 2D T_2-FSE (**b**), and fat-saturated 3D UTE (**c**) sequences. The menisci (curved arrows) in the same knee joint are imaged with 2D PD-FSE (**d**), fat-saturated 2D T_2-FSE (**e**), and fat-saturated 3D UTE (**f**) sequences. The PCL, patellar tendon, quadriceps tendon, and menisci all show low signal with the clinical sequences but high signal with the UTE sequences

Quantitative UTE Imaging of the Knee Joint: Ex Vivo Evaluation

Ex Vivo UTE-Based T_2^* (UTE-T_2^*) Imaging

Conventional clinical MRI sequences are routinely used to diagnose articular cartilage degeneration. However, these sequences have limited sensitivity to early degenerative changes such as subtle cartilage matrix alterations. UTE-T_2^* mapping is a novel imaging technology that may potentially detect cartilaginous changes during the early stages of degeneration within a tissue that appears normal on visual inspection. Williams et al. examined the sensitivity of UTE-

T_2^* mapping to collagen matrix degeneration in human articular cartilage using polarized light microscopy (PLM) as the reference standard [18]. PLM uses the optical properties of articular cartilage to reveal information about its composition and structure. Birefringence is used to assess the optical properties of anisotropically oriented macromolecules, which alter the plane of polarized light. Loss of birefringence is seen in collagenase-induced matrix disruption [28]. In Williams's study, 33 osteochondral cores were harvested from human tibial plateaus for UTE-T_2^* and standard Carr–Purcell–Meiboom–Gill (CPMG) T_2 mapping. After MRI, the same cores were harvested and bisected for hematoxylin/eosin (HE) staining for histological assessment as well as glycosaminoglycan (GAG) content assessment and picrosirius red (PSR) staining for PLM. HE and PLM images were qualitatively assessed following a scale developed by David-Vaudey et al. called the DV matrix grade [29]. UTE-T_2^* maps were correlated with collagen matrix organization. Areas of cartilage damage exhibited low UTE-T_2^* values, as shown in Fig. 31.2e, f. The deep cartilage adjacent to the subchondral bone was poorly detected with conventional clinical CPMG maps. Because of the low detectable signal, it was difficult to derive T_2 values within the tolerance of the curve-fit algorithm for many voxels (Fig. 31.2g–i). The mean CPMG-T_2 value increased with increasing matrix degeneration for DV matrix grades 0-3 but decreased for DV matrix grade 4 (Fig. 31.2k). CPMG-T_2 values did not differ significantly with DV matrix grade. In comparison, UTE-T_2^* values were significantly correlated with DV matrix grade. In addition, decreased mean UTE-T_2^* values were correlated with increasing matrix degeneration (Fig. 31.2j). Significantly decreased UTE-T_2^* values were observed in mildly (DV matrix grade 1) and severely degenerate (DV matrix grade 4) tissues compared to healthy tissues (DV matrix grade 0) [18].

Ex Vivo UTE-Based $T_{1\rho}$ (UTE-$T_{1\rho}$) Imaging

Loss of PGs or GAGs is an early sign of joint degeneration. In 1997, $T_{1\rho}$ imaging was proposed to detect PG depletion associated with OA [15]. More recent studies have suggested that $T_{1\rho}$ can detect PG loss in OA patients [16]. As a result, $T_{1\rho}$ imaging is now emerging as a potentially important noninvasive method for probing biochemical changes that may precede morphological degeneration in joints. However, $T_{1\rho}$ imaging techniques based on clinical MRI sequences are limited because short-T_2 tissues show a relatively low signal, and their $T_{1\rho}$ values often cannot be accurately measured. UTE combined with continuous wave spin-locking $T_{1\rho}$, or UTE-$T_{1\rho}$ techniques, have been developed to probe PG in short-T_2 tissues [22, 23]. The UTE-$T_{1\rho}$ sequence provides a much higher signal from short-T_2 tissues such as the Achilles tendon, which shows as a signal void with conventional FSE- or GRE-based $T_{1\rho}$ sequences. To determine the sensitivity of quantitative UTE-$T_{1\rho}$ measurements to biomechanical function, we performed indentation testing on cadaveric human menisci (Fig. 31.3). Significant correlations were found between CPMG-T_2 and UTE-$T_{1\rho}$ and indentation stiffness. The correlation was markedly stronger for UTE-$T_{1\rho}$ ($R^2 = 0.42$) compared with conventional CPMG-T_2 ($R^2 = 0.19$). Thus, UTE-$T_{1\rho}$ correlates significantly better ($p < 0.001$) with indentation stiffness than CPMG-T_2.

Ex Vivo UTE Adiabatic $T_{1\rho}$ (UTE-AdiabT$_{1\rho}$) Imaging

Continuous wave $T_{1\rho}$ imaging is sensitive to the magic angle effect [17]. The highly ordered collagen fibers in short-T_2 tissues are subjected to strong dipole–dipole interactions. Previous studies have demonstrated that $T_{1\rho}$ values can increase by more than 200% in the middle and deep zones of articular cartilage and by 300% in ligaments when the tissue fibers are reoriented from $0°$ to $55°$ relative to the B_0 field [17, 30]. The strong angular dependence of $T_{1\rho}$ makes the evaluation of tissue degeneration complicated. More recently, trains of adiabatic inversion pulses have been proposed to measure adiabatic $T_{1\rho}$ relaxation (AdiabT$_{1\rho}$) as an alternative to continuous wave $T_{1\rho}$ relaxation [24] to reduce the sensitivity to the magic angle effects [31]. A significant drawback is that AdiabT$_{1\rho}$ using conventional MRI data acquisitions is of limited value for probing PG depletion in short-T_2 tissues due to the lack of detectable signals. UTE-based AdiabT$_{1\rho}$ (UTE-AdiabT$_{1\rho}$) sequences can resolve this problem [25]. They allow magic angle-insensitive $T_{1\rho}$ mapping of both short- and long-T_2 tissues of joints on clinical scanners. The technique combines a train of adiabatic inversion pulses with UTE data acquisition to generate $T_{1\rho}$ contrast. Figure 31.4 shows representative 3D UTE-AdiabT$_{1\rho}$ images of a cadaveric human knee joint, where high signal and contrast were achieved for all the primary knee joint tissues. Excellent single-component UTE-AdiabT$_{1\rho}$ fitting was achieved for all the major knee joint tissues, providing AdiabT$_{1\rho}$ values of 24.5 ± 1.3 ms for the quadriceps tendon, 38.8 ± 3.2 ms for the PCL, 33.2 ± 1.3 ms for the meniscus, and 55.6 ± 5.2 ms for the patellar cartilage. Another study demonstrated that UTE-AdiabT$_{1\rho}$ imaging is relatively insensitive to the magic angle effect [32], which is a significant advantage over conventional continuous wave UTE-$T_{1\rho}$ imaging.

Ex Vivo UTE-Magnetization Transfer (UTE-MT) Imaging

Magnetization transfer (MT) imaging has been developed to evaluate the macromolecular proton pool in various tissues [33]. Conventional clinical MT sequences typically employ off-resonance saturation, followed by GRE or FSE data acquisitions. However, they cannot be effectively used to evaluate ultrashort-T_2 tissues in the knee joint due to the lack of detectable signals. UTE-MT sequences resolve this limitation and can be used to quantitatively evaluate macromolecular protons with extremely short-T_2^*'s of the order of ~0.01 ms, which are otherwise "invisible" with current clinical imaging sequences [26, 34, 35]. With UTE-MT imaging,

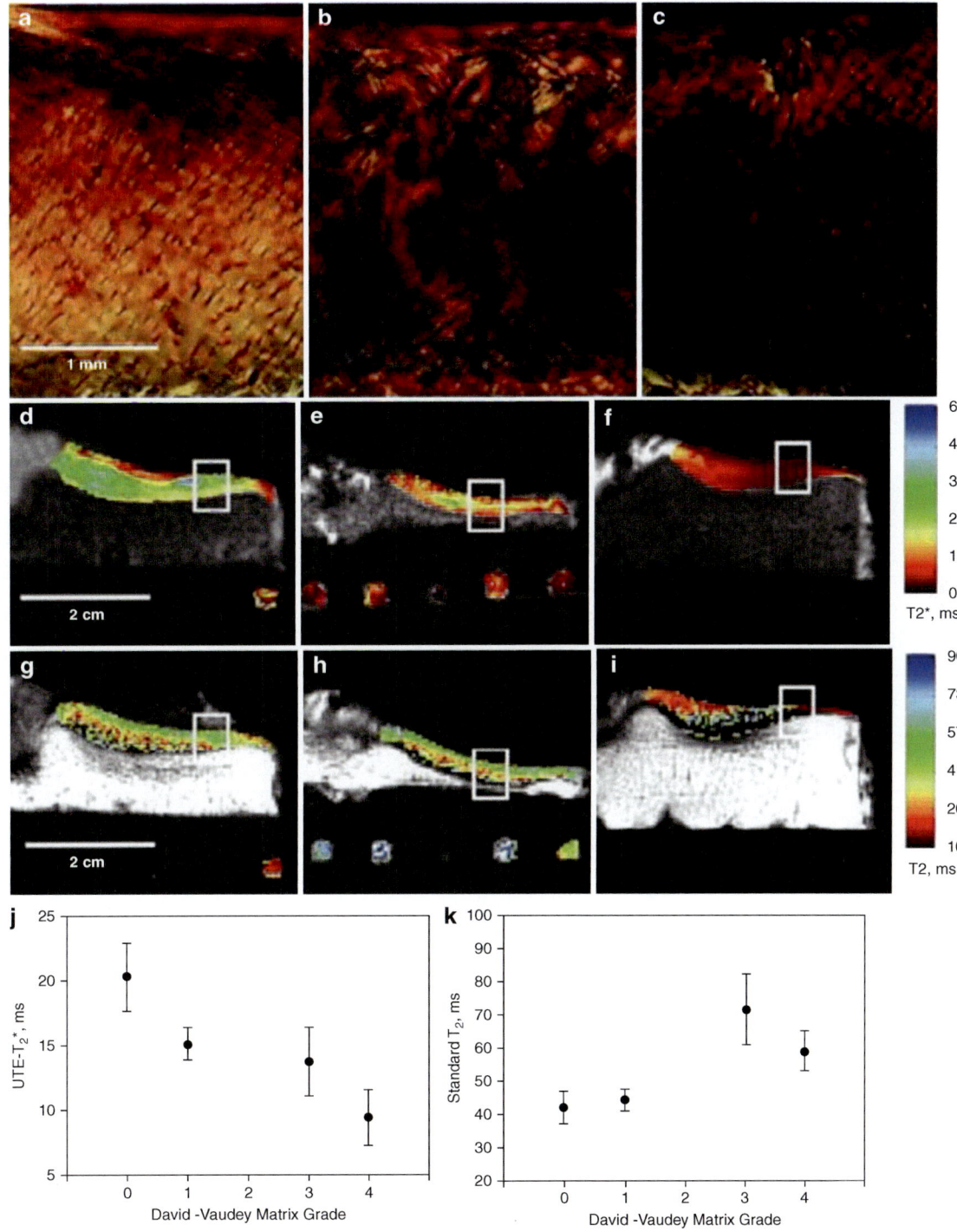

Fig. 31.2 Representative PLM, UTE-T$_2$*, and standard T$_2$ maps of articular cartilage from human tibial plateau explants. The bone–cartilage interface is poorly characterized by CPMG-T$_2$ mapping (bottom row) due to low signal but is well-characterized by UTE-T$_2$* mapping (middle row). The tissue from a healthy 18-year-old male (first column) shows an organized matrix, including a bright and intact superficial zone on the surface, a dark middle zone, and a thick and bright deep zone extending to bone (**a**), with relatively high UTE-T$_2$* values, ranging from 20 to 30 ms (**d**), and noisy CPMG-T$_2$ values, especially in the deep zone (**g**). The tissue harvested after total knee replacement surgery (second column) exhibits a disorganized matrix beneath an intact articular surface (**b**), with midrange UTE-T$_2$* values around 13 ms (**e**) and midrange CPMG-T$_2$ values (**h**). The tissue from a 76-year-old male (third column) shows articular fibrillation and a lack of deep tissue birefringence (**c**), with extremely low UTE-T$_2$* values around 3 ms (**f**) and long CPMG-T$_2$ values (**i**). The white boxes outline tissue regions corresponding to the osteochondral cores, which were sectioned for histological and compositional analyses. UTE-T$_2$* and CPMG-T$_2$ values change in opposite directions with matrix organization measured according to the David-Vaudey matrix grading scale. UTE-T$_2$* values decrease with increasing matrix degeneration ($p = 0.008$) (**j**), whereas CPMG-T$_2$ values increase but were not found to vary significantly with matrix degeneration ($p = 0.13$) (**k**). (Reproduced with permission from Williams et al. [18])

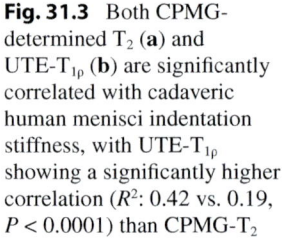

Fig. 31.3 Both CPMG-determined T_2 (**a**) and UTE-$T_{1\rho}$ (**b**) are significantly correlated with cadaveric human menisci indentation stiffness, with UTE-$T_{1\rho}$ showing a significantly higher correlation (R^2: 0.42 vs. 0.19, $P < 0.0001$) than CPMG-T_2

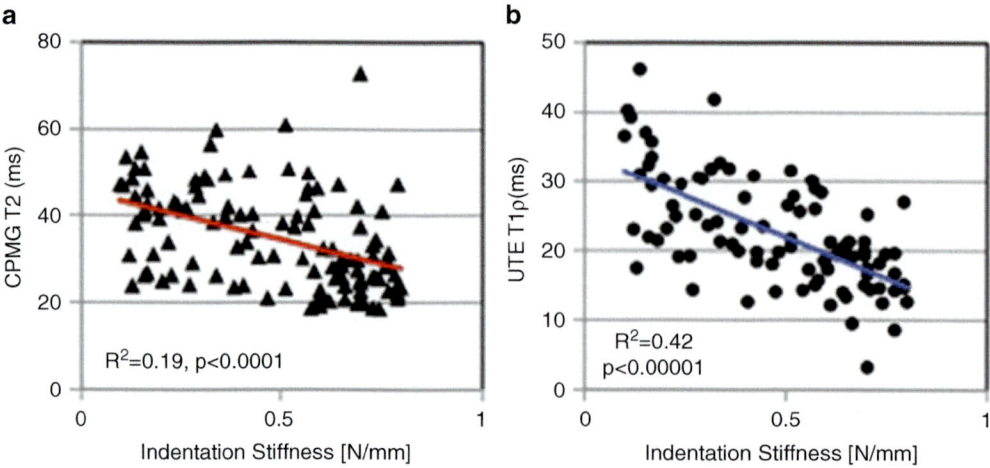

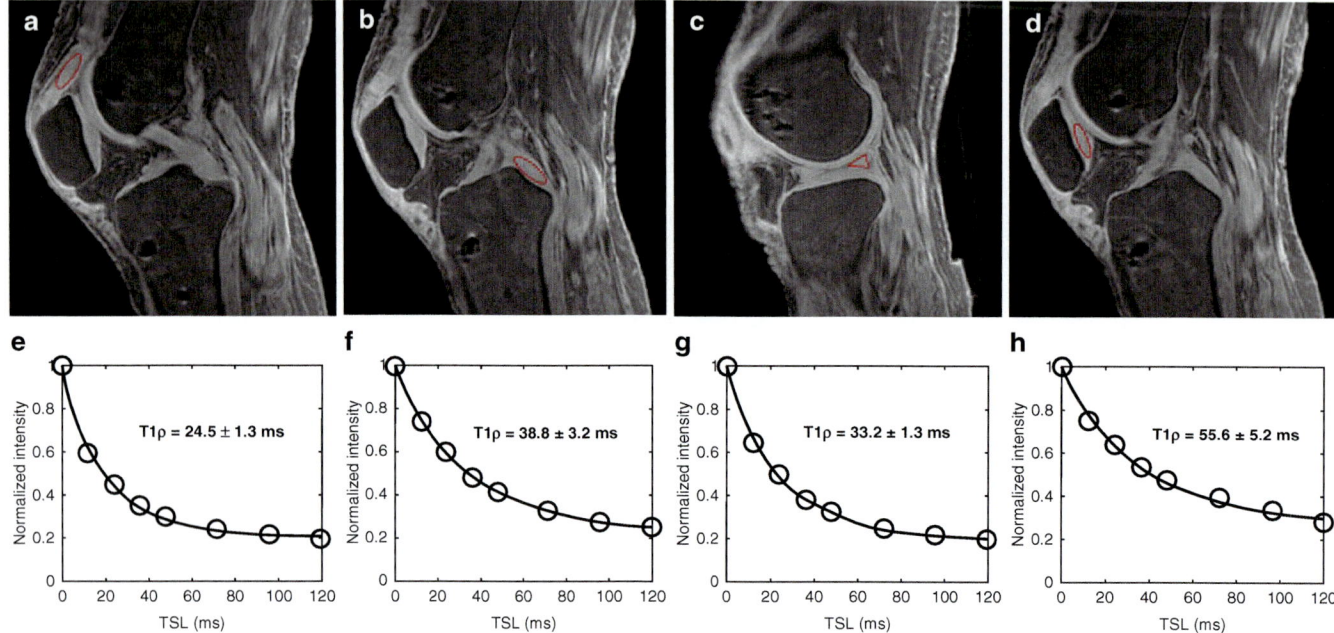

Fig. 31.4 Selected 3D UTE-Adiab$T_{1\rho}$ images of a cadaveric human knee joint of a 63-year-old female donor with regions of interest (red circles) drawn in quadriceps tendon (**a**), PCL (**b**), meniscus (**c**), and patellar cartilage (**d**) and the corresponding mono-exponential fitting curves demonstrating $T_{1\rho}$ values of 24.5 ± 1.3 ms for the quadriceps tendon (**e**), 38.8 ± 3.2 ms for the PCL (**f**), 33.2 ± 1.3 for the meniscus (**g**), and 55.6 ± 5.2 ms for the patellar cartilage (**h**), respectively. (Reproduced with permission from Ma et al. [25])

the MT pulse is placed at a frequency offset Δf away from the narrower lines of water components, and this is followed by UTE data acquisitions. The MT pulse results in saturation of macromolecular protons (mainly collagen backbone protons), which exchange with water protons, leading to a reduction in the detectable signal from short- and long-T_2 tissues in the knee joint. The MT effect can be assessed using the MT ratio (MTR), which is semiquantitative and is affected by many factors, such as hardware differences. Semiquantitative UTE-MTR has been developed to assess changes in articular cartilage and other musculoskeletal tissues [35].

More robust quantitative information can be derived through MT modeling of UTE-MT data acquired with saturation pulses at a series of off-resonance frequencies [26]. A two-pool MT model, which includes a free pool composed of water protons and a semisolid pool consisting of collagen protons, has been proposed to extract fundamental MT parameters, such as the macromolecular proton fraction (MMF), relaxation times, and exchange rates. The free pool typically has a Lorentzian line shape, whereas the semisolid pool with restricted motion has a Gaussian or super-Lorentzian line shape. A critical feature of MMF is its insensitivity to magic angle effects (<10% variation) [36, 37].

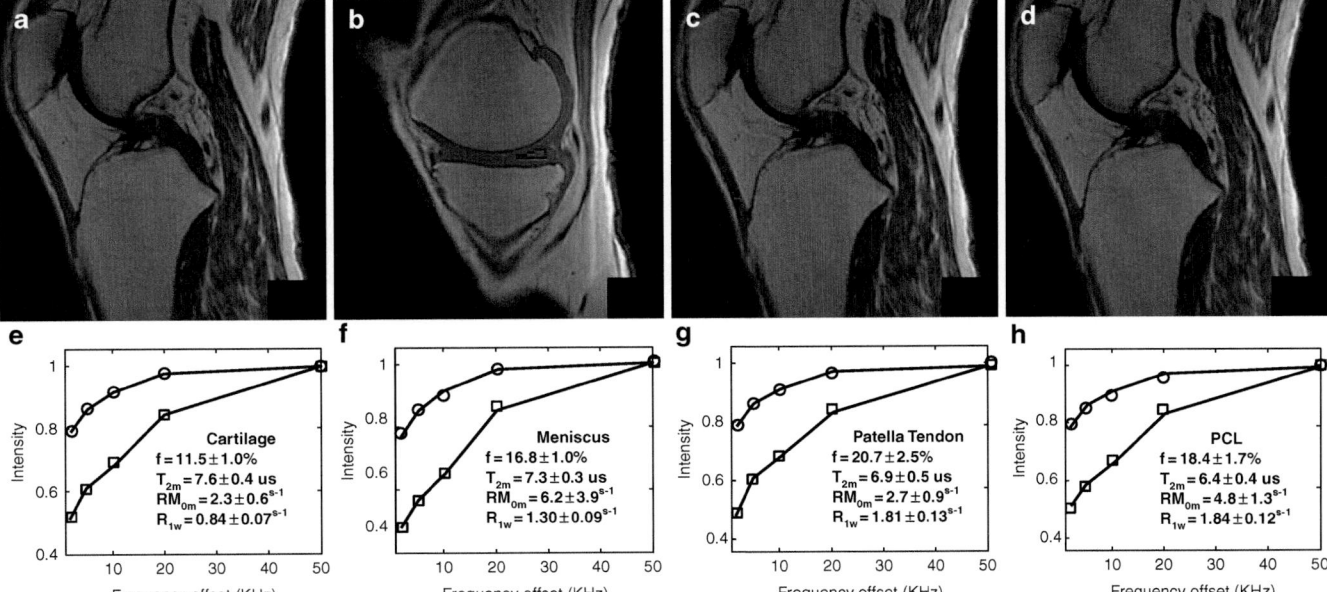

Fig. 31.5 UTE-MT imaging of a cadaveric human knee joint. This allows quantitative imaging of articular cartilage (**a, e**), meniscus (**b, f**), patellar tendon (**c, g**), and PCL (**d, h**). Excellent two-pool MT modeling is achieved for all primary knee joint tissues, demonstrating an MMF of $11.5 \pm 1.0\%$ for cartilage, $16.8 \pm 1.0\%$ for meniscus, $20.7 \pm 2.5\%$ for patellar tendon, and $18.4 \pm 1.7\%$ for the PCL

Geometrical anisotropy minimizes the orientation of the dipolar interaction between water hydrogen and macromolecular hydrogen, which, together with rotational symmetry, results in little orientational dependence on MT [38]. As a result, MMF can serve as a magic angle-insensitive biomarker for musculoskeletal tissue degeneration in situations in which MMF is reduced due to collagen damage, PG loss, and/or higher water content. Figure 31.5 shows typical UTE-MT imaging of different knee joint tissues and the corresponding two-pool MT modeling. As can be seen, excellent two-pool MT modeling is achieved for all the primary knee joint tissues, including articular cartilage, menisci, patellar tendon, and PCL. MMF values range from $11.5 \pm 1.0\%$ for cartilage, $16.8 \pm 1.0\%$ for meniscus, and $18.4 \pm 1.7\%$ for PCL, to $20.7 \pm 2.5\%$ for patellar tendon. UTE-MT sequences offer a significant advantage over conventional MT sequences, which cannot provide MMF mapping of short-T_2 tissues such as the meniscus, ligaments, tendons, and bone.

Ex Vivo Evaluation of OA with a Panel of Quantitative UTE Biomarkers

Different UTE-based quantitative biomarkers may be sensitive to different tissue components within the knee joint. Recently, Wan et al. have investigated the feasibility of using 3D UTE-based biomarkers to detect PG loss and collagen degradation induced by an enzyme in the human ex vivo cartilage [39]. The specificity of these biomarkers in cartilage imaging was also investigated. A total of 104 human knee cartilage samples were harvested in a trypsin digestion study and a sequential trypsin and collagenase digestion study, respectively. In all, 44 samples were randomly divided into a trypsin digestion group (tryp group) and a control group (phosphate-buffered saline (PBS) group) ($n = 22$ for each group) for the trypsin digestion experiment. The other 60 samples were equally divided into 4 groups for sequential trypsin and collagenase digestion, including PBS + Tris (incubated in PBS and then in Tris buffer solution), PBS + 30-U col (incubated in PBS, and then in 30-U/mL collagenase (30-U col) with Tris buffer solution), tryp +30-U col (incubated in trypsin solution and then in 30-U/mL collagenase with Tris buffer solution), and tryp + Tris (incubated in trypsin solution and then in Tris buffer solution). UTE biomarkers, including T_1, T_2^*, AdiabT$_{1\rho}$, MTR, and MMF as well as the sample weight for each cartilage sample were evaluated before and after treatment. PG and hydroxyproline assays were performed as a reference standard. All UTE biomarkers differentiated healthy and degenerate cartilage in the trypsin digestion experiment. However, only UTE-T_1 and UTE-AdiabT$_{1\rho}$ were significantly correlated with PG concentration in the digestion solution ($p = 0.004$ and $p = 0.0001$, respectively). In the sequential digestion experiment, no significant differences were found for UTE-T_1 and UTE-AdiabT$_{1\rho}$ values between the PBS + Tris and PBS + 30-U col groups ($p = 0.627$ and $p = 0.877$, respectively). UTE-T_1 and UTE-AdiabT$_{1\rho}$ values increased significantly in the tryp + Tris ($p = 0.031$ and $p = 0.024$, respectively) and tryp + 30-U col. groups (both $p < 0.0001$). Significant decreases in MMF and

MTR were found in the tryp + 30-U col group compared with the PBS + Tris group ($p = 0.002$ and $p = 0.001$, respectively). Figure 31.6 presents the correlation of the change ratio of quantitative UTE-based T_1, $T_{1\rho}$, MMF, MTR, and T_2^* after digestion with the PG concentration in the digestion solutions, which was standardized with cartilage weights. The change ratios of UTE-T_1 and UTE-AdiabT$_{1\rho}$ were positively correlated with PG concentration ($p < 0.0001$), and the correlation coefficients were 0.74 and 0.86, respectively. There was no correlation between the change ratio of UTE-MMF, UTE-MTR, and UTE-T_2^* with PG concentration, as p values were all >0.05. The Wan study suggests that UTE-AdiabT$_{1\rho}$ and UTE-T_1 have the potential to detect PG loss, whereas UTE-MMF and UTE-MTR are promising for the detection of collagen degradation in articular cartilage. This could facilitate an earlier noninvasive diagnosis of OA [39].

Different UTE-based biomarkers can be simultaneously applied to each knee joint tissue for better diagnosis of degeneration. Recently, Shao et al. have investigated the diagnostic efficacy of multiparametric quantitative UTE-MRI in evaluating human cartilage degeneration using 20 fresh anterolateral femoral condyle samples obtained from 20 patients who had undergone total knee arthroplasty [40]. The samples were imaged using UTE-MTR, UTE-AdiabT$_{1\rho}$, UTE-T_2^*, and clinical CubeQuant-T_2 sequences. UTE-MTR showed the strongest correlation with both Osteoarthritis Research Society International grade ($r = -0.709$, $P < 0.001$) and polarized light microscopy-collagen organization score

($r = 0.579$, $P < 0.001$) in all quantitative UTE-MRI metrics. The UTE-MTR and UTE-AdiabT$_{1\rho}$ values showed a significant difference between the normal group and the mild degeneration group ($P = 0.047$ and $P = 0.015$, respectively), whereas UTE-T_2^* and CubeQuant-T_2 did not. The UTE-MTR values were $15.90 \pm 1.06\%$ for normal cartilage and $14.59 \pm 1.35\%$ for mildly degenerate cartilage. The UTE-AdiabT$_{1\rho}$ values were 40.19 ± 2.87 ms for normal cartilage and 42.6 ± 2.26 ms for mildly degenerate cartilage. The receiver operating characteristic (ROC) analysis showed that UTE-MTR (area under the curve (AUC) = 0.805, $P = 0.001$; sensitivity = 73.7%; specificity = 89.5%) displayed the highest diagnostic efficacy in diagnosing mild cartilage degeneration, whereas UTE-AdiabT$_{1\rho}$ and CubeQuant-T_2 showed lower diagnostic efficacy (AUC = 0.727, $P = 0.017$ and AUC = 0.712, $P = 0.026$, respectively). Quantitative UTE-MTR and UTE-AdiabT$_{1\rho}$ biomarkers may be used to evaluate early cartilage degeneration. Combinations of quantitative UTE biomarkers will probably provide a more comprehensive evaluation of knee degeneration in the main joint tissues. The efficacy of this biomarker panel approach remains to be investigated, ideally on a series of joint tissues with histologically confirmed degeneration and detailed biochemical and biomechanical assessments. This information will also facilitate the development of new grading systems, which involve not only morphological information but also quantitative measurements of the main joint tissues for a truly "whole-organ" approach to the diagnosis of OA.

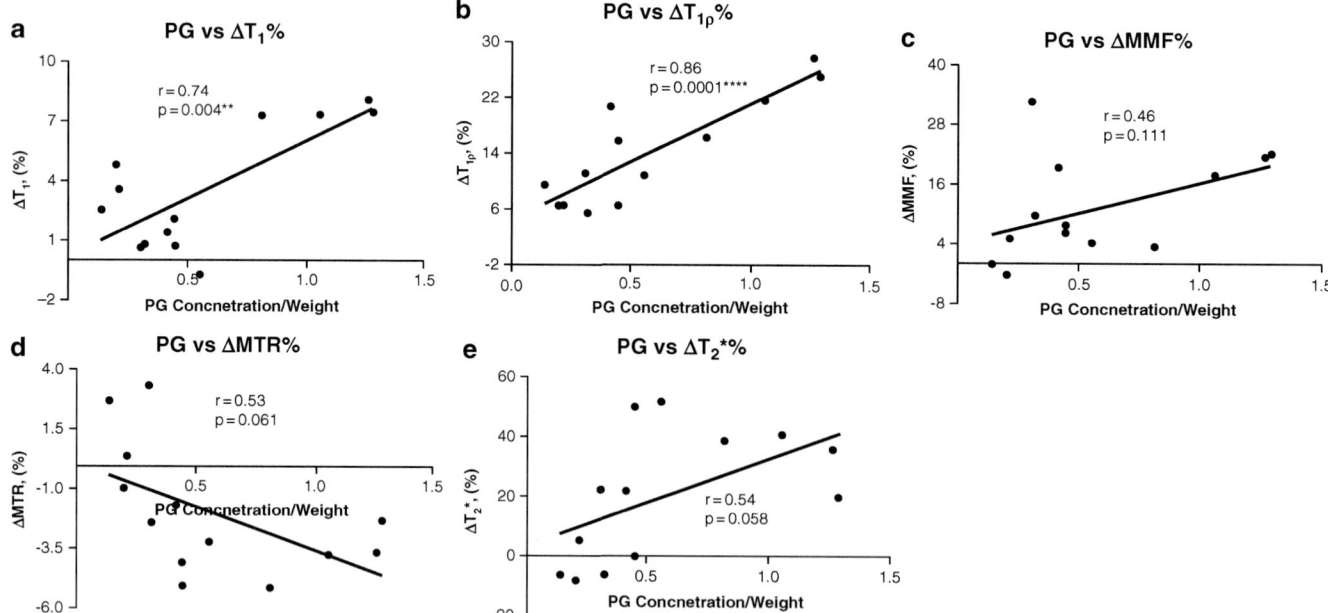

Fig. 31.6 Correlation of the change ratio of quantitative UTE-based biomarkers, T_1 (**a**), $T_{1\rho}$ (**b**), MMF (**c**), MTR (**d**), and T_2^* (**e**) after digestion, with PG concentration in the digestion solutions standardized by cartilage weights. The change ratios of T_1 and $T_{1\rho}$ are positively correlated with PG concentration ($p < 0.0001$) with correlation coefficients of 0.74 and 0.86, respectively. There is no correlation between the change ratios of UTE-based MMF, MTR, and T_2^* with PG concentration, as the p values are all >0.05. (Reproduced with permission from Wan et al. [39])

Quantitative UTE Imaging of the Knee Joint: In Vivo Evaluation

In Vivo UTE-T$_2^*$ Quantification of Knee Joint Degeneration

A previous ex vivo study demonstrated that UTE-T$_2^*$ mapping reflects collagen structural integrity and degeneration in cartilage, as confirmed by PLM [18]. Another cross-sectional clinical study of ACL-injured patients provided evidence that UTE-T$_2^*$ mapping effectively identifies subsurface injuries in menisci that are clinically intact on conventional clinical MRI and at arthroscopic surgery [41]. A more recent study by the same group has suggested that UTE-T$_2^*$ mapping is sensitive to deep subsurface matrix changes in articular cartilage after ACL tears and that it can be used to track cartilage disease status [19]. Furthermore, UTE-T$_2^*$ mapping can detect longitudinal changes in articular cartilage and menisci after anatomical ACL reconstruction [19]. Figure 31.7 shows a longitudinal study's selected UTE-T$_2^*$ data in the meniscus in ACL-reconstructed patients. Before ACL reconstruction, UTE-T$_2^*$ values were elevated compared with those of uninjured controls and increased with increasing meniscal injuries (three groups: uninjured controls, intact menisci, and torn menisci). UTE-T$_2^*$ values in torn menisci did not differ from those in intact menisci (post hoc pairwise, $P > 0.14$) before ACL reconstruction. Within the initially intact medial menisci of ACL-reconstructed patients, UTE-T$_2^*$ values decreased from 12.5 ± 2.0 to 10.4 ± 2.4 ms or 17% over 2 years to levels that did not differ from those measured in uninjured controls (Fig. 31.7d). Elevated UTE-T$_2^*$ values (14.8 ± 4.0 ms) were observed in torn medial menisci 2 years after ACL reconstruction compared to those in uninjured controls (9.8 ± 1.4 ms) and those of ACL-reconstructed patients with intact medial menisci (10.4 ± 2.4 ms) [19].

In Vivo UTE-AdiabT$_{1\rho}$ Quantification of Knee Joint Degeneration

Recent ex vivo studies have demonstrated that UTE-AdiabT$_{1\rho}$ can detect PG loss induced by enzymatic treatment in articular cartilage [39] and can differentiate between histologically confirmed normal and mildly degenerate femoral condyle samples obtained from patients who underwent total knee arthroplasty [40]. The UTE-AdiabT$_{1\rho}$ sequence also allows systematic evaluation of knee joint tissues in vivo. In a recent study, Wu et al. have investigated UTE-AdiabT$_{1\rho}$ imaging of whole knee cartilage in healthy volunteers and in patients with varying degrees of OA [42]. Both subregional and global UTE-AdiabT$_{1\rho}$ values of articular cartilage were cor-

related with Kellgren–Lawrence (KL) grade and Whole-Organ Magnetic Resonance Imaging Score (WORMS) [43], two widely used clinical tools to evaluate OA patients. The subregion cartilage was divided into two subcategories according to the extent and depth of cartilage lesions [43, 44]. The extent group included WORMS 0 (controls); WORMS 1, 2, and 2.5 (regional lesions); and WORMS 3, 4, and 5 (diffuse lesions). The depth group included WORMS 0 (controls); WORMS 1, 2, 3, and 4 (partial-thickness lesions); and WORMS 2.5 and 5 (full-thickness lesions) [44, 45]. Single-component exponential fitting was performed to generate 3D UTE-AdiabT$_{1\rho}$ values for a total of 713 cartilage subregions from 66 human subjects. Receiver operating characteristic (ROC) and area under the curve (AUC) were used to evaluate the diagnostic efficacy of UTE-AdiabT$_{1\rho}$ for the detection of doubtful-minimal OA (KL = 1–2) and mild cartilage degeneration (WORMS = 1). Figure 31.8a, b shows the boxplot of UTE-AdiabT$_{1\rho}$ values in different WORMS groups. Statistically significant differences were observed in UTE-AdiabT$_{1\rho}$ values between WORMS extent groups and depth groups. The mean UTE-AdiabT$_{1\rho}$ values were 37.3 ± 5.45 ms for normal controls, 39.1 ± 6.46 ms for doubtful-minimal OA, and 39.0 ± 6.42 ms for moderate-severe OA. Higher UTE-AdiabT$_{1\rho}$ values were observed in both larger and deeper lesions, with 44.1 ± 5.6 ms for cartilage with diffuse lesions, 46.8 ± 6.5 ms for cartilage with full-thickness lesions, and 35.5 ± 4.9 ms for normal cartilage. The diagnostic threshold value of UTE-AdiabT$_{1\rho}$ for doubtful-minimal OA was 38.5 ms with 64.5% sensitivity and 54.5% specificity. The diagnostic threshold value of UTE-AdiabT$_{1\rho}$ for mild cartilage degeneration was 39.4 ms with a higher sensitivity (80.8%) and specificity (63.5%). The AUCs of UTE-AdiabT$_{1\rho}$ for doubtful-minimal OA and mild cartilage degeneration were 0.6 and 0.8, respectively (Fig. 31.8c, d). The corresponding cutoff points were UTE-AdiabT$_{1\rho} \geq 38.5$ ms for doubtful-minimal OA and UTE-AdiabT$_{1\rho} \geq 39.4$ ms for mild cartilage degeneration [42]. The 3D UTE-AdiabT$_{1\rho}$ sequence may significantly improve the robustness of quantitative evaluation of articular cartilage degeneration. A systematic evaluation of UTE-AdiabT$_{1\rho}$ values for all the principal components in the knee joint, including the osteochondral junction, menisci, ligaments, and tendons, remains to be conducted.

In Vivo UTE-MT Imaging in Knee Joint Degeneration

The 3D multispoke UTE-MT sequence can be used for fast volumetric mapping of MMF in both short- and long-T$_2$ tissues in the knee joint, facilitating a more comprehensive diagnosis of early OA than conventional sequences, which

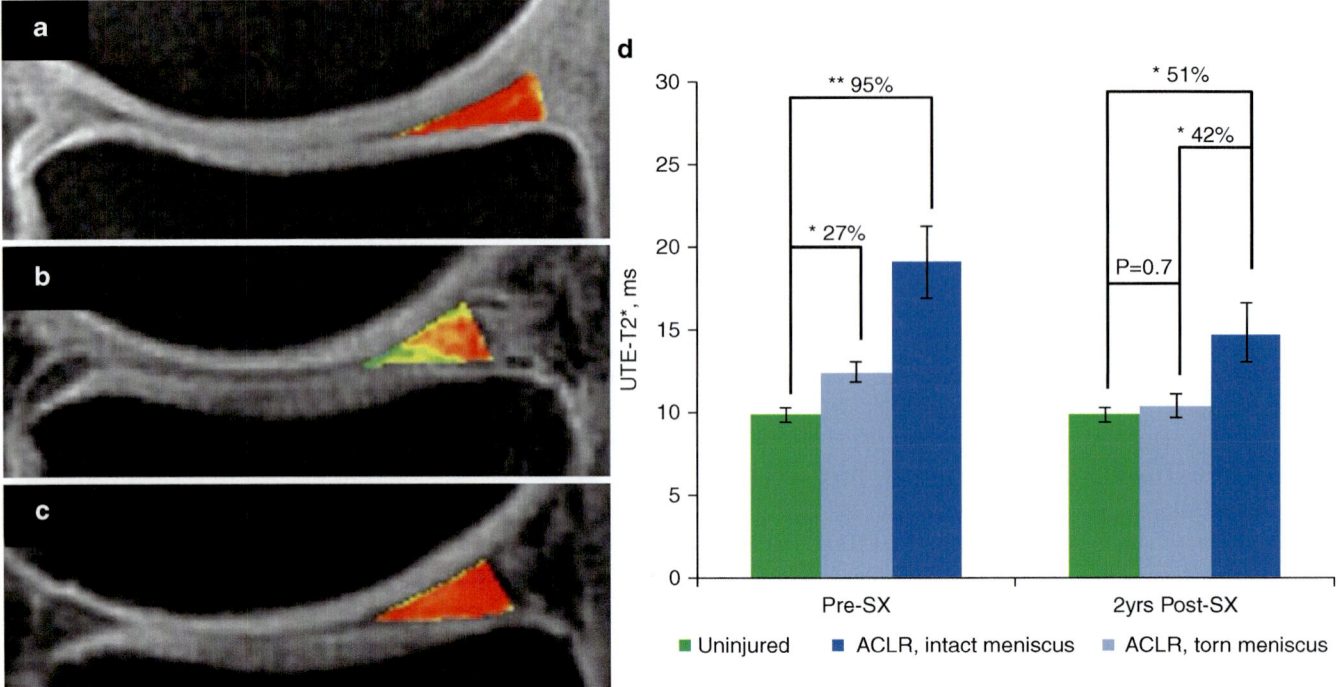

Fig. 31.7 UTE-T_2^* mapping of the posterior medial menisci from an uninjured control (**a**), an ACL-reconstructed patient with an intact medial meniscus before surgery (**b**), and the same patient 2 years after ACL reconstruction (**c**). UTE-T_2^* maps show subsurface meniscal matrix changes in intact menisci in patients with ACL injuries. UTE-T_2^* values in intact medial menisci of ACL-injured patients before ACL reconstruction were 27% higher than those observed in healthy controls ($P = 0.02$). UTE-T_2^* values in intact menisci of ACL-reconstructed joints 2 years after joint stabilization surgery decreased by 17% ($P = 0.03$) to levels that did not differ from those of asymptomatic controls ($P = 0.7$). UTE-T_2^* values in torn menisci before surgery were significantly higher (95%) than those of uninjured controls ($P < 0.01$) (**d**). ACLR = ACL-reconstructed. (Reproduced with permission from Chu et al. [19])

can only provide morphological information about long-T_2 tissues [26]. Recently, Xue et al. have investigated the feasibility of two-pool modeling of 3D UTE-MT imaging for in vivo assessment of whole knee cartilage in healthy volunteers and OA patients and have explored the relationship between MMF and clinical evaluations of OA patients as measured by the KL grade and WORMS [46]. Quantitative 3D UTE-MT sequences with 3 off-resonance pulse flip angles (500°, 1000°, and 1500°) and 5 frequency offsets (2, 5, 10, 20, and 50 kHz) were applied to 62 participants at 3 T. MMF of articular cartilage of the whole knee was quantified using a modified rectangular pulse approximation two-pool MT model based on the 3D multispoke UTE-MT images. Nine spokes were acquired after each MT preparation pulse to speed up data acquisition ninefold [26]. The closely fitting curves achieved for signal intensity versus off-resonance pulse flip angles and frequency offsets showed the benefit of using the 3D UTE-MT sequence to model MMF in articular cartilage. In addition, the test–retest repeatability of MMF derived from two healthy volunteers with three repeated scans showed a mean coefficient of variation of 3.5%, which suggests that MMF values for knee

cartilage can be reliably measured in vivo [46]. Figure 31.9 shows representative 3D UTE-MT modeling results achieved in three subjects with different KL and WORMS grades, with a mean MMF of 10.2 ± 0.6% for the healthy 20-year-old female control, a mean MMF of 9.9 ± 2.2% for the 58-year-old male in the doubtful-minimal OA group with KL = 1 and WORMS 2, and a mean MMF of 6.2 ± 1.1% for the 67-year-old female in the moderate-severe OA group with KL = 3 and WORMS 4.

MMF was also compared in different groups classified according to the condensed KL grade and WORMS score [46]. The correlations were evaluated using Spearman's correlation coefficient, whereas the diagnostic efficacy of MMF in detecting OA in its early stages was evaluated using ROC curves. MMF showed significant negative correlations with the KL grade ($r = -0.53$, $P < 0.05$) and WORMS score ($r = -0.49$, $P < 0.05$). MMF ranged from 11.8 ± 0.8% for healthy volunteers (KL = 0) to 10.6 ± 1.1% for moderate-severe OA patients (KL = 3–4). A lower MMF was observed in larger or deeper lesions in cartilage, with a mean MMF of 9.6 ± 1.7% for cartilage with diffuse lesions and 8.8 ± 1.7% for cartilage with full-thickness lesions.

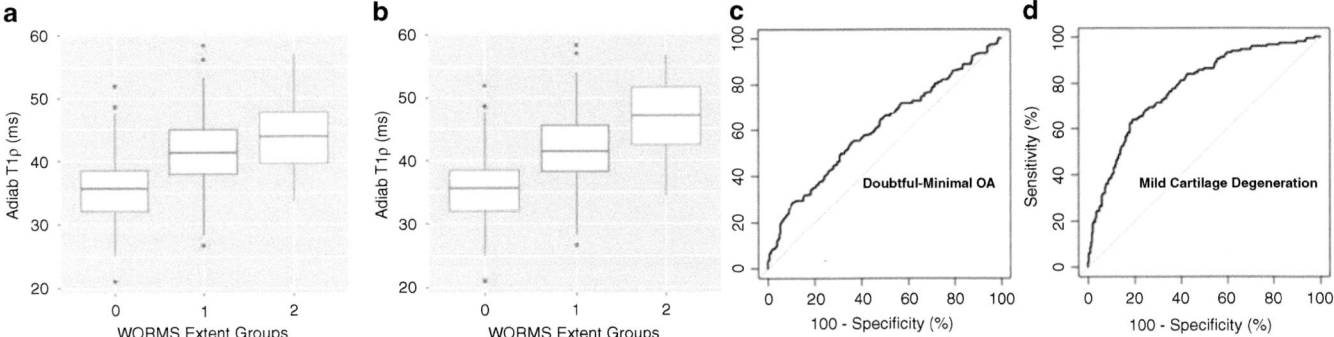

Fig. 31.8 Boxplot of 3D UTE-AdiabT$_{1\rho}$ values in different WORMS extent groups (**a**) and WORMS depth groups (**b**) for a total of 713 cartilage subregions from 66 human subjects with varying degrees of knee joint degeneration, and ROC curves of UTE-AdiabT$_{1\rho}$ for the diagnosis of doubtful-minimal OA (KL = 1–2) (**c**) and mild cartilage degeneration (WORMS = 1) (**d**). (Reproduced with permission from Wu et al. [42])

In comparison, normal cartilage had a mean MMF of 12.1 ± 1.6%. The mean MMF dropped significantly ($P < 0.05$) by 7.6% from KL = 0 to KL = 1–2 and by 10.2% from KL = 0 to KL = 3–4. Similarly, the mean MMF dropped by 9.9% from normal to regional cartilage lesions, by 20.7% from normal to diffuse cartilage lesions, by 12.4% from normal to partial-thickness cartilage lesions, and by 27.3% from normal to full-thickness cartilage lesions, which were all statistically significant with $P < 0.05$. Figure 31.10a–c shows the boxplots. MMF can also distinguish doubtful-minimal OA from normal controls and mild cartilage degeneration from normal cartilage according to the ROC curves. The AUC values of MMF for doubtful-minimal OA and mild cartilage degeneration were 0.8 and 0.7, respectively, according to the ROC curves (Fig. 31.10d, e). The diagnostic threshold value of MMF was 11.5% with a sensitivity of 82.1% for doubtful-minimal OA, and 10.5% with a specificity of 75.2% for mild cartilage degeneration [46]. This study highlights the clinical value of MMF in detecting OA in its early stages.

The meniscus plays a crucial role in the long term health of the knee joint by facilitating load transmission, stabilization, shock absorption, and lubrication [6]. Meniscal degeneration is significantly associated with the development and progression of OA [47]. Early detection of biochemical changes in the meniscus may be essential for preserving the tissue, avoiding the onset of OA, and slowing its progression. Many quantitative MRI techniques, such as T$_{1\rho}$ and T$_2$ mapping, have been developed to evaluate compositional change in meniscal tissue [19, 48]. MT imaging has also been developed for indirect evaluation of macromolecules in long-T$_2$ tissues of the knee joint to explore its value in the early diagnosis of OA. However, MT imaging has been less studied in the meniscus due to the fundamental technical challenges related to the meniscal structure [49]. The meniscus is collagen-rich and consists of distinct groups of highly organized collagen fibers, including the meshwork fibers, which cover the meniscal surfaces, lamella-like collagen fibril bundles,

which lie beneath the superficial network, radial fibers, which are located in the external circumference of the anterior and posterior segments, and circumferential fibers, which are located in the central region between the femoral and tibial surface layers [50]. The highly organized collagen fiber structure dramatically reduces T$_2$ due to strong dipole–dipole interactions. Consequently, the meniscus is largely invisible with conventional clinical MRI sequences [19].

UTE sequences allow direct imaging of short-T$_2$ tissues in the meniscus [19, 51]. This UTE-MT modeling provides comprehensive assessment of tissue properties such as the MMF [52, 53], which is largely insensitive to the magic angle effect [36, 37], making them excellent candidates for quantitative evaluation of meniscal degeneration. Recently, Zhang et al. have evaluated biomarkers derived from 3D UTE-MT imaging, including MMF and MTR, in the meniscus in healthy subjects and patients with mild and advanced OA, and have assessed the correlations with the morphological assessment of meniscal degeneration using modified WORMS [54]. Patients with mild OA ($n = 19$; 37–86 years; 10 males) or advanced OA ($n = 12$; 52–88 years; 4 males) and healthy volunteers ($n = 17$; 20–49 years; 7 males) were scanned with clinical and 3D UTE sequences. Representative T$_2$-FSE and UTE images and maps of MMF and MTR for knee menisci of a normal volunteer, a patient with mild OA, and a patient with more advanced OA, respectively, are shown in Fig. 31.11. The menisci showed near-zero signal with the T$_2$-FSE sequence but a high signal with the UTE sequence, allowing volumetric mapping of MMF and MTR for quantitative assessment of meniscal degeneration. Both MMF and MTR decreased with meniscal degeneration.

Both MMF and MTR were calculated in the anterior and posterior horns of medial and lateral menisci, respectively. They were correlated with age and meniscal WORMS scores in three groups of human subjects: healthy volunteers and patients with mild or advanced OA [54]. The diagnostic effectiveness of MMF and MTR was assessed

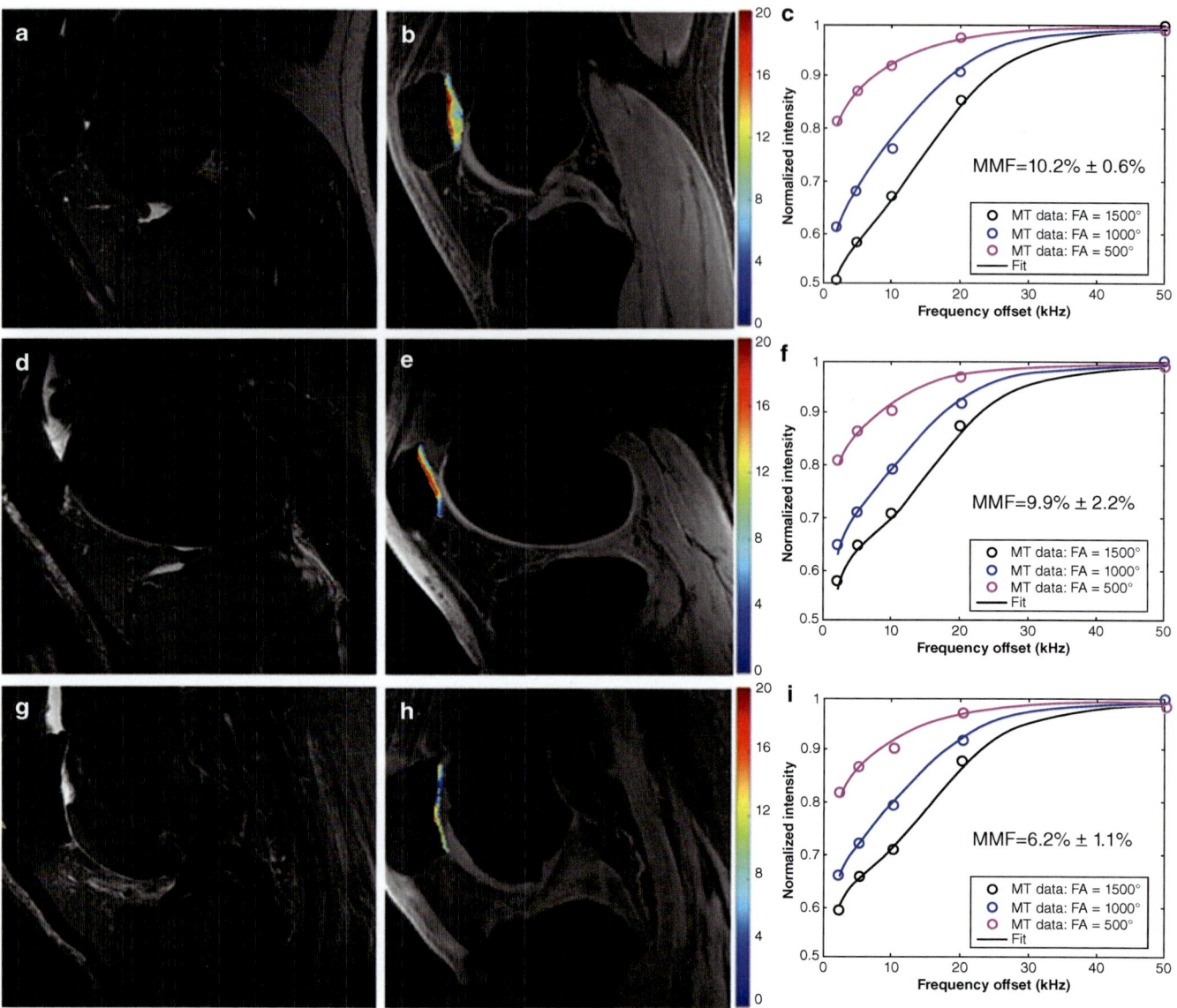

Fig. 31.9 Three representative subjects with different KL and WORMS grades and UTE-MT modeling results: a healthy 20-year-old female volunteer (first row) with normal T_2-FSE (WORMS of patella = 0, KL = 0) (**a**), an MMF map (**b**), and MT modeling curves showing a mean MMF (mean ± standard deviation (SD) of patella) of 10.2 ± 0.6% (**c**); a 58-year-old male (second row) with abnormal T_2-FSE (WORMS of the patella = 2, KL = 1) (**d**), an MMF map (**e**), and MT modeling curves showing a mean MMF of 9.9 ± 2.2% (**f**); and a 67-year-old female (third row) with abnormal T_2-FSE (WORMS of patella = 4, KL = 3) (**g**), an MMF map (**h**), and MT modeling curves showing a mean MMF of 6.2 ± 1.1% (**i**). (Reproduced with permission from Xue et al. [46])

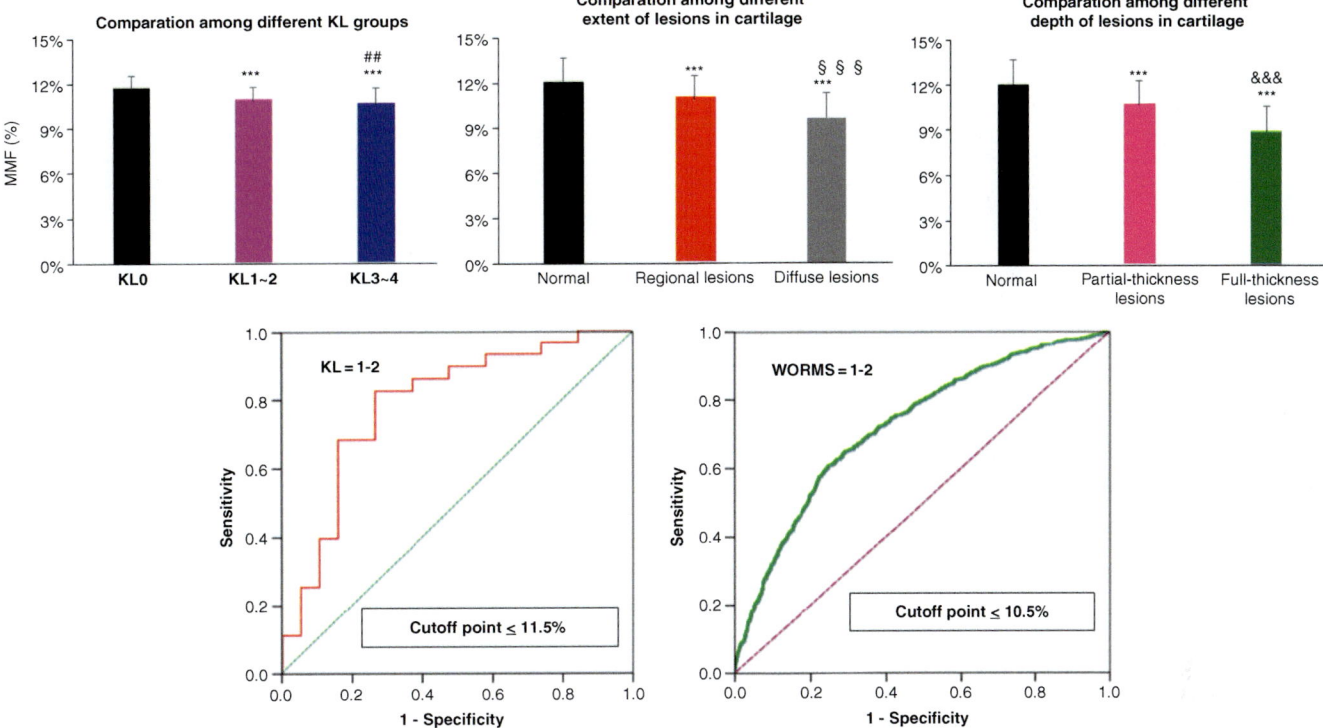

Fig. 31.10 MMF in different KL groups (***$P < 0.001$, compared to KL = 0; ## $P < 0.01$, compared to KL = 1–2) (**a**); MMF in regions differing in the extent of cartilage lesions based on WORMS (*** $P < 0.001$, compared to normal cartilage; §§§ $P < 0.001$, compared to regional lesions of cartilage) (**b**); MMF in regions differing in the depth of cartilage lesions based on WORMS (*** $P < 0.001$, compared to normal cartilage; &&& $P < 0.001$, compared to partial-thickness lesions of cartilage) (**c**); and ROC curves of MMF for the diagnosis of doubtful-minimal OA (KL = 1–2) (**d**) and mild cartilage degeneration (WORMS = 1–2) (**e**). The AUC of MMF for doubtful-minimal OA was 0.8 with a cutoff point of MMF ≤ 11.5%, whereas the AUC of MMF for mild cartilage degeneration was 0.7 with a cutoff point of MMF ≤ 10.5%. (Reproduced with permission from Xue et al. [46])

using ROC curves and AUC analyses. Significant negative correlations were observed between MMF and meniscal WORMS scores with $r = -0.769$ ($P < 0.01$) and between the MTR and meniscal WORMS scores with $r = -0.320$ ($P < 0.01$), respectively, as shown in Fig. 31.12a, b. Mild negative correlations between the MMF and age ($r = -0.438$, $P < 0.01$) and between the MTR and age ($r = -0.289$, $P < 0.01$) were also observed. The ROC curves for the MMF and MTR are shown in Fig. 31.12c, d, respectively. The AUCs of the MMF and MTR values for differentiating OA patients from healthy volunteers were 0.762 and 0.699, respectively, with a cutoff MMF ≤ 15.95% and a MTR ≤ 0.56, with sensitivities of 70.97% and 84.68% and specificities of 70.59% and 50%, respectively. Furthermore, the posterior horn meniscal MMF and MTR values were best for differentiating OA patients from healthy volunteers via ROC curve analysis with AUCs of 0.835 and 0.883, respectively, a cutoff MMF ≤ 14.86% and MTR < 0.56, with sensitivities of 67.74% and 87.10% and specificities of 94.12% and 82.35%, respectively. These results demonstrate that 3D UTE-MT biomarkers of MTR, especially MMF, can detect compositional changes in the meniscus and differentiate healthy subjects from patients with mild or advanced knee OA [54].

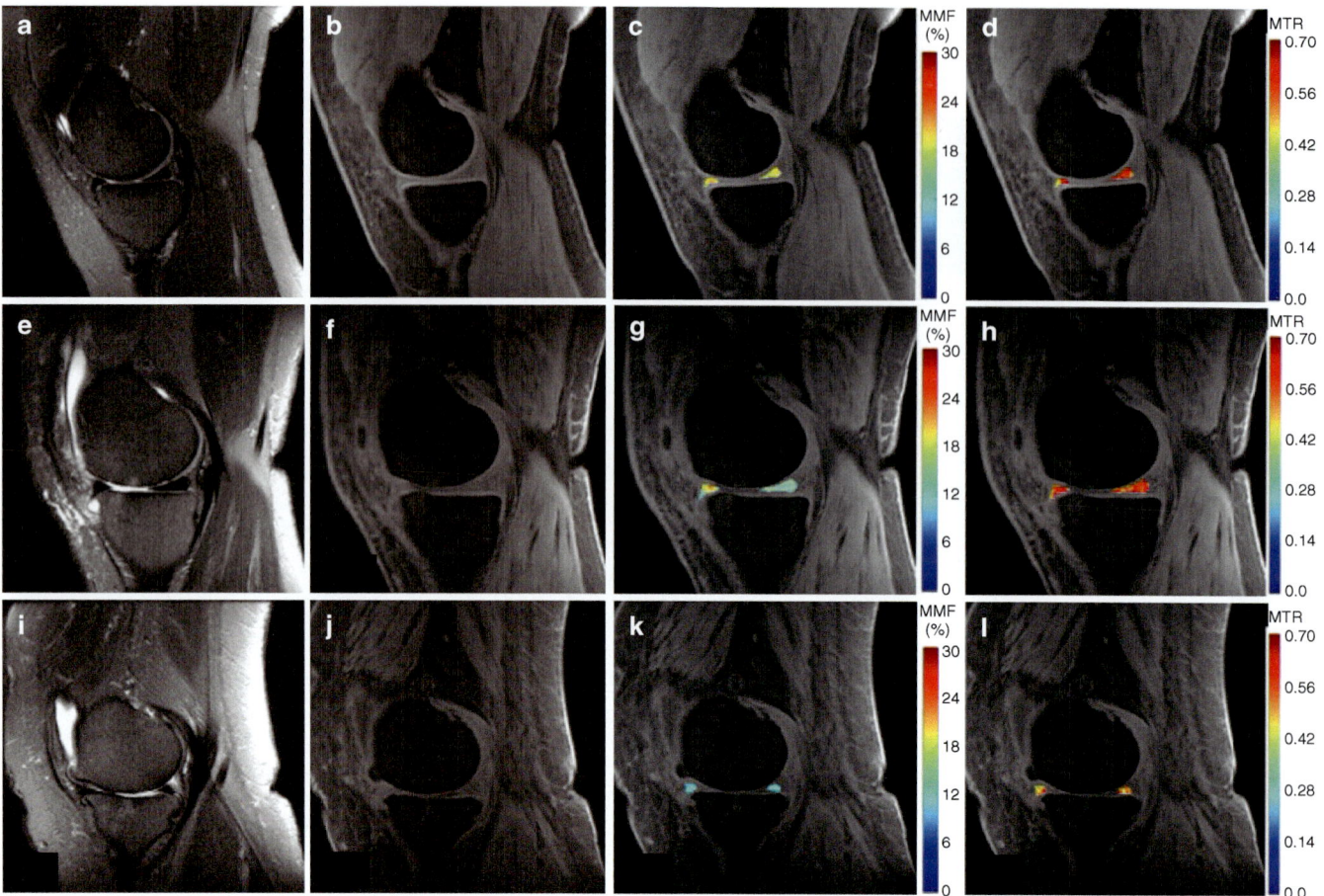

Fig. 31.11 A comparison of three human subjects, including a 23-year-old female healthy volunteer (first row) imaged with T$_2$-FSE (T$_2$-FSE) (**a**) and UTE (**b**) sequences as well as the corresponding MMF (**c**) and MTR (**d**) maps, a 58-year-old male with mild osteoarthritis (OA) (second row), imaged with T$_2$-FSE (**e**) and UTE (**f**) sequences and the cor-responding MMF (**g**) and MTR (**h**) maps, and a 68-year-old female with advanced OA (third row) imaged with T$_2$-FSE (**i**) and UTE (**j**) sequences as well as the corresponding MMF (**k**) and MTR (**l**) maps. MMF and MTR were lower in abnormal menisci than in healthy menisci. (Reproduced with permission from Zhang et al. [54])

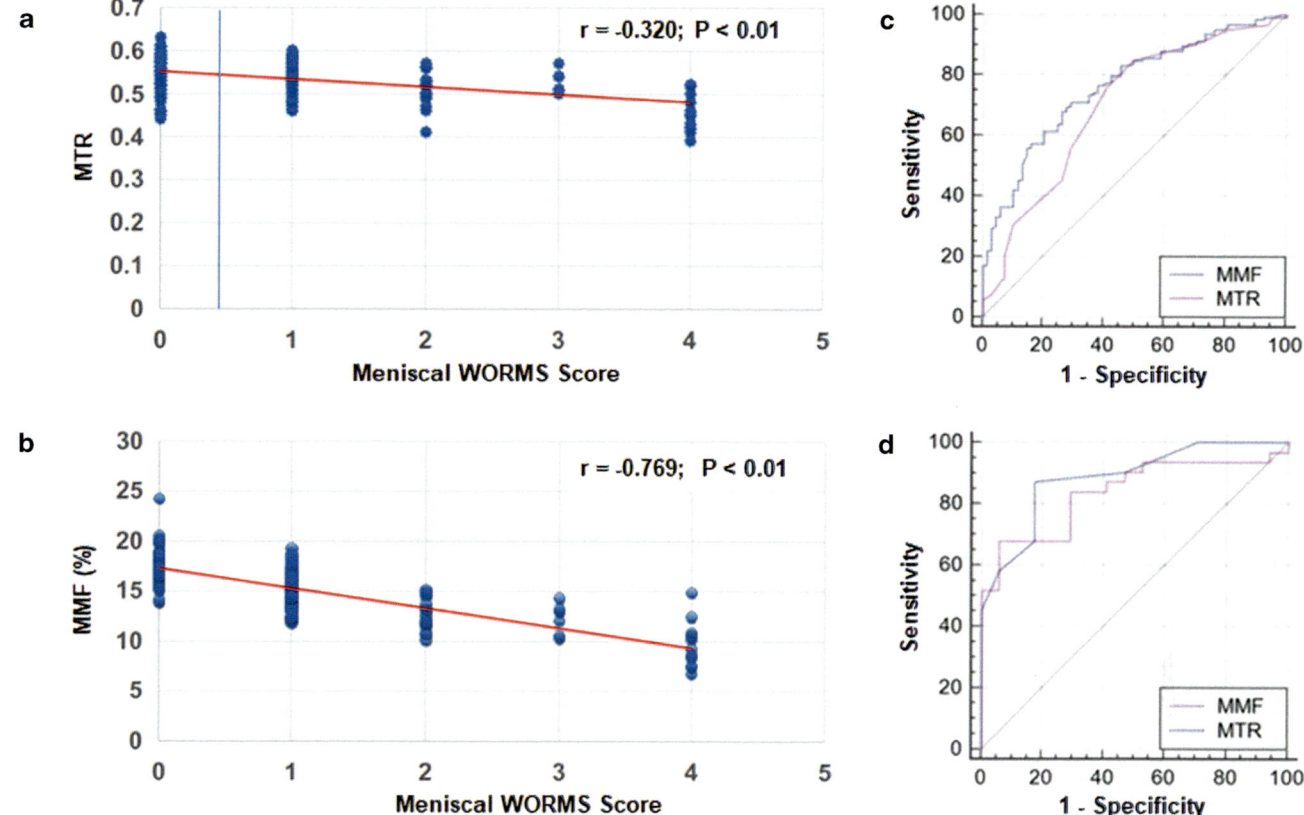

Fig. 31.12 Scatter plots showing the correlations of MTR (**a**) and MMF (**b**) with meniscal WORMS scores. The mean MTR and MMF values decreased with increased WORMS scores of menisci. The AUC values of the whole meniscal MTR and MMF values for differentiating OA patients from normal controls via ROC curve analysis were 0.699 and 0.762, respectively, with no significant difference between them ($P > 0.05$) (**c**). The AUC values of the posterior horn medial MTR and MMF values for differentiating OA patients from normal controls via ROC curve analysis were 0.883 and 0.835, respectively, with no significant difference between them ($P > 0.05$) (**d**). (Reproduced with permission from Zhang et al. [54])

Morphological and Quantitative UTE Imaging: New Directions

UTE Assessment of the Osteochondral Junction (OCJ)

OA is a degenerative disease with pathological changes typically involving all the principal tissues or tissue components of the knee [55]. There is increasing interest in the region of the OCJ, which encompasses the tissue components between deep uncalcified cartilage and trabecular bone. The OCJ consists of the deep uncalcified layer of articular cartilage, the tidemark, the calcified cartilage, and the subchondral bone plate [56]. The OCJ is the region where calcified cartilage meets subchondral bone. However, it is beneficial to consider the tissue components between superficial cartilage and subchondral bone plate as a whole group, which is concerned with the dissipation of stress in a region between semirigid and rigid tissues. While these tissue components are avascular in normal joints, in OA, osteoclasts are activated and form channels through the subchondral bone plate, allowing blood vessels and nerves to extend from marrow into deep cartilage [57, 58]. This process is associated with a cascade of abnormalities, including local inflammation, upregulation of metalloproteinase activity, extracellular matrix degradation, reduction of cartilage load-bearing capacity, and degenerative changes [56, 57, 59].

Although it is generally accepted that the initial changes of OA are degeneration and erosion starting in superficial uncalcified cartilage, some studies cannot be explained by this model [60–63]. The OCJ may play an essential role in the pathogenesis of OA [60–62]. The highly modified mineralized region of cartilage in the OCJ is 10–100 times stiffer than uncalcified cartilage but is less stiff than subchondral bone plate. Thus, the OCJ is a transition zone of intermediate stiffness between uncalcified cartilage and subchondral bone. In OA, the OCJ may become reactive and extend to adjacent uncalcified cartilage, leading to thinning of superficial uncalcified cartilage [60]. The calcified cartilage was extremely hypermineralized and twice as hard as neighboring subchondral bone plate in a study of OA human femoral heads [61]. The OCJ may function as a hard-grinding abrasive and accelerate wear rates in such a situation. Changes in the OCJ can compromise uncalcified cartilage and cause it to degenerate [62]. The hypermineralized OCJ may have shortened T_2^* and T_1s; however, its water content may also be reduced due to increased mineral content. Therefore, the MRI signal intensity of hypermineralized OCJ may be higher (if shortening of T_1 dominates) or lower (if water content reduction dominates) than that of normal OCJ.

However, the OCJ region is difficult to image with conventional MRI sequences due to its short mean transverse relaxation time, leading to little or no signal when the acquisition mode is enabled after RF excitation [64]. UTE-MRI sequences have been employed to resolve this challenge [9, 65–67]. Du et al. proposed a dual adiabatic inversion recovery UTE (dual-IR-UTE) approach for high contrast imaging of the OCJ [66, 67]. This sequence employs two long adiabatic inversion pulses to invert long-T_2 water and long-T_2 fat longitudinal magnetizations. The 2D UTE acquisition starts at a delay time of TI_1 tuned for the inverted long-T_2 water magnetization to reach the null point and TI_2 tuned for the inverted fat magnetization to reach the null point. Excellent contrast can then be generated for the OCJ with long-T_2 water, and fat signals can be efficiently suppressed without problems from susceptibility and/or chemical shift artifacts [65–67]. In addition, effacement and thickening of the OCJ region can be observed [66].

Recently, Ma et al. have reported a 3D adiabatic inversion recovery prepared UTE (3D IR-UTE) Cones sequences for volumetric imaging of the OCJ region with high spatial resolution and contrast [68]. The sequence combines a basic 3D UTE Cones sequence with an adiabatic IR preparation pulse with a duration of ~6 ms. Spokes (N_{sp}) are acquired after each IR pulse to improve the acquisition efficiency. The fat signal is suppressed with a conventional chemical shift-based fat saturation module. Figure 31.13 shows clinical and

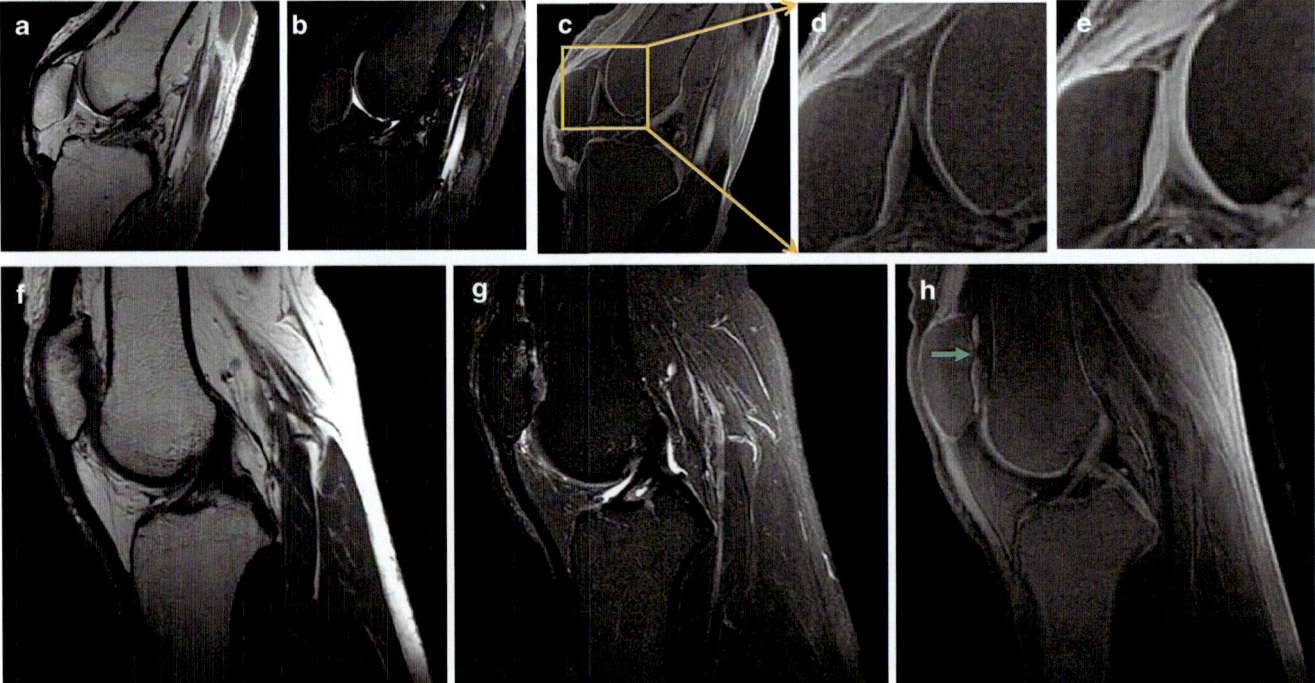

Fig. 31.13 Imaging of a normal ex vivo knee joint specimen from a 31-year-old male donor (**a–e**) and an abnormal knee joint from a 54-year-old female patient (**f–h**). The clinical PD-FSE (**a**) and T_2-FSE (**b**) sequences are used for comparison with the fat-saturated 3D IR-UTE Cones sequence (**c**). The fat-saturated IR-UTE image shows high OCJ contrast (i.e., a high signal band), which can be seen more clearly in the zoomed image (**d**). The conventional fat-saturated UTE Cones image shows a high signal but poor contrast in the OCJ region (**e**). The abnormal OCJ region (arrow) in the patient is seen with the 3D fat-saturated IR-UTE image (**h**) but not with the clinical PD-FSE (**f**) and T_2-FSE (**g**) images. (Reproduced with permission from Ma et al. [68])

UTE imaging of a normal ex vivo knee joint (Fig. 31.13a–e) and an abnormal knee joint in an OA patient (Fig. 31.13f–h). The 3D fat-saturated UTE Cones sequence shows high signals from all the main knee joint tissue components, including the OCJ, menisci, ligaments, and tendons. However, there is little contrast between the OCJ region and the more superficial layers of articular cartilage. The fat-saturated 3D IR-UTE Cones sequence shows a well-defined continuous high signal band in the patellar, femoral, and tibia cartilage of this normal knee joint adjacent to the subchondral bone plate. In distinction, the OA patient shows an ill-defined focal loss and non-visualization of the high signal band adjacent to the plate (Fig. 31.13h). The abnormal OCJ region shown with the 3D IR-UTE Cones sequence corresponds well in position with the abnormal superficial layers seen with the clinical PD- and T_2-weighted FSE sequences.

The OCJ region may play a central role in the initiation and/or progression of OA. MR imaging of the OCJ region may therefore be of critical importance in elucidating the structural and functional pathogenesis of OA, including features associated with the internal layers of cartilage without loss of cartilage in the superficial layers. More research is needed to investigate the morphology of normal vs. abnormal OCJ, including this region's normal mineralization, hypermineralization, and degeneration. Quantitative evaluation of the OCJ, including measurement of its MR relaxation times (T_1, T_2, T_2^*, and $T_{1\rho}$) and proton density, is also full of interest.

UTE Imaging for Monitoring Therapy and Recovery

Conventional MRI clearly indicates where the mesenchymal stem cells (MSCs) are located; however, it cannot detect MSCs in regions beyond the fat pad or synovial fluid. Imaging superparamagnetic iron oxide (SPIO) nanoparticle-labeled cells in joints is challenging due to the presence of dense bone and susceptibility effects associated with highly magnetic SPIOs [27]. Previous studies have raised questions over the specificity of the sequences used for SPIO nanoparticle imaging in joints due to these technical challenges [69]. UTE-MRI can be used to track SPIO nanoparticle-labeled multipotent MSCs injected into joints containing osteochondral defects, thereby providing a method for monitoring the distribution of these cells in the treatment of OA [27]. SPIOs show fast MR signal decay, making it challenging to image them in tissues, which also show fast signal decay. As a result, conventional clinical MRI techniques have difficulty tracking SPIO-labeled MSCs in joints. By reducing the TE down to 32 µs, the 3D UTE Cones sequence reduces SPIO artifact and match histology within bone, as demonstrated in Fig. 31.14 [27]. The 3D UTE images match the histological detail of the recovering osteochondral defect. Within the osteochondral defect, 3D UTE images at both free induction decay (FID) (TE = 0.03 ms) and a later echo (TE = 0.16 ms) have similar intensities to muscle, indicating a lack of SPIOs in the defects. The 3D UTE images demonstrate the anatomical features of healing defects observed in the histological images, with the highest anatomical detail being demonstrated following post-acquisition processing [27]. Subtraction of the second echo image from the first UTE image shows features that match histology and demonstrate bone, fibrous repair tissue, bone tissue formation, and cartilage (Fig. 31.14d, e). The 3D UTE images show additional details with the intermediate TEs, which are not readily apparent on histological samples (Fig. 31.14b). Kaggie et al.'s study does not show SPIOs in the defects 1 week after injection, mainly due to the limited lifespan of MSCs [27]. A longitudinal study with earlier time points to confirm whether there are earlier honing effects and longer-term effects of injected MSCs would be helpful. The superior structure detection of UTE images over conventional clinical images

TE = 0.03 ms   TE = 4.0 ms   TE = 16.1 ms $TE_{0.03} - TE_{4.0}$

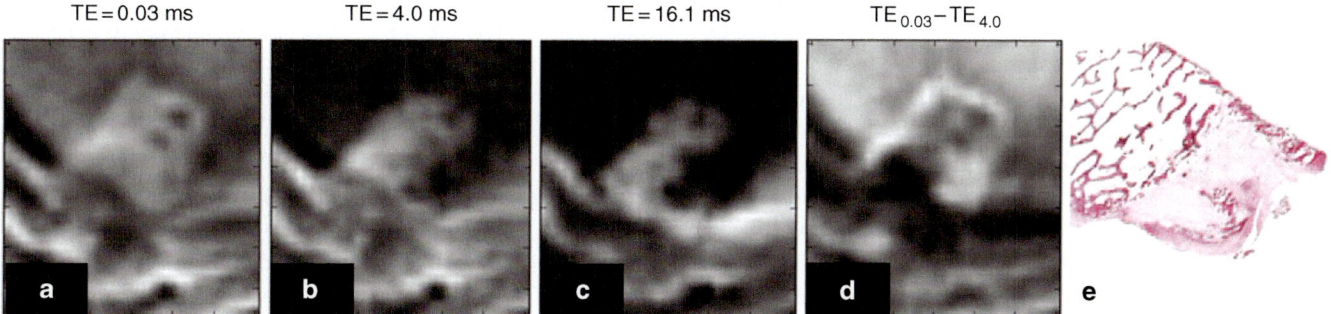

Fig. 31.14 3D UTE images of the osteochondral defect created in an ovine distal femoral condyle with TEs of 0.03 ms (**a**), 4.0 ms (**b**), and 16.1 ms (**c**), subtraction of a later echo (TE = 4 ms) image from the first (TE = 0.03 ms) image (**d**), and an HE-stained histological section of the osteochondral defect (**e**) imaged 2 weeks post-surgery and 1-week post-SPIO-labeled MSC injection. An excellent correlation exists between the 3D UTE images and the histological sections, particularly with the subtracted images (**d**). The defect shows no significant presence of SPIOS, which would be indicated by higher signal loss in a later echo (e.g., TE = 16.1 ms) images. (Reproduced with permission from Kaggie et al. [27])

is a unique strength of 3D UTE-MRI, which can be used for longitudinal monitoring of clinical and experimental joint surface defect healing [27]. The 3D UTE sequence enables further validation of biological healing of minor osteochondral defects, which are difficult to image due to their small size and the fast MRI signal decay of bone and SPIOs. The excellent correlation between 3D UTE-MRI and histology facilitates future studies monitoring MSC locations and the effects of mesenchymal stem/stromal cell healing of damaged tissues [27].

The precise mechanism by which MSCs exert an influence on healthy and diseased tissues remains to be established. Some early reports indicate that MSCs honing in on defects contributes "building blocks" for tissue regeneration [70]. However, in vivo studies using MRI tracking of SPIO-labeled MSCs have failed to provide evidence of this honing in osteoarthritic and joint defect models, with SPIO signals mainly confined to the synovium [69]. A body of evidence supports a role in modifying and mediating disease, although MSCs may not directly contribute to rebuilding the damaged tissue. Increasing evidence supports the hypothesis that MSCs exert a paracrine effect on resident cells [71], possibly via MSC-derived extracellular vesicles [72]. There is also evidence that extracellular vesicles from MSCs contain several biologically active factors that benefit the pathology [73]. If extracellular vesicles are the "active agent" of MSCs, then tracking and understanding their distribution within target tissues such as joints becomes a significant issue. Developing and validating sensitive 3D UTE-MRI methods will be crucial to understanding MSC biology [27].

Conclusions

The knee joint has many connective tissues with short- or ultrashort-T_2s such as the OCJ, menisci, ligaments, tendons, and bone. The ability of UTE sequences to directly image these short- and ultrashort-T_2 tissues may significantly change how OA is diagnosed, and could improve the classification and staging of the disease. One of the most widely used MRI scoring systems for evaluating OA, namely, WORMS/MOAKS (MRI Osteoarthritis Knee Score) incorporates 14 features: articular cartilage integrity, subarticular bone marrow abnormality, subarticular cysts, subarticular bone attrition, marginal osteophytes, medial and lateral meniscal integrity, anterior and posterior cruciate ligament integrity, medial and lateral collateral ligament integrity, synovitis/effusion, intra-articular loose bodies, and periarticular cysts/bursitis [43]. However, the 14 features are mostly related to articular cartilage, although OA is a "whole-organ disease." There are no widely accepted imaging scoring systems for the OCJ, menisci, ligaments, ten-

dons, and bone, at least in part due to the poor signal and low contrast seen with conventional clinical MRI sequences. UTE imaging of all primary knee joint tissues or tissue components may significantly improve morphological assessment of joint degeneration. With advances in UTE-MRI, including robust contrast mechanisms and accurate quantitative imaging of short-T_2 tissues, we anticipate the development of new grading systems not only for knee OA but also for other diseases such as spine degeneration, which is also a "whole-organ disease." The Pfirrmann grading system is widely used to evaluate intervertebral disk degeneration [74]. The cartilaginous endplate plays a crucial role in transporting oxygen and nutrients necessary to maintain the disk's health [75]; however, it is difficult to image with conventional clinical MRI sequences. High-contrast UTE imaging of the cartilaginous endplate is likely to improve the performance of the Pfirrmann grading system [76]. Combined morphological and quantitative UTE imaging for both short- and long-T_2 tissues facilitates more comprehensive assessment of tissue degeneration and could directly influence the development of new grading systems for musculoskeletal diseases and other conditions as well.

Summary

Morphological changes in OA typically happen during the late stage of diseases when intervention is likely to be less effective. Quantitative UTE-MRI biomarkers may be used to probe early changes in disease such as proteoglycan loss (via UTE-$T_{1\rho}$ or UTE-AdiabT$_{1\rho}$), collagen matrix degradation (via UTE-T_2^*, UTE-MTR, or UTE-MMF), and water content change (via UTE proton density mapping). UTE-T_2^* and UTE-$T_{1\rho}$ are both sensitive to the magic angle effect. UTE-AdiabT$_{1\rho}$ and UTE-MMF show little sensitivity to the magic angle effect and are expected to further improve the efficacy in diagnosing early OA.

It is likely that combined morphological and quantitative UTE imaging of both short- and long-T_2 tissues in the knee joint will provide a more comprehensive assessment of OA. This combination will require extensive data analysis involving many tissues or tissue components. Deep learning-based automatic segmentation and quantitative relaxometry could facilitate the translational study of the novel morphological and quantitative UTE-MRI techniques [77–79], and this may significantly impact the diagnosis and treatment monitoring of OA and other diseases. UTE imaging can also be used to track superparamagnetic iron oxide nanoparticle-labeled multipotent mesenchymal stem/stromal cells injected into joints containing osteochondral defects, thereby providing a method for monitoring cell location in the treatment of OA [27].

References

1. Yelin E, Weinstein S, King T. The burden of musculoskeletal diseases in the United States. Semin Arthritis Rheum. 2016;46(3):259–60.

2. Guermazi A, Roemer FW, Burstein D, Hayashi D. Why radiography should no longer be considered a surrogate outcome measure for longitudinal assessment of cartilage in knee osteoarthritis. Arthritis Res Ther. 2011;13(6):247.

3. Mankin HJ, Dorfman H, Lippiello L, Zarins A. Biochemical and metabolic abnormalities in articular cartilage from osteo-arthritic human hips. II. Correlation of morphology with biochemical and metabolic data. J Bone Joint Surg Am. 1971;53(3):523–37.

4. Eckstein F, Burstein D, Link TM. Quantitative MRI of cartilage and bone: degenerative changes in osteoarthritis. NMR Biomed. 2006;19(7):822–54.

5. Brandt KD, Radin EL, Dieppe PA, van de Putte L. Yet more evidence that osteoarthritis is not a cartilage disease. Ann Rheum Dis. 2006;65(10):1261–4.

6. Hunter DJ, Zhang YQ, Niu JB, Tu X, Amin S, Clancy M, et al. The association of meniscal pathologic changes with cartilage loss in symptomatic knee osteoarthritis. Arthritis Rheum. 2006;54(3):795–801.

7. Tan AL, Toumi H, Benjamin M, Grainger AJ, Tanner SF, Emery P, et al. Combined high-resolution magnetic resonance imaging and histological examination to explore the role of ligaments and tendons in the phenotypic expression of early hand osteoarthritis. Ann Rheum Dis. 2006;65(10):1267–72.

8. Afsahi AM, Ma Y, Jang H, Jerban S, Chung CB, Chang EY, et al. Ultrashort echo time magnetic resonance imaging techniques: met and unmet needs in musculoskeletal imaging. J Magn Reson Imaging. 2022;55(6):1597–612.

9. Chang EY, Du J, Chung CB. UTE imaging in the musculoskeletal system. J Magn Reson Imaging. 2015;41(4):870–83.

10. Gatehouse PD, Bydder GM. Magnetic resonance imaging of short T2 components in tissue. Clin Radiol. 2003;58(1):1–19.

11. Reiter DA, Lin PC, Fishbein KW, Spencer RG. Multicomponent T2 relaxation analysis in cartilage. Magn Reson Med. 2009;61(4):803–9.

12. Du J, Diaz E, Carl M, Bae W, Chung CB, Bydder GM. Ultrashort echo time imaging with bicomponent analysis. Magn Reson Med. 2012;67(3):645–9.

13. Mosher TJ, Dardzinski BJ. Cartilage MRI T2 relaxation time mapping: overview and applications. Semin Musculoskelet Radiol. 2004;8(4):355–68.

14. Mosher TJ, Zhang Z, Reddy R, Boudhar S, Milestone BN, Morrison WB, et al. Knee articular cartilage damage in osteoarthritis: analysis of MR image biomarker reproducibility in ACRIN-PA 4001 multicenter trial. Radiology. 2011;258(3):832–42.

15. Duvvuri U, Reddy R, Patel SD, Kaufman JH, Kneeland JB, Leigh JS. T1rho-relaxation in articular cartilage: effects of enzymatic degradation. Magn Reson Med. 1997;38(6):863–7.

16. Li X, Benjamin Ma C, Link TM, Castillo DD, Blumenkrantz G, Lozano J, et al. In vivo T(1rho) and T(2) mapping of articular cartilage in osteoarthritis of the knee using 3 T MRI. Osteoarthr Cartil. 2007;15(7):789–97.

17. Shao H, Pauli C, Li S, Ma Y, Tadros AS, Kavanaugh A, et al. Magic angle effect plays a major role in both T1rho and T2 relaxation in articular cartilage. Osteoarthr Cartil. 2017;25(12):2022–30.

18. Williams A, Qian Y, Bear D, Chu CR. Assessing degeneration of human articular cartilage with ultra-short echo time (UTE) T2* mapping. Osteoarthr Cartil. 2010;18(4):539–46.

19. Chu CR, Williams AA, West RV, Qian Y, Fu FH, Do BH, et al. Quantitative magnetic resonance imaging UTE-T2* mapping of cartilage and meniscus healing after anatomic anterior cruciate ligament reconstruction. Am J Sports Med. 2014;42(8):1847–56.

20. Pauli C, Bae WC, Lee M, Lotz M, Bydder GM, D'Lima DL, et al. Ultrashort-echo time MR imaging of the patella with bicomponent analysis: correlation with histopathologic and polarized light microscopic findings. Radiology. 2012;264(2):484–93.

21. Shao H, Chang EY, Pauli C, Zanganeh S, Bae W, Chung CB, et al. UTE bi-component analysis of T2* relaxation in articular cartilage. Osteoarthr Cartil. 2016;24(2):364–73.

22. Du J, Carl M, Diaz E, Takahashi A, Han E, Szeverenyi NM, et al. Ultrashort TE T1rho (UTE T1rho) imaging of the Achilles tendon and meniscus. Magn Reson Med. 2010;64(3):834–42.

23. Ma YJ, Carl M, Shao H, Tadros AS, Chang EY, Du J. Three-dimensional ultrashort echo time cones T1rho (3D UTE-cones-T1rho) imaging. NMR Biomed. 2017;30(6):e3709.

24. Casula V, Autio J, Nissi MJ, Auerbach EJ, Ellermann J, Lammentausta E, et al. Validation and optimization of adiabatic T1rho and T2rho for quantitative imaging of articular cartilage at 3 T. Magn Reson Med. 2017;77(3):1265–75.

25. Ma YJ, Carl M, Searleman A, Lu X, Chang EY, Du J. 3D adiabatic T1rho prepared ultrashort echo time cones sequence for whole knee imaging. Magn Reson Med. 2018;80(4):1429–39.

26. Ma YJ, Chang EY, Carl M, Du J. Quantitative magnetization transfer ultrashort echo time imaging using a time-efficient 3D multi-spoke cones sequence. Magn Reson Med. 2018;79(2):692–700.

27. Kaggie JD, Markides H, Graves MJ, MacKay J, Houston G, El Haj A, et al. Ultra short Echo time MRI of iron-labelled mesenchymal stem cells in an ovine osteochondral defect model. Sci Rep. 2020;10(1):8451.

28. Nieminen MT, Toyras J, Rieppo J, Hakumaki JM, Silvennoinen J, Helminen HJ, et al. Quantitative MR microscopy of enzymatically degraded articular cartilage. Magn Reson Med. 2000;43(5):676–81.

29. David-Vaudey E, Ghosh S, Ries M, Majumdar S. T2 relaxation time measurements in osteoarthritis. Magn Reson Imaging. 2004;22(5):673–82.

30. Du J, Statum S, Znamirowski R, Bydder GM, Chung CB. Ultrashort TE T1rho magic angle imaging. Magn Reson Med. 2013;69(3):682–7.

31. Hanninen N, Rautiainen J, Rieppo L, Saarakkala S, Nissi MJ. Orientation anisotropy of quantitative MRI relaxation parameters in ordered tissue. Sci Rep. 2017;7(1):9606.

32. Wu M, Ma YJ, Kasibhatla A, Chen M, Jang H, Jerban S, et al. Convincing evidence for magic angle less-sensitive quantitative T1rho imaging of articular cartilage using the 3D ultrashort echo time cones adiabatic T1rho (3D UTE cones-AdiabT1rho) sequence. Magn Reson Med. 2020;84(5):2551–60.

33. Wolff SD, Balaban RS. Magnetization transfer contrast (MTC) and tissue water proton relaxation in vivo. Magn Reson Med. 1989;10(1):135–44.

34. Chang EY, Bae WC, Shao H, Biswas R, Li S, Chen J, et al. Ultrashort echo time magnetization transfer (UTE-MT) imaging of cortical bone. NMR Biomed. 2015;28(7):873–80.

35. Springer F, Martirosian P, Machann J, Schwenzer NF, Claussen CD, Schick F. Magnetization transfer contrast imaging in bovine and human cortical bone applying an ultrashort echo time sequence at 3 Tesla. Magn Reson Med. 2009;61(5):1040–8.

36. Ma YJ, Shao H, Du J, Chang EY. Ultrashort echo time magnetization transfer (UTE-MT) imaging and modeling: magic angle independent biomarkers of tissue properties. NMR Biomed. 2016;29(11):1546–52.

37. Zhu Y, Cheng X, Ma Y, Wong JH, Xie Y, Du J, et al. Rotator cuff tendon assessment using magic-angle insensitive 3D ultrashort echo time cones magnetization transfer (UTE-cones-MT) imaging and modeling with histological correlation. J Magn Reson Imaging. 2018;48(1):160–8.

38. Henkelman RM, Stanisz GJ, Kim JK, Bronskill MJ. Anisotropy of NMR properties of tissues. Magn Reson Med. 1994;32(5):592–601.

39. Wan L, Cheng X, Searleman AC, Ma YJ, Wong JH, Meyer RS, et al. Evaluation of enzymatic proteoglycan loss and collagen degradation in human articular cartilage using ultrashort echo time-based biomarkers: a feasibility study. NMR Biomed. 2022;35(5):e4664.

40. Shao H, Yang J, Ma Y, Su X, Tang G, Jiang J, et al. Evaluation of cartilage degeneration using multiparametric quantitative ultrashort echo time-based MRI: an ex vivo study. Quant Imaging Med Surg. 2022;12(3):1738–49.

41. Williams A, Qian Y, Golla S, Chu CR. UTE-T_2 * mapping detects sub-clinical meniscus injury after anterior cruciate ligament tear. Osteoarthr Cartil. 2012;20(6):486–94.

42. Wu M, Ma YJ, Liu M, Xue Y, Gong L, Wei Z, et al. Quantitative assessment of articular cartilage degeneration using 3D ultrashort echo time cones adiabatic T1rho (3D UTE-cones-AdiabT1rho) imaging. Eur Radiol. 2022;32:6178.

43. Peterfy CG, Guermazi A, Zaim S, Tirman PF, Miaux Y, White D, et al. Whole-organ magnetic resonance imaging score (WORMS) of the knee in osteoarthritis. Osteoarthr Cartil. 2004;12(3):177–90.

44. Wang L, Chang G, Xu J, Vieira RL, Krasnokutsky S, Abramson S, et al. T_1rho MRI of menisci and cartilage in patients with osteoarthritis at 3T. Eur J Radiol. 2012;81(9):2329–36.

45. Guermazi A, Eckstein F, Hayashi D, Roemer FW, Wirth W, Yang T, et al. Baseline radiographic osteoarthritis and semi-quantitatively assessed meniscal damage and extrusion and cartilage damage on MRI is related to quantitatively defined cartilage thickness loss in knee osteoarthritis: the multicenter osteoarthritis study. Osteoarthr Cartil. 2015;23(12):2191–8.

46. Xue YP, Ma YJ, Wu M, Jerban S, Wei Z, Chang EY, et al. Quantitative 3D ultrashort Echo time magnetization transfer imaging for evaluation of knee cartilage degeneration in vivo. J Magn Reson Imaging. 2021;54(4):1294–302.

47. Antony B, Driban JB, Price LL, Lo GH, Ward RJ, Nevitt M, et al. The relationship between meniscal pathology and osteoarthritis depends on the type of meniscal damage visible on magnetic resonance images: data from the osteoarthritis initiative. Osteoarthr Cartil. 2017;25(1):76–84.

48. Rauscher I, Stahl R, Cheng J, Li X, Huber MB, Luke A, et al. Meniscal measurements of T_1rho and T_2 at MR imaging in healthy subjects and patients with osteoarthritis. Radiology. 2008;249(2):591–600.

49. Adler RS, Swanson SD, Doi K, Craig JG, Aisen AM. The effect of magnetization transfer in meniscal fibrocartilage. Magn Reson Med. 1996;35(4):591-5:591.

50. Petersen W, Tillmann B. Collagenous fibril texture of the human knee joint menisci. Anat Embryol (Berl). 1998;197(4):317–24.

51. McWalter EJ, Gold GE. UTE T_2 * mapping detects sub-clinical meniscus degeneration. Osteoarthr Cartil. 2012;20(6):471–2.

52. Jerban S, Kasibhatla A, Ma Y, Wu M, Chen Y, Guo T, et al. Detecting articular cartilage and meniscus deformation effects using magnetization transfer ultrashort Echo time (MT-UTE) modeling during mechanical load application: ex vivo feasibility study. Cartilage. 2021;13(1_suppl):665S–73S.

53. Jerban S, Ma Y, Dorthe EW, Kakos L, Le N, Alenezi S, et al. Assessing cortical bone mechanical properties using collagen proton fraction from ultrashort echo time magnetization transfer (UTE-MT) MRI modeling. Bone Rep. 2019;11:100220.

54. Zhang X, Ma YJ, Wei Z, Wu M, Ashir A, Jerban S, et al. Macromolecular fraction (MMF) from 3D ultrashort echo time cones magnetization transfer (3D UTE-cones-MT) imaging predicts meniscal degeneration and knee osteoarthritis. Osteoarthr Cartil. 2021;29(8):1173–80.

55. Loeser RF, Goldring SR, Scanzello CR, Goldring MB. Osteoarthritis: a disease of the joint as an organ. Arthritis Rheum. 2012;64(6):1697–707.

56. Mapp PI, Walsh DA. Mechanisms and targets of angiogenesis and nerve growth in osteoarthritis. Nat Rev Rheumatol. 2012;8(7):390–8.

57. Walsh DA, McWilliams DF, Turley MJ, Dixon MR, Fransès RE, Mapp PI, et al. Angiogenesis and nerve growth factor at the osteochondral junction in rheumatoid arthritis and osteoarthritis. Rheumatology. 2010;49(10):1852–61.

58. Suri S, Gill SE, Massena de Camin S, Wilson D, McWilliams DF, Walsh DA. Neurovascular invasion at the osteochondral junction and in osteophytes in osteoarthritis. Ann Rheum Dis. 2007;66(11):1423–8.

59. Findlay DM, Atkins GJ. Osteoblast-chondrocyte interactions in osteoarthritis. Curr Osteoporos Rep. 2014;12(1):127–34.

60. Anderson DD, Brown TD, Radin EL. The influence of basal cartilage calcification on dynamic juxtaarticular stress transmission. Clin Orthop Relat Res. 1993;286:298–307.

61. Ferguson VL, Bushby AJ, Boyde A. Nanomechanical properties and mineral concentration in articular calcified cartilage and subchondral bone. J Anat. 2003;203(2):191–202.

62. Oegema TR Jr, Carpenter RJ, Hofmeister F, Thompson RC Jr. The interaction of the zone of calcified cartilage and subchondral bone in osteoarthritis. Microsc Res Tech. 1997;37(4):324–32.

63. Walsh DA, McWilliams DF, Turley MJ, Dixon MR, Franses RE, Mapp PI, et al. Angiogenesis and nerve growth factor at the osteochondral junction in rheumatoid arthritis and osteoarthritis. Rheumatology (Oxford). 2010;49(10):1852–61.

64. Gold GE, Thedens DR, Pauly JM, Fechner KP, Bergman G, Beaulieu CF, et al. MR imaging of articular cartilage of the knee: new methods using ultrashort TEs. AJR Am J Roentgenol. 1998;170(5):1223–6.

65. Bae WC, Dwek JR, Znamirowski R, Statum SM, Hermida JC, D'Lima DD, et al. Ultrashort echo time MR imaging of osteochondral junction of the knee at 3 T: identification of anatomic structures contributing to signal intensity. Radiology. 2010;254(3):837–45.

66. Du J, Carl M, Bae WC, Statum S, Chang EY, Bydder GM, et al. Dual inversion recovery ultrashort echo time (DIR-UTE) imaging and quantification of the zone of calcified cartilage (ZCC). Osteoarthr Cartil. 2013;21(1):77–85.

67. Du J, Takahashi AM, Bae WC, Chung CB, Bydder GM. Dual inversion recovery, ultrashort echo time (DIR UTE) imaging: creating high contrast for short-T(2) species. Magn Reson Med. 2010;63(2):447–55.

68. Ma YJ, Jerban S, Carl M, Wan L, Guo T, Jang H, et al. Imaging of the region of the osteochondral junction (OCJ) using a 3D adiabatic inversion recovery prepared ultrashort echo time cones (3D IR-UTE-cones) sequence at 3 T. NMR Biomed. 2019;32(5):e4080.

69. Delling U, Brehm W, Ludewig E, Winter K, Julke H. Longitudinal evaluation of effects of intra-articular mesenchymal stromal cell administration for the treatment of osteoarthritis in an ovine model. Cell Transplant. 2015;24(11):2391–407.

70. Caplan AI, Bruder SP. Mesenchymal stem cells: building blocks for molecular medicine in the 21st century. Trends Mol Med. 2001;7(6):259–64.

71. Park CW, Kim KS, Bae S, Son HK, Myung PK, Hong HJ, et al. Cytokine secretion profiling of human mesenchymal stem cells by antibody array. Int J Stem Cells. 2009;2(1):59–68.

72. Raposo G, Stoorvogel W. Extracellular vesicles: exosomes, microvesicles, and friends. J Cell Biol. 2013;200(4):373–83.

73. Rani S, Ryan AE, Griffin MD, Ritter T. Mesenchymal stem cell-derived extracellular vesicles: toward cell-free therapeutic applications. Mol Ther. 2015;23(5):812–23.

74. Pfirrmann CW, Metzdorf A, Zanetti M, Hodler J, Boos N. Magnetic resonance classification of lumbar intervertebral disc degeneration. Spine (Phila Pa 1976). 2001;26(17):1873–8.

75. Fields AJ, Ballatori A, Liebenberg EC, Lotz JC. Contribution of the endplates to disc degeneration. Curr Mol Biol Rep. 2018;4(4):151–60.

76. Bae WC, Statum S, Zhang Z, Yamaguchi T, Wolfson T, Gamst AC, et al. Morphology of the cartilaginous endplates in human intervertebral disks with ultrashort echo time MR imaging. Radiology. 2013;266(2):564–74.

77. Byra M, Wu M, Zhang X, Jang H, Ma YJ, Chang EY, et al. Knee menisci segmentation and relaxometry of 3D ultrashort echo time cones MR imaging using attention U-net with transfer learning. Magn Reson Med. 2020;83(3):1109–22.

78. Xue YP, Jang H, Byra M, Cai ZY, Wu M, Chang EY, et al. Automated cartilage segmentation and quantification using 3D ultrashort echo time (UTE) cones MR imaging with deep convolutional neural networks. Eur Radiol. 2021;31(10):7653–63.

79. Kijowski R, Liu F, Caliva F, Pedoia V. Deep learning for lesion detection, progression, and prediction of musculoskeletal disease. J Magn Reson Imaging. 2020;52(6):1607–19.

Bound Water and Pore Water in Osteoporosis

32

Jeffry S. Nyman and Mark D. Does

Introduction

Osteoporosis (OP) and the resulting bone fractures are a global problem affecting millions of people. The annual costs associated with treating osteoporosis and its associated fractures were estimated at $22 billion in the United States in 2009 [1] and at €37 billion in the European Union (EU) in 2010 [2]. Importantly, the latter study identified that 95% of these costs were due to fixation of incident fractures and long term fracture care, indicating the potential to reduce costs through better diagnosis and preventative treatment. Otherwise, the costs related to bone fractures will increase as the aging population grows [3]. Despite this economic burden and negative impact on the quality of life, the clinical standard for evaluating bone health, dual-energy X-ray absorptiometry (DXA), does not fully predict increased fracture risk with age or disease. Moreover, no clinical imaging

J. S. Nyman
Institute of Image Science, Vanderbilt University Medical Center, Nashville, TN, USA

Biomedical Engineering, Vanderbilt University, Nashville, TN, USA

Department of Veterans Affairs, Tennessee Valley Healthcare System, Nashville, TN, USA

Orthopaedic Surgery and Rehabilitation, Vanderbilt University Medical Center, Nashville, TN, USA

Center for Bone Biology, Vanderbilt University Medical Center, Nashville, TN, USA
e-mail: jeffry.s.nyman@vumc.org

M. D. Does (✉)
Institute of Image Science, Vanderbilt University Medical Center, Nashville, TN, USA

Biomedical Engineering, Vanderbilt University, Nashville, TN, USA

Radiology and Radiological Sciences, Vanderbilt University Medical Center, Nashville, TN, USA

Electrical Engineering, Vanderbilt University Medical Center, Nashville, TN, USA
e-mail: mark.does@vanderbilt.edu

methods exist to probe changes in the soft tissue components of bone, which may play an important role in determining the resistance of bone to fracture. Consequently, there is a great need for improved and novel quantitative diagnostic methods for measuring bone properties that report more accurately on an individual's fracture risk. This chapter presents the rationale for and the technical descriptions of how ultrashort echo time (UTE) magnetic resonance imaging (MRI) can be used to evaluate bone fracture risk.

Beyond Bone Mineral Density (BMD)

The increased risk of bone fracture due to aging is disproportionate to the age-related decrease in bone mineral density (BMD) [4]. Likewise, clinical assessments of areal BMD (aBMD) using DXA do not necessarily identify individuals at risk of costly fractures [5, 6]. Quantitative computed tomography (CT) offers more accurate measures of BMD—volumetric, rather than areal—but BMD itself is a measure that does not explain the known decrease in mechanical properties when bone is dehydrated [7] or the known decrease in collagen integrity that accompanies age-related increase in bone brittleness [8, 9]; nor does BMD account for the deleterious effects of accumulating nonenzymatic, glycation-mediated modifications of collagen I on the biomechanical properties of bone [10]. This begs the question: beyond BMD, what measurable characteristics of bone can report a fracture risk?

Bone structure on a macroscopic scale, which can be imaged with either CT or MRI methods, likely plays an important role in determining whole-bone biomechanical properties [11–13]. To quantitatively probe a structure with imaging, one can compute simple metrics such as the cross-sectional moment of inertia [14] or cortical bone thickness [15] and correlate these with measures of fracture resistance or patient outcome. Alternatively, one can convert an entire three-dimensional (3D) image stack of bone structure into complex finite element models along with volumetric-BMD-derived moduli and assumed material behavior to simulate the response of bone to known loads [16–18]. The former approach is most likely to gain traction clinically since the necessary images and the subsequent metrics are easily computed [19, 20]. At present, full finite element modeling requires substantial dedicated computing power and expertise to implement, although the Food and Drug Administration (FDA) has recently approved one implementation of CT-derived finite element analysis (FEA) that predicts a patient's bone strength [21]. Trabecular bone volume fraction and the accompanying microarchitectural parameters acquired at distal sites (the radius and tibia) can differ between those that suffer from a fragility fracture and age-matched individuals without a history of fracture, but there is overlap in the imaging measurements between the groups [22–24]. The missing piece for accurate fracture prediction is noninvasive assessment of the material properties of bone tissue (i.e., biomechanical properties that are independent of bone structure).

In addition to structure, the material composition of cortical and trabecular bone is important in dictating fracture resistance properties of whole bone. Volumetric BMD is one such compositional measure, but, in addition to the mineral content, bone includes soft tissue components—primarily hydrated collagen I (~90% of the organic matrix) and pore water. There is good reason to believe that these components play a critical role in dissipating energy under load and so provide increased resistance to fracture because of the contribution of organic matrix to bone toughness [25]. Dry cortical bone has long been known to be more brittle than hydrated bone of equal mineral density [26], and age-related decreases in the stability of collagen [8] and collagen strength [9] have been found to correlate with loss in fracture toughness of bone. In addition, there is an inverse relationship between intracortical porosity and the apparent material strength of

bone as determined by mechanical testing of uniform, millimeter-sized specimens of human cortical bone [27]. A recent analysis of the distal radius from cadavers has indicated that most bone loss between 65 and 80 years is cortical [28] and that age-related increase in porosity (for pores >80 μm diameter) of the distal radius was correlated with a loss of strength as predicted by quantitative CT-derived finite element models [29]. It should be noted that while an increase in porosity results in a corresponding decrease in DXA-measured BMD, an observed decrease in BMD cannot be ascribed to an increase in porosity; thus, DXA cannot be used to measure changes in microstructural porosity. In contrast, clinical MRI, which measures signal from water, can directly detect the soft tissue components of bone and may, therefore, provide access to unique imaging biomarkers of fracture risk.

^{1}H Nuclear Magnetic Resonance (NMR) Signals of the Cortical Bone

Several non-imaging studies of ^{1}H relaxometry from bone specimens laid the groundwork for a better understanding of the MR signals from cortical bone [30–35]. From there, through a series of ^{1}H NMR Carr–Purcell–Meiboom–Gill (CPMG) studies of human cortical bone samples, strong relationships were established between the high-field relaxation and line width characteristics of ^{1}H NMR signals from collagen, collagen-bound water, and pore water in cortical bone [36].

Figure 32.1 shows the mean and variation across individuals of the T_2 spectrum of ^{1}H signals from cortical bone [37]. The spectrum is divided into three domains, each of which largely corresponds to a different microanatomical source of protons. The fastest relaxing signals, with $T_2 < 100$ μs, come

Fig. 32.1 Summary of ^{1}H T_2 spectra measured from 40 human cortical bone samples. All spectra exhibited a short-T_2 component, primarily derived from collagen protons, an intermediate-T_2 component, primarily derived from collagen-bound water protons, and a broad distribution of long-T_2 components, derived from a combination of PW and lipid protons. (Reproduced with permission from Horch et al. [37])

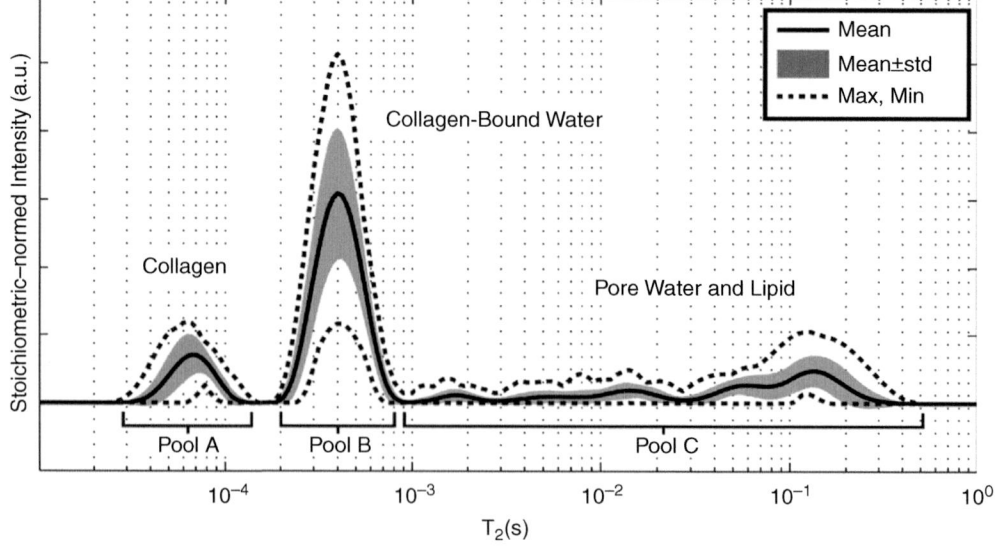

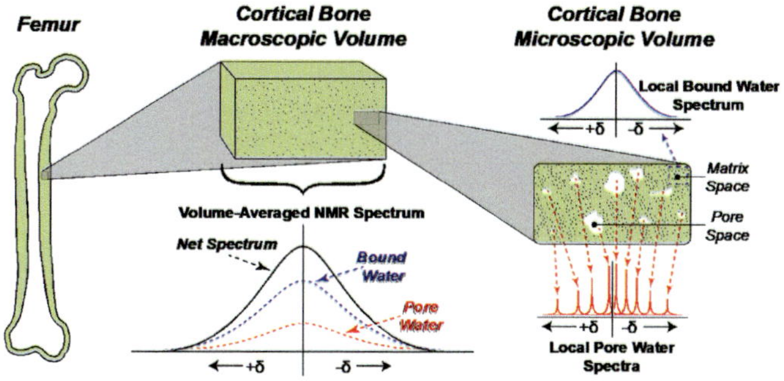

Fig. 32.2 A model of water ^1H NMR line shapes in human cortical bone. Across a macroscopic volume of cortical bone akin to an MRI voxel (middle), numerous BW and PW components are combined into a broad-net NMR spectrum with similarly broadened BW and PW contributions. On the local microscale (right), bound water in bone matrix space gives rise to a homogeneously broadened NMR spectrum. Conversely, the relatively mobile water within each pore space gives rise to a narrower NMR spectrum of varying chemical shifts (dictated by pore geometry and pore-matrix susceptibility variation). The sum of these microscale contributions gives rise to a heterogeneously broadened PW line shape across macroscopic bone volumes (middle). (Reproduced with permission from Horch et al. [52])

from collagen protons, and, for the most part, these signals decay too rapidly for most UTE-related MRI methods and will not be further discussed here. The intermediate-T_2 domain is comprised of signals from water bound to organic matrix (henceforth referred to as bound water (BW)). These signals also decay rapidly, $T_2 \approx 350$ μs, but well within times that are accessible with UTE-MRI. Lastly, the broad distribution of long lived signals, $T_2 > 1$ ms, are derived from water (and to a lesser extent, lipids) residing in the pore networks of cortical bone (henceforth referred to as pore water, PW). It is important to appreciate that these later two pools of water are physically distinct and do not exchange. The BW is trapped within bone matrix and its environment, and its relaxation characteristics do not vary much from bone to bone. In contrast, the PW relaxation rates, which are largely dictated by pore size, vary widely within and between bones [38]. Figure 32.2 provides a graphical representation of bound and pore water in bone, showing that the BW is homogeneously broadened ($T_2^* \approx T_2$), whereas the widely varied environments of PW result in it having a heterogeneously broadened signal ($T_2^* \ll T_2$).

UTE-MRI Imaging of BW and PW

Traditionally, clinical MRI has not been suitable for imaging dense tissues, such as cortical bone, because the ^1H NMR signals from such tissues decay rapidly. That is, their transverse relaxation time constant, T_2, is small compared with the time delay between signal excitation and acquisition—the so-called echo time (TE). However, in the early 2000s,

advancements in UTE-MRI led to the technique having several applications in imaging cortical bone [39–45].

With regard to the application of MRI to fracture risk assessment, the earliest studies focused on assessing trabecular bone volume and architecture, as reviewed by Wehrli [46], and this continues to be an active area of research and development [24, 47–50]. As UTE technology has improved, ever more work on cortical bone has been reported. Pioneering work by the groups at the University of Pennsylvania and the University of California, San Diego (UCSD), set the stage for quantitative UTE-MRI of human cortical bone [43, 45, 51].

With these advances and leveraging the understanding of BW and PW relaxation characteristics, two approaches, broadly speaking, have been developed to selectively image the BW and PW signals. One approach uses T_2-selective adiabatic radiofrequency (RF) pulse preparations to suppress the signal from one pool in order to directly image the signal from the other pool [52–54]. These methods are known as adiabatic inversion recovery (AIR) and double adiabatic full passage (DAFP), for BW and PW measurements, respectively. Another approach is to acquire multiple images with varied T_2^* weightings and fit these signals to a bi- or tricomponent signal model, which includes BW and PW terms [55–58]. Both approaches have been evaluated in a variety of experimental settings and show promise for clinical application. Methodological details on the bi/tri-component methods are found in Chap. 23 ("Quantitative Ultrashort Echo Time Magnetic Resonance Imaging: T_2^*"), and some details of the T_2-selective approach are provided below.

AIR and DAFP Imaging of BW and PW

To suppress the signal from pore water and selectively image bound water in cortical bone, the AIR scheme (Fig. 32.3a) is essentially an application of previous methods used to suppress signals from the surrounding tissues in UTE applications [59, 60]. The short T_2 of bound water magnetization causes it to be saturated by the adiabatic RF pulse, whereas pore water is approximately fully inverted. (It should be noted that this requires an adiabatic pulse of a relatively large bandwidth, ≈ 3 kHz, due to the heterogeneously broadened PW line width.) After an appropriate inversion delay period (inversion time, TI), the PW longitudinal magnetization reaches zero, whereas the BW magnetization is substantially recovered and is the sole contributor to a subsequent excitation and UTE readout. To selectively image pore water, the same adiabatic T_2 selectivity can be achieved by successively applying two adiabatic inversion pulses to saturate the BW magnetization while rotating the PW magnetization a full 360° back to near its equilibrium value (Fig. 32.3b). Consequently, this approach was named the double adiabatic

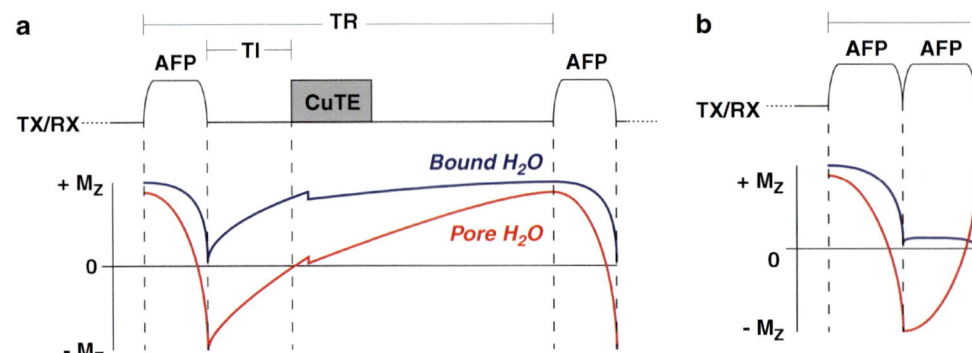

Fig. 32.3 (a) The AIR scheme nulls PW magnetization, creating a predominantly BW signal measured by the conventional UTE readout (labeled "CuTE" in this image). (b) The double adiabatic full-passage (DAFP) scheme drives bound water magnetization to saturation, leaving only PW for the UTE readout. (Reproduced with permission from Horch et al. [52])

full-passage (DAFP) preparation. More complete explanations and experimental demonstrations of the AIR and DAFP methods can be found in Horch et al. [52]. Below, we provide some important details related to their application to UTE-MRI on a clinical scanner.

Technical Challenges and Solutions

Distinguishing BW and PW signals is only part of the challenge in developing an effective MRI protocol to provide quantitative maps of BW or PW. As with any quantitative imaging method, scan times must be sufficiently short to mitigate the risk of motion artifacts but must be long enough to provide sufficient spatial resolution and signal-to-noise ratio (SNR) to allow accurate and precise BW/PW measurements. This is a particular challenge for UTE-MRI, which is often run as a 3D acquisition, and is a further challenge for adiabatic magnetization preparation schemes, which are limited (at the low end) in repetition time (TR) by specific absorption rate (SAR) considerations.

In the context of AIR and DAFP methods, two strategies have been implemented to address scan time challenges while providing sufficient spatial resolution for imaging cortical bone of the radius and the tibia. For 3D imaging, to achieve 1.2-mm (wrist) or 1.5-mm (tibia) isotropic resolution, previous work had acquired 20,000 or 33,782 radial spokes in the k-space per image [54]. To meet these sampling requirements while accommodating a relatively long TR ($\geq$400 ms), $N_{sp} = 16$ spokes of the k-space were acquired per TR, with a repetition time per spoke of $TR_A = 3.2$ ms (Fig. 32.4). To avoid amplitude modulation across these 16 spokes, a variable flip angle excitation scheme was used, with an initial excitation flip angle of 12.5° and an effective excitation angle of 60° [61].

To scan faster, increasing N_{sp} requires reduced flip angles, resulting in $SNR \approx N_s^{-1/2}$, so the choice of N_{sp} depends on the SNR and scan time requirements. The choice of N_S may also affect measurement accuracy because each spoke experiences a slightly different magnetization preparation. For the AIR sequence, each of the N_s spokes is acquired at a different TI and, therefore, includes a varying amount of non-nulled pore water signal. If the net PW signal across the N_{sp} spokes is zero, then this is not a problem, but increasing N_{sp} likely results in a greater net PW signal and corruption of the BW measurement. For the DAFP sequence, the recovery of BW magnetization increases with each spoke, so $N_{sp} \times TR_A$ should be kept small compared to the T_1 of BW.

Another approach to accelerating BW/PW imaging is to use a two-dimensional (2D) UTE acquisition. Naturally, encoding only 2D rather than 3D greatly reduces the number of spokes of the k-space that must be sampled, but 2D UTE brings about its own technical challenges. With conventional slice-selective excitation, the time needed to rephase magnetization across the slice imparts a lower limit on the achievable TE, which is likely to be beyond what is needed for UTE. An ingenious solution to this problem, devised by John Pauly, is to break the slice-selective excitation into two half-pulse excitations, each of which ends at the center of excitation k-space (i.e., magnetization within the slice is in phase). The complex signals resulting from each acquisition are added, and signals from inside the slice are added constructively, whereas the signals outside the slice are canceled [62]. No rephasing gradient is needed, and, so, the acquisition can start immediately after the excitation pulse is complete. However, the efficacy of half-pulse excitation is highly sensitive to gradient waveform inaccuracies.

Even on a well-tuned system, gradient waveform errors are likely to be large enough to introduce a significant out-of-slice signal into the image, and this error cannot be corrected

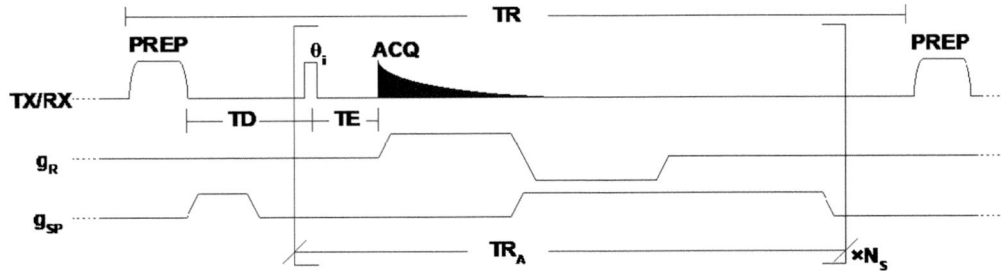

Fig. 32.4 The 3D UTE AIR or DAFP pulse sequence with multispoke acquisition. The PREP is a single adiabatic inversion pulse for AIR and two consecutive adiabatic inversion pulses for DAFP. The effective TI = TD + $TR_A \times N_{sp}/2$, where N_{sp} radial spokes are acquired with the period TR_A during each TR period. (Reproduced with permission from Manhard et al. [53])

at post-processing, even if the actual slice-selective gradient waveforms are known. One solution to this problem is to pre-distort the applied gradient waveform so that the actual gradient response closely matches the intended response [63]. A pre-distorted waveform can be computed with a constrained iterative procedure, involving repeated measurements of the actual gradient waveform and adjustments to the applied (i.e., pre-distorted) waveform [63]. This approach has been tested for axial 2D BW/PW UTE-MRI [64] and, recently, has been generalized for arbitrary slice orientations and offsets [65], making 2D BW/PW UTE-MRI a fast and versatile protocol.

In addition to scan time, care must be taken to ensure the accuracy and reproducibility of BW and PW measurements, and there are several sources of potential problems. First, a common step for quantitative MRI (qMRI) is to avoid or correct for B_1 inhomogeneity. To avoid problems with B_1^+ (transmit field) inhomogeneity, RF transmission can be performed with a body coil with the tissue of interest centrally positioned within the magnet. For signal reception, it is desirable to use a local coil to maximize SNR, but this also introduces significant variations in B_1^- (the receiver field). A relative B_1^- map can be quickly generated from the ratio of two images, one acquired with the body coil as the receiver and the other with the local coil, and this map can then be used to correct signal amplitudes of the AIR and DAFP images.

Second, another common step for qMRI, is signal amplitude normalization: cortical bone signals from an AIR or DAFP acquisition need to be normalized in order to provide a quantitatively meaningful value. One could normalize the signal amplitude from another tissue, such as nearby skeletal muscle or bone marrow, but variations in the proton density and/or T_1 within the reference tissue then contribute errors to bone measurements. A more robust approach is to use a reference water phantom, of known proton concentration and relaxation characteristics. A previous work has used a 10%/90% mixture of water (H_2O) and denatured water (D_2O) + 80 mM $CuSO_4$ to create a signal that is visible on both AIR and DAFP images [54]. For forearm and lower limb imaging, it is easy to place a phantom containing the reference fluid within the field of view.

The third step that is particular to qMRI of bone is to correct for the effect of the short T_2^* on signal amplitude. This is particularly important for the AIR imaging of BW because the BW of $T_2^* \approx 350$ μs is similar to the sampling duration of each spoke in the k-space. The relaxation-induced amplitude modulation in the k-space blurs the signal, resulting in reduction in the amplitudes of signals in voxels near bone-muscle/marrow boundaries. However, because the T_2^* of BW does not vary much across bone or between individuals, a relatively simple correction is possible. For a known image geometry, T_2^*, and k-space trajectory, the signal attenuation can be numerically estimated as follows: (1) a masked 2D bone image, $s(x, y)$ (bone signal = 1, all other signal equals 0) is Fourier-transformed to produce the k-space domain signal, $S(k_x, k_y)$; (2), $S(k_x, k_y)$ is then apodized to reflect the effect of T_2^* decay during acquisition; (3) the resulting apodized signal is inverse Fourier-transformed to produce a blurred image, $s_b(x, y)$; and, (4) the signal loss map is defined voxelwise as $\beta(x, y) \triangleq s_b(x, y)/s(x, y)$, which is then used to correct the AIR and DAFP signal intensities [53].

BW and PW as Surrogates of Cortical Bone Strength

Mechanical testing of cortical bone to determine material properties is inherently destructive and cannot be readily adapted to produce a clinical technique that assesses bone quality. Therefore, surrogate imaging markers of bone must be significantly correlated with material properties of bone if they are to inform on a patient's fracture risk. The first study to test for significant correlations between the material properties of human cortical bone (midshaft of the cadaveric femurs) and BW/PW involved low-field (0.64T) T_2^* relaxometry and quasi-static, load-to-failure tests of cortical beams in three-point bending [35]. Free induction decays were transformed by multi-exponential analysis, and concentrations of BW and PW (C_{bw} and C_{pw}, respectively) were computed from the summed signals in the $T_2^* = 0.15$–0.40 ms and $T_2^* = 1.5$–6 ms domains, respectively. C_{bw} and work-to-fracture per moment of inertia (i.e., toughness) were significantly lower for old donors (10 males between 67 and 87 years of age) compared with middle-aged donors (8 males between 47 and 59 years of age). In this cohort of male donors, C_{pw} and the ultimate stress of cortical bone in bending (i.e., bending strength) were not significantly different between the two age groups. Regardless, Pearson's correlation coefficients (r values) between C_{bw} and the two material properties were positive and significant at the 95% confidence level (toughness $r = +0.64$ and bending strength $r = +0.60$), whereas Pearson's r between C_{pw} and bending strength was negative and significant at the 90% confidence level ($r = -0.456$). C_{pw} did not significantly correlate with toughness in this initial study [35].

A subsequent study involved three-point bending tests of human cortical bone from the midshaft of cadaveric femurs (26 male and 14 female donors between 21 and 105 years of age) and multi-exponential T_2 analysis of CPMG measurements acquired at 4.7 T. Values of C_{bw} and C_{pw} were computed from summed signals in the $T_2 = 0.15$–1 ms and $T_2 = 1.0$–1000 ms, domains, respectively [37]. In this study, Pearson's r between C_{bw} and bending strength was positive and significant at a 95% confidence level ($r = +0.82$); however, unlike the previous study involving T_2^*, C_{pw} significantly and negatively correlated with bending strength ($r = -0.78$). Notably, micro-CT (μCT)-derived measurements of volumetric BMD (isotropic voxel size = 6 μm) also significantly correlated with bending strength ($r = +0.66$), but the combination of all ^{1}H signals did not. In a follow-up study, C_{bw} and C_{pw} positively and negatively, respectively, correlated with crack initiation toughness (K_{init}) as determined by R-curve testing of human cortical bone (Spearman's $r = +0.63$ and $r = -0.53$, respectively) [66]. With cortical bone samples from the midshaft of 62 cadaveric femurs (30 male and 32 female donors between 21 and 101 years of age), general linear regression models were fit to the data, including donor age. Age and C_{pw} were negative contributors and C_{bw} was a positive contributor to the prediction of K_{init} and explained 47.0% of its variance. For comparison, age (a negative contributor) and μCT-derived volumetric BMD (a positive contributor) explained 40.8% of the variance in K_{init}. Although C_{bw} was weakly correlated with C_{pw}, they were independent predictors of the fracture toughness of human cortical bone.

The previously cited studies measured C_{bw} and C_{pw} of isolated bone specimens without imaging, but since the publication of the earliest two of those studies, several MRI measures of BW and/or PW have reported correlations with bone mechanical properties. Following our T_2-derived non-imaging studies of BW and PW [37, 66], we conducted two studies comparing the mechanical properties of cortical bone to AIR and DAFP UTE-MRI measures of BW and PW, respectively [67, 68]. In the first study [67], 3D maps of C_{bw} and C_{pw} were generated from cadaveric forearms (20 male and 20 female donors between 56 and 97 years of age) using a 3 T human scanner. Subsequently, soft tissue was removed and the distal one-third of the radius was loaded to failure in three-point bending. Ultimate stress significantly correlated with the mean C_{bw} (Spearman's $r = +0.56$) and the mean C_{pw} (Spearman's $r = -0.68$), though the strength of correlation coefficients depended on the contouring of the region of interest on the endosteal surface (i.e., how cortical bone was masked from the medullary canal). Other metrics of the maps such as skewness also correlated with this measure of the bending strength of cortical bone as did both areal and volumetric BMD. In multivariable linear regression models, the median C_{pw} combined with the mean C_{bw} explained 63.5% of the variance in ultimate stress (i.e., bending strength = $-0.566 \times C_{pw} + 0.372 \times C_{bw}$, where the coefficients were standardized to convey relative contributions).

Because three-point bending of the human radius does not exactly adhere to the assumptions of beam theory that provide the equation to determine ultimate stress, we subsequently acquired AIR and DAFP UTE-MRI scans of another set of cadaveric forearms (14 male and 15 female donors between 57 and 84 years of age) for finite element analysis (FEA) and experimentally evaluated the radii with a three-point bending test [68]. Finite element models of each bone scan were generated using tetrahedral elements, and the open-source solver FEBio Studio [69] was used to simulate the same experimental three-point bending tests. The material behavior of the bone was described with an elastic, perfectly plastic stress–strain model defined by the elastic modulus, E, the yield stress, Y, and Poisson's ratio = 0.3. Simulations were run iteratively to find values for E and Y in each bone to best match experimental force vs. displacement curves, and, then, linear regression was used to relate these material properties to the mean UTE-MRI measures of C_{bw} and C_{pw} as follows:

$$E = 0.39(\pm 0.08)C_{bw} + 0.05(\pm 0.04)C_{pw} + 2.06(\pm 1.88)\,(32.1)$$

$$Y = 6.6(\pm 1.17)C_{bw} + 0.15(\pm 0.53)C_{pw} + 29.71(\pm 26.74)(32.2)$$

where E is in units of GPa, Y is in units of MPa, and both C_{pw} and C_{bw} are in units of mol ^{1}H per liter of bone. To the best of our knowledge, these are the first-described empirical relationships between UTE-MRI markers and material properties using FEA.

The FEA simulations were then rerun to predict the force vs. displacement response of each radius in three cases: (a) all elements with an elastic modulus of 8.66 GPa and yield stress of 131.88 MPa, values selected to provide the highest

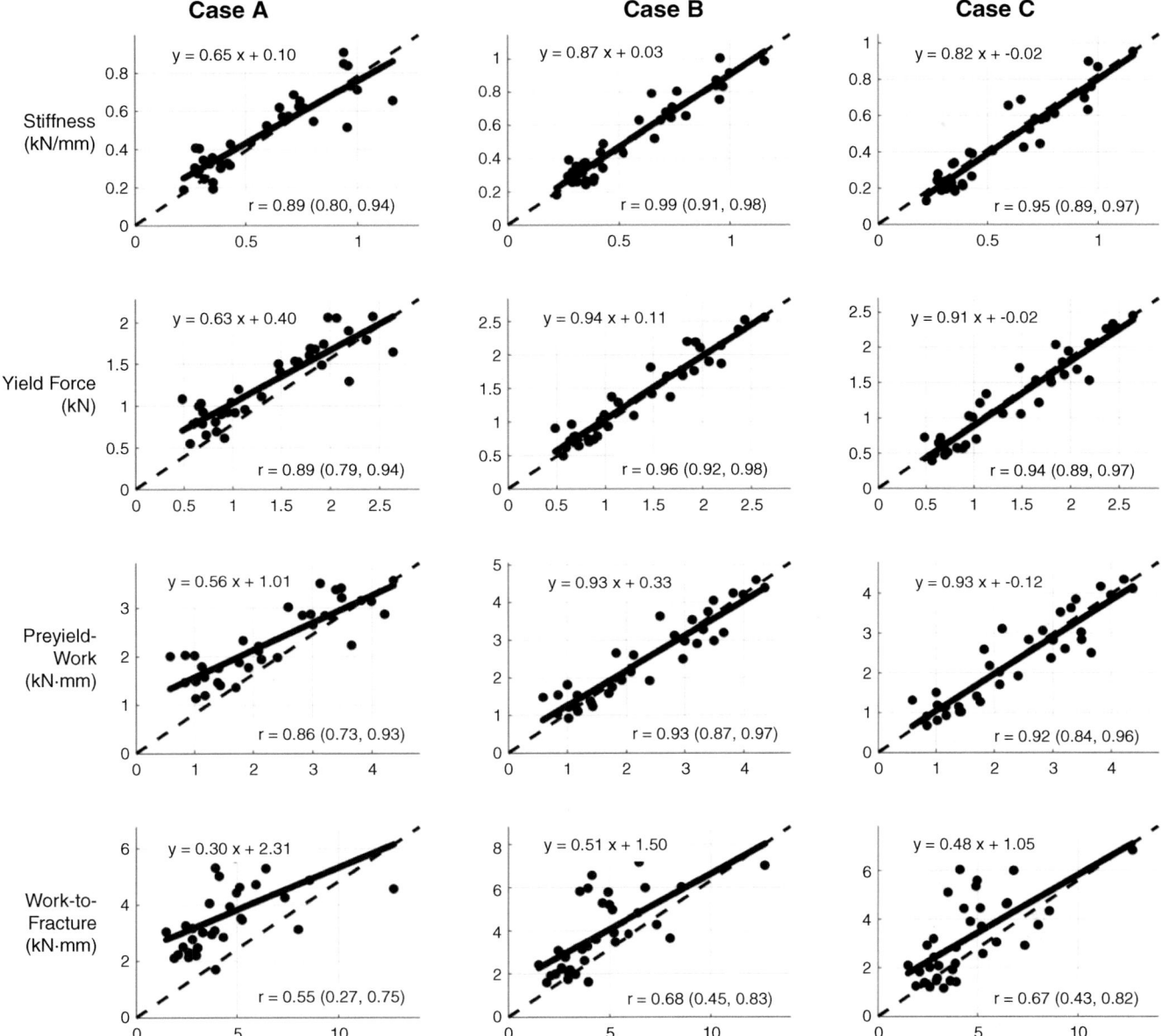

Fig. 32.5 Correlations between measured mechanical data (X-axis) and FEA-predicted mechanical data (Y-axis) in three different cases for defining the modulus and yield stress. Case A: homogeneous tissue properties; case B: homogeneous tissue properties derived from the mean values of C_{bw} and C_{pw}; and case C: heterogeneous tissue properties derived from 3D maps of C_{bw} and C_{pw}. (Reproduced with permission from Ketsiri et al. [68])

correlation between FEA and mechanical tests, on average, (b) all elements for each bone with an elastic modulus and yield stress computed from the above equations using the mean values of C_{bw} and C_{pw}, and (c) each element of each bone with its own elastic modulus and yield strength based on the same equations and 3D maps of C_{bw} and C_{pw}. For each case, FEA significantly predicted bending stiffness, yield force, pre-yield work, and work-to-fracture (Fig. 32.5). Without BW and PW informing the material properties in the FEA simulations (case A), the predictions of the structural-dependent mechanical properties of the radius departed from

unity (predicted y = actual y). Except for work-to-fracture, the predictions of the mechanical properties matched unity when the material properties were informed by BW and PW (case B and case C). However, the heterogeneous distribution of the material properties (case C) did not improve the predictions over the homogeneous distribution (case B). The inability of our UTE-derived FEA to accurately predict work-to-fracture is not surprising because the elastic, perfectly plastic model that we incorporated in the FEA does not simulate fracture (only constant stress during inelastic strain). Further studies are needed to determine whether C_{bw}

and C_{pw} can inform a damage model of the stress vs. strain behavior in FEA that simulates the failure of elements at a given inelastic strain (i.e., stress within element equals zero at BW and/or PW-derived failure strain).

Other UTE-MRI studies have used bi- and tri-component methods to relate BW/PW to the mechanical properties of bone. Upon acquiring cadaveric distal femurs and tibiae (seven male and seven female donors between 23 and 90 years of age), Bae et al. generated beams of cortical bone for bicomponent UTE-MRI (3T, whole-body scanner), µCT imaging (isotropic voxel size = 9 µm), and quasi-static, load-to-failure testing (four-point bending) [55]. The results showed that bending strength significantly correlated with C_{bw} ($r = -0.47$) but not C_{pw}. In a follow-up study by the same group, bi- (BW/PW) and tri-component (BW/PW/fat) analyses of 3D UTE-derived T_2^* signals from 135 cortical bone samples (18 male and 19 female donors) were evaluated in comparison to 4-point bending tests [70]. The results showed that bending strength significantly correlated with bicomponent BW/PW signal fractions ($r = +/-0.54$) and tricomponent BW/PW/fat signal fractions ($r = +0.62/-0.57/-0.46$). It should be noted that this latter study only reported signal fractions (i.e., sum fractions = 1) not concentrations, C_{bw} or C_{pw}. Nonetheless, both studies support the ability of UTE-MRI markers of BW and PW obtained using multi-exponential T_2^* analysis to assess the fracture resistance of bone.

Because cortical porosity is a known determinant of bone strength [71], at least two studies have evaluated indirect measures of PW content as predictors of the mechanical properties of bone. Jones et al. measured an index of porosity (ratio of images acquired at two TEs, see Chap. 34) from UTE-MRI at 3 T in cadaveric proximal femurs (10 male donors between 44 and 93 years of age and 5 female donors between 65 and 81 years) and then subjected the proximal femurs to a mechanical test that replicated a sideways fall [72]. The porosity index in a region of the proximal midshaft inferior to the lesser trochanter significantly correlated with stiffness of the femoral neck ($r = -0.82$), whereas the correlation between CT-derived volumetric BMD and stiffness resulted in a significant but lower correlation coefficient ($r = +0.58$). Moreover, although not using UTE, another recent study has measured T_1 with conventional MRI as a surrogate measure of PW content [73]. With this approach, their study of the bovine tibia found that toughness and ultimate stress significantly correlated with T_1 ($r = -0.77$ and $r = -0.71$, respectively) when measured by a variable flip angle.

Determinants of BW and PW in Cortical Bone

As described in detail in our review of the water compartments of bone [74], water resides in the vascular channels and in the lacunar–canalicular network (LCN) and includes the cellular connections of osteocytes, which are the bone-residing cells responsible for mineral homeostasis and responsiveness of bone to microdamage and changes in mechanical loading. UTE imaging markers of PW indicate the level of porosity in cortical bone. One of the first applications of ^1H NMR relaxometry to bone was the assessment of porosity [31, 32]. Since the relaxation rate of the transverse spin state of ^1H following a perturbation depends on the surface area-to-volume ratio of a given pore in which water resides, the T_2 spectrum of cortical bone is a broad distribution of peaks with LCN water relaxing faster than water in Haversian's and Volkmann's canals. Utilizing this phenomenon, Wang and Ni [32] found a strong correlation between PW and cortical porosity (Pearson's $r = +0.85$) by histomorphometry (void area per total area) for cortical bone samples from 19 cadaveric femurs (16–89 years). In their low-field NMR study using CPMG measurements of T_2 signals, "lacunar water" (void area/bone area = ~1.9%) relaxed with $T_2 = $ ~0.2–8 ms and "'Haversian water" (void area/bone area = ~5–25%) relaxed with $T_2 = 9$–200 ms. A strong correlation between PW, specifically total water minus BW, and cortical porosity, as determined by µCT, has also been observed with high-field NMR (9.4T) measurements [75].

Numerous studies involving a variety of UTE imaging markers of PW report direct correlations with CT-derived measurements of cortical porosity [67, 70, 76–80]. In addition, imaging markers of total water ^1H concentration or density also correlate with cortical porosity [81, 82]. There has been one study to date reporting significantly higher PW in patients with osteoporosis (OP) than in patients with osteoarthritis (OA). Porrelli et al. [83] used low-field NMR (0.47 T) to acquire pulsed gradient spin echo measurements, CPMG measurements, and free induction decay (FID) intensity from trabecular bone cores that were acquired from discarded proximal femurs. These patient samples came from hemiarthroplasty cases involving femoral neck fracture ($N = 35$ for the OP group) and total hip arthroplasty cases involving arthritic pain ($N = 29$ for the OA group). Their unitless measurement of PW (i.e., porosity) was significantly higher in OP (83.5 ± 12.3) than in OA (70 ± 16).

What determines BW of bone is less understood than PW [74]. BW primarily arises from hydrogen bonds between water and the hydrophilic residues of proteins, namely, collagen I, and is dependent on the amount of organic matrix in a given volume of bone. In our ex vivo manipulation study of human cortical bone, removing protein with sodium hypochlorite (96 h) removes the volume fraction of BW(V_{bw}/V_{bone}) going from an initial 10–24% to 15%–5% [84]. μCT-derived tissue mineral density did not change. In addition, post-sodium hypochlorite volume fraction strongly correlated with the remaining organic fraction (Pearson's $r = +0.970$) as determined by gravimetric measurements (100 × (air-dry mass − ash mass)/air-dry mass). In this same study, we also found that ribose incubation at 37 °C for 4 weeks to accumulate advanced glycation end products (AGEs) in cortical bone samples significantly, but modestly, decreased V_{bw}/V_{bone}, whereas thermal denaturation significantly increased V_{bw}/V_{bone} (more so than the age-related decrease). As confirmed by Raman spectroscopy, ribose incubation constricted the helical coils of collagen I, whereas thermal denaturation uncoiled the helices, exposing more hydroxyproline to hydrogen bonding with water [84].

Since glycosaminoglycans (GAGs) are negatively charged, their quantity in bone is another potential contributor to BW levels as well as to the toughness of cortical bone [85–87]. In a series of studies by Wang et al., a decrease in GAGs decreased BW; enzymatic removal of GAGs affected the in situ toughness of wet cortical bone but not dry cortical bone [85]; GAG staining, in situ toughness of wet cortical bone (femur midshaft), and low-field, T_2^*-derived BW of cortical bone decreased with donor age (young: 26 ± 6 years, middle-aged: 52 ± 5 years, and elderly: 73 ± 5 years). BW significantly correlated with the quantity of GAGs (Pearson's $r = +0.660$) [86]. Global deficiency in biglycan, a protein that binds to GAGs in Bgn knockout mice compared to wild-type mice, was associated with reduced GAG content and low-field, T_2^*-derived BW [87].

The surface of bone mineral crystals includes positive (Ca^{2+}) and negative charges (PO_4^{3-}) and, so, is also believed to interact with water [88]. In a seminal study of the physicochemical properties of cortical bone, Robinson reported that the mineralization of osteoid displaces bound water [89]. In our μCT and high-field NMR studies of rodent cortical bone, which does not experience much remodeling (i.e., turnover by the coupled actions of osteoclasts and osteoblasts), we observed an age-related increase and decrease in tissue mineral density and V_{bw}/V_{bone}, respectively, in rat femur midshaft [90] and in mouse femur [91]. While the increase in the degree of mineralization of cortical bone as rodents age from 6 to 20 or 24 months could be the reason BW decreased, pentosidine, an AGE cross-link, also increased in these studies. Our current working hypothesis is that BW concentration in adult cortical bone primarily depends on the proportions of organic matrix and GAGs but is modulated by

the degree of mineralization and collagen I helical constriction. The former is a function of bone turnover, and the latter is a balance between time-dependent, nonenzymatic, glycation-mediated posttranslational modifications (e.g., carboxymethyllysine, deamidation) and damage-induced denaturation.

References

1. Blume SW, Curtis JR. Medical costs of osteoporosis in the elderly Medicare population. Osteoporosis Int. 2011;22(6):1835–44.
2. Hernlund E, Svedbom A, Ivergård M, Compston J, Cooper C, Stenmark J, McCloskey EV, Jönsson B, Kanis JA. Osteoporosis in the European Union: medical management, epidemiology and economic burden. A report prepared in collaboration with the international osteoporosis foundation (IOF) and the European Federation of Pharmaceutical Industry Associations (EFPIA). Arch Osteoporos. 2013;8(1–2):136.
3. Gullberg B, Johnell O, Kanis JA. World-wide projections for hip fracture. Osteoporosis Int. 1997;7(5):407–13.
4. Hui SL, Slemenda CW, Johnston CC. Age and bone mass as predictors of fracture in a prospective study. J Clin Invest. 1988;81(6):1804–9.
5. Ott SM. When bone mass fails to predict bone failure. Calcified Tissue Int. 1993;53(Suppl 1):S7–S13.
6. Schuit SCE, Klift MVD, Weel AEAM, de Laet CEDH, Burger H, Seeman E, Hofman A, Uitterlinden AG, van Leeuwen JPTM, Pols HAP. Fracture incidence and association with bone mineral density in elderly men and women: the Rotterdam study. Bone. 2004;34(1):195–202.
7. Nyman JS, Roy A, Shen X, Acuna RL, Tyler JH, Wang X. The influence of water removal on the strength and toughness of cortical bone. J Biomech. 2006;39(5):931–8.
8. Zioupos P, Currey JD, Hamer AJ. The role of collagen in the declining mechanical properties of aging human cortical bone. J Biomed Mater Res. 1999;45(2):108–16.
9. Wang X, Shen X, Li X, Agrawal CM. Age-related changes in the collagen network and toughness of bone. Bone. 2002;31(1):1–7.
10. Oxlund H, Barckman M, Ørtoft G, Andreassen TT. Reduced concentrations of collagen cross-links are associated with reduced strength of bone. Bone. 1995;17(4):S365–71.
11. Manske SL, Liu-Ambrose T, Bakker PMD, Liu D, Kontulainen S, Guy P, Oxland TR, McKay HA. Femoral neck cortical geometry measured with magnetic resonance imaging is associated with proximal femur strength. Osteoporosis Int. 2006;17(10):1539–45.
12. Black DM, Bouxsein ML, Marshall LM, Cummings SR, Lang TF, Cauley JA, Ensrud KE, Nielson CM, Orwoll ES. Proximal femoral structure and the prediction of hip fracture in men: a large prospective study using QCT. J Bone Miner Res. 2008;23(8):1326–33.
13. Bouxsein ML. Technology insight: noninvasive assessment of bone strength in osteoporosis. Nat Clin Pract Rheum. 2008;4(6):310–8.
14. Augat P, Reeb H, Claes LE. Prediction of fracture load at different skeletal sites by geometric properties of the cortical shell. J Bone Miner Res. 1996;11(9):1356–63.
15. Szulc P, Duboeuf F, Schott AM, Dargent-Molina P, Meunier PJ, Delmas PD. Structural determinants of hip fracture in elderly women: re-analysis of the data from the EPIDOS study. Osteoporosis Int. 2006;17(2):231–6.
16. Keyak JH, Rossi SA, Jones KA, Skinner HB. Prediction of femoral fracture load using automated finite element modeling. J Biomech. 1997;31(2):125–33.

17. Pistoia W, Rietbergen BV, Lochmüller EM, Lill CA, Eckstein F, Rüegsegger P. Estimation of distal radius failure load with micro-finite element analysis models based on three-dimensional peripheral quantitative computed tomography images. Bone. 2002;30(6):842–8.

18. Crawford RP, Cann CE, Keaveny TM. Finite element models predict in vitro vertebral body compressive strength better than quantitative computed tomography. Bone. 2003;33(4):744–50.

19. Riggs BL, Melton LJ, Robb RA, Camp JJ, Atkinson EJ, Oberg AL, Rouleau PA, McCollough CH, Khosla S, Bouxsein ML. Population-based analysis of the relationship of whole bone strength indices and fall-related loads to age- and sex-specific patterns of hip and wrist fractures. J Bone Miner Res. 2006;21(2):315–23.

20. Bouxsein ML, Melton LJ, Riggs BL, Muller J, Atkinson EJ, Oberg AL, Robb RA, Camp JJ, Rouleau PA, McCollough CH, Khosla S. Age- and sex-specific differences in the factor of risk for vertebral fracture: a population-based study using QCT. J Bone Miner Res. 2006;21(9):1475–82.

21. Keaveny TM, Clarke BL, Cosman F, Orwoll ES, Siris ES, Khosla S, Bouxsein ML. Biomechanical computed tomography analysis (BCT) for clinical assessment of osteoporosis. Osteoporosis Int. 2020;31(6):1025–48.

22. Liu XS, Stein EM, Zhou B, Zhang CA, Nickolas TL, Cohen A, Thomas V, McMahon DJ, Cosman F, Nieves J, Shane E, Guo XE. Individual trabecula segmentation (ITS)-based morphological analyses and microfinite element analysis of HR-pQCT images discriminate postmenopausal fragility fractures independent of DXA measurements. J Bone Miner Res. 2012;27(2):263–72.

23. Nishiyama KK, Macdonald HM, Hanley DA, Boyd SK. Women with previous fragility fractures can be classified based on bone microarchitecture and finite element analysis measured with HR-pQCT. Osteoporosis Int. 2013;24(5):1733–40.

24. Chang G, Honig S, Liu Y, Chen C, Chu KK, Rajapakse CS, Egol K, Xia D, Saha PK, Regatte RR. 7 Tesla MRI of bone microarchitecture discriminates between women without and with fragility fractures who do not differ by bone mineral density. J Bone Miner Metab. 2015;33(3):285–93.

25. Zioupos P. Ageing human bone: factors affecting its biomechanical properties and the role of collagen. J Biomater Appl. 2001;15(3):187–229.

26. Sedlin ED, Hirsch C. Factors affecting the determination of the physical properties of femoral cortical bone. Acta Orthop Scand. 1966;37(1):29–48.

27. McCalden RW, McGeough JA, Barker MB, Court-Brown CM. Age-related changes in the tensile properties of cortical bone. The relative importance of changes in porosity, mineralization, and microstructure. J Bone Joint Surg Am. 1993;75(8):1193–205.

28. Zebaze RM, Ghasem-Zadeh A, Bohte A, Iuliano-Burns S, Mirams M, Price RI, Mackie EJ, Seeman E. Intracortical remodelling and porosity in the distal radius and post-mortem femurs of women: a cross-sectional study. Lancet. 2010;375(9727):1729–36.

29. Burghardt AJ, Kazakia GJ, Ramachandran S, Link TM, Majumdar S. Age- and gender-related differences in the geometric properties and biomechanical significance of intracortical porosity in the distal radius and tibia. J Bone Miner Res. 2010;25(5):983–93.

30. Fernández-Seara MA, Wehrli SL, Takahashi M, Wehrli FW. Water content measured by proton-deuteron exchange NMR predicts bone mineral density and mechanical properties. J Bone Miner Res. 2004;19(2):289–96.

31. Fantazzini P, Brown RJS, Borgia GC. Bone tissue and porous media: common features and differences studied by NMR relaxation. Magn Reson Imaging. 2003;21(3–4):227–34.

32. Wang X, Ni Q. Determination of cortical bone porosity and pore size distribution using a low field pulsed NMR approach. J Orthopaed Res. 2003;21(2):312–9.

33. Ni Q, King JD, Wang X. The characterization of human compact bone structure changes by low-field nuclear magnetic resonance. Meas Sci Technol. 2004;15(1):58.

34. Ni Q, Nyman JS, Wang X, Santos ADL, Nicolella DP. Assessment of water distribution changes in human cortical bone by nuclear magnetic resonance. Meas Sci Technol. 2007;18(3):715.

35. Nyman JS, Ni Q, Nicolella DP, Wang X. Measurements of mobile and bound water by nuclear magnetic resonance correlate with mechanical properties of bone. Bone. 2008;42(1):193–9.

36. Horch RA, Nyman JS, Gochberg DF, Dortch RD, Does MD. Characterization of 1H NMR signal in human cortical bone for magnetic resonance imaging. Magnet Reson Med. 2010;64(3):680–7.

37. Horch RA, Gochberg DF, Nyman JS, Does MD. Non-invasive predictors of human cortical bone mechanical properties: T_2-discriminated 1H NMR compared with high resolution X-ray. PLoS One. 2011;6(1):e16359.

38. Ketsiri T, Uppuganti S, Harkins KD, Gochberg DF, Nyman JS, Does MD. T_1 relaxation of bound and pore water in cortical bone. NMR Biomed. 2022;36:e4878.

39. Robson MD, Bydder GM. Clinical ultrashort echo time imaging of bone and other connective tissues. NMR Biomed. 2006;19(7):765–80.

40. Reichert ILH, Robson MD, Gatehouse PD, He T, Chappell KE, Holmes J, Girgis S, Bydder GM. Magnetic resonance imaging of cortical bone with ultrashort TE pulse sequences. Magn Reson Imaging. 2005;23(5):611–8.

41. Robson MD, Gatehouse PD, Bydder M, Bydder GM. Magnetic resonance: an introduction to ultrashort TE (UTE) imaging. J Comput Assist Tomogr. 2003;27(6):825–46.

42. Du J, Hamilton G, Takahashi A, Bydder M, Chung CB. Ultrashort echo time spectroscopic imaging (UTESI) of cortical bone. Magnet Reson Med. 2007;58(5):1001–9.

43. Techawiboonwong A, Song HK, Leonard MB, Wehrli FW. Cortical bone water: in vivo quantification with ultrashort echo-time MR imaging1. Radiology. 2008;248(3):824–33.

44. Techawiboonwong A, Song HK, Wehrli FW. In vivo MRI of sub-millisecond T_2 species with two-dimensional and three-dimensional radial sequences and applications to the measurement of cortical bone water. NMR Biomed. 2008;21(1):59–70.

45. Du J, Carl M, Bydder M, Takahashi A, Chung CB, Bydder GM. Qualitative and quantitative ultrashort echo time (UTE) imaging of cortical bone. J Magn Reson. 2010;207(2):304–11.

46. Wehrli FW. Structural and functional assessment of trabecular and cortical bone by micro magnetic resonance imaging. J Magn Reson Imaging. 2007;25(2):390–409.

47. Krug R, Carballido-Gamio J, Burghardt AJ, Kazakia G, Hyun BH, Jobke B, Banerjee S, Huber M, Link TM, Majumdar S. Assessment of trabecular bone structure comparing magnetic resonance imaging at 3 Tesla with high-resolution peripheral quantitative computed tomography ex vivo and in vivo. Osteoporosis Int. 2008;19(5):653–61.

48. Folkesson J, Goldenstein J, Carballido-Gamio J, Kazakia G, Burghardt AJ, Rodriguez A, Krug R, de Papp AE, Link TM, Majumdar S. Longitudinal evaluation of the effects of alendronate on MRI bone microarchitecture in postmenopausal osteopenic women. Bone. 2011;48(3):611–21.

49. Rajapakse CS, Leonard MB, Bhagat YA, Sun W, Magland JF, Wehrli FW. Micro–MR imaging–based computational biomechanics demonstrates reduction in cortical and trabecular bone strength after renal transplantation. Radiology. 2012;262(3):912–20.

50. Chang G, Rajapakse CS, Regatte RR, Babb J, Saxena A, Belmont HM, Honig S. 3 tesla MRI detects deterioration in proximal femur microarchitecture and strength in long-term glucocorticoid users compared with controls. J Magn Reson Imaging. 2015;42(6):1489.

51. Rad HS, Lam SCB, Magland JF, Ong H, Li C, Song HK, Love J, Wehrli FW. Quantifying cortical bone water in vivo by three-dimensional ultra-short echo-time MRI. NMR Biomed. 2011;24(7):855–64.

52. Horch RA, Gochberg DF, Nyman JS, Does MD. Clinically compatible MRI strategies for discriminating bound and pore water in cortical bone. Magnet Reson Med. 2012;68(6):1774–84.

53. Manhard MK, Horch RA, Harkins KD, Gochberg DF, Nyman JS, Does MD. Validation of quantitative bound- and pore-water imaging in cortical bone. Magnet Reson Med. 2014;71(6):2166–71.

54. Manhard MK, Horch RA, Gochberg DF, Nyman JS, Does MD. In vivo quantitative MR imaging of bound and pore water in cortical bone. Radiology. 2015;277(1):221–9.

55. Bae WC, Chen PC, Chung CB, Masuda K, D'Lima D, Du J. Quantitative ultrashort echo time (UTE) MRI of human cortical bone: correlation with porosity and biomechanical properties. J Bone Miner Res. 2012;27(4):848–57.

56. Biswas R, Bae W, Diaz E, Masuda K, Chung CB, Bydder GM, Du J. Ultrashort echo time (UTE) imaging with bi-component analysis: bound and free water evaluation of bovine cortical bone subject to sequential drying. Bone. 2012;50(3):749–55.

57. Chen J, Carl M, Ma Y, Shao H, Lu X, Chen B, Chang EY, Wu Z, Du J. Fast volumetric imaging of bound and pore water in cortical bone using three-dimensional ultrashort-TE (UTE) and inversion recovery UTE sequences. NMR Biomed. 2016;29(10):1373–80.

58. Lu X, Jerban S, Wan L, Ma Y, Jang H, Le N, Yang W, Chang EY, Du J. Three-dimensional ultrashort echo time imaging with tricomponent analysis for human cortical bone. Magnet Reson Med. 2019;82(1):348–55.

59. Larson PEZ, Conolly SM, Pauly JM, Nishimura DG. Using adiabatic inversion pulses for long-T_2 suppression in ultrashort echo time (UTE) imaging. Magnet Reson Med. 2007;58(5):952–61.

60. Du J, Bydder M, Takahashi AM, Carl M, Chung CB, Bydder GM. Short T_2 contrast with three-dimensional ultrashort echo time imaging. Magn Reson Imaging. 2011;29(4):470–82.

61. Haacke EM, Brown RW, Thompson MR, Venkatesan R. Magnetic resonance imaging: physical principles and sequence design. Wiley; 1999.

62. Pauly JM. Selective excitation for ultrashort echo time imaging. eMagRes. 2012.

63. Harkins KD, Does MD, Grissom WA. Iterative method for pre-distortion of MRI gradient waveforms. IEEE T Med Imaging. 2014;33(8):1641–7.

64. Manhard MK, Harkins KD, Gochberg DF, Nyman JS, Does MD. 30-second bound and pore water concentration mapping of cortical bone using 2D UTE with optimized half-pulses. Magnet Reson Med. 2017;77(3):945–50.

65. Harkins KD, Ketsiri T, Nyman JS, Does MD. Fast bound and pore water mapping of cortical bone with arbitrary slice oriented two-dimensional ultra-short echo time. Magn Reson Med. 2023;89(2):767–73.

66. Granke M, Makowski AJ, Uppuganti S, Does MD, Nyman JS. Identifying novel clinical surrogates to assess human bone fracture toughness. J Bone Miner Res. 2015;30(7):1290–300.

67. Manhard MK, Uppuganti S, Granke M, Gochberg DF, Nyman JS, Does MD. MRI-derived bound and pore water concentrations as predictors of fracture resistance. Bone. 2016;87:1–10.

68. Ketsiri T, Uppuganti S, Harkins KD, Gochberg DF, Nyman JS, Does MD. Finite element analysis of bone mechanical properties using MRI-derived bound and pore water concentration maps. Comput Method Biomec. 2022:1–12.

69. Maas SA, Ellis BJ, Ateshian GA, Weiss JA. FEBio: finite elements for biomechanics. J Biomech Eng. 2012;134(1):011005.

70. Jerban S, Lu X, Dorthe EW, Alenezi S, Ma Y, Kakos L, Jang H, Sah RL, Chang EY, D'Lima D, Du J. Correlations of cortical bone microstructural and mechanical properties with water proton frac-

tions obtained from ultrashort echo time (UTE) MRI tricomponent T_2* model. NMR Biomed. 2020;33(3):e4233.

71. Mirzaali MJ, Schwiedrzik JJ, Thaiwichai S, Best JP, Michler J, Zysset PK, Wolfram U. Mechanical properties of cortical bone and their relationships with age, gender, composition and microindentation properties in the elderly. Bone. 2016;93:196–211.

72. Jones BC, Jia S, Lee H, Feng A, Shetye SS, Batzdorf A, Shapira N, Noël PB, Pleshko N, Rajapakse CS. MRI-derived porosity index is associated with whole-bone stiffness and mineral density in human cadaveric femora. Bone. 2021;143:115774.

73. Talebi M, Abbasi-Rad S, Malekzadeh M, Shahgholi M, Ardakani AA, Foudeh K, Rad HS. Cortical bone mechanical assessment via free water Relaxometry at 3T. J Magn Reson Imaging. 2021;54(6):1744–51.

74. Granke M, Does MD, Nyman JS. The role of water compartments in the material properties of cortical bone. Calcified Tissue Int. 2015;97(3):292–307.

75. Ong HH, Wright AC, Wehrli FW. Deuterium nuclear magnetic resonance unambiguously quantifies pore and collagen-bound water in cortical bone. J Bone Miner Res. 2012;27(12):2573–81.

76. Li C, Seifert AC, Rad HS, Bhagat YA, Rajapakse CS, Sun W, Lam SCB, Wehrli FW. Cortical bone water concentration: dependence of MR imaging measures on age and pore volume fraction. Radiology. 2014;272(3):796–806.

77. Seifert AC, Wehrli SL, Wehrli FW. Bi-component T_2* analysis of bound and pore bone water fractions fails at high field strengths. NMR Biomed. 2015;28(7):861–72.

78. Chen J, Grogan SP, Shao H, D'Lima D, Bydder GM, Wu Z, Du J. Evaluation of bound and pore water in cortical bone using ultrashort-TE MRI. NMR Biomed. 2015;28(12):1754–62.

79. Jerban S, Ma Y, Wong JH, Nazaran A, Searleman A, Wan L, Williams J, Du J, Chang EY. Ultrashort echo time magnetic resonance imaging (UTE-MRI) of cortical bone correlates well with histomorphometric assessment of bone microstructure. Bone. 2019;123:8–17.

80. Jerban S, Ma Y, Li L, Jang H, Wan L, Guo T, Searleman A, Chang EY, Du J. Volumetric mapping of bound and pore water as well as collagen protons in cortical bone using 3D ultrashort echo time cones MR imaging techniques. Bone. 2019;127:120–8.

81. Seifert AC, Li C, Wehrli SL, Wehrli FW. A surrogate measure of cortical bone matrix density by long T_2-suppressed MRI. J Bone Miner Res. 2015;30(12):2229–38.

82. Jerban S, Ma Y, Jang H, Namiranian B, Le N, Shirazian H, Murphy ME, Du J, Chang EY. Water proton density in human cortical bone obtained from ultrashort echo time (UTE) MRI predicts bone microstructural properties. Magn Reson Imaging. 2020;67:85–9.

83. Porrelli D, Abrami M, Pelizzo P, Formentin C, Ratti C, Turco G, Grassi M, Canton G, Grassi G, Murena L. Trabecular bone porosity and pore size distribution in osteoporotic patients—a low field nuclear magnetic resonance and microcomputed tomography investigation. J Mech Behav Biomed. 2022;125:104933.

84. Nyman JS, Uppuganti S, Unal M, Leverant CJ, Adabala S, Granke M, Voziyan P, Does MD. Manipulating the amount and structure of the organic matrix affects the water compartments of human cortical bone. Jbmr Plus. 2019;3(6):e10135.

85. Wang X, Xu H, Huang Y, Gu S, Jiang JX. Coupling effect of water and proteoglycans on the in situ toughness of bone. J Bone Miner Res. 2016;31(5):1026–9.

86. Wang X, Hua R, Ahsan A, Ni Q, Huang Y, Gu S, Jiang JX. Age-related deterioration of bone toughness is related to diminishing amount of matrix glycosaminoglycans (GAGs). Jbmr Plus. 2018;2(3):164–73.

87. Hua R, Ni Q, Eliason TD, Han Y, Gu S, Nicolella DP, Wang X, Jiang JX. Biglycan and chondroitin sulfate play pivotal roles in bone toughness via retaining bound water in bone mineral matrix. Matrix Biol. 2020;94:95–109.

88. Timmins PA, Wall JC. Bone water Calc Tiss Res. 1977;23(1):1–5.
89. Robinson RA. Physicochemical structure of bone. Clin Orthop Relat R. 1975;112:263–315.
90. Uppuganti S, Granke M, Makowski AJ, Does MD, Nyman JS. Age-related changes in the fracture resistance of male Fischer F344 rat bone. Bone. 2016;83:220–32.

91. Creecy A, Uppuganti S, Girard MR, Schlunk SG, Amah C, Granke M, Unal M, Does MD, Nyman JS. The age-related decrease in material properties of BALB/c mouse long bones involves alterations to the extracellular matrix. Bone. 2020;130:115126.

Chamith S. Rajapakse and Brandon C. Jones

Introduction

Osteoporosis is a major health issue that affects an estimated 200 million people worldwide [1] and causes 2 million fractures per annum in the United States [2]. The Global Burden of Disease study found that, from 1990 to 2019, there was a 33% increase in bone fracture incidence and a 65% increase in fracture-related disability years [3], and this trend is expected to continue with aging of populations [4, 5]. Clinically, osteoporosis is diagnosed by radiographic evaluation of bone mineral density (BMD) performed via dual-energy X-ray absorptiometry (DXA) or quantitative computed tomography (QCT). However, DXA is based on two-dimensional (2D) bone projections, which fail to account for complex three-dimensional (3D) bone morphologies and heterogeneous absorption from non-osseous tissues [6]. DXA is commonly seen as a poor predictor of osteoporotic fracture and has a sensitivity for predicting a fracture event of less than 50% [6–8]. QCT volumetric BMD is more accurate and sensitive to bone quality changes from diseases or pharmaceuticals, but it requires more ionizing radiation than DXA, and this can increase risk with repeat scans in longitudinal studies [9, 10].

On the other hand, magnetic resonance imaging (MRI) can assess bone quality at any anatomic site and does not involve ionizing radiation, making it well suited for research studies and longitudinal examinations [11]. However, the apparent transverse relaxation time (T_2^*) of water protons in bone is too short to allow capture of bone signal by conventional MRI techniques. As a result, MRI assessment of bone health has traditionally focused on macroscopic morphological whole-bone evaluation and indirect assessment of trabecular bone microarchitecture by imaging fat and inferring trabecular structure using reversed contrast [12–23]. In more recent years, the development of ultrashort echo time (UTE) sequences has allowed direct assessment of proton signals in dense osseous regions, such as those in cortical bone, and this has enabled a wide range of new techniques for MRI assessment of bone health [24–26].

Cortical bone is the dense outer shell of bone, which accounts for 80% of whole-body bony mass [27]. The majority of fractures in old age occur in the nonvertebral regions of the body, which are predominantly cortical bone, and the majority of bone loss after 64 years is in cortical bone [28–30]. Moreover, cortical bone sustains half of the mechanical load in the femoral neck [31], which is the site of the most dangerous osteoporotic fractures. Cortical bone is a porous structure composed of a series of microscopic osteons, which are layered and interwoven with pores of varying length scales, including Haversian/Volkmann's canals (10–200 μm), lacunae (1–10 μm), and canaliculi (0.1–1 μm) [32, 33]. With aging, especially with osteoporosis, cortical bone loss is predominantly manifested as a drastic expansion of existing intracortical pores [34–36]. As such, cortical porosity is a crucial parameter for assessing bone health, and it has been associated with incident fracture risk independent of age, sex, height, weight, or BMD [37]. Furthermore, multiple osteoporotic medications have been shown to improve cortical porosity in vivo [38–40]. Although the majority of cortical pores are too small to be directly imaged by any noninvasive modality, various UTE methods have been proposed to indirectly probe cortical microstructure, and these are highlighted in the following sections.

C. S. Rajapakse
Department of Radiology, Perelman School of Medicine, University of Pennsylvania, Philadelphia, PA, USA

Department of Orthopaedic Surgery, Perelman School of Medicine, University of Pennsylvania, Philadelphia, PA, USA
e-mail: chamith@pennmedicine.upenn.edu

B. C. Jones (✉)
Department of Radiology, Perelman School of Medicine, University of Pennsylvania, Philadelphia, PA, USA

Department of Bioengineering, School of Engineering and Applied Sciences, University of Pennsylvania, Philadelphia, PA, USA
e-mail: bcjones@seas.upenn.edu

© The Author(s), under exclusive license to Springer Nature Switzerland AG 2023
J. Du, G. M. Bydder (eds.), *MRI of Short- and Ultrashort-T₂ Tissues*, https://doi.org/10.1007/978-3-031-35197-6_33

Cortical T₂ Species

As stated in previous chapters, the MRI-labile water protons in cortical bone exist in two pools with vastly different T_2 values [41–43]. The water protons that reside in Haversian/Volkmann's canals and the lacuna–canalicular system are relatively mobile and unrestricted, allowing for motion averaging of dipolar interactions. As a result, these water protons have longer T_2s ranging from 1–1000 ms at 3 T [41, 42]. This longer-T_2 pool is termed "pore water" since these protons exist in the larger vacuous spaces in bone. On the other hand, the water protons that are hydrogen-bound to the collagenous matrix and osteoid experience highly restricted motion, resulting in a drastically shorter T_2 of approximately 390 μs at 3 T [44]. This shorter-T_2 pool is termed "bound water" due to its tight bonds with the organic constituents of bone.

The large distribution of cortical pore size in bone (0.1–200 μm) is the cause of the extremely large range in T_2s (1–1000 ms) for pore water. More specifically, the T_2 of free water in any porous structure is inversely proportional to the surface-to-volume ratio of the pore [32]. Thus, smaller bone pores have a higher surface-to-volume ratio; therefore, the water within them has a shorter T_2 (nearer to the 1-ms mark), whereas larger bone pores have a smaller surface-to-volume ratio and much longer T_2s. The relationship between the cortical pore size and T_2 of the pore water has inspired several UTE methods to quantify cortical microarchitecture.

The Suppression Ratio

The suppression ratio (SR) was proposed by Li et al. [45] in 2014 as a biomarker of cortical porosity. Although the T_2^* of bound water is exceptionally short at 390 μs, UTE sequences with nominal TEs as short as 30–50 μs are capable of acquiring the bulk of the signal from cortical bone, including that arising from both the bound and pore water pools. Furthermore, the use of adiabatic inversion pulses with UTE sequences (inversion recovery UTE, IR-UTE) provides reliable long-T_2 signal suppression by nulling most of the signal from pore water, thus selectively isolating the bound water pool (see Chapter 14 for more information; example shown in Fig. 33.1), [46, 47]. Given this, the SR was proposed as the ratio of the magnitudes of the signals from two co-localized UTE scans, one with and one without long-T_2 signal suppression:

$$\text{Suppression ratio} = \frac{S_{\text{unsuppressed}}}{S_{\text{suppressed}}} = \frac{S_{\text{UTE}}}{S_{\text{IR-UTE}}} \approx$$
$$\frac{\text{Total water}}{\text{Bound water}} = \frac{\text{Pore water} + \text{bound water}}{\text{Bound water}} \quad (33.1)$$

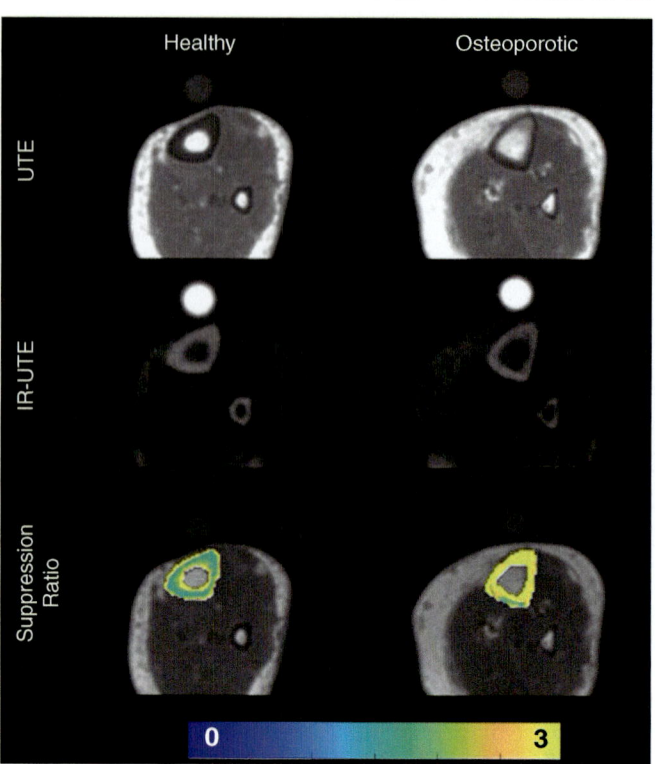

Fig. 33.1 An illustration of unsuppressed UTE (first row), long-T_2 signal-suppressed IR-UTE (second row), and SR maps (third row) in a healthy (left column) and an osteoporotic patient (right column). The healthy patient was a 67-year-old woman with a body mass index (BMI) of 23.5 and a median SR of 2.05. The osteoporotic patient was a 67-year-old woman with a BMI of 21.2 and an SR of 3.6. The cortical thinning characteristic of osteoporosis can be seen in each of osteoporotic patient's images (right column). In the second row, the IR-UTE sequence produces effective long-T_2 signal suppression, with the majority of the signal coming from the tibia, fibula, and reference phantom (although the phantom is not necessary for SR calculation) in both patients. In the third row, cortical bone in the osteoporotic patient exhibits a greater SR across the entire tibia than that in the healthy patient

The unsuppressed UTE sequence acquires signal from both pools, whereas the long-T_2-suppressed sequence predominantly acquires signal from the bound water pool. Two primary mechanisms cause the SR to increase positively with cortical porosity. First, the intracortical pore expansion arising from aging and osteoporosis causes an increase in the proton density of pore water and a concomitant decrease in the proton density of bound water as the osteoid is resorbed. This effectively increases the numerator while decreasing the denominator of Eq. (33.1), both of which cause an increase in SR. Second, as the cortical pores expand, their T_2 increases, and this improves the efficacy of the long-T_2 signal suppression of pore water with the IR-UTE sequence. So, as the pores become larger, the signal in the denominator $S_{\text{suppressed}}$ decreases, which further increases the SR.

To the best of the authors' knowledge, Li et al.'s study is the only published study to date using SR. Li et al. thoroughly validated this biomarker in 13 cadaveric tibia specimens and in human subjects [45]. The SR was strongly associated with μCT-derived porosity ($R = 0.88$) and specimen age ($R = 0.87$). The authors also evaluated SR in vivo in 34 women between 26 and 79 years of age and found that the SR was positively associated with age ($R = 0.64$) and inversely associated with volumetric bone mineral density ($R = -0.67$). The authors also showed that SR was highly reproducible in vivo, with a coefficient of variation of 1.5%.

An illustration of the SR in age-matched postmenopausal women in an as-yet unpublished study is shown in Fig. 33.1. This figure shows the UTE and IR-UTE sequence acquired in the mid-tibia of two postmenopausal women, one with BMD-diagnosed osteoporosis and the other with healthy bone density. The osteoporotic patient's tibia can be seen to have a thinner cortex and a considerably larger porosity throughout the bone.

The literature on SR is scant, and the parameter is largely unexplored, likely due to the long-T_2 UTE suppression sequence initially requiring long scan times and being limited to 2D scans [48]. More recently, the use of variable flip angle sequences combined with long-T_2 signal suppression has allowed reliable long-T_2-suppressed 3D images to be acquired in a clinically feasible scan time of 6 min [47, 49]. Although significant further work is needed to validate this parameter in vivo, it has great potential and some key advantages over other UTE cortical bone techniques. First, the SR measurement does not require specialized hardware or an external reference phantom in the scan field-of-view (FOV) and is, therefore, better suited for research studies that include multiple imaging centers. Second, the image processing is simple and does not require ill-posed curve fitting or long scan times to acquire many echoes and fit relaxation parameters. However, it requires an adiabatic long-T_2 suppression module, which may not be available on some clinical scanners. Nevertheless, SR is a promising biomarker for noninvasively assessing cortical porosity.

The Porosity Index (PI)

Shortly after the SR was proposed, in 2015, Rajapakse et al. proposed another biomarker of cortical porosity called the porosity index [48]. The porosity index (PI) is simply calculated as the ratio of the magnitude signals obtained at two different TEs using a UTE sequence [48]:

$$\text{Porosity index} = \frac{S_{\text{TElong}}}{S_{\text{TEultrashort}}} \approx \frac{\text{Pore water}}{\text{Total water}} \approx \frac{\text{Pore water}}{\text{Pore water} + \text{bound water}} \tag{33.2}$$

For best results, the ultrashort TE should be made as short as possible (30–50 μs), whereas the longer TE should be around 2 ms. The PI parameter is based on the assumption that, over the $\approx$2-ms delay, the bound water pool signal with a T_2^* of 390 μs entirely decays away. In contrast, the pore water pool, which has a much longer T_2^* (1–1000 ms), experiences negligible decay. This can be regarded as an estimate of the pore water volume fraction within a given voxel and scales positively with the cortical porosity. The PI is also aided by the same effects described previously, wherein larger cortical pores have longer-T_2 values and experience less signal decay [32], corresponding to an increase in the numerator and an increase in the PI. Conversely, smaller pores have shorter T_2s and the signal from them decays faster, resulting in a decrease in the denominator of the PI in Eq. (33.2). Additionally, the fact that both TE readouts are acquired with the same sequence means that it has self-normalizing properties that mitigate the effects of radiofrequency and static field inhomogeneities.

Rajapakse et al. validated the use of PI in cadaveric tibia specimens [48]. The PI was shown to be strongly associated with μCT-derived porosity ($R = 0.88$), average pore size ($R = 0.90$), and specimen age ($r = 0.80$), and was inversely associated with volumetric BMD ($R = -0.70$). The PI was similarly shown to be positively correlated with pore water fraction ($R = 0.79$) and pore water T_2^* ($R = 0.80$) [48]. Later, Zhao et al. demonstrated that PI has a high degree of reproducibility in vivo with a coefficient of variation of 3.8%. The authors also found that PI was inversely associated with bone mineral phosphorus density ($r = -0.71$) and, after the exclusion of an extreme outlier, was inversely correlated with bound water density ($r = -0.65$) [49]. In 2019, Hong et al. compared PI to near-infrared spectral imaging (NIRSI) and mechanical testing-derived uniaxial stiffness in cadaveric tibia specimens. The authors found that PI was inversely associated with the stiffness of the tibia ($r = -0.79$); in other words, as porosity increases, bone stiffness decreases. They also showed that PI was inversely proportional to NIRSI-derived collagen content ($r = -0.73$) and NIRSI-derived bound water content ($r = -0.95$) [50]. More recently, Jones et al. have investigated the efficacy of PI in evaluating bone health in cadaveric femur specimens. They performed mechanical testing on whole femur specimens simulating loads experienced during a sideways fall fracture. The PI was found to be inversely associated with the mechanical stiffness of the sideways fall ($r = -0.82$) of the femur, suggesting that it could evaluate bone mechanical competence [51].

Xiong et al. explored the efficacy of PI in assessing bone quality in vivo in a cohort of 95 patients with chronic kidney disease (CKD) [52]. CKD has significant deleterious effects on bone health produced by disrupting mineral metabolism and is one of many diseases that can cause "secondary osteoporosis," i.e., osteoporosis that is caused by comorbidity

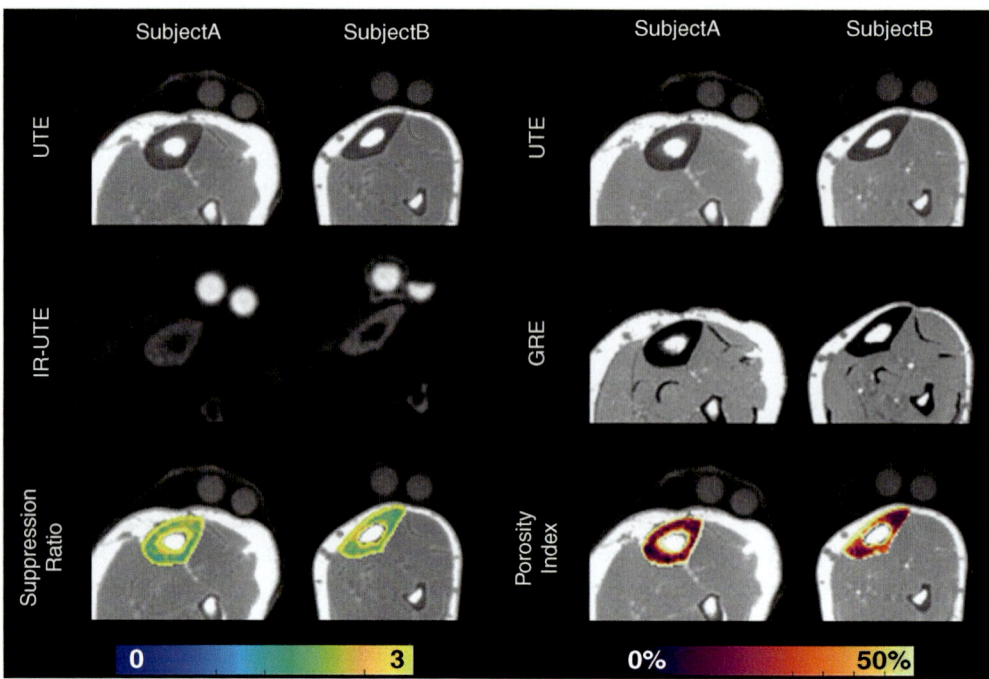

Fig. 33.2 An illustration of the SR and PI parameters in two healthy subjects. Subject A is a 26-year-old male, and subject B is a 27-year-old male. The workflow for SR calculation in both subjects is shown on the left side (first two columns) and the workflow for PI calculation for both subjects is shown on the right side (third and fourth columns). In the first two columns, standard UTE ($S_{unsuppressed}$) images are depicted in the first row, whereas long-T_2-suppressed UTE ($S_{suppressed}$) images are shown in the second row and the SR is shown in the third row. On the right side, the PI workflow is shown for both subjects. Standard UTE images are depicted in the first row (TE$_{ultrashort}$), whereas the longer TE images, denoted as GRE (TE$_{long}$), are shown in the second row and PI is shown in the third row. The color parameter maps in the third row demonstrate the spatial distribution of the cortical porosity as measured by the two techniques. Similar trends in porosity can be seen with both methods. In subject A, greater porosity is visible in the anterior part of the cortex, whereas the posterolateral side shows relatively dense, healthy cortex. In subject B, greater porosity can be seen in the thin cortex on the anterolateral side, whereas the posteromedial point shows a dense cortex with lower porosity

instead of aging-related hormonal changes [53]. Notably, PI increased with increasing severity of the CKD stage, whereas lumbar DXA did not. Moreover, significant associations between PI and several bone metabolism biomarkers were found, with PI being positively correlated with the parathyroid hormone, ß-cross-laps, total procollagen type 1 amino-terminal propeptides, and osteocalcin ($P = 0.001$) [52].

Taken together, these studies suggest that PI is a useful biomarker for assessing bone health. However, PI has not yet been investigated in any longitudinal in vivo studies, so its efficacy in long-term studies is yet to be established. Nevertheless, PI has been validated in ex vivo studies by comparison with μCT and NIRSI and has shown to be related to secondary osteoporosis in vivo and warrants further exploration. An example in vivo comparison between the PI and SR parameters is shown in Fig. 33.2 in two healthy individuals.

The PI is an especially useful biomarker for assessing bone quality in vivo because it can be derived from a single UTE sequence that is available on most MRI scanners. Additionally, since the biomarker is computed as the ratio of two images with different TEs, the processing is simple and only requires accurate segmentation to perform. Although the PI has the potential to be a powerful measure of bone quality in research studies, substantial work is still needed to further explore and validate it.

Conclusions

Both SR and PI are useful biomarkers for assessing cortical bone porosity. While the physics underlying these biomarkers is complicated, their computation and interpretation is comparatively simple and easy to replicate, even for those with limited programming and physics experience. From a practical point of view, they are, therefore, well suited for use in larger, multicenter imaging research studies and potentially for translation to the clinic. The biomarkers have been extensively validated in preclinical studies and have shown promise in a few in vivo studies, but substantial further work is needed to establish their usefulness in vivo. Specifically, future studies should investigate whether these parameters can detect impairments in porosity associated with bone diseases as well as investigate longitudinal changes following anti-osteoporotic medication or other interventions.

Additionally, most of the in vivo studies with these parameters have focused on the tibia due to technical reasons since its thicker cortex and superficial location provide a high signal-to-noise ratio (SNR). However, the most devastating osteoporotic fractures occur in the proximal femur, which has a large cortical bone content. Future studies should investigate use of these parameters in the proximal femur to provide more relevant information on bone quality and fracture risk.

Current approaches with SR and PI simply compute the median or mean within the volume of interest. However, our preliminary work indicates that these parameters capture meaningful spatial differences in cortical porosity within the tibia, which are seen with other modalities. At the moment, it is unclear how to best use the spatial data to provide further information on bone quality, but this is a highly active area of research.

Ongoing work is focused on implementing these parameters in larger clinical patient studies and comparing their porosity measurements with those from other modalities.

References

1. Sozen T, Ozisik L, Basaran NC. An overview and management of osteoporosis. Eur J Rheumatol. 2017;4(1):46–56.
2. Lewiecki EM, Ortendahl JD, Vanderpuye-Orgle J, Grauer A, Arellano J, Lemay J, et al. Healthcare policy changes in osteoporosis can improve outcomes and reduce costs in the United States. JBMR Plus. 2019;3(9):e10192.
3. Wu A-M, Bisignano C, James SL, Abady GG, Abedi A, Abu-Gharbieh E, et al. Global, regional, and national burden of bone fractures in 204 countries and territories, 1990–2019: a systematic analysis from the global burden of disease study 2019. Lancet Healthy Longev. 2021;2(9):e580–e92.
4. Wright NC, Looker AC, Saag KG, Curtis JR, Delzell ES, Randall S, et al. The recent prevalence of osteoporosis and low bone mass in the United States based on bone mineral density at the femoral neck or lumbar spine. J Bone Miner Res. 2014;29(11):2520–6.
5. Cummings SR, Melton LJ. Epidemiology and outcomes of osteoporotic fractures. Lancet (London, England). 2002;359(9319):1761–7.
6. Bolotin HH. The significant effects of bone structure on inherent patient-specific DXA in vivo bone mineral density measurement inaccuracies. Med Phys. 2004;31(4):774–88.
7. Bolotin HH. DXA in vivo BMD methodology: an erroneous and misleading research and clinical gauge of bone mineral status, bone fragility, and bone remodelling. Bone. 2007;41(1):138–54.
8. Marshall D, Johnell O, Wedel H. Meta-analysis of how well measures of bone mineral density predict occurrence of osteoporotic fractures. BMJ (Clinical research ed). 1996;312(7041):1254–9.
9. Mao SS, Li D, Syed YS, Gao Y, Luo Y, Flores F, et al. Thoracic quantitative computed tomography (QCT) can sensitively monitor bone mineral metabolism: comparison of thoracic QCT vs lumbar QCT and dual-energy X-ray absorptiometry in detection of age-relative change in bone mineral density. Acad Radiol. 2017;24(12):1582–7.
10. Bergot C, Laval-Jeantet AM, Hutchinson K, Dautraix I, Caulin F, Genant HK. A comparison of spinal quantitative computed tomography with dual energy X-ray absorptiometry in European women with vertebral and nonvertebral fractures. Calcif Tissue Int. 2001;68(2):74–82.
11. Chang G, Boone S, Martel D, Rajapakse CS, Hallyburton RS, Valko M, et al. MRI assessment of bone structure and microarchitecture. J Magn Reson Imaging. 2017;46(2):323–37.
12. Bauer JS, Monetti R, Krug R, Matsuura M, Mueller D, Eckstein F, et al. Advances of 3T MR imaging in visualizing trabecular bone structure of the calcaneus are partially SNR-independent: analysis using simulated noise in relation to micro-CT, 1.5T MRI, and biomechanical strength. J Magn Reson Imaging. 2009;29(1):132–40.
13. Baum T, Dütsch Y, Müller D, Monetti R, Sidorenko I, Räth C, et al. Reproducibility of trabecular bone structure measurements of the distal radius at 1.5 and 3.0 T magnetic resonance imaging. J Comput Assist Tomogr. 2012;36(5):623–6.
14. Baum T, Kutscher M, Muller D, Rath C, Eckstein F, Lochmuller EM, et al. Cortical and trabecular bone structure analysis at the distal radius-prediction of biomechanical strength by DXA and MRI. J Bone Miner Metab. 2013;31(2):212–21.
15. Issever AS, Link TM, Newitt D, Munoz T, Majumdar S. Interrelationships between 3-T-MRI-derived cortical and trabecular bone structure parameters and quantitative-computed-tomography-derivedbone mineral density. Magn Reson Imaging. 2010;28(9):1299–305.
16. Krug R, Carballido-Gamio J, Burghardt AJ, Kazakia G, Hyun BH, Jobke B, et al. Assessment of trabecular bone structure comparing magnetic resonance imaging at 3 Tesla with high-resolution peripheral quantitative computed tomography ex vivo and in vivo. Osteoporos Int. 2008;19(5):653–61.
17. Gomberg BG, Saha PK, Song HK, Hwang SN, Wehrli FW. Application of topological analysis to magnetic resonance images of human trabecular bone. IEEE Trans Med Imaging. 2000;19(3):166–74.
18. Carballido-Gamio J, Krug R, Huber MB, Hyun B, Eckstein F, Majumdar S, et al. Geodesic topological analysis of trabecular bone microarchitecture from high-spatial resolution magnetic resonance images. Magn Reson Med. 2009;61(2):448–56.
19. Saha P, Xu Y, Duan H, Heiner A, Liang G. Volumetric topological analysis: a novel approach for trabecular bone classification on the continuum between plates and rods. IEEE Trans Med Imaging. 2010;29(11):1821–38.
20. Wald MJ, Magland JF, Rajapakse CS, Bhagat YA, Wehrli FW. Predicting trabecular bone elastic properties from measures of bone volume fraction and fabric on the basis of micromagnetic resonance images. Magn Reson Med. 2012;68(2):463–73.
21. Benito M, Vasilic B, Wehrli FW, Bunker B, Wald M, Gomberg B, et al. Effect of testosterone replacement on bone architecture in hypogonadal men. J Bone Miner Res. 2005;20(10):1785–91.
22. Wehrli FW, Ladinsky GA, Jones C, Benito M, Magland J, Vasilic B, et al. In vivo magnetic resonance detects rapid remodeling changes in the topology of the trabecular bone network after menopause and the protective effect of estradiol. J Bone Miner Res. 2008;23(5):730–40.
23. Rajapakse CS, Leonard MB, Bhagat YA, Sun W, Magland JF, Wehrli FW. Micro-MR imaging-based computational biomechanics demonstrates reduction in cortical and trabecular bone strength after renal transplantation. Radiology. 2012;262(3):912–20.
24. Seifert AC, Wehrli FW. Solid-state quantitative (1)H and (31) P MRI of cortical bone in humans. Curr Osteoporos Rep. 2016;14(3):77–86.

25. Ma YJ, Jerban S, Jang H, Chang D, Chang EY, Du J. Quantitative ultrashort echo time (UTE) magnetic resonance imaging of bone: an update. Front Endocrinol (Lausanne). 2020;11:567417.

26. Sollmann N, Loffler MT, Kronthaler S, Bohm C, Dieckmeyer M, Ruschke S, et al. MRI-based quantitative osteoporosis imaging at the spine and femur. J Magn Reson Imaging. 2021;54(1):12–35.

27. Seeman E. Age- and menopause-related bone loss compromise cortical and trabecular microstructure. J Gerontol A Biol Sci Med Sci. 2013;68(10):1218–25.

28. Zebaze RM, Ghasem-Zadeh A, Bohte A, Iuliano-Burns S, Mirams M, Price RI, et al. Intracortical remodelling and porosity in the distal radius and post-mortem femurs of women: a cross-sectional study. Lancet. 2010;375(9727):1729–36.

29. Kanis JA, Johnell O, Oden A, Dawson A, De Laet C, Jonsson B. Ten year probabilities of osteoporotic fractures according to BMD and diagnostic thresholds. Osteoporos Int. 2001;12(12):989–95.

30. Riggs BL, Wahner HW, Dunn WL, Mazess RB, Offord KP, Melton LJ. Differential changes in bone mineral density of the appendicular and axial skeleton with aging: relationship to spinal osteoporosis. J Clin Invest. 1981;67(2):328–35.

31. Manske SL, Liu-Ambrose T, Cooper DM, Kontulainen S, Guy P, Forster BB, et al. Cortical and trabecular bone in the femoral neck both contribute to proximal femur failure load prediction. Osteoporos Int. 2009;20(3):445–53.

32. Wang X, Ni Q. Determination of cortical bone porosity and pore size distribution using a low field pulsed NMR approach. J Orthop Res. 2003;21(2):312–9.

33. Cowin SC. Bone poroelasticity. J Biomech. 1999;32(3):217–38.

34. Martin RB, Ishida J. The relative effects of collagen fiber orientation, porosity, density, and mineralization on bone strength. J Biomech. 1989;22(5):419–26.

35. McCalden RW, McGeough JA, Barker MB, Court-Brown CM. Age-related changes in the tensile properties of cortical bone. The relative importance of changes in porosity, mineralization, and microstructure. J Bone Joint Surg Am. 1993;75(8):1193–205.

36. Roschger P, Gupta HS, Berzlanovich A, Ittner G, Dempster DW, Fratzl P, et al. Constant mineralization density distribution in cancellous human bone. Bone. 2003;32(3):316–23.

37. Samelson EJ, Broe KE, Xu H, Yang L, Boyd S, Biver E, et al. Cortical and trabecular bone microarchitecture as an independent predictor of incident fracture risk in older women and men in the bone microarchitecture international consortium (BoMIC): a prospective study. Lancet Diabetes Endocrinol. 2019;7(1):34–43.

38. Hansen S, Hauge EM, Jensen JE, Brixen K. Differing effects of PTH 1-34, PTH 1-84 and zoledronic acid on bone microarchitecture and estimated strength in postmenopausal women with osteoporosis. An 18 month open-labeled observational study using HR-pQCT. J Bone Miner Res. 2013;28(4):736–45.

39. Kanis JA, Cooper C, Rizzoli R, Reginster JY. European guidance for the diagnosis and management of osteoporosis in postmenopausal women. Osteoporos Int. 2019;30(1):3–44.

40. Tsai JN, Nishiyama KK, Lin D, Yuan A, Lee H, Bouxsein ML, et al. Effects of denosumab and teriparatide transitions on bone microarchitecture and estimated strength: the DATA-switch HR-pQCT study. J Bone Miner Res. 2017;32(10):2001–9.

41. Horch RA, Nyman JS, Gochberg DF, Dortch RD, Does MD. Characterization of 1H NMR signal in human cortical bone for magnetic resonance imaging. Magn Reson Med. 2010;64(3):680–7.

42. Horch RA, Gochberg DF, Nyman JS, Does MD. Non-invasive predictors of human cortical bone mechanical properties: T(2)-discriminated H NMR compared with high resolution X-ray. PLoS One. 2011;6(1):e16359.

43. Horch RA, Gochberg DF, Nyman JS, Does MD. Clinically compatible MRI strategies for discriminating bound and pore water in cortical bone. Magn Reson Med. 2012;68(6):1774–84.

44. Seifert AC, Wehrli SL, Wehrli FW. Bi-component T_2^* analysis of bound and pore bone water fractions fails at high field strengths. NMR Biomed. 2015;28(7):861–72.

45. Li C, Seifert AC, Rad HS, Bhagat YA, Rajapakse CS, Sun W, et al. Cortical bone water concentration: dependence of MR imaging measures on age and pore volume fraction. Radiology. 2014;272(3):796–806.

46. Robson MD, Bydder GM. Clinical ultrashort echo time imaging of bone and other connective tissues. NMR Biomed. 2006;19(7):765–80.

47. Li C, Magland JF, Zhao X, Seifert AC, Wehrli FW. Selective in vivo bone imaging with long-T_2 suppressed PETRA MRI. Magn Reson Med. 2017;77(3):989–97.

48. Rajapakse CS, Bashoor-Zadeh M, Li C, Sun W, Wright AC, Wehrli FW. Volumetric cortical bone porosity assessment with MR imaging: validation and clinical feasibility. Radiology. 2015;276(2):526–35.

49. Zhao X, Song HK, Seifert AC, Li C, Wehrli FW. Feasibility of assessing bone matrix and mineral properties in vivo by combined solid-state 1H and 31P MRI. PLoS One. 2017;12(3):e0173995.

50. Hong AL, Ispiryan M, Padalkar MV, Jones BC, Batzdorf AS, Shetye SS, et al. MRI-derived bone porosity index correlates to bone composition and mechanical stiffness. Bone Rep. 2019;11:100213.

51. Jones BC, Jia S, Lee H, Feng A, Shetye SS, Batzdorf A, et al. MRI-derived porosity index is associated with whole-bone stiffness and mineral density in human cadaveric femora. Bone. 2021;143:115774.

52. Xiong Y, He T, Wang Y, Liu WV, Hu S, Zhang Y, et al. CKD stages, bone metabolism markers, and cortical porosity index: associations and mediation effects analysis. Front Endocrinol. 2021;12:775066.

53. Nickolas TL, Stein EM, Dworakowski E, Nishiyama KK, Komandah-Kosseh M, Zhang CA, et al. Rapid cortical bone loss in patients with chronic kidney disease. J Bone Miner Res. 2013;28(8):1811–20.

A UTE-Based Biomarker Panel in Osteoporosis

34

Saeed Jerban, Yajun Ma, Eric Y. Chang, Christine B. Chung, Graeme M. Bydder, and Jiang Du

Introduction

Osteoporosis (OPo) is a metabolic bone disease, which affects at least a dozen million people in the United States and leads to more than two million bone fractures every year [1]. For many patients, OPo can result in long-term disability and death. It usually results from an imbalanced bone remodeling process in which new bone volume generation by osteoblasts cannot keep pace with bone volume resorption by osteoclasts [2–4]. The World Health Organization (WHO) has defined OPo as reduction in bone mineral density (BMD) measured at the hip or spine by at least 2.5 standard deviations (SDs) from the average BMD of a young healthy population [5]. Osteopenia (OPe) is a condition that precedes OPo in which a patient's BMD is decreased one SD below the average young, healthy BMD [6].

Bone can be generally classified as cortical (compact bone) or trabecular (spongy bone). Approximately 80% of the volume of bone in the human skeletal system is cortical, which hosts the majority of the nonvertebral fractures in the elderly population [7]. However, cortical OPo always progresses in tandem with trabecular bone deterioration [8]. It is crucial to characterize and assess the underlying structure and function of cortical and trabecular bone thoroughly to understand how bone degenerates and fails during the progression of OPo. The development of noninvasive imaging techniques to characterize the structural and biochemical status of bone is a major force for achieving this.

Bone is organized in a highly complex hierarchical structure [9] composed of mineral matrix (>40% by volume), organic matrix (>30%), and water (~20%) at cortical sites [10, 11]. Bone mineral provides stiffness and strength, particularly during compressive loading, whereas collagen provides ductility and the crucial ability to absorb energy before a fracture. Bone contains more water at trabecular sites, primarily in combination with fat in bone marrow, which typically occupies more than 80% of bone volume, but sometimes occupies more than 95% of bone volume in OPo [8, 12]. In addition to the water present in marrow, a fraction of bone water called "pore water" (PW) resides in pores of various sizes at cortical and trabecular bone sites, including the Haversian canals (10–200 μm), lacunae (1–10 μm), and canaliculi (0.1–1 μm) [10, 13]. The majority of bone water, particularly in a healthy bone, is "bound water" (BW), which is bound to the organic and mineral matrices [13–19]. BW and PW contribute differently to the mechanical properties of bone [20, 21].

S. Jerban (✉)
Department of Radiology, University of California, San Diego, La Jolla, CA, USA

Department of Orthopaedic Surgery, University of California, San Diego, La Jolla, CA, USA
e-mail: sjerban@health.ucsd.edu

Y. Ma
Department of Radiology, University of California, San Diego, La Jolla, CA, USA
e-mail: yam013@health.ucsd.edu

E. Y. Chang · C. B. Chung
Department of Radiology, University of California, San Diego, La Jolla, CA, USA

Research Service, Veterans Affairs San Diego Healthcare System, San Diego, CA, USA
e-mail: e8chang@health.ucsd.edu; cbchung@health.ucsd.edu

G. M. Bydder
Department of Radiology, University of California, San Diego, La Jolla, CA, USA

Mātai Medical Research Institute, Tairāwhiti Gisborne, New Zealand
e-mail: gbydder@health.ucsd.edu

J. Du
Department of Radiology, University of California, San Diego, La Jolla, CA, USA

Research Service, Veterans Affairs San Diego Healthcare System, San Diego, CA, USA

Department of Bioengineering, University of California, San Diego, La Jolla, CA, USA
e-mail: jiangdu@health.ucsd.edu

J. Du, G. M. Bydder (eds.), *MRI of Short- and Ultrashort-T₂ Tissues*, https://doi.org/10.1007/978-3-031-35197-6_34

X-ray-based medical imaging methods such as dual-energy X-ray absorptiometry (DEXA) and quantitative computed tomography (QCT) are essential to the clinical process of evaluating bone. These methods measure BMD based on the degree of X-ray attenuation in patients' bones. The organic matrix, water, and fat, which together represent between 55 and ~80% of cortical and trabecular bone by volume, respectively, only make minor contributions to the signals obtained using standard X-ray-based techniques [22–25]. A major missing factor in bone assessment using DEXA for monitoring the clinical progression of OPo is the contribution of bone organic matrix and water to the overarching biomechanical properties of bone. Despite its widespread use in clinical practice, DEXA-based diagnosis of OPo using the WHO criterion (DEXA T-score < −2.5) often fails to predict fracture risk accurately [26–28], with reported prediction rates of between 30 and 50% when used alone [29–37]. For instance, the observed decrease in areal BMD from age 60 to 80 years accounts for a doubling of the fracture risk, but it is clinically known that the overall fracture risk increases 13-fold during this period [27, 32].

Magnetic resonance imaging (MRI) has been increasingly used to evaluate the non-mineral portions of bone and thus improve bone assessment in patients affected by OPo. Notably, cortical bone has a short apparent transverse relaxation time (T_2^*); therefore, typical conventional clinical MRI pulse sequences with echo times (TEs) of a few milliseconds cannot capture signals from bone [38, 39]. To address this shortcoming, ultrashort echo time (UTE)-MRI sequences have been developed. These provide direct imaging of bone and allow quantitative measurements that are sensitive to OPo-related bone changes [19, 40–42].

OPo-related changes in bone at different stages of OPo progression are not just limited to the mineral matrix but also involve the organic matrix, PW and BW, and fat fraction. The changes usually vary concurrently but follow different time courses and reflect different mechanical properties of bone. Employing a panel of UTE-MRI-based biomarkers to assess all the main components of bone can help provide a more comprehensive picture of disease progression than the use of BMD alone. This chapter describes different UTE-MRI techniques that can be included in a UTE-MRI biomarker panel for OPo. The techniques described are based on the bone component, which is targeted, such as total water (TW), PW, BW, fat, macromolecules in the organic matrix, and the mineral matrix.

Cortical Bone Water Content Assessment

UTE-MRI has been used in several studies to estimate the water content of cortical bone. Water content is a central component in the OPo-related biomarker panel. It is assumed that pores are occupied by water and that the increased porosity seen in cortical bone during OPo development is manifested as an increase in PW. Evaluation of this water can, in principle, provide information about OPo development.

Total Water Assessment with Basic UTE

The total water content of cortical bone can be estimated by comparing the UTE-MRI signal of bone with that of an external reference of known proton density (PD) [43–49]. The estimated content needs to be corrected for differences between the T_2^* and T_1 values of bone and the external reference standard [50]. A mixture of distilled water and deuterated water (e.g., 20% H_2O and 80% D_2O, 22 mol/L ^1H) with a matched effective T_2^* of cortical bone (e.g., $T_2^* \approx 0.4$ ms) has been the most common external reference standard described in the literature for this estimation [44, 45, 47, 49, 50]. However, rubber erasers have also been mentioned as external phantoms because their apparent proton density and MRI properties are similar to those of bone [51]. Significant correlations have been reported between the estimated TW content in cortical bone and the microstructure of bone [50, 51]. Therefore, TW content can be potentially used as an important OPo-related UTE biomarker at cortical bone sites. It is the sum of PW and BW.

For accurate estimation of TW content, we should consider the following: first, the difference between the relaxation times of cortical bone and the external standard; second, the spatial variation of coil sensitivity in the scanned field of view (FOV); and third, the duration of the radiofrequency (RF) pulse and its homogeneity (or actual flip angle (FA)) [44, 52]. Due to the short T_1 in cortical bone, the T_1 effect on TW content calculation can be neglected if one uses a relatively low FA combined with a relatively high repetition time (TR) to produce a proton density (PD)-weighted UTE sequence [51].

Bound Water Assessment with Inversion Recovery UTE

Inversion recovery UTE (IR-UTE) sequences can suppress the long-T_2 signal from PW and specifically image BW in bone [53, 54]. Comparing the IR-UTE signal from bone with that of an external reference standard can be used to estimate BW content [47–50, 55]. BW content quantification based on the IR-UTE sequence requires efficient nulling of the PW signal [44]. PW content in cortical bone can be calculated by subtracting the IR-UTE-measured BW content from the UTE-measured TW content [44, 50, 56]. As described in earlier studies, the BW signal is an exponential function of BW T_1 ($T_{1\text{-BW}}$). Higher $T_{1\text{-BW}}$ values significantly increase the estimation of BW content if appropriate T_1 compensation is not

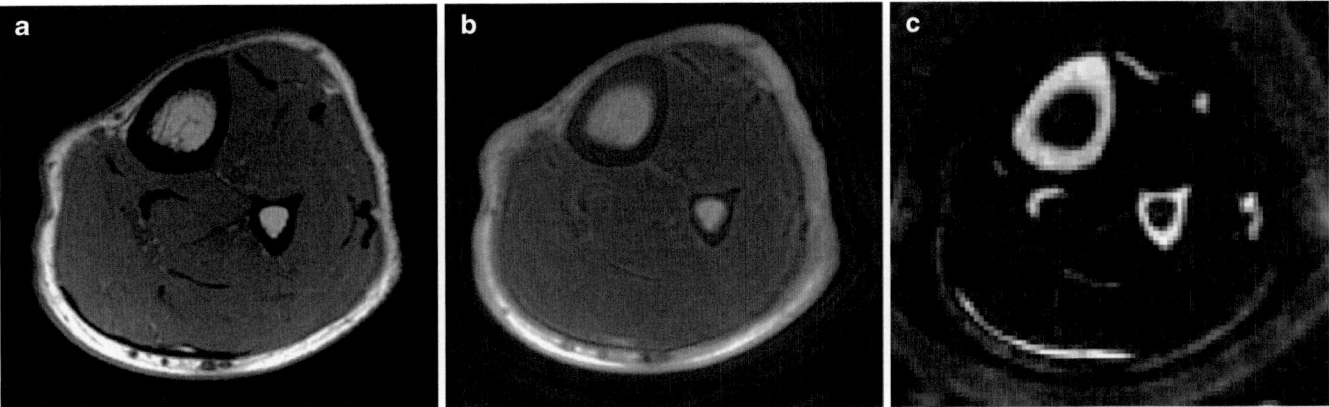

Fig. 34.1 Representative axial images of the tibial midshaft of a healthy 25-year-old female using (**a**) a clinical gradient echo (GRE) sequence, (**b**) a UTE-Cones sequence, and (**c**) an IR-UTE sequence. Suppression of long-T_2 signals in panel (**c**) highlights cortical bone in the tibia and fibula (as well as tendons and aponeuroses)

included [50]. While Tan et al. reported using a short $T_{1\text{-BW}}$ of 112 ms at 3 T in vivo [57], a value consistent with earlier reports by the same group [50, 58], other studies have reported $T_{1\text{-BW}}$ equal to 290 ms at 3 T [47, 49].

Figure 34.1 shows conventional gradient echo (GRE), basic UTE, and IR-UTE imaging of the tibial midshaft in a healthy 25-year-old female.

Figure 34.2 shows in vivo TW proton density (TWPD), BW proton density (BWPD), and PW proton density (PWPD) maps for representative subjects with healthy bone, OPe, and OPo. TWPD and PWPD were observed in the following ascending order: healthy bone < OPe < OPo. Conversely, BWPD was observed in the following ascending order: OPo < OPe < healthy bone.

Both BW and PW have also been estimated using a dual-TR UTE imaging technique using model-based UTE signal decomposition [59]. PW content has been reported to significantly correlate with subject age [59].

Pore Water Assessment with Double Adiabatic Full-Passage (DAFP) UTE

In addition to the indirect calculation of PW by subtracting the IR-UTE-measured BW content from the UTE-measured TW content, a double adiabatic full-passage (DAFP) pulse was proposed to directly image PW in cortical bone using a pulse preparation to saturate the BW signal followed by a UTE acquisition [47, 54]. This technique requires excellent nulling of the BW signal, which can be challenging. Horch et al. [54] used UTE-MRI at 4.7 T for direct imaging of both BW and PW and reported significant correlations with the mechanical properties of bone strips. Later, Manhard et al. [60] demonstrated a significant correlation between BW measured at 3 T and bone fracture toughness of cortical bone specimens.

BW and PW Estimation Using UTE Signal Fractional Indexes

Dual-echo time UTE imaging [61] can be used to calculate the porosity index (PI), which is the signal ratio between two MRI images, one with a TE ≈ 0.05 ms and one with a TE ≈ 2 ms. The first echo image represents signals from both BW and PW, and the second echo mostly represents the PW signal. Although this technique does not estimate the absolute PW content, it gives an estimate of bone porosity. The PI in the human cadaveric tibiae has shown significant correlations with microcomputed tomography (μCT)-based porosity, mechanical stiffness, donor age, and collagen estimation from near-infrared spectroscopy [61–63]. Recent in vivo studies have shown significantly higher PI in OPo and OPe patients than in healthy volunteers [63].

The suppression ratio (SR), defined as the ratio between bone UTE signal without, and with, long-T_2 signal suppression performed via dual-band saturation-prepared UTE (DB-UTE) or IR-UTE, is another UTE-MRI-based index that has been proposed for evaluation of cortical bone microstructure [46]. Bones from older subjects showed higher SR values [46]. Similarly, ex vivo investigations have shown that SR demonstrates significant correlations with bone porosity, mechanical properties, and donor age [46, 63]. Recent in vivo studies have shown significantly higher SR in OPo and OPe patients than in healthy volunteers [63].

BW and PW Assessment with Bicomponent Signal Modeling

The T_2^* of PW is roughly ten times the T_2^* of BW, and they can be distinguished from one another using UTE-MRI acquisition techniques combined with multicomponent T_2^* analysis [21, 64, 65]. Such techniques, however, do not

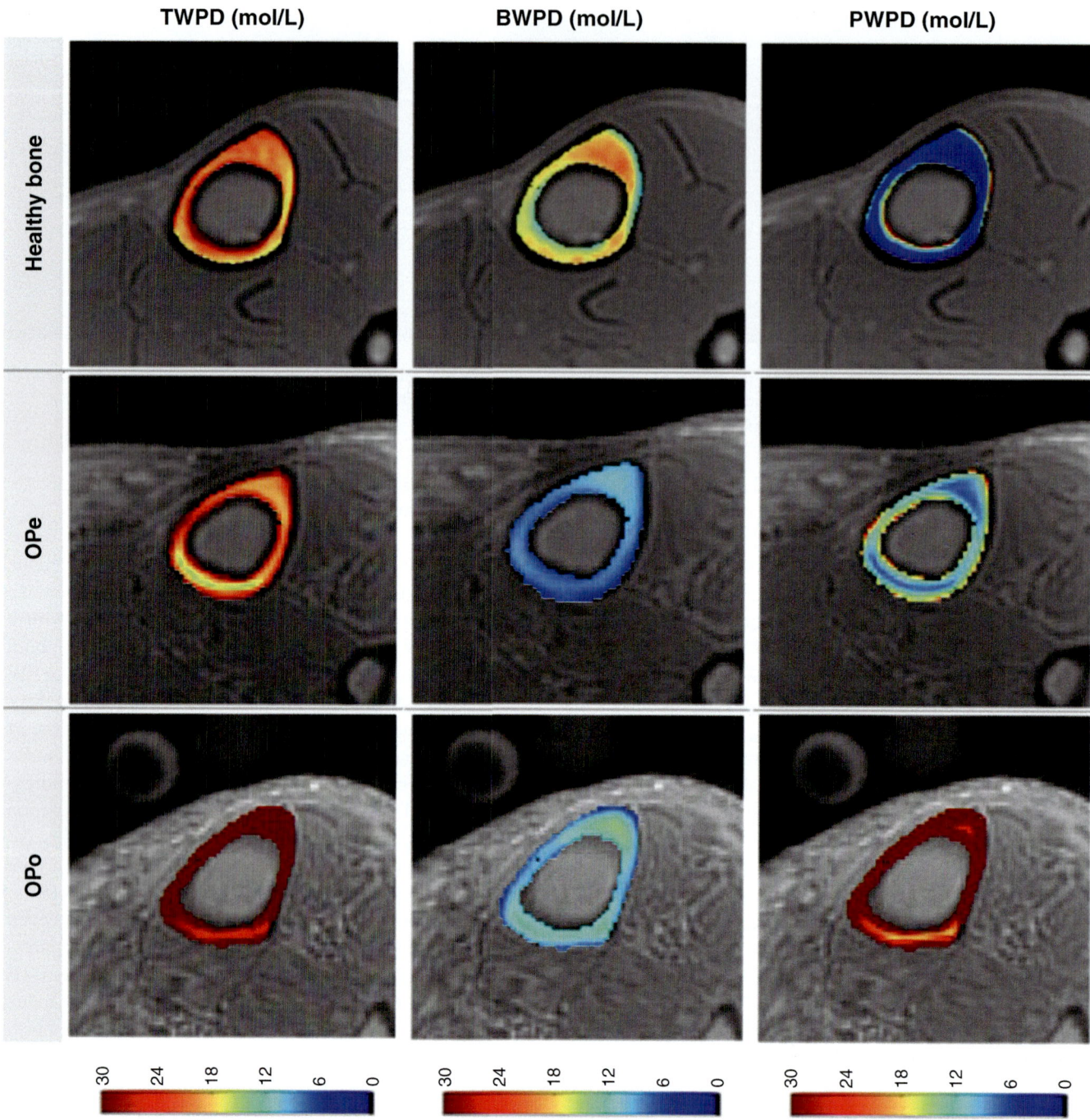

Fig. 34.2 Generated TW proton density (TWPD), BW proton density (BWPD), and PW proton density (PWPD) maps for (first row) a representative subject with healthy bone (a 35-year-old female), (second row) a representative patient with OPe (a 76-year-old female), and (third row) a representative patient with OPo (a 76-year-old female).

For these examples, TWPD and PWPD were observed in the following ascending order: healthy bone < OPe < OPo. On the contrary, BWPD was observed in the following ascending order: OPo < OPe < healthy bone

estimate the absolute water proton content. Multicomponent T_2^* fitting requires a series of MRI images with different TEs, which can extend the scanning process. Bicomponent exponential T_2^* fitting has been used in many studies to quantify BW and PW [17, 21, 66]. Both Bae et al. [21] and

Seifert et al. [67] found that BW and PW fractions obtained from bicomponent T_2^* analysis were significantly correlated with human cortical bone porosity measured using μCT. Bae et al. also reported significant correlations between bicomponent T_2^* results and mechanical properties of human cortical bone strips [21]. Recently, the efficacy of UTE-MRI bicomponent T_2^* analysis has been investigated by comparing it with histomorphometric measures of bone porosity [66]. Bicomponent T_2^* was found to be capable of detecting bone porosity, including pores below the range detectable by μCT [66].

UTE-MRI, μCT, and histological images of a representative bone specimen (a 71-year-old male) are shown in Fig. 34.3. Bone layers closer to the endosteum showed higher porosity and larger pore size. Bicomponent T_2^* fittings and the histomorphometric pore size distributions within three bone layers are depicted in the second and third row subfig-

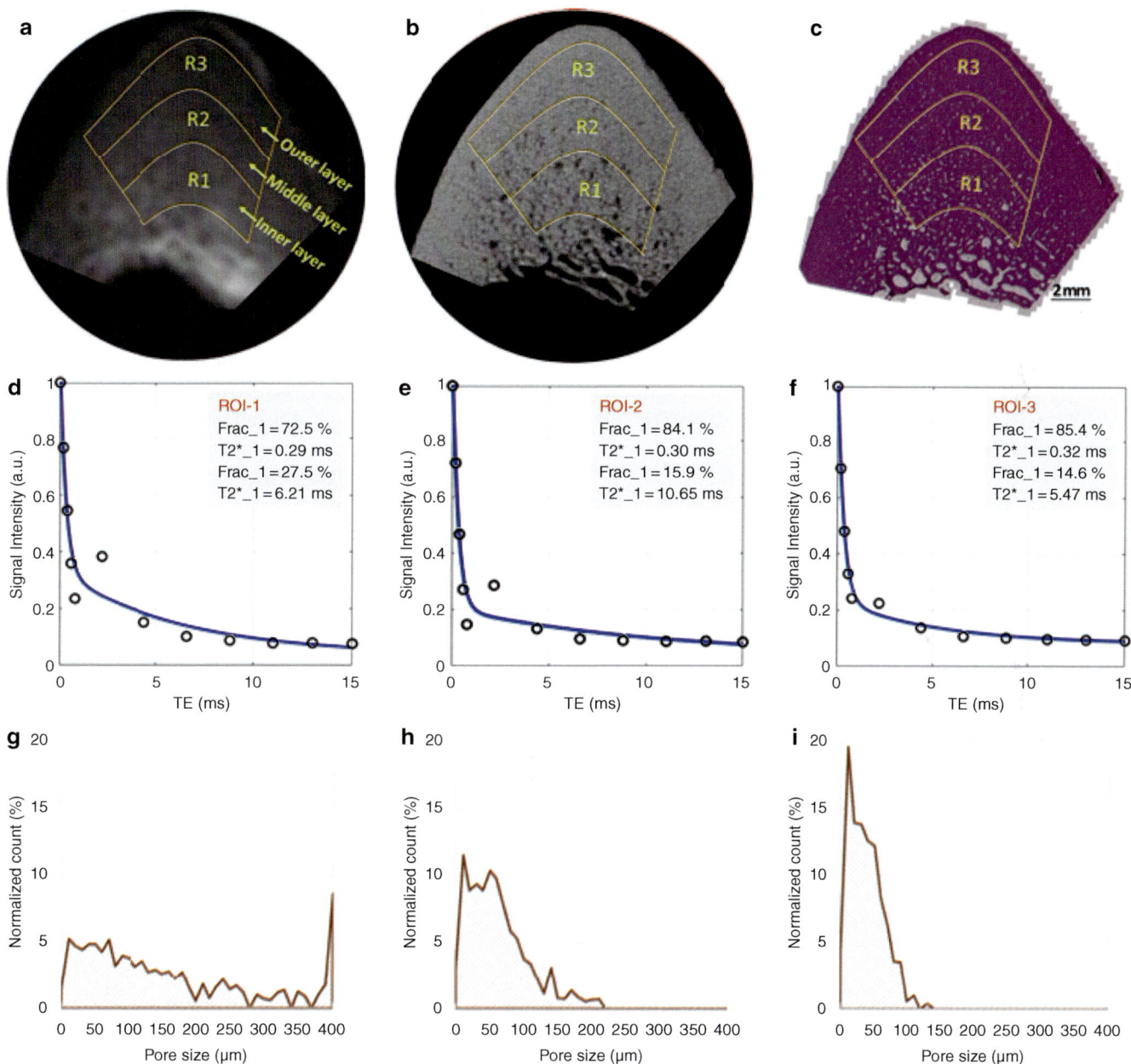

Fig. 34.3 MRI-based and histomorphometric analyses for three representative regions of interest (ROIs) in three different cortical bone layers. Selected ROIs in three different bone layers of a representative bone specimen (male, 71-year-old) illustrated on (**a**) UTE-MRI (TE = 32 μs, 250-μm pixel size), (**b**) μCT (9-μm pixel size), and (**c**) histological (hematoxylin and eosin (H&E)-stained, 0.2-μm pixel size) images. Bicomponent exponential fitting of the T_2^* decay within (**d**) ROI-1, (**e**) ROI-2, and (**f**) ROI-3. The oscillating data points indicate the presence of fat, particularly in ROI-1 and ROI-2 near the endosteum. Pore size distribution obtained from histomorphometric analyses are shown for (**g**) ROI-1, (**h**) ROI-2, and (**i**) ROI-3. The histomorphometric porosity and pore size for ROI-1 to ROI-3 are 33.1, 13.9, 7.1%, 221, 83, and 49 μm, respectively. The μCT-based porosities are 21.2, 8.2, and 1.7% for ROIs-1 to ROI-3, respectively. (Adapted with permission from Jerban et al. [66])

ures, respectively. The short-T_2 fraction (Frac1) was found to be higher in regions with lower porosity and lower pore size [66]. Peaks in pore size distributions shifted toward lower values for layers closer to the periosteum, indicating fewer large pores in the outer layers of cortical bone.

UTE bicomponent analysis was also utilized to study the effect of field strength on the T_2^* of cortical bone at 1.5 T and 3 T [68]. The BW T_2^* and PW T_2^* of human cortical bone were 21% and 68% lower, respectively, at 3 T compared with those at 1.5 T [68]. However, BW and PW fractions showed only minor changes with field strength (<4%), suggesting that UTE bicomponent analysis may provide consistent BW and PW fractions at 1.5 T and 3 T, respectively, thereby allowing field-independent comparison. Seifert et al. [67] later studied the performance of bicomponent analysis at higher magnetic fields (7 T and 9.4 T) and suggested that bicomponent analysis may fail at high magnetic fields, likely due to inaccurate fitting caused by significant decrease in the difference between the short-component T_2^* and long-component T_2^* at higher magnetic fields.

BW, PW, and Fat Content Assessment with Tri-component Signal Modeling

Human cortical bone contains considerable fat, particularly in regions near bone marrow. Different studies have observed oscillation of an average signal using multi-echo MRI in T_2 fitting analyses [16, 67, 69], a phenomenon that is most likely due to fat chemical shift [69]. To remove fat signal contamination in bone water assessment, fat suppression techniques such as chemical shift fat saturation (Fat-Sat),

soft–hard water excitation, and single-point Dixon methods have been used [70, 71]. Fat-Sat is widely used in clinical magnetic resonance (MR) sequences; however, it is not suitable for bone imaging due to the saturation of the broad spectrum of bone. A novel soft-hard pulse has been proposed to overcome this effect by utilizing a low-power soft pulse for fat excitation in the opposite direction of the following hard pulse [70]. Single-point Dixon is a post-processing method, which separates water and fat signals, thus making them available for further analysis [71].

A tri-component fitting model has been developed to include fat modeled using its nuclear magnetic resonance (NMR) spectrum [72]. This improved estimates of BW and PW fractions in cortical bone and also provided estimates of the fat content in bone. Estimation of water fraction by tri-component T_2^* fitting improved correlation with μCT-based porosity compared to bicomponent fitting [72, 73]. Tri-component analysis has also shown a higher correlation with the mechanical properties of bone [73]. The tri-component model avoids BW overestimation in the endosteal side of the cortex, which is a common error with bicomponent analysis [72, 73]. The estimated fat content using a tri-component fitting model needs to be validated before extending it to in vivo applications.

Figure 34.4a shows a UTE-MRI image of a set of cortical bone specimens with 4 mm × 2 mm cross sections placed in a 1″ birdcage coil. Figure 34.4b, c illustrates the μCT images of samples I and II with 15 and 33% average porosities, respectively [73]. Bicomponent and tri-component fitting analyses are shown in Fig. 34.4d–g for both specimens. Sample II shows a significant oscillating signal, which is well fitted using the tri-component model.

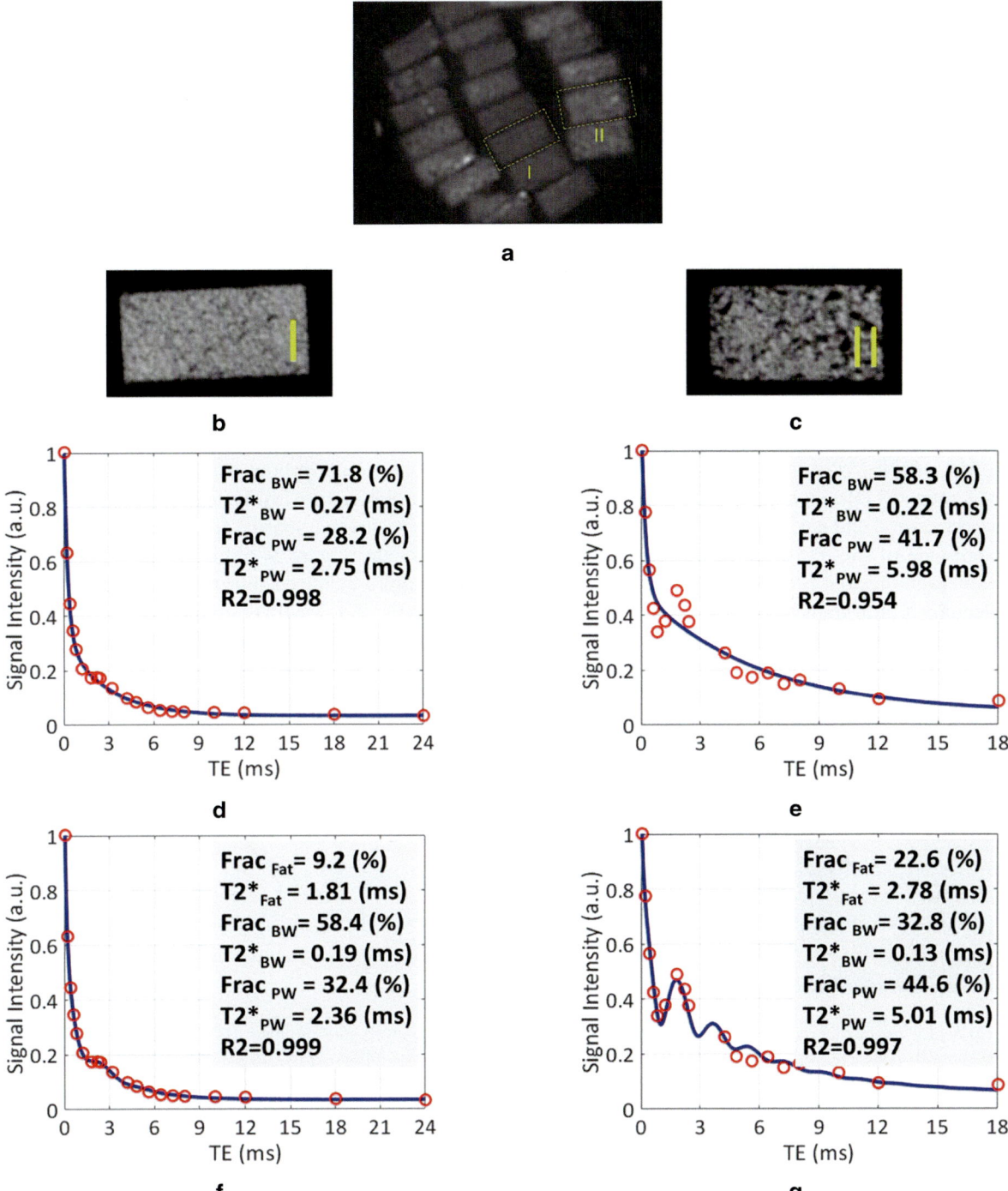

Fig. 34.4 A UTE-MRI image and µCT images of two representative cortical bone strips harvested from different donors possessing different porosities, in addition to bicomponent and tri-component T_2^* fitting results. (**a**) A UTE-MRI (TE = 0.032 ms) image of a set of cortical bone strips with approximately 4 mm × 2 mm cross sections soaked in Fomblin, which produces no signal with MRI. (**b, c**) µCT images of representative cortical bone strips from a 47-year-old male and a 57-year-old female, respectively. (**d, e**) Bicomponent T_2^* fittings for bone strips are shown in panels (**b**) and (**c**), respectively. (**f, g**) Tri-component T_2^* fitting for the bone strips are shown in panels (**a**) and (**b**), respectively. The oscillating signal decay in cortical bone specimens is better fitted by including the signal contribution of fat using the tri-component model (higher fitting R_2 values). (Adapted with permission from Jerban et al. [73])

Cortical Bone Organic Matrix Assessment

In addition to the evaluation of water components that multiple research groups have focused on, the evaluation of bone organic matrix can provide additional information about bone remodeling status and bone mechanical properties. Direct quantification of collagen backbone protons is challenging with current MRI scanners because the collagen protons possess extremely short T_2^*s [74]. Magnetization transfer (MT) imaging combined with UTE-MRI has been suggested as a method to indirectly assess protons in the collagenous matrix [75, 76]. With MT techniques, a high-power saturation RF pulse is applied with a frequency offset from the water resonance frequency to saturate the magnetization of collagen protons. Saturated magnetization is transferred from the collagen to water protons, which can then be imaged with UTE-MRI. UTE-MT assessment of collagen protons, such as MT ratio (MTR), significantly correlates with the bone's microstructural and mechanical properties [77].

The magnitude of the transferred saturation is a function of the macromolecular proton fraction (MMF). MMF, macromolecular proton transverse relaxation time (T_{2mm}), and exchange rates can be obtained with a two-pool model using UTE-MT data acquired with a series of RF pulse powers and frequency offsets [75]. MMF derived from UTE-MT modeling has shown a strong correlation with human bone microstructure measured via μCT and histomorphometry [66, 76] and with mechanical properties [50, 65, 66, 76].

Figure 34.5 shows the relationship between bone microstructure and UTE-MT modeling results [76]. Fig. 34.5a shows a zoomed μCT image of a representative tibial bone specimen focused on the anterior tibia. Porosity and BMD were measured at two selected regions in the middle and outer layers of the cortex. Two-pool MT modeling analyses of the selected regions of interest (ROIs) are shown in Fig. 34.5b, c using three MT saturation pulse powers (500°, 1000°, and 1500°) and five off-resonance frequencies (2, 5, 10, 20, and 50 kHz).

Macromolecular proton density (MMPD) can be calculated as a function of MMF and TWPD [50]. MMPD can demonstrate organic matrix density regardless of the water content density. Figure 34.6 shows in vivo MMF and MMPD maps for representative subjects with healthy bone, OPe, and OPo. MMF and MMPD are observed in the following ascending order: OPo < OPe < healthy bone.

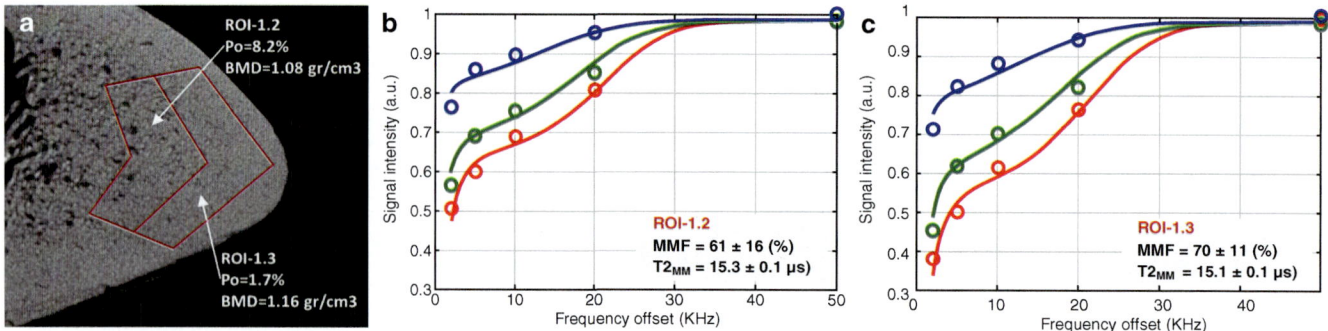

Fig. 34.5 (**a**) A μCT image of a representative tibial specimen (male, 73-year-old) focused on the anterior tibia with two selected ROIs in the middle and outer layers. The measured porosity (Po) in the middle layer (ROI-1.2) is higher than that of the outer layer (ROI-1.3). The two-pool MT model analyses in (**b**) ROI-1.2 and (**c**) ROI-1.3 used three pulse saturation powers (500° in blue, 1000° in green, and 1500° in red) and five frequency offsets (2, 5, 10, 20, and 50 kHz). MMF and T_{2mm} refer to macromolecular fraction and macromolecular T_2, respectively. (Adapted with permission from Jerban et al. [76])

Fig. 34.6 Generated MMF and macromolecular proton density (MMPD) maps for (first row) a representative participant with healthy bone (a 35-year-old female), (second row) a representative patient with OPe (a 76-year-old female), and (third row) a representative patient with OPo (a 76-year-old female). For these examples, MMF and MMPD are observed in the following ascending order: OPo < OPe < healthy bone

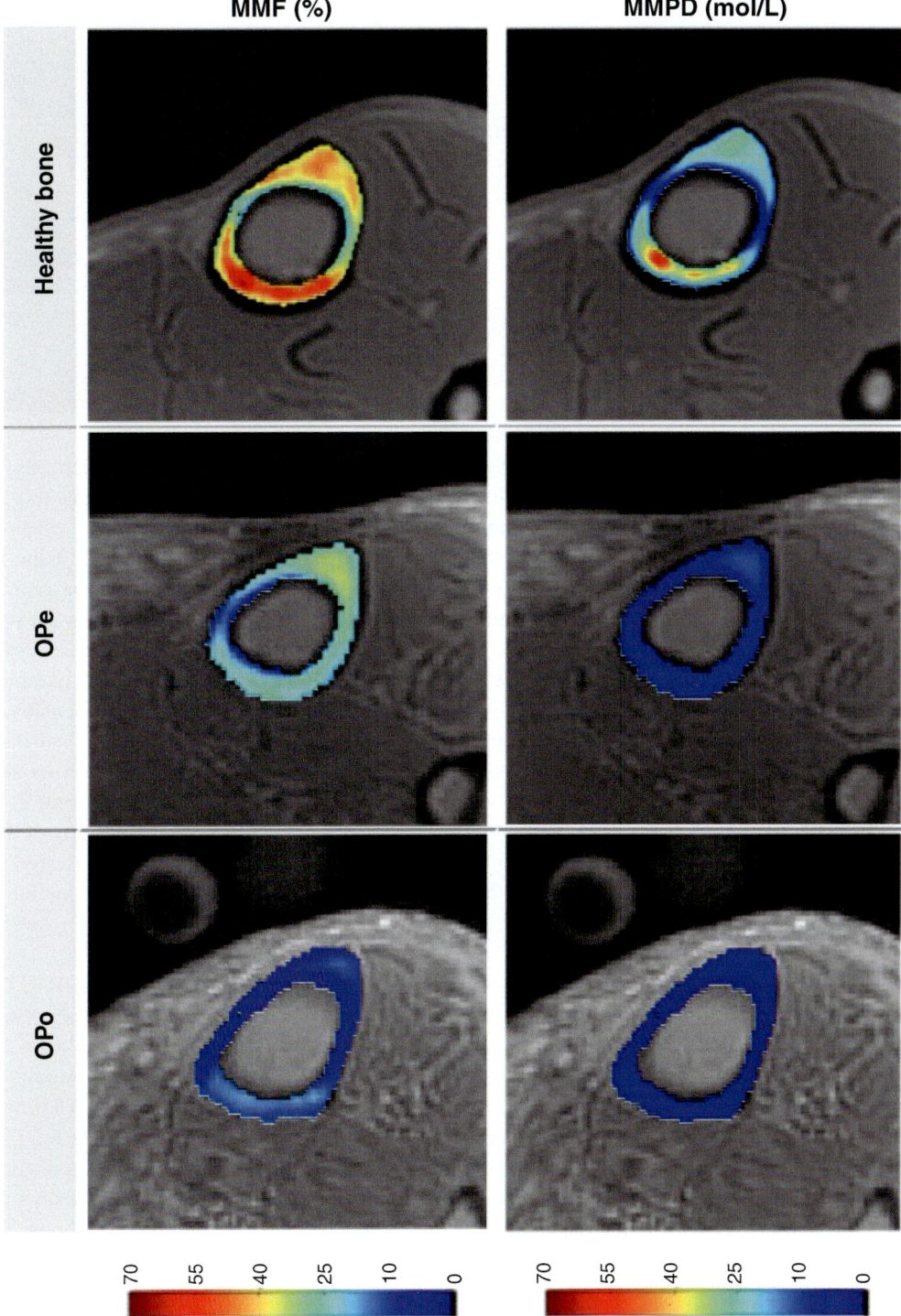

Cortical Bone Mineral Assessment

Although the X-ray-based methods (DEXA and CT) are the gold standards of bone mineral assessment, UTE-MRI shows potential to assess bone mineral. Utilizing UTE-MRI for bone mineral assessments can complete the UTE-based biomarker panel in OPo evaluation. Single modality imaging with MRI can provide information about all major bone components and potentially facilitate clinical decision-making.

Quantitative Susceptibility Mapping (UTE-QSM) for Mineral Assessment

Quantitative susceptibility mapping (QSM) deconvolves the magnetic susceptibility of tissue based on phase changes in the MR signal. Tissues with stronger magnetic susceptibilities undergo faster evolution of the phase than those with lower susceptibility. Dimov et al. [78] developed the UTE-QSM technique to detect mineral variations in the porcine

Fig. 34.7 (**a**) Quantitative susceptibility map (QSM) using Cones 3D UTE-MRI scans ($0.5 \times 0.5 \times 2$ mm^3 voxel size) of a representative tibial midshaft cortical bone sample (a 45-year-old female), (**b**) μCT-based volumetric bone mineral density (BMD) maps of the same specimen. The local maxima in the QSM map correspond to the regions of high BMD in μCT-based maps. (Adapted with permission from Jerban et al. [79])

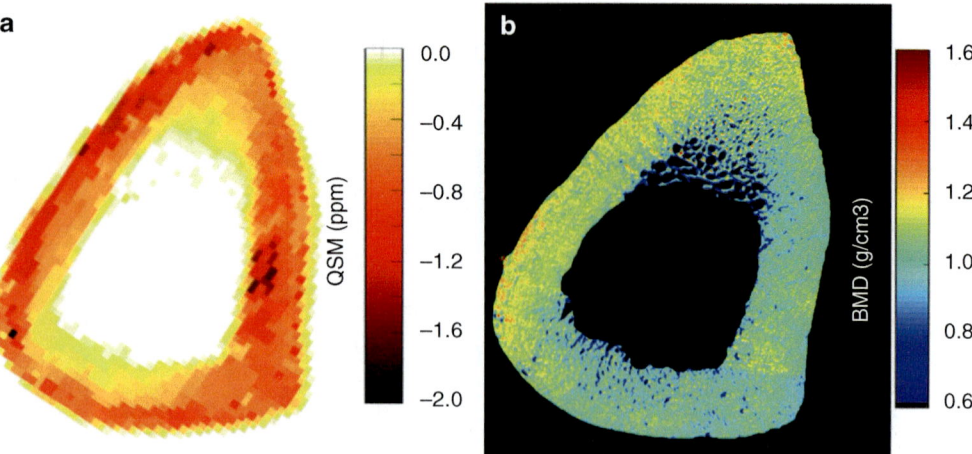

hoof and human distal femur. They reported significant correlations between radial 3D UTE-QSM values and computed tomography (CT) X-ray attenuation measured in Hounsfield units in a combined set of ROIs covering tendon, trabecular bone, and cortical bone. Recently, UTE-QSM has been investigated in human tibial cortical bone specimens, and significant correlations between QSM and BMD have been reported [79]. Figure 34.7 illustrates Cones UTE-QSM and volumetric BMD maps in a representative cortical bone specimen from the tibial midshaft. The local maxima of the QSM map qualitatively correspond to the regions of high BMD in μCT-based maps [79].

UTE ^{31}P Imaging for Assessment of Bone Minerals

Phosphorus (i.e., ^{31}P) imaging combined with UTE, water- and fat-suppressed proton projection MRI (WASPI), or zero echo time (ZTE) MR acquisitions have been employed for bone mineral estimation in several studies [48, 49, 80]. The feasibility of in vivo ^{31}P imaging in human subjects has been shown at 1.5 T using UTE-based imaging of the tibia and femoral head [81]. Phosphorus imaging can be considered a direct method of mineral imaging compared with the previously discussed UTE-QSM method, which evaluates mineral based on its magnetic susceptibility. However, the hardware adjustment necessary for phosphorus imaging has resulted in the underutilization of this technique in bone assessment even in research centers.

Trabecular Bone Quantification

Direct imaging of trabecular bone is technically challenging because of the fast signal decay of bone, as implied by its ultrashort-T_2 [38]. To create high contrast for trabecular bone with proton imaging, it is critical to suppress signals from long-T_2 tissues, particularly marrow fat. Wurnig et al. [82] used the UTE sequence to visualize trabecular bone ex vivo and to measure its T_2^* at different magnetic field strengths. This direct trabecular bone imaging was achieved with an SPIR (spectral presaturation with inversion recovery) module to suppress marrow fat signal. Investigating T_2^* values in trabecular bone regions showed significant correlations with bone microstructural parameters obtained with μCT [82]. However, the innate sensitivity of the SPIR-UTE technique to B_0 inhomogeneity and the rather complicated multipeak fat spectrum may limit its specificity in imaging trabecular bone. The relatively long T_2^* of ~2.42 ms derived from the single-component fitting of SPIR-UTE imaging of trabecular bone at 3 T, which is significantly longer than the T_2^* of ~0.3 ms for cortical bone measured with IR-UTE imaging at the same field strength, suggests incomplete long-T_2 signal suppression.

The 3D adiabatic IR-UTE-Cones (3D IR-UTE-Cones) sequence has been proposed by Ma et al. [83] to directly visualize trabecular bone and measure relaxation times [83]. A broadband adiabatic inversion pulse was used together with a short TR/inversion time (TI) combination to suppress signals from long-T_2 tissues such as muscles and marrow fat. The suppression is followed by multispoke UTE acquisition to detect signals from short-T_2 water components in trabecular bone. This technique has low sensitivity to B_1 and B_0 inhomogeneities due to the broadband adiabatic inversion pulses [83]. The technique has been applied ex vivo and in vivo at 3 T and resulted in ranges of T_2^* values (0.3–0.45 ms) and proton densities (5–9 mol/L) for trabecular bone. In vivo 3D IR-UTE-Cones images of the lumbar spine at different TEs (0.032–2.2 ms) are shown in Fig. 34.8, in addition to the corresponding T_2^* curve fitting. The fitted T_2^* is extremely close to that of cortical bone, consistent with effective suppression of signals from bone marrow fat.

Bound water proton density mapping can be achieved for trabecular bone by comparing its signal to that obtained with

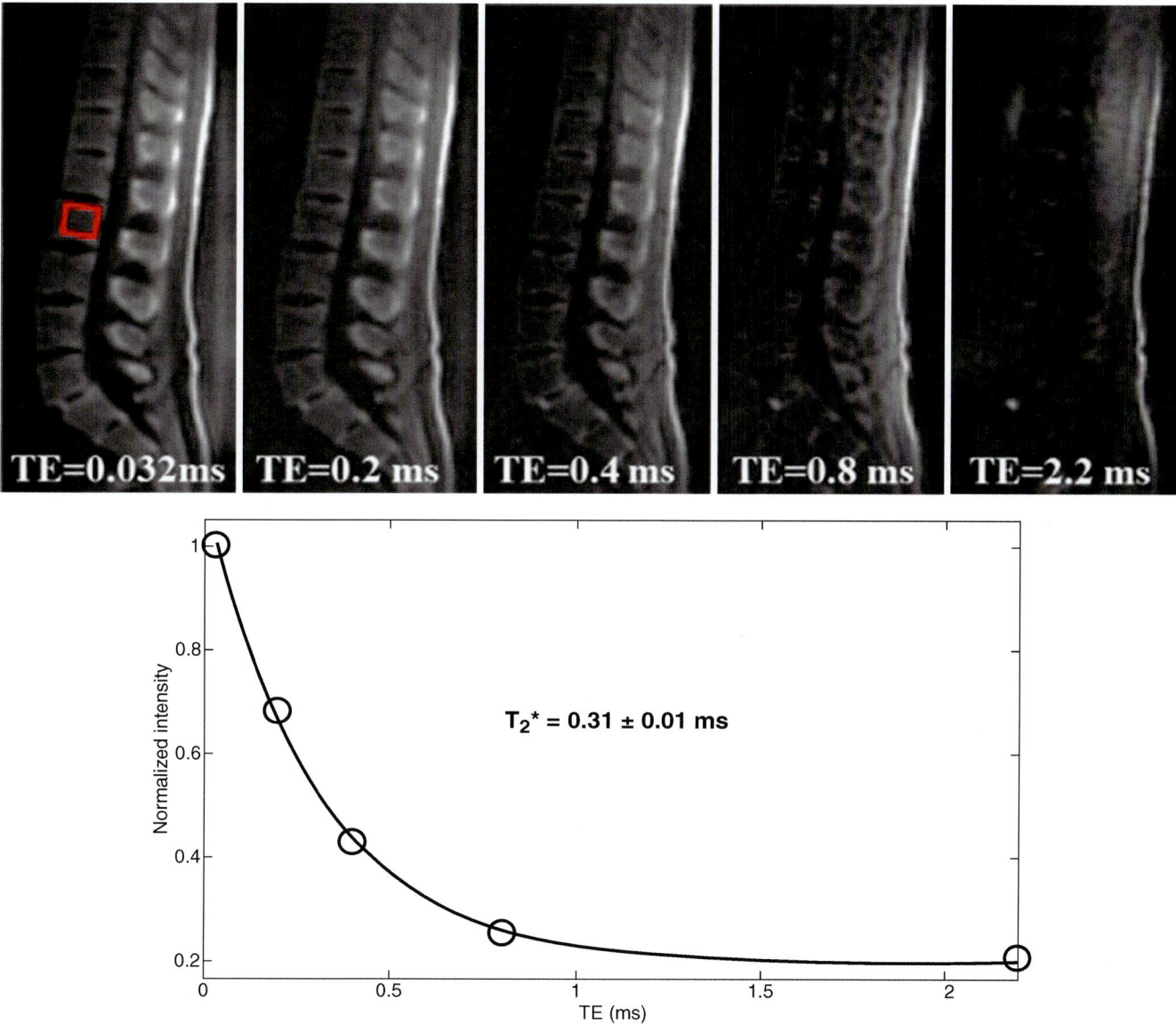

Fig. 34.8 In vivo imaging of the spine of a 36-year-old male volunteer using the 3D IR-UTE-Cones sequence with TEs of 0.032, 0.2, 0.4, 0.8, and 2.2 ms. Single-component fitting was achieved for a selected verte-bra giving a short T_2^* of 0.31 ± 0.01 ms and demonstrating that long-T_2 water and marrow fat can be effectively suppressed by the IR-UTE-Cones sequence. (Adapted with permission from Ma et al. [83])

3D IR-UTE-Cones imaging and that from an external reference standard with a known proton density similar to that previously described in cortical bone studies [83].

Conclusions

Quantification limited to bone mineral for OPo evaluation, as takes place in clinical practice, may miss major changes in other bone components such as the organic matrix, different water components (TW, BW, and PW), and fat fraction. The quantitative UTE-MRI techniques discussed in this chapter can assess all the major components of bone, and these may experience changes during OPo development that do not parallel BMD changes and may thus provide a more comprehensive evaluation of cortical bone. Basic UTE and adiabatic IR-prepared UTE (IR-UTE) sequences can quantify TW, BW, and PW. UTE tri-component T_2^* analysis distinguishes between BW and PW signals and fractions in addition to providing assessment of fat fraction. UTE-magnetization transfer (UTE-MT) sequences can quantify the organic matrix in bone, and UTE quantitative susceptibility mapping (UTE-QSM) sequences provide bone mineral assessment. Combining these UTE-based techniques after optimization to shorten their scan times may provide a comprehensive technique for OPo and OPe evaluation.

Acknowledgments The authors acknowledge the grant support from the National Institutes of Health (K01AR080257, R01AR068987, R01AR062581, R01AR075825, R01AR079484, and 5P30AR073761) and Veterans Affairs Clinical Science and Rehabilitation R&D (I01CX001388, I01RX002604, and I01CX000625).

References

1. National Institutes of Health, statement CDC. Osteoporosis prevention, diagnosis, and therapy. JAMA. 2001;285(6):785–95.
2. Teitelbaum SL. Bone resorption by osteoclasts. Science. 2000;289(5484):1504–8.
3. Atkins GJ, Findlay DM. Osteocyte regulation of bone mineral: a little give and take. Osteoporosis Int. 2012;23(8):2067–79.
4. Aubin JE, Triffitt JT. Mesenchymal stem cells and osteoblast differentiation. Principles of Bone Biol. 2002:59–81.
5. Edwards MH, Dennison EM, Aihie Sayer A, Fielding R, Cooper C. Osteoporosis and sarcopenia in older age. Bone. 2015;80:126–30.
6. Kaplan SJ, Pham TN, Arbabi S, et al. Association of radiologic indicators of frailty with 1-year mortality in older trauma patients: opportunistic screening for sarcopenia and osteopenia. JAMA Surg. 2017;152(2):e164604.
7. Zebaze RM, Ghasem-Zadeh A, Bohte A, et al. Intracortical remodelling and porosity in the distal radius and post-mortem femurs of women: a cross-sectional study. Lancet. 2010;375(9727):1729–36.
8. MacDonald HM, Nishiyama KK, Kang J, Hanley DA, Boyd SK. Age-related patterns of trabecular and cortical bone loss differ between sexes and skeletal sites: a population-based HR-pQCT study. J Bone Miner Res. 2011;26(1):50–62.
9. Ritchie RO, Buehler MJ, Hansma P. Plasticity and toughness in bone. Phys Today. 2009;62(6):41–7.
10. Cowin SC. Bone poroelasticity. J Biomech. 1999;32(3):217–38.
11. Wehrli FW, Song HK, Saha PK, Wright AC. Quantitative MRI for the assessment of bone structure and function. NMR Biomed. 2006;19(7):731–64.
12. Ott SM. Cortical or trabecular bone: what's the difference? Am J Nephrol. 2018;47(6):373–5.
13. Wang X, Ni Q. Determination of cortical bone porosity and pore size distribution using a low field pulsed NMR approach. J Orthop Res. 2003;21(2):312–9.
14. Nyman JS, Ni Q, Nicolella DP, Wang X. Measurements of mobile and bound water by nuclear magnetic resonance correlate with mechanical properties of bone. Bone. 2008;42(1):193–9.
15. Horch RA, Nyman JS, Gochberg DF, Dortch RD, Does MD. Characterization of 1H NMR signal in human cortical bone for magnetic resonance imaging. Magn Reson Med. 2010;64(3):680–7.
16. Diaz E, Chung CB, Bae WC, et al. Ultrashort echo time spectroscopic imaging (UTESI): an efficient method for quantifying bound and free water. NMR Biomed. 2012;25(1):161–8.
17. Biswas R, Bae WC, Diaz E, et al. Ultrashort echo time (UTE) imaging with bi-component analysis: bound and free water evaluation of bovine cortical bone subject to sequential drying. Bone. 2012;50(3):749–55.
18. Ong HH, Wright AC, Wehrli FW. Deuterium nuclear magnetic resonance unambiguously quantifies pore and collagen-bound water in cortical bone. J Bone Miner Res. 2012;27(12):2573–81.
19. Du J, Bydder GM. Qualitative and quantitative ultrashort-TE MRI of cortical bone. NMR Biomed. 2013;26(5):489–506.
20. Horch RA, Gochberg DF, Nyman JS, Does MD. Non-invasive predictors of human cortical bone mechanical properties: T_2-discriminated 1H NMR compared with high resolution X-ray. PLoS One. 2011;6(1):1–5.
21. Bae WC, Chen PC, Chung CB, Masuda K, D'Lima D, Du J. Quantitative ultrashort echo time (UTE) MRI of human corti-

cal bone: correlation with porosity and biomechanical properties. J Bone Miner Res. 2012;27(4):848–57.
22. Zioupos P, Currey JD, Hamer AJ. The role of collagen in the declining mechanical properties of aging human cortical bone. J Biomed Mater Res. 1999;45(2):108–16.
23. Wang X, Shen X, Li X, Mauli Agrawal C. Age-related changes in the collagen network and toughness of bone. Bone. 2002;31(1):1–7.
24. Nyman JS, Roy A, Shen X, Acuna RL, Tyler JH, Wang X. The influence of water removal on the strength and toughness of cortical bone. J Biomech. 2006;39(5):931–8.
25. Wehrli FW, Fernández-Seara MA. Nuclear magnetic resonance studies of bone water. Ann Biomed Eng. 2005;33(1):79–86.
26. Yeni YN, Brown CU, Norman TL. Influence of bone composition and apparent density on fracture toughness of the human femur and tibia. Bone. 1998;22(1):79–84.
27. De Laet CEDH, Van Hout BA, Burger H, Hofman A, Pols HAP. Bone density and risk of hip fracture in men and women: cross sectional analysis. BMJ. 1997;315(7102):11–5.
28. Trajanoska K, Schoufour JD, de Jonge EAL, et al. Fracture incidence and secular trends between 1989 and 2013 in a population based cohort: the Rotterdam study. Bone. 2018;114:116–24.
29. Cummings SR. Are patients with hip fractures more osteoporotic? Review of evidence. Am J Med. 1985;78(3):487–94.
30. Marshall D, Johnell O, Wedel H. Meta-analysis of how well measures of bone mineral density predict occurrence of osteoporotic fractures. BMJ. 1996;18(704):1254–9.
31. Faulkner KG. Bone matters: are density increases necessary to reduce fracture risk? J Bone Miner Res. 2000;15(2):183–7.
32. Schuit SCE, Van Der Klift M, Weel AEAM, et al. Fracture incidence and association with bone mineral density in elderly men and women: the Rotterdam study. Bone. 2004;34(1):195–202.
33. Sandor T, Felsenberg D, Brown E. Comments on the hypotheses underlying fracture risk assessment in osteoporosis as proposed by the World Health Organization. Calcif Tissue Int. 1999;64(3):267–70.
34. McCreadie BR, Goldstein SA. Biomechanics of fracture: is bone mineral density sufficient to assess risk? J Bone Miner Res. 2000;15(12):2305–8.
35. Homminga J, McCreadie BR, Ciarelli TE, Weinans H, Goldstein SA, Huiskes R. Cancellous bone mechanical properties from normals and patients with hip fractures differ on the structure level, not on the bone hard tissue level. Bone. 2002;30(5):759–64.
36. Kanis JA, Johnell O, Oden A, Dawson A, De Laet C, Jonsson B. Ten year probabilities of osteoporotic fractures according to BMD and diagnostic thresholds. Osteoporosis Int. 2001;12(12):989–95.
37. Russo CR, Lauretani F, Bandinelli S, et al. Aging bone in men and women: beyond changes in bone mineral density. Osteoporosis Int. 2003;14(7):531–8.
38. Robson MD, Gatehouse PD, Bydder M, Bydder GM. Magnetic resonance: an introduction to ultrashort TE (UTE) imaging. J Comput Assist Tomogr. 2003;27(6):825–46.
39. Reichert ILH, Robson MD, Gatehouse PD, et al. Magnetic resonance imaging of cortical bone with ultrashort TE pulse sequences. Magn Reson Imaging. 2005;23(5):611–8.
40. Chang EY, Du J, Chung CB. UTE imaging in the musculoskeletal system. J Magn Reson Imaging. 2015;41(4):870–83.
41. Manhard MK, Nyman JS, Does MD. Advances in imaging approaches to fracture risk evaluation. Transl Res. 2017;181:1–14.
42. Wehrli FW. Magnetic resonance of calcified tissues. J Magn Reson. 2013;229:35–48.
43. Techawiboonwong A, Song HK, Leonard MB, Wehrli FW. Cortical bone water: in vivo quantification with ultrashort echo-time MR imaging. Radiology. 2008;248(3):824–33.
44. Du J, Carl M, Bydder M, Takahashi A, Chung CB, Bydder GM. Qualitative and quantitative ultrashort echo time (UTE) imaging of cortical bone. J Magn Reson. 2010;207(2):304–11.

45. Rad HS, Lam SCB, Magland JF, et al. Quantifying cortical bone water in vivo by three-dimensional ultra-short echo-time MRI. NMR Biomed. 2011;24(7):855–64.

46. Li C, Seifert AC, Rad HS, et al. Cortical bone water concentration: dependence of MR imaging measures on age and pore volume fraction. Radiology. 2014;272(3):796–806.

47. Manhard MK, Horch RA, Gochberg DF, Nyman JS, Does MD. In vivo quantitative MR imaging of bound and pore water in cortical bone. Radiology. 2015;277(1):221–9.

48. Seifert AC, Wehrli FW. Solid-state quantitative (1)H and (31) P MRI of cortical bone in humans. Curr Osteoporos Rep. 2016;14(3):77–86.

49. Zhao X, Song HK, Seifert AC, Li C, Wehrli FW. Feasibility of assessing bone matrix and mineral properties in vivo by combined solidstate 1H and 31P MRI. PLoS One. 2017;12(3):e0173995.

50. Jerban S, Ma Y, Li L, et al. Volumetric mapping of bound and pore water as well as collagen protons in cortical bone using 3D ultrashort echo time cones MR imaging techniques. Bone. 2019;127:120–8.

51. Jerban S, Ma Y, Jang H, et al. Water proton density in human cortical bone obtained from ultrashort echo time (UTE) MRI predicts bone microstructural properties. Magn Reson Imaging. 2020;67:85–9.

52. Ma Y, Lu X, Carl M, et al. Accurate T_1 mapping of short T_2 tissues using a three-dimensional ultrashort echo time cones actual flip angle imaging-variable repetition time (3D UTE-cones AFI-VTR) method. Magn Reson Med. 2018;80(2):598–608.

53. Du J, Takahashi AM, Bae WC, Chung CB, Bydder GM. Dual inversion recovery, ultrashort echo time (DIR UTE) imaging: creating high contrast for short-T_2species. Magn Reson Med. 2010;63(2):447–55.

54. Horch RA, Gochberg DF, Nyman JS, Does MD. Clinically compatible MRI strategies for discriminating bound and pore water in cortical bone. Magn Reson Med. 2012;68(6):1774–84.

55. Du J, Chiang AJT, Chung CB, et al. Orientational analysis of the achilles tendon and enthesis using an ultrashort echo time spectroscopic imaging sequence. Magn Reson Imaging. 2010;28(2):178–84.

56. Chen J, Grogan SP, Shao H, et al. Evaluation of bound and pore water in cortical bone using ultrashort-TE MRI. NMR Biomed. 2015;28(12):1754–62.

57. Guo T, Ma Y, Jerban S, et al. T1 measurement of bound water in cortical bone using 3D adiabatic inversion recovery ultrashort echo time (3D IR-UTE) cones imaging. Magn Reson Med. 2020;84(2):634–45.

58. Chen J, Chang EY, Carl M, et al. Measurement of bound and pore water T1 relaxation times in cortical bone using three-dimensional ultrashort echo time cones sequences. Magn Reson Med. 2016;77(6):2136–45.

59. Abbasi-Rad S, Saligheh RH. Quantification of human cortical bone bound and free water in vivo with ultrashort echo time MR imaging: a model-based approach. Radiology. 2017;283(3):862–72.

60. Manhard MK, Uppuganti S, Granke M, Gochberg DF, Nyman JS, Does MD. MRI-derived bound and pore water concentrations as predictors of fracture resistance. Bone. 2016;87:1–10.

61. Rajapakse CS, Bashoor-Zadeh M, Li C, Sun W, Wright AC, Wehrli FW. Volumetric cortical bone porosity assessment with MR imaging: validation and clinical feasibility. Radiology. 2015;276(2):526–35.

62. Hong AL, Ispiryan M, Padalkar MV, et al. MRI-derived bone porosity index correlates to bone composition and mechanical stiffness. Bone Rep. 2019;11:100213.

63. Jerban S, Ma Y, Moazamian D, et al. MRI-based porosity index (PI) and suppression ratio (SR) in the tibial cortex show significant differences between normal, osteopenic, and osteoporotic female subjects. Front. Endocrinol. 2023;14:1148345. https://doi.org/10.3389/fendo.2023.1148345.

64. Du J, Hermida JC, Diaz E, et al. Assessment of cortical bone with clinical and ultrashort echo time sequences. Magn Reson Med. 2013;70(3):697–704.

65. Jerban S, Ma Y, Dorthe EW, et al. Assessing cortical bone mechanical properties using collagen proton fraction from ultrashort echo time magnetization transfer (UTE-MT) MRI modeling. Bone Rep. 2019;11:100220.

66. Jerban S, Ma Y, Wong JH, et al. Ultrashort echo time magnetic resonance imaging (UTE-MRI) of cortical bone correlates well with histomorphometric assessment of bone microstructure. Bone. 2019;123:8–17.

67. Seifert AC, Wehrli SL, Wehrli FW. Bi-component T_2^* analysis of bound and pore bone water fractions fails at high field strengths. NMR Biomed. 2015;28(7):861–72.

68. Li S, Chang EY, Bae WC, et al. Ultrashort echo time bi-component analysis of cortical bone—a field dependence study. Magn Reson Med. 2014;71(3):1075–81.

69. Li S, Ma L, Chang EY, et al. Effects of inversion time on inversion recovery prepared ultrashort echo time (IR-UTE) imaging of bound and pore water in cortical bone. NMR Biomed. 2015;28(1):70–8.

70. Ma Y, Jerban S, Jang H, Chang EY, Du J. Fat suppression for ultrashort echo time imaging using a novel soft-hard composite radiofrequency pulse. Magn Reson Med. 2019;82(6):2178–87.

71. Jang H, Carl M, Ma Y, et al. Fat suppression for ultrashort echo time imaging using a single point Dixon method. NMR Biomed. 2019;32(5):e4069.

72. Lu X, Jerban S, Wan L, et al. Three dimensional ultrashort echo time imaging with tri-component analysis for human cortical bone. Magn Reson Med. 2019;82(1):348–55.

73. Jerban S, Lu X, Dorthe EW, et al. Correlations of cortical bone microstructural and mechanical properties with water proton fractions obtained from ultrashort echo time (UTE) MRI tricomponent T_2^* model. NMR Biomed. 2020;33(3):e4233.

74. Ma Y, Chang EY, Bydder GM, Du J. Can ultrashort-TE (UTE) MRI sequences on a 3-T clinical scanner detect signal directly from collagen protons: freeze-dry and D2O exchange studies of cortical bone and achilles tendon specimens. NMR Biomed. 2016;29(7):912–7.

75. Ma Y, Chang EY, Carl M, Du J. Quantitative magnetization transfer ultrashort echo time imaging using a time-efficient 3D multispoke cones sequence. Magn Reson Med. 2017;79(2):692–700.

76. Jerban S, Ma Y, Wan L, et al. Collagen proton fraction from ultrashort echo time magnetization transfer (UTE-MT) MRI modelling correlates significantly with cortical bone porosity measured with micro-computed tomography (μCT). NMR Biomed. 2019;32(2):e4045.

77. Chang EY, Bae WC, Shao H, et al. Ultrashort echo time magnetization transfer (UTE-MT) imaging of cortical bone. NMR Biomed. 2015;28(7):873–80.

78. Dimov AV, Liu Z, Spincemaille P, Prince MR, Du J, Wang Y. Bone quantitative susceptibility mapping using a chemical species-specific R_2^* signal model with ultrashort and conventional echo data. Magn Reson Med. 2017;79(1):121–8.

79. Jerban S, Lu X, Jang H, et al. Significant correlations between human cortical bone mineral density and quantitative susceptibility mapping (QSM) obtained with 3D cones ultrashort echo time magnetic resonance imaging (UTE-MRI). Magn Reson Imaging. 2019;62:104–10.

80. Seifert AC, Li C, Rajapakse CS, et al. Bone mineral (31)P and matrix-bound water densities measured by solid-state (31)P and (1) H MRI. NMR Biomed. 2014;27(7):739–48.

81. Robson MD, Gatehouse PD, Bydder GM, Neubauer S. Human imaging of phosphorus in cortical and trabecular bone in vivo. Magn Reson Med. 2004;51(5):888–92.

82. Wurnig MC, Calcagni M, Kenkel D, et al. Characterization of trabecular bone density with ultra-short echo-time MRI at 1.5, 3.0 and 7.0 T—comparison with micro-computed tomography. NMR Biomed. 2014;27(10):1159–66.

83. Ma YJ, Chen Y, Li L, et al. Trabecular bone imaging using a 3D adiabatic inversion recovery prepared ultrashort TE cones sequence at 3T. Magn Reson Med. 2020;83(5):1640–51.

Noah B. Bonnheim, Misung Han, Aaron J. Fields, Cynthia Chin, and Roland Krug

Introduction

The clinical value of the conventional magnetic resonance imaging (MRI) examination in the spine is controversial, in part due to its relatively low and variable diagnostic specificity for identifying probable anatomic causes of back pain. For example, degenerative structural changes observed in the spine using clinical T_1- and T_2-weighted sequences—such as disc degeneration, disc herniation, endplate damage, spondylolisthesis, stenosis, and facet arthropathy, among other common imaging findings—tend to be associated with pain in some patients but also occur (with varying prevalence) in asymptomatic individuals [1–3]. The link between degenerative pathologies seen on clinical imaging and individual clinical outcomes is further obscured by evidence demonstrating that new episodes of low back pain are unlikely to be accompanied by new imaging findings [4] and that imaging findings are unreliable predictors of treatment outcomes [5]. The unclear associations between conventional MRI-based assessment of spinal structures and individual clinical outcomes have motivated the development of new imaging techniques to enhance the diagnostic value of MRI in the spine and to improve our fundamental understanding of degenerative spinal conditions [6, 7].

Several new MRI techniques enable researchers to probe pathologies of the spine with quantitative and objective measurements of the physical and biochemical processes occuring in spinal tissues. For example, techniques now enable measurement of metabolic activity in the intervertebral disc with magnetic resonance spectroscopy (MRS) [8], molecular diffusion in the disc and vertebral bone marrow with diffusion-weighted imaging (DWI) [6], and spatial maps of water and fat content in the paraspinal muscles and vertebral bone marrow with chemical shift imaging (CSI) [9, 10]. One class of quantitative MRI techniques that is gaining increasing interest and applicability in the spine involves multi-echo imaging to compute spatial maps of tissue relaxation times, such as T_2, T_2^*, T_1, and $T_{1\rho}$, [11] since such relaxation time values can provide quantitative and continuous biomarkers—i.e., objective and quantitative indicators of normal physiological or pathogenic processes [12]—that reflect tissue biochemical composition. Ultrashort echo time (UTE) imaging represents a major methodological advance in spinal imaging by enabling both morphological and quantitative assessments of tissues with short-T_2 relaxation times; such tissues are found throughout the spine and are implicated in pathologies associated with back pain.

Many tissues in the spine, including the vertebral cartilage endplate (CEP), the ligaments and tendons connecting the vertebrae with each other and with the spinal musculature, and the mineralized bone tissues comprising the vertebral body and its posterior elements, are composed of a majority of short-T_2 components (with the T_2 values approximately <10 ms) [13]. The transverse magnetization from these short-T_2 tissues is largely decayed at the time of signal acquisition using conventional T_1- and T_2-weighted sequences (with prescribed echo times (TEs) typically ranging from 10 to 80 ms), causing these tissues to appear as signal voids without internal contrast or conspicuity [14]. The rapid T_2 signal decay of bone, CEP, tendons, and ligaments relates to relatively strong dipolar interactions between protons bound within solid structures (such as the crystalline component of bone) or bound to proteins (such as water molecules bound to collagen fibers) [12]. In the case of tissues with highly aligned collagen, including cartilage, tendons, and ligaments, the strength of these dipolar interactions depends on the macroscopic orientation of the collagen fibers relative to the static magnetic field (B_0) [15]. Thus, the signal intensity generated by such tissues and their T_2 relax-

N. B. Bonnheim (✉) · A. J. Fields
Department of Orthopaedic Surgery, University of California, San Francisco, CA, USA
e-mail: noah.bonnheim@ucsf.edu; aaron.fields@ucsf.edu

M. Han · C. Chin · R. Krug
Department of Radiology and Biomedical Imaging, University of California, San Francisco, CA, USA
e-mail: misung.han@ucsf.edu; cynthia.t.chin@ucsf.edu; roland.krug@ucsf.edu

ation times are sensitive to in situ orientation to B_0 during imaging, a topic discussed in more detail below.

The rest of this chapter describes applications of UTE imaging in the spine with a focus on the vertebral endplate and also includes the ligaments, facet joints, vertebral bone, and sacroiliac joints (SIJs). The CEP is a primary focus due to recent discoveries emphasizing the important role of CEP quality in disc degeneration and low back pain [16–18]. Finally, we discuss technical aspects of UTE-MRI in the spine and several practical considerations related to spine imaging.

The Vertebral Cartilage Endplate (CEP)

The vertebral CEP is a thin layer of hyaline-like cartilage that, along with the abutting osseous endplate, separates the vertebral body from the intervertebral disc [19, 20]. Like articular cartilage, the CEP consists of an extracellular matrix of proteoglycans, water, and collagen, which is remodeled by chondrocytes residing within lacunae interspersed throughout the extracellular matrix [17, 21]. Unlike articular cartilage, which has depth-wise zones of varying collagen organization [22], the collagen fibers in the CEP are mainly aligned parallel to the surface of the endplate [23, 24] and are not highly integrated into the underlying osseous endplate [17, 19]. Typically, the CEP is approximately 0.5–1.0-mm-thick, and its thickness can vary with location and spinal level, being thinnest centrally and at the upper spinal levels [25].

In addition to resisting mechanical forces from intradiscal pressure [26], the CEP is a semipermeable barrier that enables nutrient transport from the vertebral capillaries into the avascular disc [27–29]. The permeability of the CEP is much lower than that of the abutting osseous endplate and is thus considered to be the primary barrier to nutrient transport. Many nutrients that nourish cells in the nucleus pulposus (NP) pass from the vertebral capillaries, across the CEP, and into the disc; conversely, metabolic waste from NP cells travels in the opposite direction: from the disc, across the CEP, and into the vertebral bone marrow [28, 30]. The permeability of the CEP is influenced by aspects of its biochemical composition, including the relative amounts of collagen and aggrecan [28, 30], and deficits in CEP permeability are believed to be one etiological factor contributing to poor disc nutrition and, subsequently, disc degeneration [16, 30–34]. Deficits in CEP permeability are also believed to contribute to heterogeneous treatment outcomes following intradiscal biological therapy, an emerging class of therapies for chronic low back pain [35–39]. By design, such therapies increase intradiscal nutrient demands, and hence therapeutic efficacy likely depends on CEP permeability [30, 35–38]. The importance of the CEP in disc degeneration and regeneration moti-

vates noninvasive assessment of CEP health using MRI, as such assessments could help elucidate the etiology of disc degeneration and help identify patients who may be likely to benefit from biological therapies.

Endplate pathologies are also associated with low back pain independent of their role in disc degeneration. Structural damage to the endplates co-locate with elevated levels of innervation and chemical sensitization factors [17, 40–43], suggesting that sensitization of nociceptors originating at the endplate could cause low back pain. Endplate damage can also expose the underlying vertebral bone marrow to intervertebral disc tissue, which can stimulate an inflammatory immune response since the disc is normally immune-privileged (i.e., sequestered from the systemic circulation and treated as a foreign substance by leukocytes in the bone marrow) [43]. Vertebral endplate bone marrow lesions, which occur adjacent to structural endplate damage, are observed on T_1- and T_2-weighted MRI as signal intensity abnormalities and are classified as "Modic changes" [44]. These endplate bone marrow lesions are associated with neoinnervation, inflammation, high bone turnover, fibrosis, and low back pain [41, 43–45]. Vascularized granulation tissue signaling inflammation and/or regional conversion of hematopoietic marrow to fat in these lesions can generate hypo- and hyperintense signals and contrast within the vertebral body adjacent to damaged endplates, which are visible using conventional clinical T_1- and T_2-weighted sequences; however, the endplate damage itself (particularly, damage to the CEP), may be difficult to discern. Although there is strong evidence to support the role of endplate damage in low back pain, the diagnostic value of these observations is limited by a lack of conspicuity and contrast of the endplate on conventional clinical MRI.

Endplate Assessment with UTE-MRI

UTE-MRI provides a tool for visualizing the CEP (Fig. 35.1) and thus for elucidating its role in degenerative pathologies associated with low back pain [46–48]. The intermediate-to-high signal intensity observed in the CEP on UTE images is attributable to the bilayer of calcified and uncalcified endplate cartilage [46]; this bilayer is distinguishable on UTE images acquired at a sufficiently high spatial resolution. Studies using UTE imaging have found that changes in CEP morphology, including focal thinning, diffuse thickening, irregular damage, and signal discontinuity, co-locate with lesions in the underlying osseous endplate and are associated with disc degeneration [25, 49, 50]. Such morphological changes have been detected using UTE with substantial levels of interobserver reliability (Cohen's kappa range: 0.67–0.78 across studies) and strongly correspond to CEP morphology measured using histology [25, 46, 47].

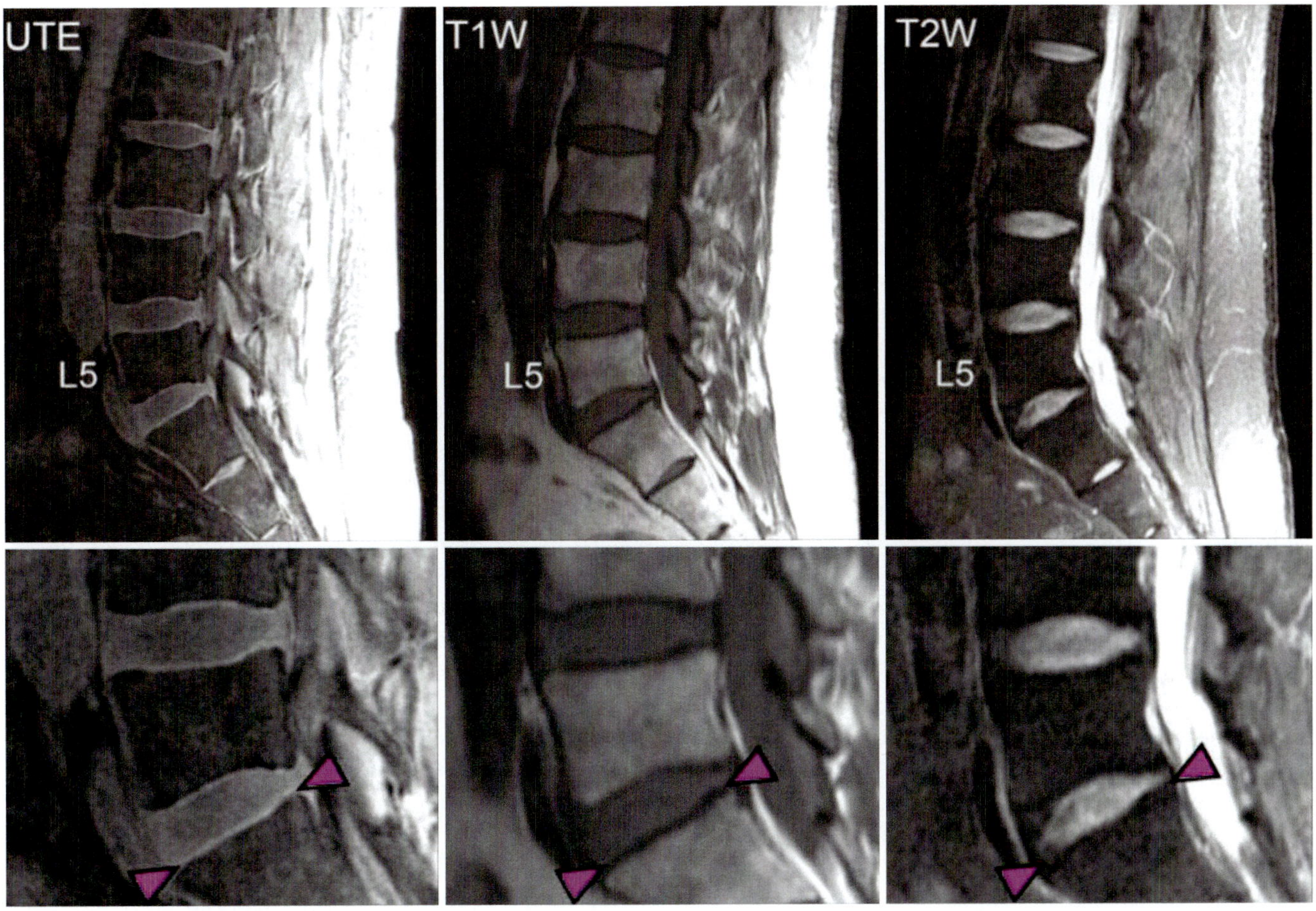

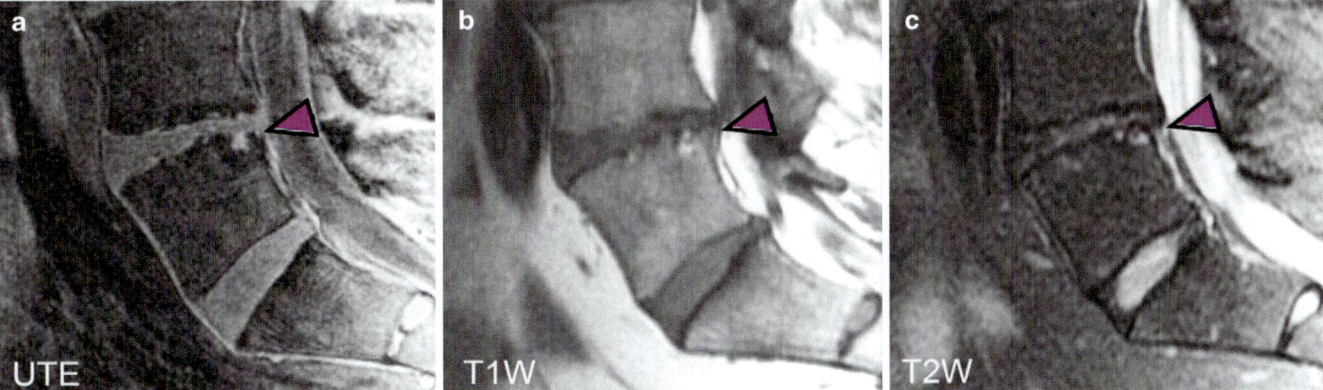

Fig. 35.1 Mid-sagittal images of the lumbar spine (upper row) with insets centered on the L5 vertebral body (lower row) from UTE-MRI (left column; echo time (TE) = 0.248 ms) and clinical fast spin echo images with T_1 and T_2-weighting (middle and right columns; TE = 15 and TE = 60 ms for T_1 and T_2-weighting, respectively). The CEP appears hyperintense on UTE images and hypointense on T_1- and T_2-weighted images (arrowheads annotate the inferior L5–S1 CEP region)

Fig. 35.2 The morphology of vertebral endplate damage at L5 (arrowheads) is more clearly defined on (**a**) UTE images than (**b**) on conventional T_1-weighted or (**c**) T_2-weighted images

Endplate defects observed using UTE imaging have also been shown to be strongly associated with chronic low back pain independent of endplate bone marrow lesions (Modic changes) [51], likely due to elevated levels of innervation in the damaged endplates [41]. Importantly, many endplate defects that are conspicuous on UTE images are not detected using T_1- or T_2-weighted images (Fig. 35.2) [17, 41]. Some endplate pathologies, such as tidemark avulsions in which the outer annulus fibrosus separates from the vertebra, may be more pronounced on T_2-weighted images than on UTE images due to high T_2 contrast from fluid/gas accumulation [52]. UTE imaging thus provides a powerful complementary (but not alternative) technique to conventional clinical imaging techniques in examining endplate pathologies.

In addition to CEP evaluation, UTE imaging has also been used to assess the intervertebral disc [49, 53–57], particularly through visualization of its short-T_2 components in relation to its longer-T_2 components (which can be observed using conventional T_2-weighted MRI). For example, the echo subtraction technique (see Chapter 11: Echo Subtraction) has been used to observe interindividual differences in the organization of the collagenous structures in the annulus fibrosus, which can be visualized as striated patterns in that region [49].

T_2^* Mapping

Multi-echo UTE imaging enables measurement of T_2^* relaxation times in the CEP. Spatial maps of CEP T_2^* values (Fig. 35.3) can be generated via voxel-by-voxel relaxometry from images acquired at several TEs spanning the normal T_2^* decay time (TEs spaced between approximately 0.1 and 25.0 ms) [16, 48, 58, 59]. Typically with this technique, the signal decay of each voxel is fitted to a mono-exponential decay function of the form: $SI_i(TE) = S_0 e^{TE/T2_i^*}$, where SI_i denotes the signal intensity of voxel i (see Chap. 22: T_2^* Quantification). Bi- and tri-component decay functions have been used to distinguish bound water from pore water and fat in cortical bone [60], though the extent to which this is possible in the CEP or vertebral bone is unclear.

T_2^* relaxation times measured in lumbar CEP tissue in situ (mean ± SD = 19.6 ± 5.3 ms, range = 1.3–32.0 ms) are age-dependent [16, 59] and are associated with aspects of CEP biochemical composition, including its water and glycosaminoglycan (GAG) contents and collagen-to-GAG

ratios [58]. Since the relative amounts of these biochemical constituents influence the CEP's permeability to nutrients [30, 33], T_2^* values can provide a quantitative assay of CEP composition and serve as a proxy for its permeability. Moreover, since deficits in CEP permeability can limit nutrient supply to and metabolite transport from cells in the intervertebral disc, measurement of CEP T_2^* values with UTE-MRI represents a powerful new diagnostic technique for probing the role of nutrient transport in disc degeneration [48]. Similarly, the technique could theoretically be used to elucidate the role of nutrient transport in disc regeneration following anabolic therapies, since the therapeutic efficacy of such therapies requires an adequate nutrient supply [48].

A limited number of studies have used UTE-based CEP T_2^* biomarkers in clinical cohorts to elucidate the role of the CEP in disc degeneration [16, 59]. For example, a biomarker defined by the mean T_2^* value in the central region of the CEP was associated with more severe intervertebral disc degeneration in patients with chronic low back pain after adjusting for age, which demonstrates the potential utility and clinical relevance of UTE-based T_2^* biomarkers [16, 48]. Overall, assessing CEP health using UTE-measured T_2^* relaxation time is a nascent technique that shows great promise for identifying phenotypes of disc degeneration and guiding therapeutic treatments for chronic low back pain.

Ligaments, Tendons, and Entheses

Like the CEP, the ligaments, tendons, and entheses (sites of attachment of tendons, ligaments, and joint capsules with bone) contain a high proportion of short-T_2 components (2–10 ms), which are not visible with conventional clinical pulse sequences and TEs [13]. UTE imaging can enhance signal and contrast in these tissues relative to conventional MRI; altering tissue orientation in the static magnetic field—

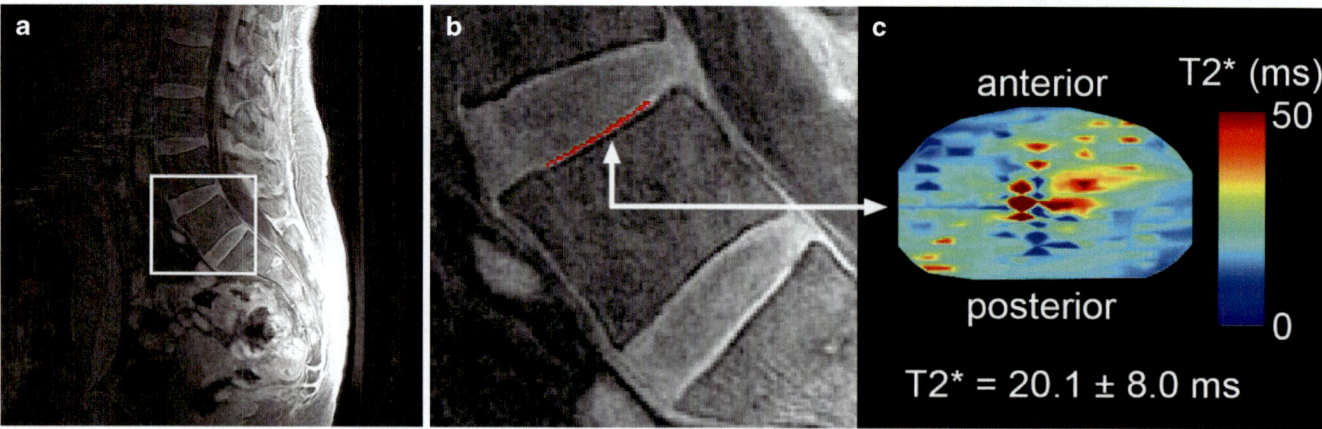

Fig. 35.3 (a) A mid-sagittal lumbar UTE image (TE = 0.248 ms). (b) Inset centered on the L5 vertebral body showing the segmentation of the inferior L4–L5 CEP (red) and (c) transverse CEP T_2^* map. The mean ± standard deviation (SD) CEP T_2^* was computed in the central CEP

referred to as magic angle imaging (see "Technical Considerations" below)—can also be used to enhance ligamentous contrast in UTE imaging [13, 61–63]. Computation of T_2^* relaxation times has been described for the Achilles tendon and enthesis [63] and could facilitate quantitative evaluation of spinal tissues with similar compositions.

In the spine, UTE imaging has been shown to enhance visualization of the anterior and posterior longitudinal ligaments, the ligamentum flavum, and the interspinous ligaments (Fig. 35.4) [13, 61]. For example, ligamentous hypertrophy and ossification associated with degeneration have been shown to appear with greater conspicuity on UTE images compared with conventional MR images [61, 64]. To date, only a few clinical studies have included UTE imaging to assess pathologies of spinal ligaments, tendons, and enthesis, and the potential benefits of UTE in both research and routine clinical settings are yet to be fully explored.

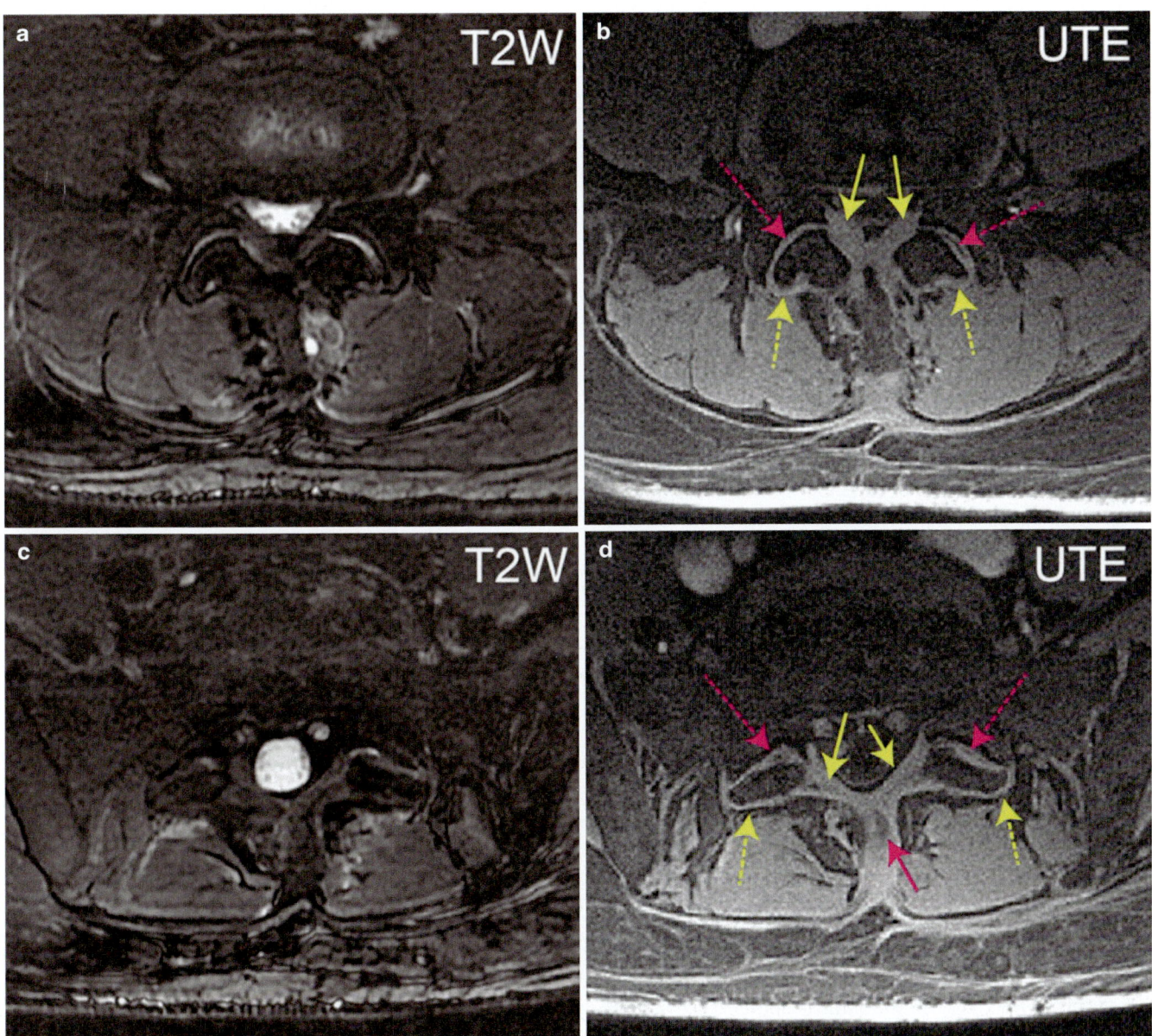

Fig. 35.4 Axial T_2-weighted two-dimensional (2D) fast spin echo images (**a**, **c**) and fat-suppressed UTE images (**b**, **d**) of the facet joints at L4–L5 (**a**, **b**) and L5–S1 (**c**, **d**) from a patient with low back pain. Broad disc bulges and facet arthropathy are observed at both levels. UTE images better depict a thickened ligamentum flavum (yellow solid arrows), dorsal capsule (yellow and pink dashed arrows), and interspinal ligament (pink solid arrow) compared with T_2-weighted images. Images courtesy of Emma Bahroos, MSc, and Sharmila Majumdar, PhD

The Facet Joints

The facet joints are synovial joints located between the superior and inferior articular processes of adjacent vertebrae (part of the posterior elements). Contact between hyaline-cartilage-covered bony protuberances helps transmit rotational, compressive, and shear loads between adjacent spinal levels, and the capsular ligaments help resist tensile forces that can develop in forward flexion [65]. Disc degeneration may increase facet loading and contribute to facet arthropathy, a painful arthritic condition. The facet joints are innervated by the medial branch nerves, and facet arthropathy constitutes a common source of low back pain [66].

Clinical imaging of the facet joints typically involves computed tomography (CT) and/or T_1- and T_2-weighted MRI to evaluate joint space narrowing, hypertrophy of articular processes, cartilage thinning, synovial and subchondral cysts, and redundancy of the surrounding ligaments. Although CT has been the preferred method for assessing the facet joints due to its ability to depict osseous details [67, 68], UTE imaging may be advantageous due to its ability to simultaneously evaluate the bone, cartilage, and the surrounding ligamentous structures without radiation [62, 69]. For example, UTE images can depict a thickened ligamentum flavum, dorsal synovial capsule, and interspinal ligaments with greater levels of detail and contrast compared to T_2-weighted MRI (Fig. 35.4). The ability to delineate the facet joints and the connections between the facet synovial membrane, joint capsule, ligamentum flavum, and interspinous ligament could help characterize degenerative structural changes, for example, by helping to identify contact between adjacent spinous processes (Baastrup's disease), which is a contributor to low back pain that is likely underdiagnosed [70].

Bone

Zero echo time (ZTE) imaging (see Chapter 5: ZTE-MRI) has emerged as a method to image bone morphology, mineralization (calcification and ossification), and fractures [71]. Using ZTE in combination with post-processing techniques such as coil inhomogeneity correction and signal inversion, CT-like images with high bony contrast can be generated. In the spine, evidence suggests that the sensitivity and specificity of using UTE/ZTE imaging to assess vertebral and facet-joint morphology in the lumbar and cervical regions are commensurate with CT [72]. For example, detection of vertebral fractures with UTE imaging has been demonstrated with a sensitivity, specificity, and accuracy of 0.91, 0.96, and 0.91, respectively, and an inter-reader agreement of 0.52–1.00 (substantial to excellent) [71]. UTE imaging has also

been used to assess the biochemical composition and failure properties of human cortical bone in the distal femur and tibia [73]; however, it remains unclear whether these parameters can also be measured in vertebral bone.

The Sacroiliac Joints (SIJs)

SIJ pathologies are believed to be important contributors to low back pain and are difficult to diagnose with conventional clinical imaging [74]. UTE imaging of the SIJs provides high signal and contrast of hard and soft tissues (Fig. 35.5), representing a promising imaging modality for assessing SIJ pathologies that associate with pain. For example, in patients with axial spondyloarthropathy, UTE imaging has been shown to detect bony erosions in the SIJs with higher specificity than conventional MRI [75]. T_2^* mapping of the SIJ cartilage has also been proposed as a method for assessing cartilage health and sacroiliitis [76]; however, the factors influencing T_2^* relaxation times in SIJ cartilage, and the dependence of measurement orientation on SIJ T_2^* values owing to magic angle effects (see "Technical Considerations below"), remain unknown.

Technical Considerations

Optimal assessment of spinal structures requires high spatial resolution, particularly for imaging thin tissues such as the CEP, bony endplate, or vertebral cortex (each approximately ≤1-mm thick). Ideally for UTE imaging in the spine, a 3.0 T scanner is recommended over a 1.5T scanner due to improved

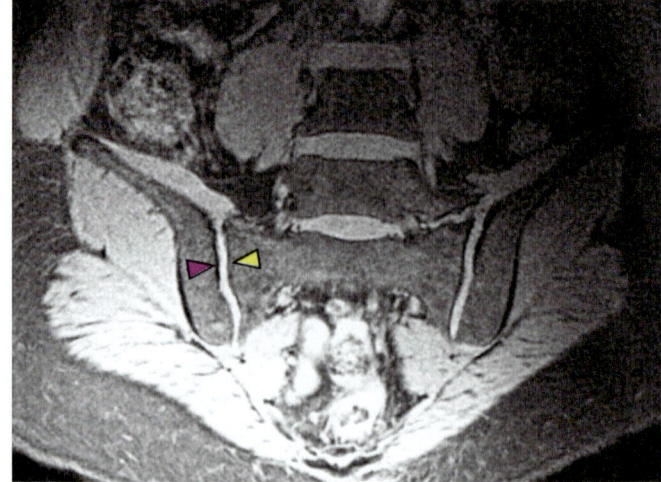

Fig. 35.5 A coronal UTE image (TE = 0.264 ms) of the SIJs. The cartilaginous and osseous boundaries between the sacrum (yellow arrowhead) and ilium (pink arrowhead) are depicted with high signal and contrast

signal-to-noise ratio (SNR). As with conventional MRI sequences, there are trade-offs between spatial resolution, SNR, and scan time. Since the spine is located deep within the body and the radiofrequency (RF) signal attenuates with depth, sufficient SNR is critical for UTE imaging of the spine.

UTE in the lumbar spine was first described using a two-dimensional (2D) sequence [61]; however, modern applications typically utilize three-dimensional (3D) imaging due to higher SNR efficiency, decreased sensitivity to eddy current effects, and the ability to image thinner slices. In particular, Cones [77] and stack-of-spiral [78] trajectories are frequently used as efficient k-space trajectories for 3D UTE imaging, as these techniques reduce oversampling and provide a significantly shortened scan time and higher SNR efficiency compared to radial trajectories. At 3.0 T, a six-echo sagittal 3D UTE Cones T_2^* mapping acquisition of the lumbar spine with a planar voxel resolution of 0.5 mm (28-cm field of view, 3-mm-slice thickness, 28 slices, TE range: 0.248–25.2 ms) requires approximately 13 min [16].

An additional advantage of the radial/Cones/spiral imaging trajectories frequently used for 3D UTE imaging is their relatively low sensitivity to motion artifacts (e.g., from respiration) owing to their oversampling of low k-space regions and motion averaging. In clinical imaging of the lumbar spine, an anterior coil array is not normally used so as to limit artifacts from respiratory motion; however, in UTE imaging of the lumbar spine, an anterior coil array may be used in addition to a posterior coil array to enhance SNR.

Imaging trajectories used for UTE imaging are sensitive to signals emanating from outside of the prescribed field of view, which can degrade image quality by producing streak artifacts (Fig. 35.6). Because of the large spatial coverage of the posterior array coils typically used for spinal imaging, slab-selective UTE imaging [79] can be used to limit such artifacts. Patient positioning with respect to coil elements, and appropriate selection of coil elements (when manual coil element selection is possible), can also help limit streak artifacts and/or ensure that artifacts do not obscure the spinal regions of interest.

Many spinal tissues, including the CEP and tendons/ligaments, have organized and anisotropic collagen structures; such tissues are subjected to dipolar interactions between collagen-bound water molecules whose strength depends on the orientation (θ) of the collagen fibers relative to the externally applied magnetic field (B_0) [58, 80]. These dipole–dipole interactions are minimized when $\theta = 54.7°$ (commonly approximated as 55°), the so-called "magic angle" [15]. When imaged at the magic angle, tissues with ordered collagen structures such as the CEP display maximal signal intensity and T_2^* relaxation times; at other

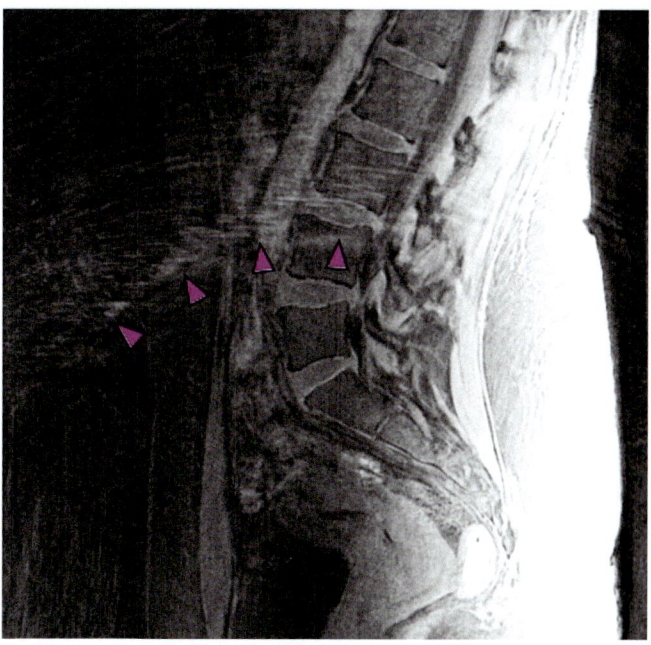

Fig. 35.6 Streak artifacts (pink arrowheads) can degrade UTE image quality in the spine and cause nonuniformly distributed image noise

angles, signal intensity and T_2^* relaxation times are artificially depressed.

The magic angle phenomenon in UTE imaging has been used advantageously as a mechanism of contrast enhancement [13, 63]; however, the phenomenon also confounds quantitative analysis of T_2^* biomarkers [16, 48, 59]. For example, when imaged at the magic angle, UTE-measured CEP T_2^* values have been shown to be significantly associated with GAG content, collagen-to-GAG ratios, and hydration of the CEP (these compositional factors influence the amount of free or mobile water in the CEP, affecting spin–spin relaxation) [58]. However, the associations between T_2^* and biochemical composition disappear when T_2^* values are measured in CEPs oriented at 0° or 90°. The effects of measurement angle on CEP T_2^* values are not well-understood, introducing errors in the assessment of CEP health for those CEPs not oriented near the magic angle in situ (i.e., most spinal levels—coincidently, CEPs located at the L5–S1 level tend to be oriented at the magic angle when a patient is imaged in a supine position). Research is needed to elucidate the effects of the magic angle on CEP T_2^* biomarkers to enable assessment of CEP composition throughout the spine.

Sequence availability is currently a limiting factor for widespread clinical use of UTE imaging in the spine, as the major MRI vendors (e.g., GE, Philips, Siemens) do not yet provide clinically available UTE sequences. The promising applications of UTE imaging in both clinical research and clinical practice will likely help accelerate the commercialization and availability of UTE imaging.

Conclusions

UTE imaging represents a major methodological advance in spinal imaging by enabling both morphological and quantitative assessments of tissues with short-T_2 relaxation times, including the cartilage and hard tissue found throughout the spine. In particular, the CEP and osseous endplates, vertebrae, facet joints, spinal ligaments, and SIJs—each of which exhibit pathologies implicated in low back pain—are comprised of short-T_2 components, which appear without contrast or conspicuity on conventional MRI. UTE imaging can overcome this limitation by generating signal and contrast from the short-T_2 components of such tissues and thus has profound implications for understanding, diagnosing, and treating painful pathologies of the spine.

Acknowledgments The authors acknowledge Dr. Zehra Akkaya for helpful discussions regarding the chapter contents. This work was supported by the National Institute of Arthritis and Musculoskeletal and Skin Diseases of the National Institutes of Health under award numbers UH2AR076719, UH3AR076719, U19AR076737, and F32AR081139 and through R01AR070198. The content is solely the responsibility of the authors and does not necessarily represent the official views of the National Institutes of Health.

References

1. Panagopoulos J, Magnussen JS, Hush J, Maher CG, Crites-Battie M, Jarvik JG, et al. Prospective comparison of changes in lumbar spine MRI findings over time between individuals with acute low back pain and controls: an exploratory study. AJNR Am J Neuroradiol. 2017;38(9):1826–32.
2. Brinjikji W, Diehn FE, Jarvik JG, Carr CM, Kallmes DF, Murad MH, et al. MRI findings of disc degeneration are more prevalent in adults with low back pain than in asymptomatic controls: a systematic review and meta-analysis. AJNR Am J Neuroradiol. 2015;36(12):2394–9.
3. Brinjikji W, Luetmer PH, Comstock B, Bresnahan BW, Chen LE, Deyo RA, et al. Systematic literature review of imaging features of spinal degeneration in asymptomatic populations. AJNR Am J Neuroradiol. 2015;36(4):811–6.
4. Carragee E, Alamin T, Cheng I, Franklin T, van den Haak E, Hurwitz E. Are first-time episodes of serious LBP associated with new MRI findings? Spine J. 2006;6(6):624–35.
5. Djurasovic M, Carreon LY, Crawford CH, Zook JD, Bratcher KR, Glassman SD. The influence of preoperative MRI findings on lumbar fusion clinical outcomes. Eur Spine J. 2012;21(8):1616–23.
6. Mallio CA, Vadalà G, Russo F, Bernetti C, Ambrosio L, Zobel BB, et al. Novel magnetic resonance imaging tools for the diagnosis of degenerative disc disease: a narrative review. Diagnostics (Basel). 2022;12(2):420.
7. de Mello R, Ma Y, Ji Y, Du J, Chang EY. Quantitative MRI musculoskeletal techniques: an update. AJR Am J Roentgenol. 2019;213(3):524–33.
8. Gornet MG, Peacock J, Claude J, Schranck FW, Copay AG, Eastlack RK, et al. Magnetic resonance spectroscopy (MRS) can identify painful lumbar discs and may facilitate improved clinical outcomes of lumbar surgeries for discogenic pain. Eur Spine J. 2019;28(4):674–87.
9. Sollmann N, Bonnheim NB, Joseph GB, Chachad R, Zhou J, Akkaya Z, et al. Paraspinal muscle in chronic low back pain: comparison between standard parameters and chemical shift encoding-based water-fat MRI. J Magn Reson Imaging. 2022;56(5):1600–8.
10. Fields AJ, Ballatori A, Han M, Bailey JF, McCormick ZL, O'Neill CW, et al. Measurement of vertebral endplate bone marrow lesion (Modic change) composition with water–fat MRI and relationship to patient-reported outcome measures. Eur Spine J. 2021;30(9):2549–56.
11. Bonnheim NB, Lazar AA, Kumar A, Akkaya Z, Zhou J, Guo X, et al. ISSLS Prize in Bioengineering Science 2023: Age- and sexrelated differences in lumbar intervertebral disc degeneration between patients with chronic low back pain and asymptomatic controls. Eur Spine J. 2023;32(5):1517–24.
12. Siriwanarangsun P, Statum S, Biswas R, Bae WC, Chung CB. Ultrashort time to echo magnetic resonance techniques for the musculoskeletal system. Quant Imaging Med Surg. 2016;6(6):731–43.
13. Robson MD, Gatehouse PD, Bydder M, Bydder GM. Magnetic resonance: an introduction to ultrashort TE (UTE) imaging. J Comput Assist Tomogr. 2003;27(6):825–46.
14. Chang EY, Du J, Chung CB. UTE imaging in the musculoskeletal system. J Magn Reson Imaging. 2015;41(4):870–83.
15. Erickson S, Prost R, Timins M. The "magic angle" effect: background physics and clinical relevance. Radiology. 1993;188(1):23–5.
16. Bonnheim NB, Wang L, Lazar AA, Zhou J, Chachad R, Sollmann N, et al. The contributions of cartilage endplate composition and vertebral bone marrow fat to intervertebral disc degeneration in patients with chronic low back pain. Eur Spine J. 2022;31(7):1866–72.
17. Lotz JC, Fields AJ, Liebenberg EC. The role of the vertebral end plate in low back pain. Global Spine J. 2013;3(3):153–63.
18. Fields AJ, Ballatori A, Liebenberg EC, Lotz JC. Contribution of the endplates to disc degeneration. Curr Mol Biol Rep. 2018;4(4):151–60.
19. Roberts S, Menage J, Urban JPG. Biochemical and structural properties of cartilage end-plate and relation to the intervertebral disc. Spine (Phila Pa 1976). 1989;14(2):166–74.
20. Moore RJ. The vertebral end-plate: what do we know? Eur Spine J. 2000;9(2):92–6.
21. Roberts S, Menage J, Duance V, Wotton S, Ayad S. Collagen types around the cells of the intervertebral disc and cartilage endplate: an immunolocalization study. Spine (Phila Pa 1976). 1991;16(9):1030–8.
22. Huber M, Trattnig S, Lintner F. Anatomy, biochemistry, and physiology of articular cartilage. Investig Radiol. 2000;35(10):573–80.
23. Aspden RM, Hickey DS, Hukins DWL. Determination of collagen fibril orientation in the cartilage of vertebral end plate. Connect Tissue Res. 1981;9(2):83–7.
24. Paietta RC, Burger EL, Ferguson VL. Mineralization and collagen orientation throughout aging at the vertebral endplate in the human lumbar spine. J Struct Biol. 2013;184(2):310–20.
25. Berg-Johansen B, Han M, Fields AJ, Liebenberg EC, Lim BJ, Larson PEZ, et al. Cartilage endplate thickness variation measured by ultrashort echo-time MRI is associated with adjacent disc degeneration. Spine (Phila Pa 1976). 2018;43(10):E592–600.
26. Berg-Johansen B, Fields AJ, Liebenberg EC, Li A, Lotz JC. Structure-function relationships at the human spinal disc-vertebra interface. J Orthop Res. 2018;36(1):192–201.
27. Nachemson A, Lewin T, Maroudas A, Freeman MAR. In vitro diffusion of dye through the end-plates and the annulus fibrosus of human lumbar inter-vertebral discs. Acta Orthop Scand. 1970;41(6):589–607.
28. Roberts S, Urban J, Evans H, Einsten S. Transport properties of the human cartilage endplate in relation to its composition and calcification. Spine (Phila Pa 1976). 1996;21(4):415–20.

29. Holm S, Maroudas A, Urban JPG, Selstam G, Nachemson A. Nutrition of the intervertebral disc: solute transport and metabolism. Connect Tissue Res. 1981;8(2):101–19.

30. Wong J, Sampson S, Bell-Briones H, Ouyang A, Lazar A, Lotz J, et al. Nutrient supply and nucleus pulposus cell function: effects of the transport properties of the cartilage endplate and potential implications for intradiscal biologic therapy. Osteoarthr Cartil. 2019;27(6):956–64.

31. Shirazi-Adl A, Taheri M, Urban JPG. Analysis of cell viability in intervertebral disc: effect of endplate permeability on cell population. J Biomech. 2010;43(7):1330–6.

32. Rajasekaran S, Babu JN, Arun R, Armstrong BRW, Shetty AP, Murugan S. ISSLS prize winner: a study of diffusion in human lumbar discs: a serial magnetic resonance imaging study documenting the influence of the endplate on diffusion in normal and degenerate discs. Spine (Phila Pa 1976). 2004;29(23):2654–67.

33. Dolor A, Sampson S, Lazar A, Lotz J, Szoka F, Fields A. Matrix modification for enhancing the transport properties of the human cartilage endplate to improve disc nutrition. PLoS One. 2019;14(4):e0215218.

34. Sampson SL, Sylvia M, Fields AJ. Effects of dynamic loading on solute transport through the human cartilage endplate. J Biomech. 2019;83:273–9.

35. Binch A, Fitzgerald J, Growney E, Barry F. Cell-based strategies for IVD repair: clinical progress and translational obstacles. Nat Rev Rheumatol. 2021;17(3):158–75.

36. Huang YC, Urban JPG, Luk KDK. Intervertebral disc regeneration: do nutrients lead the way? Nat Rev Rheumatol. 2014;10(9):561–6.

37. Vedicherla S, Buckley CT. Cell-based therapies for intervertebral disc and cartilage regeneration-current concepts, parallels, and perspectives. J Orthop Res. 2017;35(1):8–22.

38. Moriguchi Y, Alimi M, Khair T, Manolarakis G, Berlin C, Bonassar LJ, et al. Biological treatment approaches for degenerative disk disease: a literature review of in vivo animal and clinical data. Global Spine J. 2016;6(5):497–518.

39. Ju DG, Kanim LE, Bae HW. Is there clinical improvement associated with intradiscal therapies? A comparison across randomized controlled studies. Global Spine J. 2022;12(5):756–64.

40. Brown MF, Hukkanen MVJ, McCarthy ID, Redfern DRM, Batten JJ, Crock HV, et al. Sensory and sympathetic innervation of the vertebral endplate in patients with degenerative disc disease. J Bone Joint Surg Br. 1997;79(1):147–53.

41. Fields A, Liebenberg E, Lotz J. Innervation of pathologies in the lumbar vertebral end plate and intervertebral disc. Spine J. 2014;14(3):513–21.

42. Antonacci MD, Mody DR, Rutz K, Weilbaecher D, Heggeness MH. A histologic study of fractured human vertebral bodies. J Spinal Disord Tech. 2002;15(2):118–26.

43. Dudli S, Fields A, Samartzis D, Karppinen J, Lotz J. Pathobiology of Modic changes. Eur Spine J. 2016;25(11):3723–34.

44. Modic MT, Steinberg PM, Ross JS, Masaryk TJ, Carter JR. Degenerative disk disease: assessment of changes in vertebral body marrow with MR imaging. Radiology. 1988;166:193–9.

45. Jensen TS, Karppinen J, Sorensen JS, Niinimäki J, Leboeuf-Yde C. Vertebral endplate signal changes (Modic change): a systematic literature review of prevalence and association with non-specific low back pain. Eur Spine J. 2008;17(11):1407–22.

46. Bae WC, Statum S, Zhang Z, Yamaguchi T, Wolfson T, Gamst AC, et al. Morphology of the cartilaginous endplates in human intervertebral disks with ultrashort echo time MR imaging. Radiology. 2013;266(2):564–74.

47. Jin RC, Huang YC, Luk KDK, Hu Y. A computational measurement of cartilaginous endplate structure using ultrashort time-to-echo MRI scanning. Comput Methods Prog Biomed. 2017;143:49–58.

48. Bonnheim NB, Wang L, Lazar AA, Chachad R, Zhou J, Guo X, et al. Deep-learning-based biomarker of spinal cartilage endplate health using ultra-short echo time magnetic resonance imaging. Quant Imaging Med Surg. 2023;13(5):2807–21.

49. Chen KC, Tran B, Biswas R, Statum S, Masuda K, Chung CB, et al. Evaluation of the disco-vertebral junction using ultrashort time-to-echo magnetic resonance imaging: inter-reader agreement and association with vertebral endplate lesions. Skelet Radiol. 2016;45(9):1249–56.

50. Law T, Anthony MP, Chan Q, Samartzis D, Kim M, Cheung KMC, et al. Ultrashort time-to-echo MRI of the cartilaginous endplate: technique and association with intervertebral disc degeneration. J Med Imaging Radiat Oncol. 2013;57(4):427–34.

51. Bailey JF, Fields AJ, Ballatori A, Cohen D, Jain D, Coughlin D, et al. The relationship between endplate pathology and patient-reported symptoms for chronic low back pain depends on lumbar paraspinal muscle quality. Spine (Phila Pa 1976). 2019;44(14):1010–7.

52. Berg-Johansen B, Jain D, Liebenberg E, Fields A, Link T, O'Neill C, et al. Tidemark avulsions are a predominant form of endplate irregularity. Spine (Phila Pa 1976). 2018;43(16):1095–101.

53. Pang H, Bow C, Cheung J, Zehra U, Borthakur A, Karppinen J, et al. The UTE disc sign on MRI. Spine (Phila Pa 1976). 2018;43(7):503–11.

54. Tang P, Xu J, Liu W, Li Y, Fan W, Huang X. Study of the feasibility of conventional MR images and magnetic resonance (MR)/ultra-short echo time (UTE) technique in the evaluation of lumbar disc degeneration in the axial plane. J Med Imaging Health Inform. 2021;11(3):817–21.

55. Zehra U, Cheung J, Bow C, Crawford R, Luk K, Lu W, et al. Spinopelvic alignment predicts disc calcification, displacement, and Modic changes: evidence of an evolutionary etiology for clinically-relevant spinal phenotypes. JOR Spine. 2020;3(1):e1083.

56. Zehra U, Bow C, Cheung JPY, Pang H, Lu W, Samartzis D. The association of lumbar intervertebral disc calcification on plain radiographs with the UTE disc sign on MRI. Eur Spine J. 2018;27(5):1049–57.

57. Hall-Craggs MA, Porter J, Gatehouse PD, Bydder GM. Ultrashort echo time (UTE) MRI of the spine in thalassaemia. Br J Radiol. 2004;77(914):104–10.

58. Fields A, Han M, Krug R, Lotz J. Cartilaginous end plates: quantitative MR imaging with very short echo times-orientation dependence and correlation with biochemical composition. Radiology. 2015;274(2):482–9.

59. Wang L, Han M, Wong J, Zheng P, Lazar A, Krug R, et al. Evaluation of human cartilage endplate composition using MRI: spatial variation, association with adjacent disc degeneration, and in vivo repeatability. J Orthop Res. 2020;39(7):1470–8.

60. Lu X, Jerban S, Wan L, Ma Y, Jang H, Le N, et al. Three-dimensional ultrashort echo time imaging with tricomponent analysis for human cortical bone. Magn Reson Med. 2019;82(1):348–55.

61. Gatehouse PD, He T, Hughes SPF, Bydder GM. MR imaging of degenerative disc disease in the lumbar spine with ultrashort TE pulse sequences. MAGMA. 2004;16(4):160–6.

62. Benjamin M, Bydder GM. Magnetic resonance imaging of entheses using ultrashort TE (UTE) pulse sequences. J Magn Reson Imaging. 2007;25(2):381–9.

63. Du J, Pak BC, Znamirowski R, Statum S, Takahashi A, Chung CB, et al. Magic angle effect in magnetic resonance imaging of the achilles tendon and enthesis. Magn Reson Imaging. 2009;27(4):557–64.

64. Azuma M, Khant ZA, Yoneyama M, Ikushima I, Hamanaka H, Yokogami K, et al. Evaluation of cervical ossification of the posterior longitudinal ligament with 3D broadband IR-prepared ultrashort echo-time imaging: a pilot study. Jpn J Radiol. 2021;39(5):487–93.

65. White A, Panjabi M. Physical properties and functional biomechanics of the spine. In: In: clinical biomechanics of the spine. 2nd ed. Philadelphia, PA: J.B. Lippincott Company; 1990. p. 1–83.

66. Gellhorn AC, Katz JN, Suri P. Osteoarthritis of the spine: the facet joints. Nat Rev Rheumatol. 2013;9(4):216–24.

67. Berg L, Thoresen H, Neckelmann G, Furunes H, Hellum C, Espeland A. Facet arthropathy evaluation: CT or MRI? Eur Radiol. 2019;29(9):4990–8.

68. Weishaupt D, Zanetti M, Hodler J, Boos N. MR imaging and CT in osteoarthritis of the lumbar facet joints. Skelet Radiol. 1999;28(4):215–9.

69. Sanal HT, Mett T, Statum S, Du J, Znamirowski R, Bydder G, et al. Evaluation of articular cartilage of lumbar facet joints with UTE MR imaging and multi-echo SE T_2 mapping techniques. Proc Intl Soc Mag Reson Med. 2009:79.

70. Filippiadis DK, Mazioti A, Argentos S, Anselmetti G, Papakonstantinou O, Kelekis N, et al. Baastrup's disease (kissing spines syndrome): a pictorial review. Insights Imaging. 2015;6(1):123–8.

71. Schwaiger BJ, Schneider C, Kronthaler S, Gassert FT, Böhm C, Pfeiffer D, et al. CT-like images based on T_1 spoiled gradient-echo and ultra-short echo time MRI sequences for the assessment of vertebral fractures and degenerative bone changes of the spine. Eur Radiol. 2021;31(7):4680–9.

72. Hou B, Liu C, Li Y, Xiong Y, Wang J, Zhang P, et al. Evaluation of the degenerative lumbar osseous morphology using zero echo time magnetic resonance imaging (ZTE-MRI). Eur Spine J. 2022;31(3):792–800.

73. Bae WC, Chen PC, Chung CB, Masuda K, D'Lima D, Du J. Quantitative ultrashort echo time (UTE) MRI of human cortical bone: correlation with porosity and biomechanical properties. J Bone Miner Res. 2012;27(4):848–57.

74. Barros G, Mcgrath L, Gelfenbeyn M. Sacroiliac joint dysfunction in patients with low back pain. Fed Pract. 2019;36(8):370–5.

75. Hahn S, Song JS, Choi EJ, Cha JG, Choi Y, Ju Song Y, et al. Can bone erosion in axial spondyloarthropathy be detected by ultrashort echo time imaging? A comparison with computed tomography in the sacroiliac joint. J Magn Reson Imaging. 2022;56(5):1580–90.

76. Wong TT, Quarterman P, Duong P, Rasiej MJ, Wang R, Jaramillo D, et al. A pilot study on feasibility of ultrashort echo time T_2^* cartilage mapping in the sacroiliac joints. J Comput Assist Tomogr. 2021;45(5):717–21.

77. Gurney P, Hargreaves B, Nishimura D. Design and analysis of a practical 3D cones trajectory. Magn Reson Med. 2006;55(3):575–82.

78. Qian Y, Boada FE. Acquisition-weighted stack of spirals for fast high-resolution three-dimensional ultra-short echo time MR imaging. Magn Reson Med. 2008;60(1):135–45.

79. Afsahi AM, Lombardi AF, Wei Z, Carl M, Athertya J, Masuda K, et al. High-contrast lumbar spinal bone imaging using a 3D slab-selective UTE sequence. Front Endocrinol (Lausanne). 2022;12:800398.

80. Fullerton GD, Rahal A. Collagen structure: the molecular source of the tendon magic angle effect. J Magn Reson Imaging. 2007;25(2):345–61.

MRI of Tendinopathy Using Ultrashort TE (UTE) Sequences

Stephan J. Breda and Edwin H. G. Oei

Introduction

Tendons are connective tissue structures of the human body that usually connect muscle to bone [1]. In the lower leg, the muscle–tendon unit consists of the quadriceps muscles, quadriceps tendon, and patellar tendon—examples of the so-called positional tendons—and their function is to transmit the force of muscle contraction to the lower leg in order to extend the knee. Tendons, such as the Achilles tendon, can also function as springs by storing energy during deceleration and releasing it during acceleration [2]. This is referred to as elastic strain energy storage because energy is stored in a structural manner as a result of elastic deformation [3]. An example demonstrating the use of this capacity of tendons to store energy is that humans typically jump higher when a preparatory countermovement precedes their takeoff. Unlike positional tendons, energy-storing tendons must be able to withstand highly repetitive tensile forces.

Tendons are sparsely populated with cells (tenocytes). These secrete and build up the largest component of the tendon, the extracellular matrix (ECM) [4]. Moreover, tendons are only slightly vascularized, although tendon sheaths have a richer blood supply. The ECM of a tendon is composed of type I collagen, which accounts for about 80% of the dry weight of tendons [5]. Collagen fibers are highly organized and grouped into fascicles, fibers, and fibrils. This organization imparts tensile strength and provides the tendon with its unique structural and functional properties.

Although water is widely present within tendons, it is often overlooked as a factor affecting tendon properties [6]. Water may comprise more than 80% of the total tendon weight [7] and is tightly bound to the collagen fibers and large water-attracting molecules called proteoglycans and their associated glycosaminoglycan (GAG) side chains within the ECM [8]. The interaction of proteoglycans with water and collagen contributes to the mechanical properties of tendon tissue by increasing stiffness and resistance against shear and compressive forces [9]. Proteoglycans are generally large and highly negatively charged molecules that consist of a core protein that is highly glycosylated [10]. They are an essential part of the ECM and so are part of the most abundant tissue in the human body.

Among the significant global burden of musculoskeletal disorders, tendinopathy is an important contributor, with a high prevalence in both the generally sedentary population and athletic individuals [11]. Common sites of tendinopathy include the patellar tendon, Achilles tendon, rotator cuff tendons around the shoulder (in particular, the supraspinatus tendon), and the flexor and extensor tendons around the elbow. This chapter is mainly focused on patellar tendinopathy (PT) in line with the authors' expertise. PT or "jumper's knee" is a common and often chronic overuse injury of the patellar tendon [12]. Athletes performing repetitive jumping and landing activities, such as basketball and volleyball players, are most commonly affected. Prevalence rates of 45% for elite volleyball players and 32% for elite basketball players have been reported [13]. PT is also seen in soccer players and athletes performing track-and-field activities [14, 15]. Athletes with PT experience pain at the inferior patellar pole, where the patellar tendon attaches to patellar bone [16]. Pain is related to highly demanding loads, such as high jumps or explosive cutting maneuvers [17]. Typically, pain is worse during warm-up of the knee extensor muscles but eases with activity. Pain forces most athletes with PT to diminish their participation in training and performance. It even leads to stopping sports participation in more than half the athletes [18]. It has also been shown that 58% of patients with PT encounter problems with participation in physically demanding work [19]. The concerns, frustrations, and impact on quality of life and daily functioning in individuals with tendinopathy have been well-described [20]. The cornerstone in

S. J. Breda · E. H. G. Oei (✉)
Department of Radiology and Nuclear Medicine, Erasmus MC University Medical Center, Rotterdam, The Netherlands
e-mail: s.breda@erasmusmc.nl; e.oei@erasmusmc.nl

the treatment of tendinopathy is exercise therapy, of which progressive tendon-loading exercises are the best available conservative therapy for PT [21].

Imaging of Tendons

Tendinopathy is a clinical diagnosis, characterized by pain localized to the tendon attachment or mid-portion and load-related pain that increases with demand [22]. In clinical practice, the role of imaging in tendinopathy is to assist in differential diagnosis as a complementary examination and to confirm the presence of characteristic findings that support the clinical diagnosis [23]. These findings are often initially assessed with ultrasound as an easily accessible and relatively cheap imaging tool and include the observation of tendon thickening with hypoechoic areas and/or increased Doppler flow [24, 25]. Tendon abnormalities visualized using ultrasound in asymptomatic tendons are predictive of future tendinopathy, with an increased relative risk varying from four for PT to seven for Achilles tendinopathy [26]. However, differences in response to therapeutic exercises in tendinopathy are not explained by changes in tendon structure [27]. The role of magnetic resonance imaging (MRI) is often to rule out mimickers of tendinopathy, such as chondral changes in the patellofemoral joint [28]. When the healing response to overuse injury is impeded by recurring microtrauma, the tissue alterations in tendinopathy are considered to be degenerative and are associated with compromised function [4].

MRI of tendons is often challenging because of the rapid decay of the free induction decay signal from water in the tendons, due to strong spin–spin interactions [29]. Because tendon consists of a high fraction of collagen, which mainly has short (1–10 ms) and ultrashort (0.1–1 ms) transverse relaxation times, signals from tendon are poorly detected using clinically available

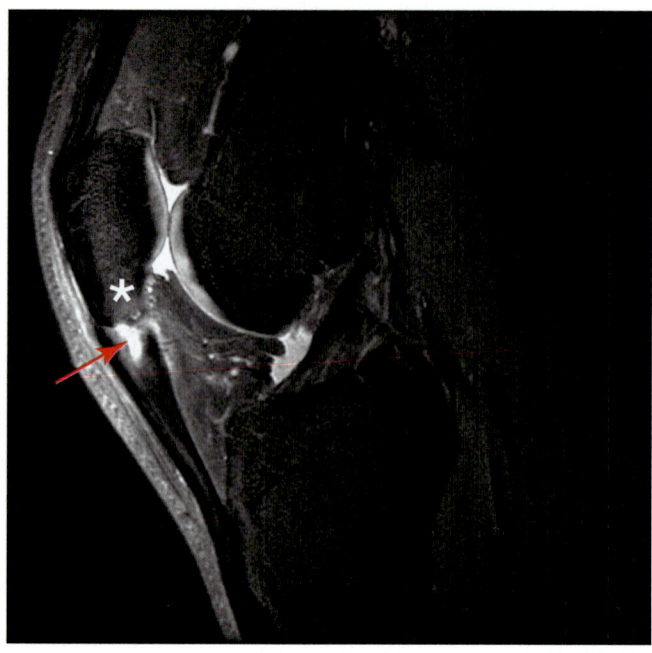

Fig. 36.1 A sagittal 3D proton density (PD)-weighted fat-saturated (FS) fast spin echo (FSE) image of the knee of an athlete with PT. A high signal (red arrow) is seen in the proximal tendon and its attachment to the inferior pole of the patella (white asterisk) (TE = 30 ms, repetition time (TR) = 1200 ms)

sequences that employ long echo times (TEs) [30]. Therefore, a significant amount of information regarding these ultrashort- and short-T_2 components is lost using conventional sequences, hampering their use for tissue quantification. Figure 36.1 shows a sagittal magnetic resonance (MR) image of the knee in an athlete with PT. Axial UTE images of the knee at TEs of 0.032 ms and 0.97 ms are depicted in Fig. 36.2.

Characteristic findings in PT on MRI are thickening of the proximal patellar tendon and increased signal intensity at its attachment to the inferior patellar border. The increased signal intensity reflects degenerative change with increased tissue-free water components.

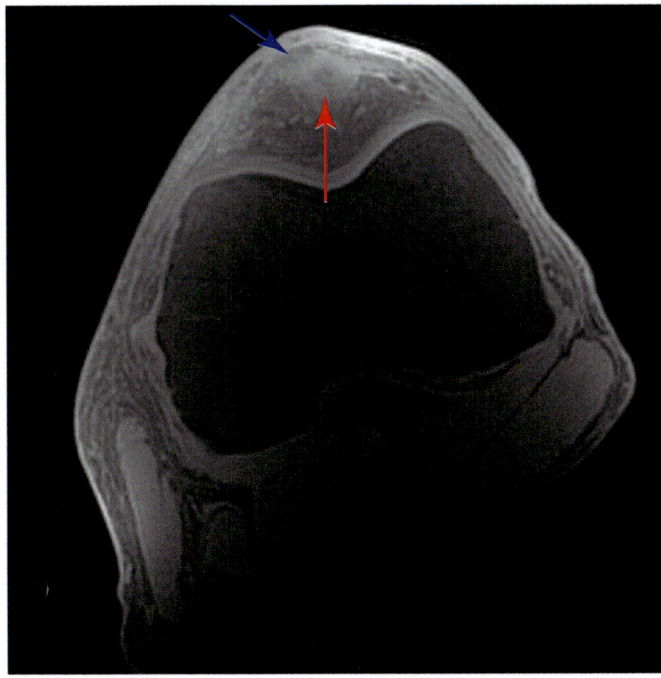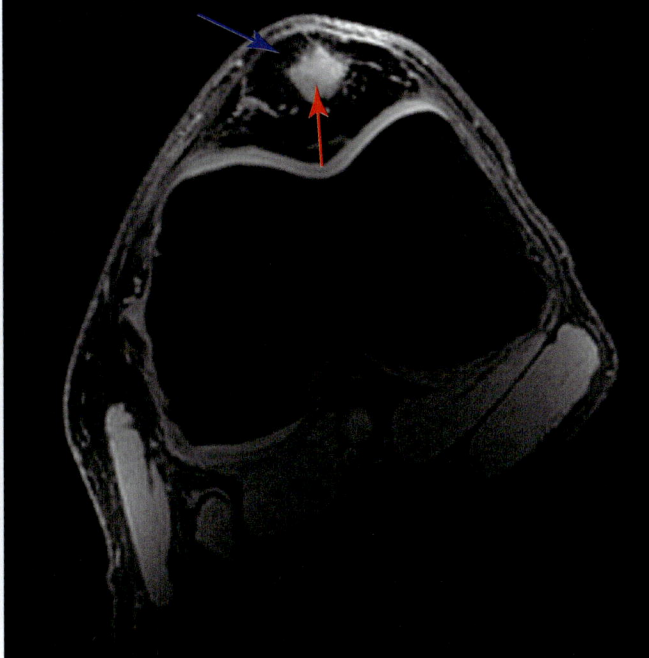

Fig. 36.2 Axial UTE images at TE = 0.032 ms (left) and TE = 0.97 ms (right) at a constant TR of 83.4 ms, illustrating the fast free induction decay of aligned collagen in the patellar tendon (blue arrows). The remaining high signal that is observed in the dorsal aspect of the patellar tendon reflects degenerative change with an increased tissue water content (red arrows)

Quantitative MRI in Tendinopathy

UTE sequences have been developed to encode signals from tissues with extremely rapid signal decays such as tendons [31]. UTE sequences enable quantitative analysis of tendons (T_2^* mapping) and have the potential to detect structural abnormalities earlier than conventional morphological sequences [32].

T_2^*s can be calculated using a mono-exponential decay model. However, the structural complexity of the ECM and the interaction of water protons with glycoproteins (proteoglycans and glycosaminoglycans) result in different components with different T_2^*s within tendon [33]. Because of this, the transverse signal decay is more complex than that described by a mono-exponential model. Multi-exponential models may provide additional information regarding the decay of these different components, either using a single echo train or by combining two or more interleaved multi-echo scans. The biexponential model is able to provide T_2^*s of two different water fractions, namely, bound and free water. The bound fraction is regarded as water protons that are influenced by the macromolecules in the tendon, such as collagen and proteoglycans. Biexponential analysis of T_2^*s has been successfully employed to sample both short- and long-T_2^* components in biological tissues [34]. UTE-MRI has been implemented mostly for tendons, such as the patellar tendon [35] and Achilles tendon [32], but also for rotator cuff tendons [36], bone [37], articular cartilage [38], menisci [39] and intervertebral disks [40]. Using bicomponent analyses on UTE-acquired transverse relaxometry data, significantly higher T_2^*s have been found in patients with tendinopathy (patellar, Achilles, and rotator cuff) than in healthy subjects [32, 35, 36].

An Example of UTE-MRI Implementation in a Clinical Trial of Patellar Tendinopathy

UTE-MRI has been sparsely applied as an outcome measure in clinical trials, but one example is the JUMPER study, which was a randomized controlled clinical trial comparing the effect of progressive tendon-loading exercises to eccentric exercise therapy in 76 athletes with PT (ClinicalTrials.gov ID: NCT02938143) [21]. In the trial, a 3D UTE-MRI technique was longitudinally implemented to assess the association between T_2^* changes and clinical outcomes. MRI was performed at baseline, after 12 weeks, and after 24 weeks of follow-up in athletes performing exercise therapy for PT.

Image Acquisition

Imaging was performed using a 3.0 T system (Discovery MR750, GE Healthcare) with a 16-channel flexible coil (NeoCoil, Pewaukee). A 3D gradient echo-based multi-echo UTE-T_2 mapping sequence described as 3D-UTE-Cones (GE Healthcare) was used. This utilized a k-space sampling scheme with a center-out, twisted, 3D cone trajectory that allowed a minimal nominal TE of 0.03 ms [41]. With the relatively long examination time that was needed for typical UTE-MRI acquisitions to provide large volumetric coverage, it was important to ensure a stable and comfortable position of the anatomy of interest. In this study, the knee was positioned in 30° flexion, using a cylindrical tube and foam padding [42]. A total of 16 echoes (0.032, 0.49, 0.97, 2.92, 4.87, 6.82, 8.77, 10.72, 12.67, 14.62, 16.57, 18.52, 20.47, 22.42, 24.37, and 26.32 ms) were acquired using 4 multi-echo sequences with a constant repetition time of 83.4 ms (Fig. 36.3). The axial 3D UTE Cones sequence parameters were acquisition time = 13:15 min per multi-echo sequence, field of view (FOV) = 15 cm, matrix size = 252 × 252, voxel size = 0.6 × 0.6 × 1.5 mm³, number of slices = 60, number of excitations (NEX) = 1, readout bandwidth = 125 kHz, and flip angle = 17°. Echoes were scanned in interleaved order using four fat-saturated (FS) multi-echo acquisitions with a total scan time of 53 min [42]. Because the patellar tendon is adjacent to fat in the knee (Hoffa's infrapatellar fat pad), fat signal suppression was used to reduce the long-T_2 signals from fat and minimize chemical shift artifacts that can contaminate T_2^* quantification. To increase scan efficiency, up to two UTE k-space spokes were acquired per fat saturation pulse. Fat saturation pulses could alter the available longitudinal magnetization prior to UTE excitation, particularly for short-T_2 tissues [43]. Therefore, the bandwidth of the fat saturation pulse was decreased from 633 to 333 Hz in order to minimize the effects of fat saturation on measured short-T_2^* values.

Image Preparation

For the purpose of robust and efficient image analysis, image registration was performed to allow spatial one-to-one mapping of voxels across the three longitudinal UTE acquisitions at baseline, 12 weeks, and 24 weeks. After initial rigid registration of the entire knee volume (with correction for rotation and translation between multi-echo acquisitions and different examinations), a groupwise nonlinear refinement registration was performed [44, 45].

Image Analysis

As mentioned above, T_2^*s can be calculated from UTE-MRI using mono-exponential or biexponential decay models. In this trial, the T_2^* relaxometry data from the three visits were fitted to registered UTE images using both mono-exponential and biexponential models. Evaluation of longitudinal change in T_2^* was performed using a method that allowed separate analysis of changes in different regions of the patellar tendon. This method was designed to overcome the high spatial anisotropy of T_2^* in tendinopathy [42]. The fraction of short-T_2^* components, a parameter resulting from biexponential fitting, was used to define three subregions. The first subregion was identified by selecting voxels with mostly short T_2^*s (60–100% short-T_2^* components) and was considered to represent normal aligned collagen. The second subregion was identified by selecting the voxels with mostly long T_2^*s (0–30% short-T_2^* components) and was believed to represent degenerate tissue. The last subregion (30–60% short-T_2^* components) was the interface that separated the two subregions mentioned above. Voxels were automatically selected, based on thresholding the percentage of short-T_2^* components within a manual region of interest covering the outer margins of the proximal patellar tendon on ten consecutive slices. In the three subregions identified with biexponential fitting, the longitudinal change in T_2^* was calculated using mono-exponential fitting.

Results

Figure 36.4 illustrates an example of this image analysis method in one patient of the JUMPER study. Among all athletes, a significant decrease in T_2^* was found in the voxels that represented the degenerated tissue in the patellar tendon, from 14 ± 3 ms at baseline to 13 ± 4 ms at 24 weeks (adjusted mean difference (95% confidence interval (95% CI):= 1 ms (1–2))). The T_2^* decrease in the tissue compartment that corresponded with degenerate tissue was significantly associated with an improvement in the severity of symptoms as measured with the Victorian institute of sports assessment for patellar tendons (VISA-P) score, a validated clinical outcome score in PT [46] (main effect, −1.2 (95% CI: −2.0 to −0.4)). There was no association with clinical outcome in the other tissue compartments.

Limitations

There are, unfortunately, several limitations of T_2^* mapping using UTE-MRI. The orientational dependence of transverse relaxation times in tendons is potentially the most important

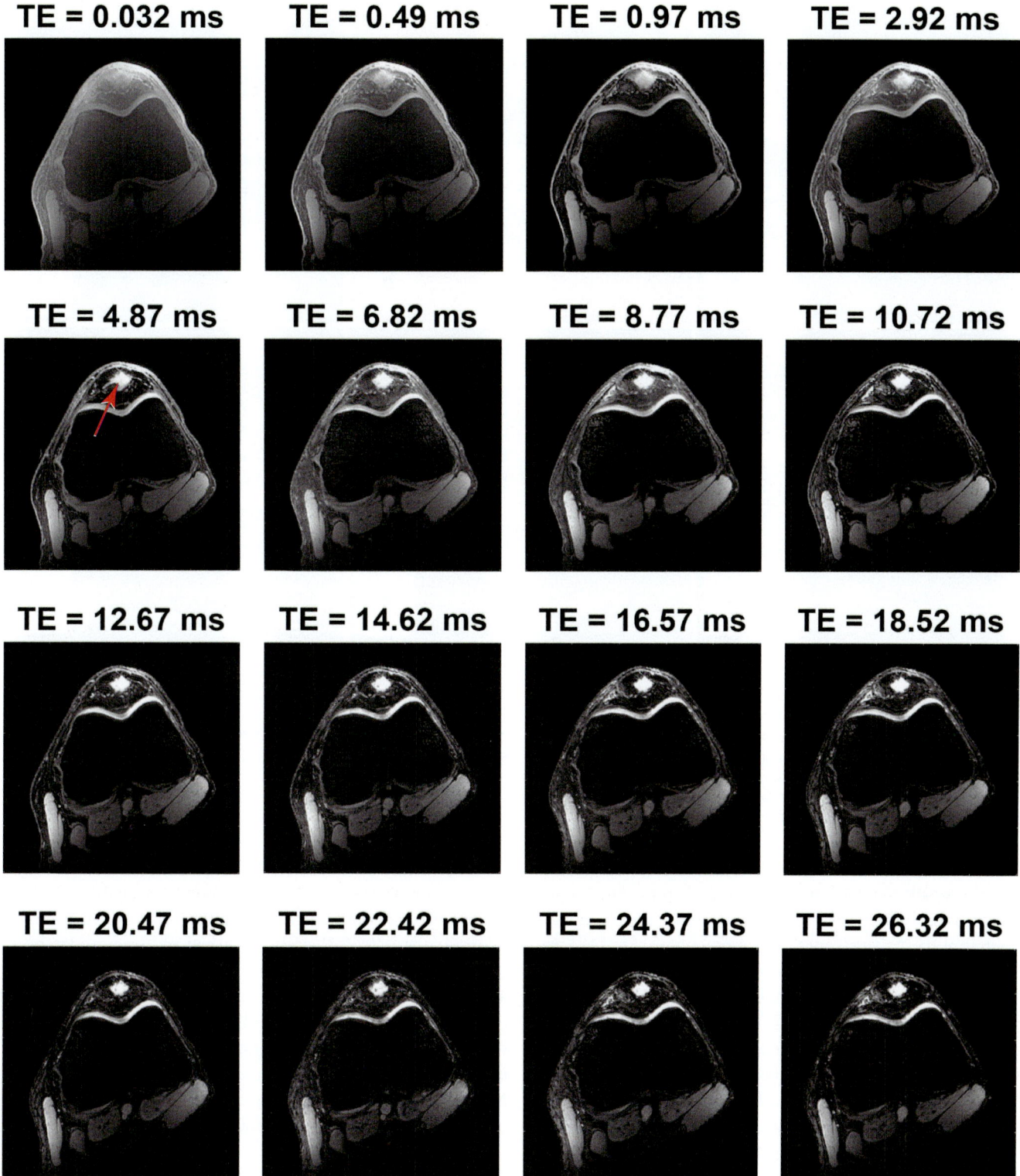

Fig. 36.3 Axial 3D UTE Cones images of the knee with different TEs in a patient with PT, showing a rounded area of increased signal intensity located posteriorly within the normally aligned collagen of the proximal patellar tendon (red arrow). The abnormality is barely apparent at TE = 0.032 ms but becomes obvious at longer TEs

limitation of quantitative T_2^* mapping and is also difficult to mitigate in clinical studies. In addition to altering the water proton fractions, anisotropy of T_2^* also directly affects T_2^* measurements [47]. The collagen fiber orientation of tendons with respect to the static magnetic field and the restriction of translational motion of the water molecules lead to a variety of intramolecular dipolar interactions of protons in collagen-rich tissues that are surrounded by water molecules. This mainly affects transverse relaxation times (T_2 and T_2^*), leading to orientation dependence of T_2^* values in tendon. Due to

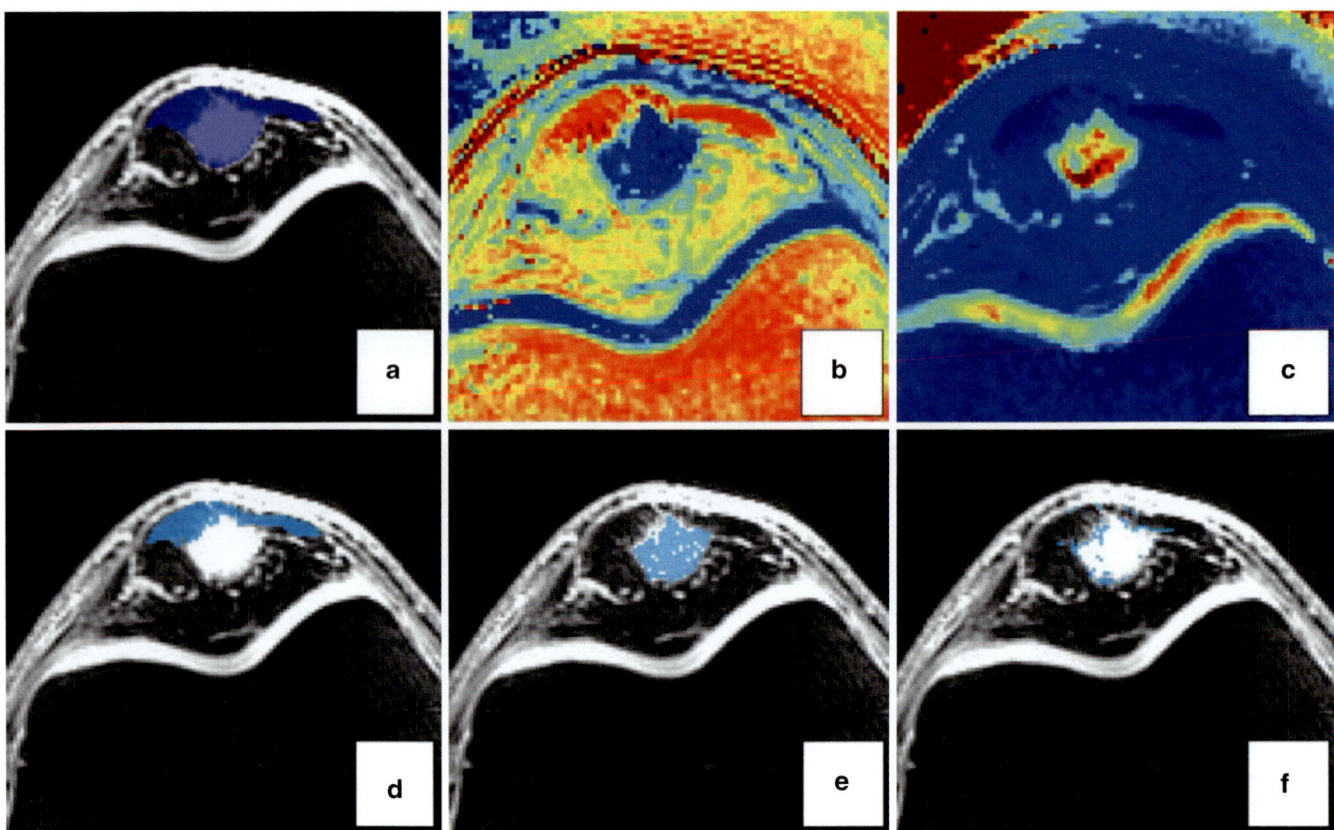

Fig. 36.4 Illustration of T_2^* analysis in PT using 3D UTE-MRI. (**a**) For image analysis, a mask that covered the outer margins of the patellar tendon was manually drawn on ten consecutive slices. (**b**) A biexponential fitting map, displaying the percentage of short-T_2^* components on a scale from dark blue (0% short components) to red (100% short-T_2^* components). (**c**) A mono-exponential fitting map, on a scale from dark blue (short T_2^*) to red (long T_2^*). (**d**) Voxels selected based on a thresh-old of 60–100% short-T_2^* components (representing aligned collagen), $T_2^* = 3$ ms. (**e**) Voxels selected based on a threshold of 0–30% short-T_2^* components (representing the degenerate tissue), $T_2^* = 14$ ms. (**f**) Voxels selected based on a threshold of 30–60% short-T_2^* components (representing the interface between panels (**d**) and (**e**), $T_2^* = 7.5$ ms)

anisotropy, T_2^* is considerably shortened with fibers parallel to B_0 as a result of additional dephasing of spins. The longest T_2s are found where the dipolar interactions are the lowest, which is at the "magic" angle of approximately 55° [48]. For free water, relaxation is comparable to the relaxation of a protein solution. A recent study has demonstrated the relationship between T_2^* decay, T_2^* anisotropy, and tendon heterogeneity and that a difference of only 10° (from 30° to 40° knee flexion) of tendon fibers can change T_2^* by about 100% [48]. This study showed that the difference that was observed in comparing healthy and degenerate Achilles tendons (3.35 ms vs. 6.65 ms, respectively) [32] could be the result of a change in fiber-to-field angle of only 10°. This seriously complicates interpretation of the results. In tendons with a more complex course, such as the supraspinatus tendon at the shoulder joint, this effect can easily lead to misinterpretation of serial measurements due to different positioning of the tendon in the scanner. Second, there may be large spatial variability in T_2^*s within tendons due to the heterogeneous structure of the tissue; however, analysis in most studies is based on the assumption that tendons are homogeneous. In the JUMPER study, a method was proposed to overcome these problems with T_2^* anisotropy [42]. Third, the assumption that only two fractions can describe all fractions of water proton relaxation in collagen, as in the biexponential model, is most likely not correct. However, sampling of more than two fractions as suggested by nonlocalized spectroscopy MR [49] is highly challenging due to the introduction of fitting errors and the unrealistically high signal-to-noise ratio (SNR) required to characterize the different fractions [34]. The reliability of biexponential fitting parameters is relatively poor when compared to a mono-exponential model, making them less attractive for clinical follow-up studies. Finally, the time-consuming acquisition protocols and post-processing that are presently involved in UTE-MRI preclude its large-scale application in routine clinical practice.

Future Perspectives

Although it has been shown that T_2^* mapping of the tendons with UTE-MRI has the potential to detect degenerative changes and possibly even subtle changes in T_2^* over time, the limitations of the technique, many of which cannot be easily overcome, likely mitigate against application of the technique in routine clinical practice. However, the technique currently has the potential to investigate microstructural tissue properties in a noninvasive manner in clinical research and therefore can contribute to deeper understanding of the structural changes that occur in healthy tendons due to aging, tendon overload in athletes, and response to therapy in tendinopathy.

References

1. Benjamin M, Kaiser E, Milz S. Structure-function relationships in tendons: a review. J Anat. 2008;212(3):211–28.
2. Biewener AA. Muscle-tendon stresses and elastic energy storage during locomotion in the horse. Comp Biochem Physiol B Biochem Mol Biol. 1998;120(1):73–87.
3. Anderson FC, Pandy MG. Storage and utilization of elastic strain energy during jumping. J Biomech. 1993;26(12):1413–27.
4. Samiric T, Parkinson J, Ilic MZ, Cook J, Feller JA, Handley CJ. Changes in the composition of the extracellular matrix in patellar tendinopathy. Matrix Biol. 2009;28(4):230–6.
5. Hudson DM, Archer M, Rai J, Weis M, Fernandes RJ, Eyre DR. Age-related type I collagen modifications reveal tissue-defining differences between ligament and tendon. Matrix Biol plus. 2021;12:100070.
6. Lozano PF, Scholze M, Babian C, et al. Water-content related alterations in macro and micro scale tendon biomechanics. Sci Rep. 2019;9(1):7887.
7. Eriksen CS, Svensson RB, Gylling AT, Couppé C, Magnusson SP, Kjaer M. Load magnitude affects patellar tendon mechanical properties but not collagen or collagen cross-linking after long-term strength training in older adults. BMC Geriatr. 2019;19(1):30.
8. Khan KM, Cook JL, Bonar F, Harcourt P, Astrom M. Histopathology of common tendinopathies. Update and implications for clinical management. Sports Med. 1999;27(6):393–408.
9. Thorpe CT, Birch HL, Clegg PD, Screen HRC. The role of the non-collagenous matrix in tendon function. Int J Exp Pathol. 2013;94(4):248–59.
10. Chen D, Smith LR, Khandekar G, et al. Distinct effects of different matrix proteoglycans on collagen fibrillogenesis and cell-mediated collagen reorganization. Sci Rep. 2020;10(1):19065.
11. Safiri S, Kolahi AA, Cross M, et al. Global, regional, and national burden of other musculoskeletal disorders 1990-2017: results from the global burden of disease study 2017. Rheumatology (Oxford). 2021;60(2):855–65.
12. Scott A, Squier K, Alfredson H, et al. ICON 2019: international scientific tendinopathy symposium consensus: clinical terminology. Br J Sports Med. 2020;54(5):260–2.
13. Lian OB, Engebretsen L, Bahr R. Prevalence of jumper's knee among elite athletes from different sports: a cross-sectional study. Am J Sports Med. 2005;33(4):561–7.
14. Docking SI, Rio E, Cook J, Orchard JW, Fortington LV. The prevalence of Achilles and patellar tendon injuries in Australian foot-

ball players beyond a time-loss definition. Scand J Med Sci Sports. 2018;28(9):2016–22.
15. Zwerver J, Bredeweg SW, van den Akker-Scheek I. Prevalence of Jumper's knee among nonelite athletes from different sports. Am J Sports Med. 2011;39(9):1984–8.
16. Cook JL, Khan KM, Kiss ZS, Purdam CR, Griffiths L. Reproducibility and clinical utility of tendon palpation to detect patellar tendinopathy in young basketball players. Victorian Institute of Sport tendon study group. Br J Sports Med. 2001;35(1):65–9.
17. Rudavsky A, Cook J. Physiotherapy management of patellar tendinopathy (jumper's knee). J Physiother. 2014;60(3):122–9.
18. van der Worp H, van Ark M, Roerink S, Pepping G-J, van den Akker-Scheek I, Zwerver J. Risk factors for patellar tendinopathy: a systematic review of the literature. Br J Sports Med. 2011;45(5):446–52.
19. De Vries AJ, Koolhaas W, Zwerver J, et al. The impact of patellar tendinopathy on sports and work performance in active athletes. Res Sport Med. 2017;25(3):253–65.
20. Turner J, Malliaras P, Goulis J, McAuliffe S. "It's disappointing and it's pretty frustrating, because it feels like it's something that will never go away." A qualitative study exploring individuals' beliefs and experiences of Achilles tendinopathy. PLoS One. 2020;15(5):e0233459.
21. Breda SJ, Oei EHG, Zwerver J, et al. Effectiveness of progressive tendon-loading exercise therapy in patients with patellar tendinopathy: a randomised clinical trial. Br J Sports Med. 2021;55(9):501–9.
22. Malliaras P, Cook J, Purdam C, Rio E. Patellar tendinopathy: clinical diagnosis, load management, and advice for challenging case presentations. J Orthop Sport Phys Ther. 2015;45(11):887–98.
23. Rabello LM, van den Akker-Scheek I, Brink MS, Maas M, Diercks RL, Zwerver J. Association between clinical and imaging outcomes after therapeutic loading exercise in patients diagnosed with achilles or patellar tTendinopathy at short- and long-term follow-up. Clin J Sport Med. 2020;30(4):390–403.
24. Davies SG, Baudouin CJ, King JB, Perry JD. Ultrasound, computed tomography and magnetic resonance imaging in patellar tendinitis. Clin Radiol. 1991;43(1):52–6.
25. Weinberg EP, Adams MJ, Hollenberg GM. Color doppler sonography of patellar tendinosis. AJR Am J Roentgenol. 1998;171(3):743–4.
26. McAuliffe S, McCreesh K, Culloty F, Purtill H, O'Sullivan K. Can ultrasound imaging predict the development of Achilles and patellar tendinopathy? A systematic review and meta-analysis. Br J Sports Med. 2016;50(24):1516–23.
27. Drew BT, Smith TO, Littlewood C, Sturrock B. Do structural changes (eg, collagen/matrix) explain the response to therapeutic exercises in tendinopathy: a systematic review. Br J Sports Med. 2014;48(12):966–72.
28. Docking SI, Ooi CC, Connell D. Tendinopathy: is imaging telling us the entire story? J Orthop Sports Phys Ther. 2015;45(11):842–52.
29. Krasnosselskaia LV, Fullerton GD, Dodd SJ, Cameron IL. Water in tendon: orientational analysis of the free induction decay. Magn Reson Med. 2005;54(2):280–8.
30. Privalov PL, Crane-Robinson C. Role of water in the formation of macromolecular structures. Eur Biophys J. 2017;46(3):203–24.
31. Chang EY, Du J, Chung CB. UTE imaging in the musculoskeletal system. J Magn Reson Imaging. 2015;41(4):870–83.
32. Juras V, Apprich S, Szomolanyi P, Bieri O, Deligianni X, Trattnig S. Bi-exponential T_2 analysis of healthy and diseased Achilles tendons: an in vivo preliminary magnetic resonance study and correlation with clinical score. Eur Radiol. 2013;23(10):2814–22.
33. Peto S, Gillis P, Henri VP. Structure and dynamics of water in tendon from NMR relaxation measurements. Biophys J. 1990;57(1):71–84.
34. Du J. Quantitative ultrashort TE (UTE) imaging of short T2 tissues. In: Encyclopedia of magnetic resonance. Chichester, UK: Wiley; 2012.

35. Kijowski R, Wilson JJ, Liu F. Bicomponent ultrashort echo time T_2^* analysis for assessment of patients with patellar tendinopathy. J Magn Reson Imaging. 2017;46(5):1441–7.

36. Ashir A, Ma Y, Jerban S, et al. Rotator cuff tendon assessment in symptomatic and control groups using quantitative MRI. J Magn Reson Imaging. 2020;52(3):864–72.

37. Du J, Bydder GM. Qualitative and quantitative ultrashort-TE MRI of cortical bone. NMR Biomed. 2013;26(5):489–506.

38. Pauli C, Bae WC, Lee M, et al. Ultrashort–echo time MR imaging of the patella with bicomponent analysis: correlation with histopathologic and polarized light microscopic findings. Radiology. 2012;264(2):484–93.

39. Williams A, Qian Y, Golla S, Chu CR. UTE-T_2^* mapping detects sub-clinical meniscus injury after anterior cruciate ligament tear. Osteoarthr Cartil. 2012;20(6):486–94.

40. Bae WC, Statum S, Zhang Z, et al. Morphology of the cartilaginous endplates in human intervertebral disks with ultrashort echo time MR imaging. Radiology. 2013;266(2):564–74.

41. Gurney PT, Hargreaves BA, Nishimura DG. Design and analysis of a practical 3D cones trajectory. Magn Reson Med. 2006;55(3):575–82.

42. Breda SJ, Poot DHJ, Papp D, et al. Tissue-specific T_2^* biomarkers in patellar tendinopathy by subregional quantification

using 3D ultrashort echo time MRI. J Magn Reson Imaging. 2020;52(2):420–30.

43. Carl M, Nazaran A, Bydder GM, Du J. Effects of fat saturation on short T_2 quantification. Magn Reson Imaging. 2017;43:6–9.

44. Klein S, Staring M, Murphy K, Viergever MA, Pluim JPW. Elastix: a toolbox for intensity-based medical image registration. IEEE Trans Med Imaging. 2010;29(1):196–205.

45. Huizinga W, Poot DHJ, Guyader J-M, et al. PCA-based groupwise image registration for quantitative MRI. Med Image Anal. 2016;29:65–78.

46. Hernandez-Sanchez S, Hidalgo MD, Gomez A. Responsiveness of the VISA-P scale for patellar tendinopathy in athletes. Br J Sports Med. 2014;48(6):453–7.

47. Momot KI, Pope JM, Wellard RM. Anisotropy of spin relaxation of water protons in cartilage and tendon. NMR Biomed. 2010;23(3):313–24.

48. Hager B, Schreiner MM, Walzer SM, et al. Transverse relaxation anisotropy of the Achilles and patellar tendon studied by MR microscopy. J Magn Reson Imaging. 2022;56(4):1091–103.

49. Henkelman RM, Stanisz GJ, Kim JK, Bronskill MJ. Anisotropy of NMR properties of tissues. Magn Reson Med. 1994;32(5):592–601.

Hemophilic Arthropathy

Soo Hyun Shin, Annette von Drygalski, Sam Sedaghat,
Jiang Du, Eric Y. Chang, and Hyungseok Jang

Introduction

Hemophilia is an X-linked bleeding disorder characterized by deficiencies in clotting factors VIII or IX [1]. Patients with hemophilia suffer from frequent spontaneous joint bleeds, leading to debilitating hemophilic arthropathy (HA) [2–8]. Prophylaxis with clotting factor replacement has been used to prevent joint bleeding. However, the cost of this is $250k–$500k per year per patient, which makes hemophilia one of the most costly chronic diseases to treat on a per-patient basis in the United States [8–11]. Asymptomatic and silent bleeds as well as unnoticed microhemorrhages generate hemosiderin deposits that are the primary cause of joint degeneration in HA [2–7]. Sensitive and reliable measures to assess individual response to therapy and the general efficacy of treatment are of critical importance. Noninvasive imaging of hemosiderin and the subsequent damage it causes to cartilage and subchondral bone could be invaluable for

S. H. Shin · S. Sedaghat · H. Jang (✉)
Department of Radiology, University of California, San Diego,
La Jolla, CA, USA
e-mail: shs033@health.ucsd.edu; ssedaghat@health.ucsd.edu;
h4jang@health.ucsd.edu

A. von Drygalski
Department of Medicine, University of California, San Diego,
La Jolla, CA, USA
e-mail: avondrygalski@health.ucsd.edu

J. Du
Department of Radiology, University of California, San Diego,
La Jolla, CA, USA

VA San Diego Healthcare System, San Diego, CA, USA

Department of Bioengineering, University of California, San
Diego, La Jolla, CA, USA
e-mail: jiangdu@health.ucsd.edu

E. Y. Chang
Department of Radiology, University of California, San Diego,
La Jolla, CA, USA

VA San Diego Healthcare System, San Diego, CA, USA
e-mail: e8chang@health.ucsd.edu

optimizing costly treatment plans and monitoring disease progression [8, 12].

Physical examination, even by an experienced observer, has only limited reliability in assessing HA [13]. Radiography only shows late osseous changes and is insensitive to soft tissue abnormalities such as synovitis and cartilage degeneration [14–17]. Computed tomography (CT) is sensitive to bony changes but cannot evaluate synovitis or cartilage degeneration [17]. Ultrasound has the advantages of low cost, short examination duration, and high reliability for detecting synovitis but suffers from limited acoustic windows and penetration, which preclude complete evaluation of inner joint structures, as well as poor sensitivity to hemosiderin [18–29].

Magnetic resonance imaging (MRI) is the only validated gold standard available for precise evaluation of joints [25–40]. Although it provides excellent soft tissue contrast and high sensitivity to both iron deposition and structural changes in cartilage, it still has significant limitations, including imprecise, semiquantitative evaluation of hemosiderin deposition and the inability to detect early iron deposition and degeneration in both cartilage and subchondral bone.

This chapter reviews the promise and feasibility of ultrashort echo time (UTE) imaging techniques to provide quantitative assessment of hemosiderin in HA.

Current MRI Techniques in HA

Existing clinical MRI techniques fail to quantify intra-articular hemosiderin deposits resulting from recurrent joint bleeds, which are the hallmark of hemophilia [4–7]. Iron from red blood cells catalyzes radical hydroxyl production that triggers a cascade of degradative enzymes and cytokines (e.g., interleukin-1 (IL-1) and tumor necrosis factor-α (TNF-α)) produced by macrophages and leads to oxygen metabolite generation by chondrocytes and inhibition of proteoglycan (PG) synthesis [41]. Cartilage damage may be directly induced by blood that subsequently causes an inflammatory response over and above that caused by hemosiderin itself. Since joint bleeds can be asymptomatic and go unnoticed, it is critical to monitor hemosiderin levels and distribution after joint bleeds [4–7]. However, clinical MRI tends to overestimate hemosiderin levels and underestimate synovial hypertrophy due to the "blooming artifact" associated with high iron concentrations [26–29]. Furthermore, none of the current MRI techniques can quantitatively map hemosiderin levels, which may be extremely helpful in guiding treatment.

Conventional clinical MRI fails to detect the initial manifestation of cartilage degeneration resulting from repeated episodes of intra-articular bleeding [25–29]. Monitoring early cartilage degeneration is the focus of current research. However, clinical MRI can only detect structural changes, which are seen during the irreversible late stage of the disease. Early changes in HA involve iron deposition and associated inhibition of PG synthesis and collagen degradation [4–7]. T_2^* has been shown to be sensitive to iron deposition in cartilage [42]. $T_{1\rho}$ is sensitive to PG depletion [43–49], whereas T_2 is sensitive to collagen degradation [50, 51]. The principal confounding factor in T_2^*, T_2, and $T_{1\rho}$ measures is the magic angle effect [52–58], which may result in spurious several-fold increases in the values of these tissue properties. These far exceed changes produced by disease (e.g., ~10–30% in osteoarthritis (OA)) [59] and make interpretation of elevated $T_{1\rho}$s and T_2^*/T_2s difficult or impossible. Furthermore, since a single joint bleed can have devastating effects on all joint components [6], techniques are needed to evaluate changes not only in articular cartilage but in other joint tissues as well, such as the osteochondral junction (OCJ), menisci, ligaments, and tendons. These tissues have short T_2s and are "invisible" when imaged with conventional clinical MRI sequences [60, 61], which is a significant limitation because joint degeneration is a "whole-organ" disease involving all the primary joint tissues.

The candidate sites for changes that precede cartilage degradation are invisible with conventional MRI. Recurrent bleeds lead to bony changes that are clinically characterized by cyst formation, subchondral sclerosis, osteophyte formation, epiphyseal enlargement, and osteoporosis (OP) [12, 62]. Subchondral bone cysts are a prominent feature of HA. Some recent studies have found that the OCJ, rather than the more superficial uncalcified cartilage, is the site of the initial changes that lead to cartilage degradation [63–79]. In adults without OA, the OCJ becomes quiescent, but, in adults with OA, the OCJ becomes reactive and calcifies adjacent unmineralized cartilage. This can lead to relative thinning of uncalcified cartilage and a concomitant increase in the force gradient across cartilage, resulting in further damage [65]. To better understand its involvement in iron-induced cartilage degeneration, it is essential to develop noninvasive imaging techniques to evaluate the OCJ. However, current conventional MRI techniques cannot image the OCJ due to its ultrashort T_2^*.

Potential of UTE-MRI in HA

UTE techniques may provide comprehensive evaluation of blood-induced joint damage and so improve the diagnosis and treatment monitoring of HA.

For morphological imaging of HA, UTE imaging is expected to be more robust to susceptibility artifacts (i.e., blooming artifacts) caused by highly concentrated hemosiderin than conventional MRI techniques. Figure 37.1 shows three-dimensional (3D) UTE and gradient echo (GRE) imaging of the hemophiliac knee of a 48-year-old patient. UTE imaging shows dramatically reduced blooming artifacts in the synovium compared with GRE imaging and is expected to provide a more accurate measure of the synovial volume. Moreover, UTE sequences can directly detect signals from OCJ. The adiabatic inversion pulse provides robust suppression of signals from the adjacent layers of cartilage, fat, and muscle, enabling high contrast inversion recovery UTE (IR-UTE) imaging of the OCJ [80]. This is likely to be important in elucidating the role of the OCJ in different stages of cartilage degeneration and in understanding the evolution of HA induced by recurrent bleeding. UTE-MRI sequences can directly detect signals from hemosiderin-laden synovium, OCJ, deep cartilage, menisci, ligaments, tendons, and bone. The IR-UTE sequence provides high contrast imaging of the OCJ and hemosiderin-laden synovium. Bony changes can be directly visualized with excellent contrast.

UTE-based techniques also offer robust volumetric mapping of T_1, T_2^*, susceptibility, PG, and collagen in all primary joint tissues. Quantitative UTE imaging techniques are expected to assess hemosiderin deposition and early cartilage destruction, including PG depletion, collagen degradation, bony erosions, and cysts using a single modality. UTE-based T_2^* and quantitative susceptibility mapping (QSM) have recently shown feasibility for detecting hemosiderin in hemophilic joints.

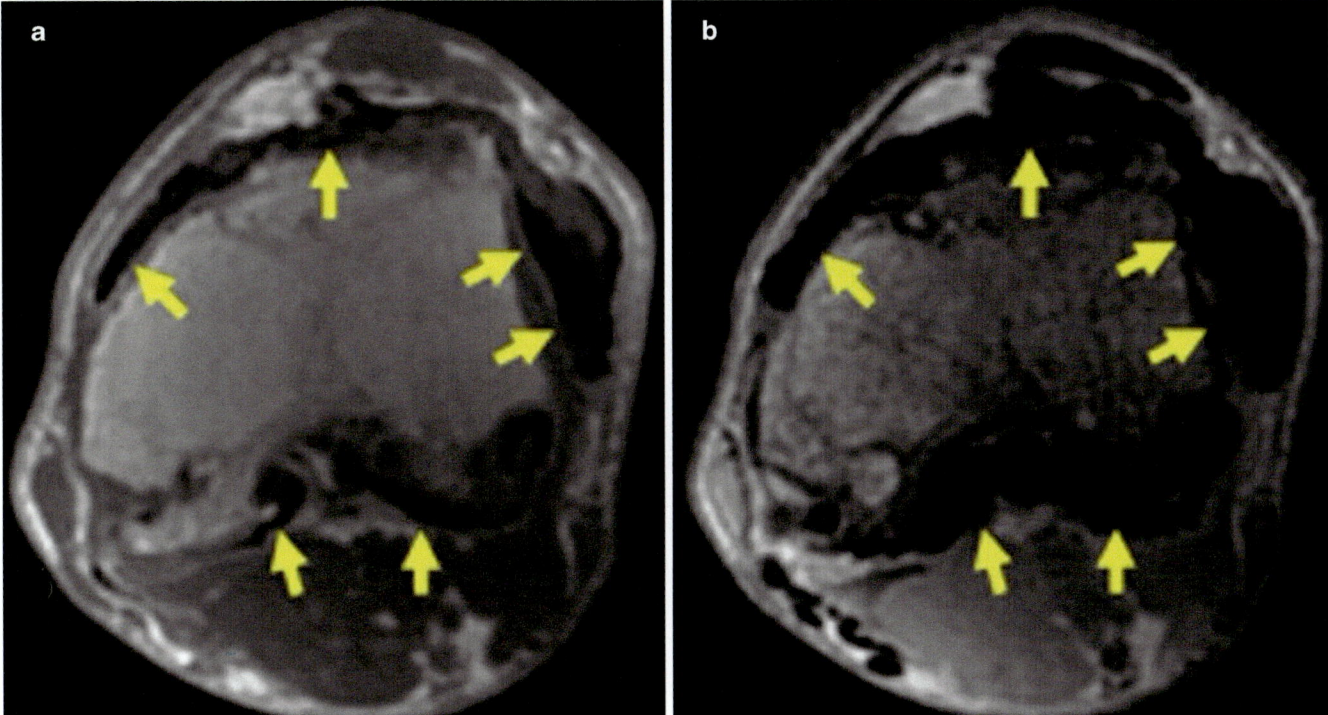

Fig. 37.1 A blooming artifact in (**a**) three-dimensional (3D) UTE (echo time (TE) = 0.032 ms) and (**b**) 3D gradient echo (GRE) imaging (TE = 4.4 ms). UTE imaging shows dramatically decreased blooming artifacts (yellow arrows)

UTE-T_2^* Mapping in HA

von Drygalski et al. investigated the feasibility of UTE-based T_2^* mapping in cartilage from the knee joints of patients with hemophilia A and hemophilia B [42]. In this study, 23 adult hemophilic patients were recruited and underwent 3D UTE imaging as well as clinical T_1- and T_2-weighted MRI in their elbows ($n = 7$), ankles ($n = 7$), and knees ($n = 9$). With 3D UTE imaging for T_2^* mapping, four images were obtained at TEs ranging from 0 to 9 ms using a 3 T clinical magnetic resonance (MR) scanner. In this study, most target joints in the elbow showed a near-complete loss of cartilage and OCJ and were therefore excluded from the quantitative analysis of cartilage. The knees and ankles were included in the analysis ($n = 16$). Figure 37.2 shows two examples from two hemophilic patients

(Fig. 37.2a: severe hemophilia A, Fig. 37.2b: mild hemophilia A). The T_2^* of patellar cartilage was measured as 3 ms in the patient with severe hemophilia, whereas that in the patient with mild hemophilia was measured as 12.1 ms. Due to the accumulation of iron, T_2^* was much shorter with severe hemophilia. In all patients, the mean T_2^* in the knee and ankle joint cartilages was 9.2 ms (range 3.0–14.6 ms), as shown in Fig. 37.3a. Figure 37.3b shows the scatter plot between the hemophilia joint health scores (HJHSs, with 0 being the best and 20 being the worst) and UTE-based T_2^*s in all patients, and Spearman's rank correlation, which exhibited a strong negative correlation (r_s) of −0.81 with $P < 0.001$. The conventional MRI International Prophylaxis Study Group (IPSG) score only showed a moderate negative correlation with the HJHSs ($r_s = -0.52$, $P = 0.037$) (Fig. 37.3c).

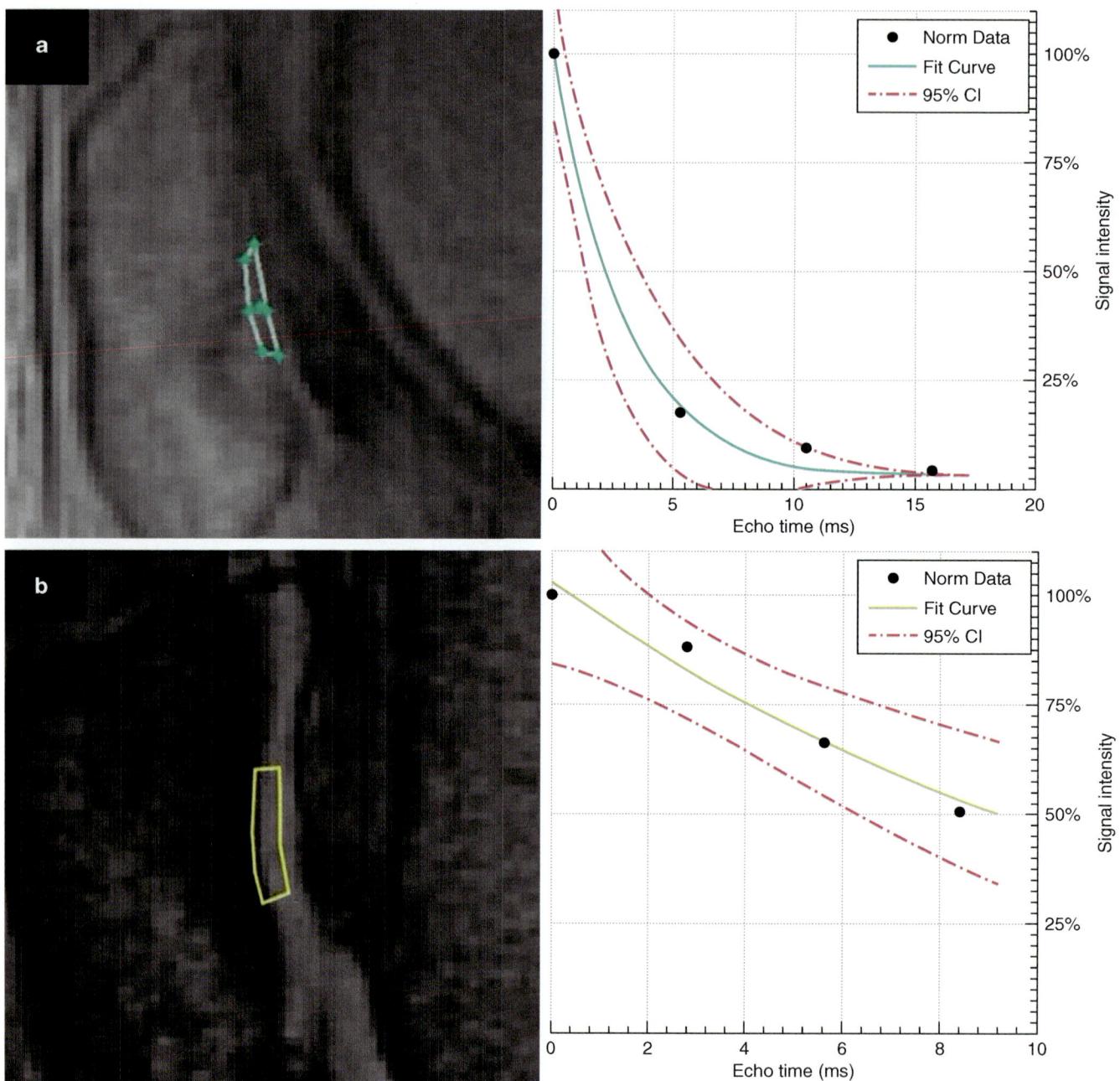

Fig. 37.2 T_2^* decay in the patellar cartilage from two hemophilic patients ((**a**) severe hemophilia and (**b**) mild hemophilia). The signal shows rapid decay in the patient with severe hemophilia, where the estimated T_2^* was 3.0 ms due to iron deposition in cartilage. In comparison, cartilage signal from the patient with mild hemophilia showed a much longer T_2^* of 12.1 ms. (Adapted with permission from von Drygalski et al. [42])

Fig. 37.3 UTE-T_2^* in HA. (a) Measured T_2^* in all patients, (b) a scatter plot for T_2^* vs. HJHS, and (c) a scatter plot for T_2^* vs. the International Prophylaxis Study Group (IPSG) score. (Adapted with permission from von Drygalski et al. [42])

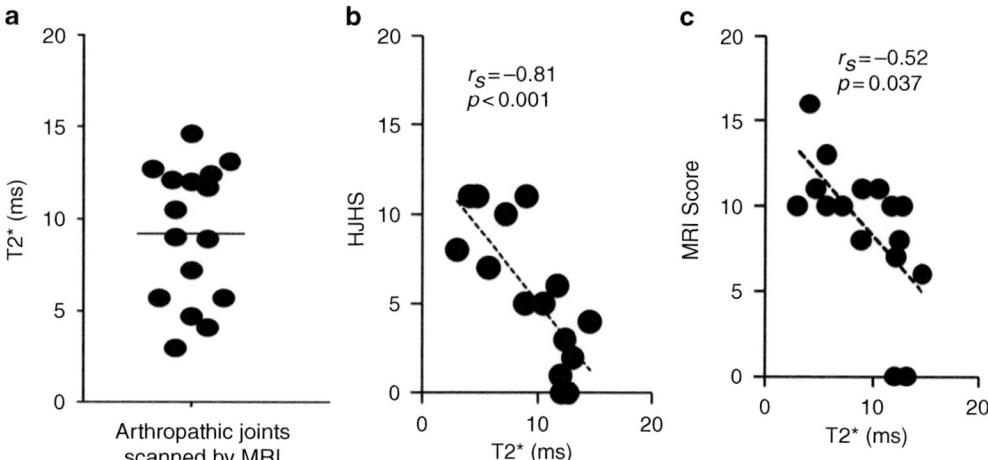

UTE Quantitative Susceptibility Mapping (UTE-QSM) in HA

QSM is utilized to quantify iron levels based on its paramagnetic susceptibility [81–84]. This may provide a more reliable assessment of hemosiderin than conventional susceptibility-weighted imaging (SWI). However, clinical MRI sequences cannot image critically important regions of highly concentrated hemosiderin due to the marked shortening of T_2^* that occurs with increased iron content. As an alternative, UTE sequences with TEs ~100 times shorter than clinical TEs have been investigated to detect signals directly from short-T_2 tissues, including hemosiderin-enriched synovium [85–88].

Jang et al. have demonstrated the feasibility of UTE-based QSM (UTE-QSM) to evaluate susceptibilities of highly concentrated iron and so accurately map hemosiderin distribution and content in hemophilic joints [85]. In their study, a 3D UTE sequence with a Cones trajectory was utilized to obtain multiple images at six different TEs, including short and long TEs (0.032, 0.2, 0.4, 2.8, 3.6, and 4.4 ms), and capture signals from both short-T_2^* tissues (e.g., hemosiderin, tendon, ligament, and meniscus) and long-T_2 tissues (muscle, cartilage, and fat). Phase and magnitude images were processed with a QSM algorithm based on morphology-enabled dipole inversion (MEDI) [89]. One major issue is that the off-resonant fat signal complicates the estimation of tissue susceptibility in UTE-QSM. To address this issue, a fat signal model was used, which takes into account chemical shift of fat in the total B_0 field map estimation, similar to m-point Dixon or iterative decomposition of water and fat with echo asymmetry and least squares estimation (IDEAL) [90]. The total field map produced in this way was processed with a projection onto a dipole field (PDF) algorithm to remove the background field map and thus achieve a local tissue field map. Then, a tissue susceptibility map was obtained using the MEDI algorithm.

Figure 37.4 shows in vivo UTE-QSM results in three patients with HA. In the conventional T_1- and T_2-weighted fast spin echo (FSE) imaging, hemosiderin deposition is shown as a dropout of signal but not depicted with anatomical detail. UTE-QSM provides more precise detection of hemosiderin. Patient A with more severe HA (HJHS 12) shows a higher level of hemosiderin deposition in the joint than patient C with milder HA (HJHS 4). Figure 37.5 shows the susceptibility map from patient A obtained using UTE-QSM (left) and the corresponding histological images with Perls' Prussian blue iron staining (right) from the tissue harvested after total knee arthroplasty performed following the MRI examination. The measured susceptibility with UTE-QSM is 4.5 ± 1.8 ppm for tissue A and 2.7 ± 1.1 ppm for tissue B, which agrees with histological observations showing higher iron concentration in tissue A compared with tissue B.

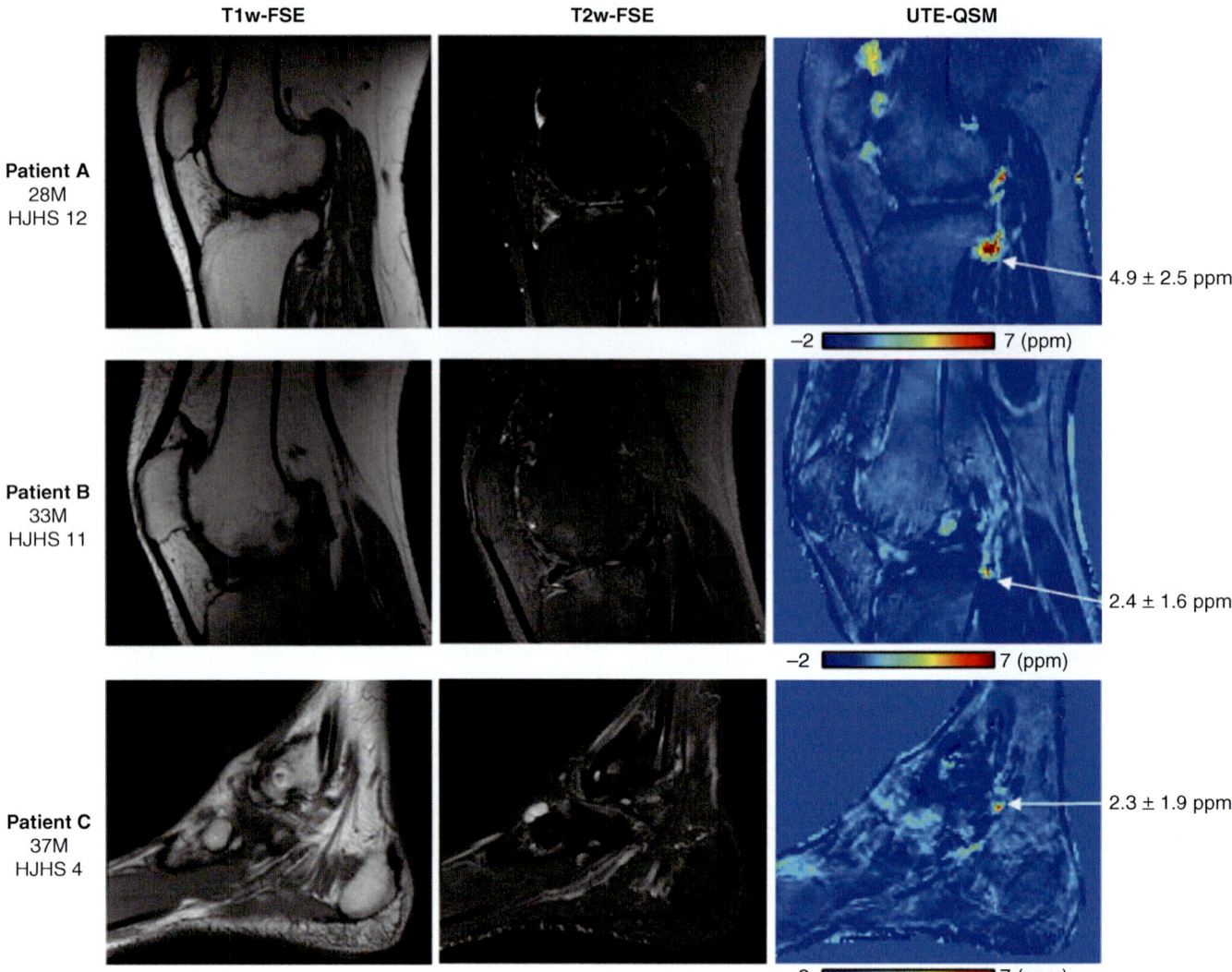

Fig. 37.4 In vivo UTE-QSM in three patients with HA. Accumulated hemosiderin appears as low signal on the clinical MR images (T_1w-fast spin echo (FSE) and T_2w-FSE). These images do not provide specific information about tissues with low signals (e.g., tendon, meniscus, and bone). UTE-QSM yields a volumetric susceptibility map, which is more specific to paramagnetic hemosiderin. The estimated susceptibility values were 4.9 ± 2.5 ppm (parts per million), 2.4 ± 1.6 ppm, and 2.3 ± 1.9 ppm in the regions indicated by white arrows in patients A, B, and C, respectively. (Adapted with permission from Jang et al. [85])

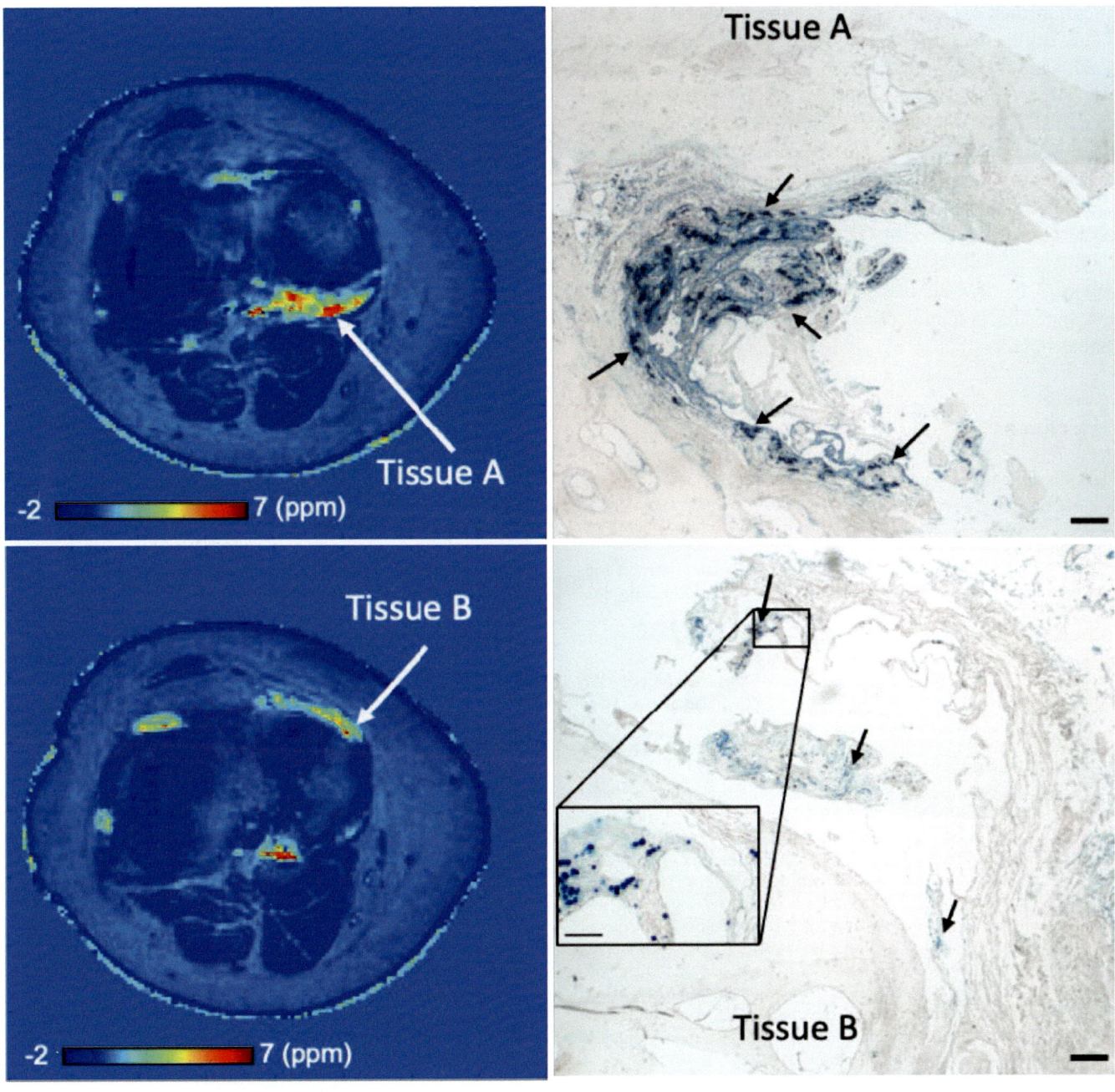

UTE-QSM **Histology**

Fig. 37.5 Osteochondral tissues from a 28-year-old patient with HA (HJHS = 12). UTE-QSM (left) shows high susceptibility in regions with accumulated hemosiderin in synovium and the OCJ. This patient underwent total knee arthroplasty (TKA) after MRI, and the joint tissues were harvested. The histological images (right) are from osteochondral tissues taken after the TKA stained with Perls' Prussian blue and red hematoxylin counterstain. On histology, tissue A shows higher iron content. The bars represent 200 μm in the full-field images and 50 μm in the insets. The corresponding susceptibility from UTE-QSM was 4.5 ± 1.8 ppm for tissue A and 2.7 ± 1.1 ppm for tissue B, which agrees with the histological observations. (Adapted with permission from Jang et al. [85])

Conclusions

UTE imaging is a promising technique for assessing HA because it captures signals from short-T_2 tissues such as hemosiderin, tendon, ligament, meniscus, and bone, and this may provide more reliable diagnostic information about the major tissues in the joint than conventional MRI. UTE-T_2^* and UTE-QSM have shown their efficacy in quantifying hemosiderin. Although UTE-QSM is more technically demanding, it can provide more accurate quantification than UTE-T$_2^*$, which is more susceptible to the magic angle effect. Moreover, UTE-T$_2^*$ cannot discriminate paramagnetic compounds from diamagnetic compounds (e.g., iron from calcium) and is a less specific biomarker than UTE-QSM. However, UTE-QSM is still at an early stage of development and needs further improvement, for example, to reduce streak artifacts. A complete study with a panel of quantitative UTE techniques, including IR-UTE, UTE-magnetization transfer (UTE-MT), UTE-T$_1$, and UTE-T$_{1\rho}$, as well as UTE-QSM and UTE-T$_2^*$, in a larger cohort of hemophilic patients and healthy controls, would elucidate the potential clinical benefit of the UTE techniques in HA.

References

1. Scott JP, Montgomery RR. Hereditary clotting factor deficiencies (bleeding disorders). In: Kliegman RM, Stanton BF, St. Gem III JW, et al., editors. Essentials of pediatrics. Philadelphia, PA: Saunders; 2011. p. 1699–702.
2. Arnold WD, Hilgartner MW. Hemohpilic arthropathy, current concepts of pathogenesis and management. J Bone Joint Surg Am. 1977;59(3):287–305.
3. Soreff J. Joint debridement in the treatment of advanced hemophilic knee arthropathy. Clin Orthop Relat Res. 1984;191:179–84.
4. Roosendaal G, TeKoppele JM, Vianen ME, Van Den Berg HM, Lafeber FPJG, Bijlsma JWJ. Blood-induced joint damage: a canine in vivo study. Arthritis Rheum. 1999;42(5):1033–9.
5. van Meegeren MER, Roosendaal G, Jansen NWD, Lafeber FPJG, Mastbergen SC. Blood-induced joint damage: the devastating effects of acute joint bleeds versus micro-bleeds. Cartilage. 2013;4(4):313–20.
6. van Vulpen LFD, van Meegeren MER, Roosendaal G, et al. Biochemical markers of joint tissue damage increase shortly after a joint bleed: an explorative human and canine in vivo study. Osteoarthr Cartil. 2015;23(1):62–9.
7. Valentino LA. Blood-induced joint disease: the pathophysiology of hemophilic arthropathy. J Thromb Haemost. 2010;8(9):1895–902.
8. Srivastava A, Brewer AK, Mauser-Bunschoten EP, Key NS, Kitchen S, Llinas A, Ludlam CA, Mahlangu JN, Mulder K, Poon MC, Street A. Treatment guidelines working group on behalf of the world federation of hemophilia. Guidelines for the management of hemophilia. Haemophilia. 2013;19(1):e1–47.
9. Manco-Johnson MJ, Abshire TC, Shapiro AD, et al. Prophylaxis versus episodic treatment to prevent joint disease in boys with severe hemophilia. New Engl J Med. 2007;357(6):535–44.
10. Blankenship CS. To manage costs of hemophilia, patients need more than clotting factor. Biotechnol Healthc. 2008;5(4):34–40.
11. Zhou ZY, Koerper MA, Johnson KA, Riske B, Baker JR, Ullman M, Curtis RG, Poon JL, Lou M, Nichol MB. Burden of illness: direct and indirect costs among persons with hemophilia A in the United States. J Med Econ. 2015;18(6):457–65.
12. van Vulpen LFD, Holstein K, Martinoli C. Joint disease in haemophilia: pathophysiology, pain and imaging. Haemophilia. 2018;24(Suppl 6):44–9.
13. Guzman J, Burgos-Vargas R, Duarte-Salazar C, Gomez-Mora P. Reliability of the articular examination in children with juvenile rheumatoid arthritis: interobserver agreement and sources of disagreement. J Rheumatol. 1995;22(12):2331–6.
14. Fischer K, Nijdam A, Holmström M, Petrini P, Ljung R, van der Schouw YT, Berntorp E. Evaluating outcome of prophylaxis in hae-

mophilia: objective and self-reported instruments should be combined. Haemophilia. 2016;22(2):e80–6.
15. Pergantou H, Matsinos G, Papadopoulos A, Platokouki H, Aronis S. Comparative study of validity of clinical, X-ray and magnetic resonance imaging scores in evaluation and management of haemophilic arthropathy in children. Haemophilia. 2006;12(3):241–7.
16. Poonnoose PM, Hilliard P, Doria AS, Keshava SN, Gibikote S, Kavitha ML, Feldman BM, Blanchette V, Srivastava A. Correlating clinical and radiological assessment of joints in haemophilia: results of a cross sectional study. Haemophilia. 2016;22(6):925–33.
17. Yu W, Lin Q, Guermazi A, Yu X, Shang W, Zhu H, Meng W, Xu R, Zhao Y. Comparison of radiography, CT and MR imaging in detection of arthropathies in patients with haemophilia. Haemophilia. 2009;15(5):1090–6.
18. Foppen W, van der Schaaf IC, Beek FJA, Mali WPTM, Fischer K. Diagnostic accuracy of point-of-care ultrasound for evaluation of early blood-induced joint changes: comparison with MRI. Haemophilia. 2018;24(6):971–9.
19. Keshava SN, Gibikote SV, Mohanta A, Poonnoose P, Rayner T, Hilliard P, Lakshmi KM, Moineddin R, Ignas D, Srivastava A, Blanchette V, Doria AS. Ultrasound and magnetic resonance imaging of healthy paediatric ankles and knees: a baseline for comparison with haemophilic joints. Haemophilia. 2015;21(3):e210–22.
20. Bakeer N, Shapiro AD. Merging into the mainstream: the evolution of the role of point-of-care musculoskeletal ultrasound in hemophilia. F1000Res. 2019;8:F1000.
21. Plut D, Kotnik BF, Zupan IP, Kljucevsek D, Vidmar G, Snoj Z, Martinoli C, Salapura V. Diagnostic accuracy of haemophilia early arthropathy detection with ultrasound (HEAD-US): a comparative magnetic resonance imaging (MRI) study. Radiol Oncol. 2019;53(2):178–86.
22. Di Minno MND, Iervolino S, Soscia E, Tosetto A, Coppola A, Schiavulli M, Marrone E, Ruosi C, Salvatore M, Di Minno G. Magnetic resonance imaging and ultrasound evaluation of "healthy" joints in young subjects with severe haemophilia A. Haemophilia. 2013;19(3):e167–73.
23. von Drygalski A, Moore RE, Nguyen S, Barnes RFW, Volland LM, Hughes TH, Du J, Chang EY. Advanced hemophilic arthropathy: sensitivity of soft tissue discrimination with musculoskeletal ultrasound. J Ultrasound Med. 2018;37(8):1945–56.
24. Nguyen S, Lu X, Ma Y, Du J, Chang EY, von Drygalski A. Musculoskeletal ultrasound for intra-articular bleed detection: a highly sensitive imaging modality compared with conventional magnetic resonance imaging. J Thromb Haemost. 2018;16(3):490–9.
25. Cross S, Vaidya S, Fotiadis N. Hemophilic arthropathy: a review of imaging and staging. Semin Ultrasound CT MRI. 2013;34(6):516–24.
26. Soliman M, Daruge P, Dertkigil SSJ, De Avila Fernandes E, Negrao JR, de Aguiar Vilela Mitraud S, Sakuma ETI, Fernandes ARC, Zhang N, Huo A, Li YJ, Zhou F, Rodrigues BM, Mohanta A, Blanchette VS, Doria AS. Imaging of haemophilic arthropathy in growing joints: pitfalls in ultrasound and MRI. Haemophilia. 2017;23(5):660–72.
27. Doria AS. State-of-the-art imaging techniques for the evaluation of haemophilic arthropathy: present and future. Haemophilia. 2010;16(Suppl 5):107–14.
28. Hermann G, Gilbert MS, Abdelwahab IF. Hemophilia: evaluation of musculoskeletal involvement with CT, sonography, and MR imaging. AJR Am J Roentgenol. 1992;158(1):119–23.
29. Keshava SN, Gibikote S, Doria AS. Imaging evaluation of hemophilia: musculoskeletal approach. Semin Thromb Hemost. 2015;41(8):880–93.
30. Yulish BS, Bryan J, Lieberman M, Mulopolos P, Stnandjord SE, Modic T. hemophilic arthropathy: assessment with MR imaging. Radiology. 1987;164(3):759–62.

31. Kraft J, Blanchette V, Babyn P, Feldman B, Cloutier S, Israels S, Pai M, Rivard GE, Gomer S, McLimont M, Moineddin R, Doria AS. Magnetic resonance imaging and joint outcomes in boys with severe hemophilia A treated with tailored primary prophylaxis in Canada. J Thromb Haemost. 2012;10(12):2494–502.

32. Eerdekens M, Peerlinck K, Staes F, Pialat JB, Hermans C, Lobet S, Deschamps K. Clinical gait features are associated with MRI findings in patients with haemophilic ankle arthropathy. Haemophilia. 2020;26(2):333–9.

33. Doria AS, Zhang N, Lundin B, Hilliard P, Man C, Weiss R, Detzler G, Blanchette V, Moineddin R, Eckstein F, Sussman MS. Quantitative versus semiquantitative MR imaging of cartilage in blood-induced arthritic ankles: preliminary findings. Pediatr Radiol. 2014;44(5):576–86.

34. Foppen W, Van Der Schaaf IC, Beek FJA, Mali WPTM, Fischer K. MRI predicts 5-year joint bleeding and development of arthropathy on radiographs in hemophilia. Blood Adv. 2020;4(1):113–21.

35. den Uijl IEM, De Schepper AMA, Camerlinck M, Grobbee DE, Fischer K. Magnetic resonance imaging in teenagers and young adults with limited haemophilic arthropathy: baseline results from a prospective study. Haemophilia. 2011;17(6):926–30.

36. Oldenburg J, Zimmermann R, Katsarou O, Zanon E, Kellermann E, Lundin B, Ellinghaus P. Potential biomarkers of haemophilic arthropathy: correlations with compatible additive magnetic resonance imaging scores. Haemophilia. 2016;22(5):760–4.

37. Lundin B, Berntorp E, Pettersson H, Wirestam R, Jonsson K, Ståhlberg F, Ljung R. Gadolinium contrast agent is of limited value for magnetic resonance imaging assessment of synovial hypertrophy in hemophiliacs. Acta Radiol. 2007;48(5):520–30.

38. Hong W, Raunig D, Lundin B. SPINART study: validation of the extended magnetic resonance imaging scale for evaluation of joint status in adult patients with severe haemophilia A using baseline data. Haemophilia. 2016;22(6):e519–26.

39. Hemke R, Kuijpers TW, Van Den Berg JM, van Veenendaal M, Dolman KM, van Rossum MA, Maas M. The diagnostic accuracy of unenhanced MRI in the assessment of joint abnormalities in juvenile idiopathic arthritis. Eur Radiol. 2013;23(7):1998–2004.

40. Oldenburg J, Zimmermann R, Katsarou O, Theodossiades G, Zanon E, Niemann B, Kellermann E, Lundin B. Controlled, cross-sectional MRI evaluation of joint status in severe haemophilia A patients treated with prophylaxis vs. on demand. Haemophilia. 2015;21(2):171–9.

41. Roosendaal G, Vianen ME, Wenting MJ, van Rinsum AC, van den Berg HM, Lafeber FP, Bijlsma JW. Iron deposits and catabolic properties of synovial tissue from patients with haemophilia. J Bone Joint Surg Br. 1998;80(3):540–5.

42. von Drygalski A, Barnes RFW, Jang H, Ma Y, Wong JH, Berman Z, Du J, Chang EY. Advanced magnetic resonance imaging of cartilage components in haemophilic joints reveals that cartilage hemosiderin correlates with joint deterioration. Haemophilia. 2019;25(5):851–8.

43. Duvvuri U, Reddy R, Patel SD, Kaufman JH, Kneeland JB, Leigh JS. T1rho-relaxation in articular cartilage: effects of enzymatic degradation. Magn Reson Med. 1997;38(6):863–7.

44. Duvvuri U, Charagundla SR, Kudchodkar SB, Kaufman JH, Kneeland JB, Rizi R, Leigh JS, Reddy R. Human knee: in vivo $T_1\rho$-weighted MR imaging at 1.5 T—preliminary experience. Radiology. 2001;220(3):822–6.

45. Regatte RR, Akella SVS, Borthakur A, Kneeland JB, Reddy R. In vivo proton MR three-dimensional $T_1\rho$ mapping of human articular cartilage: initial experience. Radiology. 2003;229(1):269–74.

46. Regatte RR, Akella SVS, Lonner JH, Kneeland JB, Reddy R. T-1ρ relaxation mapping in human osteoarthritis (OA) cartilage: comparison of T-1ρ with T2. J Magn Reson Imaging. 2006;23(4):547–53.

47. Li X, Han ET, Ma B, Link TM, Newitt DC, Majumdar S. In vivo 3T spiral imaging based multi-slice $T_1\rho$ mapping of knee cartilage in osteoarthritis. Magn Reson Med. 2005;54(4):929–36.

48. Li X, Ma CB, Link TM, Castillo D-D, Blumenkrantz G, Lozano J, Carballido-Gamio J, Ries M, Majumdar S. In vivo $T_1\rho$ and T_2 mapping of articular cartilage in osteoarthritis of the knee using 3T MRI. Osteoarthr Cartil. 2007;15(7):789–97.

49. Li X, Han ET, Ma B, Busse RF, Majumdar S. In vivo T1ρ mapping in cartilage using 3D magnetization-prepared angle-modulated partitioned k-space spoiled gradient echo snapshots (3D MAPPS). Magn Reson Med. 2008;59(2):298–307.

50. Nieminen MT, Rieppo J, Toyras J, Hakumaki JM, Silvennoinen J, Hyttinen MM, Helminen HJ, Jurvelin JS. T_2 relaxation reveals spatial collagen architecture in articular cartilage: a comparative quantitative MRI and polarized light microscopy study. Magn Reson Med. 2001;46(3):487–93.

51. Mosher TJ, Dardzinski BJ. Cartilage MRI T_2 relaxation time mapping: overview and applications. Semin Musculoskelet Radiol. 2004;8(4):355–68.

52. Erickson SJ, Cox IH, Hyde JS, Carrera GF, Strandt JA, Estkowski LD. Effect of tendon orientation on MR imaging signal intensity: a manifestation of the "magic angle" phenomenon. Radiology. 1991;181(2):389–92.

53. Rubenstein JD, Kim JK, Morova-Prozner I, Stanchev PL, Henkelman RM. Effects of collagen orientation on MR imaging characteristics of bovine articular cartilage. Radiology. 1993;188(1):219–26.

54. Henkelman RM, Staniz GJ, Kim JK, Bronskill MJ. Anisotropy of NMR properties of tissues. Magn Reson Med. 1994;32(5):592–601.

55. Xia Y, Farquhar T, Burton-Wurster N, Lust G. Origin of cartilage laminae in MRI. J Magn Reson Imaging. 1997;7(5):887–94.

56. Mosher TJ, Smith H, Dardzinski BJ, Schmithorst VJ, Smith MB. MR imaging and T_2 mapping of femoral cartilage: in vivo determination of the magic angle effect. AJR Am J Roentgenol. 2001;177(3):665–9.

57. Mlynárik V, Szomolányi P, Toffanin R, Vittur F, Trattnig S. Transverse relaxation mechanisms in articular cartilage. J Magn Reson. 2004;169(2):300–7.

58. Shao H, Pauli C, Li S, Ma Y, Tadros AS, Kavanaugh A, Chang EY, Tang G, Du J. Magic angle effect plays a major role in both T_1rho and T_2 relaxation in articular cartilage. Osteoarthr Cartil. 2017;25(12):2022–30.

59. Mosher TJ, Zhang Z, Reddy R, Boudhar S, Milestone BN, Morrison WB, Kwoh CK, Eckstein F, Witschey WR, Borthakur A. Knee articular cartilage damage in osteoarthritis: analysis of MR image biomarker reproducibility in ACRIN-PA 4001 multicenter trial. Radiology. 2011;258(3):832–42.

60. Gold GE, Thedens DR, Pauly JM, Fechner KP, Bergman G, Beaulieu CF, Macovski A. MR imaging of articular cartilage of the knee: new methods using ultrashort TEs. AJR Am J Roentgenol. 1998;170(5):1223–6.

61. Robson MD, Gatehouse PD, Bydder M, Bydder GM. Magnetic resonance: an introduction to ultrashort TE (UTE) imaging. J Comput Assist Tomogr. 2003;27(6):825–46.

62. Pettersson H, Ahlberg A, Nilsson IM. A radiologic classification of hemophilic arthropathy. Clin Orthop Relat Res. 1980;149:153–9.

63. Burr DB, Schaffler MB. The involvement of subchondral mineralized tissues in osteoarthrosis: quantitative microscopic evidence. Microsc Res Tech. 1997;37(4):343–57.

64. Burr DB. Anatomy and physiology of the mineralized tissues: role in the pathogenesis of osteoarthrosis. Osteoarthr Cartil. 2004;12(Suppl A):S20–30.

65. Anderson DD, Brown TD, Radin EL. The influence of basal cartilage calcification on dynamic juxtaarticular stress transmission. Clin Orthop Relat Res. 1993;286:298–307.

66. Lane LB, Villacin A, Bullough PG. The vascularity and remodeling of subchondral bone and calcified cartilage in adult human femoral and humeral heads. J Bone Joint Surg. 1997;59(3):272–8.

67. Howell DS. Osteoarthritis: speculations on some biochemical factors of possible aetiological nature including cartilage mineralization. In: Nuki K, editor. The aetiopathogenesis of osteoarthrosis. Kent, Pitman Medical; 1979. p. 93–104.

68. Brown TD, Radin EL, Martin RB, Burr DB. Finite element studies of some juxtarticular stress changes due to localized subchondral stiffening. J Biomech. 1984;17(1):11–24.

69. Revell PA, Pirie C, Amir G, Rashad S, Walker F. Metabolic activity in the calcified zone of cartilage: observations on tetracycline labeled articular cartilage in human osteoarthritic hips. Rheumatol Int. 1990;10(4):143–7.

70. Oegema TR, Johnson SL, Meglitsch T, Carpenter RJ. Prostaglandins and the zone of calcified cartilage in osteoarthritis. Am J Ther. 1996;3(2):139–49.

71. Miller LM, Novatt JT, Hamerman D, Carlson CS. Alternations in mineral composition observed in osteoarthritic joints of cynomolgus monkeys. Bone. 2004;35(2):498–506.

72. Li B, Marshall D, Roe M, Aspden R. The electron microscope appearance of the subchondral bone plate in the human femoral head in osteoarthritis and osteoporosis. J Anat. 1999;195:101–10.

73. Frisbie DD, Oxford JT, Southwood L, Trotter GW, Rodkey WG, Steadman JR, Goodnight JL, McIlwraith CW. Early events in cartilage repair after subchondral bone microfracture. Clin Orthop Relat Res. 2003;407:215–27.

74. Mente PL, Lewis JL. Elastic modulus of calcified cartilage is an order of magnitude less than that of subchondral bone. J Orthop Res. 1994;12(5):637–47.

75. Thambyah A, Broom N. On how degeneration influences load-bearing in the cartilage—bone system: a microstructural and micromechanical study. Osteoarthr Cartil. 2007;15(12):1410–23.

76. Ferguson VL, Bushby AJ, Boyde A. Nanomechanical properties and mineral concentration in articular calcified cartilage and subchondral bone. J Anat. 2003;203(2):191–9.

77. Arkill KP, Winlove CP. Solute transport in the deep and calcified zones of articular cartilage. Osteoarthr Cartil. 2008;16(6):708–14.

78. Lyons TJ, McClure SF, Stoddart RW, McClure J. The normal human chondro-osseous junctional region: evidence for contact of uncalcified cartilage with subchondral bone and marrow spaces. BMC Musculoskelet Disord. 2006;7(1):52.

79. Frisbie DD, Morisset S, Ho CP, Rodkey WG, Steadman JR, McIlwraith CW. Effects of calcified cartilage on healing of chondral defects treated with microfracture in horses. Am J Sports Med. 2006;34(11):1824–31.

80. Ma Y, Jerban S, Carl M, Wan L, Guo T, Jang H, Bydder GM, Chang EY, Du J. Imaging of the region of the osteochondral junction (OCJ) using a 3D adiabatic inversion recovery prepared ultrashort echo time cones (3D IR-UTE cones) sequence at 3T. NMR Biomed. 2019;32(5):e4080.

81. Liu T, Khalidov I, de Rochefort L, Spincemaille P, Liu J, Tsiouris AJ, Wang Y. A novel background field removal method for MRI using projection onto dipole fields (PDF). NMR Biomed. 2011;24(9):1129–36.

82. Li W, Wu B, Liu C. Quantitative susceptibility mapping of human brain reflects spatial variation in tissue composition. NeuroImage. 2011;55:1645–56.

83. Liu J, Liu T, De Rochefort L, Ledoux J, Khalidov I, Chen W, Tsiouris AJ, Wisnieff C, Spincemaille P, Prince MR, Wang Y. Morphology enabled dipole inversion for quantitative susceptibility mapping using structural consistency between the magnitude image and the susceptibility map. NeuroImage. 2012;59(3):2560–8.

84. Li W, Wang N, Yu F, Han H, Cao W, Romero R, Tantiwongkosi B, Duong TQ, Liu C. A method for estimating and removing streaking artifacts in quantitative susceptibility mapping. NeuroImage. 2015;108:111–22.

85. Jang H, Drygalski A, Wong J, et al. Ultrashort echo time quantitative susceptibility mapping (UTE-QSM) for detection of hemosiderin deposition in hemophilic arthropathy: a feasibility study. Magn Reson Med. 2020;84(6):3246–55.

86. Jang H, Lu X, Searleman A, Jerban S, Ma Y, von Drygalski A, Chang EY, Du J. True phase quantitative susceptibility mapping using continuous single point imaging: a feasibility study. Magn Reson Med. 2019;81(3):1907–14.

87. Lu X, Ma Y, Chang EY, He Q, Searleman A, von Drygalski A, Du J. Simultaneous quantitative susceptibility mapping (QSM) and R_2^* for high iron concentration quantification with 3D ultrashort echo time sequences: an echo dependence study. Magn Reson Med. 2018;79(4):2315–22.

88. Lu X, Jang H, Ma Y, Jerban S, Chang EY, Du J. Ultrashort echo time quantitative susceptibility mapping (UTE-QSM) of highly concentrated magnetic nanoparticles: a comparison study about different sampling strategies. Molecules. 2019;24(6):1143.

89. Liu J, Liu T, De Rochefort L, et al. Morphology enabled dipole inversion for quantitative susceptibility mapping using structural consistency between the magnitude image and the susceptibility map. NeuroImage. 2012;59(3):2560–8.

90. Reeder SB, Pineda AR, Wen Z, Shimakawa A, Yu H, Brittain JH, Gold GE, Beaulieu CH, Pelc NJ. Iterative decomposition of water and fat with echo asymmetry and least-squares estimation (IDEAL): application with fast spin-echo imaging. Magn Reson Med. 2005;54(3):636–44.

Rotator Cuff Injury

Aria Ashir and Eric Y. Chang

Introduction

Shoulder pain is an exceedingly common musculoskeletal problem with reported annual incidences as high as 14.7 per 1000 patients and a lifetime prevalence of 70% [1, 2]. Rotator cuff pathology is the most common cause of shoulder pain, with studies finding that rotator cuff tendon disease is the cause of 70% of primary care shoulder pain visits [3, 4]. This chapter focuses on rotator cuff anatomy, rotator cuff tendinopathy, imaging pitfalls in assessing rotator cuff tendinopathy, recent magnetic resonance imaging (MRI) advances for evaluating this disease entity, and potential future investigations of the role of quantitative MRI in assessing additional rotator cuff disease.

Anatomy

The rotator cuff is composed of four muscles and their respective tendons. These muscles include supraspinatus, infraspinatus, teres minor, and subscapularis. The supraspinatus, infraspinatus, and teres minor muscles originate from the posterior surface of the scapula and insert on the greater tuberosity of the humerus with supraspinatus inserting most superiorly, followed by infraspinatus and then teres minor.

A. Ashir
Department of Radiology, University of California, San Diego, La Jolla, CA, USA

Research Service, VA San Diego Healthcare System, San Diego, CA, USA

Santa Barbara Cottage Hospital, Santa Barbara, USA

E. Y. Chang (✉)
Department of Radiology, University of California, San Diego, La Jolla, CA, USA

Research Service, VA San Diego Healthcare System, San Diego, CA, USA

The subscapularis muscle originates from the anterior surface of the scapula and inserts on the lesser tuberosity of the humerus. The subscapularis fibers continue and join the transverse ligament of the humerus, which passes from the lesser tuberosity to the greater tuberosity. This ligament houses the long head of the biceps tendon in the bicipital groove.

Rotator Cuff Tendinopathy

Rotator cuff disease may be due to various factors, including inflammation, degeneration, trauma, or impingement, and MRI is the gold standard for evaluating most rotator cuff diseases. This chapter will focus on rotator cuff tendinopathy, as this is an important condition that is difficult to evaluate. Ultrashort echo time (UTE) MRI techniques have been successfully applied in the study of this disease entity. Rotator cuff tendinopathy or tendinosis can be classified as tendon degeneration and inflammation believed to be due to factors including traumatic insult, overload, and impingement by the surrounding structures, the most common of which is subacromial impingement on the supraspinatus tendon. Rotator cuff tendinopathy is a significant source of pain and has an incidence of 0.3–0.5% and an annual prevalence of 0.5–7.4% [5]. Many patients with rotator cuff tendinopathy state that their symptoms cause less restful sleep, difficulty with work and life activities, and loss of baseline abilities [6].

MRI Challenges

MRI is the gold standard for imaging many shoulder derangements, including rotator cuff tendinopathy [7, 8]. The appearance of rotator cuff tendinosis on MRI is a typically increased signal within the tendon on fluid-sensitive sequences (e.g.,

T_2-weighted fat-suppressed sequences), which is not as intense as fluid, and a diffuse increased signal on low-to-intermediate echo time (TE) sequences. Additional findings include tendon thickening, or fraying, where the tendon margins are indistinct, but there is no gap within the tendon fibers as is seen in tears. In contrast, healthy rotator cuff tendons should appear dark on all conventional sequences.

The clinical appearance of rotator cuff tendinopathy has been shown to be somewhat unreliable, as studies have found increased T_2 signal or increased diffuse signal on intermediate TE sequences in up to 89% of supraspinatus tendons in young, asymptomatic volunteers. This may represent a normal tendon with signal increase due to artifacts or a pathological tendon such as degeneration [9].

The challenges in evaluating rotator cuff tendinopathy are due to multiple factors. Tendons have many organized collagen fibrils, which, in turn, result in short T_2s. The best studied tendon is the Achilles tendon, whose T_2 values are as short as 1–2 ms [10]. The resultant low signal on conventional MRI sequences, which typically use TEs of several milliseconds or longer, may pose challenges in the evaluation of rotator cuff tendinopathy. Conventional MRI demonstrates a low sensitivity of 13–50% for rotator cuff tendinopathy compared with surgical findings with exceedingly poor interobserver reliability [11]. A low signal also creates challenges when making quantitative MRI measurements. One solution to this problem is to shorten the pulse sequence TE so that more signal is detected [10]. Another challenge is that the anisotropic nature of tendons causes remarkably large changes in MRI signal intensity, or T_2 values, with differences in orientation (Fig. 38.1). This is known as the "magic angle effect" and is due to unaveraged dipolar interactions of proton nuclear spins [12]. As tissue fiber orientation approaches approximately 54.78° relative to the main magnetic field, signal intensity is at its greatest, and this may be falsely interpreted as rotator cuff tendinopathy. Unlike the Achilles tendon, which has a more constant orientation in clinical imaging, the rotator cuff tendon orientation is varied and always passes through the magic angle. In histologically normal rotator cuff tendons, up to a sixfold change in signal intensity has been reported at 3 T purely due to different orientations of the shoulder [13]. In the following section, we will discuss MRI methods that help maximize signals while minimizing confounding magic angle effects when evaluating rotator cuff tendinopathy.

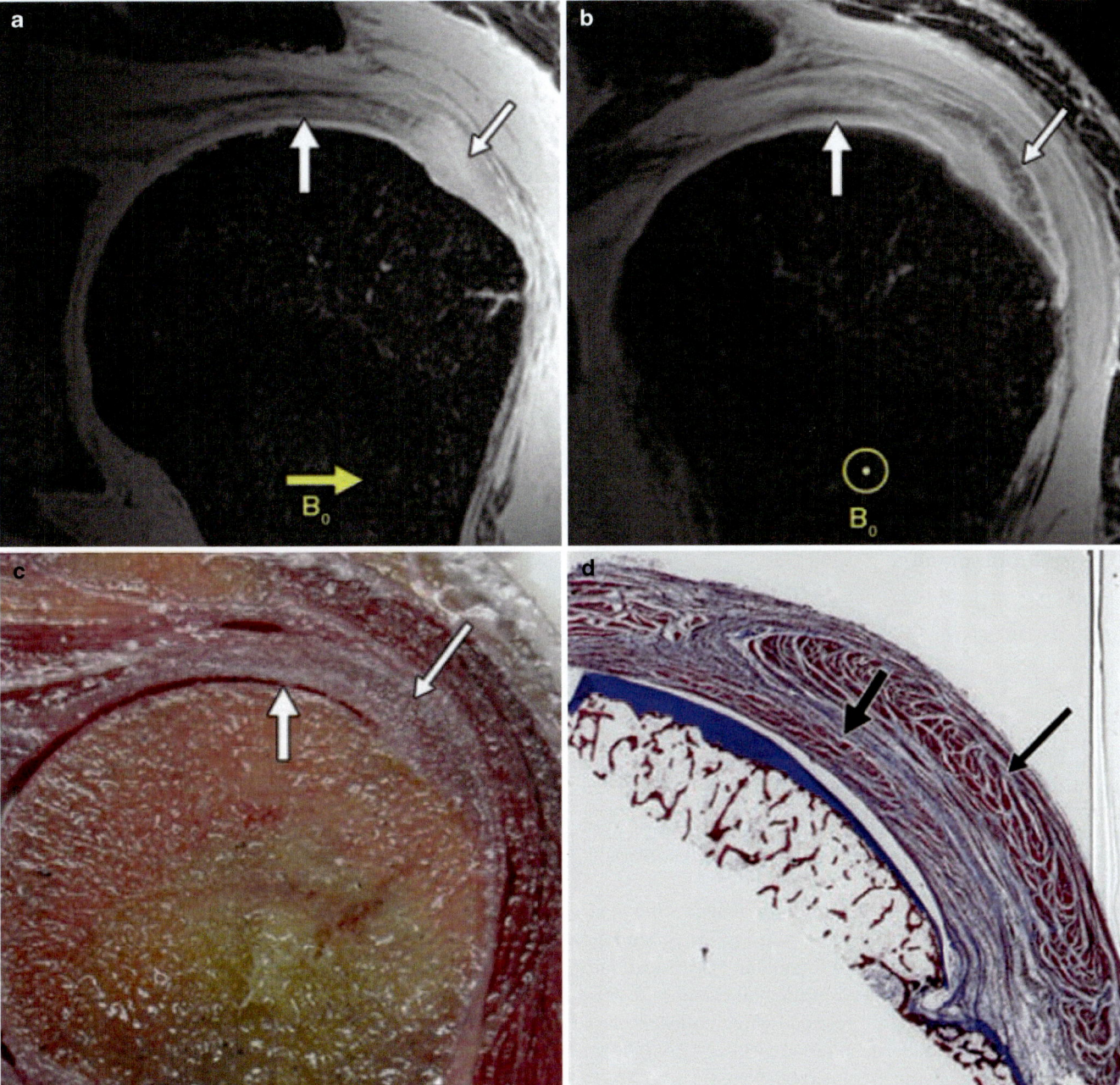

Fig. 38.1 MR images and anatomic section with Masson trichrome staining of the shoulder in a male 53-year-old cadaver. (**a** and **b**) Coronal 3D gradient echo images with the specimen oriented at 90° relative to the main magnetic field, corresponding to the placement of central tendon of supraspinatus parallel to the external magnetic field (B_0) (yellow arrow, **a**) and with a rotator cable oriented along the main magnetic field (B_0 courses in and out of the plane of the image) (yellow circle, **b**) show infraspinatus (thin arrows) and rotator cable (thick arrows) contributions to the rotator cuff, which are best shown in panel (**b**). (**c** and **d**) The infraspinatus (thin arrows) and rotator cable (thick arrows) are confirmed on anatomic section (**c**) and photomicrograph using Masson trichrome staining (**d**). (Adapted with permission from Chang et al. [13])

Recent MRI Advances

Ultrashort TE (UTE) MRI sequences have been used to better capture the signal from short-T_2 tissues like the rotator cuff tendons. Furthermore, UTE-magnetization transfer (UTE-MT) techniques have been shown to provide magic angle-independent biomarkers of tissue properties in cadaveric Achilles tendons with analysis including biomarkers such as the macromolecular fraction (MMF) [14, 15]. This Achilles tendon study paved the way for subsequent research focusing on the rotator cuff, with confirmation of the finding of magic angle-independent biomarkers of tissue properties (Fig. 38.2).

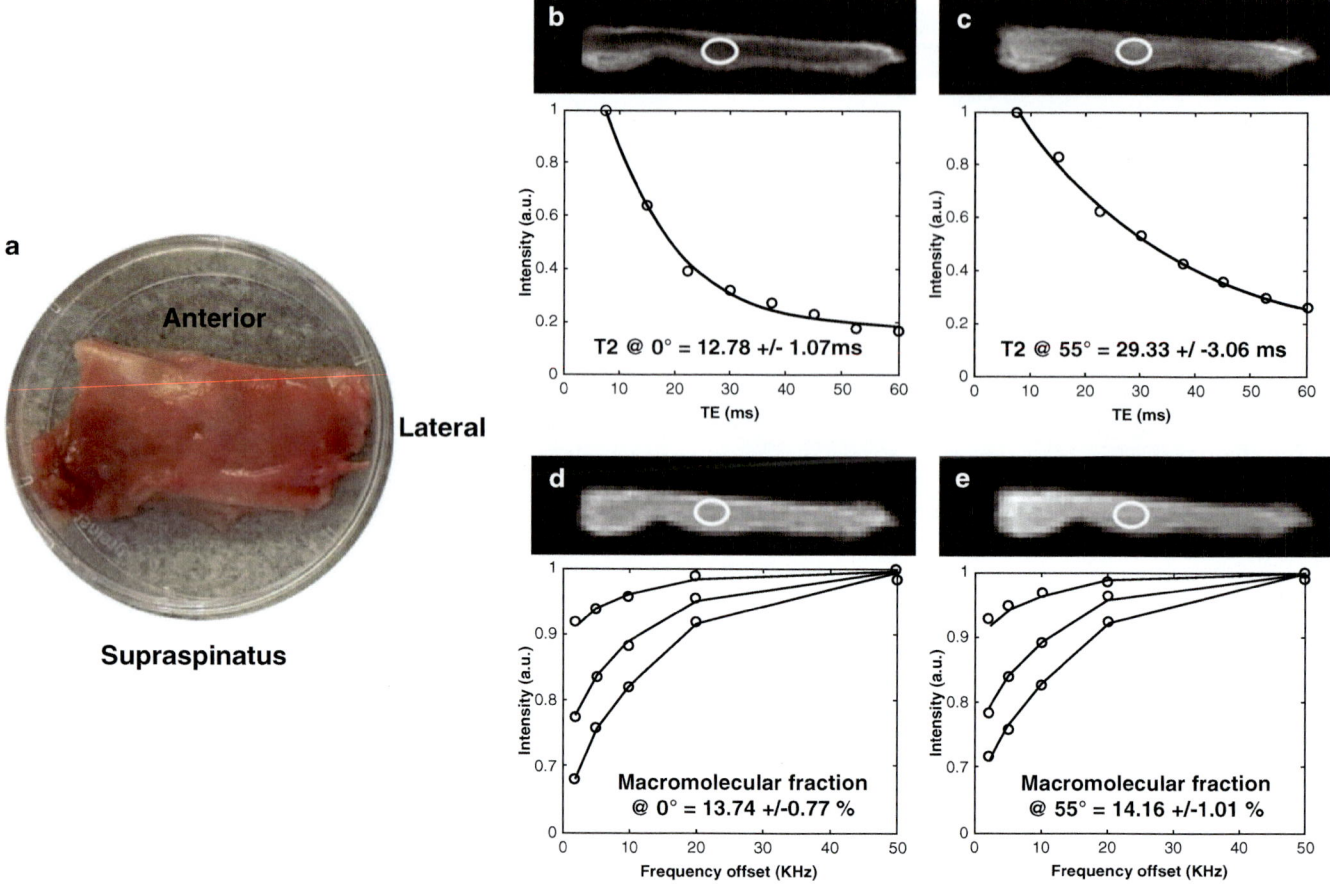

Fig. 38.2 A supraspinatus tendon from an 87-year-old. (**a**) The tendon as viewed from the bursal side, cut from the myotendinous junction to the footprint. Spin echo images with T_2 curves at (**b**) $0°$ and (**c**) $55°$ demonstrate marked signal intensity change and a 129% increase in T_2 between the two orientations. UTE-Cones-MT images with two-pool modeling curves in (**d**) $0°$ and (**e**) $55°$ demonstrate a stable high signal and a 3% difference in the macromolecular fraction between the two orientations. (Adapted with permission from Zhu et al. [17])

MMF can be a surrogate measure for collagen. Guo et al. removed collagen from cadaveric supraspinatus tendons using enzymes (collagenase) and found that MMF, adiabatic $T_{2\rho}$, and T_2* were useful in determining the extent of degeneration. MMF strongly correlated with collagen loss ($r = -0.81$; 95% confidence interval (95% CI): -0.90 to -0.66), whereas adiabatic $T_{2\rho}$ ($r = 0.66$; 95% CI: 0.42–0.81) and T_2* ($r = 0.58$; 95% CI: 0.31–0.76) moderately correlated with collagen loss [16]. Studies have confirmed that MFF values obtained with the 3D-UTE-Cones-MT technique decreased, whereas T_2 values increased in histologically proven severe tendinopathic tendons when compared to mildly tendinopathic samples (Figs. 38.3 and 38.4). When these histological samples were analyzed in different orientations to the magnetic field, the results were statistically significant for differences in both T_2 values and MMF values when compared with the mild and severely diseased tendons. However, at $55°$ relative to the magnetic field, the T_2 values failed to show a difference between the groups, whereas the MFF values continued to be significantly different [17]. These findings further support the notion that MMF measurements obtained using UTE-MRI sequences are particularly useful for tendons due to their relative insensitivity to magic angle effects.

Additional investigation has been conducted in vivo. Ashir et al. utilized the UTE-MT technique on symptomatic rotator cuff tendinopathy patients and control groups [18]. Symptomatic rotator cuff tendons showed significantly lower MMF values and higher T_2 values when compared to control patients. This study found that MMF values were superior to T_2 values when specifically assessing the lateral portion of the rotator cuff tendon, which is the portion that courses

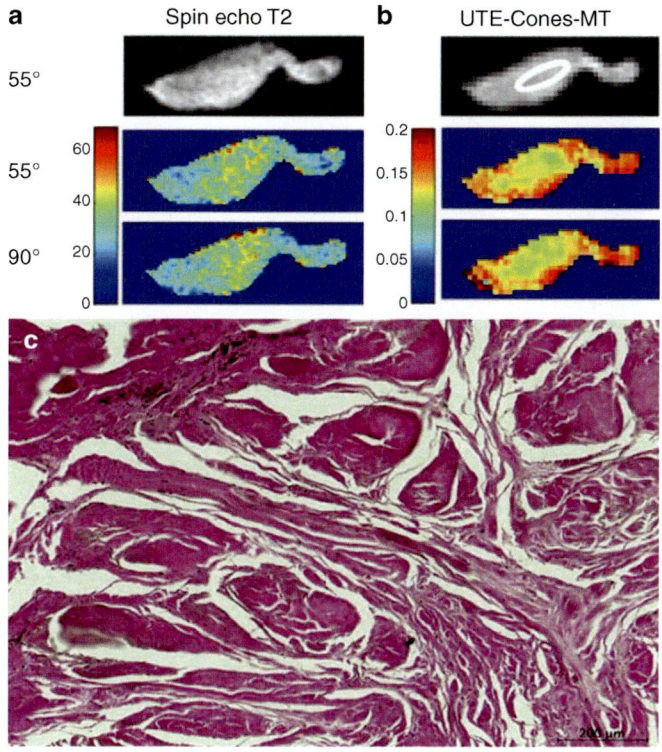

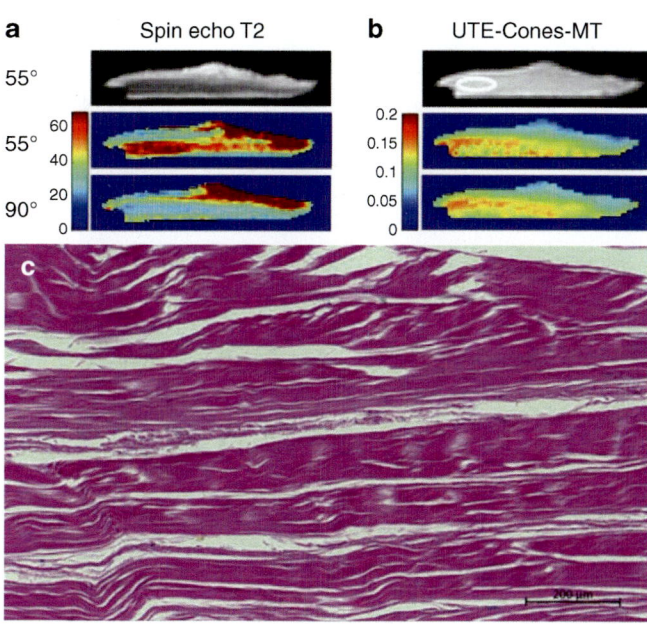

Bonar Score = 7
Mean Macromolecular Fraction = 10.88%

Fig. 38.3 Infraspinatus tendon region of interest (ROI) with severe tendinosis. (**a**) A sample spin echo image and T_2 pixel maps at 55° and 90° demonstrate little variability in signal and T_2 values between orientations, indicative of little anisotropy. For the ROI shown, the T_2 values ranged from 31.25 to 34.80 ms, with an 11% change between the two orientations. (**b**) A sample UTE-Cones-MT image with macromolecular fraction pixel maps at 55° and 90° shows stable values at the two orientations. For the ROI shown, the macromolecular fractions ranged from 10.08 to 11.74%, representing a 16% change between orientations. (**c**) A hematoxylin and eosin (H&E)-stained slide demonstrates a Bonar score of 7 (abnormal cells with a score of 2, disrupted collagen with a score of 2, and high vascularity with a score of 3). (Adapted with permission from Zhu et al. [17])

Bonar Score = 1
Mean Macromolecular Fraction = 14.76%

Fig. 38.4 Infraspinatus tendon ROI with mild tendinosis. (**a**) A sample spin echo image and T_2 pixel maps at 55° and 90° demonstrate tremendous variability in T_2 values between orientations. For the ROI shown, the T_2 values ranged from 17.09 to 68.19 ms, representing a 299% change between the two orientations. (**b**) A sample UTE-Cones-MT image with macromolecular fraction pixel maps at 55° and 90°, which show stable values between orientations. For the ROI shown, the macromolecular fractions ranged from 14.16 to 15.08%, representing a 6% change between orientations. (**c**) A H&E-stained slide demonstrates a total Bonar score of 1 (normal cells and collagen with scores of 0 and mildly abnormal vascularity with a score of 1). (Adapted with permission from Zhu et al. [17])

closest to the magic angle and is frequently involved in rotator cuff tendinosis (Fig. 38.5). In addition, this study found that in patients with unilateral shoulder pain, the symptomatic and asymptomatic shoulders showed decreased MMF and increased T_2 values when compared to control shoulders in asymptomatic individuals. Thus, the contralateral shoulder may show asymptomatic tendinopathy, and this can be assessed with quantitative UTE-MRI [18]. Involvement of the contralateral shoulder in tendinopathy may be expected as studies have shown that patients with rotator cuff tears have been found to have high rates of tears in the contralateral shoulder [19].

These studies demonstrate the potential use of quantitative UTE-MRI in analyzing rotator cuff tendinopathy in the clinical setting. With these techniques, there is no need for additional hardware for scanners. However, further investigation is required to validate biomarkers, evaluate larger sample sizes, and shorten the time required to run these sequences to facilitate throughput and decrease costs.

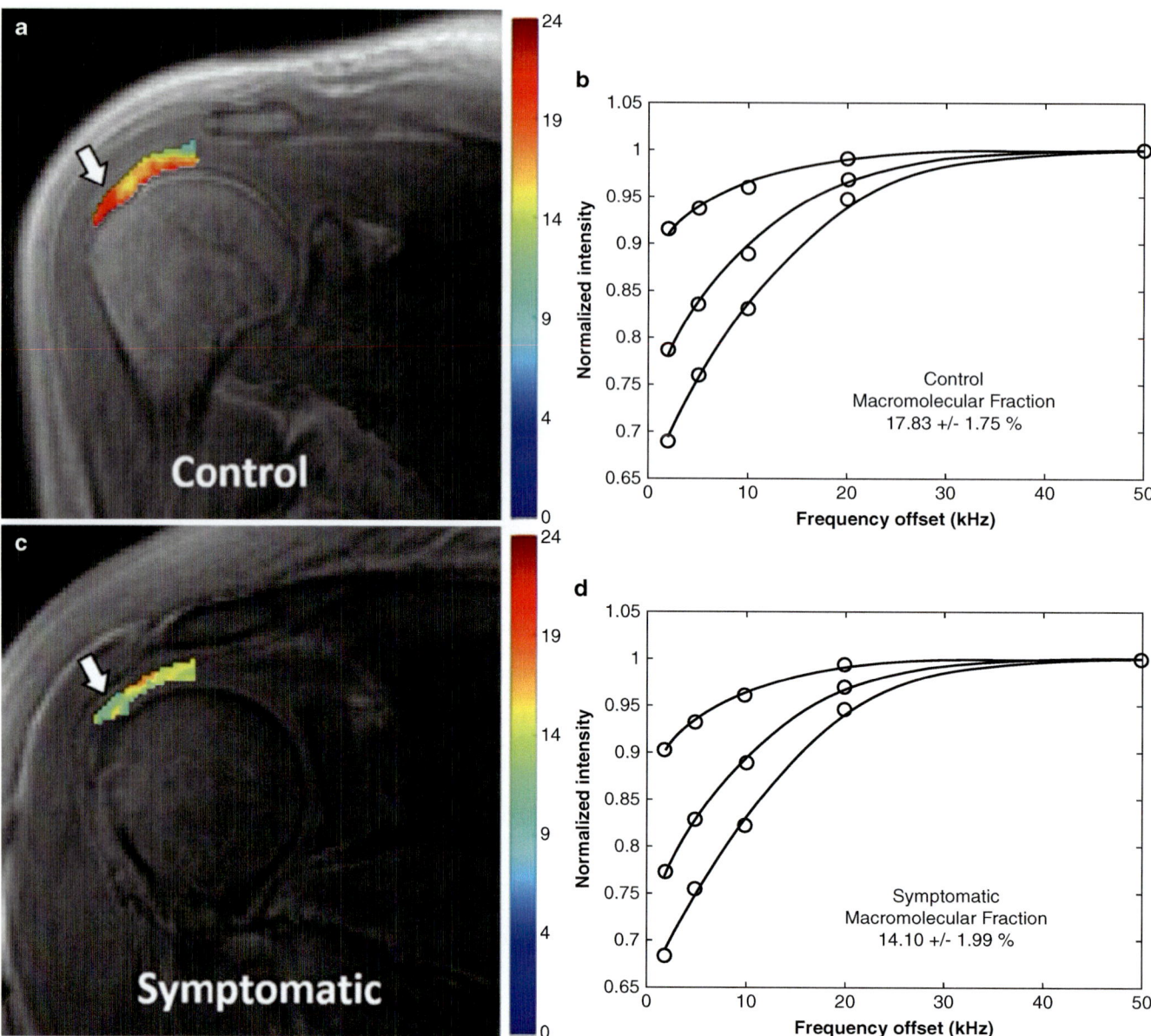

Fig. 38.5 Coronal oblique UTE-Cones-MT images with pixel maps from two-pool MT modeling for the superior rotator cuff tendon and fitting curves. (**a**) A pixel map overlay from a 31-year-old control subject demonstrates the ROI used for tendon analysis, from which six segments were delineated. (**b**) The fitting curve from the entire ROI, including all six segments in this slice, shows an excellent fit with a mean MMF of 17.83%. (**c**) A pixel map overlay from a 29-year-old symptomatic patient demonstrates areas of visibly lower MMF values compared with panel (**a**) (white arrows). (**d**) The fitting curve from the entire ROI, including all six segments on this slice, shows an excellent fit with a mean MMF of 14.10%. (Adapted with permission from Ashir et al. [18])

Future Studies

The utility of quantitative MRI and UTE techniques needs to be further investigated both in terms of evaluating rotator cuff tendinopathy and other rotator cuff diseases. One potential use for these techniques is the evaluation of the rotator cuff tendon status prior to, and following, surgical repair. For example, following a full-thickness rotator cuff tear, the preoperative status of the torn tendon stump is of particular interest. Quantitative MRI may be a noninvasive means of

evaluating the tendon stump and providing prognostic information to the clinician prior to surgery. In the case that there is significant fibrotic change in the stump, the surgical team may choose to carry out a resection of the tendon. To our knowledge, there is little work currently published investigating these techniques, although there have been some studies looking at UTE-T_2* values in patients following arthroscopic repair, in which decreased T_2 values seemed to correlate with healing, and 12 months after repair were shown to be comparable to T_2* values in controls [20]. A similar study looking at quantitative T_2 mapping of rotator cuff tendons following arthroscopic repair found decreased T_2 values with increased healing and improved clinical outcome over time during a 1-year follow-up period [21].

An additional area of interest where quantitative MRI may be useful is in the assessment of the rotator cuff muscles. In various disease processes, a muscle may atrophy and/or show compositional changes with increased fat and fibrosis. UTE-MRI may be particularly helpful in cases of pronounced fibrosis, where the tissue displays shortened T_2 characteristics and therefore may show an increased signal-to-noise ratio with shorter TE sequences. Although a few studies have quantified the fat content of the rotator cuff muscles using Dixon-based fat quantification or chemical shift-based fat quantification, to our knowledge, there are no studies looking at rotator cuff muscle fibrosis and degeneration using quantitative UTE-MRI [22, 23]. Evaluation of muscle fibrosis is an application where UTE-MRI may prove useful.

References

1. Luime JJ, Koes BW, Hendriksen IJ, Burdorf A, Verhagen AP, Miedema HS, et al. Prevalence and incidence of shoulder pain in the general population; a systematic review. Scand J Rheumatol. 2004;33(2):73–81.
2. van der Windt DA, Koes BW, de Jong BA, Bouter LM. Shoulder disorders in general practice: incidence, patient characteristics, and management. Ann Rheum Dis. 1995;54(12):959–64.
3. Cadogan A, Laslett M, Hing WA, McNair PJ, Coates MH. A prospective study of shoulder pain in primary care: prevalence of imaged pathology and response to guided diagnostic blocks. BMC Musculoskelet Disord. 2011;12:119.
4. Piper CC, Hughes AJ, Ma Y, Wang H, Neviaser AS. Operative versus nonoperative treatment for the management of full-thickness rotator cuff tears: a systematic review and meta-analysis. J Shoulder Elb Surg. 2018;27(3):572–6.
5. Littlewood C, May S, Walters S. Epidemiology of rotator cuff tendinopathy: a systematic review. Shoulder & Elbow. 2013;5(4):256–65.
6. Ulack C, Suarez J, Brown L, Ring D, Wallace S, Teisberg E. What are people that seek Care for Rotator Cuff Tendinopathy Experiencing in their daily life? J Patient Exp. 2022;9:23743735211069811.
7. Expert Panel on Musculoskeletal I, Amini B, Beckmann NM, Beaman FD, Wessell DE, Bernard SA, et al. ACR appropriateness criteria((R)) shoulder pain-traumatic. J Am Coll Radiol. 2018;15(5S):S171–S88.
8. Expert Panel on Musculoskeletal I, Small KM, Adler RS, Shah SH, Roberts CC, Bencardino JT, et al. ACR appropriateness criteria((R)) shoulder pain-atraumatic. J Am Coll Radiol. 2018;15(11S):S388–402.
9. Neumann CH, Holt RG, Steinbach LS, Jahnke AH Jr, Petersen SA. MR imaging of the shoulder: appearance of the supraspinatus tendon in asymptomatic volunteers. AJR Am J Roentgenol. 1992;158(6):1281–7.
10. Chang EY, Du J, Chung CB. UTE imaging in the musculoskeletal system. J Magn Reson Imaging. 2015;41(4):870–83.
11. Robertson PL, Schweitzer ME, Mitchell DG, Schlesinger F, Epstein RE, Frieman BG, et al. Rotator cuff disorders: interobserver and intraobserver variation in diagnosis with MR imaging. Radiology. 1995;194(3):831–5.
12. Berendsen HJC. Nuclear magnetic resonance study of collagen hydration. J Chem Phys. 1962;36(12):3297–305.
13. Chang EY, Szeverenyi NM, Statum S, Chung CB. Rotator cuff tendon ultrastructure assessment with reduced-orientation dipolar anisotropy fiber imaging. AJR Am J Roentgenol. 2014;202(4):W376–8.
14. Ma YJ, Shao H, Du J, Chang EY. Ultrashort echo time magnetization transfer (UTE-MT) imaging and modeling: magic angle independent biomarkers of tissue properties. NMR Biomed. 2016;29(11):1546–52.
15. Ma YJ, Chang EY, Carl M, Du J. Quantitative magnetization transfer ultrashort echo time imaging using a time-efficient 3D multi-spoke cones sequence. Magn Reson Med. 2018;79(2):692–700.
16. Guo T, Ma YJ, High RA, Tang Q, Wong JH, Byra M, et al. Assessment of an in vitro model of rotator cuff degeneration using quantitative magnetic resonance and ultrasound imaging with biochemical and histological correlation. Eur J Radiol. 2019;121:108706.
17. Zhu Y, Cheng X, Ma Y, Wong JH, Xie Y, Du J, et al. Rotator cuff tendon assessment using magic-angle insensitive 3D ultrashort echo time cones magnetization transfer (UTE-cones-MT) imaging and modeling with histological correlation. J Magn Reson Imaging. 2018;48(1):160–8.
18. Ashir A, Ma Y, Jerban S, Jang H, Wei Z, Le N, et al. Rotator cuff tendon assessment in symptomatic and control groups using quantitative MRI. J Magn Reson Imaging. 2020;52(3):864–72.
19. Ranebo MC, Bjornsson Hallgren HC, Adolfsson LE. Patients with a long-standing cuff tear in one shoulder have high rates of contralateral cuff tears: a study of patients with arthroscopically verified cuff tears 22 years ago. J Shoulder Elb Surg. 2018;27(3):e68–74.
20. Xie Y, Liu S, Qu J, Wu P, Tao H, Chen S. Quantitative magnetic resonance imaging UTE-T2* mapping of tendon healing after arthroscopic rotator cuff repair: a longitudinal study. Am J Sports Med. 2020;48(11):2677–85.
21. Xie Y, Liu S, Qiao Y, Hu Y, Zhang Y, Qu J, et al. Quantitative T2 mapping-based tendon healing is related to the clinical outcomes during the first year after arthroscopic rotator cuff repair. Knee Surg Sports Traumatol Arthrosc. 2021;29(1):127–35.
22. Nardo L, Karampinos DC, Lansdown DA, Carballido-Gamio J, Lee S, Maroldi R, et al. Quantitative assessment of fat infiltration in the rotator cuff muscles using water-fat MRI. J Magn Reson Imaging. 2014;39(5):1178–85.
23. Kalin PS, Huber FA, Hamie QM, Issler LS, Farshad-Amacker NA, Ulbrich EJ, et al. Quantitative MRI of visually intact rotator cuff muscles by multiecho Dixon-based fat quantification and diffusion tensor imaging. J Magn Reson Imaging. 2019;49(1):109–17.

Aurea Mohana-Borges, Jiyo Athertya, Hyungseok Jang,
Yajun Ma, Eric Y. Chang, Jiang Du, and Christine B. Chung

Introduction

The temporomandibular joint (TMJ) is an anatomically and biomechanically complex structure that plays a crucial role in jaw movements related to mastication and speech [1]. Temporomandibular disorders (TMDs) are common and affect up to one-third of all adults at some stage in their life [2]. The symptoms include clickings, limitation of oral aperture, and pain, which increase at more advanced ages [3]. TMD symptoms have a higher incidence in females, with female-to-male ratios ranging between 2:1 to 8:1 [4–6]. TMDs are generally categorized into those of muscular origin (myogenic) and those that primarily involve the joint (arthrogenous) (Fig. 39.1). In the latter, intra-articular components can undergo structural and functional failure, leading to internal derangement. Internal derangement denotes a mechanical fault in the joint with damage to articular tissues and biomechanical failure [7].

Disc displacement has been established as the most common cause of internal derangement [8]. The natural progression of TMJ internal derangement is believed to involve deformity and degeneration of the disc that may be followed by perforation [9]. The structural breakdown of the intra-articular tissues, such as disc and articular cartilage, induces a low-grade joint inflammation, which can ultimately lead to the development of osseous changes [3]. These have been reported to be significantly more common in the condyle than in the temporal bone [10]. The classic findings of articular surface remodeling, subchondral sclerosis, and osteophytosis are the harbingers of osteoarthritis (OA).

TMJ disorders are quite challenging from a clinical perspective, with various abnormalities presenting similar signs and symptoms. In 1992, a panel of TMD experts published the "Research Diagnostic Criteria for Temporomandibular Disorders" (RDC/TMD), which was validated and updated in 2014 and renamed the "Diagnostic Criteria for TMD" (DC/TMD). The DC/TMD included magnetic resonance imaging (MRI) as the gold standard for the definitive diagnosis of the displaced TMJ disc [11, 12]. Studies have shown that physical examination alone can be inaccurate in determining the status of the joint and that the accuracy of the clinical diagnosis varies between 43% and 83% using MRI as the gold standard [13].

A. Mohana-Borges · J. Athertya · H. Jang · Y. Ma
Department of Radiology, University of California, San Diego,
La Jolla, CA, USA
e-mail: amohanaborges@health.ucsd.edu; jathertya@health.ucsd.edu; h4jang@health.ucsd.edu; yam013@health.ucsd.edu

E. Y. Chang · C. B. Chung (✉)
Department of Radiology, University of California, San Diego,
La Jolla, CA, USA

VA San Diego Healthcare System, San Diego, CA, USA
e-mail: e8chang@health.ucsd.edu; cbchung@health.ucsd.edu

J. Du
Department of Radiology, University of California, San Diego,
La Jolla, CA, USA

VA San Diego Healthcare System, San Diego, CA, USA

Department of Bioengineering, University of California, San
Diego, La Jolla, CA, USA
e-mail: jiangdu@health.ucsd.edu

TMJ Anatomy

The TMJ is a unique articulation in several aspects. Its condylar and temporal bone components are maintained in apposition by muscles, ligaments, and the joint capsule. The osseous articulating surfaces of the joint are covered by fibrocartilage rather than hyaline cartilage, presumably related to the forces to which they are subjected [14, 15]. The fibrocartilaginous disc of the TMJ is considered the most critical anatomic structure of the joint and is situated between the mandibular condyle and the temporal bone. Figure 39.2 demonstrates a normal articular disc viewed from above, with its capsular attachment seen posteriorly and the intimate relationship with the lateral pterygoid muscle shown anteriorly. Figure 39.3 shows the TMJ's

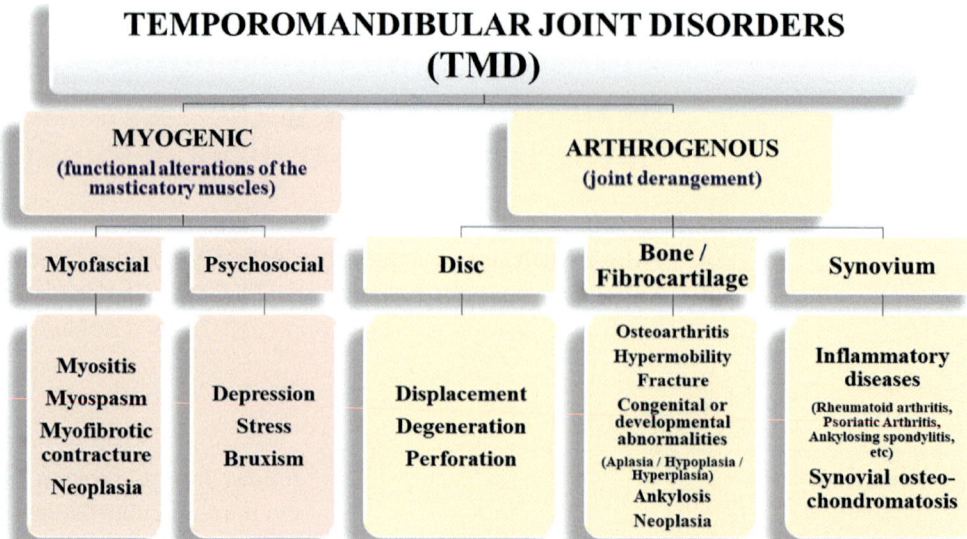

main components in a lateral view diagram with a companion magnetic resonance (MR) image, both in the sagittal plane.

The articular disc has a biconcave appearance in the sagittal plane with a thin intermediate zone and thick anterior and posterior bands [6]. It is firmly attached to the head of the condyle medially and laterally where it blends with the capsule [16]. As a result, the disc divides the joint into large superior and small inferior compartments [14]. Rotational movements of the condyle occur in the lower joint compartment in the first few millimeters of jaw opening, whereas condylar gliding with translation occurs in the upper joint compartment as jaw opening continues [16]. A synovial membrane lines each of the two joint spaces, except along the articulating surfaces [6].

The prominent posterior fibrous attachments (bilaminar retrodiscal zone) consist of two distinct laminae. The superior lamina is composed of a loose fibroelastic tissue, whereas the inferior lamina consists of a more taut fibrous connective tissue [17]. The superior lamina attaches to the postglenoid process and prevents disc slippage during wide opening of the mouth. The inferior lamina curves downward onto the posterior surface of the mandibular neck, where it fuses with the posterior capsule to prevent excessive rotation of the disc over the condyle [17]. There are small neurovascular structures between both laminae, and these are wrapped in loose elastic fibers. The anterior fibrous attachment of the disc attaches to the temporal bone and anterior surface of the condyle (Figs. 39.2 and 39.3).

The TMJ disc has structural characteristics in common with the meniscus of the knee, including its overall composition as well as its distribution of collagen I and II, glycosami-

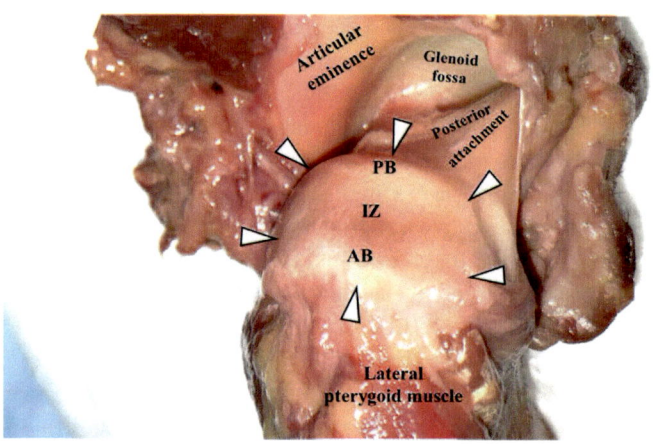

Fig. 39.2 TMJ dissection with a wide joint opening. It should be noted that the articular disc can be viewed from above (arrowheads), which has a slightly oblique anteroposterior orientation. The disc has a thin intermediate zone (IZ) and thick anterior and posterior bands (AB and PB, respectively). The disc capsular attachment is seen posteriorly, and the intimate relationship with the lateral pterygoid muscle is seen anteriorly

noglycans, and water [18]. Unlike the knee meniscus, however, the TMJ disc has a significant proportion of elastic fibers that varies with age and structural alteration within the disc [19, 20]. This distinct structural composition is relevant to understanding the TMJ disc imaging features assessed with ultrashort echo time (UTE) techniques as demonstrated later in this chapter.

The muscles of mastication are an extremely common source of TMD pain. They mainly consist of the masseter, medial and lateral pterygoid, and temporalis muscles [21]. These muscles are innervated by the mandibular division of the trigeminal nerve.

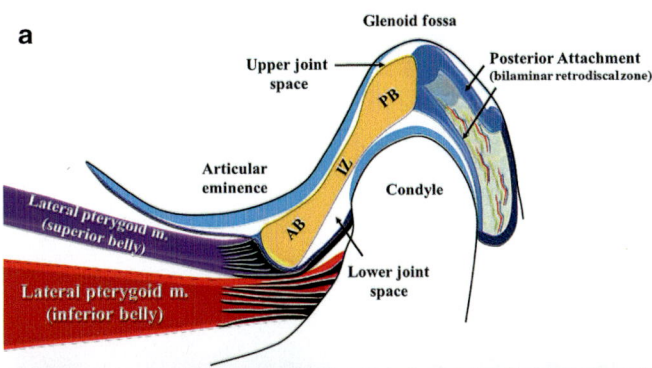

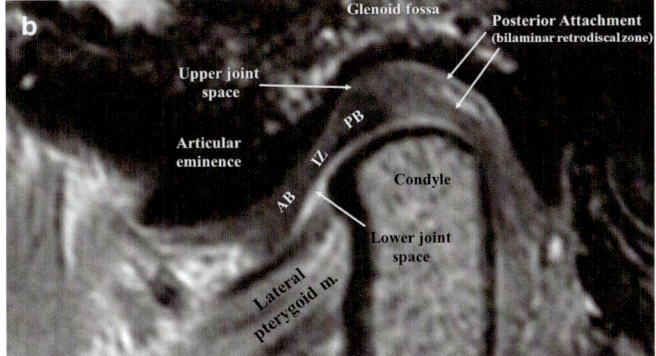

Fig. 39.3 (**a**) A diagram of a lateral view of the sagittal plane demonstrating the main components of the TMJ. (**b**) Companion MR image in a cadaveric specimen obtained with a proton density (PD)-weighted sequence (echo time (TE) = 29 ms, repetition time (TR) = 3353 ms, and acquisition matrix = 320 × 256). AB anterior band; IZ intermediate zone; PB posterior band

TMJ MRI

Due to its excellent soft tissue contrast and multiplanar imaging capabilities, MRI has revolutionized the understanding of TMJ pain and dysfunction. Before the advent of MRI, TMJ diagnosis was largely a syndromic exercise. With MRI, the radiologist has a window to assess the structures of the TMJ and provide specific anatomic diagnoses.

The basic MR evaluation of the TMJ is primarily focused on the disc, including characterizing its morphology, position with an open and a closed mouth, and, to a lesser degree, its intrinsic signal intensity (Figs. 39.4 and 39.5). With regard to disc morphology and position, standard clinical MR sequences at 1.5 T appear to be effective in accurate characterization [22–24]. This has been debated in a study questioning the level of evidence in the past literature (from 1988 to 2005) on the efficacy of MRI in the diagnosis of disc position and configuration, among other things [25]. The authors emphasized the need for high-quality studies of the diagnostic efficacy of MR in TMD evaluation. Similarly, debate exists about the significance of the signal intensity of the TMJ disc. Some authors consider variation in signal intensity of the TMJ disc similar to

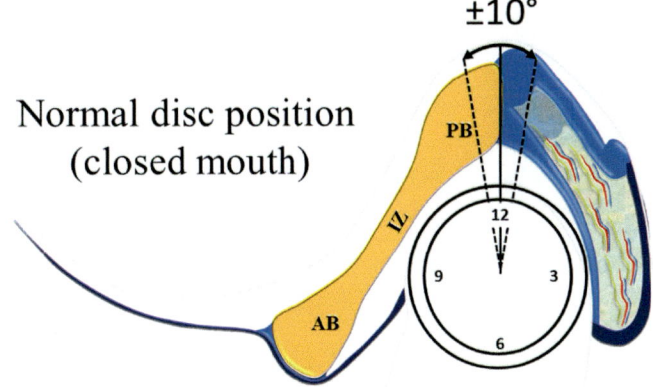

Fig. 39.4 A diagram of normal disc position with the mouth closed. The posterior band normally lies immediately above the condyle near the 12 o'clock position, with a variation of ±10°. Some authors consider anterior disc displacement of up to 30° normal as this provides better correlation of disc displacement with clinical symptoms in TMD

that of the knee meniscus and others to that of the intervertebral disc. For instance, it has been reported that the normal TMJ disc has low signal intensity throughout and that as the TMJ disc degenerates it becomes high signal intensity in the same way as the knee meniscus does [26, 27]. Other reports describe the normal TMJ disc as intermediate-to-high signal intensity on T_1-weighted MR images with a decreased signal as it degenerates, similar to the intervertebral disc [28]. Most recently, the posterior band of the TMJ disc has been addressed [29]. In the setting of tissue degeneration, an increase in signal intensity within the posterior band was demonstrated on proton density (PD)-weighted fat-suppressed and T_1-weighted sequences [29].

For some time, little novel MRI has been reported for TMJ evaluation on the technical side. Exploration of diffusion-weighted MRI parameters has been proposed in the literature for the characterization of the stages of inflammation [31]. Although MRI provided the initial steps toward noninvasive evaluation of the structural components of the TMJ, its tissue characterization has not been specific. The fibrocartilaginous nature of the articular surfaces and disc suggests that these tissues have a relatively short T_2, making them incompletely detectable with standard clinical sequences, and their T_2s unable to be accurately quantified with standard T_2 measurement techniques.

UTE pulse sequences with nominal TEs less than 0.1 ms allow signals from short- and ultrashort-T_2 tissues to be detected and allow quantitative assessment of tissues with predominantly short-T_2 tissue components in the clinical setting. UTE sequences provide high-resolution morphological imaging of the TMJ condylar articular surface and disc, which typically appear as a low signal with conventional gra-

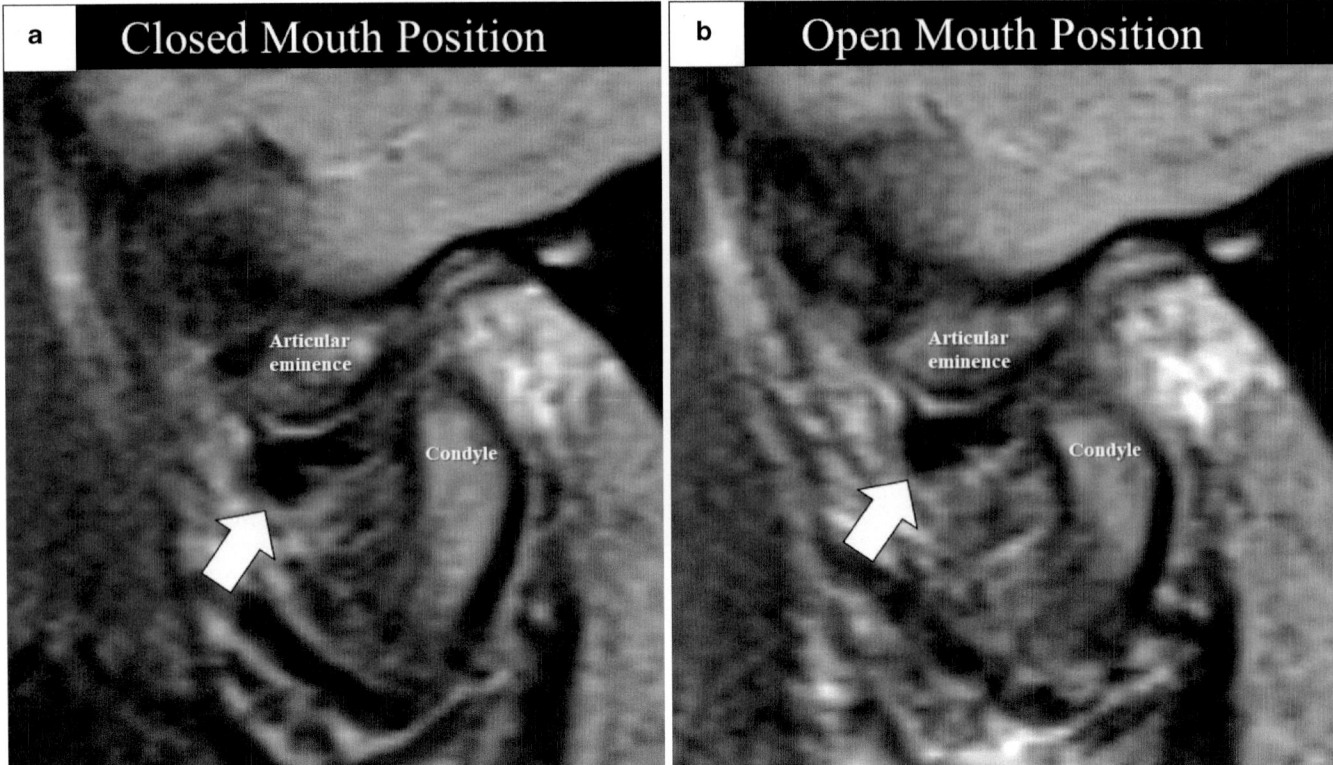

Fig. 39.5 Conventional MRI with (**a**) closed and (**b**) open mouth positions with a PD-weighted sequence (TR = 2500 ms, TE = 41 ms) in the sagittal plane. This case illustrates (**a**) anterior disc displacement (**b**) without reduction with the opening of the mouth (white arrows). The abnormal disc morphology in both positions should be noted. The dislocated disc interferes with smooth joint movement and causes biomechanical failure

dient echo and spin echo sequences. UTE sequences also allow quantification of T_1, T_2, T_2^*, $T_{1\rho}$, magnetization transfer, and diffusion in the TMJ disc and other joint tissues. These biomarkers can potentially be used for systematic structural and functional assessment of TMDs. A summary of UTE strategies for TMJ imaging to be described in this chapter is shown as a flowchart in Fig. 39.6.

Morphological UTE Imaging

Both two-dimensional (2D) and three-dimensional (3D) UTE sequences have been developed for high-resolution imaging of the TMJ [32–35]. The 2D UTE sequence employs an initial slice-selective radiofrequency (RF) half excitation, which is followed by radial imaging of the *k*-space from the center out [36, 37]. This is followed by a second half excitation with the slice-selective gradient polarity reversed and repeated radial mapping. The two sets of data are added to give a single line of *k*-space, and the process is repeated through 360° in 256 or 512 steps. The data are mapped onto a Cartesian grid (e.g., 512 x 512) and reconstructed by inverse 2D Fourier transformation (FT) to produce a gradient

echo-like image. Alternatively, 3D imaging can be performed with a nonselective (hard) excitation pulse followed by a 3D radial acquisition [38].

Figure 39.7 shows a representative 2D UTE imaging of a cadaveric TMJ joint with a nominal TE of 8 μs. A chemical shift-based saturation pulse was used to reduce the signal from bone marrow fat. Conventional clinical T_1- and PD-weighted fast spin echo (FSE) sequences were also applied to this sample. On visual inspection, the disc tissue appeared predominantly low in signal intensity on the T_1- and PD-weighted sequences (Fig. 39.7b, c). On the UTE-MR image (Fig. 39.7a), the tissue had a high signal (bright appearance), allowing it to be distinguished from the surrounding tissues and providing morphological characterization.

Higher contrast can be achieved for the TMJ disc using dual-echo UTE spin echo (UTE-SE) sequences, where the first UTE free induction decay (FID) data acquisition detects signals from both short- and long-T_2 tissues, whereas the second SE data acquisition only detects signals from long-T_2 tissues. TMJ imaging is subjected to strong susceptibility artifacts from the adjacent mastoids and air–tissue interface, leading to much reduced T_2^*'s for the condylar fibrocartilage

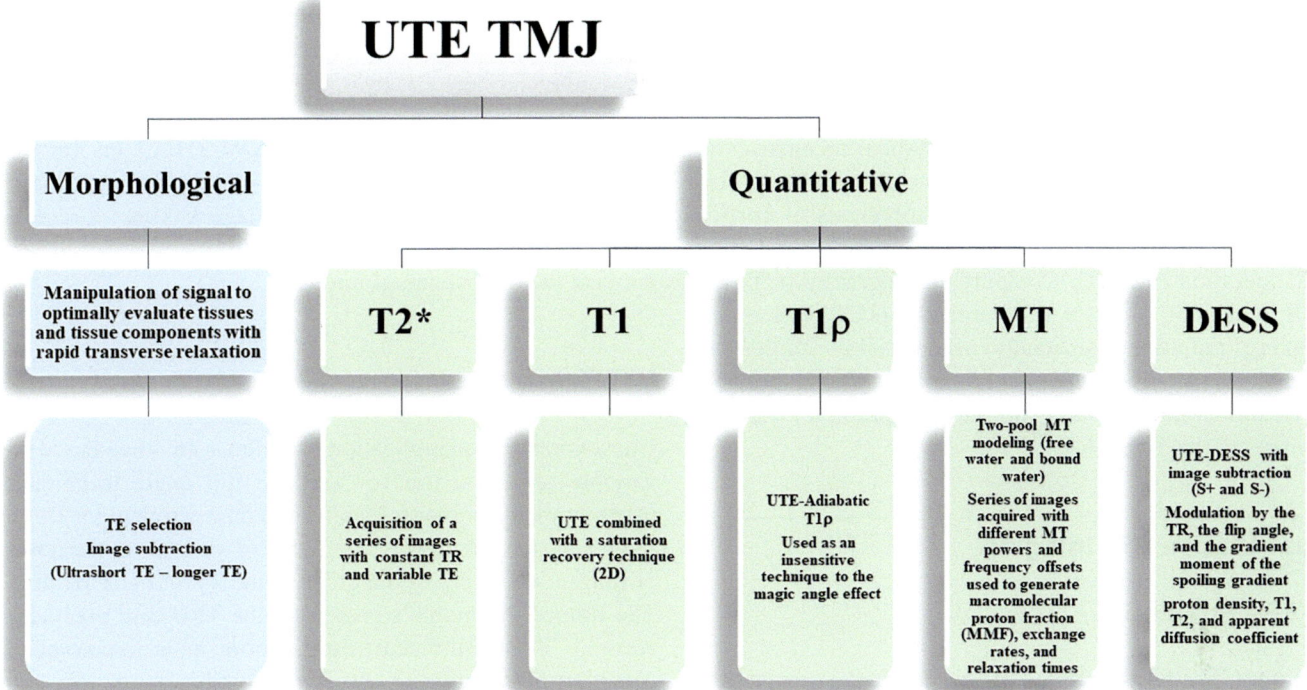

Fig. 39.6 A flowchart of UTE strategies for TMJ imaging. DESS double echo steady state; MT magnetization transfer; S⁺ free induction decay-like signal; S⁻ echo-like signal; TE echo time; TR repetition time

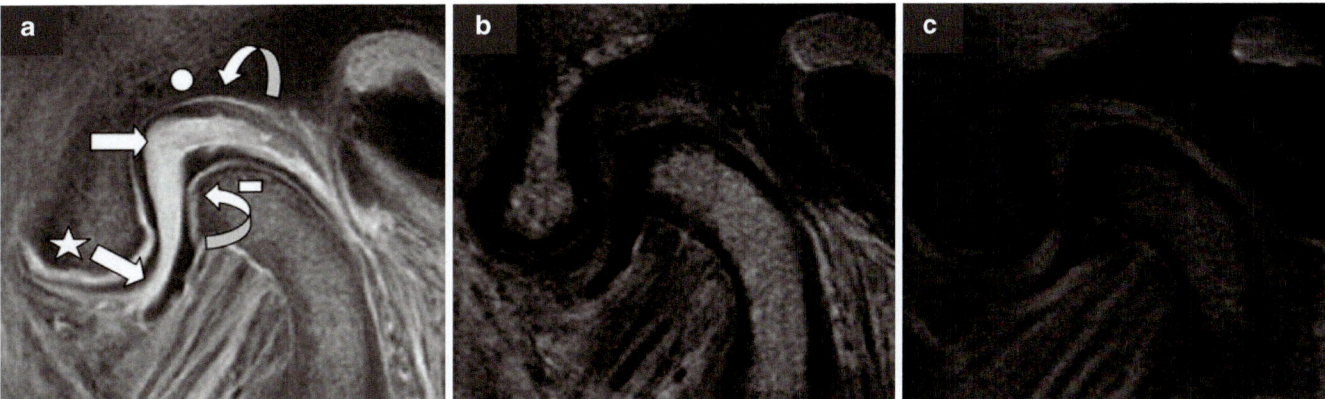

Fig. 39.7 (**a**) UTE, (**b**) T₁-weighted, and (**c**) PD-weighted fat-suppressed MR images of the TMJ in a cadaveric specimen show the high signal in the TMJ disc (straight arrows) situated between the condylar eminence (star), condylar fossa (circle), and mandibular condyle (rectangle) on the UTE-MR image. The fibrocartilaginous articular surfaces (curved arrows) of the condyle (rectangle) and condylar fossa (circle) are also characterized by linear high signal intensity. The UTE-MR sequence facilitates the identification of these short-T₂ tissues by acquiring signals from them. They are not apparent on the two standard clinical sequences (**b, c**). (Adapted with permission from Sanal et al.[35])

and other tissues surrounding the TMJ disc. SE sequences can greatly minimize susceptibility artifact, leading to much improved depiction of the short-T₂* (using UTE-SE) and long-T₂ tissues surrounding the TMJ disc. The TMJ disc is well depicted using a UTE-FID data acquisition but shows a low signal on the second SE image. Subtraction of the sec-

ond SE image from the first UTE-FID image provides high contrast imaging of the TMJ disc, as shown in Fig. 39.8c.

Zero TE (ZTE) sequences have similarities to the UTE group of sequences, but, unlike conventional UTE, the readout gradients are enabled prior to the RF pulse excitation [38, 39]. The ZTE acquisition method uses a short rectangular hard pulse excitation and a small flip angle with gradual reorientation of the gradients in three directions [40]. Similar to UTE acquisitions, k-space is filled with a 3D radial center-out method and then transformed by gridding and inverse FT [40]. There is a data gap at the center of k-space, and this is compensated for using an oversampled acquisition and mathematical reconstruction [41]. ZTE has several applications, including, but not limited to, detection of ultrashort-T_2 components of cortical bone and dentine, morphometric bone analysis, and silent MR operation [42, 43]. Computed tomography (CT)-like ZTE images of bone are an alternative to CT. This avoids ionizing radiation, especially when serial studies are needed. Substantial agreement has been found between ZTE and cone-beam CT in the evaluation of osseous changes in the TMJ [44].

Quantitative UTE Imaging

UTE-T_2^* Imaging

The TMJ disc has structural similarities to the meniscus of the knee joint, with collagen fibers accounting for approximately 80% of its dry weight [18–20]. This highly organized fiber structure leads to strong dipole–dipole interactions and, subsequently, a short T_2^* [32–35, 45]. As a result, the disc typically shows little or no signal when imaged with clinical MRI sequences [30, 46]. The T_2^* value for the TMJ disc can be reliably measured with UTE-type sequences, where the TMJ disc and surrounding joint tissues can be depicted with high spatial resolution and high signal. Figure 39.7 shows 2D UTE imaging of a cadaveric human TMJ sample using a constant TR of 400 ms and a series of TEs of 0.1, 0.5, 1.0, 1.5, 2, 4, 8, 15, and 25 ms. UTE images taken at multiple TEs

were analyzed by the exponential fitting of signal intensity to $S(\mathrm{TE}) = S_0 \cdot \exp(-\mathrm{TE}/T_2^*)$. Regions of interest (ROIs) were drawn in the TMJ disc (curved arrow in Fig. 39.9a) and condylar fibrocartilage (straight arrow in Fig. 39.9a), respectively. Excellent mono-exponential fitting was achieved, demonstrating short-T_2^* values of 6.97 ± 0.12 ms for the TMJ disc and 3.21 ± 0.16 ms for condylar fibrocartilage (Fig. 39.9). The condylar fibrocartilage has an extremely short T_2^*, likely to be affected by strong susceptibility differences at the osteochondral interface.

UTE-T_1 Imaging

Conventional T_1 quantification techniques are often based on variable repetition time or variable flip angle techniques using gradient echo or fast spin echo data acquisition. These sequences have relatively long TEs of several milliseconds or longer, which are of the order of the T_2^* of the TMJ disc. The limited detectable signal from the TMJ disc precludes accurate T_1 measurement. Furthermore, it is important to consider the duration of the RF excitation, saturation, and inversion pulses, which may not be negligible for short-T_2 tissues, leading to considerable transverse relaxation during the application of the RF pulses. It is easier to saturate than to invert the longitudinal magnetizations of short-T_2 tissues. UTE-based saturation recovery techniques with progressively increasing saturation recovery times (TSRs) have been proposed for T_1 quantification of short-T_2 tissues [47]. Figure 39.10 shows 2D UTE-TSR imaging of a cadaveric human TMJ sample. A series of UTE images were acquired with a constant TE of 12 μs and a series of TSRs of 10, 50, 100, 200, 400, 800, 1600, and 3200 ms. Mono-exponential signal recovery curve fitting was used to measure T_1 values

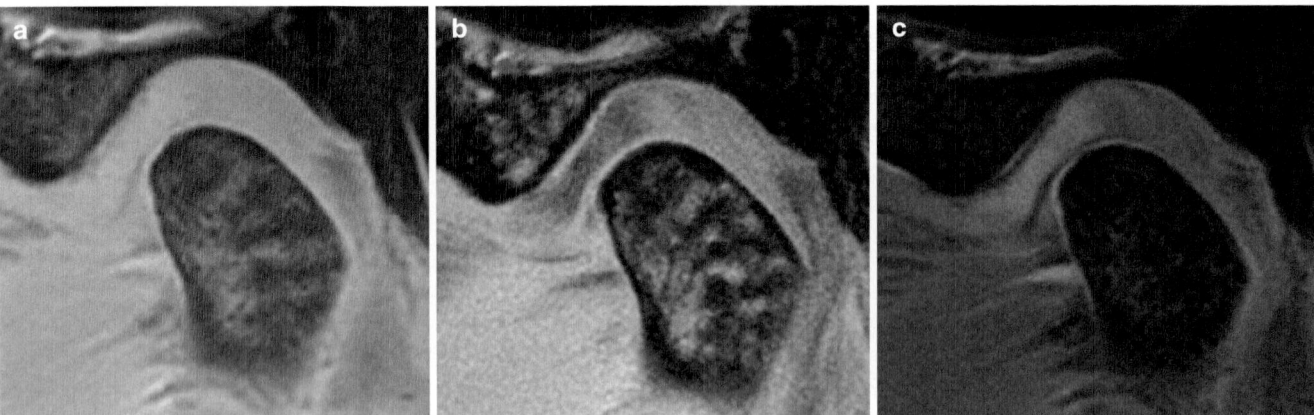

Fig. 39.8 Dual-echo UTE-SE imaging of the TMJ disc. The first UTE-FID acquisition shows high signal from TMJ tissues, including the condylar fibrocartilage and tissues surrounding the TMJ disc (**a**). The second SE data acquisition shows high signals from the condylar fibrocartilage and tissues surrounding the TMJ disc due to their longer T_2s but lower signal from the TMJ disc due to its short T_2 (**b**). Subtraction of the second SE image from the first UTE-FID image provides high contrast for the TMJ disc (**c**)

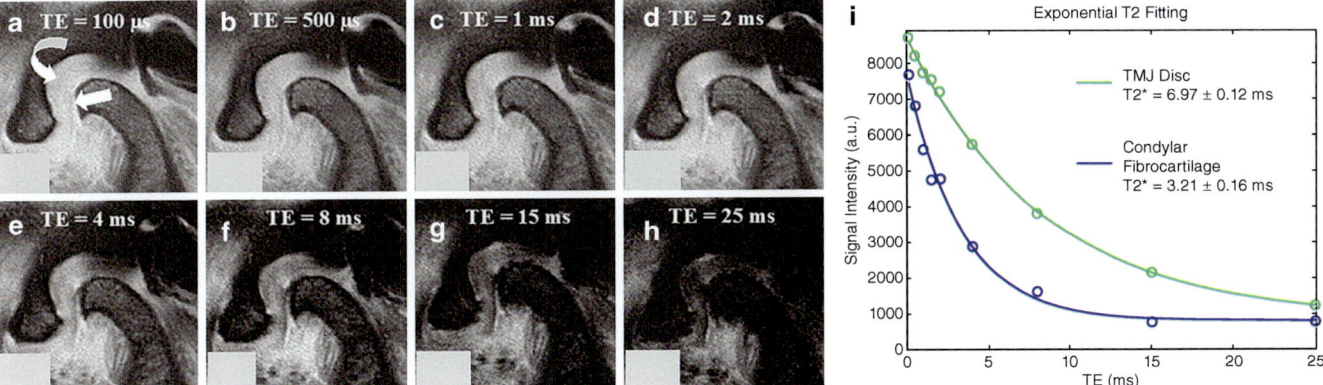

Fig. 39.9 2D UTE images acquired with a TR of 400 ms and a series of TEs of 0.1 (**a**), 0.5 (**b**), 1 (**c**), 2 (**d**), 4 (**e**), 8 (**f**), 15 (**g**), and 25 ms (**h**) as well as mono-exponential T_2^* fitting (**i**), which demonstrates short-T_2^* values of 6.97 ± 0.12 ms for the TMJ disc (curved arrow in panel **a**) and 3.21 ± 0.16 ms for condylar fibrocartilage (straight arrow in panel **a**), respectively

for the condylar fibrocartilage and the TMJ disc. As expected, the TMJ disc has a relatively short T_1 of 658 ± 34 ms, whereas the condylar fibrocartilage has a longer T_1 of 927 ± 86 ms (Fig. 39.10).

UTE-$T_{1\rho}$ Imaging

The spin–lattice relaxation in the rotating frame ($T_{1\rho}$) has emerged as an important noninvasive method for detecting biochemical changes that may precede morphological degeneration in musculoskeletal tissues [48]. $T_{1\rho}$ imaging techniques based on conventional MR sequences have limited value for evaluation of short-T_2 tissues, which show little or low signal when the TEs are of the order of, or even longer than, the T_2^* values. UTE-based $T_{1\rho}$ (UTE-$T_{1\rho}$) imaging has been developed to measure $T_{1\rho}$ of short-T_2 tissues [49, 50]. However, $T_{1\rho}$ imaging is sensitive to the magic angle effect, whereby the $T_{1\rho}$ values may be greatly increased when the direction of collagen fibers is reoriented from parallel to B_0 to near 54° to B_0 [51, 52]. More recently, UTE adiabatic $T_{1\rho}$ (UTE-Adiab$T_{1\rho}$) sequences have been developed for robust $T_{1\rho}$ mapping of both short- and long-T_2 tissues on clinical scanners [53, 54]. The UTE-Adiab$T_{1\rho}$ sequence is much less sensitive to the magic angle effect [55] and can distinguish mild cartilage degeneration from normal cartilage, with higher UTE-Cones-Adiab$T_{1\rho}$ values seen in the more degenerate cartilage [56].

The UTE-Adiab$T_{1\rho}$ sequence has also been employed to evaluate normal and degenerate cadaveric TMJs, as shown in Fig. 39.11. Unlike the articular cartilage, UTE-Adiab$T_{1\rho}$ demonstrates a substantially lower value of 31.3 ± 7.1 ms in the degenerate TMJ disc compared to 40.3 ± 12.3 ms in normal disc, possibly representing higher proteoglycan in the degenerate tissue. $T_{1\rho}$ values are inversely related to proteoglycan content in the tissue, as evidenced by Safranin O

evaluation, which shows a disorganized fibrillar pattern and increased Safranin O staining in the degenerate TMJ disc compared to the normal TMJ disc. Similarly, progressive increase in the proteoglycan levels was observed in the intervertebral disc in the early stages of the annulus fibrosus degeneration before an eventual decrease in the severely degenerate tissues [57]. Increased proteoglycan in the TMJ disc has been described as a pathological and adaptive response to mechanical loading [58].

UTE-MT Imaging

Magnetization transfer or MT imaging has been used to indirectly assess macromolecules with restricted motion and extremely short T_2s [59]. In this technique, a saturation pulse is placed at a frequency offset from the narrow line of free water to saturate macromolecular protons that exchange with water protons, leading to a reduced detectable signal in free water. The MT effect is typically evaluated using the magnetization transfer ratio (MTR), which is calculated as the percentage change in signal with and without a saturation pulse. MTR is only semiquantitative and has limitations such as hardware dependence and variability with the scan protocol [60].

MT modeling is employed to provide more reliable quantitative information. The most widely used two-pool quantitative MT model assumes a free pool composed of water protons and a semisolid pool consisting of collagen protons [61]. A series of images acquired with different MT RF powers and frequency offsets are subjected to two-pool modeling to generate macromolecular proton fractions (MMFs), exchange rates, and relaxation times. However, clinical MT sequences based on conventional data acquisitions cannot be used to evaluate short-T_2 tissues due to the lack of detectable signals. UTE-based MT (UTE-MT) sequences can directly

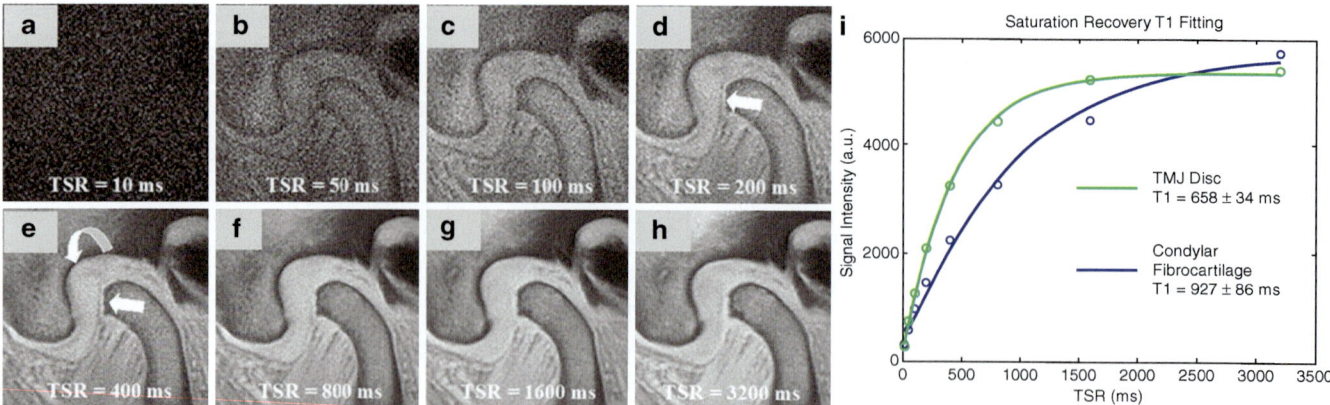

Fig. 39.10 UTE-TSR images and T_1 fitting for the TMJ disc (curved arrow) and condylar fibrocartilage (arrow) using the saturation recovery technique with a series of saturation recovery times (TSRs) of 10 (**a**), 50 (**b**), 100 (**c**), 200 (**d**), 400 (**e**), 800 (**f**), 1600 (**g**), and 3200 ms (**h**), as well as mono-exponential recovery curve fitting (**i**), which shows fitted T_1 values of 658 ± 34 ms for the disc and 927 ± 86 ms for the condylar fibrocartilage

detect signals from water components in short-T_2 tissues and can be used to indirectly probe MMF in cortical bone, menisci, ligaments, tendons, cartilage, the rotator cuff, and many other musculoskeletal tissues [62–69]. Most importantly, the UTE-MT modeling-derived MMF is insensitive to the magic angle effect [64] and is highly correlated with tissue biomechanical properties and degeneration [65–67]. UTE-MT-derived MMF also shows a strong correlation with degeneration, with decreased MMF for cartilage and knee meniscus in mild and advanced osteoarthritis compared to healthy subjects [68, 69].

UTE-MT modeling has also been used to evaluate normal and degenerate cadaveric TMJs. Figure 39.12 shows MMF mapping of the normal versus degenerate TMJ disc with the quantitative UTE-MT technique, with a mean MMF of 11.2 ± 1.8% for the normal disc and 9.8 ± 2.6% for the degenerate disc. Percentage MMF was calculated using MT modeling from data with MT pulse flip angles of 500° and 1500° and frequency offsets of 2, 5, 10, 20, and 50 kHz. The signal of all tissue components in the disc can be detected and quantified with this sequence. The ability of the 3D UTE-MT sequence to interrogate macromolecular protons with detailed analysis of free pool protons and semisolid pool protons provides a more robust evaluation of tissue structure and change with disease state than conventional T_2 and T_2^* measurements.

UTE-DESS Imaging

Double echo steady-state MRI or DESS-MRI has been proposed for fast, high-resolution, diffusion-weighted imaging of musculoskeletal tissues such as articular cartilage [70]. More recently, UTE-based DESS (UTE-DESS) imaging has been specifically introduced for short-T_2 tissues, such as the deep articular cartilage, menisci, ligaments, and tendons [71, 72]. In this technique, free induction decay-like signal (S^+) and echo-like signal (S^-) are acquired with a pair of balanced readout and read-in gradients separated by a trapezoidal spoiling gradient. Figure 39.13 shows 3D UTE-DESS imaging of a cadaveric human TMJ sample. The first S^+ image is capable of visualizing the TMJ disc and condylar fibrocartilage, whereas the S^- image shows little signal from the TMJ disc due to its fast signal decay. Subtraction of the S^- image from the S^+ image provides high contrast imaging of the TMJ disc in the echo subtraction image (Fig. 39.13d).

The S^+ and S^- signals include the contribution from the current RF excitation and the stimulated echoes from the preceding RF excitations [70]. Compared to S^+ images, S^- images have more T_2 and diffusion weighting. These are modulated by the repetition time, the flip angle, and the gradient moment of the spoiling gradient. Higher diffusion weighting is achieved using a longer TR, a lower flip angle, and a higher gradient moment. The signal model used for DESS can be directly applied to UTE-DESS imaging [70, 72]. Four parameters, including proton density, T_1, T_2, and apparent diffusion coefficient (ADC), can be estimated by fitting the signal intensity of both S^+ and S^- using this signal model. The quantitative 3D UTE-DESS sequence can be applied to normal and degenerate cadaveric TMJ, to produce T_2 and ADC maps, as shown in Fig. 39.14. A higher mean T_2 value of 17.14 ± 3.2 ms was observed in the degenerate TMJ disc, whereas a lower mean T_2 value of 15.84 ± 5.27 ms was observed in the normal disc. The same trend is observed in

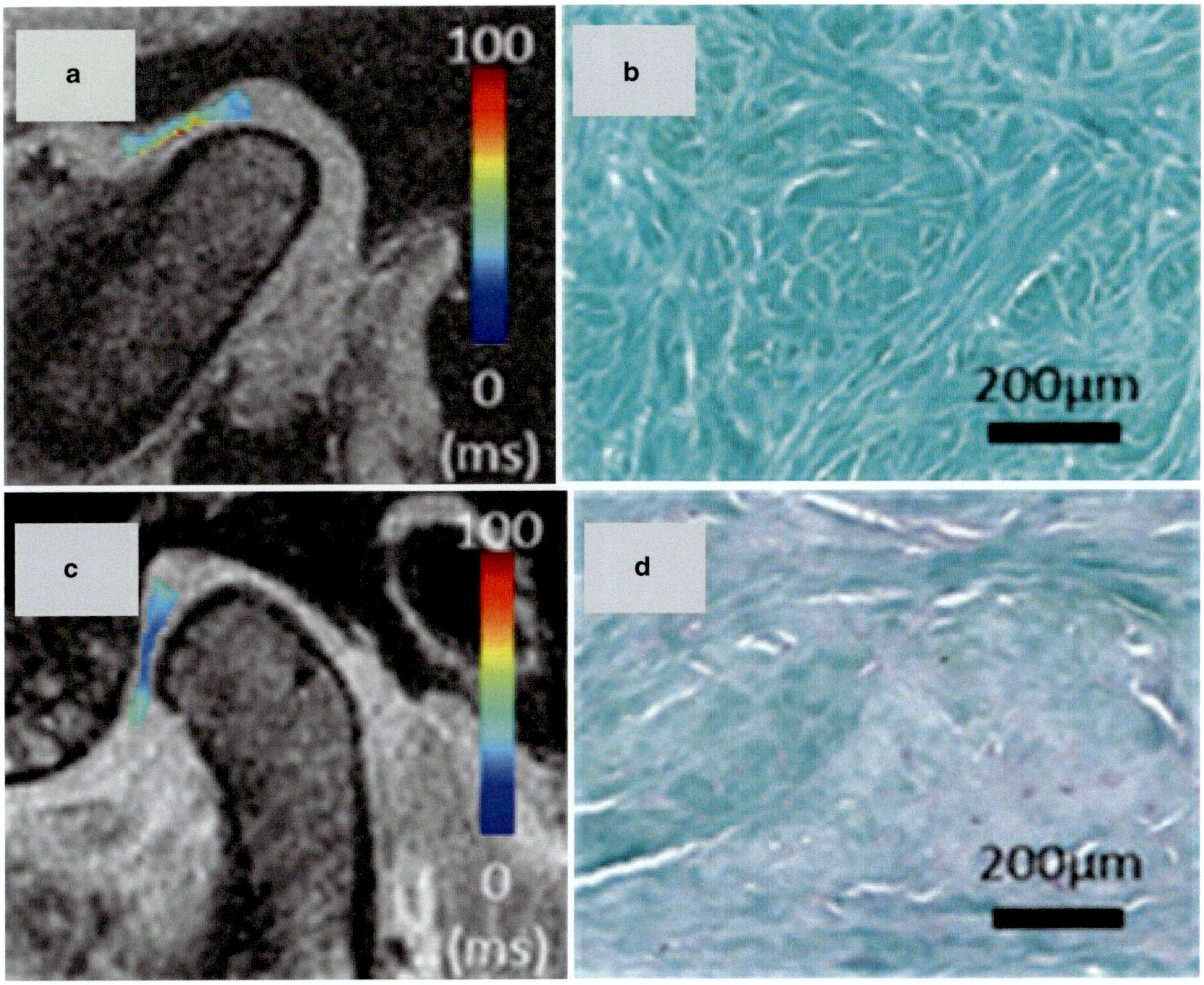

Fig. 39.11 Sagittal 3D UTE-AdiabT$_{1\rho}$ mapping in the normal (**a**) and degenerate (**b**) TMJ demonstrates a measurable quantitative decrease in T$_{1\rho}$ in the degenerate TMJ disc compared to the normal disc. Corresponding Safranin O staining in the normal (**c**) and degenerate (**d**)

TMJ discs. Safranin O staining confirms increased proteoglycan content (**d**) in the degenerate TMJ disc compared to the normal disc. These findings can represent early stages of disc degeneration

Fig. 39.12 MMF mapping of the normal (**a**) and degenerate (**b**) TMJ discs using 3D UTE-MT imaging in the sagittal plane and two-pool signal modeling, with a mean MMF of 11.2 ± 1.8% for the normal disc and 9.8 ± 2.6% for the degenerate disc

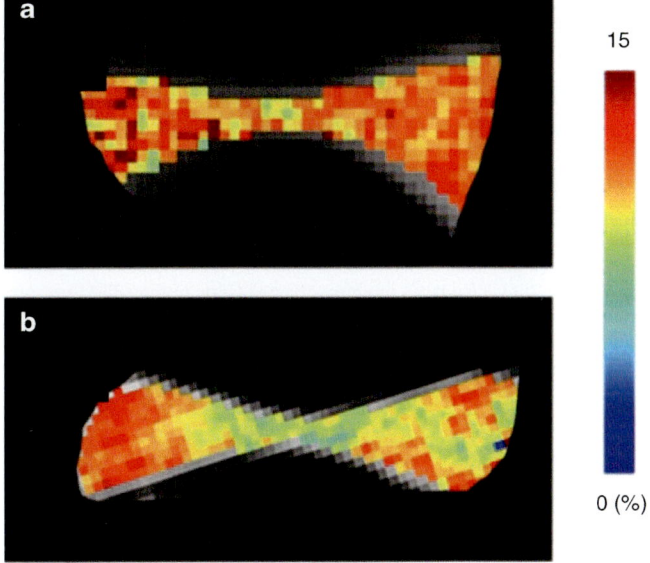

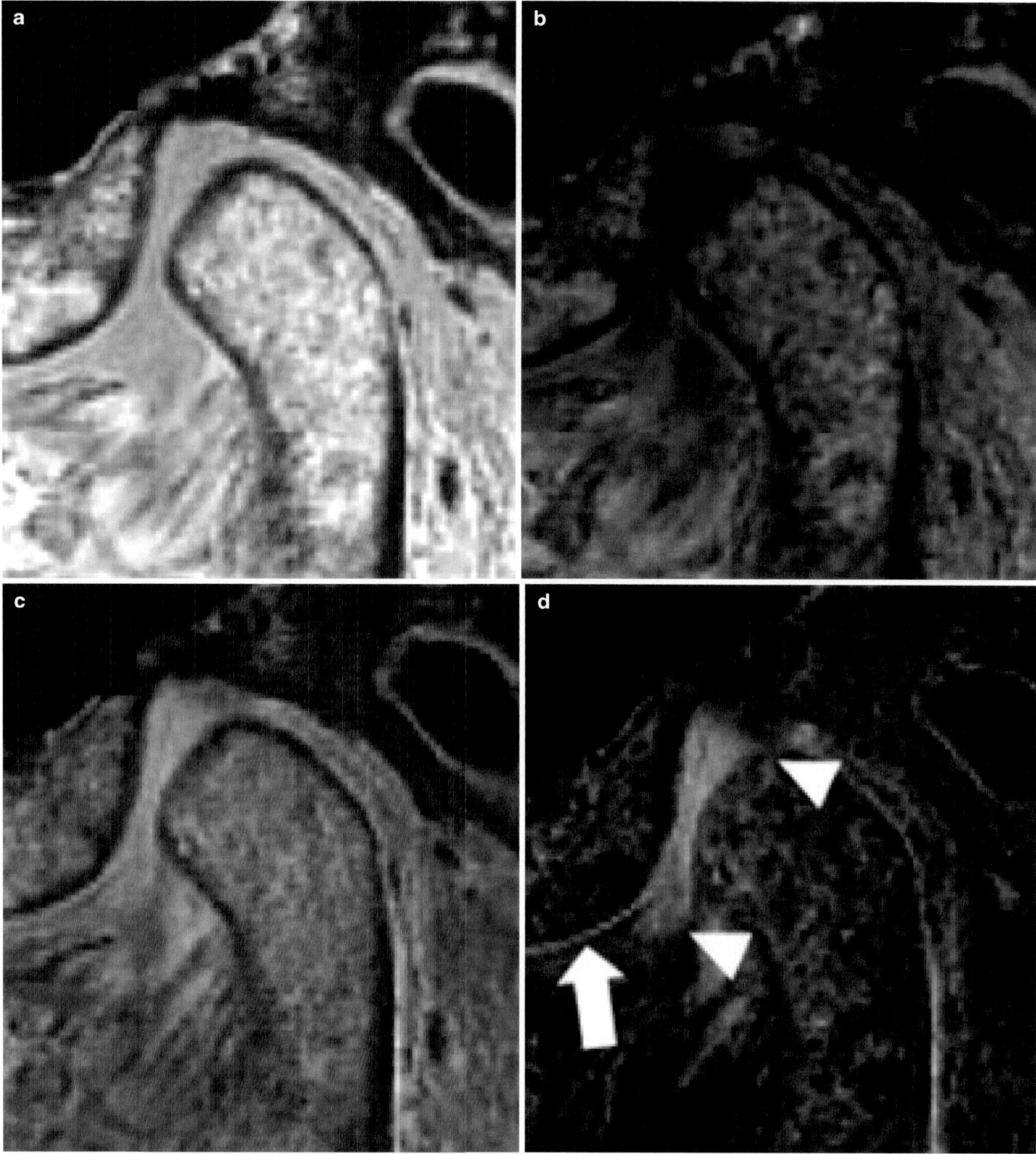

Fig. 39.13 3D UTE-DESS imaging of a cadaveric human TMJ sample shows high signal for all joint tissues in the S⁺ image (**a**), low signal in the TMJ disc in the S⁻ image (**b**), good contrast for the TMJ disc in the subtraction image (**c**), and much improved contrast for the TMJ disc (arrowheads) and articular fibrocartilage (arrow) in the echo subtraction image (**d**)

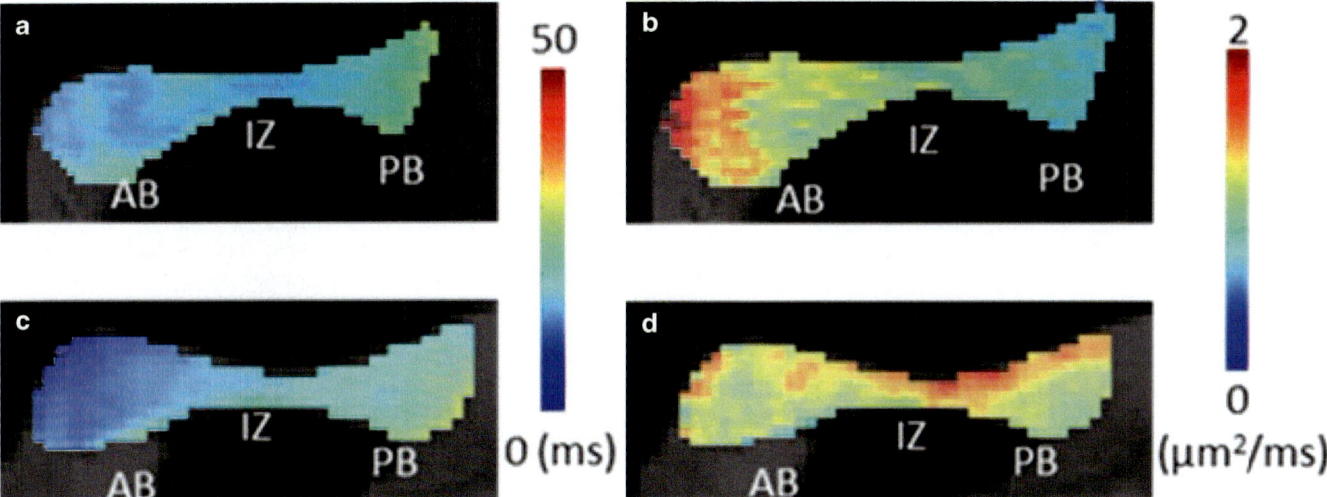

Fig. 39.14 Sagittal 3D UTE-DESS imaging of normal (**a**, **b**) and degenerate (**c**, **d**) cadaveric human TMJ discs. Both the T_2 (**a**, **c**) and ADC (**b**, **d**) values are increased in the degenerate TMJ disc

ADC values, with a higher ADC of 1.25 ± 0.17 $\mu m^2/ms$ for the degenerate TMJ disc and a lower ADC of 1.10 ± 0.29 $\mu m^2/ms$ for the normal disc. The added advantage of the 3D UTE-DESS map is its high spatial resolution (0.6 mm in-plane), which is not possible with conventional echo planar imaging (EPI)-based diffusion imaging.

Conclusions

UTE is a relatively novel MRI technique for the assessment of TMJ. In vitro studies with cadaveric joints have demonstrated that it is feasible and allows direct imaging of TMJ structures. UTE provides not only high spatial resolution but also quantitative compositional information on the articular disc, mandibular condyle, and surrounding soft tissues. Morphological imaging can be obtained with both 2D and 3D sequences and dual-echo UTE sequences, which provide a wide range of disc information, from "bright disc" to "black disc." ZTE has emerged as an alternative to serial CT studies aimed at the evaluation of bone morphology, with potential applications in cases of OA and rheumatic diseases, particularly when affecting young individuals.

In the field of quantitative imaging, UTE has been used to access non-visible early damage by assessing changes in the macromolecules of collagen, proteoglycan, and water content associated with tissue degeneration. T_2^*, T_1, $T_{1\rho}$, and MT UTE sequences have proven their worth in the assessment of TMJ disc and articular fibrocartilage. While the T_2^* of the TMJ disc can be reliably measured using UTE imaging with variable TEs, T_1 can be quantified with saturation recovery UTE imaging with variable TSRs. The 3D UTE-AdiabT$_{1\rho}$ sequence provides magic angle-insensitive $T_{1\rho}$ mapping, and

UTE-MT modeling allows orientation-independent MMF mapping of the TMJ disc and surrounding long-T_2 tissues. More recently, the UTE-DESS sequence has allowed T_2 and ADC mapping of the TMJ disc, muscle, and other soft tissues with high spatial resolution compared to conventional EPI-based MRI for diffusion.

The future direction of UTE in TMJ is toward the translation of the knowledge presented in this chapter to clinical applications. One fundamental step is the promotion of studies dedicated to TMDs in which structures with short-T_2 components play a role in the pathogenesis, such as in myofascial pain syndromes, osteoarthritis related to disc displacement, peripheral nerve diseases, and inflammatory enthesopathies. In addition, technical improvements are needed to allow dynamic imaging of the TMJ and masticatory musculature with UTE, opening a whole new window for the visualization of the biomechanics of mastication. The UTE and ZTE groups of sequences will probably provide more systematic and comprehensive evaluation of the TMJ disorders than conventional sequences, and this is likely to lead to better diagnosis and patient care of TMDs.

References

1. Tamimi D, Jalali E, Hatcher D. Temporomandibular joint imaging. Radiol Clin N Am. 2018;56(1):157–75.
2. Greene CS, Marbach JJ. Epidemiologic studies of mandibular dysfunction: a critical review. J Prosthet Dent. 1982;48(2):184–90.
3. Tanaka E, Detamore MS, Mercuri LG. Degenerative disorders of the temporomandibular joint: etiology, diagnosis, and treatment. J Dent Res. 2008;87(4):296–307.
4. Warren MP, Fried JL. Temporomandibular disorders and hormones in women. Cells Tissues Organs. 2001;169(3):187–92.

5. Martins-Júnior RL, Palma AJG, Marquardt EJ, de Barros Gondin TM, de Carvalho Kerber F. Temporomandibular disorders: a report of 124 patients. J Contemp Dent Pract. 2010;11(5):71–8.

6. Behzadi F, Mandell JC, Smith SE, Guenette JP. Temporomandibular joint imaging: current clinical applications, biochemical comparison with the intervertebral disc and knee meniscus, and opportunities for advancement. Skelet Radiol. 2020;49(8):1183–93.

7. Warburton G. Oral and maxillofacial surgery for the clinician. In: Bonanthaya K, Panneerselvam E, Manuel S, Kumar VV, Rai A, editors. Oral Maxillofac Surg Clin. Singapore: Springer Singapore; 2021. p. 1361–80.

8. Li DTS, Leung YY. Temporomandibular disorders: current concepts and controversies in diagnosis and management. Diagnostics (Basel). 2021;11(3):459.

9. Wilkes CH. Surgical treatment of internal derangements of the temporomandibular joint: a long-term study. Arch Otolaryngol Neck Surg. 1991;117(1):64–72.

10. Emshoff R, Brandlmaier I, Schmid C, Bertram S, Rudisch A. Bone marrow edema of the mandibular condyle related to internal derangement, osteoarthrosis, and joint effusion. J Oral Maxillofac Surg. 2003;61(1):35–40.

11. Dworkin SF, LeResche L. Research diagnostic criteria for temporomandibular disorders: review, criteria, examinations and specifications, critique. J Craniomandib Disord. 1992;6(4):301–55.

12. Schiffman E, Ohrbach R, Truelove E, Look J, Anderson G, Goulet J-P, et al. Diagnostic criteria for temporomandibular disorders (DC/TMD) for clinical and research applications: recommendations of the international RDC/TMD consortium network* and orofacial pain special interest group†. J Oral Facial Pain Headache. 2014;28(1):6–27.

13. Üşümez S, Öz F, Güray E. Comparison of clinical and magnetic resonance imaging diagnoses in patients with TMD history. J Oral Rehabil. 2004;31(1):52–6.

14. Griffin CJ, Hawthorn R, Harris R. Anatomy and histology of the human temporomandibular joint. Monogr Oral Sci. 1975;4:1–26.

15. Helland MM. Anatomy and function of the temporomandibular joint. J Orthop Sport Phys Ther. 1980;1(3):145–52.

16. Rayne J. Functional anatomy of the temporomandibular joint. Br J Oral Maxillofac Surg. 1987;25(2):92–9.

17. Salamon NM, Casselman JW. Temporomandibular joint disorders: a pictorial review. Semin Musculoskelet Radiol. 2020;24(5):591–607.

18. Detamore MS, Orfanos JG, Almarza AJ, French MM, Wong ME, Athanasiou KA. Quantitative analysis and comparative regional investigation of the extracellular matrix of the porcine temporomandibular joint disc. Matrix Biol. 2005;24(1):45–57.

19. Clément C, Bravetti P, Plénat F, Foliguet B, El HA, Gaudy JF, et al. Quantitative analysis of the elastic fibres in the human temporomandibular articular disc and its attachments. Int J Oral Maxillofac Surg. 2006;35(12):1120–6.

20. Leonardi R, Villari L, Bernasconi G, Caltabiano M. Histochemical study of the elastic fibers in pathologic human temporomandibular joint discs. J Oral Maxillofac Surg. 2001;59(10):1186–92.

21. Akita K, Sakaguchi-Kuma T, Fukino K, Ono T. Masticatory muscles and branches of mandibular nerve: positional relationships between various muscle bundles and their innervating branches. Anat Rec. 2019;302(4):609–19.

22. Benbelaïd R, Fleiter B, Zouaoui A, Gaudy JF. Proposed graphical system of evaluating disc-condyle displacements of the temporomandibular joint in MRI. Surg Radiol Anat. 2005;27(5):361–7.

23. Foucart JM, Carpentier P, Pajoni D, Marguelles-Bonnet R, Pharaboz C. MR of 732 TMJs: anterior, rotational, partial and sideways disc displacements. Eur J Radiol. 1998;28(1):86–94.

24. Schmitter M, Kress B, Ludwig C, Koob A, Gabbert O, Rammeisberg P. Temporomandibular joint disk position assessed at coronal MR imaging in asymptomatic volunteers. Radiology. 2005;236(2):559–64.

25. Limchaichana N, Petersson A, Rohlin M. The efficacy of magnetic resonance imaging in the diagnosis of degenerative and inflammatory temporomandibular joint disorders: a systematic literature review. Oral Surg Oral Med Oral Pathol Oral Radiol Endod. 2006;102(4):521–36.

26. Katzberg RW, Bessette RW, Tallents RH, Plewes DB, Manzione JV, Schenck JF, et al. Normal and abnormal temporomandibular joint: MR imaging with surface coil. Radiology. 1986;158(1):183–9.

27. Schellhas KP, Fritts HM, Heithoff KB, Jahn JA, Wilkes CH, Omlie MR. Temporomandibular joint: MR fast scanning. Cranio J Craniomandib Pract. 1988;6(3):209–16.

28. Helms CA, Kaban LB, McNeill C, Dodson T. Temporomandibular joint: morphology and signal intensity characteristics of the disk at MR imaging. Radiology. 1989;172(3):817–20.

29. Orhan K, Nishiyama H, Tadashi S, Murakami S, Furukawa S. Comparison of altered signal intensity, position, and morphology of the TMJ disc in MR images corrected for variations in surface coil sensitivity. Oral Surg Oral Med Oral Pathol Oral Radiol Endod. 2006;101(4):515–22.

30. Tomas X, Pomes J, Berenguer J, Quinto L, Nicolau C, Mercader JM, et al. MR imaging of temporomandibular joint dysfunction: a pictorial review. Radiographics. 2006;26(3):765–81.

31. Otonari T, Wakoh M, Sano T, Yamamoto M, Ohkubo M, Harada T. Parameters for diffusion weighted magnetic resonance imaging for temporomandibular joint. Bull Tokyo Dent Coll. 2006;47(1):5–12.

32. Bae WC, Tafur M, Chang EY, Du J, Biswas R, Kwack K-S, et al. High-resolution morphologic and ultrashort time-to-echo quantitative magnetic resonance imaging of the temporomandibular joint. Skelet Radiol. 2016;45(3):383–91.

33. Geiger D, Bae WC, Statum S, Du J, Chung CB. Quantitative 3D ultrashort time-to-echo (UTE) MRI and micro-CT (μCT) evaluation of the temporomandibular joint (TMJ) condylar morphology. Skelet Radiol. 2014;43(1):19–25.

34. Bae WC, Biswas R, Statum S, Sah RL, Chung CB. Sensitivity of quantitative UTE MRI to the biomechanical property of the temporomandibular joint disc. Skelet Radiol. 2014;43(9):1217–23.

35. Sanal HT, Bae WC, Pauli C, Du J, Statum S, Znamirowski R, et al. Magnetic resonance imaging of the temporomandibular joint disc: feasibility of novel quantitative magnetic resonance evaluation using histologic and biomechanical reference standards. J Orofac Pain. 2011;25(4):345–53.

36. Bergin CJ, Pauly JM, Macovski A. Lung parenchyma: projection reconstruction MR imaging. Radiology. 1991;179(3):777–81.

37. Weiger M, Pruessmann KP. Short-T2 MRI: principles and recent advances. Prog Nucl Magn Reson Spectrosc. 2019;114-115:237–70.

38. Chang EY, Du J, Chung CB. UTE imaging in the musculoskeletal system. J Magn Reson Imaging. 2015;41(4):870–83.

39. Larson PEZ, Han M, Krug R, Jakary A, Nelson SJ, Vigneron DB, et al. Ultrashort echo time and zero echo time MRI at 7T. MAGMA. 2016;29(3):359–70.

40. Mastrogiacomo S, Dou W, Jansen JA, Walboomers XF. Magnetic resonance imaging of hard tissues and hard tissue engineered bio-substitutes. Mol Imaging Biol. 2019;21(6):1003–19.

41. Jerban S, Chang DG, Ma Y, Jang H, Chang EY, Du J. An update in qualitative imaging of bone using ultrashort echo time magnetic resonance. Front Endocrinol (Lausanne). 2020;11:1–12.

42. Aydıngöz Ü, Yıldız AE, Ergen FB. Zero echo time musculoskeletal MRI: technique, optimization, applications, and pitfalls. Radiographics. 2022;42(5):1398–414.

43. Ljungberg E, Damestani NL, Wood TC, Lythgoe DJ, Zelaya F, Williams SCR, et al. Silent zero TE MR neuroimaging: current state-of-the-art and future directions. Prog Nucl Magn Reson Spectrosc. 2021;123:73–93.

44. Lee C, Jeon KJ, Han SS, Kim YH, Choi YJ, Lee A, et al. CT-like MRI using the zero-TE technique for osseous changes of the TMJ. Dentomaxillofac Radiol. 2020;49(3):20190272.

45. Carl M, Sanal HT, Diaz E, Du J, Girard O, Statum S, et al. Optimizing MR signal contrast of the temporomandibular joint disk. J Magn Reson Imaging. 2011;34(6):1458–64.

46. Emshoff R, Innerhofer K, Rudisch A, Bertram S. Clinical versus magnetic resonance imaging findings with internal derangement of the temporomandibular joint: An evaluation of anterior disc displacement without reduction. J Oral Maxillofac Surg. 2002;60(1):36–41.

47. Du J, Carl M, Bydder M, Takahashi A, Chung CB, Bydder GM. Qualitative and quantitative ultrashort echo time (UTE) imaging of cortical bone. J Magn Reson. 2010;207(2):304–11.

48. Duvvuri U, Reddy R, Patel SD, Kaufman JH, Kneeland JB, Leigh JS. T_1rho-relaxation in articular cartilage: effects of enzymatic degradation. Magn Reson Med. 1997;38(6):863–7.

49. Du J, Carl M, Diaz E, Takahashi A, Han E, Szeverenyi NM, et al. Ultrashort TE T_1rho (UTE T_1rho) imaging of the Achilles tendon and meniscus. Magn Reson Med. 2010;64(3):834–42.

50. Ma YJ, Carl M, Shao H, Tadros AS, Chang EY, Du J. Three-dimensional ultrashort echo time cones $T_1\rho$ (3D UTE-cones-$T_1\rho$) imaging. NMR Biomed. 2017;30(6):10.1002/nbm.3709.

51. Shao H, Pauli C, Li S, Ma Y, Tadros AS, Kavanaugh A, et al. Magic angle effect plays a major role in both T_1rho and T_2 relaxation in articular cartilage. Osteoarthr Cartil. 2017;25(12):2022–30.

52. Du J, Statum S, Znamirowski R, Bydder GM, Chung CB. Ultrashort TE $T_1\rho$ magic angle imaging. Magn Reson Med. 2013;69(3):682–7.

53. Ma Y-J, Carl M, Searleman A, Lu X, Chang EY, Du J. 3D adiabatic $T_1\rho$ prepared ultrashort echo time cones sequence for whole knee imaging. Magn Reson Med. 2018;80(4):1429–39.

54. Wu M, Zhao W, Wan L, Kakos L, Li L, Jerban S, et al. Quantitative three-dimensional ultrashort echo time cones imaging of the knee joint with motion correction. NMR Biomed. 2020;33(1):e4214.

55. Wu M, Ma Y, Wan L, Jerban S, Jang H, Chang EY, et al. Magic angle effect on adiabatic $T_1\rho$ imaging of the Achilles tendon using 3D ultrashort echo time cones trajectory. NMR Biomed. 2020;33(8):e4322.

56. Wu M, Ma Y-J, Kasibhatla A, Chen M, Jang H, Jerban S, et al. Convincing evidence for magic angle less-sensitive quantitative $T_1\rho$ imaging of articular cartilage using the 3D ultrashort echo time cones adiabatic $T1\rho$ (3D UTE cones-AdiabT1ρ) sequence. Magn Reson Med. 2020;84(5):2551–60.

57. Cs-Szabo G, Ragasa-San Juan D, Turumella V, Masuda K, Thonar EJMA, An HS. Changes in mRNA and protein levels of proteoglycans of the anulus fibrosus and nucleus pulposus during intervertebral disc degeneration. Spine (Phila Pa 1976). 2002;27(20):2212–9.

58. Nakao Y, Konno-Nagasaka M, Toriya N, Arakawa T, Kashio H, Takuma T, et al. Proteoglycan expression is influenced by mechanical load in TMJ discs. J Dent Res. 2015;94(1):93–100.

59. Wolff SD, Balaban RS. Magnetization transfer contrast (MTC) and tissue water proton relaxation in vivo. Magn Reson Med. 1989;10(1):135–44.

60. Sinclair CDJ, Samson RS, Thomas DL, Weiskopf N, Lutti A, Thornton JS, et al. Quantitative magnetization transfer in in vivo healthy human skeletal muscle at 3 T. Magn Reson Med. 2010;64(6):1739–48.

61. Henkelman RM, Huang X, Xiang Q-S, Stanisz GJ, Swanson SD, Bronskill MJ. Quantitative interpretation of magnetization transfer. Magn Reson Med. 1993;29(6):759–66.

62. Ma Y-J, Chang EY, Carl M, Du J. Quantitative magnetization transfer ultrashort echo time imaging using a time-efficient 3D multispoke cones sequence. Magn Reson Med. 2018;79(2):692–700.

63. Ma Y, Tadros A, Du J, Chang EY. Quantitative two-dimensional ultrashort echo time magnetization transfer (2D UTE-MT) imaging of cortical bone. Magn Reson Med. 2018;79(4):1941–9.

64. Ma YJ, Shao H, Du J, Chang EY. Ultrashort echo time magnetization transfer (UTE-MT) imaging and modeling: magic angle independent biomarkers of tissue properties. NMR Biomed. 2016;29(11):1546–52.

65. Zhu Y, Cheng X, Ma Y, Wong JH, Xie Y, Du J, et al. Rotator cuff tendon assessment using magic-angle insensitive 3D ultrashort echo time cones magnetization transfer (UTE-cones-MT) imaging and modeling with histological correlation. J Magn Reson Imaging. 2018;48(1):160–8.

66. Jerban S, Ma Y, Wan L, Searleman AC, Jang H, Sah RL, et al. Collagen proton fraction from ultrashort echo time magnetization transfer (UTE-MT) MRI modelling correlates significantly with cortical bone porosity measured with micro-computed tomography (µCT). NMR Biomed. 2018;5(6):e4045.

67. Jerban S, Ma Y, Nazaran A, Dorthe EW, Cory E, Carl M, et al. Detecting stress injury (fatigue fracture) in fibular cortical bone using quantitative ultrashort echo time-magnetization transfer (UTE-MT): an ex vivo study. NMR Biomed. 2018;31(11):e3994.

68. Xue YP, Ma YJ, Wu M, Jerban S, Wei Z, Chang EY, et al. Quantitative 3D ultrashort echo time magnetization transfer imaging for evaluation of knee cartilage degeneration in vivo. J Magn Reson Imaging. 2021;54(4):1294–302.

69. Zhang X, Ma YJ, Wei Z, Wu M, Ashir A, Jerban S, et al. Macromolecular fraction (MMF) from 3D ultrashort echo time cones magnetization transfer (3D UTE-cones-MT) imaging predicts meniscal degeneration and knee osteoarthritis. Osteoarthr Cartil. 2021;29(8):1173–80.

70. Bieri O, Ganter C, Scheffler K. Quantitative in vivo diffusion imaging of cartilage using double echo steady-state free precession. Magn Reson Med. 2012;68(3):720–9.

71. Chaudhari AS, Sveinsson B, Moran CJ, McWalter EJ, Johnson EM, Zhang T, et al. Imaging and T_2 relaxometry of short-T_2 connective tissues in the knee using ultrashort echo-time double-echo steady-state (UTEDESS). Magn Reson Med. 2017;78(6):2136–48.

72. Jang H, Ma Y, Carl M, Jerban S, Chang EY, Du J. Ultrashort echo time cones double echo steady state (UTE-cones-DESS) for rapid morphological imaging of short T_2 tissues. Magn Reson Med. 2021;86(2):881–92.

Jiang Du, Yajun Ma, Chun Zeng, Sam Sedaghat, Hyungseok Jang, and Graeme M. Bydder

Introduction

Multiple sclerosis (MS) is a disabling demyelinating disease of the central nervous system (CNS) and is the most common cause of neurological disability in young adults [1]. Magnetic resonance imaging (MRI) has been formally included in the diagnosis of MS since 2001 [2]. Conventional MRI techniques, including T_1- and T_2-weighted structural imaging [3–5], gadolinium enhancement [6], diffusion-weighted imaging (DWI) [7], diffusion tensor imaging (DTI) [8], and magnetization transfer (MT) [9], have all been employed to detect tissue abnormalities in patients with MS. T_1-weighted imaging often shows MS lesions as isointense, but lesions can be hypointense in the presence of a chronic tissue injury or severe inflammatory edema [3]. T_2-weighted imaging usu-

ally shows lesions as hyperintense [5]. Gadolinium-enhanced imaging highlights active lesions [6]. DTI provides information on the microstructure of nerve fibers [8], and the MT ratio (MTR) can provide an indirect marker of myelin disorder in regions of the white matter (WM) [10].

However, conventional MRI correlates only modestly with disability as assessed by the Expanded Disability Status Scale (EDSS) [11–16]. For example, a T_2 lesion load is modestly correlated with disability ($R^2 = 0.04$–0.25) in several cross-sectional studies [11–14]. Gadolinium-enhancing lesions show moderate correlation with the EDSS in the first 6 months with poor prediction of changes in disability in the following 1–2 years [15]. According to a recent large-scale multicenter study, EDSS has been poorly correlated with normalized brain volume ($R^2 = 0.03$), cross-sectional area ($R^2 = 0.07$), MTR of the whole-brain tissue ($R^2 = 0.03$), and MTR of the gray matter (GM) ($R^2 = 0.03$) with no significant correlation with other magnetic resonance (MR) metrics [16]. GM atrophy shows slightly increased correlation with the EDSS ($R^2 = 0.13$–0.26) and the Multiple Sclerosis Functional Composite (MSFC) measure ($R^2 = 0.24$) [17, 18].

Conventional MRI sequences lack specificity in evaluation of the heterogeneous pathological substrates of MS disease and cannot accurately estimate damage in areas of the brain outside of focal lesions [19]. Most conventional MRI techniques have difficulty distinguishing the cardinal pathological substrates of MS, namely, demyelination, remyelination, inflammation, edema, axonal loss, and gliosis [20–22], which largely explains their poor performance in assessing disability. Myelin integrity plays a key role in the normal function of the nervous system [23–31], but conventional MRI sequences cannot accurately evaluate myelin changes in the brain, leading to underestimation of its role in MS.

Myelin is an insulating layer consisting of lipids and proteins that wrap around axons. It increases the axon's membrane electrical resistance and decreases the membrane capacitance, facilitating fast propagation of action potentials along nerve axons. More specifically, myelin can increase action potential transmission speed by ~100-fold and

J. Du (✉)
Department of Radiology, University of California, San Diego, La Jolla, CA, USA

Department of Bioengineering, University of California, San Diego, La Jolla, CA, USA

VA San Diego Healthcare System, San Diego, CA, USA
e-mail: jiangdu@health.ucsd.edu

Y. Ma · S. Sedaghat · H. Jang
Department of Radiology, University of California, San Diego, La Jolla, CA, USA
e-mail: yam013@health.ucsd.edu; ssedaghat@health.ucsd.edu; h4jang@health.ucsd.edu

C. Zeng
Department of Radiology, University of California, San Diego, La Jolla, CA, USA

Department of Radiology, The First Affiliated Hospital of Chongqing Medical University, Chongqing, China
e-mail: c3zeng@health.ucsd.edu

G. M. Bydder
Department of Radiology, University of California, San Diego, La Jolla, CA, USA

Mātai Medical Research Institute, Tairāwhiti, Gisborne, New Zealand
e-mail: gbydder@health.ucsd.edu

decrease refractory time by ~30-fold, which together increase brain "connectivity" or the information-processing capacity of the brain by ~3000-fold [23–25]. The neuron signal transmission speed is directly related to the thickness of the myelin wrapping and the neuronal myelin content. Generation of oligodendrocytes and myelin is required for learning complex motor skills [26–28], and myelin is indispensable for the development and maintenance of elaborate cognitive functions. On the other hand, myelin impairment disrupts axonal transport, integrity, and plasticity, leading to massive reductions in neuronal signal transduction [29–31]. Demyelination of axons removes saltatory conduction, physical protection, and metabolic support, resulting in a variety of neurodegenerative pathologies, including MS [1]. It is of critical importance to develop clinically feasible methods to quantitatively evaluate myelin and to accurately capture the demyelination and remyelination process for personalized treatment in MS.

Direct assessment of the integrity of myelin in the white matter (WM) and gray matter (GM) of the brain may be important for more accurate diagnosis and assessment of prognosis in MS [32–36]. However, the nonaqueous protons in myelin have ultrashort T_2s (less than 1 ms) [33–36]. Conventional MRI sequences with echo times (TEs) of several milliseconds or longer cannot directly detect useful signals from myelin protons, precluding quantitative assessment of myelin properties such as its T_1 and T_2^* as well as phase information and proton density (PD) [37]. Two-dimensional (2D) and three-dimensional (3D) ultrashort TE (UTE) sequences with minimum nominal TEs of 8–50 μs, which are 100~1000 times shorter than the TEs of conventional clinical sequences, allow direct detection of signals from myelin protons using clinical MRI scanners [35–41]. A series of data acquisition strategies and contrast mechanisms as well as quantitative imaging techniques have been developed for ex vivo and in vivo imaging of myelin. Applications of these in MS have been investigated in preliminary studies.

UTE Imaging of Myelin: Phantom Studies

Direct MRI of nonaqueous myelin protons has proven to be technically challenging. Several groups have investigated the MR properties of myelin. Broad-line proton spectro-scopic studies have shown that myelin is in a liquid–crystalline state [42]. Multicomponent analysis of spin echo or free induction decay (FID) of WM samples has shown a broad range of short-T_2/T_2^* values for myelin protons (e.g., ~50 μs [43], 7.5–101 μs [44], 50–1000 μs [33], 150–250 μs [45], etc.). Nuclear magnetic resonance (NMR) spectrometric studies have found a wide distribution of T_2^* values ranging from 8 μs to 26 ms in the spinal cord [34]. These studies indicate that myelin can be directly imaged with UTE sequences using high-performance NMR spectrometers. However, myelin imaging using whole-body scanners is more challenging due to their much lower radiofrequency (RF) power and weaker gradient systems. The excitation efficiency is lower on clinical scanners than on spectrometers, as myelin magnetization may experience significant transverse relaxation during the excitation process on whole-body scanners. Significant signal loss is also expected during the spatial encoding due to the relatively weak gradient system and long data acquisition time on clinical scanners.

The capability of UTE-MRI for direct imaging of myelin has been demonstrated through a series of phantom studies on a clinical 3T scanner [36]. Figure 40.1 shows UTE imaging of a purified lyophilized bovine myelin extract powder (type 1 bovine brain lipid extract, Sigma-Aldrich B1502, St. Louis, MO, USA), which is an organophilic extract of predominantly myelin-related brain lipids. Clinical gradient echo and spin echo sequences cannot detect any signal from lyophilized bovine myelin powder. In comparison, UTE sequences provide high signals from the myelin phantoms, with excellent single-component exponential curve fitting demonstrating a short T_2^* of 152 ± 4 μs. This ultrashort-T_2^* value explains why nonaqueous myelin protons are "invisible" with conventional MRI sequences. UTE sequences also show a high signal for the lyophilized bovine myelin powders suspended in 99.9% denatured water (D_2O) (Sigma-Aldrich) to form a paste-like phantom, which is again "invisible" with conventional clinical MRI sequences [36]. The myelin–D_2O paste phantom shows a short T_2^* of 242 ± 13 μs, which is slightly longer than the T_2^* of myelin powder likely due to the greater susceptibility of myelin in powder form.

Although bovine myelin powders are organophilic extracts of predominantly myelin-related brain lipids, they

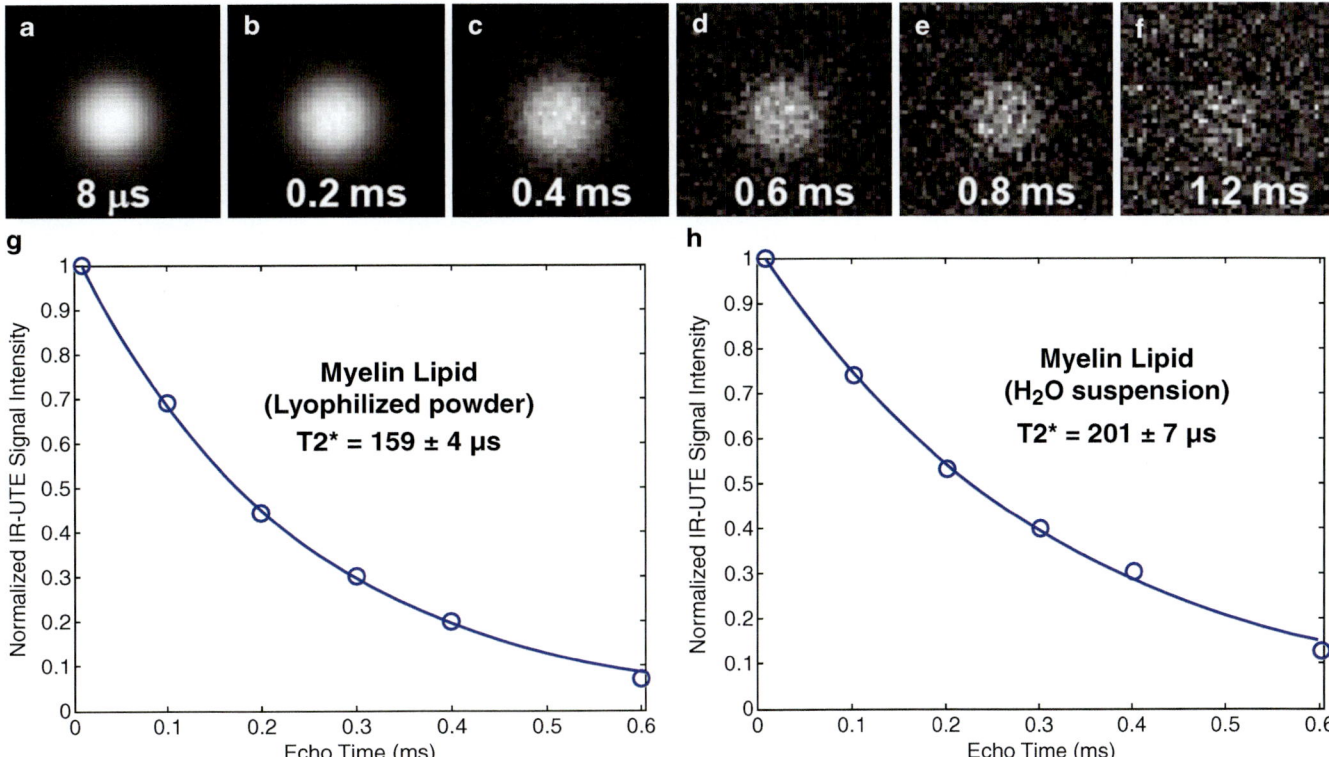

Fig. 40.1 UTE imaging of myelin powder with TEs of 8 μs (**a**), 0.2 (**b**), 0.4 (**c**), 0.6 (**d**), 0.8 (**e**), and 1.2 ms (**f**) demonstrates a T_2^* of 152 ± 4 μs (**g**). Myelin lipid–D_2O paste shows a T_2^* of 242 ± 13 μs (**h**). (Reproduced with permission from Sheth et al. [36])

might not have myelin's typical physiological bilayer structure. To demonstrate the capability of UTE sequences for direct imaging of structured myelin protons, myelin with its membrane architecture preserved was isolated from porcine WM by mechanical homogenization [40]. Myelin vesicles obtained in this way were further purified using discontinuous sucrose gradient ultracentrifugation [46]. The myelin vesicles were thoroughly washed out to get rid of residual sucrose and then resuspended twice in deuterated tris-Cl buffer to remove residual H_2O. Finally, the intact myelin vesicles were subjected to conventional and UTE imaging on a clinical 3 T scanner in the forms of lyophilized powders and D_2O paste. The phantoms were "invisible" with conventional sequences but showed a high signal with UTE imaging, which demonstrated an ultrashort T_2^* of 225 ± 7 μs and a short T_1 of 367 ± 4 ms for the myelin vesicles [40], as shown in Fig. 40.2.

The capability of quantitative UTE imaging for determining myelin PD was demonstrated on a series of myelin phantoms consisting of lyophilized myelin lipid powders resuspended in D_2O at concentrations of 6%, 9%, 12%, 18%, and 24% [41]. The diluted myelin pastes were put into different syringes along with a D_2O-only control (0% myelin) prior to imaging. Figure 40.3 shows the normalized UTE signal intensity after correction for coil sensitivity, with a highly linear increase in signal with myelin concentration ($R^2 = 0.99$). This high linearity is similar to the result obtained using a 9.4-T spectrometer with a UTE or zero echo time (ZTE) sequence, where the MR signal amplitudes were linearly correlated with myelin concentration with an R^2 of 0.98–0.99 [34, 47]. The results demonstrate the detectability of nonaqueous myelin protons not only with high-performance spectrometers but also with clinical whole-body scanners and their potential for in vivo myelin imaging.

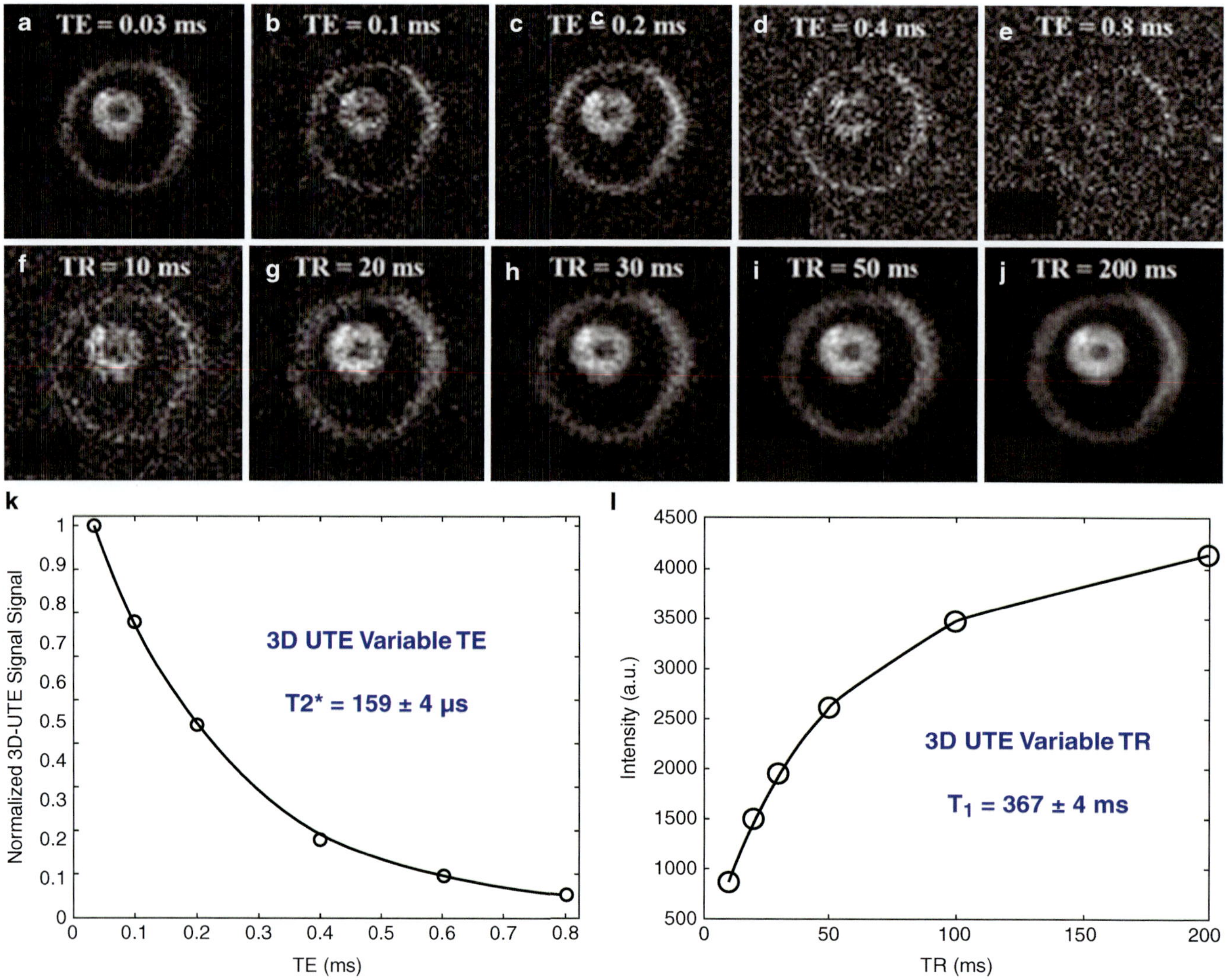

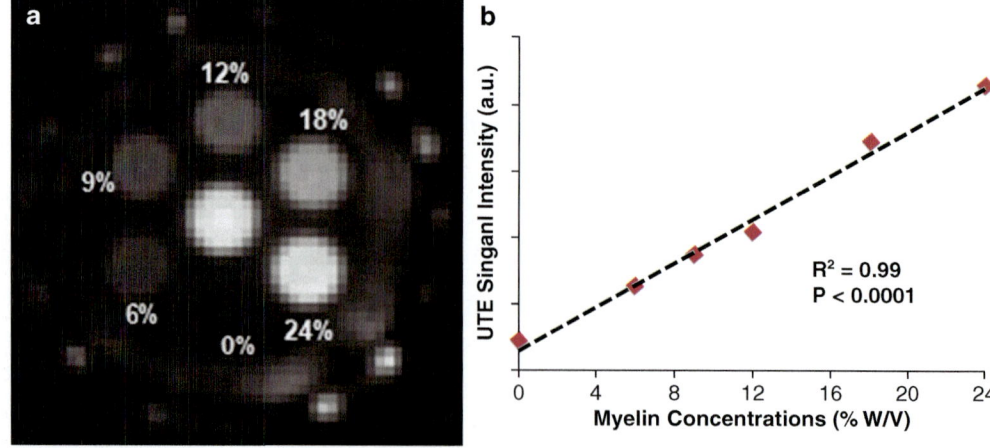

Fig. 40.2 UTE imaging of intact myelin vesicles with a constant repetition time (TR) of 100 ms but varying TEs of 0.03 ms (**a**), 0.1 ms (**b**), 0.2 ms (**c**), 0.4 ms (**d**), and 0.8 ms (**e**) and a constant TE of 0.03 ms but varying TRs of 10 ms (**f**), (20 ms (**g**), 30 ms (**h**), 50 ms (**i**), and 200 ms (**j**) as well as single-component exponential signal decay fitting, which shows a T_2^* of 225 ± 7 µs (**k**), and single-component exponential signal recovery fitting, which shows a T_1 of 367 ± 4 ms (**l**). The central black hole is hard plastic ("invisible" in UTE imaging). (Reproduced with permission from Ma et al. [40])

Fig. 40.3 (**a**) UTE imaging of myelin–D_2O phantoms with myelin concentrations ranging from 0 to 24% weight/volume (W/V). (**b**) A high linear correlation was observed between UTE signal intensity and myelin concentration ($R^2 = 0.99$; $P < 0.0001$), demonstrating that the UTE sequence can directly image and quantify myelin using a clinical whole-body 3 T scanner. (Reproduced with permission from Ma et al. [41])

UTE Imaging of Myelin: Contrast Mechanisms

The phantom studies described above demonstrate that the basic UTE sequence can detect signals directly from the non-aqueous myelin protons. However, myelin only represents a small fraction of the total UTE signal from the brain, with the dominant signal coming from the long-T_2 white matter (WM_L) and the long-T_2 gray matter (GM_L) [45]. It is essential to suppress the long-T_2 water signals (i.e., intra/extracellular water, myelin water, and cerebrospinal fluid (CSF)) to generate high-contrast images of myelin. A series of contrast mechanisms have been developed to effectively suppress signals from long-T_2 water components while leaving ultrashort-T_2 myelin components to be detected. Details of these contrast mechanisms are described below.

Long-T_2-Saturated UTE

In this approach, a long-duration, low-amplitude 90° pulse is used to flip the long-T_2 magnetization into the transverse plane, where it is eventually spoiled by a large crusher gradient [48, 49]. The short-T_2 magnetization experiences significant transverse relaxation during the long saturation process, leading to it having largely unchanged longitudinal magnetization, which is subsequently detected after RF excitation by UTE data acquisition (Fig. 40.4a) [49]. Long-T_2-saturated UTE imaging has been applied to short- and ultrashort-T_2 components in the musculoskeletal system (e.g., the Achilles tendon and menisci) and the brain (e.g., myelin) [48]. In long-T_2-saturated UTE imaging, a key parameter is the time bandwidth product of the saturation pulse. Rectangular pulses, single-band pulses, and dual-band pulses have all

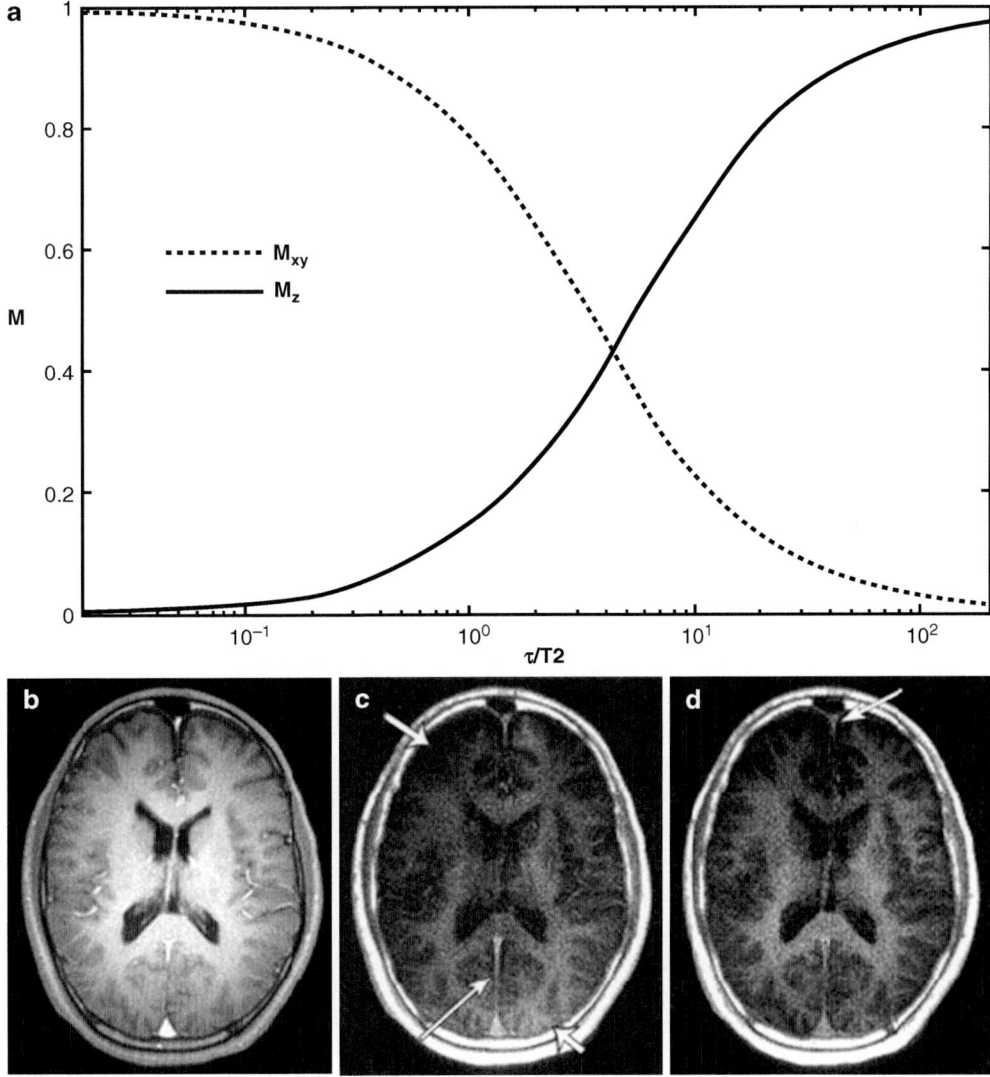

Fig. 40.4 Simulation of longitudinal (M_z) and transverse (M_{xy}) magnetizations as a function of τ/T_2, where τ is the duration of a simple rectangular 90° saturation pulse (**a**) and selected UTE MR images of the brain in a healthy volunteer without long-T_2 suppression (**b**), with a 16-ms rectangular suppression pulse (**c**) and with a single-band suppression pulse (duration = 40 ms, time–bandwidth product = 2.4) (**d**). Short- and ultrashort-T_2 myelin components in the WM and the falx cerebri (long, thin arrows in panels **c** and **d**) are highlighted only after the application of the long-T_2 suppression pulses. More robust long-T_2 signal suppression is achieved with the single-band pulse (**d**) than with the rectangular pulse, which produces variable long-T_2 signal suppression across the slice (shorter, wider arrows) (**c**). (Reproduced with permission from Larson et al. [48] and Sussman et al. [49])

been systematically investigated to study the relationship between long-T_2 suppression efficiency and spectral profile sharpness. Figure 40.4b–d shows UTE imaging of the brain in a healthy volunteer both with and without long-T_2 saturation. The regular UTE sequence is T_1-weighted and shows a high signal from all tissue components with relatively short T_1s (CSF has a long T_1 and its signal is low). The ultrashort-T_2 components in the WM are only specifically highlighted after the application of long-T_2 saturation pulses. This ultrashort-T_2 component is lost in patients with MS [48]. A major limitation of the long-T_2 saturation pulse is its sensitivity to off-resonance effects, which can lead to incomplete long-T_2 signal suppression. Another limitation is its sensitivity to short-T_1 contamination. The short-T_2 contrast may be degraded due to fast signal recovery during the saturation recovery period from tissues with long T_2s but short T_1s such as fat. The long-T_2 saturation technique is also sensitive to B_1 inhomogeneity, which may lead to significant residual long-T_2 signals, which compromise short- and ultrashort-T_2 contrast.

Off-Resonance Saturated UTE

In this approach, a high-power saturation pulse is placed a few kilohertz (kHz) away from the water peak, followed by regular UTE data acquisition [50]. The nonaqueous myelin protons with ultrashort T_2s have much broader spectral absorption line shapes than long-T_2 water components in the brain and are therefore more sensitive to effects from appropriately placed off-resonance irradiation. The saturation pulse can preferentially saturate signals from myelin and leave long-T_2 water signals largely unaffected. Signals from the various water components can be effectively suppressed by subtraction of UTE images with and without off-resonance irradiation, thereby creating high contrast imaging of myelin [50]. Off-resonance saturation can also create high phase contrast for myelin. Myelin contributes minimally to phase contrast in conventional clinical MRI due to the lack of detectable signals. There is little phase contrast between the GM and WM in regular UTE imaging. However, off-resonance saturated UTE imaging can provide high phase contrast in the brain even at a nominal TE of 106 µs [50]. Figure 40.5 shows off-resonance saturated UTE imaging, which provides reversed phase contrast between the GM and WM when compared to conventional MRI [50]. Both magnitude and phase UTE images of the saturated components were calculated using complex subtraction, where the saturated signal component of combined GM and CSF has a positive phase shift, whereas that of the WM primarily shows

a negative phase shift [50]. CSF has a similar positive phase shift with both UTE and conventional gradient echo phase images, but WM shows the opposite shift. As a result, off-resonance saturated UTE phase images can potentially improve the characterization of tissue microstructure in the brain by indirectly accessing myelin, thus providing a new way of demonstrating phase contrast in the brain [50].

Inversion Recovery UTE (IR-UTE)

In this approach (Fig. 40.6), a long-duration adiabatic inversion pulse (Silver-Hoult, ~8 ms in duration) is used to invert the longitudinal magnetizations of long-T_2 components in the white matter (WM$_L$) and the gray matter (GM$_L$) [32]. Nonaqueous myelin protons have ultrashort T_2 or T_2*s, and, therefore, their longitudinal magnetizations are largely saturated by the adiabatic inversion pulse due to fast transverse relaxation during the long inversion process [51]. Signals from myelin are selectively detected when UTE data acquisitions start at the inversion time (TI) necessary for the inverted longitudinal magnetization of WM$_L$ to reach its null point. There are some residual signals from the GM$_L$ due to its longer T_1. These are detected by a dual-echo initial UTE FID and later gradient echo data acquisitions. As the myelin signal quickly decays to near zero, the second echo only acquires signals from the non-nulled GM$_L$. Subtraction of the second echo image from the first one selectively detects signals from myelin in the WM [37]. Details of this contrast mechanism are shown in Fig. 40.6a, b. Myelin has an ultrashort T_2 of sub-milliseconds, which is far shorter than the duration of the adiabatic inversion pulse. Its longitudinal magnetization is largely saturated by the long adiabatic inversion pulse and, subsequently, recovers relatively quickly because of its short T_1 [52]. As a result, at the null point, the WM signal mainly comes from myelin. In the GM, the signal changes are more complicated. On the UTE FID image, in the GM, the positive longitudinal magnetization from myelin and the negative longitudinal magnetization from the GM$_L$ produce a net reduction in the magnitude of the transverse magnetization. At the second echo (e.g., TE ~ 2 ms), the myelin signal in the GM decays to zero, whereas the signal from the GM$_L$ largely remains unchanged due to its much longer T_2*. Therefore, the detected magnitude signal of the GM is greater at the second echo than at the FID. As a result, the GM has a higher magnitude signal at the second echo than at the FID (Fig. 40.6b). Subtraction of the second echo from the FID generates a positive signal for myelin in the WM but a negative signal for myelin in the GM, thus creating high myelin contrast between the two tissues (Fig. 40.6e).

Fig. 40.5 The off-resonance saturated UTE sequence. This employs two consecutive 180° adiabatic RF pulses for off-resonance saturation, a minimum-phase RF pulse for signal excitation, and 3D radial sampling with multiple spokes acquired after each saturation pulse for improved acquisition efficiency (**a**). Selected magnitude (**b**) and phase (**c**) UTE images of the saturated signal components obtained with a TE of 106 μs and a saturation frequency of −1.2 kHz. The UTE phase images demonstrate negative phase shifts in the WM and positive phase shifts in CSF (**c**). (Reproduced with permission from Wei et al. [50])

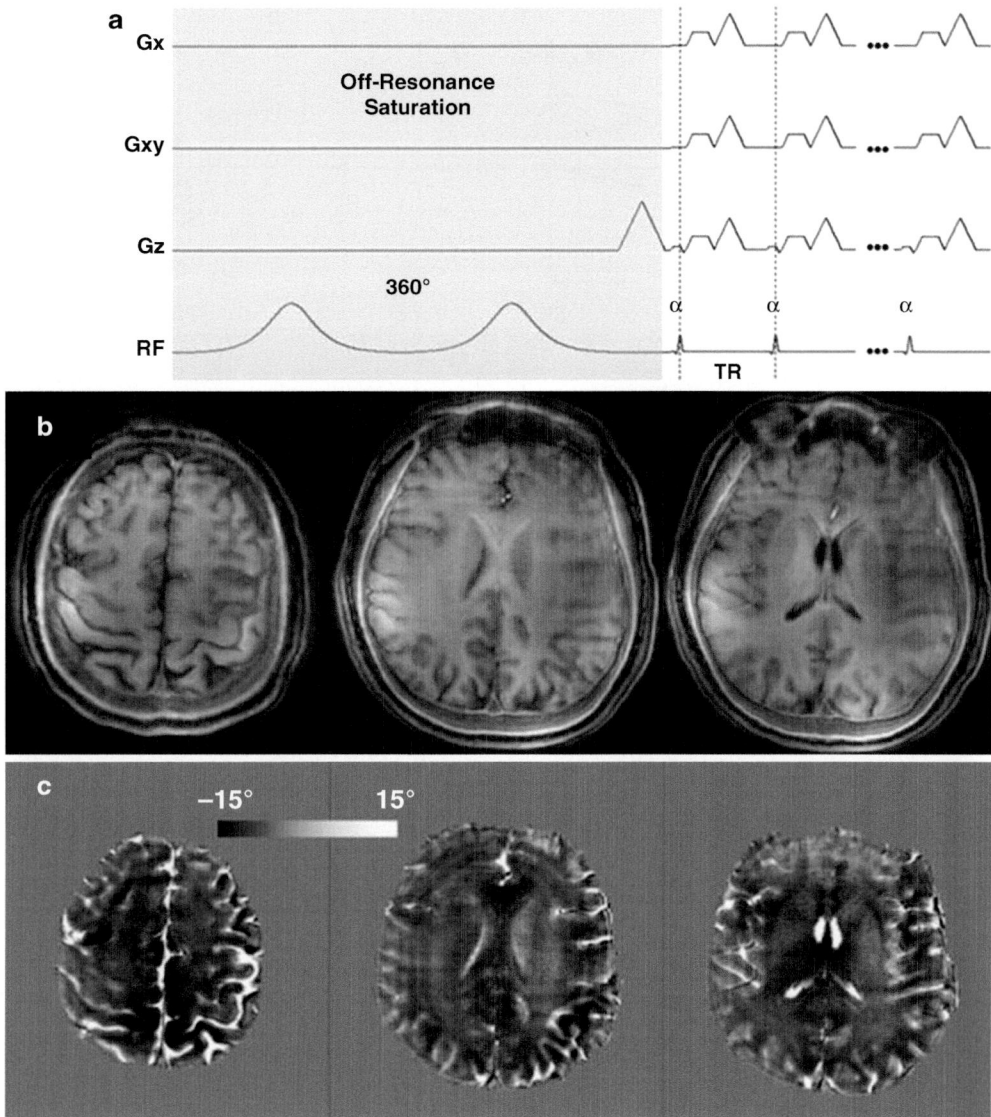

Double Echo Sliding Inversion Recovery UTE (DESIRE-UTE)

In this approach (Fig. 40.7a), a train of 3D dual-echo UTE spokes (e.g., a total number of N_{sp}) are acquired after a single adiabatic IR preparation [40]. There are four key components in DESIRE-UTE imaging. First, a sufficient number of continuous image spokes (e.g., 71) are sequentially acquired to cover a wide range of TIs, including all potential null points for long-T_1 and long-T_2 tissues or tissue components, such as WM_L and GM_L; second, random gradient encoding is used so that any number of spokes can cover the 3D k-space as uniformly as possible; third, dual-echo UTE data are acquired for each spoke; and fourth, an advanced sliding window image reconstruction technique together with parallel imaging and/or compressed sensing (CS) is used to reduce undersampling artifacts. To find TI_{null}

accurately, a series of images with different TIs are generated. Acquisition spokes are grouped together by a window with a fixed size of N_w, and these N_w spokes are in the window that is subsequently used to generate a single image (Fig. 40.7a). The window starts sliding from the very first N_w spokes with the shortest TI and then slides one spoke each time to generate a new image with a slightly longer effective TI. The total number (N) of groups or images is equal to $N_{sp} - N_w + 1$. This sliding window technique generates a series of images with different T_1-dependent contrasts with the goal of using these individual images to determine the best nulling TI for WM_L and GM_L. The TI_{null} can be found when the signal in the WM reaches a minimum, or the noise level in the second echo image, where the long-T_2 components are nulled and the myelin signal decays to zero. The optimal nulling point can be achieved for each pixel, and voxel-based subtraction of the second

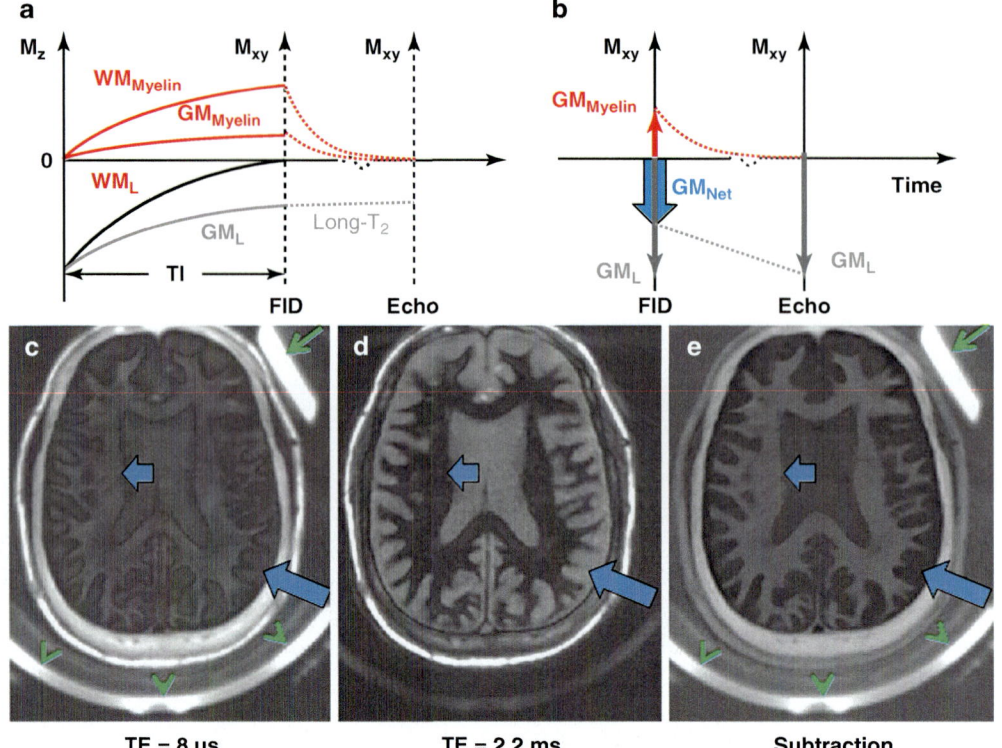

Fig. 40.6 The contrast mechanism in IR-UTE imaging of myelin in the white matter (WM_{myelin}) (**a**), where UTE data acquisition starts at a TI set to null signals from the long-T_2 white matter (WM_L), with a negative longitudinal magnetization from the long-T_2 gray matter (GM_L) due to its longer T_1. The myelin magnetization is largely saturated by the adiabatic inversion pulse due to its ultrashort T_2 ($T_2 << 1$ ms). At the null point, the GM signal includes the positive myelin (GM_{Myelin}) and the negative GM_L. At the second echo, the myelin signal decays to near zero with little change in the GM_L. Subtraction of the magnitude second echo from the magnitude first one produces high positive contrast for WM_{myelin} but negative contrast for the GM (**b**). IR-UTE imaging of the brain in a healthy volunteer with TEs of 8 μs (**c**) and 2.2 ms (**d**) as well as the echo subtraction image with a positive myelin signal (short thick arrows) in the WM and a negative myelin signal in the GM (long thick arrows) (**e**). Rubber (long thin arrow) and pads (arrow heads) have short T_2s and are readily seen with the UTE images (**c** and **e**) but are invisible on the second echo image (**d**)

echo image from the first one provides myelin imaging with optimal suppression of WM_L and GM_L. Different subjects may have different TI_{null}s due to the T_1 variations among volunteers and patients. Even different regions within the same brain may have significant T_1 variations. T_1 variation across the different brain regions or due to aging or pathological changes is a major challenge in single IR-UTE imaging where the optimal nulling point cannot be achieved for all brain regions, leading to significant long-T_2 signal contamination. The DESIRE-UTE sequence addresses this challenge and minimizes water signal contamination, thus providing more accurate myelin mapping across the whole brain [40]. DESIRE-UTE imaging of the brain of a healthy volunteer is shown in Fig. 40.7a–d. The normalized signal intensity curves for a region of interest (ROI) drawn in a WM region (yellow circle) for both the first echo image and the second echo image, respectively, are also displayed (Fig. 40.7e). The TI_{null} for WM_L can be accurately deter-

mined by choosing the signal nulling point for the second echo ($N_{img} = 26$ in this case), as indicated by the arrow. The dual-echo images and the corresponding subtraction images close to the WM_L nulling point are also displayed. A N_{img} of 26 provides the highest myelin contrast with the most complete water suppression. For shorter TIs (i.e., $N_{img} < 26$), a lower myelin signal is observed because of the cancelation of positive magnetization from myelin and negative magnetization from WM_L. For longer TIs (i.e., $N_{img} > 26$), a higher myelin signal is observed because of the residual positive magnetization from WM_L, which adds to that of myelin, leading to a higher signal level. DESIRE-UTE detected myelin loss in MS lesions ex vivo and in vivo that have been shown with clinical T_1- and T_2-weighted sequences, respectively [40]. Histological validation of quantitative myelin loss and clinical evaluation of the 3D DESIRE-UTE technique for volumetric myelin mapping remain to be investigated.

Fig. 40.7 The DESIRE-UTE contrast mechanism (**a**), in which a single adiabatic inversion pulse is followed by a train of 3D dual-echo UTE spokes (*N*). A sliding window reconstruction technique is used to generate a series of images with gradually increasing TIs. Spokes within a window size are used to generate a single image. The window starts at the beginning and slides forward one spoke each time to generate a new image. The spokes are randomly ordered for data sampling to ensure that each group of spokes is uniformly distributed in the *k*-space. Selected 3D DESIRE-UTE images of the brain of a healthy volunteer for the first echo (Echo1) (**b**), the second echo (Echo2) (**c**), the echo subtraction images (**d**), and the signal intensity curves as a function of the reconstructed DESIRE-UTE image numbers (corresponding to different TIs) for an ROI in the WM for the first echo (red curve) and the second echo (green curve) (**e**). Selective myelin images are achieved when the second echo signal reaches the minimum (complete nulling of long-T_2 signal components). (Reproduced with permission from Ma et al. [40])

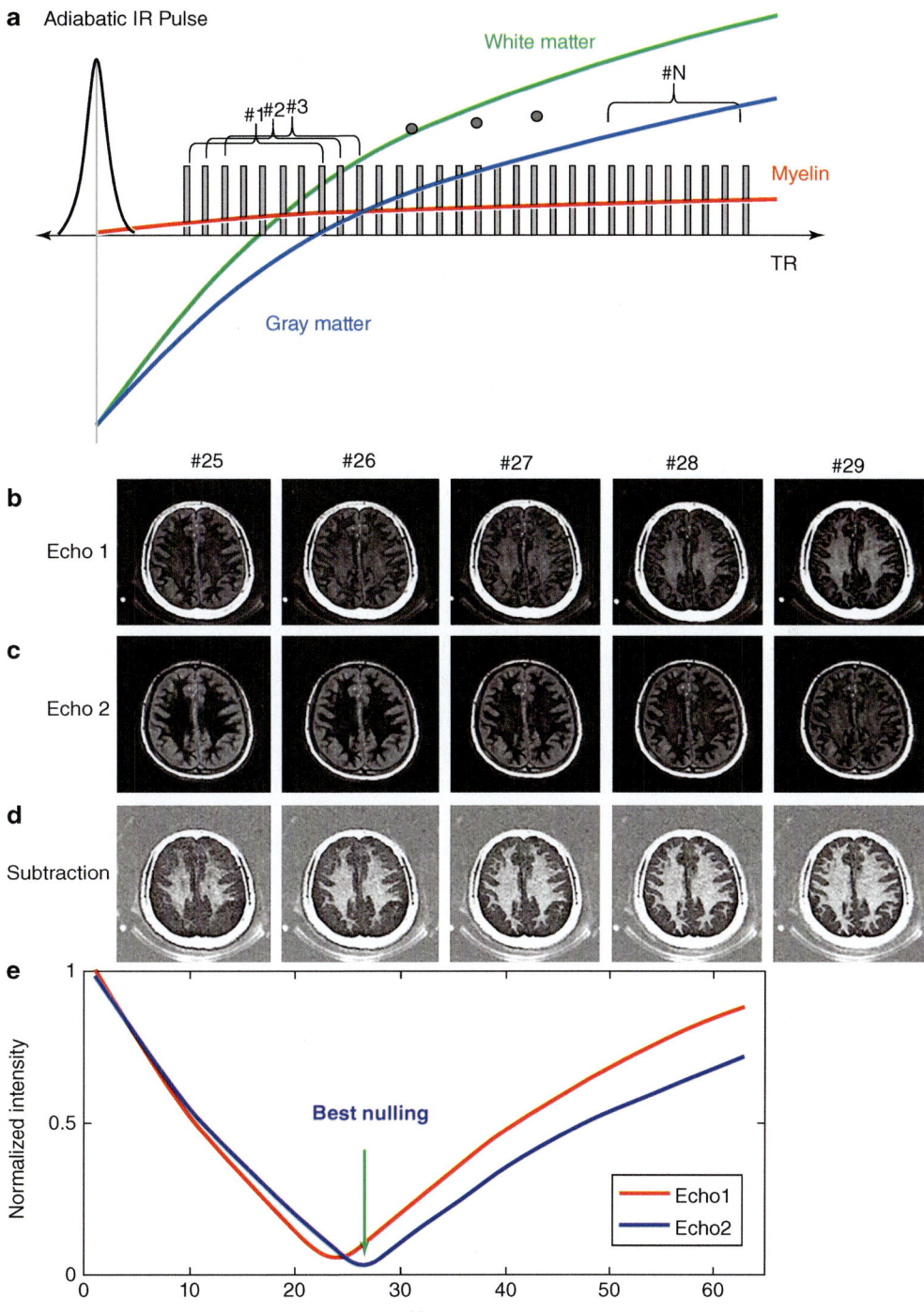

Short TR Adiabatic Inversion Recovery UTE (STAIR-UTE)

In this approach (Fig. 40.8a), a short TR and a high flip angle are used together with 3D IR-UTE imaging [38]. It is similar to regular IR-UTE imaging, but the TR is kept as short as possible and the flip angle is kept as high as possible within limits imposed by the specific absorption rate (SAR)

allowed for clinical imaging. The use of an extremely short TR and TI combination maximizes the suppression of signals from long-T_2 tissues with T_1s greater than a threshold [38]. This is extremely important as the brain WM and GM have various water components, including intra/extracellular water ($T_2 \sim 40$–130 ms, $T_1 \sim 800$–1800 ms), myelin-bound water (or myelin water, $T_2 \sim 10$–20 ms, $T_1 \sim 200$ ms), and CSF ($T_2 > 200$ ms, $T_1 > 3000$ ms), all of which have

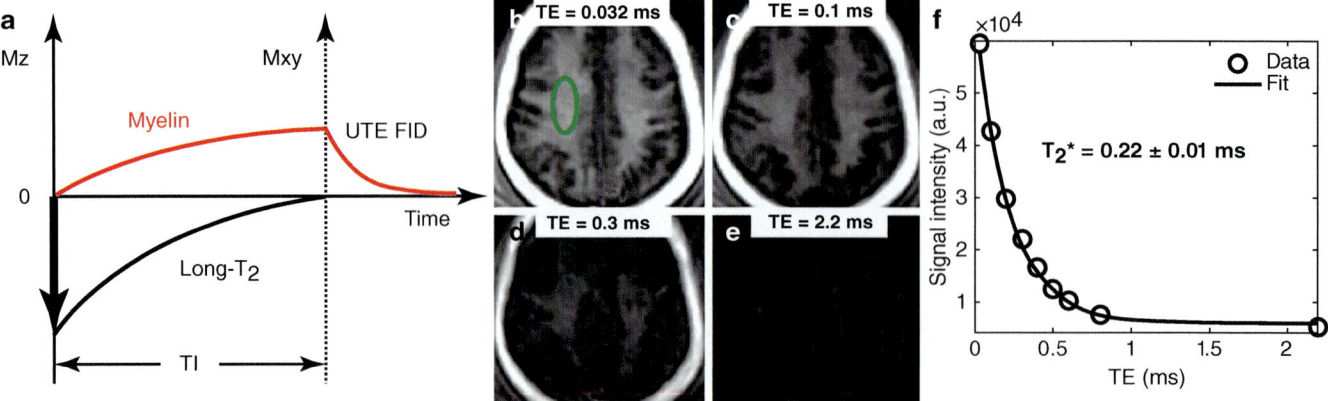

Fig. 40.8 The 3D STAIR-UTE sequence uses a short TR (e.g., TR ~ 150 ms or shorter) and a short TI (e.g., ~64 ms) to suppress long-T_2 signals (**a**). Its efficacy is demonstrated by STAIR-UTE imaging of the brain in a 29-year-old volunteer with TEs of 0.032 (**b**), 0.1 (**c**), 0.3 (**d**), and 2.2 ms (**e**) as well as by exponential fitting of the STAIR-UTE signal for the WM, which shows a T_2^* of 0.22 ± 0.01 ms (**f**), consistent with effective long-T_2 signal suppression. (Reproduced with permission from Ma et al. [38])

higher proton densities than myelin [53–56]. The various water components in the normal-appearing white matter (NAWM), normal-appearing gray matter (NAGM), and lesions have an even wider range of T_1s due to pathology, which make it difficult to null all water signals using a single inversion pulse when regular IR-UTE imaging is used. By shortening the TR, the nulling points for different T_1s approach each other, making it possible to suppress all water components above a certain minimum T_1. Numerical simulation shows that efficient water signal suppression can be achieved with TRs shorter than 150 ms [38]. The highest flip angle allowed by SAR requirements should be used in STAIR-UTE imaging as myelin has a shorter T_1 than water components, and T_1 weighting increases myelin contrast [52]. Multiple spokes can be acquired after each adiabatic inversion pulse to speed up data acquisition. This provides fast volumetric imaging of myelin across the whole brain. Figure 40.8b–f shows selected 3D STAIR-UTE images of the brain in a 29-year-old female volunteer at different TEs [38]. Long-T_2 water signals from the WM, GM, and CSF are all efficiently suppressed, leaving ultrashort-T_2^* signals from the skull and nonaqueous myelin protons to be detected. The excellent single-component exponential fitting of the STAIR-UTE signal decay shows an ultrashort T_2^* of 0.22 ± 0.01 ms, which is extremely close to the T_2^*s of lyophilized myelin powder and intact myelin vesicles, suggesting that myelin is being selectively imaged [38].

Hybrid Filling Zero Echo Time (HYFI-ZTE)

In this approach (Fig. 40.9a), ZTE with multiple radial readouts at full and lowered gradient strengths and single-point imaging (SPI) strategies are combined to efficiently sample 3D k-space with a minimized timing delay [44].

Maximal short-T_2 sensitivity is achieved by performing RF excitation only after ramping up the readout gradient. The central k-space data missed during the RF dead-time are filled with the hybrid filling (HYFI) strategy, which uses a combination of multiple radial readouts at a lowered gradient strength and SPI. Figure 40.9b, c further illustrates the time of acquisition for different k-space radii. The extremely central k-space data are acquired with SPI after a Δt or TE of 15 μs. Later acquisition is allowed within a certain duration t_{acq} during the radial HYFI parts. The ZTE data are collected during an acquisition range T_k at full gradient strength G. The HYFI strategy improves the scan efficiency in ZTE imaging with large dead-time gaps for direct imaging of myelin. Two HYFI datasets can be acquired with TEs of 15 μs and 460 μs, respectively. Subtraction of the two sets of data provides excellent long-T_2 signal suppression and creates high contrast for myelin. Figure 40.9d shows in vivo myelin images of a healthy volunteer, in which high contrast imaging of myelin is achieved by subtracting the HYFI-ZTE images with a TE of 460 μs from those with a TE of 15 μs. Short-T_2 blurring is minimized using a high-performance gradient insert with an extremely high slew rate of 600 mT/m/ms and a maximum gradient amplitude of 200 mT/m [44]. A challenge in HYFI-ZTE imaging of myelin lies in potential signal contamination from short-T_2 water components (e.g., myelin water, which has a relatively short T_2^* and T_1). Myelin water may experience significant signal decay during the longer TE, leading to signal contamination in the subtraction images. The HYFI-ZTE sequence may also be sensitive to B_1 inhomogeneity, leading to spatially dependent myelin water signal contamination. More myelin water contamination is expected in regions with stronger B_1s and thus higher HYFI-ZTE signal intensity. Long-T_2 suppression schemes, especially adiabatic IR preparation such as DESIRE or STAIR, can be

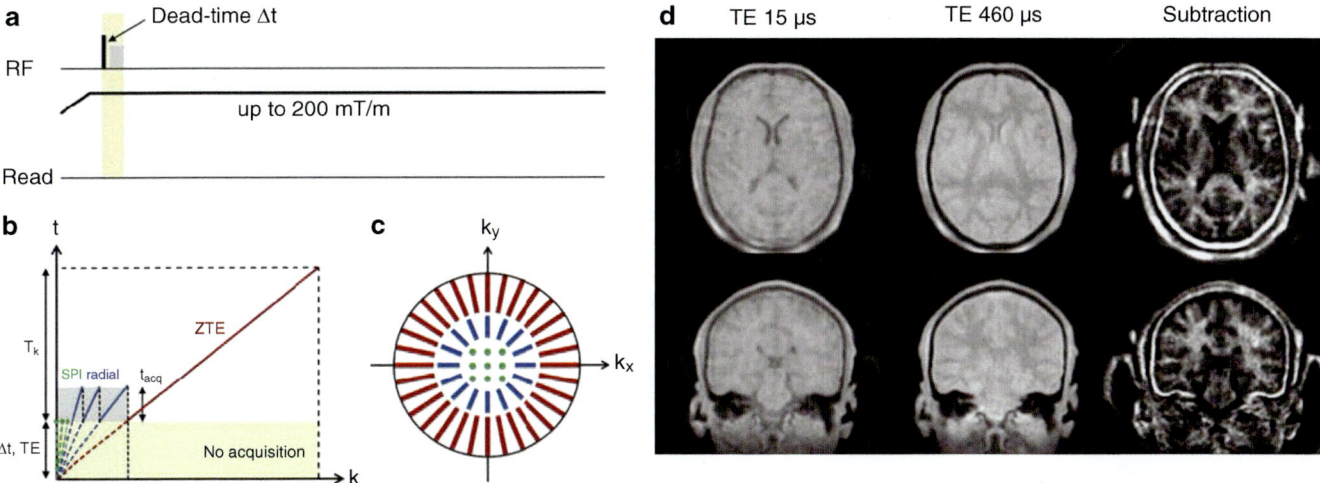

Fig. 40.9 The HYFI-ZTE sequence. This employs a short RF pulse for signal excitation after the readout gradient of amplitude up to 200 mT/m to minimize short-T_2 decay (**a**). Additional data for the central k-space locations missed during the RF dead-time between excitation and acquisition are efficiently collected with a combination of multiple radial acquisitions at lower gradient strength and SPI (**b**), where the time of acquisition t of the data is plotted as a function of the k-space radius k. Radial center-out encoding is performed, and data are acquired at the earliest time possible after the RF dead-time Δt. Data missed during Δt (yellow-shaded range, dashed lines) lead to a gap in the central k-space, which is filled with multiple sets of ZTE readouts of decreasing gradient amplitudes followed by SPI readouts at the very center. The acquisition duration t_{acq} of HYFI (gray-shaded region) is chosen based on a compromise between scan efficiency and the maximum decay acceptable for a targeted short T_2. The sampling duration T_k is an indicator of the resolution loss expected for a given T_2. A diagram of the k-space acquisition pattern is illustrated in panel (**c**), where colors indicate the different parts of the acquisition described in panel (**b**). In vivo imaging of ultrashort-T_2 tissue components in the human brain using the hybrid filling (HYFI) technique with TEs of 15 μs and 460 μs, respectively, and the subtraction images are shown in panel (**d**). The images acquired with a TE of 15 μs and a short acquisition range of 29 μs show little GM–WM contrast. A longer TE of 460 μs leads to a visibly reduced signal in the WM. Subtraction of the two datasets largely removes the long-T_2 signal and shows predominantly ultrashort-T_2 components (presumably myelin) with clear contrast between the GM and WM. Other short-T_2 signals visible in the images are from the skull, skin, and earmuffs. (Reproduced with permission from Weiger et al. [44])

combined with HYFI-ZTE for more robust suppression of long-T_2 signals and so potentially reduce water signal contamination.

Inversion Recovery Interleaved Hybrid Encoding (IR-IHE)

In this approach (Fig. 40.10a–c), dual-echo hybrid encoding datasets are acquired following a long adiabatic pulse preparation [57]. In hybrid encoding, readout gradients are applied before the RF coil dead-time to optimize the encoding time. The missing k-space due to the dead-time (blind time during RF transmit/receive switching) is filled by utilizing the SPI strategy. Zero gradient excitation-based hybrid encoding is employed to allow slab selection to reduce aliasing/streaking artifacts, utilizing a Shinnar–Le Roux pulse (pulse width = 1132 μs, bandwidth = 16 kHz) with minimum phase, isodelay, and variable-rate selective excitation (VERSE) specially designed for UTE imaging [58]. Due to the long scan time associated with 3D UTE imaging of myelin with efficient long-T_2 signal suppression, it is essential to acquire multiple spokes after each inversion pulse preparation for time-efficient data acquisition. However, there is a trade-off in this approach as the myelin image contrast is degraded due to spokes acquired at suboptimal TIs for WM signal suppression. A strategy of interleaving SPI encodings between radial frequency encodings is employed to address this issue. In conventional hybrid encoding techniques such as pointwise encoding time reduction with radial acquisition (PETRA) [59] and ramped hybrid encoding (RHE) [60], the radial frequency encoding and the SPI encoding are performed separately, one after the other. However, this approach is not suitable for multispoke IR imaging because the central k-space is encoded by SPI, which may significantly compromise the myelin contrast due to using suboptimal TIs. The IR-IHE approach addresses this limitation by interleaving SPI encodings in the time slot near the optimal TI so that the data in the central region of the k-space are acquired with the best nulling TIs. As a result, the IR-IHE sequence provides more efficient suppression of the long-T_2 water signals. Figure 40.10d shows a comparison between regular IR-prepared hybrid encoding (IR-HE) and IR-IHE imaging in a 30-year-old male volunteer [57]. The strategy of inter-

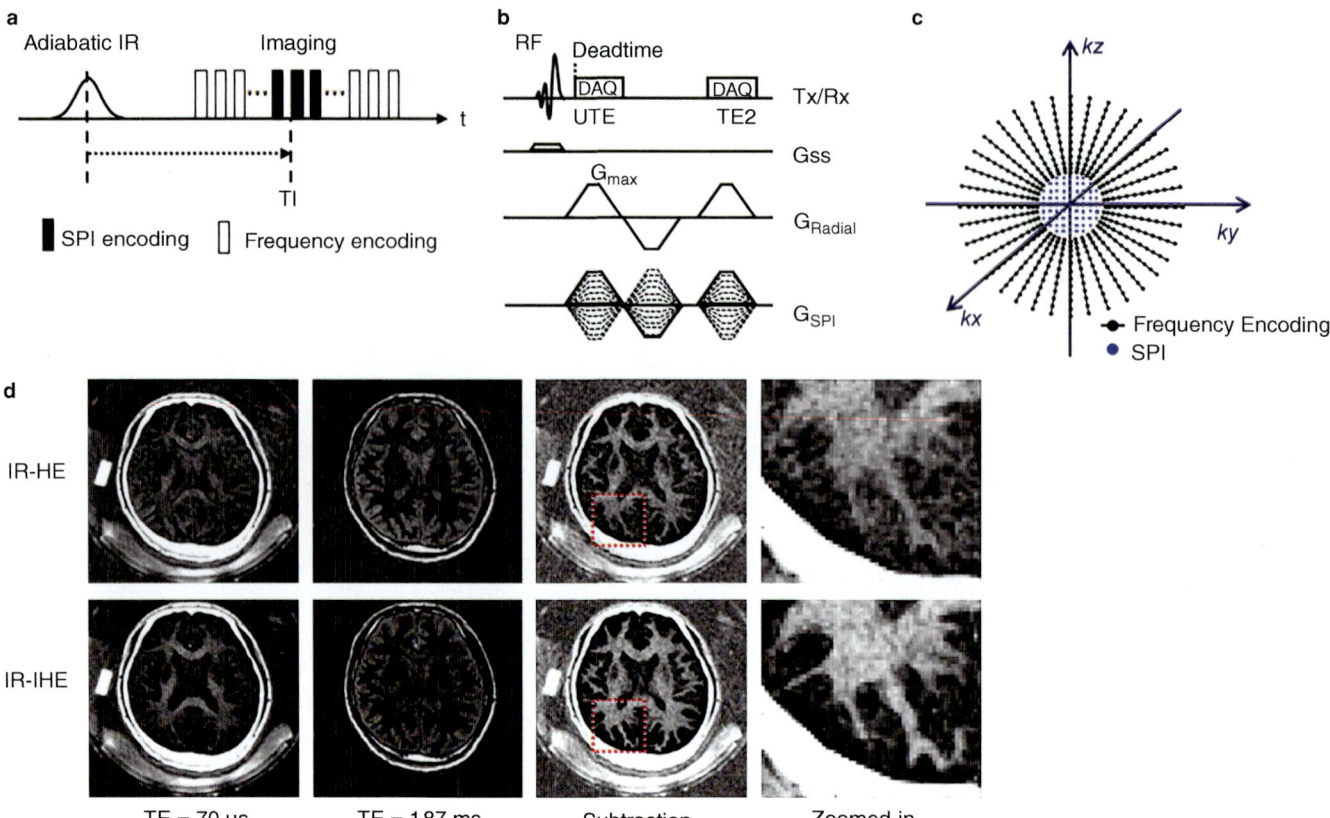

Fig. 40.10 The IR-IHE sequence employs an adiabatic inversion pulse for long-T_2 signal suppression, followed by interleaved multispoke sampling (**a**), with dual-echo hybrid encoding used for data sampling (**b**). The central k-space is sampled with the SPI strategy, and the outer k-space is sampled with radial frequency encoding (**c**). The SPI encoding is interleaved near the optimal TI for more efficient suppression of signals from long-T_2 WM. IR-HE and IR-IHE imaging of a 30-year-old healthy male volunteer with a first TE of 70 µs and a second TE of 1.87 ms and echo subtraction that shows the efficacy of interleaving SPI encoding in reducing water contamination and imaging artifacts, thereby improving myelin contrast (**d**). (Reproduced with permission from Jang et al. [57])

leaving SPI in the IR-IHE dramatically improves the myelin contrast as can be seen in the zoomed-in view, with the contrast-to-noise ratio (CNR) between myelin and the surrounding tissues more than doubled. This improvement has been confirmed by computer simulation [57]. The IR-IHE sequence also provides high contrast imaging of myelin loss in patients with MS in lesions identified with clinical magnetization-prepared rapid gradient echo (MP-RAGE) and T_2-weighted fluid attenuated IR (T_2-FLAIR) sequences [57].

UTE Imaging of Myelin: Further Validation

Animal Validation Study

Cuprizone treatment provides a frequently used toxicant-induced model of MS [61]. Cuprizone causes rapid demyelination and gliosis or rapid proliferation of glia subtypes when administered orally in mice. The cuprizone mouse model captures several aspects of MS pathology and bypasses the autoimmune component present in other preclinical models. In the model used in this study, male C57BL/6 mice at 6–9 weeks of age were fed a diet of chow mixed with 0.2% cuprizone over the course of 6 weeks. Acute demyelination was observed in the corpus callosum by the third week. Demyelination reached a maximum in the sixth week. When mice were returned to a normal diet, robust remyelination occurred in the corpus callosum, and this reached completion after ~4 weeks. The cuprizone mouse model has been widely used to study demyelination and remyelination in MS. In a preliminary study, six C57BL/6 mice, three treated with 0.2% cuprizone chow for 5 weeks and three controls, were scanned with conventional 2D T_2-FSE and 3D IR-UTE sequences on a Bruker 7 T scanner. Advanced Normalization Tools (ANTs) were used to create a common template from the control brains [62]. The treated brains were registered to this common template. Figure 40.11a–c shows coronal 2D T_2-FSE and 3D IR-UTE imaging of a control mouse. The cortical bone in the skull and myelin in the WM are depicted with a high signal and contrast on IR-UTE imaging but are "invisible" in conventional FSE imaging. Figure 40.11d–f shows the registered naïve littermates and 5-week cuprizone-

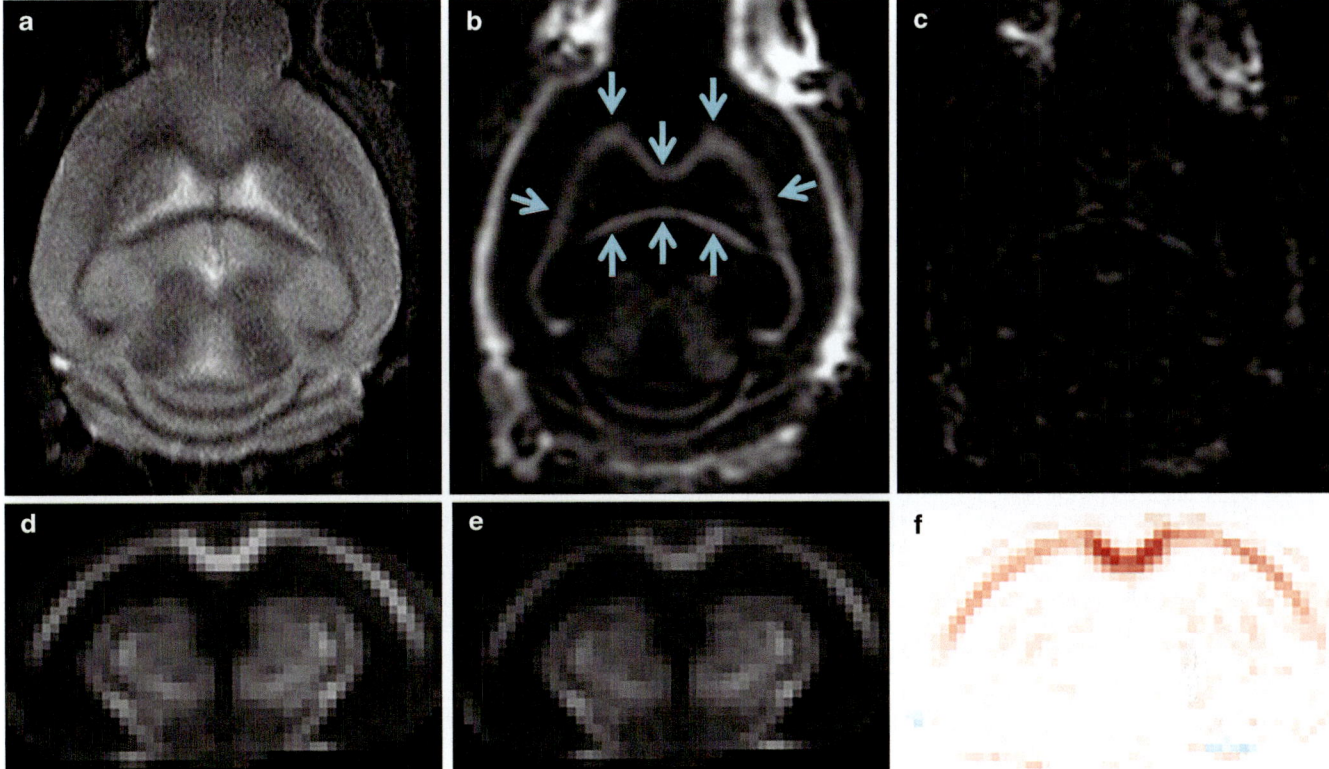

Fig. 40.11 A C57BL/6 mouse imaged with T_2-FSE (**a**), IR-UTE sequences at a TE of 0.020 ms (**b**) and 2 ms (windowed 10×) (**c**), where myelin (arrows) signals dropped to the noise level. The mean IR-UTE signal from untreated (**d**) and cuprizone-treated (**e**) mice. The IR-UTE images were registered to a common template (**f**). Coronal images at the level of splenium corpus callosum (**d–f**) show obvious myelin loss in treated mice as confirmed by Luxol fast blue (LFB) staining (results not shown)

treated mice, demonstrating obvious loss of myelin in treated mice, as confirmed by histology (results not shown). These results show that 3D IR-UTE sequences can directly image myelin and detect its loss in mice.

Cadaveric Human Brain Validation Study

UTE imaging of myelin was further validated on a cadaveric human head (a 45-year-old male donor) obtained from a nonprofit whole-body donation company (United Tissue Network, Phoenix, AZ, USA). The head specimen was initially stored at −80 °C, thawed in water at 4 °C overnight, and then thawed for 18 hours in gently agitated water at room temperature before the MRI examination. The whole head was then scanned with conventional clinical magnetization prepared rapid gradient echo (MP-RAGE) and T_2-FSE as well as 3D IR-UTE sequences. After MRI, the specimen was refrozen at −80 °C and then cut into 1.0-cm axial sections using a band saw (B16, Butcher Boy Machines, Selmer, TN, USA). ROIs were identified on review of the MR images, located on the gross slice of brain, and resected. Samples were fixed in zinc formalin (Anatech, Battle Creek, MI) for 1 week, paraffin-embedded, and sectioned at 5- and 10-μm thicknesses. Slides were stained overnight in LFB at 60 °C and briefly counterstained with neutral red. Figure 40.12 shows comparisons of selected clinical and 3D IR-UTE images of this MS brain specimen [41]. The bright signals in 3D IR-UTE images have T_2*s around ~0.20 ms, which is close to the T_2* of myelin powder phantoms shown in Fig. 40.1 and intact myelin vesicles shown in Fig. 40.2, suggesting that the signal source is from nonaqueous myelin protons. MS lesions identified in the MP-RAGE and T_2-FSE images show myelin signal loss in the corresponding regions on the IR-UTE images, with representative lesions subsequently confirmed by histology as demyelinated (Fig. 40.12b). Similar results have also been confirmed with 3D DESIRE-UTE and STAIR-UTE imaging, showing that myelin can be selectively imaged ex vivo.

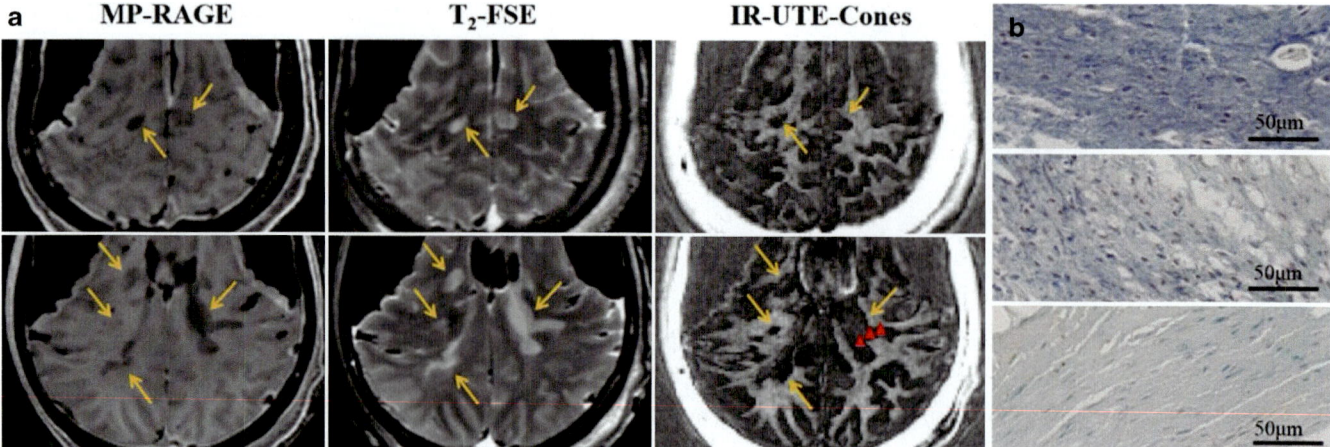

Fig. 40.12 A brain specimen from a 45-year-old male donor with confirmed MS was scanned using clinical T₁-weighted MP-RAGE, T₂-weighted FSE, and 3D IR-UTE sequences (**a**). The 3D IR-UTE sequence shows signal loss in the MS lesion (yellow arrows). Tissue blocks used for histology were chosen based on 3D MP-RAGE images, at sites where MS lesions and NAWM could be accurately located. Representative histological images of a sample MS lesion using LFB as a myelin stain, counterstained with neutral red, are shown in panel (**b**). The three histological images from top to bottom were obtained from locations indicated by the red arrowheads from top to bottom in the respective 3D IR-UTE images, corresponding to regions of the NAWM (top), lesion edge (middle), and within the lesion (bottom), with specific loss of myelin demonstrated in the MS lesion (**b**). (Reproduced with permission from Ma et al. [41])

UTE Imaging of Myelin in Multiple Sclerosis

Morphological UTE Imaging of Myelin in Multiple Sclerosis

MRI is of paramount importance for imaging in MS due to its high diagnostic performance in detecting lesions, monitoring disease progression, and evaluating treatment effects [19]. In the routine clinical setting, T₂-weighted fluid attenuated IR (T₂-FLAIR), T₂-weighted FSE, and T₁-weighted MP-RAGE sequences are used for detecting focal WM lesions in MS [3–5]. MS mainly presents with multiple focal lesions with a low signal on T₁-weighted MP-RAGE images and a high signal on T₂-FLAIR and T₂-weighted FSE images. Figure 40.13 shows representative clinical and 2D IR-UTE images of the brain from a 28-year-old female donor with confirmed MS. Areas of the NAWM show a high signal on the 2D IR-UTE subtracted images, and areas of presumed myelin loss show a low signal. Lesions seen on the 2D IR-UTE images correspond to hyperintense areas on conventional T₂-weighted FSE images or hypointense areas on MP-RAGE images. However, some lesions show more extensive changes on 2D IR-UTE images with abnormalities (partial demyelination) extending into the NAWM (e.g., thick arrow). These regions appear normal on MP-RAGE and T2-FSE images and could only be detected with the IR-UTE sequence.

Figure 40.14 shows clinical MP-RAGE and T₂-FLAIR images as well as 3D IR-UTE images in two representative MS patients [41]. Myelin signal loss in MS lesions shows as a high signal in T₂-FLAIR images but a low signal in MP-RAGE and 3D IR-UTE images. Compared to the MP-RAGE images, the 3D IR-UTE images show higher contrast and specificity for myelin, as all water components are well suppressed by the adiabatic inversion pulse.

More robust myelin imaging can be achieved with the DESIRE-UTE and STAIR-UTE sequences, where water components with varied T₁s can be more efficiently suppressed than with the single adiabatic IR-prepared UTE sequence. Figure 40.15 shows representative MP-RAGE, T₂-FLAIR, and DESIRE-UTE images of a 45-year-old patient with MS [40]. The DESIRE-UTE sequence provides extremely high contrast for myelin with excellent water suppression. Selective myelin imaging can be achieved even in regions with varying T₁s due to pathology (e.g., edema and iron deposition). MS lesions outlined in yellow circles can be easily identified. The normalized DESIRE-UTE signal for the NAWM is about four times higher than that for MS lesions, which is consistent with myelin loss in the lesions. High contrast myelin imaging can also be achieved with the 3D STAIR-UTE sequence, which provides robust volumetric myelin mapping across the whole brain.

Quantitative UTE Imaging of Myelin in Multiple Sclerosis

The myelin signal intensity derived from IR-, DESIRE-, or STAIR-UTE imaging can be used as a biomarker for evaluating MS lesions. In a study of 12 MS patients and 12 healthy controls, UTE and T₂-FLAIR signal measurements indicate excellent reproducibility with intraclass correlation

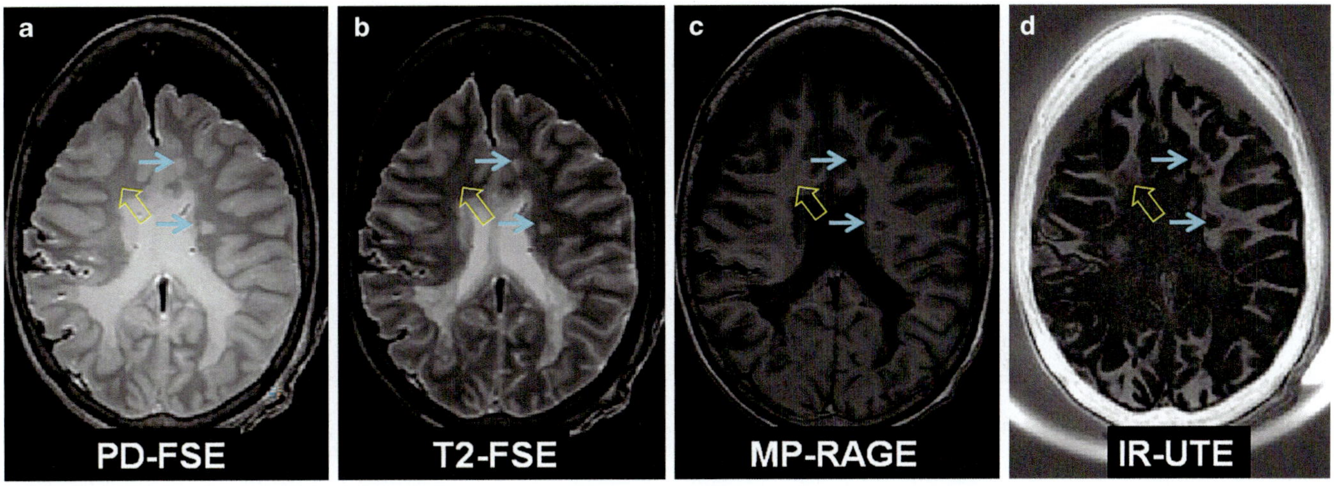

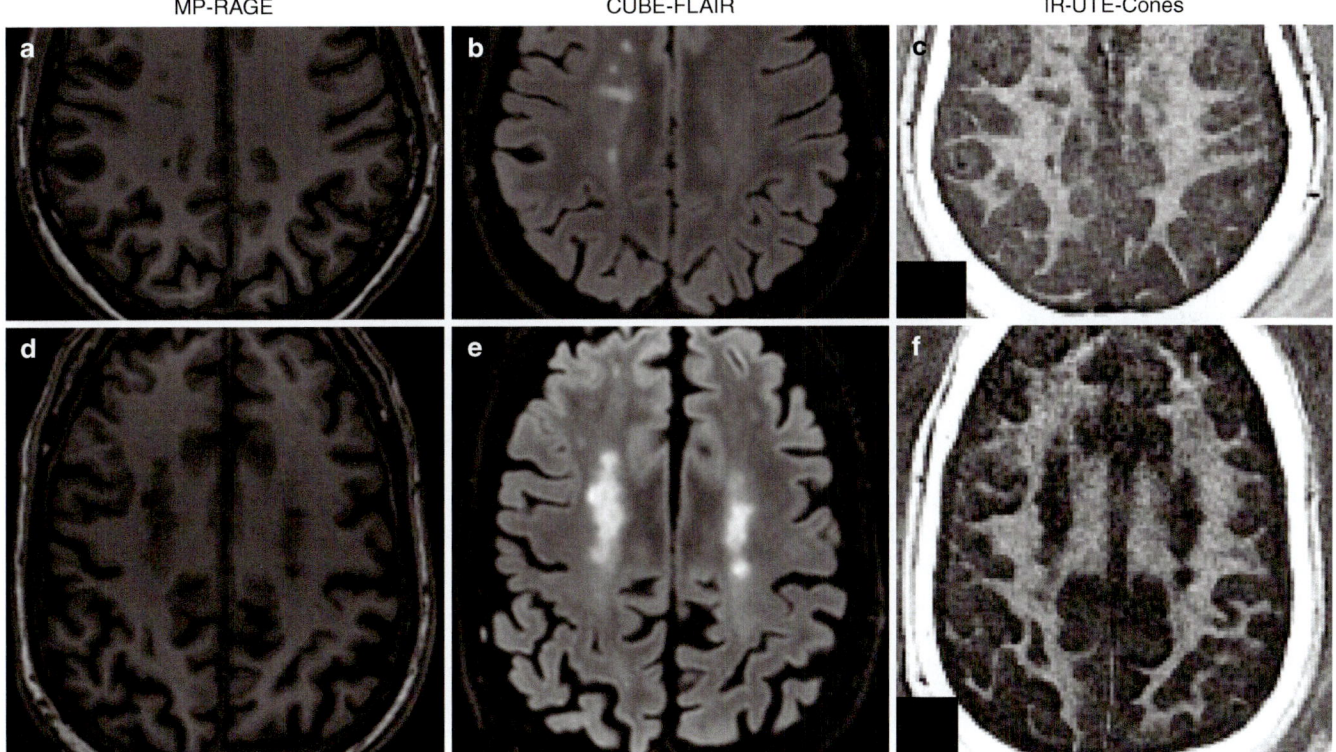

Fig. 40.13 An MS brain from a 28-year-old female donor was imaged with the 2D PD-FSE (**a**), 2D T$_2$-FSE (**b**), 3D MP-RAGE (**c**), and 2D IR-UTE sequences (**d**). Lesions (thin arrows) are hypointense with MP-RAGE, hyperintense with FSE, and low signal with IR-UTE. Partial demyelination (thick arrow) is only seen with IR-UTE but not clinical FSE and MP-RAGE sequences. (Reproduced with permission from Sheth et al. [36])

Fig. 40.14 Clinical T$_1$-weighted MR-RAGE (**a, d**), T$_2$-weighted CUBE-FLAIR (**b, e**), and 3D IR-UTE (**c, f**) imaging of two representative MS patients, including a 62-year-old female (first row) and a 62-year-old male (second row). The 3D IR-UTE sequence shows signal loss in the MS lesions identified with MP-RAGE and CUBE-FLAIR. (Reproduced with permission from Ma et al. [41])

coefficients of 0.965 and 0.947, respectively [41]. The signal intensity correlation between 3D IR-UTE and T$_2$-FLAIR was excellent, with $R^2 = 0.597$ (Fig. 40.16a). Both the IR-UTE and T$_2$-FLAIR measurements show significant dif-

ferences in normal white matter (NWM) in healthy volunteers and in the NAWM in MS patients, and in MS lesions ($p < 0.001$). This demonstrates that both the 3D IR-UIE and clinical T$_2$-FLAIR sequences can detect MS lesions accu-

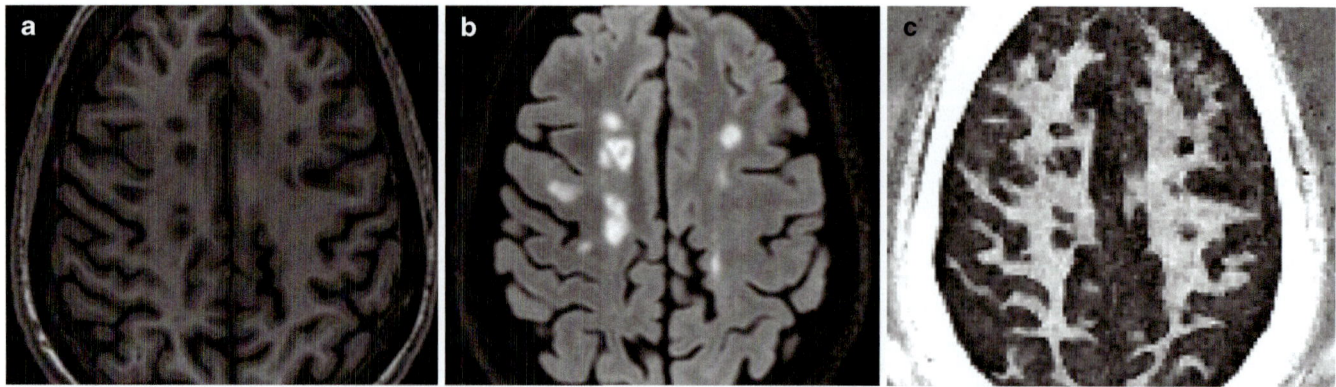

Fig. 40.15 A 45-year-old MS patient imaged with the clinical MP-RAGE (**a**), T_2-FLAIR (**b**), and 3D DESIRE-UTE (**c**) sequences. MS lesions outlined with ellipses on the MP-RAGE and T_2-FLAIR images are shown as signal voids on DESIRE-UTE images, consistent with myelin loss. (Reproduced with permission from Ma et al.[40])

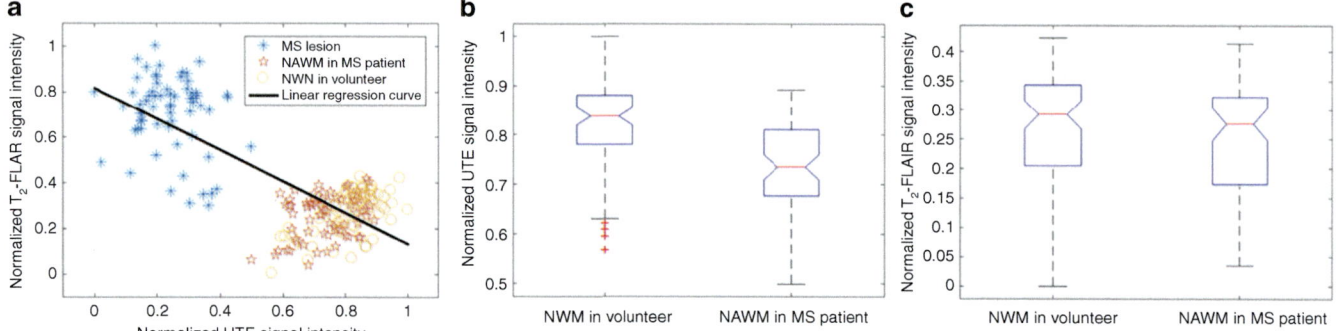

Fig. 40.16 Statistical analysis for quantitative signal intensity measurements of the WM acquired with the 3D IR-UTE and clinical T_2-FLAIR sequences, respectively. The signal intensity of the IR-UTE image shows a good correlation ($R^2 = 0.597$) with the signal intensity of the T_2-FLAIR image (**a**). The measured IR-UTE signals show significant difference in the NWM of healthy volunteers and in the NAWM of MS patients ($P < 0.001$) (**b**), which is not observed in clinical T_2-FLAIR measurements ($P = 0.204$) (**c**). The central mark in boxplots (**b**, **c**) indicates the median, and the bottom and top edges of the boxes indicate the 25th and 75th percentiles, respectively. The "+" symbol refers to outliers. (Reproduced with permission from Ma et al. [41])

rately. The signal intensity showed no statistically significant difference in T_2-FLAIR images between the NWM of healthy volunteers and the NAWM of MS patients ($p = 0.204$) (Fig. 40.16c). In comparison, the 3D IR-UTE signal intensity showed a significant difference between the two groups ($p < 0.001$) (Fig. 40.16b). These results show that the 3D IR-UTE sequence provides more useful information in the early detection of demyelination in MS patients compared with the conventional clinical T_2-FLAIR sequence.

More accurate myelin density maps can be generated by comparing the IR-, DESIRE-, or STAIR-UTE signal with that of a calibration phantom after correction for T_1, T_2^*, and coil sensitivity effects [35–41]. The phantom can be a piece of rubber eraser or water doped with D_2O and $MnCl_2$ so that its T_2^* is approximately that of myelin, minimizing errors due to signal loss during RF excitation and sampling. Figure 40.17 shows STAIR-UTE results in a 69-year-old female patient with MS. Clinical MP-RAGE and T_2-FLAIR images are also shown for comparison [39]. Lesions detected with the two clinical sequences show signal loss on the STAIR-UTE first echo images as well as the magnitude and complex echo subtracted images (Fig. 40.17c–e). Both GM and MS lesions show higher contrast on the magnitude first echo images and the magnitude echo subtracted images compared with the complex echo subtracted images. Although complex echo subtraction showed the lowest image contrast, it is the most accurate method for ultrashort-T_2 quantification because of its minimal water contamination, as confirmed by numerical simulations [39].

Figure 40.18a–d shows 3D STAIR-UTE myelin PD maps in a healthy 28-year-old female volunteer. The NWM has a myelin PD of ~9 mol/L, whereas the normal gray matter (NGM) has a myelin PD of ~5 mol/L, largely consistent with the literature. Also shown are myelin PD maps in a 45-year-old female MS patient. Myelin loss in the lesions is obvious. However, there is also widespread myelin loss across the whole brain in the NAWM, suggesting that a systematic evaluation of MS should not solely focus on the focal lesions but also include the NAWM elsewhere in the brain.

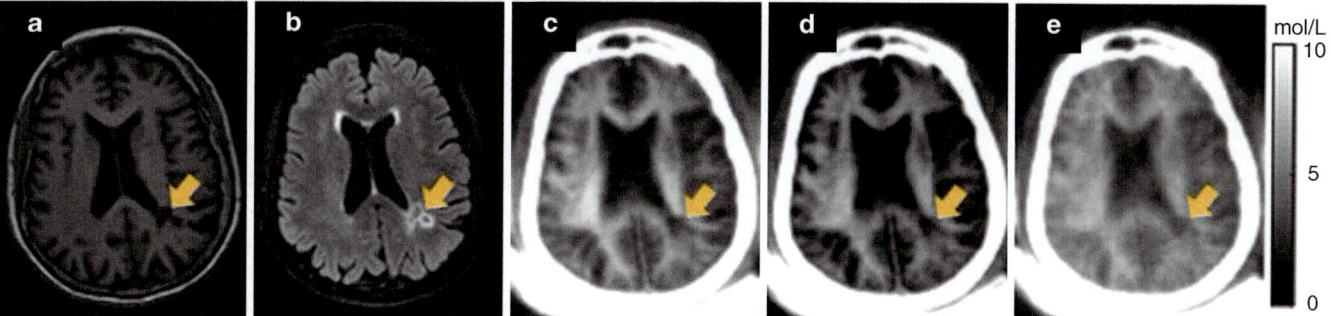

Fig. 40.17 Representative MP-RAGE (**a**), T$_2$-FLAIR (**b**), and STAIR-UTE (**c**–**e**) images of a 69-year-old female patient with MS. MS lesions (yellow arrows) appeared hypointense on the MP-RAGE image and hyperintense on the T$_2$-FLAIR image. The lesions also show signal loss on the magnitude images in the first echo images (**c**), magnitude echo subtracted images (**d**), and complex echo subtracted images (**e**) derived from the STAIR-UTE sequence. (Reproduced with permission from Ma et al. [39])

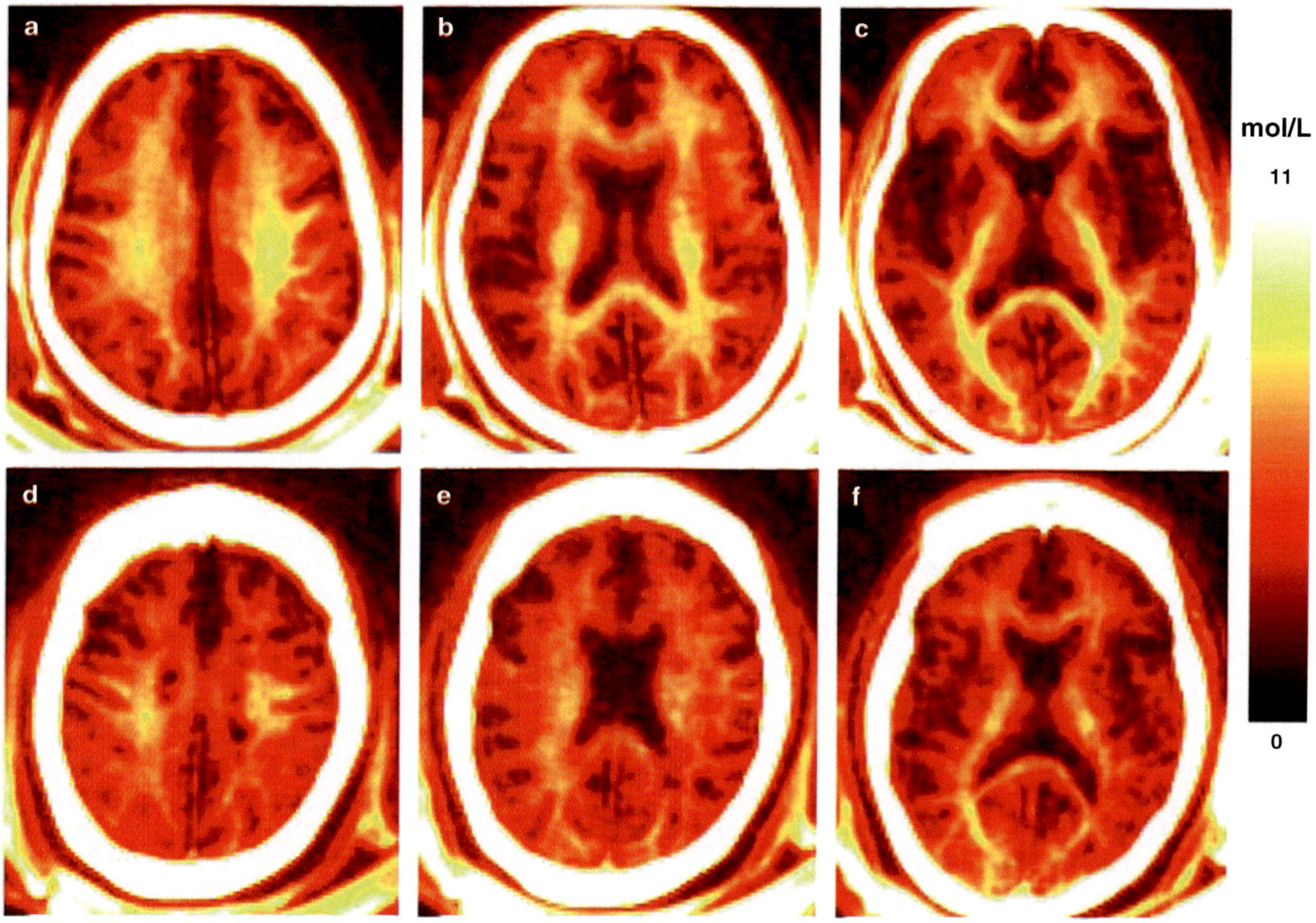

Fig. 40.18 Selected myelin PD maps in the WM and GM are generated from 3D STAIR-UTE imaging of a 28-year-old female healthy volunteer (**a**–**c**) and a 45-year-old female MS patient (**d**–**f**). Reduced myelin density is observed in the brain of the MS patient

More recently, Ma et al. have introduced a novel biomarker called ultrashort-T$_2$ proton fraction (USPF) to calculate myelin PD [39]. USPF is defined as the voxel-based ratio of the transverse magnetization of the ultrashort-T$_2$ component (presumably myelin) to the total transverse magnetization of the brain. The ultrashort-T$_2$ signal intensity map

and an image with both ultrashort-T$_2$ components and water signals present (i.e., without long-T$_2$ signal suppression) are produced to generate an USPF map. The ultrashort-T$_2$ signal is derived from STAIR-UTE imaging where the detected signal is from myelin. The total image signal is derived from UTE imaging where the detected signal is from both myelin

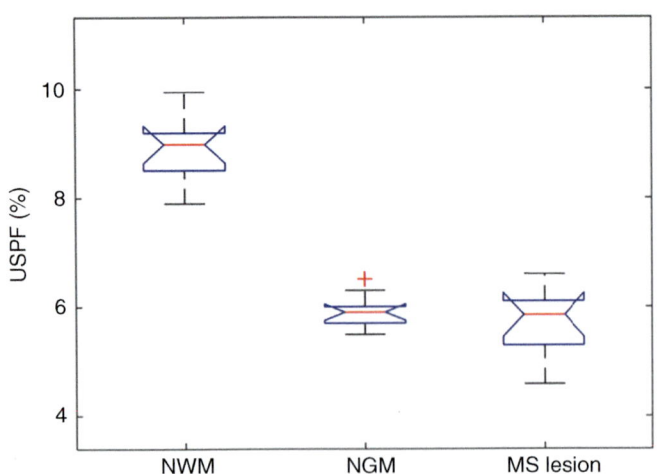

Fig. 40.19 Statistical analysis for STAIR-UTE-based USPF measurement. A lower mean USPF of 5.7 ± 0.7% is seen in lesions in MS patients compared with 8.9 ± 0.6% for the NWM in healthy volunteers ($p < 0.0001$). A mean USPF value of 5.9 ± 0.3% is seen in the NGM in healthy volunteers. The central mark in each boxplot indicates the median, whereas the bottom and top edges of each box indicate the 25th and 75th percentiles, respectively. (Reproduced with permission from Ma et al. [39])

and water components. In a representative normal brain (a 21-year-old male volunteer), USPF values range from 3.1% for the GM to 11.5% for the WM, which are consistent with the reported values of ~10% for the WM [39]. In preliminary test–retest experiments (three repeated scans), the maximum USPF difference ratio in WM regions (i.e., the left and right centrum semiovale, subcortical WM and periventricular region, and the splenium and genu of the corpus callosum) was less than 2%, demonstrating excellent repeatability of this technique [39]. Figure 40.19 shows a lower mean USPF value of 5.7 ± 0.7% for the lesions in four MS patients (49–69 years of age, all females) than that of 8.9 ± 0.6% for the NWM in four healthy volunteers (21–47 years of age, three males, one female) [39]. The normal gray matter (NGM) has a mean USPF value of 5.9 ± 0.3%. All the mean USPF differences were statistically significant ($p < 0.0001$). These results suggest that the STAIR-UTE-measured USPF is a useful biomarker for determining the ultrashort-T_2 content in MS lesions. The clinical significance remains to be investigated for MS diagnosis and treatment monitoring.

Conclusions

Myelin integrity is of critical importance for the normal functioning of the nervous system. It is important to develop advanced MRI techniques to directly measure myelin content and its MR properties such as T_1 and T_2^* relaxation times. UTE-based techniques can directly detect signals from nonaqueous myelin protons, as supported by the series

of myelin phantom studies. Advanced long-T_2 suppression techniques, especially the IR-based DESIRE-UTE and STAIR-UTE techniques, provide effective suppression of signals from various water components in the brain. This allows whole-brain myelin mapping, as evidenced by the animal and cadaveric human brain studies with histological confirmation. In vivo whole-brain myelin mapping is also feasible with the IR-UTE, DESIRE-UTE, and STAIR-UTE sequences. Measured myelin T_2^*s are close to those of myelin phantoms and intact myelin vesicles, further demonstrating the signal source from nonaqueous myelin protons rather than water components. Reduced myelin signal and myelin density as well as USPF are observed in MS lesions, consistent with clinical findings. However, UTE-based measurements are more specific to myelin than are conventional MRI measurements as the signal is directly received from myelin. Other UTE-type sequences, such as ZTE [47, 63], PETRA [59], RHE [57], sweep imaging with Fourier transformation (SWIFT) [64], SPI, and HYFI [44], can also be used for direct imaging of myelin when appropriate contrast mechanisms are employed to suppress signals from water components.

There are no imaging biomarkers currently in clinical use that demonstrate high sensitivity or specificity for myelin or have strong correlations with the clinical features of MS [11–16, 65]. This highlights the importance and need to develop novel direct imaging techniques for myelin. Furthermore, remyelination therapy is one of the principal focuses of current treatments in MS [65–68]. There are more than 20 ongoing clinical trials of remyelination treatments, which have been detailed in a recent comprehensive review by Cunniffe et al. [67]. UTE-type direct imaging techniques can potentially provide more accurate evaluation of demyelination and remyelination as well as partial myelin loss and myelin regeneration and so provide more accurate diagnosis and treatment monitoring of MS. Finally, UTE-type imaging sequences may also play an important role in the diagnosis and management of not only MS but also other neurological diseases, including Alzheimer's disease [69], Parkinson's disease [70], traumatic brain injury [71], epilepsy [72], and Huntington's disease [73].

References

1. Noseworthy JH, Lucchinetti C, Rodriguez M, Weinshenker BG. Multiple sclerosis. N Engl J Med. 2000;343(13):938–52.
2. McDonald WI, Compston A, Edan G, Goodkin D, Hartung HP, Lublin FD, et al. Recommended diagnostic criteria for multiple sclerosis: guidelines from the international panel on the diagnosis of multiple sclerosis. Ann Neurol. 2001;50(1):121–7.
3. Truyen L, van Waesberghe JH, van Walderveen MA, van Oosten BW, Polman CH, Hommes OR, et al. Accumulation of hypointense lesions ("black holes") on T1 spin-echo MRI correlates with disease progression in multiple sclerosis. Neurology. 1996;47(6):1469–76.

4. Paty DW, Li DK, Oger JJ, Kastrukoff L, Koopmans R, Tanton E, et al. Magnetic resonance imaging in the evaluation of clinical trials in multiple sclerosis. Ann Neurol. 1994;36(Suppl):S95–6.

5. Thompson AJ, Kermode AG, MacManus DG, Kendall BE, Kingsley DP, Moseley IF, et al. Patterns of disease activity in multiple sclerosis: clinical and magnetic resonance imaging study. BMJ. 1990;300(6725):631–4.

6. Grossman RI, Braffman BH, Brorson JR, Goldberg HI, Silberberg DH, Gonzalez-Scarano F. Multiple sclerosis: serial study of gadolinium-enhanced MR imaging. Radiology. 1988;169(1):117–22.

7. Filippi M, Inglese M. Overview of diffusion-weighted magnetic resonance studies in multiple sclerosis. J Neurol Sci. 2001;186(Suppl 1):S37–43.

8. Basser PJ, Mattiello J, LeBihan D. Estimation of the effective self-diffusion tensor from the NMR spin echo. J Magn Reson B. 1994;103(3):247–54.

9. Schmierer K, Scaravilli F, Altmann DR, Barker GJ, Miller DH. Magnetization transfer ratio and myelin in postmortem multiple sclerosis brain. Ann Neurol. 2004;56(3):407–15.

10. Chen JT, Collins DL, Atkins HL, Freedman MS, Arnold DL, Canadian MSBMTSG. Magnetization transfer ratio evolution with demyelination and remyelination in multiple sclerosis lesions. Ann Neurol. 2008;63(2):254–62.

11. Gawne-Cain ML, O'Riordan JI, Coles A, Newell B, Thompson AJ, Miller DH. MRI lesion volume measurement in multiple sclerosis and its correlation with disability: a comparison of fast fluid attenuated inversion recovery (fFLAIR) and spin echo sequences. J Neurol Neurosurg Psychiatry. 1998;64(2):197–203.

12. Nijeholt GJ, van Walderveen MA, Castelijns JA, van Waesberghe JH, Polman C, Scheltens P, et al. Brain and spinal cord abnormalities in multiple sclerosis. Correlation between MRI parameters, clinical subtypes and symptoms. Brain. 1998;121(Pt 4):687–97.

13. Li DK, Held U, Petkau J, Daumer M, Barkhof F, Fazekas F, et al. MRI T_2 lesion burden in multiple sclerosis: a plateauing relationship with clinical disability. Neurology. 2006;66(9):1384–9.

14. Charil A, Zijdenbos AP, Taylor J, Boelman C, Worsley KJ, Evans AC, et al. Statistical mapping analysis of lesion location and neurological disability in multiple sclerosis: application to 452 patient data sets. NeuroImage. 2003;19(3):532–44.

15. Kappos L, Moeri D, Radue EW, Schoetzau A, Schweikert K, Barkhof F, et al. Predictive value of gadolinium-enhanced magnetic resonance imaging for relapse rate and changes in disability or impairment in multiple sclerosis: a meta-analysis. Gadolinium MRI Meta-analysis Group Lancet. 1999;353(9157):964–9.

16. Rovaris M, Judica E, Sastre-Garriga J, Rovira A, Sormani MP, Benedetti B, et al. Large-scale, multicentre, quantitative MRI study of brain and cord damage in primary progressive multiple sclerosis. Mult Scler. 2008;14(4):455–64.

17. Sanfilipo MP, Benedict RH, Sharma J, Weinstock-Guttman B, Bakshi R. The relationship between whole brain volume and disability in multiple sclerosis: a comparison of normalized gray vs. white matter with misclassification correction. NeuroImage. 2005;26(4):1068–77.

18. Rudick RA, Lee JC, Nakamura K, Fisher E. Gray matter atrophy correlates with MS disability progression measured with MSFC but not EDSS. J Neurol Sci. 2009;282(1–2):106–11.

19. Filippi M, Rocca MA. MR imaging of multiple sclerosis. Radiology. 2011;259(3):659–81.

20. Schmierer K, Wheeler-Kingshott CA, Tozer DJ, Boulby PA, Parkes HG, Yousry TA, et al. Quantitative magnetic resonance of postmortem multiple sclerosis brain before and after fixation. Magn Reson Med. 2008;59(2):268–77.

21. Dousset V, Grossman RI, Ramer KN, Schnall MD, Young LH, Gonzalez-Scarano F, et al. Experimental allergic encephalomyelitis and multiple sclerosis: lesion characterization with magnetization transfer imaging. Radiology. 1992;182(2):483–91.

22. Newcombe J, Hawkins CP, Henderson CL, Patel HA, Woodroofe MN, Hayes GM, et al. Histopathology of multiple sclerosis lesions detected by magnetic resonance imaging in unfixed postmortem central nervous system tissue. Brain. 1991;114(2):1013-23.

23. Filley CM, Fields RD. White matter and cognition: making the connection. J Neurophysiol. 2016;116(5):2093–104.

24. Waxman SG. Conduction in myelinated, unmyelinated, and demyelinated fibers. Arch Neurol. 1977;34(10):585–9.

25. Felts PA, Baker TA, Smith KJ. Conduction in segmentally demyelinated mammalian central axons. J Neurosci. 1997;17(19):7267–77.

26. Funfschilling U, Supplie LM, Mahad D, Boretius S, Saab AS, Edgar J, et al. Glycolytic oligodendrocytes maintain myelin and long-term axonal integrity. Nature. 2012;485(7399):517–21.

27. Gibson EM, Purger D, Mount CW, Goldstein AK, Lin GL, Wood LS, et al. Neuronal activity promotes oligodendrogenesis and adaptive myelination in the mammalian brain. Science. 2014;344(6183):1252304.

28. McKenzie IA, Ohayon D, Li H, de Faria JP, Emery B, Tohyama K, et al. Motor skill learning requires active central myelination. Science. 2014;346(6207):318–22.

29. Sinha K, Karimi-Abdolrezaee S, Velumian AA, Fehlings MG. Functional changes in genetically dysmyelinated spinal cord axons of shiverer mice: role of juxtaparanodal Kv1 family K+ channels. J Neurophysiol. 2006;95(3):1683–95.

30. Lee Y, Morrison BM, Li Y, Lengacher S, Farah MH, Hoffman PN, et al. Oligodendroglia metabolically support axons and contribute to neurodegeneration. Nature. 2012;487(7408):443–8.

31. Chabas D, Baranzini SE, Mitchell D, Bernard CC, Rittling SR, Denhardt DT, et al. The influence of the proinflammatory cytokine, osteopontin, on autoimmune demyelinating disease. Science. 2001;294(5547):1731–5.

32. Waldman A, Rees JH, Brock CS, Robson MD, Gatehouse PD, Bydder GM. MRI of the brain with ultra-short echo-time pulse sequences. Neuroradiology. 2003;45(12):887–92.

33. Horch RA, Gore JC, Does MD. Origins of the ultrashort-T_2 1H NMR signals in myelinated nerve: a direct measure of myelin content? Magn Reson Med. 2011;66(1):24–31.

34. Wilhelm MJ, Ong HH, Wehrli SL, Li C, Tsai PH, Hackney DB, et al. Direct magnetic resonance detection of myelin and prospects for quantitative imaging of myelin density. Proc Natl Acad Sci U S A. 2012;109(24):9605–10.

35. Du J, Ma G, Li S, Carl M, Szeverenyi NM, VandenBerg S, et al. Ultrashort echo time (UTE) magnetic resonance imaging of the short T_2 components in white matter of the brain using a clinical 3T scanner. NeuroImage. 2014;87:32–41.

36. Sheth V, Shao H, Chen J, Vandenberg S, Corey-Bloom J, Bydder GM, et al. Magnetic resonance imaging of myelin using ultrashort Echo time (UTE) pulse sequences: phantom, specimen, volunteer and multiple sclerosis patient studies. NeuroImage. 2016;136:37–44.

37. Ma YJ, Jang H, Chang EY, Hiniker A, Head BP, Lee RR, et al. Ultrashort echo time (UTE) magnetic resonance imaging of myelin: technical developments and challenges. Quant Imaging Med Surg. 2020;10(6):1186–203.

38. Ma YJ, Jang H, Wei Z, Cai Z, Xue Y, Lee RR, et al. Myelin imaging in human brain using a short repetition time adiabatic inversion recovery prepared ultrashort Echo time (STAIR-UTE) MRI sequence in multiple sclerosis. Radiology. 2020;297(2):392–404.

39. Ma YJ, Jang H, Wei Z, Wu M, Chang EY, Corey-Bloom J, et al. Brain ultrashort T_2 component imaging using a short TR adiabatic inversion recovery prepared dual-echo ultrashort TE sequence with complex echo subtraction (STAIR-dUTE-ES). J Magn Reson. 2021;323:106898.

40. Ma YJ, Searleman AC, Jang H, Wong J, Chang EY, Corey-Bloom J, et al. Whole-brain myelin imaging using 3D double-Echo slid-

ing inversion recovery ultrashort Echo time (DESIRE UTE) MRI. Radiology. 2020;294(2):362–74.

41. Ma YJ, Searleman AC, Jang H, Fan SJ, Wong J, Xue Y, et al. Volumetric imaging of myelin in vivo using 3D inversion recovery-prepared ultrashort echo time cones magnetic resonance imaging. NMR Biomed. 2020;33(10):e4326.

42. Lecar H, Ehrenstein G, Stillman I. Detection of molecular motion in lyophilized myelin by nuclear magnetic resonance. Biophys J. 1971;11(2):140–5.

43. MacKay A, Laule C, Vavasour I, Bjarnason T, Kolind S, Madler B. Insights into brain microstructure from the T_2 distribution. Magn Reson Imaging. 2006;24(4):515–25.

44. Weiger M, Froidevaux R, Baadsvik EL, Brunner DO, Rosler MB, Pruessmann KP. Advances in MRI of the myelin bilayer. NeuroImage. 2020;217:116888.

45. Fan SJ, Ma Y, Zhu Y, Searleman A, Szeverenyi NM, Bydder GM, et al. Yet more evidence that myelin protons can be directly imaged with UTE sequences on a clinical 3T scanner: Bicomponent T_2^* analysis of native and deuterated ovine brain specimens. Magn Reson Med. 2018;80(2):538–47.

46. Larocca JN, Norton WT. Isolation of myelin. Curr Protoc Cell Biol. 2007;Chapter 3:Unit3 25.

47. Seifert AC, Li C, Wilhelm MJ, Wehrli SL, Wehrli FW. Towards quantification of myelin by solid-state MRI of the lipid matrix protons. NeuroImage. 2017;163:358–67.

48. Larson PE, Gurney PT, Nayak K, Gold GE, Pauly JM, Nishimura DG. Designing long-T_2 suppression pulses for ultrashort echo time imaging. Magn Reson Med. 2006;56(1):94–103.

49. Sussman MS, Pauly JM, Wright GA. Design of practical T2-selective RF excitation (TELEX) pulses. Magn Reson Med. 1998;40(6):890–9.

50. Wei H, Cao P, Bischof A, Henry RG, Larson PEZ, Liu C. MRI gradient-echo phase contrast of the brain at ultra-short TE with off-resonance saturation. NeuroImage. 2018;175:1–11.

51. Larson PE, Conolly SM, Pauly JM, Nishimura DG. Using adiabatic inversion pulses for long-T_2 suppression in ultrashort echo time (UTE) imaging. Magn Reson Med. 2007;58(5):952–61.

52. Du J, Sheth V, He Q, Carl M, Chen J, Corey-Bloom J, et al. Measurement of T1 of the ultrashort T_2^* components in white matter of the brain at 3T. PLoS One. 2014;9(8):e103296.

53. Lancaster JL, Andrews T, Hardies LJ, Dodd S, Fox PT. Three-pool model of white matter. J Magn Reson Imaging. 2003;17(1):1–10.

54. Helms G, Hagberg GE. In vivo quantification of the bound pool T1 in human white matter using the binary spin-bath model of progressive magnetization transfer saturation. Phys Med Biol. 2009;54(23):N529–40.

55. Labadie C, Lee JH, Rooney WD, Jarchow S, Aubert-Frecon M, Springer CS Jr, et al. Myelin water mapping by spatially regularized longitudinal relaxographic imaging at high magnetic fields. Magn Reson Med. 2014;71(1):375–87.

56. Schyboll F, Jaekel U, Petruccione F, Neeb H. Dipolar induced spin-lattice relaxation in the myelin sheath: a molecular dynamics study. Sci Rep. 2019;9(1):14813.

57. Jang H, Ma Y, Searleman AC, Carl M, Corey-Bloom J, Chang EY, et al. Inversion recovery UTE based volumetric myelin imaging in human brain using interleaved hybrid encoding. Magn Reson Med. 2020;83(3):950–61.

58. Jang H, Liu F, Bradshaw T, McMillan AB. Rapid dual-echo ramped hybrid encoding MR-based attenuation correction (dRHE-MRAC) for PET/MR. Magn Reson Med. 2018;79(6):2912–22.

59. Grodzki DM, Jakob PM, Heismann B. Ultrashort echo time imaging using pointwise encoding time reduction with radial acquisition (PETRA). Magn Reson Med. 2012;67(2):510–8.

60. Jang H, Wiens CN, McMillan AB. Ramped hybrid encoding for improved ultrashort echo time imaging. Magn Reson Med. 2016;76(3):814–25.

61. Blakemore WF, Franklin RJ. Remyelination in experimental models of toxin-induced demyelination. Curr Top Microbiol Immunol. 2008;318:193–212.

62. Tustison NJ, Cook PA, Klein A, Song G, Das SR, Duda JT, et al. Large-scale evaluation of ANTs and FreeSurfer cortical thickness measurements. NeuroImage. 2014;99:166–79.

63. Jang H, Carl M, Ma Y, Searleman AC, Jerban S, Chang EY, et al. Inversion recovery zero echo time (IR-ZTE) imaging for direct myelin detection in human brain: a feasibility study. Quant Imaging Med Surg. 2020;10(5):895–906.

64. Idiyatullin D, Corum C, Park JY, Garwood M. Fast and quiet MRI using a swept radiofrequency. J Magn Reson. 2006;181(2):342–9.

65. Mallik S, Samson RS, Wheeler-Kingshott CA, Miller DH. Imaging outcomes for trials of remyelination in multiple sclerosis. J Neurol Neurosurg Psychiatry. 2014;85(12):1396–404.

66. Munzel EJ, Williams A. Promoting remyelination in multiple sclerosis-recent advances. Drugs. 2013;73(18):2017–29.

67. Cunniffe N, Coles A. Promoting remyelination in multiple sclerosis. J Neurol. 2021;268(1):30–44.

68. Keough MB, Yong VW. Remyelination therapy for multiple sclerosis. Neurotherapeutics. 2013;10(1):44–54.

69. Dean DC 3rd, Jerskey BA, Chen K, Protas H, Thiyyagura P, Roontiva A, et al. Brain differences in infants at differential genetic risk for late-onset Alzheimer disease: a cross-sectional imaging study. JAMA Neurol. 2014;71(1):11–22.

70. Dean DC 3rd, Sojkova J, Hurley S, Kecskemeti S, Okonkwo O, Bendlin BB, et al. Alterations of myelin content in Parkinson's disease: a cross-sectional neuroimaging study. PLoS One. 2016;11(10):e0163774.

71. Armstrong RC, Mierzwa AJ, Marion CM, Sullivan GM. White matter involvement after TBI: clues to axon and myelin repair capacity. Exp Neurol. 2016;275(Pt 3):328–33.

72. Drenthen GS, Fonseca Wald ELA, Backes WH, Debeij-Van Hall M, Hendriksen JGM, Aldenkamp AP, et al. Lower myelin-water content of the frontal lobe in childhood absence epilepsy. Epilepsia. 2019;60(8):1689–96.

73. Bartzokis G, Lu PH, Tishler TA, Fong SM, Oluwadara B, Finn JP, et al. Myelin breakdown and iron changes in Huntington's disease: pathogenesis and treatment implications. Neurochem Res. 2007;32(10):1655–64.

Myelin Bilayer Imaging

41

Emily Louise Baadsvik and Markus Weiger

Introduction

After the advent of magnetic resonance imaging (MRI) in the 1970s, the modality quickly gained momentum for the diagnostic workup and therapeutic monitoring of patients. By the early 1980s, it was clear that MRI offered significant advantages over computed tomography (CT) in detecting brain pathology due to its superior soft tissue contrast [1]. These advantages were particularly relevant in the evaluation of demyelinating disorders such as multiple sclerosis (MS), in which the insulating sheath surrounding axons is damaged or lost [2, 3]. By the end of the 1980s, MRI was the preferred imaging technique for the diagnosis of diseases of this type [4].

Initially, MRI techniques employing inversion recovery, spin echo, and gradient echo sequences were used to generate myelin-related contrast based on differences in the relaxation times T_1 and T_2 [5]. However, the resulting contrast was not specific for demyelination because other pathologies such as edema, infarction, and inflammation produced similar contrast [4]. This low specificity for myelin prompted exploration of alternative MRI techniques that would provide greater certainty in evaluating myelin integrity.

A critical obstacle to myelin-specific MRI was the extremely rapid T_2 decay of magnetic resonance (MR) signals originating from the myelin lipid–protein bilayer itself. These signals could not be captured with the imaging systems available during the infancy of myelin MRI. To address this problem, techniques for accessing myelin content or intactness through myelin-related properties of water signals were developed, most notably relaxation-, magnetization transfer-, and diffusion-based methods [6].

In parallel to the progress of "indirect" myelin imaging techniques (i.e., those based on water signal measurements), the field of short-T_2 imaging has advanced significantly [7],

warranting reconsideration of the prospects for direct imaging of myelin (i.e., myelin bilayer imaging). In this chapter, we introduce the various features of myelin bilayer imaging and summarize the current state of research in this field. Furthermore, we address the potential role of myelin bilayer imaging in clinical and research settings, albeit with reservations about drawing conclusions at this early stage in the development of the technique.

This chapter is divided into three parts: The first part (see section "Background and Fundamental Concepts") provides a general overview of myelin and covers the main aspects of myelin MRI, including myelin bilayer signal behavior. It then delves into the fundamental concepts of short-T_2 imaging and associated hardware considerations and concludes with a discussion about the applicability of short-T_2 imaging techniques to visualize the myelin bilayer. The second part (see section "Current State of Myelin Bilayer Imaging") covers the current state of myelin bilayer imaging. The third part (see section "Future Directions") presents an outlook on the future of myelin bilayer imaging and, in particular, how such methods could fit in with the existing arsenal of MRI techniques.

Background and Fundamental Concepts

Myelin

Function and Overview

The nervous system consists of a network of neurons that communicate with each other by sending electrical impulses along connecting fibers known as axons. In vertebrates, axons are often surrounded by an insulating layer known as myelin, which increases the conduction velocity of the electrical impulses and decreases energy expenditure. Myelin achieves these favorable properties by altering the electrical environment of the axon so that instead of the impulses traveling along the fiber in a continuous manner, they jump

E. L. Baadsvik · M. Weiger (✉)
Institute for Biomedical Engineering, ETH Zurich and University of Zurich, Zurich, Switzerland
e-mail: baadsvik@biomed.ee.ethz.ch; weiger@biomed.ee.ethz.ch

© The Author(s), under exclusive license to Springer Nature Switzerland AG 2023
J. Du, G. M. Bydder (eds.), *MRI of Short- and Ultrashort-T₂ Tissues*, https://doi.org/10.1007/978-3-031-35197-6_41

between unmyelinated focal points called the nodes of Ranvier (a mechanism known as saltatory conduction) [8].

The nervous system is split into two parts, the central nervous system (CNS), comprising the brain and spinal cord, and the peripheral nervous system (PNS), comprising peripheral nerves, which constitute a relay between the CNS and the body. Both the CNS and the PNS contain myelin, but the myelination processes, chemical composition, and cell types vary between the two parts [9, 10]. In the present context, we limit our considerations to CNS myelin.

The CNS can be classified into white matter (WM) and gray matter (GM). GM mostly consists of neuronal cell bodies and contains only small amounts of myelin, whereas WM is rich in myelin (50% of dry weight), and this is responsible for its "white" macroanatomical appearance [9].

CNS myelin is a tightly compacted extension of the cell membrane of oligodendrocytes. The oligodendrocyte membrane wraps concentrically around the axon, trapping layers of intra- and extracellular water between layers of the membrane. Several proteins are involved in this process [11], and the end product is a myelin sheath consisting of trapped water pools collectively referred to as myelin water as well as a characteristic lipid–protein bilayer [6, 12]. A schematic of CNS myelin is provided in Fig. 41.1.

Role in CNS Disorders

Damage to myelin (demyelination) and errors in the development of myelin (dysmyelination) can disrupt the efficient transmission of electrical impulses between neurons [8]. Consequently, myelin disorders are frequently associated with clinical disability in affected individuals [13, 14].

One of the most prominent myelin disorders is MS, with more than 2.8 million cases reported worldwide in 2020 [15]. Many people with MS suffer from progressive motor and cognitive impairment [14], and MS is a leading cause of nontraumatic disability in young adults [16]. The disease is characterized by multiple inflammatory and demyelinating foci in the CNS known as MS lesions or plaques. MS lesions occur most notably in WM, although there is increasing evidence that GM is also commonly affected and that GM lesions play an important role in MS disease progression [17].

Other, much rarer neuroinflammatory demyelinating diseases of the CNS include acute disseminated encephalomyelitis (ADEM), neuromyelitis optica (NMO) [18], viral or metabolic demyelinating encephalopathies [19], and inherited disorders (adrenoleukodystrophies) [20]. Furthermore, de- or dysmyelination can be associated with common neurological disorders such as Alzheimer's disease [21], epilepsy [22], and stroke [23], and atypical myelination may play a role in mental disorders such as autism [24] and schizophrenia [25].

Composition

The myelin lipid–protein bilayer is distinct from most other cell membranes in that it contains an unusually large ratio of lipids to proteins: lipids constitute 70–85% of its dry

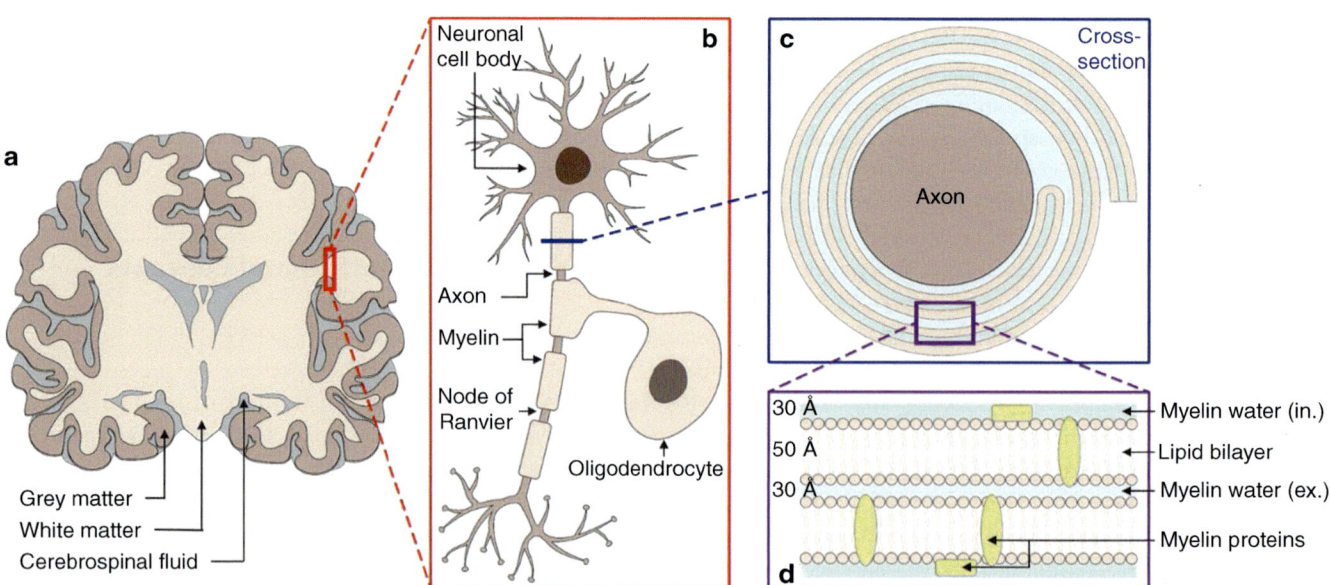

Fig. 41.1 Schematic of CNS myelin (not to scale). (**a**) GM and WM in a coronal view of the brain. (**b**) A magnified view of a neuron with a myelinated axon, including an oligodendrocyte (the myelin-forming cell). (**c**) A cross-sectional view of a myelinated axon segment. (**d**) A magnified view of the myelin sheath showing the lipid bilayer structure of the oligodendrocyte membrane and embedded myelin proteins. Myelin water compartments (extracellular (ex.) and intracellular (in.)) are also shown. Approximate spacings are given in angstroms (Å) [9]

weight, with proteins making up the remaining 15–30% [9]. As for the overall tissue composition, WM consists of around 55% lipids and 40% proteins, whereas GM comprises around 33% lipids and 55% proteins (all values by dry weight). GM has a higher water content (82%) than WM (72%), and the myelin sheath has a relatively low water content (44%) [26].

Of the total lipid content, myelin contains roughly 40–45% phospholipids, 30% galactolipids, and 25–30% cholesterol. There are no myelin-specific lipids, but the lipid most characteristic of myelin is cerebroside. Other major lipids include ethanolamine and choline phosphoglycerides [26].

In contrast to lipids, nearly all myelin proteins are unique to myelin. The two most common myelin proteins are proteolipid protein, which accounts for 50% of the total protein content, and myelin basic protein, which accounts for 30–35% of the total protein content. Other myelin proteins include myelin-associated glycoprotein and myelin oligodendrocyte glycoprotein [26].

Myelin MRI

Due to the critical consequences of demyelination and its spatially localized manifestations, it is of great interest to attain noninvasive access to maps of myelin content, a task particularly suited to MRI.

MR users have the option of choosing which nuclei to probe as long as the nuclei have nonzero spin. ^1H nuclei (i.e., protons) are by far the most common choice due to their abundance in biological tissues. In myelin MR, ^{31}P nuclei are also of relevance due to the high phospholipid content of myelin [27, 28], and ^{13}C nuclei have garnered some interest due to the central role of carbon in organic compounds [29]. However, only ^1H methods will be considered here due to the scarce usage and general limitations of methods targeting other nuclei.

MR signals are produced by exciting spins using a radiofrequency (RF) pulse, and, because relaxation mechanisms subsequently return the spins to their equilibrium state, the signals have a limited lifetime. In a simplified view, MR signals decay exponentially with time constant T_2, and nuclei in more motionally restricted molecules yield signals with shorter T_2s. Based on T_2 values, ^1H MR signals from myelin generally fit into two distinctive categories: signals of an aqueous origin (relatively weak motional restrictions, i.e., long T_2) and signals of a nonaqueous origin (relatively strong motional restrictions, i.e., short T_2).

The distinction between accessing signals of aqueous and nonaqueous origins defines the two main categories of myelin MRI techniques mentioned earlier, that is, "indirect" and "direct" methods, respectively. Indirect myelin imaging techniques are not the focus here, and only a brief overview of such methods is provided; readers are referred to the reviews by Laule et al. [6] and Piredda et al. [30] for details. Direct myelin imaging techniques, on the other hand, are the topic of this chapter, and this section introduces the MR signal properties of the myelin bilayer. In addition, the question of achievable myelin specificity of indirect and direct myelin imaging techniques is discussed.

Indirect Myelin Imaging Techniques

Signals from protons in the myelin bilayer decay so rapidly that they are invisible with standard MRI techniques; instead, access to myelin content can be gained through observation of water signals. Several MRI contrast options are sensitive to myelin in some way, including relaxation, diffusion, susceptibility, and magnetization transfer.

A popular method for myelin quantification based on the detection of water signals is myelin water imaging [31]. Due to the tightly compacted structure of the myelin sheath, myelin water (i.e., the water trapped between layers of myelin bilayer) experiences much stronger motional restrictions than free intra- or extracellular water and therefore exhibits more rapid relaxation. By observing the signal evolution over time, it is possible to separate the signal components based on relaxation times and thus to separate myelin water signals from free water signals. Myelin water content, the parameter extracted from such experiments, quantifies myelin content under the assumption that the two are invariably closely linked.

Another common technique is magnetization transfer imaging, in which exchange interactions between aqueous and nonaqueous protons modulate water signal intensity, an effect dependent on the amount of nonaqueous protons partaking in the interaction. In particular, the inhomogeneous magnetization transfer imaging method [32] is of interest for myelin quantification because the underlying physical model offers increased specificity to nonaqueous protons in the myelin sheath.

Myelin Bilayer Signal Properties

Apart from their decay behavior, the signal components in MRI are characterized by their chemical shift, that is, their resonance frequency with respect to a reference frequency. Both properties depend on the immediate chemical environment of the given nuclei. Consequently, the ^1H MR signal components of the myelin bilayer represent specific chemical groups that contain hydrogen nuclei, such as CH_2 and CH_3 groups, rather than entire lipids or proteins.

Myelin lipids yield four signal components [29], properties of which are provided in Table 41.1. Due to the specific configuration of the myelin sheath, its lipid components exhibit super-exponential decay (i.e., a super-Lorentzian lineshape), which corresponds to a spectrum of T_2 values characterized by the minimum decay component $T_{2,min}$ [33, 34]. Figure 41.2a–d illustrates the behavior of a single super-Lorentzian signal component.

By adding the T_2 spectra of the four myelin components in Table 41.1 according to their relative contributions (see Fig. 41.2e–f), it becomes evident why myelin signals are

Table 41.1 Signal components of myelin lipids, derived from nuclear magnetic resonance (NMR) experiments at 9.4T presented by Wilhelm et al. [29]

Component	Relative contribution	Decay constant ($T_{2,min}$)	Chemical shift
General alkyl chain methylene protons (CH_2)	74%	8.6 µs	1.5 ppm
Terminal methyl protons (CH_3)	12%	30 µs	0.9 ppm
Choline methyl protons (CH_3)	11%	108 µs	3.2 ppm
Cholesterol alkyl chain methylene protons (CH_2)	2%	265 µs	1.3 ppm

invisible with standard MRI techniques: around 75% of the signals exhibit decay constants below 100 µs [35]. In contrast, myelin water signals (which are considered to decay rapidly compared to free water signals) exhibit T_2 values of tens of milliseconds [36].

Because proteins comprise significantly less of the total myelin content and contain much more chemical heterogeneity than lipids [29, 37], myelin protein MR signal components have not (to our knowledge) been characterized. That said, many of the same chemical groups are involved in both lipids and proteins and they experience similar motional restrictions; as such, the overall signal behavior of myelin proteins is not expected to differ significantly from that of myelin lipids.

The Question of Myelin Specificity

Techniques that probe myelin content through measurements of water signals provide increased myelin specificity compared to traditional MRI techniques, but their indirect nature inherently puts them at risk of specificity loss should the relation between the water-based measure and myelin

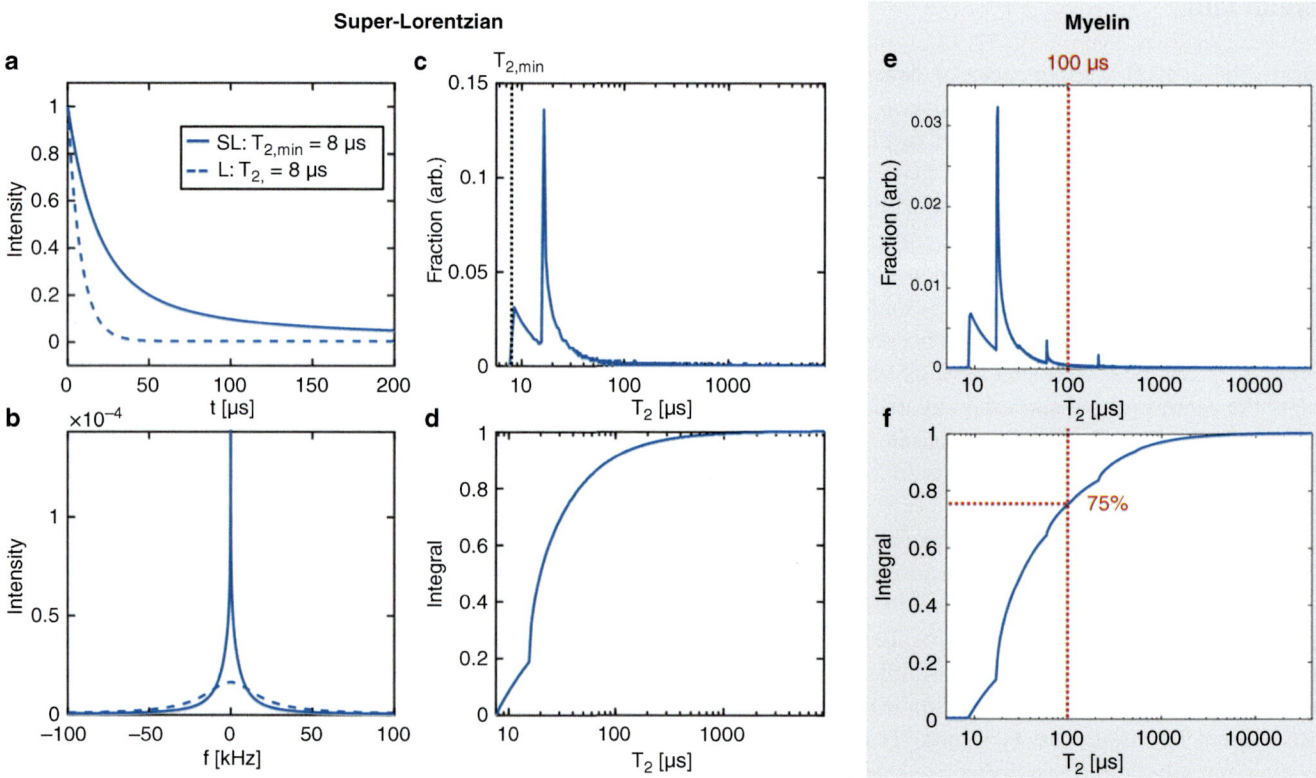

Fig. 41.2 Properties of the super-Lorentzian line shape (**a–d**) and T_2 behavior of the myelin bilayer as defined by combining the four super-Lorentzian lipid components provided in Table 41.1 (**e–f**). (**a**) Time-domain decay of a super-Lorentzian (SL) component with a $T_{2,min}$ of 8 µs (solid line) compared to a Lorentzian (L) component with a T_2 of 8 µs (dashed line). (**b**) Frequency-domain lineshape of the components from panel (**a**). (**c**) T_2 distribution of the super-Lorentzian component from panels (**a**) and (**b**). The distribution exhibits peaks at $T_{2,min}$ and $2T_{2,min}$. (**d**) Cumulative T_2 distribution obtained by integrating over the data in panel (**c**), showing the fraction of signals from the component that exhibit T_2 below a given value. (**e**) The same as panel (**c**) but for myelin bilayer lipids. It should be noted that the fractions are not comparable between panels (**c**) and (**e**). (**f**) The same as panel (**d**) but for myelin bilayer lipids. (Panels (**e**) and (**f**) modified with permission from Weiger et al. [35])

content break down. It is also conceivable that the specificity of such techniques is intrinsically suboptimal compared to what could be achieved from direct measurement of myelin bilayer content.

In native tissue, the myelin bilayer signals are superimposed on signals from water protons and non-myelin non-aqueous protons. There are ways of isolating the nonaqueous signals from the water signals [38, 39], but resolving individual myelin signal components and separating them from potentially similar non-myelin nonaqueous signal components is challenging. Ultimately, the success of nonaqueous signal component separation strategies will determine the achievable myelin specificity of myelin bilayer imaging methods.

Short-T_2 Imaging

In order to image rapidly decaying signals such as those stemming from the myelin bilayer, there are two fundamental requirements that must be met. The first and most obvious is that the signals must be captured during their lifetimes. Early signal capture translates to comparatively strong signals and, consequently, higher sensitivity to the signal source, which ideally is the tissue of interest. The second requirement is that the acquisition range (T_k), defined as the range in time after excitation over which the data are collected, must be sufficiently short in relation to the T_2s of the signals. Capturing rapidly decaying signals without adequate encoding speed leads to image blurring, which can seriously degrade image resolution and counteract the benefit of capturing the signals in the first place.

In this section, we cover the concepts of signal capture, spatial encoding, and data acquisition in the context of short-T_2 MRI. In essence, these topics concern the timing of the imaging sequence and associated hardware requirements. For a more extensive discussion of the concepts covered here and short-T_2 imaging in general, we refer the reader to the review by Weiger and Pruessmann [7].

Signal Capture

Sequence

In order to capture rapidly decaying signals, it is imperative that the imaging sequence allows the signal readout to start as soon as possible after signal generation. That is, data acquisition should follow RF excitation with minimal delay, targeting a minimal value for the echo time (TE).

This strict timing requirement has several implications. First, there is limited time to prepare magnetization between excitation and readout, and standard procedures like slice selection and phase encoding should therefore be avoided. Hence, short-T_2 imaging sequences are usually three-dimensional (3D), and some of the contrast options available with standard MRI are not available with short-T_2 MRI. Second, each k-space point should be accessible in the shortest possible time, which is achieved with radial center-out encoding geometry. Third, because the encoding gradient cannot ramp up instantaneously, the fastest way to reach a given k-space point is to ramp up the gradient before RF excitation and thereby traverse k-space at full speed.

Only a few basic sequence designs are capable of achieving sufficiently short TE to be considered short-T_2 techniques; the two most promising are known as ultrashort echo time (UTE) [40] and zero echo time (ZTE) [41]. Both designs use pure frequency encoding to acquire radial k-space spokes, but in UTE the gradient is ramped up after RF excitation and begins simultaneously with data acquisition, whereas in ZTE the gradient is ramped up before RF excitation so that it is fully operational over the entire acquisition range.

Another useful sequence is single-point imaging (SPI) [42], in which each k-space point is individually acquired using pure phase encoding. As with ZTE, the gradient is ramped up before RF excitation. The benefits of SPI are that each k-space point is acquired at the same time after excitation (TE), making the sequence immune to T_2 blurring effects, and that the radial directions can be chosen so that the data points are placed on a Cartesian grid. On the other hand, acquiring only one k-space point per excitation is inefficient both in terms of the shortest possible scan time and signal-to-noise ratio (SNR), rendering SPI generally unsuitable for *in vivo* imaging.

Rudimentary ZTE, UTE, and SPI sequences are displayed in Fig. 41.3.

RF Dead-Time

Due to the finite duration of the RF pulse and hardware switching from transmit to receive operations, there is a dead-time between signal excitation and data acquisition. In UTE, this dead-time represents the minimum TE. In ZTE, because the gradient is already operational during excitation, TE (defined as the time from the magnetic center of the excitation pulse to the center of the k-space) is theoretically zero. However, due to the RF dead-time, it is not possible to begin data acquisition immediately and thus the dead-time translates to a data gap in the central k-space, which must be handled appropriately (see later section).

The dead-time does not impact the SPI sequence because, with pure phase encoding, the minimum TE is given by the time at which the outermost k-space point (k_{max}) can be reached, which, in practice, is usually longer than the dead-time.

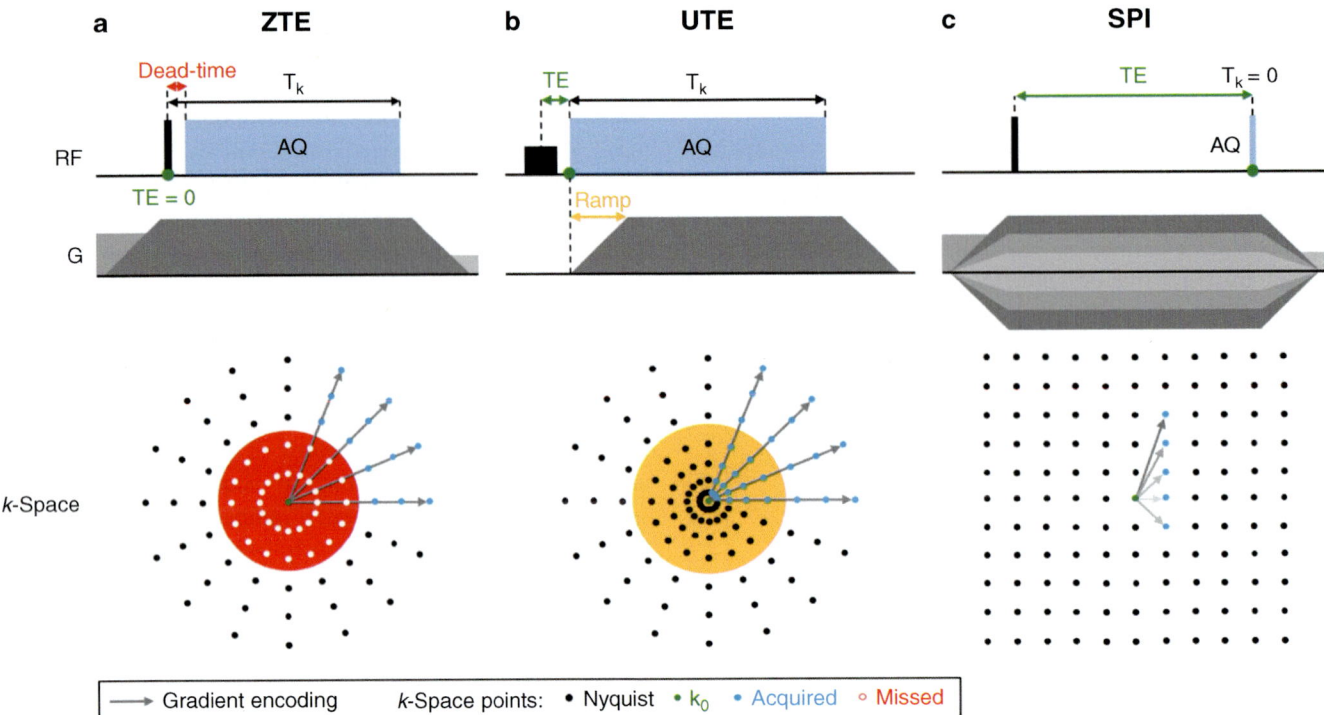

Fig. 41.3 Sequence diagrams (top row) and k-space sampling patterns (bottom row) of the ZTE (**a**), UTE (**b**), and SPI (**c**) imaging sequences. In ZTE and UTE, the acquisition range T_k represents the time required to travel from k_0 to k_{max}, where k_0 is the center of k-space and k_{max} is the k-space radius. In ZTE, the RF dead-time leads to a data gap in central k-space that contributes to the acquisition range if the data points are recovered using algebraic reconstruction [43]. In UTE, the central k-space is acquired with a nonuniform radial density due to gradient ramping. In SPI, the gradient strength is altered at each repetition time (TR) to reach each k-space point at time TE. In ZTE and SPI, encoding gradients operate continuously but change direction at each TR, as illustrated by the rectangular gradients preceding and succeeding the gradient ramps. Abbreviations: AQ acquisition; G encoding gradient. (Modified with permission from Weiger and Pruessmann [7])

Spatial Encoding and Data Acquisition

Signal decay during the acquisition range is equivalent to signal modulation by an exponential function whose width reflects the time constant of the decay. More rapid decay gives a narrower modulation function, which, in the frequency domain, translates to a wider convolution kernel. As such, signal decay that is rapid with respect to the acquisition range results in image blurring and the degree of blurring increases with more rapid signal decay.

A demonstration of the importance of early signal capture and a short acquisition range for short-T_2 imaging is provided in Fig. 41.4. As a rule of thumb, the acquisition range should be approximately equal to the T_2 of the signals to achieve near-nominal image resolution while retaining the SNR benefits of longer acquisitions [44]. Acquisition ranges shorter than T_2 avoid resolution degradation but compromise the SNR.

The acquisition range in frequency-encoded radial center-out encoding schemes is governed by the time required to traverse k-space radially from the center (k_0) to k_{max}. Because the k-space radius is proportional to the integral of the gradient over time, the only way to reach k_{max} in a shorter time is to increase the gradient amplitude, that is, use a stronger gradient.

Because the gradient is ramped up after excitation in UTE, the integral of the gradient over a given time and given maximum gradient strength is necessarily smaller than with ZTE, in which the gradient is continuously operated at full strength. The acquisition range penalty for UTE compared to ZTE corresponds to half the duration of the gradient ramp. While a longer acquisition range theoretically offers SNR benefits, UTE spends the added time in central k-space, which is already densely oversampled due to the way the radial encoding scheme fulfills the Nyquist sampling criterion at k_{max}.

In SPI, the gradient strength determines the minimum TE, but because each k-space point is individually acquired, the acquisition range is negligible.

Hardware Considerations

In summary, the requirements for successful short-T_2 imaging are as follows:

1. The RF dead-time and/or the TE, depending on the sequence, must be sufficiently short so that the targeted signals are captured with reasonable magnitude. There is no hard rule for when this condition is met, and it is up to the user to ensure that the targeted signals, based on their known characteristics such as decay behavior, can be cap-

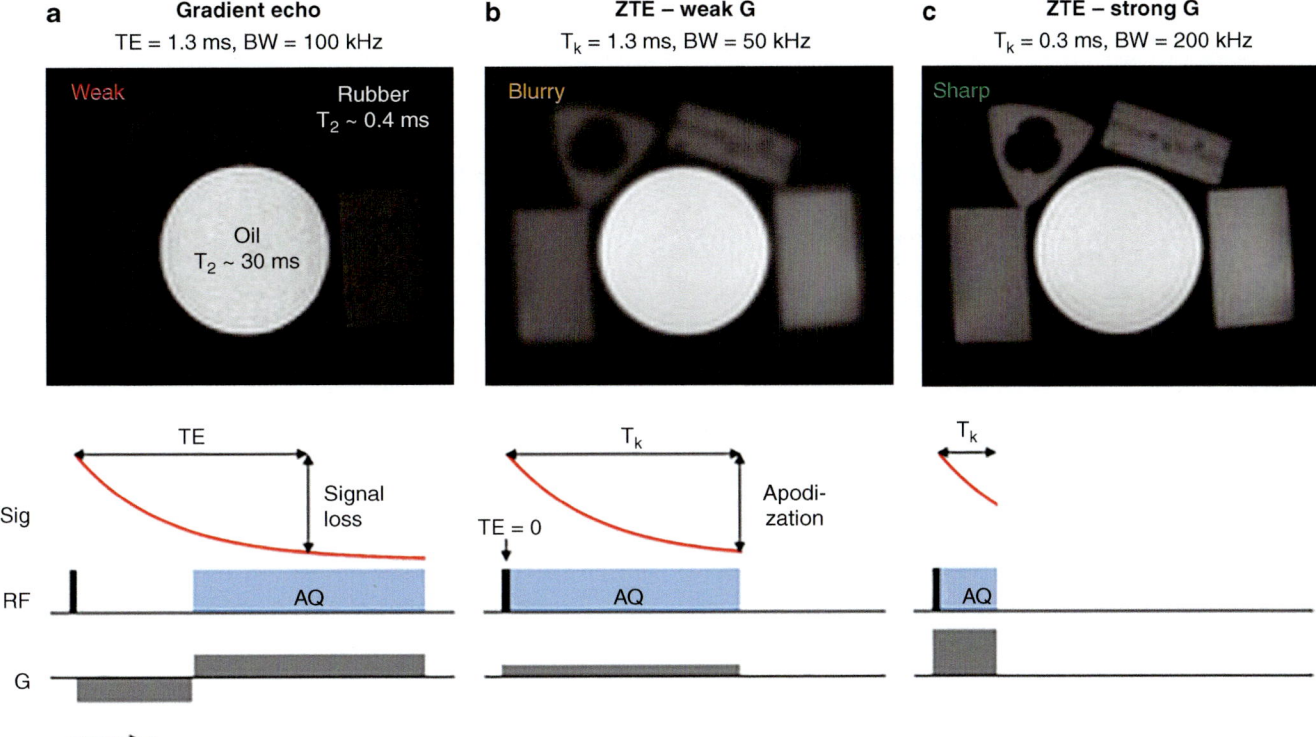

Fig. 41.4 Demonstration of the importance of early signal capture and rapid encoding/acquisition for short-T_2 imaging. (**a**) A standard gradient echo protocol, with which the short-T_2 (~400 μs) rubber phantoms are barely visible in the image. (**b**) A ZTE protocol with a weak gradient, for which the early signal capture (TE = 0) allows the short-T_2 phantoms to be visualized. However, due to signal decay during readout (apodization), the short-T_2 phantoms are blurred. (**c**) A ZTE protocol with a strong gradient, for which the rapid readout results in a sharp image. Abbreviations: AQ acquisition; G encoding gradient/gradient strength; Sig signal; T_k acquisition range. (Modified with permission from Weiger and Pruessmann [7])

tured with sufficient SNR using the available sequence and hardware.

2. The acquisition range must be approximately equal to, or less than, the T_2 of the signals to achieve near-nominal image resolution. In tissues such as myelin, in which signal decay is determined by a spectrum of T_2 values, acceptable acquisition ranges can be empirically determined by observing the level of blurring in images (in which only the short-T_2 components are included) or through simulations.

Details regarding the RF dead-time and strategies to minimize this can be found in Chap. 5 ("ZTE-MRI"). Overall, the minimum RF dead-time can be reduced to just a few microseconds depending on which technique is employed.

The constraint on the acquisition range entirely concerns gradient performance, which is covered in detail in this section. There are certain additional considerations imposed by the particularities of short-T_2 imaging that we also cover here.

The Gradient System

The magnetic field gradient is commonly characterized by its strength and slew rate. Currently, clinical gradient systems provide a maximum strength of up to 80 mT/m and a maximum slew rate of around 200 mT/m/ms.

Another important gradient specification is the duty cycle, for which 100% corresponds to continuous operation (it should be noted that MRI manufacturers may use different definitions). Running ZTE imaging sequences efficiently requires a full gradient duty cycle due to the way the gradient direction is switched from one TR to the next.

At 100% duty cycle, the maximum gradient strength of clinical systems is only around 30 mT/m. In contrast, current custom-built gradient systems can reach a strength of more than 200 mT/m at full duty cycle with a slew rate of 600 mT/m/ms by choosing targeted anatomy (typically the head or an extremity) rather than whole-body coverage [45].

The use of a strong gradient is a requirement for short-T_2 imaging regardless of the sequence. The gradient achieves spatial encoding by spreading the precession frequencies of the spins across the field of view (FOV); the stronger the gradient, the more the spin frequencies are spread out. The spread of frequencies across the FOV is equivalent to the image bandwidth (BW), such that use of a strong gradient corresponds to high-BW imaging.

The ZTE acquisition range is given by

$$T_k = \left(2\Delta r \, \gamma \, G\right)^{-1} \qquad (41.1)$$

and the image BW is given by

$$BW = \gamma G \, FOV \qquad (41.2)$$

where G denotes the gradient strength, γ is the gyromagnetic ratio, and Δr is the spatial resolution. For an isotropic FOV of 260 mm, which would accommodate head imaging, and spatial resolution of 1.5 mm, a maximum gradient strength of 40 mT/m yields an acquisition range of almost 200 μs and a BW of 0.44 MHz. With a gradient strength of 200 mT/m, the acquisition range is reduced to under 40 μs and the BW is increased to 2.2 MHz.

For UTE, a finite gradient slew rate lengthens the acquisition range compared to ZTE. Even with a slew rate of 600 mT/m/ms to reach the maximum gradient strength of 200 mT/m, the acquisition range in UTE is almost 170 μs longer than that in ZTE. That said, the acquisition range in UTE poses a different optimization problem than in ZTE because a stronger gradient does not simply speed up the encoding but also prolongs the gradient ramp. In fact, for a slew rate of 600 mT/m/ms, the minimum UTE acquisition range occurs for a gradient strength of roughly 100 mT/m. However, this optimal regime still yields an acquisition range of more than 160 μs. Even if a slew rate of 2500 mT/m/ms could be reached, for which the optimal UTE gradient strength approaches 200 mT/m, the acquisition range (80 μs) would still be twice that of ZTE for the same gradient strength.

Unwanted Signals

In addition to acquiring signals from the target tissue, short-T_2 imaging systems capture signals from materials in the vicinity of the imaging volume. This includes general setup items such as ear plugs and cushions as well as the housing of the RF coil and materials in the scanner bore.

Any encoded signals must be included in the FOV to avoid aliasing, which (particularly for 3D volumes) can result in increased encoding efforts and unfavorable imaging conditions.

Depending on the setup and imaging sample, there may be signals that decay too rapidly to encode. In such cases, it is often preferable to exclude these signals to avoid image blurring. If the signal source is not removable (for example, by adapting or using alternative hardware), signals can be excluded by delaying data acquisition past the RF dead-time

in order to allow the troublesome signals to decay away. Perhaps counterintuitively, it can even be necessary to exclude signals with particularly short T_2s stemming from tissue. This solution is also applicable to coil ringdown and other transients in the acquisition chain.

The most effective hardware solution to remove unwanted signals and limit the FOV to the object under examination is to employ ^{1}H-free RF coils. Currently, such coils are typically custom-built using materials such as glass and Teflon [46, 47].

Signals originating in the scanner bore can be excluded by passive shielding. Signals from cushions and similar items are generally not problematic because these items are available in many forms and can be chosen so that they fit inside the desired FOV.

RF Excitation BW

In ZTE and SPI, the gradient is already fully operational during RF excitation; therefore, the excitation pulse BW must match the image BW in order to excite the whole object. Consequently, because short-T_2 imaging implies a high image BW, high-BW RF pulses that are capable of reaching the desired flip angle are required. Options and considerations for excitation pulses can be found in Chap. 5 ("ZTE-MRI").

Handling the RF Dead-Time Gap

In most cases, the RF dead-time is effectively fixed in duration. In ZTE, in which the dead-time leads to a data gap in central k-space, the application of a strong gradient means that k-space is traversed faster, and, consequently, the dead-time gap covers a larger k-space radius than it would with a weaker gradient.

In conventional ZTE, the data gap is handled by algebraic reconstruction, in which oversampling is used to recover the missing data points [43]. However, this approach breaks down for gap sizes spanning more than a few Nyquist dwells [41].

When the image BW for which algebraic reconstruction is feasible is exceeded, the missing data points can be obtained using additional acquisitions with reduced gradient strength. There are several strategies for sampling the central k-space in this manner, with the most notable employing SPI (techniques known as pointwise encoding time reduction with radial acquisition (PETRA) [48] and ramped hybrid encoding (RHE) [49]), radial acquisitions (a technique known as water- and fat-suppressed proton projection MRI (WASPI) [50]), or a combination of the two (a technique known as hybrid filling (HYFI) [51]). We will not cover these strategies in further detail, but an important point to note is that, although a large dead-time gap does not, in principle, restrict imaging, the additional acquisitions required to fill the gap reduce the SNR efficiency, shift TE to finite values (for PETRA, RHE, and HYFI), and can make images more susceptible to short-T_2 artifacts (in particular, for WASPI) [52].

Myelin Bilayer Imaging Prospects

Myelin bilayer imaging has the potential to offer improved myelin specificity compared to methods relying on the detection of water signals. To exploit this potential, even the most rapidly decaying signals stemming from the myelin bilayer must be captured and spatially encoded. In this section, we discuss the ability of the UTE, ZTE, and SPI sequence designs to achieve such ultrashort-T_2 imaging.

UTE is a popular technique for myelin bilayer imaging. Although UTE can offer attractive TEs without the data gap inherent to ZTE, the gradient ramp (even with impressive slew rate specifications) prolongs the acquisition range beyond what is reasonable for spatial encoding of the bulk of myelin bilayer signals. Based on the presented calculations and previous simulations [35], UTE is most appropriate for imaging of tissues exhibiting T_2s in the hundreds of microseconds range. While this range includes the tail of the myelin bilayer T_2 distribution (see Fig. 41.2e–f), there are several non-myelin sources of signals with similar characteristics [35], rendering such measurements relatively unspecific for myelin.

ZTE, on the other hand, utilizes immediate full encoding speed to minimize the acquisition duration. As such, this technique offers a framework compatible with *in vivo* imaging of tissues exhibiting T_2s down to the tens of microseconds range [53], which includes the vast majority of myelin bilayer signals.

SPI also benefits from immediate full encoding speed, and the technique has the advantage of immunity to signal decay across the *k*-space. However, spatial resolution and TE are coupled through the available gradient strength, and SNR efficiency is low. Consequently, SPI is not advisable for *in vivo* myelin bilayer imaging but can be advantageous in *ex vivo* studies.

Even with ZTE or SPI approaches, imaging the myelin bilayer poses significant challenges and is only feasible with advanced gradient and RF hardware capable of performing high-BW imaging.

Current State of Myelin Bilayer Imaging

MR experiments sensitive to myelin bilayer signals broadly fit into two categories, namely those assessing signal properties and those producing myelin images, be it quantitative maps or contrast-weighted images. Several studies analyzing myelin bilayer signals have been performed because they

can be readily conducted using nuclear magnetic resonance (NMR) methods [29, 54–56], but imaging poses significant challenges.

So far, most studies imaging the myelin bilayer have been based on UTE approaches, which provide good SNR and data quality within moderate scan times [57–67]. The decay constants reported for multi-TE UTE investigations in the CNS consistently confirm the conclusion that UTE is primarily sensitive to tissues exhibiting T_2s in the hundreds of microseconds range, which only covers the tail of the myelin distribution shown in Fig. 41.2e–f. Consequently, it is believed that most of the signals captured in the reported UTE studies are not from myelin and that the myelin specificity in these studies is likely limited.

Initial studies utilizing ZTE approaches for myelin bilayer imaging have also been reported [55, 68, 69]; however, these studies used only moderate image BWs and, as such, their acquisition ranges were too long (hundreds of microseconds) to fully exploit the potential of ZTE.

In the interest of pursuing optimal myelin sensitivity and specificity, the focus of this part is on studies conducted using imaging techniques and hardware specifications that allow the capture and encoding of the ultrashort-T_2 signals stemming from the myelin bilayer. For practical reasons, these studies employed SPI or ZTE approaches. The two techniques have been used to address distinct research questions, and, therefore, the experiments utilizing them are described in separate sections.

SPI: Signal Analysis and Quantitative Mapping

Because certain signal components of the myelin bilayer can be said to be specific to myelin, such as the component representing the CH_2 protons on general alkyl chains (see Table 41.1), while others do not contribute significantly or distinctly enough to be distinguishable from non-myelin signals, signal component separation is an important factor in myelin specificity.

Imaging poses much stronger experimental restrictions than NMR spectroscopy and affects the ability of techniques to separate different signal components. Multi-TE SPI experiments, which provide practically voxel-wise free induction decay (FID) measurements and thus conceptually represent spatially localized NMR experiments, offer unique insights into the translation between the underlying signal components and the signal components detectable in imaging experiments.

Nonaqueous signal analysis relies on some form of water signal removal; otherwise, the aqueous signals dominate and the nonaqueous signals become much harder to characterize and/or visualize. In *ex vivo* experiments, water signals can be eliminated by performing D_2O exchange, in which the ^1H nuclei of H_2O are replaced with ^2H, resulting in free water signals with a different resonance frequency that are invisible with ^{1}H MR.

All myelin bilayer SPI experiments have been performed *ex vivo* using the same dedicated short-T_2 imaging system, and, in each experiment, the TE started at just over 30 μs. Samples from porcine [35], healthy human [70], and MS brains [71] have been studied.

In all the experiments, two nonaqueous (super-Lorentzian) signal components were identified, one in the 5–10 μs $T_{2,min}$ range and one in the 100–200 μs $T_{2,min}$ range. These components are in agreement with the results reported in NMR studies [29, 55, 56]. Figure 41.5a contains an example of myelin bilayer signal analysis in which fitting a complex three-component signal model to multi-TE WM data from a D_2O-exchanged sample enables characterization of the signal components.

The shorter nonaqueous signal component is considered to represent the general alkyl chain CH_2 protons in the myelin bilayer, and, therefore, voxel-wise fitted amplitudes of this component effectively constitute a quantitative myelin map. Despite matching the smaller myelin lipid components provided in Table 41.1, the longer component is not considered to be myelin specific.

A crucial outcome of the *ex vivo* SPI experiments is that, after identifying the signal components in D_2O-exchanged samples, taking these components as prior knowledge allows robust component mapping also in samples with native H_2O content. Myelin maps are shown in Fig. 41.5b for both a D_2O-exchanged sample and a non-exchanged sample.

An important distinction concerns the interpretation of signal components in GM compared to WM. In WM, in which myelin is abundant, it is much easier to claim myelin

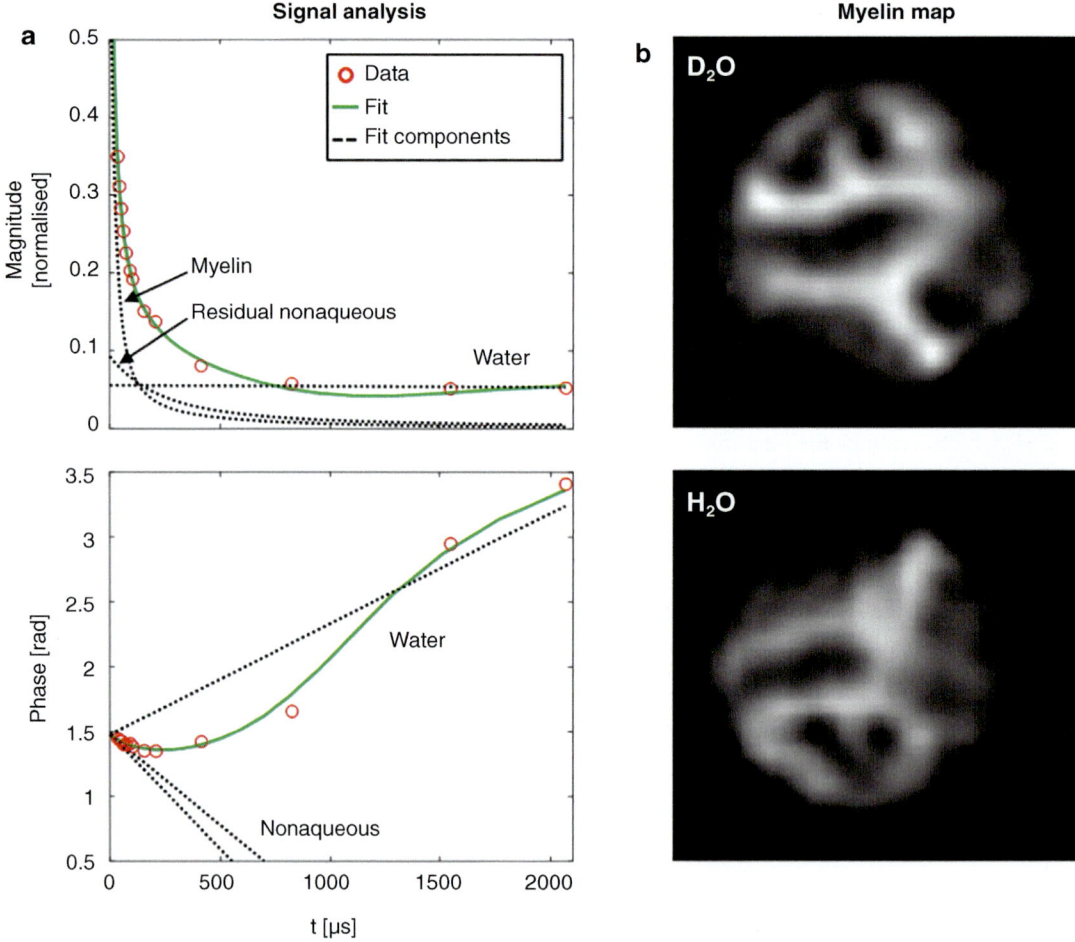

Fig. 41.5 *Ex vivo* myelin mapping results (porcine brain). (**a**) Analysis of WM signal behavior (averaged over a large region of interest) in a D_2O-exchanged sample. Three signal components were identified: myelin ($T_{2,min}$ = 7.5 μs, chemical shift = 1.4 ppm), residual nonaqueous content ($T_{2,min}$ = 101 μs, chemical shift = 1.9 ppm), and water (T_2 = 50 ms, chemical shift = 4.7 ppm). (**b**) Amplitude maps of the myelin signal component in a D_2O-exchanged sample (top row) and a non-exchanged sample (bottom row, labeled H_2O), showing larger amplitudes in WM than in GM. (Modified with permission from Weiger et al.[35])

specificity of (appropriate) signal components than in GM, in which the nonaqueous content is primarily non-myelin. The shortest nonaqueous component, which is assigned to myelin in the WM, can therefore not be considered myelin-specific in GM without further inspection.

Myelin bilayer imaging in GM is a relatively unexplored topic, and its feasibility will have to be assessed separately from the WM case. That said, GM signals exhibit similar behavior to WM signals [70], and, as such, the signal components can be mapped using the same procedure for both tissue types.

ZTE: Myelin-Weighted Imaging

The dedicated short-T_2 imaging system used for the SPI experiments covered in the previous section has also been employed to obtain myelin-weighted ZTE-based images. Notably, the combination of ZTE approaches and advanced MR hardware has allowed *in vivo* myelin bilayer imaging with an acquisition range below 30 µs [35].

In vivo, D_2O exchange for background water removal is not feasible. Instead, an image in which background water signals are largely removed can be produced by acquiring an additional image at a comparatively long TE (thus containing predominantly long-T_2 contributions) and subtracting it from the short-TE image. A limitation of this method is that some water signals (for example, from myelin water) may decay non-negligibly between the TEs of the two images and thus be inadequately removed in the subtraction procedure. Alternatively, inversion pulses can be used [55, 59], but they require accommodated sequence timing.

ZTE approaches have also been applied *ex vivo* to produce high-resolution anatomical reference images for use in conjunction with SPI experiments [35, 70, 71]. In both the *in vivo* and *ex vivo* experiments, images heavily weighted for short-T_2 tissue components were presented (using dual-TE subtraction for *in vivo* and D_2O exchange for *ex vivo* experiments). This contrast clearly differentiates WM and GM but is not fully specific to myelin, thus limiting quantitative interpretation.

In the *in vivo* experiment, a human head was imaged with a scan time of 46 minutes and an isotropic resolution of 1.7 mm; the results are shown in Fig. 41.6. Spatial resolution in such experiments is limited by the available gradient strength, SNR, and total scan time; the last two limitations could be addressed by improved RF coil hardware or increased main magnetic field strength.

Compromising Between Myelin Specificity and Technique Complexity

So far, the knowledge gained from multi-TE SPI experiments has not been utilized to improve myelin specificity in ZTE approaches. There are several hurdles to overcome when moving from *ex vivo* to *in vivo*, even given an imaging system that can technically handle both.

In principle, it is feasible to acquire a multi-TE protocol *in vivo*, although the number of TEs would be limited by scan time considerations. To improve *in vivo* myelin specificity compared to the simpler dual-TE subtraction approach, the ZTE-based multi-TE protocol would need to provide sufficient data points and data quality to extract the myelin-specific signal component seen in *ex vivo* SPI experiments. Even with such a protocol, the frequency-encoded nature of ZTE introduces differences in the time after excitation at which each k-space point is sampled, and, as such, each reconstructed image does not accurately represent a single TE, which may impact the fitting results.

The error introduced by assuming a fixed TE may prove negligible, but it could also prove necessary to account for the k-space time evolution; either way, this point must be addressed. Ultimately, errors accumulated across various aspects of the imaging protocol and reconstruction/analysis pipeline will determine the achievable myelin specificity, and optimal myelin bilayer imaging *in vivo* will likely be a compromise between the SPI multi-TE fitting and ZTE dual-TE subtraction approaches.

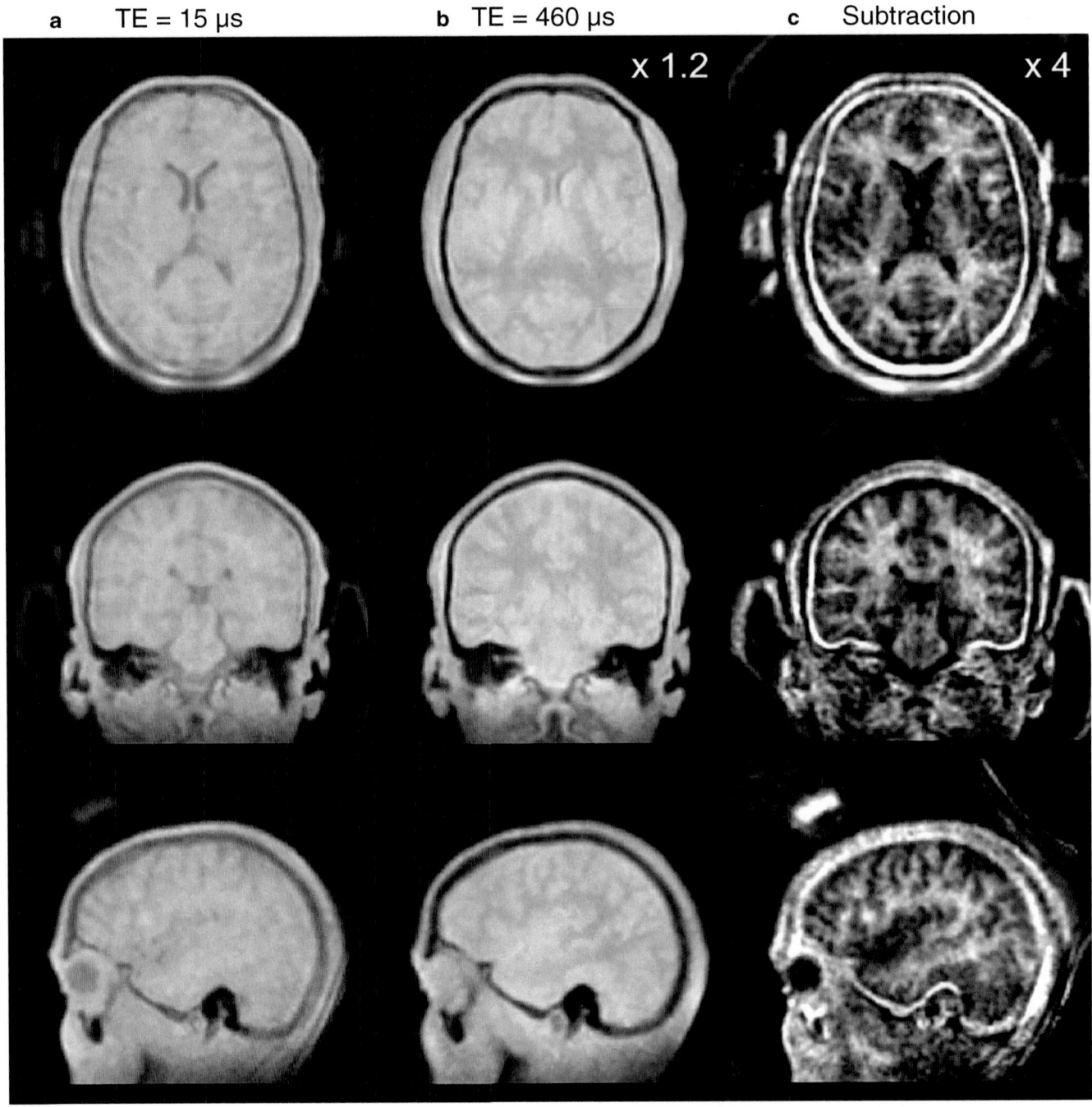

Fig. 41.6 *In vivo* myelin imaging results (human head). A long-TE image (**b**) is subtracted from a short-TE image (**a**), yielding an image depicting mainly short-T_2 tissues (**c**). The short-TE image was acquired using the PETRA variant of ZTE, and the long-TE image was acquired using the HYFI variant of ZTE. (Modified with permission from Weiger et al.[35])

Future Directions

Myelin bilayer imaging is still at an early stage in its development. So far, research has focused on *ex vivo* studies, with *in vivo* application still contending with several barriers; it is therefore difficult to speculate on the "final" state of myelin bilayer imaging. That said, it is possible to identify the main challenges facing the widespread use of myelin bilayer imaging techniques and reflect on how these techniques fit into the broader picture of clinical assessment and medical research.

Early Stages

Before pushing a technique toward widespread use and requesting support from manufacturers, the technique must be sufficiently validated to conclude that it is worthy of serious pursuit.

For myelin bilayer imaging, this primarily concerns ensuring that the proposed approaches can visualize the myelin bilayer with improved accuracy and specificity. It might also entail identifying diseases or pathological mechanisms that particularly benefit from increased myelin specificity, such as cases in which the connection between an indirect myelin measure and the underlying myelin content breaks down.

On a related note, myelin bilayer imaging should undergo thorough comparison with more established myelin MRI techniques such as myelin water imaging. In the interest of fairness, such a comparison would need to account for the discrepancy in the stage of development of the techniques; given time to mature, myelin bilayer imaging methods may well look different from today's versions.

Later Stages

The most pressing challenges of short-T_2 MRI are technical. Standard RF and gradient hardware do not meet the strict timing requirements for short-T_2 imaging, especially for the range of T_2s present in the myelin bilayer. For myelin bilayer imaging to be feasible at multiple sites and in wider studies, manufacturers would have to provide hardware such as ^{1}H-free RF coils, strong encoding gradients, and fast, high-power transmit–receive switches. The most realistic form of such a system is a dedicated head scanner, for which the primary downside would be the exclusion of spinal cord studies.

It would also be necessary to ensure that scan times are feasible for larger studies on volunteers and patients. Longer duration scans increase problems with subject motion and may require motion correction strategies. It is hard to say how long an *in vivo* protocol for myelin bilayer imaging would be, but, with the inherent SNR penalty of high-BW imaging, it is expected that the limits of acceptable scan time will be pushed. As such, it is of interest to explore scan time reduction, for instance, through undersampling strategies for gap-filled variants of ZTE.

Another topic to consider is image reconstruction speed, which, depending on the complexity of the employed signal model, could become limiting. Clinical users expect images to be available almost immediately following image acquisition, but time delays could be acceptable depending on how the myelin maps would be used. In research studies, long reconstruction times are not unusual. At the current stage of myelin bilayer imaging, optimizing processing times is not a priority.

Possible Uses

Ultimately, the utility of myelin bilayer imaging will depend on how well the obstacles to its implementation can be overcome. If the necessary technical system specifications are available, then there is no reason why large scale studies cannot be performed. If studies conclude that myelin bilayer imaging offers advantages over other available techniques, the benefits and challenges of the different methods can be weighed against each other to determine the optimal approach for a given application.

Due to the significant technical challenges and the time-consuming nature of myelin bilayer imaging techniques, it is not yet clear whether or not they will enter the realm of routine clinical imaging. It is also unclear how the availability of myelin maps will impact diagnostic practice because demyelination is a feature of many CNS disorders and is therefore not specific to any one disorder.

That said, it is plausible that myelin bilayer imaging could add significant value to the long term monitoring of patients with CNS disorders by providing accurate information about relative changes in myelin content. Such information could be used to evaluate disease progression, study the relationship between clinical symptoms and local myelin content, and understand the mechanisms involved in demyelination and myelin repair. Myelin bilayer imaging could also be useful in drug trials directed at demyelinating diseases, for which an accurate assessment of myelin content would be a valuable measure of therapeutic response.

References

1. Bydder GM, Steiner RE, Young IR, Hall AS, Thomas DJ, Marshall J, et al. Clinical NMR imaging of the brain: 140 cases. Am J Neuroradiol. 1982;3(5):459–80.
2. Lukes SA, Crooks LE, Aminoff MJ, Kaufman L, Panitch HS, Mills C, et al. Nuclear magnetic resonance imaging in multiple sclerosis. Ann Neurol. 1983;13(6):592–601.
3. Sheldon JJ, Siddharthan R, Tobias J, Sheremata WA, Soila K, Viamonte M. MR imaging of multiple sclerosis: comparison with clinical and CT examinations in 74 patients. Am J Neuroradiol. 1985;6(5):683–90.
4. Asbury AK, Herndon RM, McFarland HF, McDonald WI, Paty DW, Prineas JW, et al. Use of magnetic resonance imaging in the diagnosis of multiple sclerosis. Policy statement of the National Multiple Sclerosis Society, New York. Magn Reson Med. 1986;3(5):821–2.
5. Valk J, Van Der Knaap MS. Basic principles of magnetic resonance imaging and its application in myelin disorders. In: Magnetic resonance of myelin, myelination, and myelin disorders. Berlin Heidelberg: Springer; 1989. p. 22–5.
6. Laule C, Vavasour IM, Kolind SH, Li DKB, Traboulsee TL, Moore GRW, et al. Magnetic resonance imaging of myelin. Neurotherapeutics. 2007;4(3):460–84.
7. Weiger M, Pruessmann KP. Short-T_2 MRI: principles and recent advances. Prog Nucl Magn Reson Spectrosc. 2019;114-115:237–70.
8. Waxman SG, Bangalore L. Electrophysiologic consequences of myelination. In: Lazzarini RA, editor. Myelin biology and disorders. Elsevier; 2004. p. 117–41.
9. Rasband MN, Macklin WB. Myelin structure and biochemistry. In: Brady ST, Siegel GJ, Albers RW, Price DL, editors. Basic neurochemistry. 8th ed. Elsevier; 2012. p. 180–99.
10. Salzer JL, Zalc B. Myelination. Curr Biol. 2016;26(20):R971–5.
11. Baron W, Hoekstra D. On the biogenesis of myelin membranes: sorting, trafficking and cell polarity. FEBS Lett. 2010;584(9):1760–70.

12. Stadelmann C, Timmler S, Barrantes-Freer A, Simons M. Myelin in the central nervous system: structure, function, and pathology. Physiol Rev. 2019;99(3):1381–431.

13. World Health Organization. Neurological disorders: public health challenges. 2006.

14. Reich DS, Lucchinetti CF, Calabresi PA. Multiple sclerosis. N Engl J Med. 2018;378(2):169–80.

15. Multiple Sclerosis International Federation. Atlas of MS. 3rd edition. Part 1: Mapping multiple sclerosis around the world: key epidemiology findings. 2020.

16. Dobson R, Giovannoni G. Multiple sclerosis—a review. Eur J Neurol. 2019;26(1):27–40.

17. Calabrese M, Favaretto A, Martini V, Gallo P. Grey matter lesions in MS. Prion. 2013;7(1):20–7.

18. Popescu BFG, Lucchinetti CF. Pathology of demyelinating diseases. Annu Rev Pathol. 2012;7(1):185–217.

19. Love S. Demyelinating diseases. J Clin Pathol. 2006;59(11):1151–9.

20. Perlman SJ, Mar S. Leukodystrophies. In: Ahmad SI, editor. Neurodegenerative diseases. 2012. p. 154–71.

21. Nasrabady SE, Rizvi B, Goldman JE, Brickman AM. White matter changes in Alzheimer's disease: a focus on myelin and oligodendrocytes. Acta Neuropathol Commun. 2018;6(1):22.

22. Drenthen GS, Backes WH, Aldenkamp AP, Vermeulen RJ, Klinkenberg S, Jansen JFA. On the merits of non-invasive myelin imaging in epilepsy, a literature review. J Neurosci Meth. 2020;338:108687.

23. Jia W, Kamen Y, Pivonkova H, Káradóttir RT. Neuronal activity-dependent myelin repair after stroke. Neurosci Lett. 2019;703:139–44.

24. Zikopoulos B, Barbas H. Changes in prefrontal axons may disrupt the network in autism. J Neurosci. 2010;30(44):14595–609.

25. Stedehouder J, Kushner SA. Myelination of parvalbumin interneurons: a parsimonious locus of pathophysiological convergence in schizophrenia. Mol Psychiatry. 2017;22(1):4–12.

26. Van der Knaap MS, Valk J. Myelin and white matter. Magnetic resonance of myelination and myelin disorders: Springer Science & Business Media; 2005.

27. Kwee IL, Nakada T. Phospholipid profile of the human brain: 31P NMR spectroscopic study. Magn Reson Med. 1988;6(3):296–9.

28. Kilby PM, Bolas NM, Radda GK. 31P-NMR study of brain phospholipid structures in vivo. Biochim Biophys Acta. 1991;1085(2):257–64.

29. Wilhelm MJ, Ong HH, Wehrli SL, Li C, Tsai PH, Hackney DB, et al. Direct magnetic resonance detection of myelin and prospects for quantitative imaging of myelin density. Proc Natl Acad Sci U S A. 2012;109(24):9605–10.

30. Piredda GF, Hilbert T, Thiran JP, Kober T. Probing myelin content of the human brain with MRI: a review. Magn Reson Med. 2021;85(2):627–52.

31. MacKay A, Whittall K, Adler J, Li D, Paty D, Graeb D. In vivo visualization of myelin water in brain by magnetic resonance. Magn Reson Med. 1994;31(6):673–7.

32. Varma G, Duhamel G, de Bazelaire C, Alsop DC. Magnetization transfer from inhomogeneously broadened lines: a potential marker for myelin. Magn Reson Med. 2015;73(2):614–22.

33. Wennerström H. Proton nuclear magnetic resonance lineshapes in lamellar liquid crystals. Chem Phys Lett. 1973;18(1):41–4.

34. Bloom M, Burnell EE, Valic MI, Weeks G. Nuclear magnetic resonance line shapes in lipid bi-layer model membranes. Chem Phys Lipids. 1975;14(2):107–12.

35. Weiger M, Froidevaux R, Baadsvik EL, Brunner DO, Rösler MB, Pruessmann KP. Advances in MRI of the myelin bilayer. NeuroImage. 2020;217:116888.

36. MacKay AL, Laule C. Magnetic resonance of myelin water: an in vivo marker for myelin. Brain Plast. 2016;2(1):71–91.

37. Littlemore L. NMR studies on myelin basic protein. II. 1H N.M.R. studies of the protein and constituent peptides in aqueous solutions. Aust J Chem. 1978;31(11):2387:2387.

38. Waldman A, Rees J, Brock C, Robson M, Gatehouse P, Bydder G. MRI of the brain with ultra-short echo-time pulse sequences. Neuroradiology. 2003;45(12):887–92.

39. Gatehouse P, Bydder G. Magnetic resonance imaging of short T_2 components in tissue. Clin Radiol. 2003;58(1):1–19.

40. Robson MD, Gatehouse PD, Bydder M, Bydder GM. Magnetic resonance: an introduction to ultrashort TE (UTE) imaging. J Comput Assist Tomogr. 2003;27(6):825–46.

41. Weiger M, Pruessmann KP. MRI with zero echo time. eMagRes. 1. Chichester, UK: Wiley; 2012. p. 311–22.

42. Balcom BJ, MacGregor RP, Beyea SD, Green DP, Armstrong RL, Bremner TW. Single-point ramped imaging with T_1 enhancement (SPRITE). J Magn Reson Ser A. 1996;123(1):131–4.

43. Kuethe DO, Caprihan A, Lowe IJ, Madio DP, Gach HM. Transforming NMR data despite missing points. J Magn Reson. 1999;139(1):18–25.

44. Rahmer J, Börnert P, Groen J, Bos C. Three-dimensional radial ultrashort echo-time imaging with T_2 adapted sampling. Magn Reson Med. 2006;55(5):1075–82.

45. Weiger M, Overweg J, Rösler MB, Froidevaux R, Hennel F, Wilm BJ, et al. A high-performance gradient insert for rapid and short-T_2 imaging at full duty cycle. Magn Reson Med. 2018;79(6):3256–66.

46. Weiger M, Brunner DO, Schmid T, Froidevaux R, Rösler MB, Gross S, et al. A virtually 1H-free birdcage coil for zero echo time MRI without background signal. Magn Reson Med. 2017;78(1):399–407.

47. Rösler MB, Weiger M, Brunner DO, Froidevaux R, Schmid T, Pruessmann KP. An eight-channel array coil for zero echo time imaging. Proc Intl Soc Mag Reson Med. 2019:438.

48. Grodzki DM, Jakob PM, Heismann B. Ultrashort echo time imaging using pointwise encoding time reduction with radial acquisition (PETRA). Magn Reson Med. 2012;67(2):510–8.

49. Jang H, Wiens CN, McMillan AB. Ramped hybrid encoding for improved ultrashort echo time imaging. Magn Reson Med. 2016;76(3):814–25.

50. Wu YT, Dai GP, Ackerman JL, Hrovat MI, Glimcher MJ, Snyder BD, et al. Water- and fat-suppressed proton projection MRI (WASPI) of rat femur bone. Magn Reson Med. 2007;57(3):554–67.

51. Froidevaux R, Weiger M, Rosler MB, Brunner DO, Pruessmann KP. HYFI: hybrid filling of the dead-time gap for faster zero echo time imaging. NMR Biomed. 2021;34(6):e4493.

52. Froidevaux R, Weiger M, Brunner DO, Dietrich BE, Wilm BJ, Pruessmann KP. Filling the dead-time gap in zero echo time MRI: principles compared. Magn Reson Med. 2018;79(4):2036–45.

53. Froidevaux R, Weiger M, Rösler MB, Brunner DO, Dietrich BE, Reber J, et al. High-resolution short-T_2 MRI using a high-performance gradient. Magn Reson Med. 2020;84(4):1933–46.

54. Horch RA, Gore JC, Does MD. Origins of the ultrashort-T_2 1H NMR signals in myelinated nerve: a direct measure of myelin content? Magn Reson Med. 2011;66(1):24–31.

55. Seifert AC, Li C, Wilhelm MJ, Wehrli SL, Wehrli FW. Towards quantification of myelin by solid-state MRI of the lipid matrix protons. NeuroImage. 2017;163:358–67.

56. Manning AP, Mackay AL, Michal CA. Understanding aqueous and non-aqueous proton T1 relaxation in brain. J Magn Reson. 2021;323:106909.

57. Nayak KS, Pauly JM, Gold GE, Nishimura DG. Imaging ultra-short T_2 species in the brain. Proc Intl Soc Mag Reson Med. 2000:509.

58. Ercan E, Boernert P, Webb A, Ronen I. Whole-brain tissue-based assessment of the ultrashort T_2 component using 3D UTE MRI relaxometry. Proc Intl Soc Mag Reson Med. 2012:4279.

59. Du J, Ma G, Li S, Carl M, Szeverenyi NM, VandenBerg S, et al. Ultrashort echo time (UTE) magnetic resonance imaging of the

short T_2 components in white matter of the brain using a clinical 3T scanner. NeuroImage. 2014;87:32–41.

60. Sheth V, Shao H, Chen J, Vandenberg S, Corey-Bloom J, Bydder GM, et al. Magnetic resonance imaging of myelin using ultrashort Echo time (UTE) pulse sequences: phantom, specimen, volunteer and multiple sclerosis patient studies. NeuroImage. 2016;136:37–44.

61. Fan SJ, Ma Y, Chang EY, Bydder GM, Du J. Inversion recovery ultrashort echo time imaging of ultrashort T_2 tissue components in ovine brain at 3 T: a sequential D2O exchange study. NMR Biomed. 2017;30(10):e3767.

62. Boucneau T, Cao P, Tang S, Han M, Xu D, Henry RG, et al. In vivo characterization of brain ultrashort-T_2 components. Magn Reson Med. 2018;80(2):726–35.

63. Fan SJ, Ma Y, Zhu Y, Searleman A, Szeverenyi NM, Bydder GM, et al. Yet more evidence that myelin protons can be directly imaged with UTE sequences on a clinical 3T scanner: bicomponent T_2* analysis of native and deuterated ovine brain specimens. Magn Reson Med. 2018;80(2):538–47.

64. Ma YJ, Searleman AC, Jang H, Fan SJ, Wong J, Xue Y, et al. Volumetric imaging of myelin in vivo using 3D inversion recovery-prepared ultrashort echo time cones magnetic resonance imaging. NMR Biomed. 2020;33(10):e4326.

65. Ma Y-J, Jang H, Wei Z, Cai Z, Xue Y, Lee RR, et al. Myelin imaging in human brain using a short repetition time adiabatic inversion recovery prepared ultrashort echo time (STAIR-UTE) MRI sequence in multiple sclerosis. Radiology. 2020;297(2):392–404.

66. Muller M, Egger N, Sommer S, Wilferth T, Meixner CR, Laun FB, et al. Direct imaging of white matter ultrashort T_2* components at 7 tesla. Magn Reson Imaging. 2022;86:107–17.

67. Shen X, Özen AC, Sunjar A, Ilbey S, Sawiak S, Shi R, et al. Ultrashort T2 components imaging of the whole brain using 3D dual-echo UTE MRI with rosette k-space pattern. Magn Reson Med. 2023;89(2):508–21.

68. Seifert AC, Umphlett M, Hefti M, Fowkes M, Xu J. Formalin tissue fixation biases myelin-sensitive MRI. Magn Reson Med. 2019;82(4):1504–17.

69. Jang H, Carl M, Ma Y, Searleman AC, Jerban S, Chang EY, et al. Inversion recovery zero echo time (IR-ZTE) imaging for direct myelin detection in human brain: a feasibility study. Quant Imaging Med Surg. 2020;10(5):895–906.

70. Baadsvik EL, Weiger M, Froidevaux R, Faigle W, Ineichen BV, Pruessmann KP. Mapping the myelin bilayer with short-T_2 MRI: methods validation and reference data for healthy human brain. Magn Reson Med. 2023;89(2):665–77.

71. Baadsvik EL, Weiger M, Froidevaux R, Faigle W, Ineichen BV, Pruessmann KP. Quantitative magnetic resonance mapping of the myelin bilayer reflects pathology in multiple sclerosis brain tissue. Science Advances. 2023;9:eadi0611.

Peder Larson

Introduction

Challenges and Opportunities for Magnetic Resonance Imaging (MRI) of the Lungs

Cross-sectional imaging of the lungs, or pulmonary imaging, has proven to be an incredibly valuable tool in a wide range of pulmonary diseases. The vast majority of lung imaging is performed with computed tomography (CT), as it is fast enough to freeze respiratory motion and provides high spatial resolution to visualize the fine structure of the lungs (e.g., airways, blood vessels, and lung parenchyma).

MRI of the lungs is inherently challenging due to the presence of large local magnetic field gradients, relatively low proton density, and motion. The lungs consist of airways, blood vessels, and parenchyma that includes microscopic air sacs called alveoli. There is a relatively large difference in magnetic susceptibility between air and lung tissue, which leads to large gradients in the magnetic field within the lung. This, in turn, leads to relatively short transverse relaxation times, T_2 and T_2^*. T_2^* is particularly short ($T_2^* = 0.8$ ms at 3 T and 2.1 ms at 1.5 T [1]) because of the intravoxel dephasing caused by the large tissue gradients in the magnetic field. T_2^* lengthens significantly at lower field strengths ($T_2^* = 8$–10 ms at 0.55T [2, 3]), an emerging opportunity discussed in this chapter. The proton density in lung parenchyma is also much lower than those of other soft tissues, as much of the parenchymal space is filled with air. Furthermore, the lungs are always moving, making motion a key challenge in performing lung MRI.

The benefits of performing MRI for lung imaging include no ionizing radiation, opportunities for multiple contrasts, and integration with other MRI scans. MRI requires no ionizing radiation compared to CT and positron emission tomography (PET)/single-photon emission computed tomography (SPECT), in which exposure increases the lifetime risk of cancer [4]. This makes MRI desirable in populations of patients, such as those in pediatrics and obstetrics, where radiation sensitivity is a particular issue. This is especially true when repeated lung imaging scans are required. MRI also offers the opportunity to obtain multiple tissue contrasts. The most common lung MRI techniques are structural T_1-weighted scans but also emerging are functional contrasts such as ventilation and perfusion as well as other MRI contrast mechanisms, including T_2-weighting and diffusion weighting. Finally, lung MRI can be combined with other MRI scanning techniques, including cardiac MRI, abdominal MRI, whole-body MRI, and PET/MRI, for increasing examination efficiency by only requiring a single scan session and providing more comprehensive assessment that includes evaluation of the pulmonary system.

Why Use UTE for MRI of the Lungs?

Ultrashort echo time (UTE) MRI has emerged as the leading approach for lung MRI due to two key advantages. First, and arguably the most significant advantage, is that it can efficiently capture rapidly decaying short-T_2^* signals from lung tissue. The other advantage of UTE-MRI is motion management. It is inherently less likely to produce motion artifacts, it includes information for motion tracking, and it is also extremely well suited to motion-compensated and motion-corrected reconstructions. This advantage comes from using center-out k-space trajectories, where repeated measurements of the center of k-space can be used both to monitor motion and to alleviate potential artifacts.

P. Larson (✉)
Department of Radiology and Biomedical Imaging, University of California, San Francisco, CA, USA
e-mail: Peder.Larson@ucsf.edu

J. Du, G. M. Bydder (eds.), *MRI of Short- and Ultrashort-T₂ Tissues*, https://doi.org/10.1007/978-3-031-35197-6_42

Methods for UTE Lung MRI

This section describes three-dimensional (3D) UTE pulse sequences; however, other pulse sequences, such as zero echo time (ZTE), two-dimensional (2D) UTE, and other gradient echo sequences can be used as well.

Pulse Sequences

One of the most successful UTE pulse sequences is shown in Fig. 42.1. It is a 3D sequence consisting of a slab-selective excitation and a center-out 3D k-space trajectory [5]. The slab selection reduces spatial encoding requirements and artifacts originating outside of the lungs. Because of its short refocusing gradient, it does not introduce any significant increase in TE. 2D UTE sequences are less common because they provide limited spatial coverage, and the half-pulse excitations they require are extremely sensitive to system delays and eddy currents.

The *k*-Space Trajectory

A large group of 3D non-Cartesian k-space trajectories has been successfully used for UTE lung MRI, with their most important features being the repeated center of k-space sampling, the ability to undersample for accelerated scanning, and the ability to perform pseudorandom temporal ordering for retrospective motion correction (Fig. 42.2). 3D radial trajectories, also known as koosh ball trajectories or projection reconstruction, are the simplest trajectories. They also cover the smallest k-space area per repetition time (TR) and suffer from reduced signal-to-noise ratio (SNR) efficiency due to their high sampling density at the center of k-space, although this concern can be greatly alleviated with variable density readouts [5]. 3D spiral trajectories such as twisted projections [6], cones [7], and FLORET (Fermat

looped, orthogonally encoded trajectories) [8] cover greater areas of k-space per TR and can be flexibly designed for given readout durations and undersampling. The radial cones trajectory has the advantage of providing excellent control of undersampling [9]. Stack-of-stars and stack-of-spirals trajectories also provide efficient 3D coverage [10], but Cartesian encoding creates increased likelihood of motion artifacts in the stack dimension.

Motion Management

Strategies for motion management can be approximately divided into prospective methods such as breath-holding or gating and retrospective methods that sort data based on some estimation of respiratory motion.

Breath-holding is effective and clinically common but must be completed in 10–20 seconds, which limits the achievable spatial resolution and coverage.

Free-breathing scanning with prospective gating aims to acquire data only during the quiescent phase of respiration and allows increased spatial resolution and coverage compared to breath-holding. It relies on real-time measurement of respiratory motion (e.g., bellows belt, navigators, pilot tone) to trigger data acquisition. The main disadvantages are that it does not continuously acquire data, which reduces SNR efficiency and any irregular motion (e.g., bulk motion, coughing, shallow vs. deep breathing) may lead to additional artifacts.

Free breathing with retrospective gating uses continuous data acquisition and, upon completion, assigns data to bins for reconstruction. Using continuous acquisitions allows reconstruction of multiple respiratory phases. Continuous acquisitions can also improve SNR efficiency. In addition, retrospective motion estimations can be more accurate than prospective methods, particularly for irregular motion. It requires sufficiently dispersed temporal ordering of the sampling (e.g., golden angle-type methods) for retrospective binning of data based on estimated respiratory motion. When a subset of the data is retrospectively binned based on the respiratory motion, it should be relatively evenly distributed in k-space.

The methods for estimation of motion include k-space center signal (also known as direct current or DC component) navigators—here, the repeated center of k-space ($k = 0$) signal is used, typically with some signal processing, to estimate respiratory motion over time [13]; one-dimensional (1D) navigators—these are most common in stack-of-stars or stack-of-spirals, where applying 1D Fourier transform (FT) to data in the stack dimension provides a 1D image that can be processed to estimate respiratory motion [14, 15]; and image-based navigators—these methods use a larger area around the center of k-space to produce low-resolution dynamic images from which motion can be estimated. This has a distinct advantage in depicting different motion patterns and bulk motion [16–18] (Fig. 42.3).

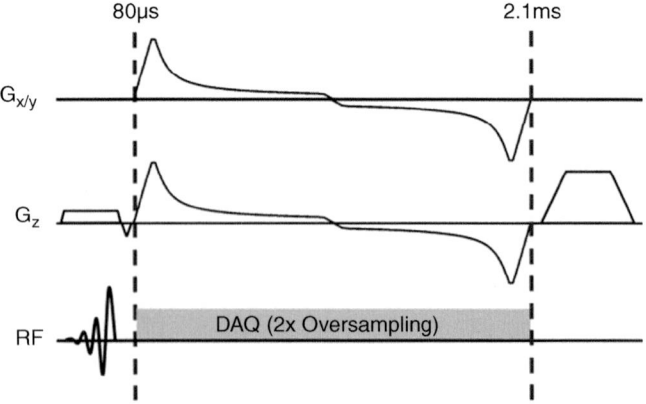

Fig. 42.1 An example 3D UTE pulse sequence for lung MRI featuring slab excitation and a variable-density, arc length-optimized, out-and-back radial readout. (Reproduced with permission from Johnson et al. [5])

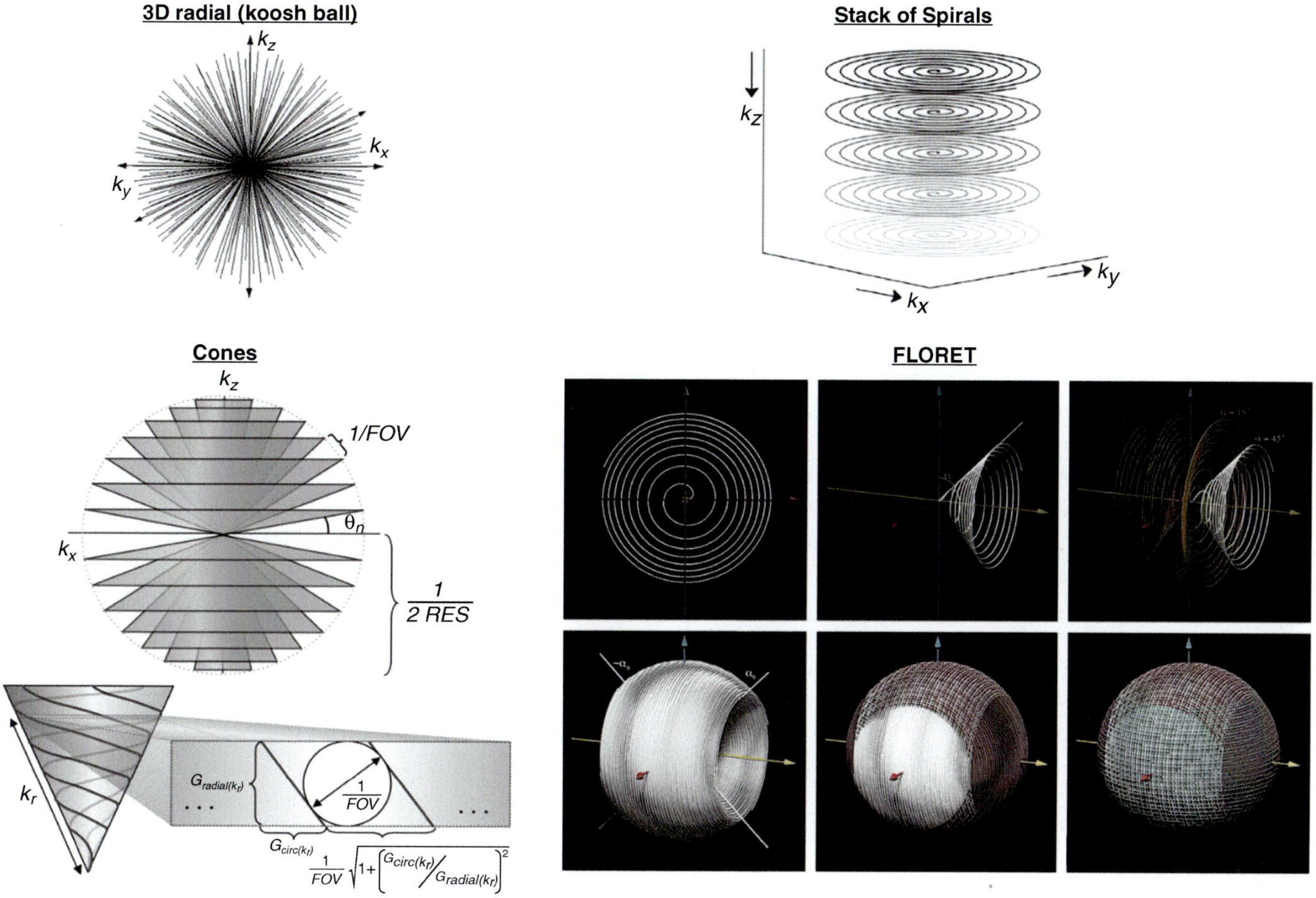

3D radial (koosh ball)

Stack of Spirals

Cones

FLORET

Fig. 42.2 3D center-out k-space trajectories that have been the most successful for UTE lung MRI, including 3D radial or koosh ball sampling, 3D cones [7], stack-of-spirals [11], and FLORET [12]. (Adapted with permission from Gurney et al. [7], Weng et al. [11], and Robison et al. [12])

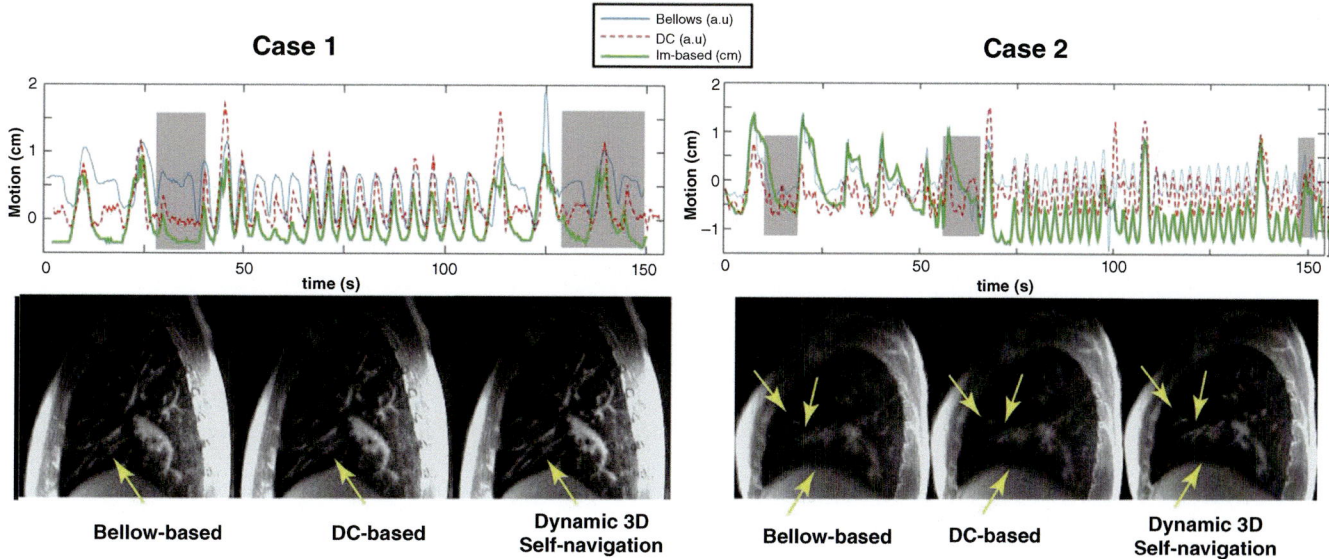

Fig. 42.3 Comparison of bellows belt, DC (k-space center), and image-based navigation for UTE lung MRI. Case 1 is a cystic fibrosis patient with mildly irregular breathing, whereas case 2 is a cystic fibrosis patient with highly irregular breathing. All motion management methods perform similarly in case 1, but the ability of image-based navigators to capture the more variable and complex motion in case 2 leads to significant improvement in image quality as shown by the arrows. (Reproduced with permission from Jiang et al. [16])

Image Reconstruction

The 3D non-Cartesian k-space trajectories used for UTE-MRI require non-Cartesian image reconstruction methods. The most straightforward and fastest methods are gridding and the use of nonuniform fast FT (FFT), but the current state-of-the-art is based on iterative reconstructions that include capabilities for parallel imaging and compressed sensing acceleration. 3D non-Cartesian trajectories are well suited to these types of accelerations as they can be uniformly or pseudorandomly undersampled.

Advanced iterative image reconstructions can also improve the image quality, motion management, and the information provided by UTE lung MRI and are typically used with free breathing and retrospectively gated acquisitions. One approach to improve image quality is to use motion-compensated reconstructions [19, 20]. These require data to be binned and images to be reconstructed for different respiratory states. These different images are then aligned using deformable image registration, allowing the data from all respiratory states to be combined into a single image. Using data from the entire scan time, these approaches are more SNR-efficient and thus can provide improved SNR and resolution.

Free-breathing data can also be reconstructed into multiple respiratory states, creating motion-resolved images that improve motion management and also provide dynamic images of respiration that can be used to measure tissue motion and ventilation. The quality of motion-resolved reconstructions is improved by jointly reconstructing all respiratory state images. This can be performed with a sparsity or low-rank penalty across the state dimension in an iterative reconstruction [14]. These are often referred to as eXtra-Dimensional or XD reconstructions (Fig. 42.4).

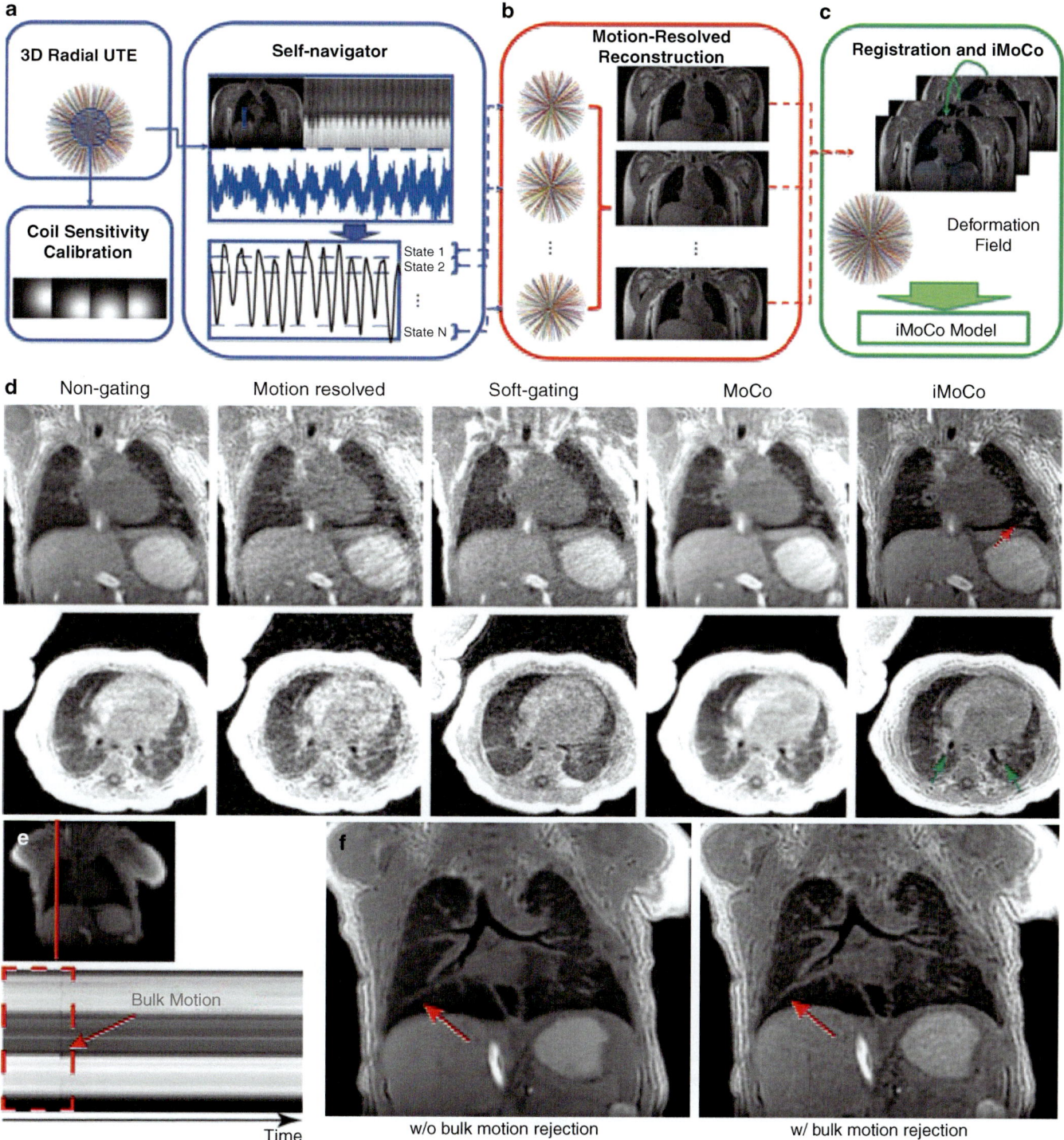

Fig. 42.4 Illustration of advanced image reconstruction methods for UTE lung MRI and example results. The depicted technique is iterative motion compensation (iMoCo) reconstruction, which includes a motion state identification with self-navigation, a motion-resolved (XD) reconstruction, and a motion-compensated reconstruction (**a–c**). Results in a 10-week-old infant (**d–f**) show progressive improvements in image quality, where iMoCo efficiently takes advantage of all the acquired data. In this example, it should be noted that a dynamic image navigator identified a period of bulk motion that could be removed to further improve image quality. (Reproduced with permission from Zhu et al. [19])

Contrast Mechanisms with UTE-MRI

T$_1$-Weighting

3D UTE-MRI nominally provides T$_1$-weighted contrast, as it uses short TRs and typically flip angles tuned to the optimal Ernst angle for lung parenchymal signal. This provides clear delineation of parenchyma, vessels, and airways within the lungs as well as well-defined borders between surrounding tissues and other organs.

Non-contrast Ventilation

Ventilation refers to the circulation and exchange of gasses in the lungs and is a critical component of lung function. It can be assessed by measuring the change in lung tissue density or volume during respiration, and this forms the basis of non-contrast ventilation imaging (Fig. 42.5) [14, 21, 22].

With UTE-MRI, non-contrast ventilation can be measured from motion-resolved reconstructed images, where the respiratory states are aligned using deformable image registration. After alignment, the change in signal amplitude can be measured as the so-called "specific ventilation," and

regional changes in volume can be measured as the so-called "regional ventilation."

Oxygen-Enhanced Ventilation

Pure oxygen is paramagnetic, whereas most tissue is diamagnetic. Due to this magnetic susceptibility difference, breathing in 100% O$_2$ results in a shortening of T$_1$ in the lung parenchyma compared to breathing room air [23–25]. This change is easily observed with typical T$_1$-weighted 3D UTE sequences. Ventilation can then be measured by comparing T$_1$-weighted images or T$_1$ values between breathing room air and 100% O$_2$ (Fig. 42.6).

New Frontiers

Recently, mid-/low-field (<1T) MRI scanners have been revisited for cost-efficiency benefits. Lower field strengths are advantageous for lung MRI because T$_2$* is increased due to the reduced effect of magnetic susceptibility differences between air and lung tissue (e.g., T$_2$* = 8–10 ms at 0.55T [2, 3]). This allows longer readouts and more SNR-efficient

Fig. 42.5 Example of UTE lung ventilation maps, showing more inhomogeneous ventilation patterns in the cystic fibrosis (CF) subject on the right. In this work, similar results were found, irrespective of whether ventilation was calculated based on signal intensity changes or tissue volume changes. (Reproduced with permission from Heidenreich et al. [22])

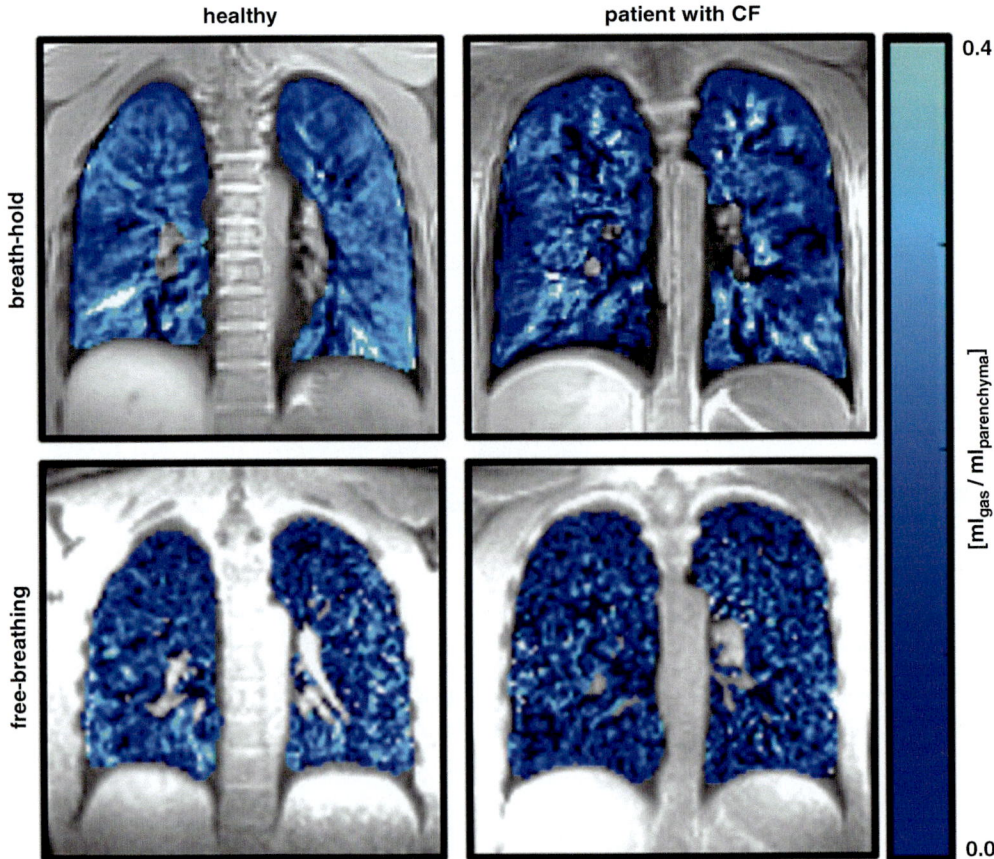

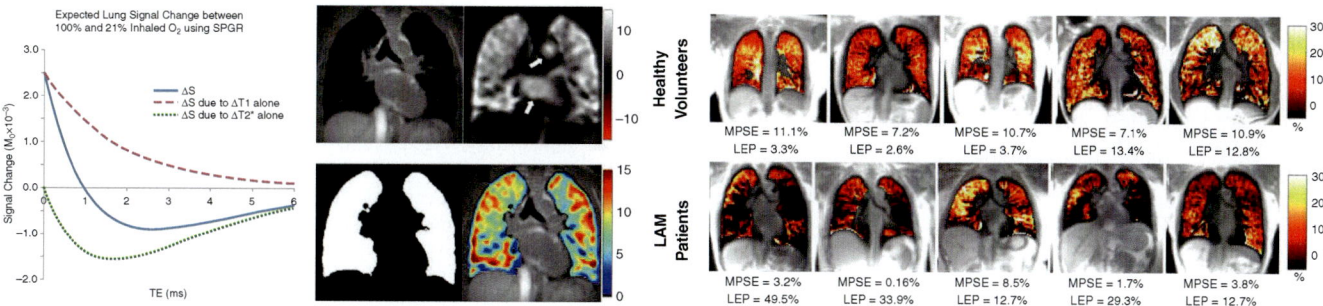

Fig. 42.6 Oxygen-enhanced ventilation imaging. (left) With UTE, theory predicts that the signal increase between room air and 100% O_2 is due to T_1 shortening without sensitivity to signal loss due to T_2^* shortening effects. (middle) UTE datasets from breathing room air and 100% O_2 are subtracted to show the ventilation effect, which can be mapped onto the lung anatomy but oxygen enhancement in the aorta and ventricles (arrows) is also visible. (right) Examples of UTE oxygen-enhanced ventilation maps in healthy volunteers and lymphangioleiomyomatosis (LAM) patients acquired at 0.55T. (Reproduced with permission from Kruger et al. [23] and Bhattacharya et al. [26])

acquisitions that can offset some of the losses due to reduced polarization at lower magnetic fields [27]. It also opens up a greater range of contrasts and reduces the need for UTE pulse sequences.

Zero echo time (ZTE) pulse sequences have also been applied for lung MRI, as they can also efficiently capture rapidly decaying signals [28]. However, they have typically not performed as well as UTE-MRI. One reason is the lack of slab selection, which, in turn, requires encoding of much larger fields of view (FOVs) and also increased susceptibility to motion artifacts from abdominal organs. ZTE-MRI also has a more limited range of available flip angles than UTE, especially over larger FOVs [29]. This also limits the SNR efficiency of ZTE.

Ventilation and perfusion measurements in the lung have been achieved using fast 2D scanning, with techniques such as Fourier decomposition [30] and phase-resolved functional lung (PREFUL) imaging [31]. Ventilation is measured using the non-contrast ventilation strategies described above. Perfusion imaging is achieved by binning the images by cardiac state and measuring changes in lung signal intensity. Using 2D scanning creates time-of-flight enhancement of inflowing spins and thus perfusion contrast. These approaches can be used with fast 2D gradient echo pulse sequences.

Conclusions

MRI has advantages compared to CT for cross-sectional lung imaging, such as no ionizing radiation, a broader range of contrasts, and integration with MRI of other tissues. UTE has greatly advanced lung MRI because it provides increased SNR for the short-T_2^* lung parenchyma and is well suited to manage motion. Recent advances in lung MRI have included ventilation and perfusion mapping and the use of <1-T MRI scanners where T_2^* is much longer.

Resources

We have gathered software resources for performing lung MRI in the following GitHub Organization: https://github.com/PulmonaryMRI/, which largely includes image reconstruction methods. All major MRI vendors now provide UTE and/or ZTE-MRI pulse sequences for lung MRI, primarily as works-in-progress packages, enabling more research in this area.

References

1. Yu J, Xue Y, Song HK. Comparison of lung T_2^* during free-breathing at 1.5 T and 3.0 T with ultrashort echo time imaging. Magn Reson Med. 2011;66(1):248–54.
2. Campbell-Washburn AE, Ramasawmy R, Restivo MC, Bhattacharya I, Basar B, Herzka DA, Hansen MS, Rogers T, Bandettini WP, McGuirt DR, Mancini C, Grodzki D, Schneider R, Majeed W, Bhat H, Xue H, Moss J, Malayeri AA, Jones EC, Koretsky AP, Kellman P, Chen MY, Lederman RJ, Balaban RS. Opportunities in interventional and diagnostic imaging by using high-performance low-field-strength MRI. Radiology. 2019;293(2):384–93.
3. Li B, Lee NG, Cui SX, Nayak KS. Lung parenchyma transverse relaxation rates at 0.55 T. Magn Reson Med. 2022;89(4):1522–30.
4. Miglioretti DL, Johnson E, Williams A, Greenlee RT, Weinmann S, Solberg LI, Feigelson HS, Roblin D, Flynn MJ, Vanneman N, Smith-Bindman R. The use of computed tomography in pediatrics and the associated radiation exposure and estimated cancer risk. JAMA Pediatr. 2013;167(8):700–7.
5. Johnson KM, Fain SB, Schiebler ML, Nagle S. Optimized 3D ultrashort echo time pulmonary MRI. Magn Reson Med. 2013;70(5):1241–50.

6. Boada FE, Gillen JS, Shen GX, Chang SY, Thulborn KR. Fast three dimensional sodium imaging. Magn Reson Med. 1997;37(5):706–15.

7. Gurney PT, Hargreaves BA, Nishimura DG. Design and analysis of a practical 3D cones trajectory. Magn Reson Med. 2006;55(3):575–82.

8. Willmering MM, Robison RK, Wang H, Pipe JG, Woods JC. Implementation of the FLORET UTE sequence for lung imaging. Magn Reson Med. 2019;82(3):1091–100.

9. Johnson KM. Hybrid radial-cones trajectory for accelerated MRI. Magn Reson Med. 2017;77(3):1068–81.

10. Dournes G, Yazbek J, Benhassen W, Benlala I, Blanchard E, Truchetet ME, Macey J, Berger P, Laurent F. 3D ultrashort echo time MRI of the lung using stack-of-spirals and spherical k-space coverages: evaluation in healthy volunteers and parenchymal diseases. J Magn Reson Imaging. 2018;48(6):1489–97.

11. Weng AM, Heidenreich JF, Metz C, Veldhoen S, Bley TA, Wech T. Deep learning-based segmentation of the lung in MR-images acquired by a stack-of-spirals trajectory at ultra-short echo-times. BMC Med Imaging. 2021;21(1):79.

12. Robison RK, Anderson AG, Pipe JG. Three-dimensional ultrashort echo-time imaging using a FLORET trajectory. Magn Reson Med. 2017;78(3):1038–49.

13. Boucneau T, Fernandez B, Besson FL, Menini A, Wiesinger F, Durand E, Caramella C, Darrasse L, Maître X. AZTEK: adaptive zero TE k-space trajectories. Magn Reson Med. 2021;85(2):926–35.

14. Feng L, Delacoste J, Smith D, Weissbrot J, Flagg E, Moore WH, Girvin F, Raad R, Bhattacharji P, Stoffel D, Piccini D, Stuber M, Sodickson DK, Otazo R, Chandarana H. Simultaneous evaluation of lung anatomy and ventilation using 4D respiratory-motion-resolved UTE sparse MRI. J Magn Reson Imaging. 2019;49(2):411–22.

15. Feng L, Axel L, Chandarana H, Block KT, Sodickson DK, Otazo R. XD-GRASP: Golden-angle radial MRI with reconstruction of extra motion-state dimensions using compressed sensing. Magn Reson Med. 2016;75(2):775–88.

16. Jiang W, Ong F, Johnson KM, Nagle SK, Hope TA, Lustig M, Larson PEZ. Motion robust high resolution 3D free-breathing pulmonary MRI using dynamic 3D image self-navigator. Magn Reson Med. 2018;79(6):2954–67.

17. Ong F, Zhu X, Cheng JY, Johnson KM, Larson PEZ, Vasanawala SS, Lustig M. Extreme MRI: large-scale volumetric dynamic imaging from continuous non-gated acquisitions. Magn Reson Med. 2020;84(4):1763–80.

18. Addy NO, Ingle RR, Luo J, Baron CA, Yang PC, Hu BS, Nishimura DG. 3D image-based navigators for coronary MR angiography. Magn Reson Med. 2017;77(5):1874–83.

19. Zhu X, Chan M, Lustig M, Johnson KM, Larson PEZ. Iterative motion-compensation reconstruction ultra-short TE (iMoCo UTE)

for high-resolution free-breathing pulmonary MRI. Magn Reson Med. 2020;83(4):1208–21.

20. Ding Z, Cheng Z, She H, Liu B, Yin Y, Du YP. Dynamic pulmonary MRI using motion-state weighted motion-compensation (MostMoCo) reconstruction with ultrashort TE: a structural and functional study. Magn Reson Med. 2022;88(1):224–38.

21. Mendes Pereira L, Wech T, Weng AM, Kestler C, Veldhoen S, Bley TA, Köstler H. UTE-SENCEFUL: first results for 3D high-resolution lung ventilation imaging. Magn Reson Med. 2019;81(4):2464–73.

22. Heidenreich JF, Veldhoen S, Metz C, Mendes Pereira L, Benkert T, Pfeuffer J, Bley TA, Köstler H, Weng AM. Functional MRI of the lungs using single breath-hold and self-navigated ultrashort echo time sequences. Radiol Cardiothorac Imaging. 2020;2(3):e190162.

23. Kruger SJ, Fain SB, Johnson KM, Cadman RV, Nagle SK. Oxygen-enhanced 3D radial ultrashort echo time magnetic resonance imaging in the healthy human lung. NMR Biomed. 2014;27(12):1535–41.

24. Sá RC, Cronin MV, Cortney Henderson A, Holverda S, Theilmann RJ, Arai TJ, Dubowitz DJ, Hopkins SR, Buxton RB, Kim PG. Vertical distribution of specific ventilation in normal supine humans measured by oxygen-enhanced proton MRI. J Appl Physiol (1985). 2010;109(6):1950–9.

25. Triphan SMF, Breuer FA, Gensler D, Kauczor HU, Jakob PM. Oxygen enhanced lung MRI by simultaneous measurement of T_1 and T_2* during free breathing using ultrashort TE. J Magn Reson Imaging. 2015;41(6):1708–14.

26. Bhattacharya I, Ramasawmy R, Javed A, Chen MY, Benkert T, Majeed W, Lederman RJ, Moss J, Balaban RS, Campbell-Washburn AE. Oxygen-enhanced functional lung imaging using a contemporary 0.55 T MRI system. NMR Biomed. 2021;34(8):e4562.

27. Javed A, Ramasawmy R, O'Brien K, Mancini C, Su P, Majeed W, Benkert T, Bhat H, Suffredini AF, Malayeri A, Campbell-Washburn AE. Self-gated 3D stack-of-spirals UTE pulmonary imaging at 0.55T. Magn Reson Med. 2022;87(4):1784–98.

28. Bae K, Jeon KN, Hwang MJ, Lee JS, Park SE, Kim HC, Menini A. Respiratory motion–resolved four-dimensional zero echo time (4D ZTE) lung MRI using retrospective soft gating: feasibility and image quality compared with 3D ZTE. Eur Radiol. 2020;30(9):5130–8.

29. Grodzki DM, Jakob PM, Heismann B. Correcting slice selectivity in hard pulse sequences. J Magn Reson. 2012;214(1):61–7.

30. Bauman G, Bieri O. Matrix pencil decomposition of time-resolved proton MRI for robust and improved assessment of pulmonary ventilation and perfusion. Magn Reson Med. 2017;77(1):336–42.

31. Voskrebenzev A, Gutberlet M, Klimeš F, Kaireit TF, Schönfeld C, Rotärmel A, Wacker F, Vogel-Claussen J. Feasibility of quantitative regional ventilation and perfusion mapping with phase-resolved functional lung (PREFUL) MRI in healthy volunteers and COPD, CTEPH, and CF patients. Magn Reson Med. 2018;79(4):2306–14.

Axel J. Krafft, Ralf B. Loeffler, and Claudia M. Hillenbrand

Introduction

Assessment of Hepatic Iron Overload

Accumulation of iron in the body, or systemic iron overload, results from a range of pathological conditions that disrupt systemic iron homeostasis [1]. These include anemias caused by iron deficiency or defective iron traffic, hereditary hemochromatosis, chronic blood transfusions [2], inherited or acquired hemolytic anemias [1], and hematological malignancies [3]. Mild iron overload may be secondary to chronic liver diseases such as hepatitis, alcoholic and nonalcoholic fatty liver disease [1, 4], and metabolic syndrome [5]. The body cannot naturally excrete iron and accumulates excess iron primarily in the liver but can also deposit iron in other organs such as the pancreas, spleen, kidneys, endocrine glands, and the heart. Iron is toxic, and, if left untreated, iron overload can lead to organ dysfunction and even death, predominantly from liver or heart failure [6, 7].

The concentration of iron in the liver is linearly correlated with total body iron (TBI) stores and is therefore considered to be a reliable marker of TBI [8, 9]. Historically, hepatic iron content (HIC) has been assessed by nontargeted percutaneous needle biopsy followed by atomic absorption spectrophotometry of the tissue sample [10, 11]. Grading the severity of iron overload is based on HIC. HIC values of up to 1.8 mg Fe/g dry weight are considered normal [12, 13]. Mild iron overload, without apparent adverse effects in some patient populations [14, 15], spans from 3.2 to 7 mg/g dry weight. HIC levels from 7 to 15 mg Fe/g are generally regarded as moderate iron overload and are associated with an increased risk of hepatic fibrosis and diabetes mellitus [16–20]. Patients with HIC >15 mg Fe/g are severely or massively iron-overloaded and have a greatly increased risk for developing liver fibrosis, cirrhosis, and hepatocellular carcinoma as well as fatal cardiac disease, arrythmia, and myocardial infarction [7, 21–24]. This massively iron-overloaded group, for whom end-organ damage must be prevented at all costs, underscores the pressing need for frequent, hence noninvasive, and accurate HIC evaluation to monitor the efficacy and guide the intensity of essential iron extraction therapy.

In most patients at risk for iron overload, the treatment goal is to maintain normal or mildly overloaded/elevated HIC and to prevent iron from accumulating to critically high, organ-damaging levels. This is accomplished by regularly monitoring HIC early on and delivering a moderate regimen of phlebotomy or chelation therapy [25]. The lower range of HIC for optimal chelation therapy is between 1.8 and 3.2 mg Fe/g dry weight and the upper range is between 3.2 and 7 mg Fe/g [26].

Emerging Role of Magnetic Resonance Imaging (MRI) in Noninvasive Iron Quantification

A liver biopsy comes with risks due to its invasiveness, is costly, suffers from a large sampling error [27], and is not suited for frequent repeat measurements that are necessary to guide chelation therapy. MRI is highly sensitive to iron deposition in tissues and has been emerging as a noninvasive alternative to liver biopsy over the past two decades. Iron accelerates T_2 and T_2^* signal decays in both spin echo and gradient echo (GRE) pulse sequences, leading to a loss of signal intensity in liver parenchyma that correlates with the concentration of iron in the organ (Fig. 43.1). T_2 or T_2^* can be

A. J. Krafft
Siemens Healthcare GmbH, Erlangen, Germany
e-mail: axeljoachim.krafft@siemens-healthineers.com

R. B. Loeffler · C. M. Hillenbrand (✉)
Research Imaging NSW, Division of Research and Enterprise, University of New South Wales, Sydney, NSW, Australia
e-mail: ralf.loeffler@unsw.edu.au;
claudia.hillenbrand@unsw.edu.au

J. Du, G. M. Bydder (eds.), *MRI of Short- and Ultrashort-T_2 Tissues*, https://doi.org/10.1007/978-3-031-35197-6_43

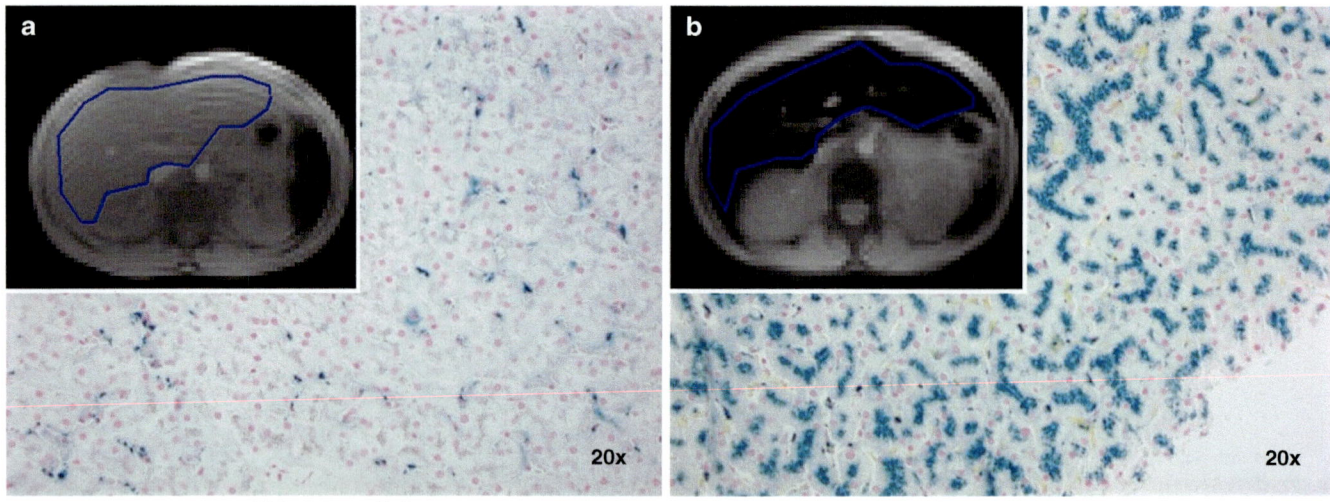

HIC: 4.2 mg Fe/g   HIC: 21.3 mg Fe/g

Fig. 43.1 Perls' iron stain histology at 20-fold magnification of (**a**) mild and (**b**) high liver iron overload. Inserts represent conventional axial GRE images at an echo time (TE) of about 1 ms and indicate the relation between iron content and MR signal levels. The loss of signal in the liver parenchyma in panel (**b**) due to increased iron deposition that greatly accelerated T_2^* decay compared to the mild iron overload case in panel (**a**) should be noted

determined by modeling the signal decay in liver parenchyma obtained at multiple echo times (TEs).

Alternatively, the liver-to-muscle signal intensity ratio (SIR) between several regions of interest (ROIs) in the liver and ROIs in paraspinal muscle in the same acquisition slice is calculated [28] in the SIR method for each TE and liver ROI at 2–5 TEs [29–31]. The paraspinal muscle serves as a reference tissue since its signal intensity is not affected by iron deposition, and the liver-to-muscle SIR is therefore a measure of the severity of hepatic iron load. The liver-to-muscle values obtained at the measured TEs have been calibrated against HIC by biopsy, and conversion algorithms have been developed [28–31] and freely shared [28].

It is, however, more common to report iron overload based on the rate of signal decay $R_2 = 1/T_2$ or $R_2^* = 1/T_2^*$ because both R_2 and R_2^* increase with iron concentration.

Limitations of Current Biopsy Calibrations and MR Methods

Biopsy-calibrated R_2^*-HIC studies have reported an excellent linear correlation between HIC and R_2^* [31–35]. With increasing HIC levels >25 mg Fe/g, these studies show that reduced precision and R_2^*-based HIC measurements eventually fail because of the inability to capture rapidly decaying signals with conventional GRE imaging techniques [32, 33, 36, 37]. Published R_2^*-HIC calibrations [31–35] are based on GRE sequences, which typically achieve minimum TEs of about 1 ms and become degraded when measuring T_2^* times ≤1 ms (corresponding to HIC levels ≥25 mg Fe/g at 1.5 T [32, 33, 35, 38, 39]).

As with R_2^*-based HIC measurements, SIR-based HIC assessment methods use GRE sequences and employ TEs of 4 ms and longer [29, 30]. Consequently, SIR-based HIC assessment also fails for high and severe HIC because the detectable signal eventually drops to the noise floor and renders SIR derivations inaccurate.

R_2-based biopsy-calibrated HIC methods [12, 40, 41] rely on spin echoes for signal generation. Although not susceptible to the accelerated T_2^* decay, the liver signal still diminishes relatively fast with T_2 in severe iron overload. Taking further into account the nonlinear relationship between R_2 and HIC by biopsy [12], the precision of R_2 relaxometry also greatly lessens at HIC levels ≥20 mg Fe/g [42]. The ability to reliably measure high and massive HIC levels via both R_2^* and R_2 relaxometry becomes even more problematic at 3 T because of the approximately twofold shortened relaxation processes [38, 39]. Therefore, ultrashort echo time (UTE) imaging sequences with their ability to achieve minimum TEs far below 1 ms have the potential to overcome the intrinsic limitations of conventional GRE and SE techniques and, in this way, extend the clinically useful range of R_2^*-, R_2- and SIR-based HIC measurements.

UTE Imaging for Iron Overload Assessment

2D Vs. 3D UTE

UTE imaging for iron overload assessment can be accomplished via 2D or 3D approaches. Both strategies have intrinsic benefits and disadvantages. For example, 2D UTE imaging requires fewer encoding steps compared to 3D, which results in shorter scan times. Particularly when working with imaging protocols that employ a high number of echoes for R_2^* relaxometry over a wide range of T_2^*s, 3D UTE imaging may lead to excessively long scan times because of the need for longer repetition times (TRs) together with a larger number of encoding steps. Having the ability to use one imaging protocol to detect a wide range of T_2^* values accurately and precisely is an important aspect of clinical applicability. Published R_2^*-HIC calibrations have shown variability [35] partly because the underlying GRE imaging protocols used in different calibration studies exhibit slight variations (e.g., with minimum TE and echo spacing). Consequently, two imaging protocols that are tailored for low-mid and high-severe HIC ranges would need to be available and with two corresponding biopsy calibrations. This might be less useful in clinical practice in comparison to a single R_2^*-HIC calibration, which covered the entire range from low to severe HICs.

In contrast to 3D UTE strategies, 2D approaches provide limited spatial coverage and require repeated acquisitions of multiple slices to cover the entire liver. As 2D UTE imaging makes use of half-pulse radiofrequency (RF) excitations (see Chap. 3 in this volume) [43, 44], the pulse sequence implementation is less straightforward than with 3D UTE imaging, which typically uses simple, nonselective RF pulses. In comparison to nonselective RF pulses, half-pulse excitation schemes are more sensitive to system imperfections [43] and require correction and compensation as outlined below. Lastly, 3D UTE imaging comes with a signal-to-noise ratio (SNR) benefit over 2D approaches but usually requires a compromise in spatial resolution and other sequence parameters to maintain clinically acceptable scan times.

2D UTE

The first study on UTE imaging for liver diseases (e.g., cirrhosis, hemochromatosis, fibrosis, and hepatocellular carcinomas) was published by Chappell et al. in 2003 [45] and showed the general feasibility and applicability of UTE-based R_2^* measurements for iron overload assessment. In this study, half-pulse excitations (TE$_{min}$ = 0.08 ms) were used together with radial k-space sampling to acquire axial cross sections of the liver in about 8.5 min. However, the study had a broader clinical scope and did not focus on investigating UTE imaging in high and severe iron overload.

The first implementation of a 2D UTE sequence, specifically aimed at providing reliable hepatic R_2^* quantification in patients with high or severe iron overload, was published by Krafft et al. in 2017. The sequence used half-pulse excitations to acquire two radially sampled multi-echo data readouts with the second utilizing reversed slice-selective gradient polarity but otherwise identical scan parameters. The acquisitions were then combined in the complex domain to obtain the desired slice profile as described by John Pauly in 1989 [46]. Although half-pulse excitations yield proper slice selectivity in theory [43, 46], they are sensitive to system imperfections, e.g., delays in gradient vs. RF timing, and eddy current effects, which impair the desired slice profile [47–52]. This can result in insufficient cancellation of out-of-slice signal components, which adversely affects quantitative R_2^* measurements and degrades HIC assessment. Krafft et al. integrated simple, readily available sequence modules to mitigate these unwanted effects [53]: specifically, the sequence used spatially selective, truncated sinc-shaped saturation pulses to suppress out-of-slice signals similar to the principles presented by Josan et al. [51] for improved half-pulse selectivity. In addition, chemically selective, truncated Gaussian saturation pulses were implemented for fat suppression to reduce streaking artifacts that may emerge from high signal intensities at the periphery of the images [54] as seen with subcutaneous fat. These are especially noticeable when surface coils are used for signal reception. Finally, the proposed sequence achieved dense temporal sampling of rapid signal decay curves via interleaving radially sampled multi-echo readout trains (5 multi-echo readout trains with 12 echoes each and respective ΔTE shifts of 0.25 ms, with TE$_{min}$ = 0.1 ms). The sequence utilized the motion insensitivity of radial sampling [55] in a free-breathing data collection of axial 2D slices of the liver lasting approximately 1:40 min. A schematic of the sequence concept is illustrated in Fig. 43.2 together with a clinical example in Fig. 43.3 comparing R_2^* measurements based on conventional breath-holding GRE and free-breathing UTE acquisitions at 3 T in a patient with Diamond–Blackfan anemia whose biopsy confirmed a high iron overload. A highly inhomogeneous distribution of T_2^* values is seen with the GRE sequence, whereas the free-breathing UTE sequences yield a uniform T_2^* distribution in the entire liver, which enables meaningful R_2^* assessment. Further examples of the clinical applicability of the proposed free-breathing UTE sequence concept are provided in Fig. 43.4.

As mentioned above, radial data sampling makes the free-breathing multi-echo UTE sequence less sensitive to breathing-related motion artifacts. Therefore, the sequence might

Fig. 43.2 A schematic timing diagram of the 2D UTE imaging concept described by Krafft et al. [53] for quantitative R_2^* measurements in patients with iron overload. Spatial saturation bands (oriented parallel to the imaging slice) and fat suppression pulses are applied prior to each half-pulse RF excitation. Radially sampled (center-out trajectories, including ramp sampling) multi-TE readout trains are acquired in an interleaved manner to achieve dense temporal sampling for fast T_2^* decays. (Reproduced with permission from Krafft et al. [53])

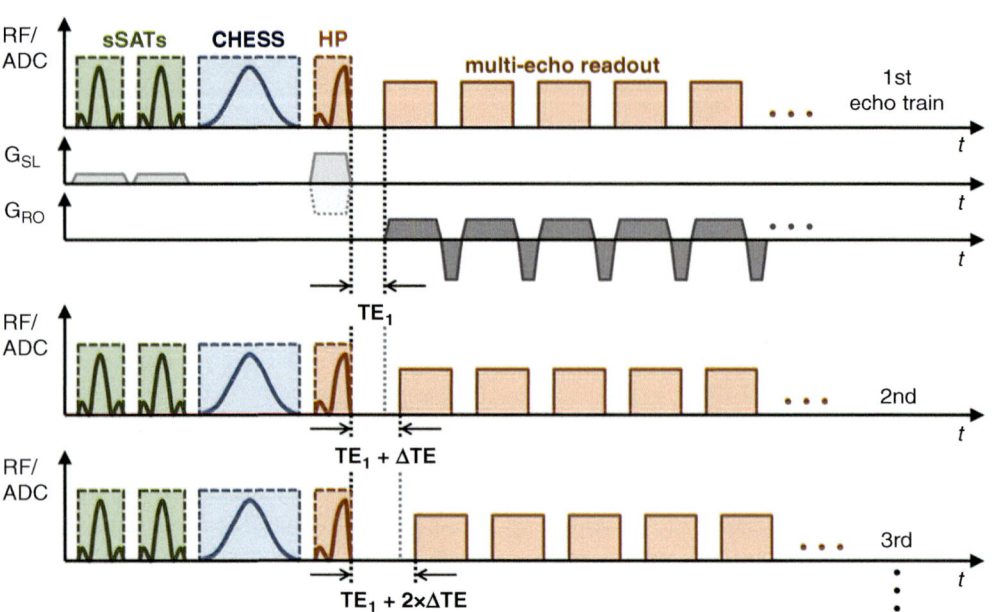

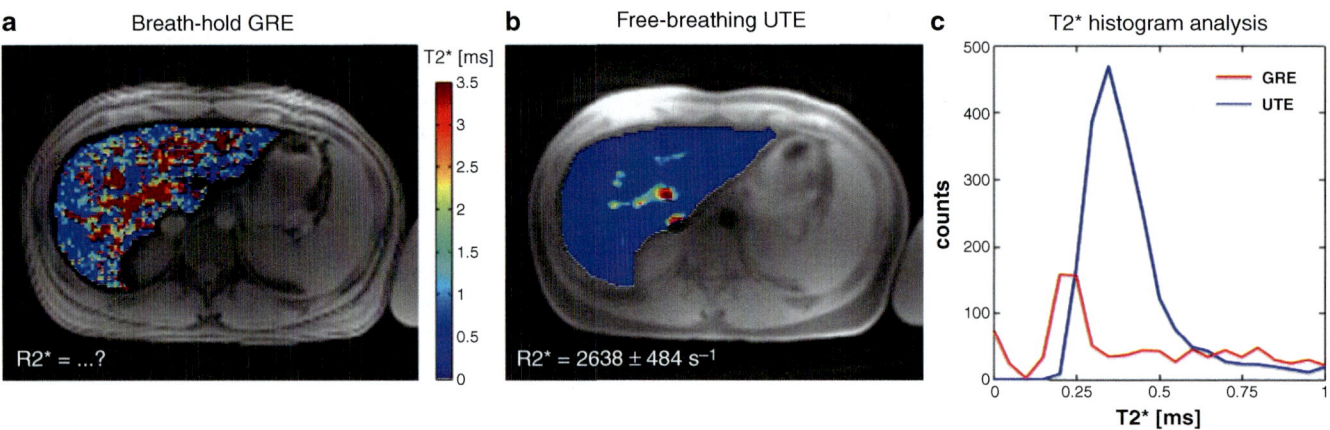

Fig. 43.3 R_2^* measurement based on (**a**) conventional breath-holding GRE versus (**b**) free-breathing UTE as described in Krafft et al. [53] for HIC assessment in a 17-year-old male patient with Diamond–Blackfan anemia (>>12 transfusions of packed red blood cells over lifetime) at 3 T. Severe iron overload was confirmed in liver biopsy with HIC = 29.7 mg Fe/g dry weight liver tissue. (**c**) The T_2^* histogram displays a well-defined peak with the free-breathing UTE sequence in contrast to the breath-holding GRE sequence, which precludes a reliable R_2^* measurement

also be suited for R_2^* screening in patients with impaired ability to hold their breath (Fig. 43.5), e.g., children and sedated patients [56].

3D UTE

3D UTE imaging for high HIC assessment was first described and studied in detail by Doyle et al. [57] where center-out, stack-of-stars radial sampling was used to collect a set of seven single-echo datasets with varying TEs ($TE_{min} = 0.19$ ms). As with 2D UTE imaging, the center-out radial trajectory allows data collection very soon after RF

excitation without the need for additional gradient encoding and therefore allows a substantial reduction in TE compared to conventional Cartesian 3D GRE imaging. The TEs of the 3D UTE sequence were selected with approximate log spacing to maximize the dynamic range for R_2^* measurements. Like other studies with 3D radial non-UTE [58] and UTE [59] imaging, the radial data sampling strategy with its robustness against respiratory motion artifacts permits data collection in free breathing, in this case with a total scan time of 35 seconds [57]. This approach also facilitates clinical applicability. A clinical example comparing this 3T UTE sequence with GRE imaging is shown in Fig. 43.6.

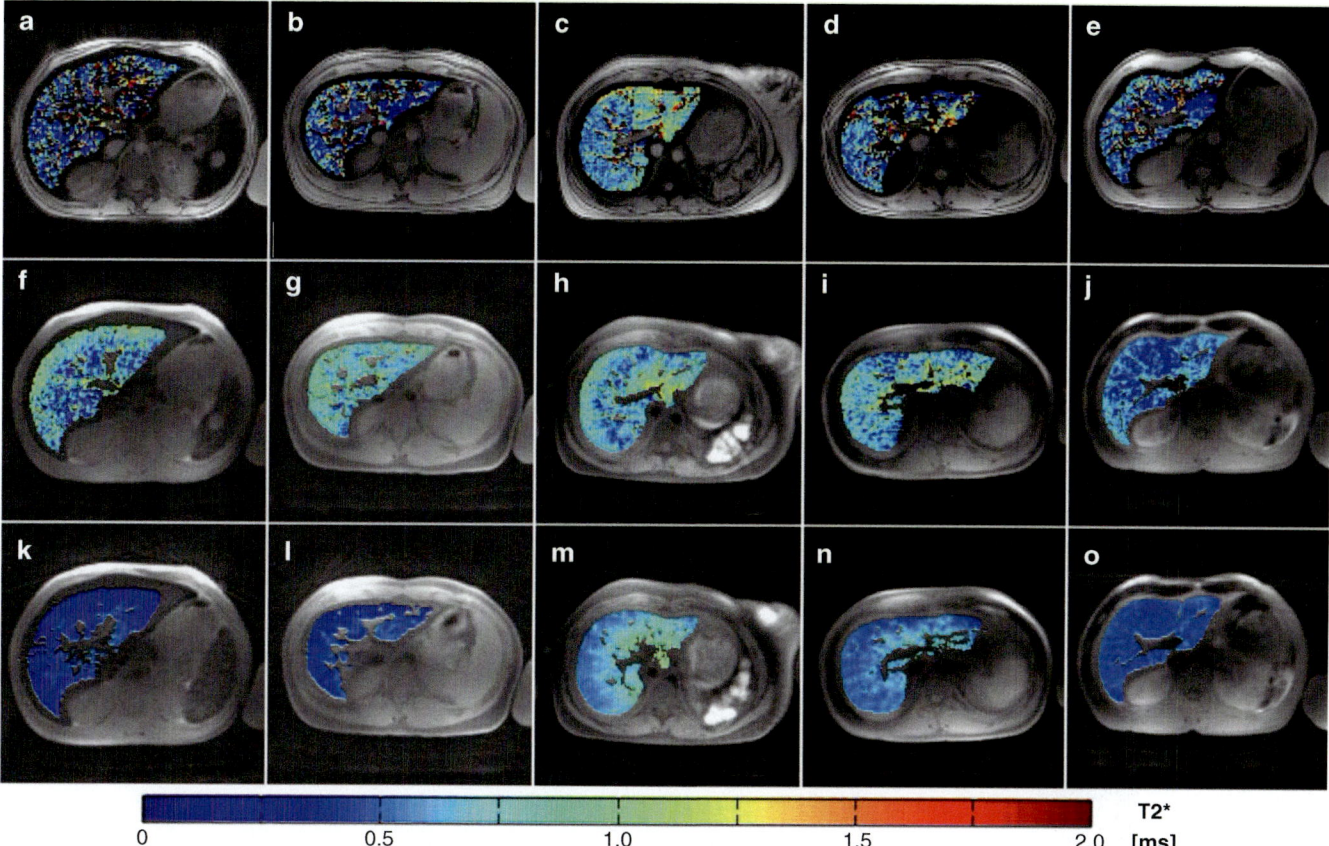

Fig. 43.4 In vivo results with (**a–e**) breath-holding GRE, (**f–j**) breath-holding UTE, and (**k–o**) free-breathing UTE sequences in five subjects diagnosed with sickle cell disease ($N = 4$) and Diamond–Blackfan anemia ($N = 1$) and a lifetime cumulative number of packed red blood cell units ≥ 90 with biopsy-confirmed severe HIC (25.4–35.4 mg Fe/g dry weight liver tissue) at 3 Tesla. The colored overlays show pixel-wise T_2^* fitting within the liver parenchyma after exclusion of unwanted struc-

tures such as the blood vessels. T_2^* maps extracted from the GRE images (top row) appear extremely noisy and preclude reliable R_2^* assessment. In contrast, T_2^* maps measured with the 2D free-breathing UTE sequence [53] acquisitions (**f–o**) appear smooth within the entire liver parenchyma, enabling meaningful measurement of the mean hepatic R_2^* values ranging from about 1500 to 3200 s^{-1}. (Reproduced with permission from Krafft et al. [53])

3D UTE imaging has also been used in a recent study by Zhu et al. [60] to study short-T_2^* signal components in the liver by incorporating a multicomponent reconstruction to extract multiple signal amplitudes and T_2^*s. The sequence makes use of an approach previously proposed by Johnson et al. [61] for optimized 3D UTE imaging (Fig. 43.7). First, the sequence uses short, minimum-phase Shinnar–Le Roux (SLR) RF pulses [62], which provide both high bandwidth and a minimum imparted phase for imaging large excitation slabs. Second, variable-density readout gradients are used to compensate for the SNR loss [63, 64], which occurs as a result of nonuniform k-space density when using conventional trapezoidal gradients (this was previously applied to sodium imaging by Nagel et al.) [65]. Last, the sequence also incorporates respiratory gating based on analyzing the signal from breathing bellows. This further improves image quality by dealing with respiratory drift and irregular breathing patterns. Zhu et al. [60] used the 3D UTE sequence with a minimum TE of 0.1 ms to acquire several densely sampled

single-echo acquisitions (up to 11 single-TE acquisitions in total) with free breathing in about 30–35 mins [60].

Based on the multicomponent reconstruction, Zhu et al. [60] reported a short-T_2^* signal component in the liver (Fig. 43.8), which was consistently observed even in healthy volunteers and was shown to confound liver fat quantification when using sequences with TE < 1 ms [60]. The authors concluded that future studies were needed to characterize these short-T_2^* components by identifying their origin and to develop strategies that mitigated their impact on liver fat fraction quantification using chemical shift-encoded approaches [60].

Kee et al. [66] have recently proposed a 3D UTE imaging technique for motion-robust, ungated, free-breathing R_2^* mapping of hepatic iron overload in children. This approach addresses two major challenges of liver R_2^* assessment: respiratory motion and rapid T_2^* decay. As studied by Tipirneni-Sajja et al. [56], improper breath-holding causes motion-related ghosting artifacts in Cartesian GRE imaging,

Magnitude Image

R2* Map

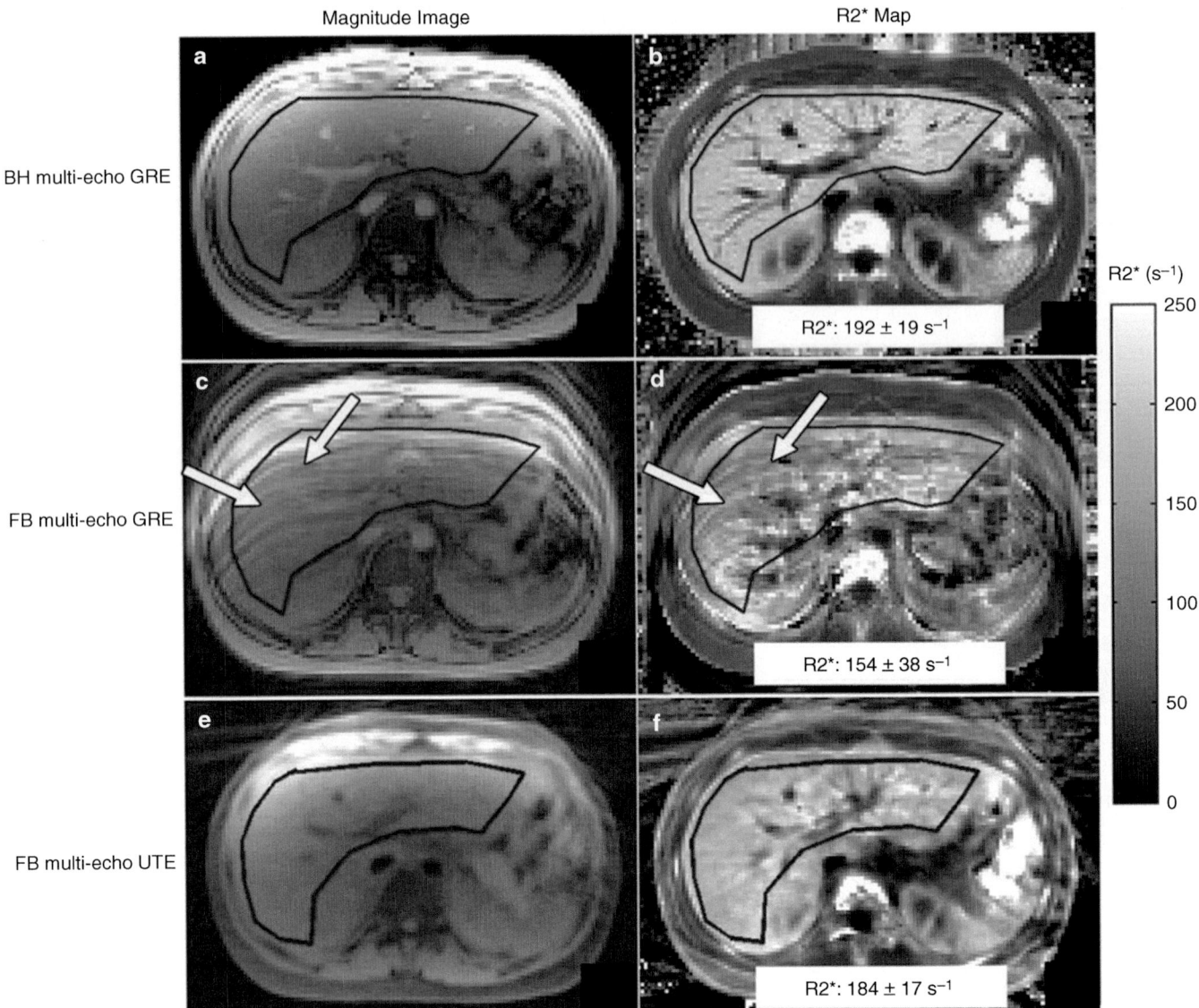

Fig. 43.5 Comparison of (**a**, **b**) breath-holding (BH) and (**c**–**f**) free-breathing (FB) sequences in a 13-year-old girl with sickle cell disease and mild iron overload. Typical motion artifacts (white arrows) are seen in the FB Cartesian GRE acquisition (**c**, **d**) in contrast to the FB images acquired with the radially sampled UTE sequence (**e**, **f**). It should be noted that the R_2^* values obtained with FB UTE imaging are in close agreement with those from BH GRE (**a**, **b**) imaging, suggesting that accurate R_2^* measurements can be obtained using UTE imaging under FB conditions (right column). (Reproduced with permission from Tipirneni-Sajja et al. [56])

and these impair R_2^* measurements. The rapid T_2^* decay in patients with high and severe HIC, particularly at 3 T, makes R_2^* measurements with conventional GRE sequences unreliable, as shown in the studies by Krafft et al. [53] and Doyle et al. [57].

The proposed sequence is based on a previously published GRE sequence using a 3D Cone trajectory [67] and uses the same Cones gradient trajectory to achieve ultrashort TEs very soon after RF excitation. Spiral-like cone interleaves starting from the center of the k-space and rewinding back to the k-space center using time-optimized gradient waveforms enable the use of multiple excitations in a time-

interleaved manner (Fig. 43.9). The 3D Cones trajectory with repeated sampling of the k-space center makes the sequence less sensitive to motion. Robustness against respiratory motion artifacts is further improved by permutation of the sequentially ordered 3D Cone interleaves in the golden ratio [68]. The sequence achieves a minimum TE of 0.036 ms and collects a total of six echoes (three echoes per echo train, two shots) in free breathing within approximately 3–6.5 min, depending on the exact sequence parameters.

A clinical example of the 3D multi-echo UTE Cones strategy is shown in Fig. 43.10. The 3D Cones trajectory shows its insensitivity to respiratory motion artifacts. It also

Fig. 43.6 Example images comparing image quality and associated R_2^* maps of 3D UTE (top) and GRE (bottom) images in a subject with high HIC at 3 T. The GRE protocol fails to capture sufficient signals to perform reliable R_2^* assessment. (Reproduced with permission from Doyle et al. [57])

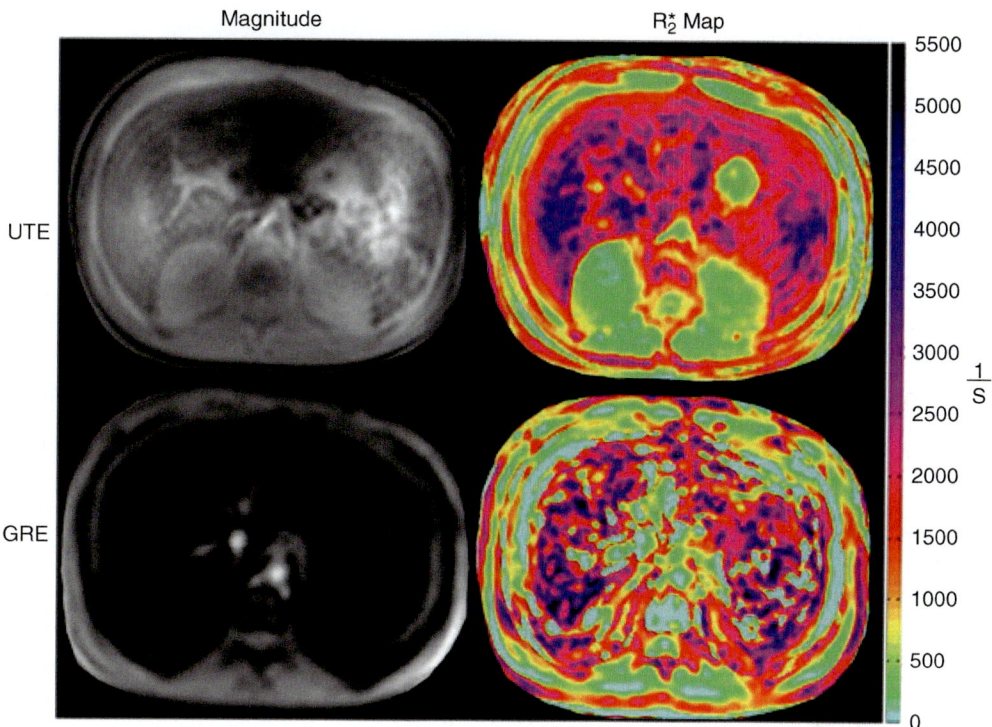

Fig. 43.7 The sequence proposed by Johnson et al. [61] for optimized 3D UTE pulmonary imaging and adopted by Zhu et al. [60] for advanced hepatic 3D UTE imaging using a minimum-phase SLR pulse and variable-density gradients. (Reproduced with permission from Johnson et al. [61])

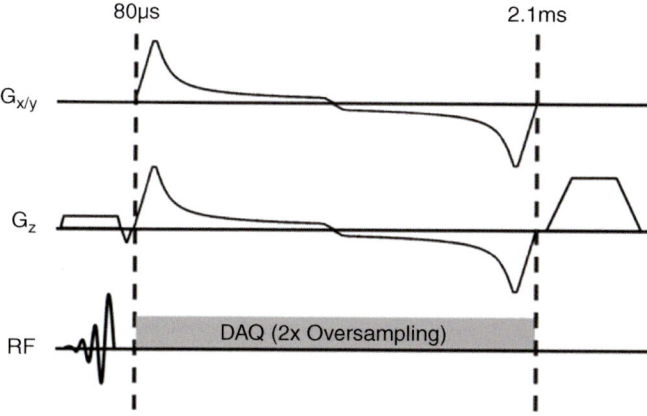

offers more efficient k-space sampling compared to 3D radial trajectories. The 3D Cones UTE concept has great potential for clinical application as it provides high spatial coverage and the ability to measure R_2^*—also for patients with high and severe HIC levels—in clinically acceptable scan times.

R_2^* Quantification and Confounding Effects

In general, hepatic R_2^* measurements are based on multi-echo acquisitions and subsequent application of image post-processing, i.e., T_2^* fitting. Although hepatic R_2^* relaxometry has shown good reproducibility, care must be taken when converting R_2^* into HIC values as the underlying R_2^*-HIC calibrations may have been established with different protocols and T_2^* post-processing methods [13]. However, it is beyond the scope of this chapter to elaborate on the general methodology, clinical acceptance, and availability of R_2^*-based iron overload assessment. Nevertheless, it is important to mention that fat is one of the main confounding factors in the quantification of liver R_2^* values from multi-echo acquisitions (and vice versa). There are a number of post-processing techniques on confounder-corrected relaxometry and fat fraction estimation in the liver, and the reader is referred to the pertinent literature for a detailed description of the techniques [69–74]. In principle, these techniques can be applied to multi-echo UTE acquisitions in the same way as they are used for multi-echo GRE acquisitions. See Fig. 43.11 for an example of the post-processing pipeline as proposed in the study by Kee et al. [66]).

However, the presence of fat in the liver of patients with iron overload varies with their primary medical condition

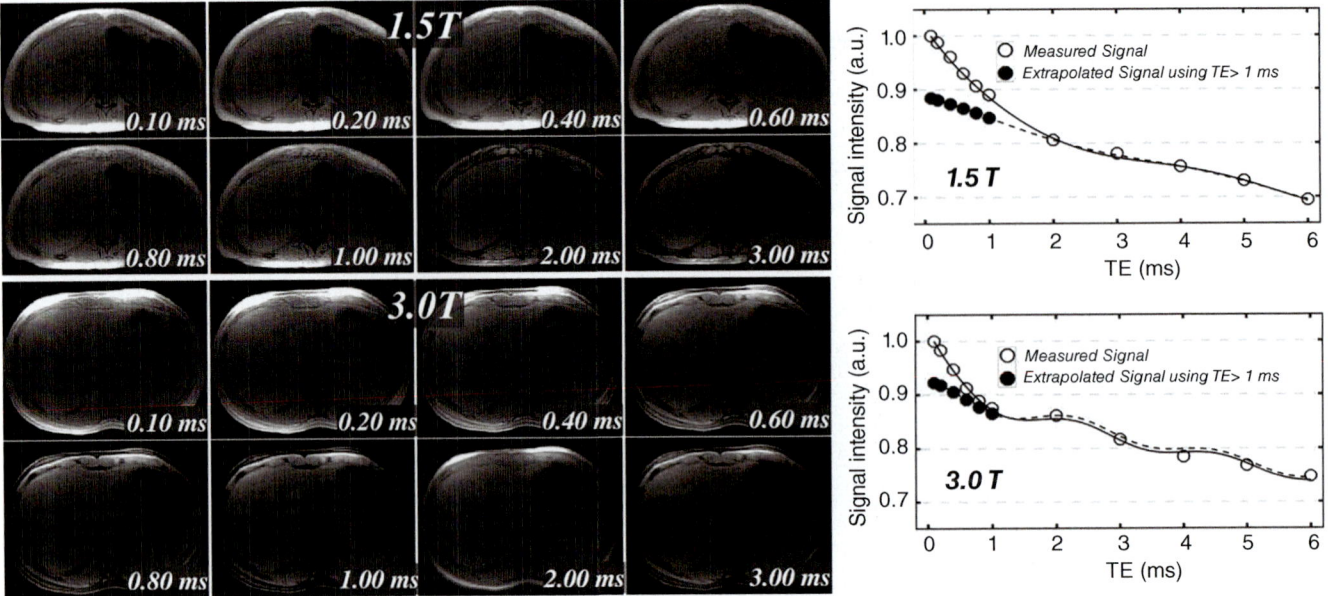

Fig. 43.8 Axial cross sections of the liver of two healthy volunteers obtained with 3D UTE imaging using multiple TEs (upper left: 1.5 T, lower left: 3.0 T). The associated signal decay curves (panels on the right) show dramatically faster decay rates at TEs < 1 ms compared to the decays of water and fat signals obtained with TEs > 1 ms at both 1.5 T (upper right) and 3.0 T (lower right). This shows the presence of an unknown liver signal component with a short or ultrashort T_2^*. (Reproduced with permission from Zhu et al. [60])

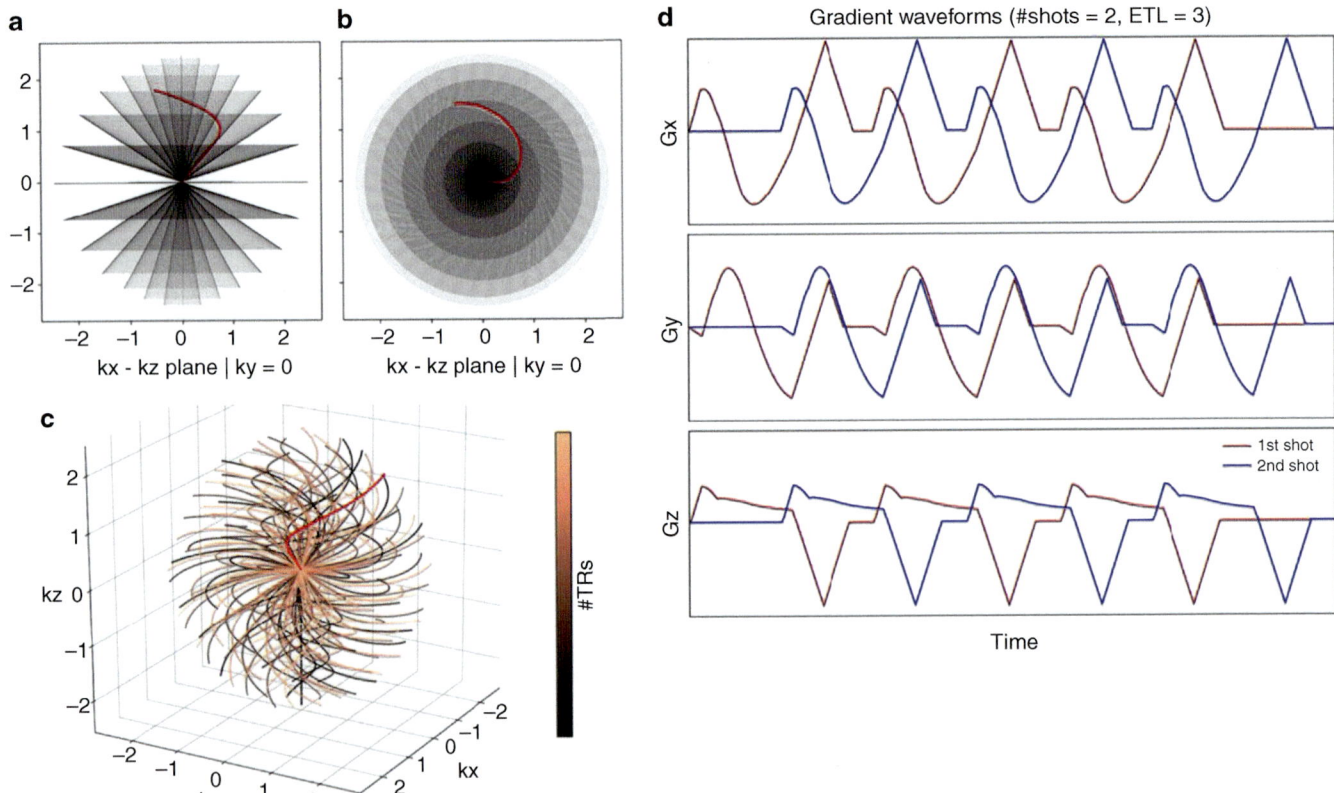

Fig. 43.9 3D UTE imaging sequence as proposed by Kee et al. [66] using multi-echo Cones trajectories (**a–c**). Here, the gradient waveforms (**d**) are illustrated to sample three TEs per echo train and acquire two shots providing six TEs for confounder-corrected R_2^* measurements via nonlinear least squares fitting of the complex-valued source images together with six-peak fat modeling, which produces fat-corrected R_2^*, B_0 field, and proton density fat fraction maps [69]. (Reproduced with permission from Kee et al. [66])

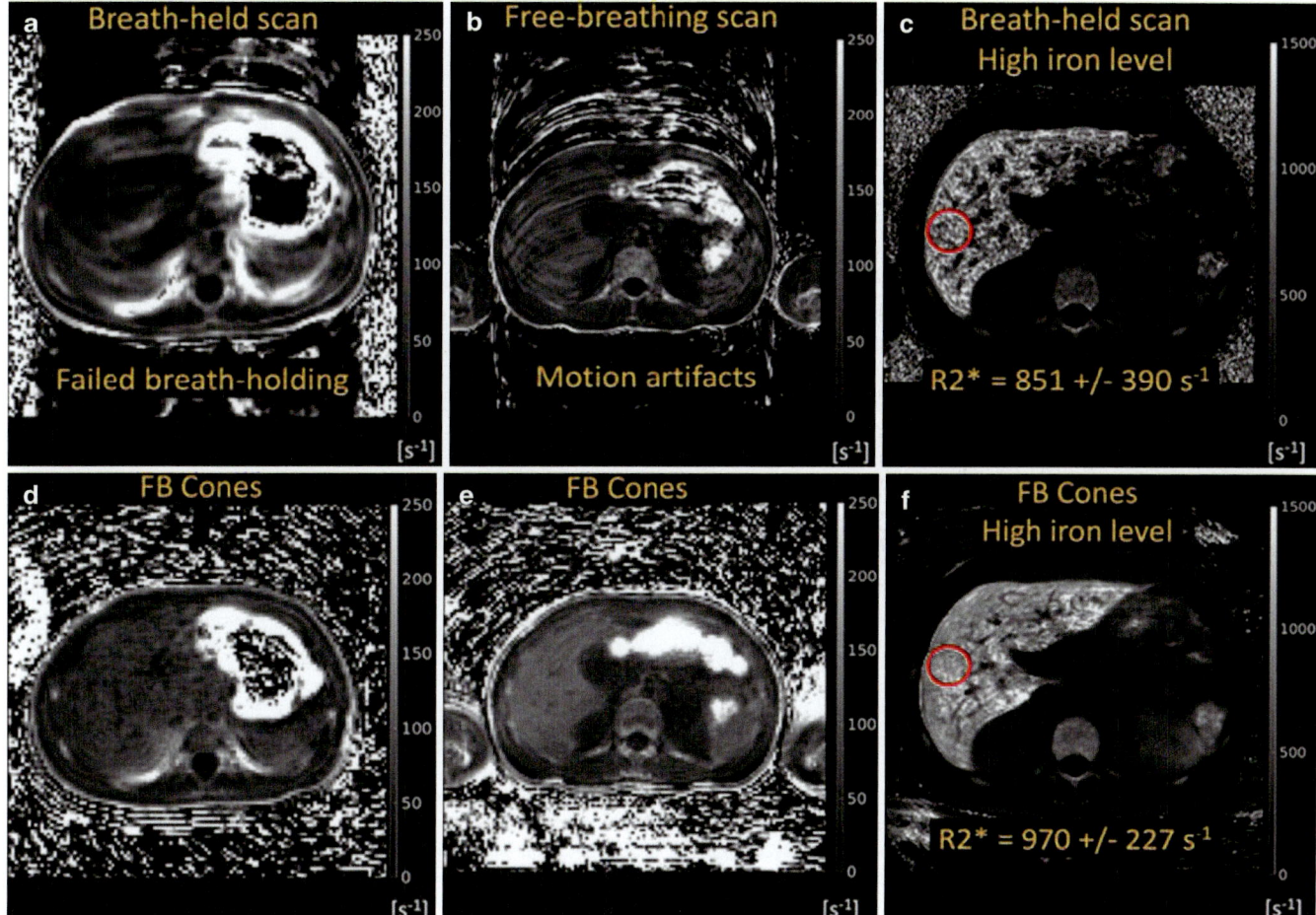

Fig. 43.10 Challenges in conventional Cartesian MRI of high R_2^* liver and comparison with free-breathing Cones. Top row: Images acquired with Cartesian GRE are shown with a single breath-holding in panel (**a**) and with signal averaging that enables free breathing in panel (**b**). Degraded image quality from respiratory motion artifacts is seen in both panels (**a**) and (**b**). Bottom row images with free-breathing Cones: images (**d**) and (**e**) show no ghosting artifacts and the R_2^* map (**f**) also appears artifact-free. Breath-held R_2^* measurements of a patient with iron overload shown in panel (**c**) appear noisy and have a larger uncertainty compared with R_2^* measurements obtained with the free-breathing Cones acquisition (**f**). (Reproduced with permission from Kee et al. [66])

[75]. Moreover, further studies will be required to investigate the performance of confounder-corrected R_2^* relaxometry in patients with high and severe HIC. The extremely rapid signal decays ($T_2^* < 1$ ms) seen in such cases might hamper extraction of multiple signal model parameters such as signal amplitudes, T_2^*, and B_0 values due to overfitting.

However, even with less complicated signal models, accurate T_2^* fitting is crucial to prevent under- or overestimation of HIC levels. Various approaches based on different T_2^* fitting models [32, 33, 76, 77] have been described in the literature to extract hepatic R_2^* values from (multiple) local regions of interest and across entire liver cross sections [13, 35, 75]. Tipirneni-Sajja et al. [78] systematically investigated the accuracy and precision of R_2^*-HIC acquisitions for various GRE and UTE protocols (Fig. 43.12). The authors found that UTE protocols with $TE_{min} = 0.1$ ms, $TE_{max} \geq 10.1$ ms, and $\Delta TE \leq 0.5$ ms can yield accurate R_2^* estimates over the entire clinically relevant R_2^* range $25 \leq R_2^* \leq 2000$ s^{-1}. Furthermore, mono-exponential T_2^* fitting with noise subtraction appears to be the most robust signal model with respect to changes in UTE scan parameters and achieves the highest R_2^* accuracy and precision.

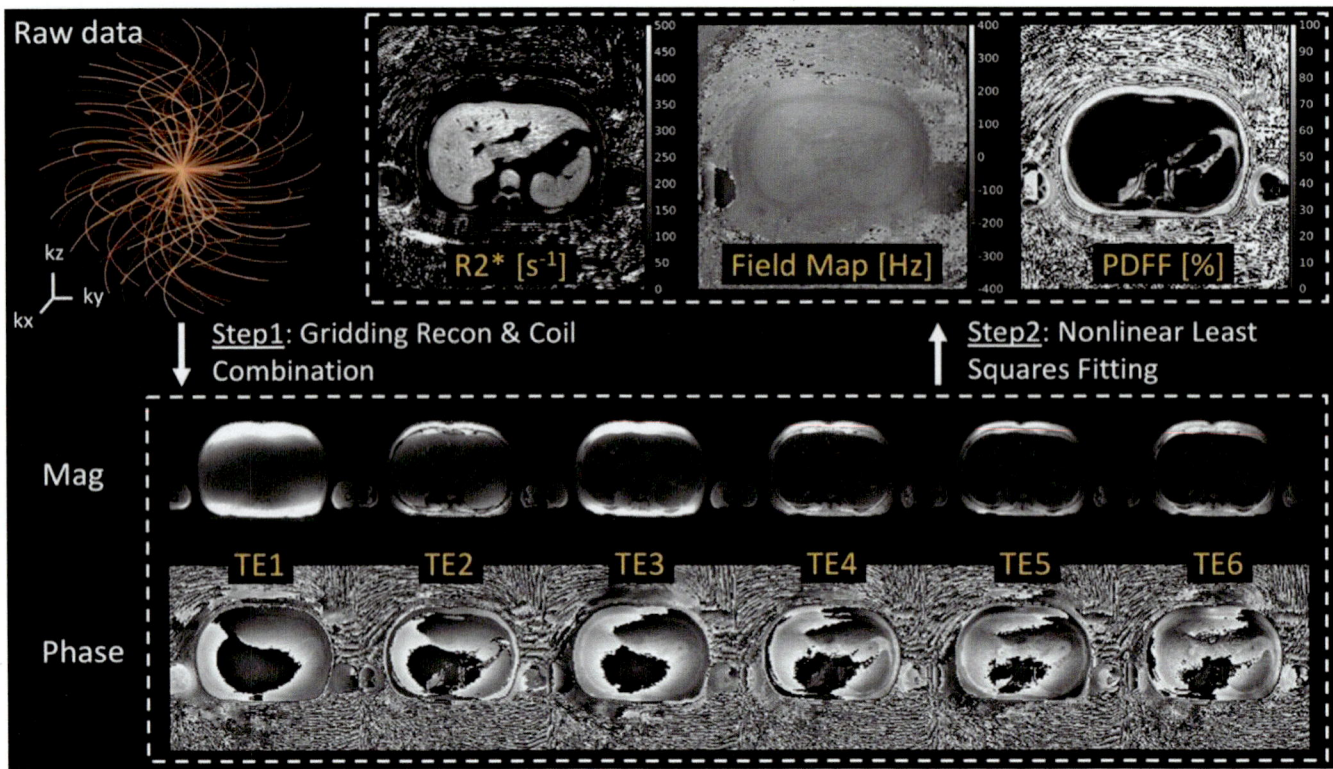

Fig. 43.11 Image reconstruction and R_2^* extraction pipeline as used by Kee et al. with their 3D multi-echo UTE sequence. First, gridding reconstruction and coil combination are performed to generate multi-echo complex-valued source images (magnitude and phase) from the *k*-space raw data. Second, these source images are processed with confounder-corrected R_2^* mapping (nonlinear least squares fitting), which deals with the presence of fat and B_0 field inhomogeneity (step 2). (Reproduced with permission from Kee et al. [66])

Besides effects related to UTE sequence parameters and T_2^* post-processing techniques, there may be other effects confounding UTE-based HIC assessment. By its nature, UTE imaging is capable of measuring signals from tissue components with extremely short decay times, which are not detected by conventional imaging sequences, such as GRE, with $TE_{min} > 1$ ms. As stated above, Zhu et al. [60] reported a short-T_2^* signal component in the liver of healthy volunteers, patients with cirrhotic liver disease,

and patients with hepatic steatosis with their 3D UTE sequence. Such a short-T_2^* component could confound estimation of hepatic fat fraction when using UTE imaging protocols. The effect and presence of this short-T_2^* component in patients with high or massive iron overload has not been studied so far. The question remains whether the short-T_2^* component could be separated from the overall T_2^* shortening caused by high HIC levels. This requires further study.

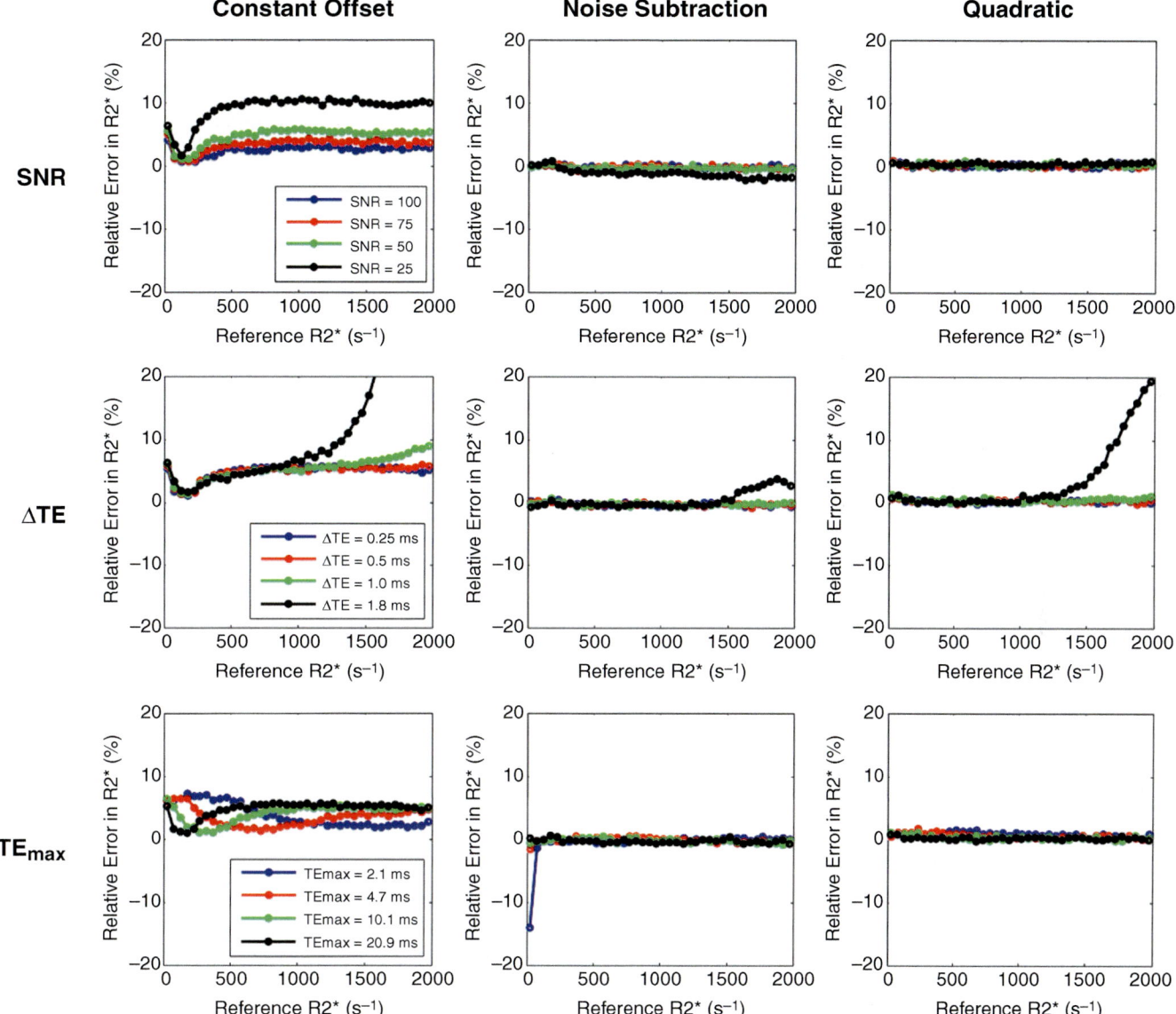

Fig. 43.12 Comparison of the relative R_2^* error for three signal models with different UTE acquisition parameters, namely, TE_{min} (= 0.1 ms) as a function of SNR (top row), ΔTE (middle row), and TE_{max} (bottom row). The SNR was held at 50 for varying ΔTE and TE_{max}. Noise subtraction and quadratic models showed high accuracy for varying acquisition parameters, except with high R_2^* values derived from the longest ΔTE of 1.8 ms. The constant offset model overestimated R_2^* for the lowest SNR and for high R_2^* values obtained using the longer ΔTEs (≥1 ms). (Reproduced with permission from Tipirneni-Sajja et al. [78])

Limitations

Despite their proven potential for reliable R_2^* assessment in patients with high and severe HIC, and in situations where breath-holding is challenging, UTE sequences are still not part of the clinical routine. A principal reason is their limited commercial availability. UTE sequences are mostly available in research sequence packages and therefore generally lack regulatory clearance. Even as research prototypes, their implementation is not straightforward and requires advanced technical expertise in MRI sequence programming. 2D UTE imaging requires nonstandard excitation schemes, which come with various challenges because of their sensitivity to various system imperfections [43, 44, 46, 47]. These require correction and need to be compensated for, to obtain reliable hepatic R_2^* quantification as outlined above in the example of the use of the 2D UTE approach by Krafft et al. [53]. Moreover, non-Cartesian readout strategies are also prone to system imperfections, e.g., gradient time delays, which make their implementation nontrivial, too. Such effects can be corrected for either by manual time delay adjustments or during data sampling and/or image reconstruction to ensure high fidelity between collected data and the underlying k-space trajectory [67, 79–83]. Further challenges in UTE imaging relate to image artifacts stemming from non-Cartesian data sampling, e.g., streaking, which requires the use of appropriate image reconstruction techniques. At the same time, more advanced reconstruction techniques might increase the potential to shorten associated scan times via data undersampling and, in this way, help in the translation of UTE imaging for iron overload assessment from research to clinical routine. The final adoption of UTE imaging in clinical routine for hepatic R_2^* measurements might also necessitate new or extended R_2^*-HIC calibration studies. Variability in existing R_2^*-HIC calibrations is seen [31–35] because of differences in the underlying GRE sequence protocols, T_2^* fitting approaches, and other effects (e.g., different patient populations) so that these R_2^*-HIC calibrations will probably not be directly applicable to R_2^* measurements extracted with UTE sequences.

Summary and Conclusions

UTE imaging in the liver for iron overload assessment can be accomplished. Various sequence concepts based on 2D and 3D UTE imaging have been used to reliably measure R_2^*. Current UTE sequences are mainly in the research domain and require nonstandard image reconstruction and T_2^* post-processing. While the implementation of such sequences is not straightforward, UTE imaging addresses a clinically relevant problem in the management of patients with high and severe iron overload in situations in which conventional GRE-based, R_2^*-HIC assessment fails. The clinical applicability of UTE sequences has been demonstrated in technical proof-of-concept studies, but further studies toward clinical translation of these advanced imaging concepts will be needed for their adoption in daily disease management. Recent advances in image reconstruction to improve image quality and to achieve shorter scan times may also help establish UTE imaging in clinical routine for iron overload assessment.

References

1. Sebastiani G, Pantopoulos K. Disorders associated with systemic or local iron overload: from pathophysiology to clinical practice. Metallomics. 2011;3(10):971–86.
2. Shander A, Cappellini MD, Goodnough LT. Iron overload and toxicity: the hidden risk of multiple blood transfusions. Vox Sang. 2009;97(3):185–97.
3. Eng J, Fish JD. Insidious iron burden in pediatric patients with acute lymphoblastic leukemia. Pediatr Blood Cancer. 2011;56(3):368–71.
4. Pietrangelo A. Iron in NASH, chronic liver diseases and HCC: how much iron is too much? J Hepatol. 2009;50(2):249–51.
5. Dongiovanni P, Fracanzani AL, Fargion S, Valenti L. Iron in fatty liver and in the metabolic syndrome: a promising therapeutic target. J Hepatol. 2011;55(4):920–32.
6. Assis-Mendonca GR, Cunha-Silva M, Fernandes MF, Torres LD, de Almeida Verissimo MP, Okano MTN, et al. Massive iron overload and acute-on-chronic liver failure in a patient with Diamond-Blackfan anaemia: a case report. BMC Gastroenterol. 2020;20(1):332.
7. Kirk P, Roughton M, Porter JB, Walker JM, Tanner MA, Patel J, et al. Cardiac T_2^* magnetic resonance for prediction of cardiac complications in thalassemia major. Circulation. 2009;120(20):1961–8.
8. Pippard MJ. Measurement of iron status. Prog Clin Biol Res. 1989;309:85–92.
9. Angelucci E, Brittenham GM, McLaren CE, Ripalti M, Baronciani D, Giardini C, et al. Hepatic iron concentration and total body iron stores in thalassemia major. N Engl J Med. 2000;343(5):327–31.
10. Barry M, Sherlock S. Measurement of liver-iron concentration in needle-biopsy specimens. Lancet. 1971;1(7690):100–3.
11. Edwards CQ, Carroll M, Bray P, Cartwright GE. Hereditary hemochromatosis. Diagnosis in siblings and children. N Engl J Med. 1977;297(1):7–13.
12. St Pierre TG, Clark PR, Chua-anusorn W, Fleming AJ, Jeffrey GP, Olynyk JK, et al. Noninvasive measurement and imaging of liver iron concentrations using proton magnetic resonance. Blood. 2005;105(2):855–61.
13. Henninger B, Alustiza J, Garbowski M, Gandon Y. Practical guide to quantification of hepatic iron with MRI. Eur Radiol. 2020;30(1):383–93.
14. Olivieri NF. Progression of iron overload in sickle cell disease. Semin Hematol. 2001;38(1 Suppl 1):57–62.
15. Cartwright GE, Edwards CQ, Kravitz K, Skolnick M, Amos DB, Johnson A, et al. Hereditary hemochromatosis. Phenotypic expression of the disease. N Engl J Med. 1979;301(4):175–9.
16. Nottage K, Gurney JG, Smeltzer M, Castellanos M, Hudson MM, Hankins JS. Trends in transfusion burden among long-term survivors of childhood hematological malignancies. Leuk Lymphoma. 2013;54(8):1719–23.
17. Risdon RA, Barry M, Flynn DM. Transfusional iron overload: the relationship between tissue iron concentration and hepatic fibrosis in thalassaemia. J Pathol. 1975;116(2):83–95.
18. Merkel PA, Simonson DC, Amiel SA, Plewe G, Sherwin RS, Pearson HA, et al. Insulin resistance and hyperinsulinemia in patients with thalassemia major treated by hypertransfusion. N Engl J Med. 1988;318(13):809–14.
19. Olivieri NF, Brittenham GM. Iron-chelating therapy and the treatment of thalassemia. Blood. 1997;89(3):739–61.
20. Haap M, Machann J, von Friedeburg C, Schick F, Stefan N, Schwenzer NF, et al. Insulin sensitivity and liver fat: role of iron load. J Clin Endocrinol Metab. 2011;96(6):E958–61.
21. Adams PC, Speechley M, Kertesz AE. Long-term survival analysis in hereditary hemochromatosis. Gastroenterology. 1991;101(2):368–72.
22. Olivieri NF, Brittenham GM, Matsui D, Berkovitch M, Blendis LM, Cameron RG, et al. Iron-chelation therapy with oral deferiprone in patients with thalassemia major. N Engl J Med. 1995;332(14):918–22.
23. Adams PC, Deugnier Y, Moirand R, Brissot P. The relationship between iron overload, clinical symptoms, and age in 410 patients with genetic hemochromatosis. Hepatology. 1997;25(1):162–6.
24. Crownover BK, Covey CJ. Hereditary hemochromatosis. Am Fam Physician. 2013;87(3):183–90.
25. Vichinsky E. Oral iron chelators and the treatment of iron overload in pediatric patients with chronic anemia. Pediatrics. 2008;121(6):1253–6.

26. Bassett ML, Halliday JW, Powell LW. Value of hepatic iron measurements in early hemochromatosis and determination of the critical iron level associated with fibrosis. Hepatology. 1986;6(1):24–9.

27. Villeneuve JP, Bilodeau M, Lepage R, Cote J, Lefebvre M. Variability in hepatic iron concentration measurement from needle-biopsy specimens. J Hepatol. 1996;25(2):172–7.

28. Gandon Y. Principle of joint quantification of iron and hepatic fat by MR. https://imagemed.univ-rennes1.fr/en/mrquantif/quantif/.

29. Gandon Y, Olivie D, Guyader D, Aube C, Oberti F, Sebille V, et al. Non-invasive assessment of hepatic iron stores by MRI. Lancet. 2004;363(9406):357–62.

30. Alustiza JM, Artetxe J, Castiella A, Agirre C, Emparanza JI, Otazua P, et al. MR quantification of hepatic iron concentration. Radiology. 2004;230(2):479–84.

31. d'Assignies G, Paisant A, Bardou-Jacquet E, Boulic A, Bannier E, Laine F, et al. Non-invasive measurement of liver iron concentration using 3-Tesla magnetic resonance imaging: validation against biopsy. Eur Radiol. 2018;28(5):2022–30.

32. Hankins JS, McCarville MB, Loeffler RB, Smeltzer MP, Onciu M, Hoffer FA, et al. R_2^* magnetic resonance imaging of the liver in patients with iron overload. Blood. 2009;113(20):4853–5.

33. Wood JC, Enriquez C, Ghugre N, Tyzka JM, Carson S, Nelson MD, et al. MRI R_2 and R_2^* mapping accurately estimates hepatic iron concentration in transfusion-dependent thalassemia and sickle cell disease patients. Blood. 2005;106(4):1460–5.

34. Garbowski MW, Carpenter JP, Smith G, Roughton M, Alam MH, He T, et al. Biopsy-based calibration of T_2^* magnetic resonance for estimation of liver iron concentration and comparison with R_2 Ferriscan. J Cardiovasc Magn Reson. 2014;16(1):40.

35. Henninger B, Zoller H, Rauch S, Finkenstedt A, Schocke M, Jaschke W, et al. R_2^* relaxometry for the quantification of hepatic iron overload: biopsy-based calibration and comparison with the literature. Rofo. 2015;187(6):472–9.

36. Hernando D, Levin YS, Sirlin CB, Reeder SB. Quantification of liver iron with MRI: state of the art and remaining challenges. J Magn Reson Imaging. 2014;40(5):1003–21.

37. Sirlin CB, Reeder SB. Magnetic resonance imaging quantification of liver iron. Magn Reson Imaging Clin N Am. 2010;18(3):359–ix.

38. Alam MH, Auger D, McGill LA, Smith GC, He T, Izgi C, et al. Comparison of 3 T and 1.5 T for T_2^* magnetic resonance of tissue iron. J Cardiovasc Magn Reson. 2016;18(1):40.

39. Storey P, Thompson AA, Carqueville CL, Wood JC, de Freitas RA, Rigsby CK. R_2^* imaging of transfusional iron burden at 3T and comparison with 1.5T. J Magn Reson Imaging. 2007;25(3):540–7.

40. St Pierre TG, Clark PR, Chua-Anusorn W. Single spin-echo proton transverse relaxometry of iron-loaded liver. NMR Biomed. 2004;17(7):446–58.

41. St Pierre TG, Clark PR, Chua-Anusorn W. Measurement and mapping of liver iron concentrations using magnetic resonance imaging. Ann N Y Acad Sci. 2005;1054:379–85.

42. Labranche R, Gilbert G, Cerny M, Vu KN, Soulieres D, Olivie D, et al. Liver iron quantification with MR imaging: a primer for radiologists. Radiographics. 2018;38(2):392–412.

43. Robson MD, Gatehouse PD, Bydder M, Bydder GM. Magnetic resonance: an introduction to ultrashort TE (UTE) imaging. J Comput Assist Tomogr. 2003;27(6):825–46.

44. Pauly JM. Selective excitation for ultrashort echo time imaging. eMagRes. 2012;1(2):381–8.

45. Chappell KE, Patel N, Gatehouse PD, Main J, Puri BK, Taylor-Robinson SD, et al. Magnetic resonance imaging of the liver with ultrashort TE (UTE) pulse sequences. J Magn Reson Imaging. 2003;18(6):709–13.

46. Pauly JM, Conolly S, Nishimura D, Macovski A, editors. Slice-selective excitation for very short T_2 species. Proc Soc Mag Reson Med. 1989:28.

47. Tyler DJ, Robson MD, Henkelman RM, Young IR, Bydder GM. Magnetic resonance imaging with ultrashort TE (UTE) PULSE sequences: technical considerations. J Magn Reson Imaging. 2007;25(2):279–89.

48. Wansapura JP, Daniel BL, Pauly J, Butts K. Temperature mapping of frozen tissue using eddy current compensated half excitation RF pulses. Magn Reson Med. 2001;46(5):985–92.

49. Lu A, Daniel BL, Pauly JM, Pauly KB. Improved slice selection for R_2^* mapping during cryoablation with eddy current compensation. J Magn Reson Imaging. 2008;28(1):190–8.

50. Josan S, Pauly JM, Daniel BL, Pauly KB. Double half RF pulses for reduced sensitivity to eddy currents in UTE imaging. Magn Reson Med. 2009;61(5):1083–9.

51. Josan S, Kaye E, Pauly JM, Daniel BL, Pauly KB. Improved half RF slice selectivity in the presence of eddy currents with out-of-slice saturation. Magn Reson Med. 2009;61(5):1090–5.

52. Harkins KD, Horch RA, Does MD. Simple and robust saturation-based slice selection for ultrashort echo time MRI. Magn Reson Med. 2015;73(6):2204–11.

53. Krafft AJ, Loeffler RB, Song R, Tipirneni-Sajja A, McCarville MB, Robson MD, et al. Quantitative ultrashort echo time imaging for assessment of massive iron overload at 1.5 and 3 tesla. Magn Reson Med. 2017;78(5):1839–51.

54. Block KT, Chandarana H, Milla S, Bruno M, Mulholland T, Fatterpekar G, et al. Towards routine clinical use of radial stack-of-stars 3D gradient-echo sequences for reducing motion sensitivity. J Korean Soc Magn Reson Med. 2014;18(2):87–106.

55. Glover GH, Pauly JM. Projection reconstruction techniques for reduction of motion effects in MRI. Magn Reson Med. 1992;28(2):275–89.

56. Tipirneni-Sajja A, Krafft AJ, McCarville MB, Loeffler RB, Song R, Hankins JS, et al. Radial ultrashort TE imaging removes the need for breath-holding in hepatic iron overload quantification by R_2^* MRI. AJR Am J Roentgenol. 2017;209(1):187–94.

57. Doyle EK, Toy K, Valdez B, Chia JM, Coates T, Wood JC. Ultrashort echo time images quantify high liver iron. Magn Reson Med. 2018;79(3):1579–85.

58. Rohani SC, Morin CE, Zhong X, Kannengiesser S, Shrestha U, Goode C, et al. Hepatic iron quantification using a free-breathing 3D radial gradient echo technique and validation with a 2D biopsy-calibrated R_2^* relaxometry method. J Magn Reson Imaging. 2022;55(5):1407–16.

59. Gai ND, Malayeri A, Agarwal H, Evers R, Bluemke D. Evaluation of optimized breath-hold and free-breathing 3D ultrashort echo time contrast agent-free MRI of the human lung. J Magn Reson Imaging. 2016;43(5):1230–8.

60. Zhu A, Hernando D, Johnson KM, Reeder SB. Characterizing a short T_2^* signal component in the liver using ultrashort TE chemical shift-encoded MRI at 1.5T and 3.0T. Magn Reson Med. 2019;82(6):2032–45.

61. Johnson KM, Fain SB, Schiebler ML, Nagle S. Optimized 3D ultrashort echo time pulmonary MRI. Magn Reson Med. 2013;70(5):1241–50.

62. Pauly J, Le Roux P, Nishimura D, Macovski A. Parameter relations for the Shinnar-Le Roux selective excitation pulse design algorithm [NMR imaging]. IEEE Trans Med Imaging. 1991;10(1):53–65.

63. Star-Lack JM. Optimal gradient waveform design for projection imaging and projection reconstruction echoplanar spectroscopic imaging. Magn Reson Med. 1999;41(4):664–75.

64. Mir R, Guesalaga A, Spiniak J, Guarini M, Irarrazaval P. Fast three-dimensional k-space trajectory design using missile guidance ideas. Magn Reson Med. 2004;52(2):329–36.

65. Nagel AM, Laun FB, Weber MA, Matthies C, Semmler W, Schad LR. Sodium MRI using a density-adapted 3D radial acquisition technique. Magn Reson Med. 2009;62(6):1565–73.

66. Kee Y, Sandino CM, Syed AB, Cheng JY, Shimakawa A, Colgan TJ, et al. Free-breathing R_2^* mapping of hepatic iron overload in children using 3D multi-echo UTE cones MRI. Magn Reson Med. 2021;85(5):2608–21.

67. Gurney PT, Hargreaves BA, Nishimura DG. Design and analysis of a practical 3D cones trajectory. Magn Reson Med. 2006;55(3):575–82.

68. Zucker EJ, Cheng JY, Haldipur A, Carl M, Vasanawala SS. Free-breathing pediatric chest MRI: performance of self-navigated golden-angle ordered conical ultrashort echo time acquisition. J Magn Reson Imaging. 2018;47(1):200–9.

69. Hernando D, Kellman P, Haldar JP, Liang ZP. Robust water/fat separation in the presence of large field inhomogeneities using a graph cut algorithm. Magn Reson Med. 2010;63(1):79–90.

70. Hernando D, Kramer JH, Reeder SB. Multipeak fat-corrected complex R_2^* relaxometry: theory, optimization, and clinical validation. Magn Reson Med. 2013;70(5):1319–31.

71. Kuhn JP, Hernando D, Mensel B, Kruger PC, Ittermann T, Mayerle J, et al. Quantitative chemical shift-encoded MRI is an accurate method to quantify hepatic steatosis. J Magn Reson Imaging. 2014;39(6):1494–501.

72. Yokoo T, Serai SD, Pirasteh A, Bashir MR, Hamilton G, Hernando D, et al. Linearity, bias, and precision of hepatic proton density fat fraction measurements by using MR imaging: a meta-analysis. Radiology. 2018;286(2):486–98.

73. Hines CD, Frydrychowicz A, Hamilton G, Tudorascu DL, Vigen KK, Yu H, et al. T_1 independent, T_2^* corrected chemical shift based fat-water separation with multi-peak fat spectral modeling is an accurate and precise measure of hepatic steatosis. J Magn Reson Imaging. 2011;33(4):873–81.

74. Hernando D, Cook RJ, Qazi N, Longhurst CA, Diamond CA, Reeder SB. Complex confounder-corrected R_2^* mapping for liver iron quantification with MRI. Eur Radiol. 2021;31(1):264–75.

75. Loeffler RB, Sharma SD, Hillenbrand CM. Iron mapping techniques and applications. In: Seiberlich N, Gulani V, Calamante F, Campbell-Washburn A, Doneva M, Hu HH, et al, editors. Advances in magnetic resonance technology and applications. 2020. p. 779–803.

76. He T, Gatehouse PD, Smith GC, Mohiaddin RH, Pennell DJ, Firmin DN. Myocardial T_2^* measurements in iron-overloaded thalassemia: an in vivo study to investigate optimal methods of quantification. Magn Reson Med. 2008;60(5):1082–9.

77. Feng Y, He T, Gatehouse PD, Li X, Harith Alam M, Pennell DJ, et al. Improved MRI R_2^* relaxometry of iron-loaded liver with noise correction. Magn Reson Med. 2013;70(6):1765–74.

78. Tipirneni-Sajja A, Loeffler RB, Krafft AJ, Sajewski AN, Ogg RJ, Hankins JS, et al. Ultrashort echo time imaging for quantification of hepatic iron overload: comparison of acquisition and fitting methods via simulations, phantoms, and in vivo data. J Magn Reson Imaging. 2019;49(5):1475–88.

79. Peters DC, Derbyshire JA, McVeigh ER. Centering the projection reconstruction trajectory: reducing gradient delay errors. Magn Reson Med. 2003;50(1):1–6.

80. Moussavi A, Untenberger M, Uecker M, Frahm J. Correction of gradient-induced phase errors in radial MRI. Magn Reson Med. 2014;71(1):308–12.

81. Kramer M, Biermann J, Reichenbach JR. Intrinsic correction of system delays for radial magnetic resonance imaging. Magn Reson Imaging. 2015;33(4):491–6.

82. Harkins KD, Does MD, Grissom WA. Iterative method for predistortion of MRI gradient waveforms. IEEE Trans Med Imaging. 2014;33(8):1641–7.

83. Duyn JH, Yang Y, Frank JA, van der Veen JW. Simple correction method for k-space trajectory deviations in MRI. J Magn Reson. 1998;132(1):150–3.

Ryan E. Breighner and Hollis G. Potter

Introduction

Zero echo time (ZTE) imaging is a magnetic resonance imaging (MRI) technique that facilitates the discrimination of tissues with ultrashort transverse relaxation times (T_2s), such as bone. Like other imaging techniques discussed in this book, it employs a radial k-space sampling strategy; however, ZTE differs from ultrashort echo time (UTE) imaging, in that the readout gradient is set prior to the application of the radiofrequency (RF) pulse, enabling near-instantaneous acquisition of signals. It is "near"-instantaneous as the RF pulse is of finite duration, and this is followed by a brief delay wherein the coil is switched from transmit to receive mode following RF excitation. Although this fast switching capability was a technical challenge [1], it has been overcome in recent generations of 3T and 1.5T scanners and is commercially available. Although nominally zero, the echo time (TE) is on the order of microseconds (~8 µs). An added benefit of the gradients being active prior to signal acquisition is that there is no need to cycle them on and off, as the gradients are merely incrementally swept through the imaged volume, appreciably reducing acoustic noise experienced by the patient.

Another surmounted challenge to the clinical application of ZTE pulse sequences is the finite duration of the RF pulse, which results in the omission of sampling of the center of the k-space. This has been addressed via radial oversampling of the center of the k-space, reconstruction techniques, and extrapolation [1]. The applicability of ZTE to imaging bone is predicated on the sparse proton density (PD) of bone tissue due to its limited water content, scarcity of free water, and its ultrashort-T_2^* values of 420–500 µs [2]. Specifically, the T_2 value of bone is several orders of magnitude shorter than those of soft tissues, facilitating clear delineation of cortical margins. As acquired, ZTE images display bone as hypointense and surrounding tissues (e.g., muscle, ligament, and tendon) with intermediate-to-high signals. This contrast facilitates inversion of the acquired images (discussed later in this chapter) to render the relative intensities of bone and soft tissue similar to computed tomography (CT). Before delving into the specifics of clinical ZTE image acquisition, post-processing, and applications, it is important to first discuss the specific motivations for why ZTE is clinically useful and necessary, amidst an ever-growing alphabet soup of pulse sequences and acronyms.

Although MRI is modality of choice for diagnosing an array of musculoskeletal injuries and disorders, particularly of soft tissues, a principal limitation of conventional magnetic resonance (MR) pulse sequences is inadequate rendering of bone. This inability to sufficiently visualize osseous tissue often necessitates the use of a multimodal imaging approach for pathologies involving both bone and soft tissue, wherein the former is imaged via radiography or CT and the latter is visualized with MRI. Although this multimodal approach often affords adequate diagnostic information, it has several drawbacks.

The chief limitation of utilizing a complementary imaging modality for bone is that most of these modalities impart ionizing radiation to the patient in the form of X-rays. Although consideration of the stochastic risks to patients from ionizing radiation is always weighed against the diagnostic utility of imaging and clinical need, we must strive to reduce this radiation burden wherever possible, particularly for patients at elevated risk, e.g., infants, juveniles, pregnant women, women of child-bearing age, and those requiring long term or serial imaging.

Beyond radiation dose concerns, the need for supplementary imaging necessitates scheduling additional appointments. It carries additional monetary and time costs of the imaging procedure(s) as well as additional burdens for scheduling and transportation. From an institutional perspective, the need for multiple imaging modalities for radiological workup of a single condition or injury consumes

R. E. Breighner (✉) · H. G. Potter
Department of Radiology and Imaging, Hospital for Special Surgery, New York, NY, USA
e-mail: breighnerr@HSS.EDU; potterh@hss.edu

© The Author(s), under exclusive license to Springer Nature Switzerland AG 2023
J. Du, G. M. Bydder (eds.), *MRI of Short- and Ultrashort-T₂ Tissues*, https://doi.org/10.1007/978-3-031-35197-6_44

additional physical resources as well as radiologist, technologist, and administrative time.

A further limitation of utilizing multiple modalities is the lack of temporal and spatial concurrence of the multiple exams. Differences in patient positioning between exams make co-localization of anatomical and pathological features between images from different modalities difficult. Although image fusion techniques exist to facilitate the alignment of image sets from multiple modalities, they are not universally available and are not the norm for routine exams. Conditions in which the abutment of soft tissue and bone is a critical feature (e.g., impingement syndromes or foraminal stenosis), contemporaneous imaging of both soft and osseous tissues may be more diagnostically useful than imaging using separate modalities.

An additional motivation for direct visualization of bone with MRI is that conventional MR pulse sequences typically afford indirect visualization of osseous defects through fluid ingress into fractures and avulsions or via edema patterns underlying a fracture rather than directly by showing cortical discontinuity. Direct visualization of bone enables more facile interpretation of images by non-radiologist clinicians and may ease the localization of defects via intraoperative fluoroscopic imaging. For the above reasons, bone imaging with ZTE has been investigated at numerous anatomical sites for orthopedic applications, as discussed later in this chapter.

ZTE Image Acquisition and Post-processing

We now turn to an overview of the process of ZTE imaging of bone. This section is divided into acquisition considerations (pulse sequence parameters, coil selection and placement, patient positioning, and prescription guidelines) and post-processing (bias field correction, contrast inversion, and background segmentation).

Image Acquisition

Where not specifically addressed below, it is advisable to follow general best practices for MRI acquisitions when acquiring ZTE. The following subsections provide guidance as a starting point for acquiring ZTE bone images, and they should be adapted to specific applications and considerations of the scanner and clinical need. As with all MRI pulse sequences, the determination of scan parameters is ultimately about acceptable trade-offs between scan time and image quality. A "good" ZTE acquisition should produce images with a tolerable level of noise, relatively flat contrast of soft tissues, and sufficient spatial resolution for the diagnostic task. The following guidelines assume that a 1.5 T or

a 3 T scanner capable of ZTE acquisition is used and that a ZTE pulse sequence is available.

Coil Selection

The ZTE pulse sequence is compatible with both transmit-receive and receive-only coils, with the only limitation on coil selection being the capacity for fast switching between transmit and receive modes [3]. In practice, commercially available implementations of ZTE enforce this restriction onboard the scanner/host computer. The selection of coils should thus be predominantly guided by their ability to transmit and recover signal uniformly around the anatomy of interest. The motivation for this guidance is to ensure adequate signal from the anatomy of interest and to minimize surface coil flare and its resulting signal intensity bias field. Although techniques are employed to reduce these effects during post-processing, proper coil selection and placement minimize the magnitude of these effects and will result in easier post-processing.

A secondary consideration in coil selection is the coil element or channel count. Although no strict lower bound on channel count exists, more acquired channels generally result in a better signal-to-noise ratio (SNR). Owing to the sparse signal that ZTE seeks to recover from bone, coil arrays with variable channel/element counts (e.g., posterior spine/head–neck–spine arrays) should enable coverage marginally greater than that required for conventional MR imaging of the same anatomy. Lastly, in keeping with maximizing signal/minimizing bias, scans of the hips and spine benefit from adding an anterior coil array to improve SNR and minimize bias/surface coil flare. Although a common practice in hip imaging, this is a departure from standard practice in the spine with conventional MRI. One should bear in mind that this also applies to the cervical spine, wherein the anterior array of the head portion of a head–neck–spine coil may be necessary to minimize bias and signal loss in the anterior region of the neck.

Sequence Parameters

As the name implies, for ZTE sequences, TE should be set to zero. Repetition time (TR) should be minimized. However, when relying on the scanner to compute the minimum TR, this should be determined after prescription of other parameters to ensure that TR is truly the minimum achievable. In practice, it will likely need to be set by the technologist at the time of scanning if deviations from a fixed sequence/protocol are made.

The flip angle is a sequence parameter of importance to the resulting contrast in ZTE images and is limited to the acquisition of relatively small values (generally $<5°$). Higher flip angles may prevent complete recovery during readout. Although compatible with acquisition and tempting because of their increased SNR, flip angles larger than 1–2° should be avoided, as they increase T_1 contrast in soft tissues. Receiver bandwidth is another parameter that can influence the contrast of ZTE images. Specifically, higher receiver bandwidths are recommended (62.5–83.3 kHz) to mitigate chemical shift artifacts, although this comes at some expense to the SNR. Additional strategies such as "perfect in-phase ZTE" [4] and shifting the center frequency have been shown to address chemical shift artifacts in ZTE.

The image matrix is solely parameterized by frequency encodes, as ZTE uses radial sampling. Matrix size (frequency encodes per radial spoke) should be considered with the field of view (FOV) size, slice thickness, and SNR to optimize sampling. Although not a requirement, it is often advantageous to acquire scans isotropically for multiplanar reformation (MPR). Thus, slice thickness should be chosen to match or closely approximate the field of view (FOV) size divided by the number of frequency encodes per spoke. In practice, we generally maximize the frequency encodes and optimize slice thickness based on this; however, for smaller anatomies, this may result in insufficient SNR, and sampling isotropy may not be possible without decreasing the number of frequency encodes, i.e., lowering the in-plane resolution.

If images of a given size are required, then a spatial interpolation schema can be employed during image reconstruction, such as zero interpolation filling (ZIP) to standard image sizes (512 × 512) or to finer slice thicknesses (below the acquired slice thickness). While these interpolative approaches improve the apparent resolution of the resulting images (their "nominal" resolution), intrinsic spatial resolution (the ability to resolve distinct anatomic features of a given size and contrast) is constrained by the acquired slice thickness, matrix, and FOV sizes.

Lastly, the number of excitations (NEX) should be specified. This refers to the number of acquisitions that will be averaged, thus increasing the SNR with each additional NEX. Depending on the anatomy and coil selection, this will likely be between 2 and 4. Scan time increases linearly with NEX, so the SNR should be optimized with other parameters before increasing NEX to achieve a greater SNR. Some implementations of ZTE (such as GE's oZTEo sequence) allow for the specification of fractional NEX, facilitating greater optimization of this sequence parameter.

Slab Prescription Considerations and Field of View (FOV)

Given its radial sampling, ZTE generally does not suffer from phase wrap (aliasing artifact), as wrapped data are diffuse, and thus frequency direction is not of critical importance when prescribing acquisitions. FOV size should be selected to afford adequate coverage of the anatomy of interest, surrounding soft tissue, and a small amount of the background (air) around the anatomy. A margin of air around

the surrounding soft tissue is recommended within the FOV, as this facilitates debiasing and background segmentation during post-processing. Some anatomies and/or acquisition planes such as axial acquisitions of the shoulder preclude this margin around the scanned anatomy (Fig. 44.1). In such instances, margins should be provided on as many sides as possible.

The imaging plane should be chosen to minimize the slice count. When assessing osseous defects, the plane should be oriented orthogonal to the defect (e.g., shoulder scans for instability and dislocation should be performed in the axial plane, as Bankart and Hill–Sachs lesions both present roughly orthogonal to the transverse plane). The matrix, FOV, slice thickness, and the number of required sequences should also be considered to reduce scan times to acceptable durations. Acquisition of a single, high quality isotropic acquisition may eliminate the need for subsequent acquisitions in different anatomic planes. The number of slices and scan durations for axial acquisitions of long bones are prohibitively large, and thus coronal and sagittal acquisitions are preferable for these anatomies if spatial resolution is sufficient for the given FOV, matrix, and clinical concern.

Post-processing of ZTE Images

Once acquired, several post-processing steps are necessary to reformat and rescale ZTE images to obtain CT-like contrast. In general, these steps include bias field correction, contrast inversion, and background segmentation. While machine learning approaches exist for generating CT-like contrast (e.g., "pseudo-CT" or "simulated CT") from MR images via various pulse sequences (including ZTE) [5], the direct inversion of ZTE contrast is sufficient for many anatomies and applications.

Intensity Correction

Signal inhomogeneities in acquired ZTE images exist due to varying proximities between the scanned anatomy and the coil and present as smooth contrast gradient fields with increased signal intensity on the surface of the skin ("surface coil flare" or "surface coil inhomogeneities"). Several pulse sequence agnostic schemes have been devised to correct these artifacts, such as "surface coil intensity correction" or SCIC. As parallel imaging is not utilized in ZTE, a priori techniques for bias field correction are not applicable.

In ZTE acquisition, it is recommended that available on-scanner intensity correction techniques be enabled during scan prescription. Moreover, post-processing intensity correction can be applied if significant bias fields persist in reconstructed images. In particular, the N4ITK bias field correction algorithm [6] has been frequently used in the

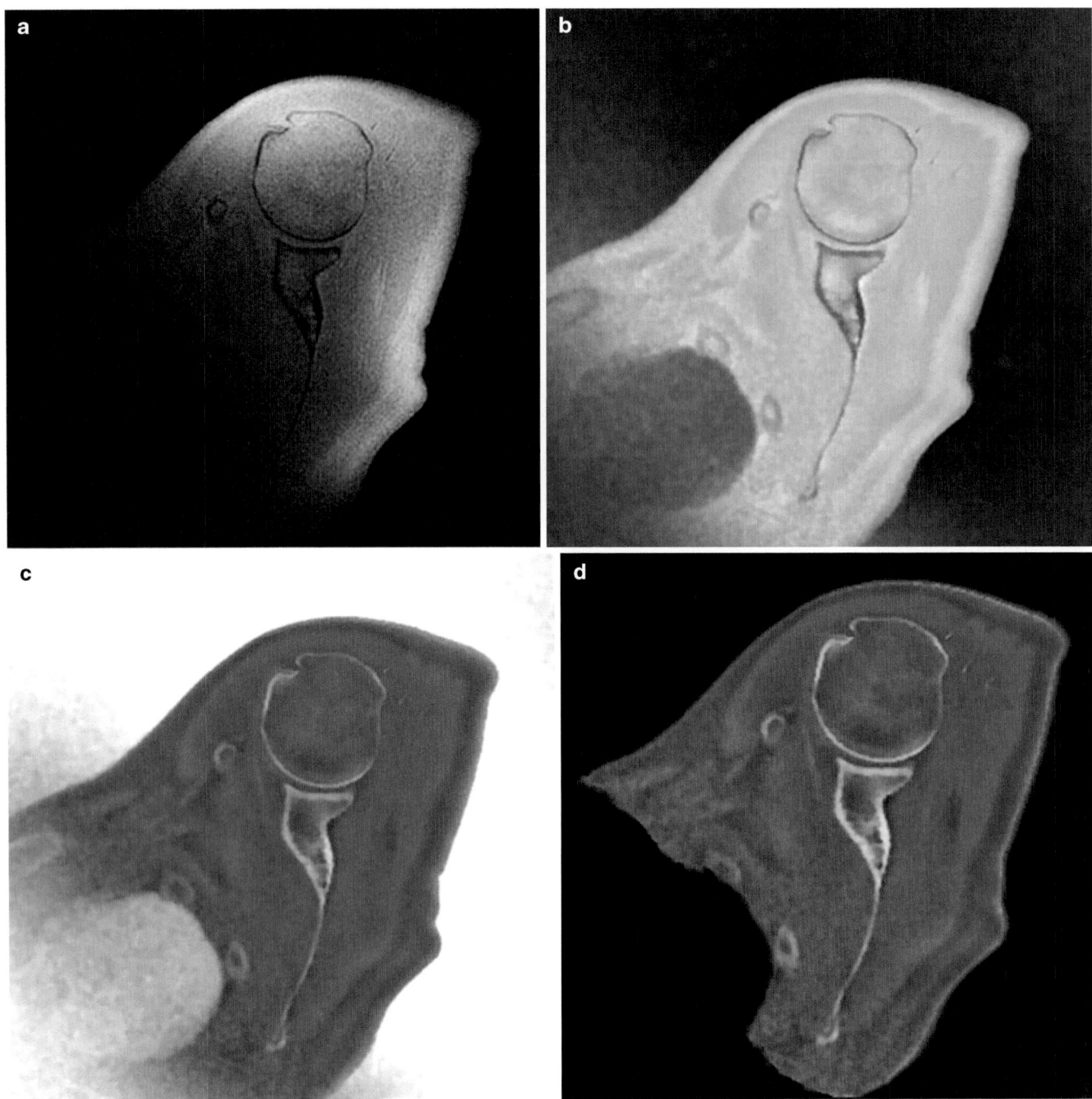

Fig. 44.1 ZTE post-processing steps: (**a**) acquired ZTE (axial shoulder), (**b**) intensity correction (N4ITK), (**c**) inverse-logarithmic intensity correction, and (**d**) background segmentation

intensity correction of ZTE images (Fig. 44.1b) [7–9]. In practice, most ZTE acquisitions require some bias field/intensity correction.

Contrast Inversion

Once images are adequately uniform in signal intensity, contrast inversion is performed to yield positive contrast for bone to mimic the appearance of CT images. Rather than

simple inversion of the contrast (image to image), an inverse-logarithmic rescaling (i.e., log(image)) approach is utilized. The logarithmic aspect of rescaling results in an image with a greater dynamic range of hypointense signals from the source image (bone) and decreases ("flattens") the dynamic range of hyperintense signals (soft tissue). An alternative approach of dividing −1 by the image (i.e., the negative reciprocal of the image) yields a similar effect on the dynamic range. Both approaches require subsequent rescaling to a useful range of intensities (in practice, we rescale to 0–4095).

Background Segmentation

Contrast inversion produces images with a bright background as air surrounding the anatomy of interest forms a largely flat field of high intensity around the object (Fig. 44.1c). General morphological image processing operations (thresholding, region growing, etc.) can be employed to segment out the background of the image (Fig. 44.1d). It is worth noting that the unprocessed source image may be more useful in segmenting the background, as the contrast inversion/rescaling results in a broader range of signal intensities in the background air (compare Fig. 44.1a and b). In addition to making the images appear more "CT-like," background segmentation improves the apparent contrast perceived by the viewer. Lastly, background segmentation facilitates volume rendering as the presence of a hyperintense background would preclude windowing the image volume in a manner that would preserve soft tissue and/or bone contrast.

Orthopedic Applications of ZTE-MRI

The earliest demonstration of ZTE-MRI for the imaging of bone in live volunteers utilized 7 T MRI, a proprietary coil, and examined the head, ankle, wrist, and knee [1]. Since this foray, applications of ZTE-MRI have been investigated in numerous orthopedic anatomical contexts and for different pathologies at the more widely available field strengths of 3 T and 1.5 T. The following sections will summarize these applications to date and their findings.

The Cranium

Owing to the pressing need for attenuation correction in positron emission tomography (PET)/MR, some of the earliest ZTE bone imaging exploring a specific clinical application at 3 T was of the cranium [10]. To this end, Wiesinger et al. demonstrated an approximate linear relationship between Hounsfield units (HU) in CT images and the corresponding inverse-logarithmic rescaled ZTE images. An important caveat to this work is that attenuation of gamma rays (PET) and X-rays (CT) in the cranium is almost entirely a product of cortical bone, and the ascertained CT–ZTE relationship does not hold for osseous structures with significant trabecular compartments (i.e., vertebral bodies or epiphyses of long bones). Although not inherently orthopedic, this study demonstrated the viability of ZTE at a more widely available

field strength (3 T) and also directly suggested the application of ZTE to orthopedic imaging.

Subsequent orthopedic/neuroradiological applications were explored in the cranium. Comparative case series by Cho et al. [11] and Lu et al. [5] examined cranial trauma ($N = 13$) and a varied cohort of craniofacial pathologies ($N = 14$), respectively. Both studies compared ZTE to concurrent CT imaging as case series looking at agreement between the modalities. Cho's study compared both image quality and direct measurement of cranial thickness and observed strong intermodal agreement between CT and ZTE. Cases from these studies included cranial and facial trauma as well as (in Lu's) postoperative assessments of shunting and fixation hardware, atraumatic craniocervical and intracranial deformities, craniosynostosis, and choanal stenosis. Agreement was noted between CT and ZTE. Figure 44.2 shows an example unprocessed ZTE image as well as the anterior and posterior views of the skull using volume rendering.

Notably, toward the prior stated motivation of mitigating ionizing radiation dose in vulnerable individuals, the Lu study examined infants as young as 2-months-old. Reduction of radiation dose is important in these patients due to their stage of development and the presence of radiosensitive tissues within the scanned anatomy.

The Shoulder

Our site's first study of ZTE imaging considered shoulder pathologies [7]. This study compared ZTE with CT in the assessment of shoulder instability morphologies (Hill–Sachs and Bankart lesion sizes) as well as measures pertinent to shoulder arthroplasty such as glenoid version and vault depth. Additionally, the Walch classification of glenoid erosion was assessed as well as the presence of intraosseous cysts in the glenoid and humeral head. Agreement of continuous measurements (glenoid morphology and lesion sizes) and in classification and nominal/ordinal grading (Walch classification, cyst presence, traumatic lesion presence) were assessed and agreed substantially between modalities and raters. Exemplar images of concurrent, coregistered MPRs of en face views of the glenoid in ZTE and CT are shown in Fig. 44.3, demonstrating a readily apparent Bankart lesion. It should be noted that some limited background (soft tissue) contrast remains in both CT and ZTE. In addition to the study's primary measurement and validation objectives, ZTE's potential to be used for three-dimensional (3D) volume rendering and generation of 3D meshes and models of bone surfaces was also demonstrated (Fig. 44.4).

A subsequent study by de Mello et al. [12] utilized such 3D volume renderings for the 3D measurement of glenoid

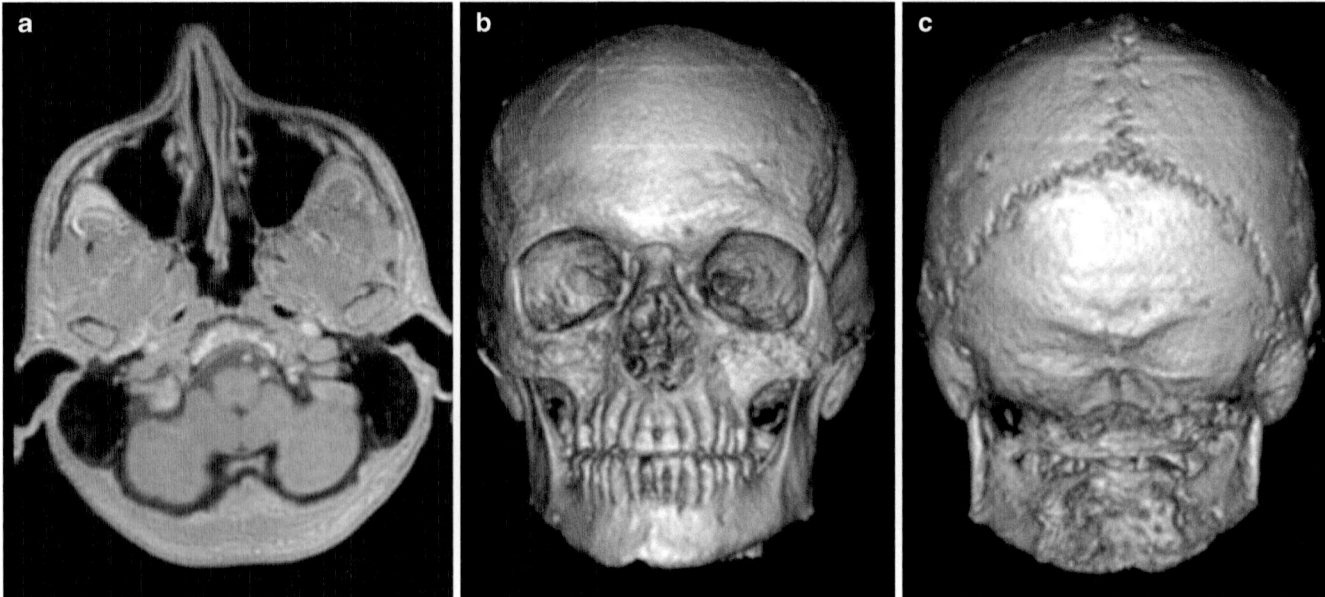

Fig. 44.2 ZTE of the head. Axial ZTE (**a**, un-post-processed) and anterior (**b**) and posterior (**c**) volume renderings for deep learning-based pseudo-CT conversion of ZTE images. Images courtesy of Mai-Lan Ho, Sven Bambach, and Bhavani Selvaraj, Nationwide Children's Hospital, Columbus, Ohio, USA

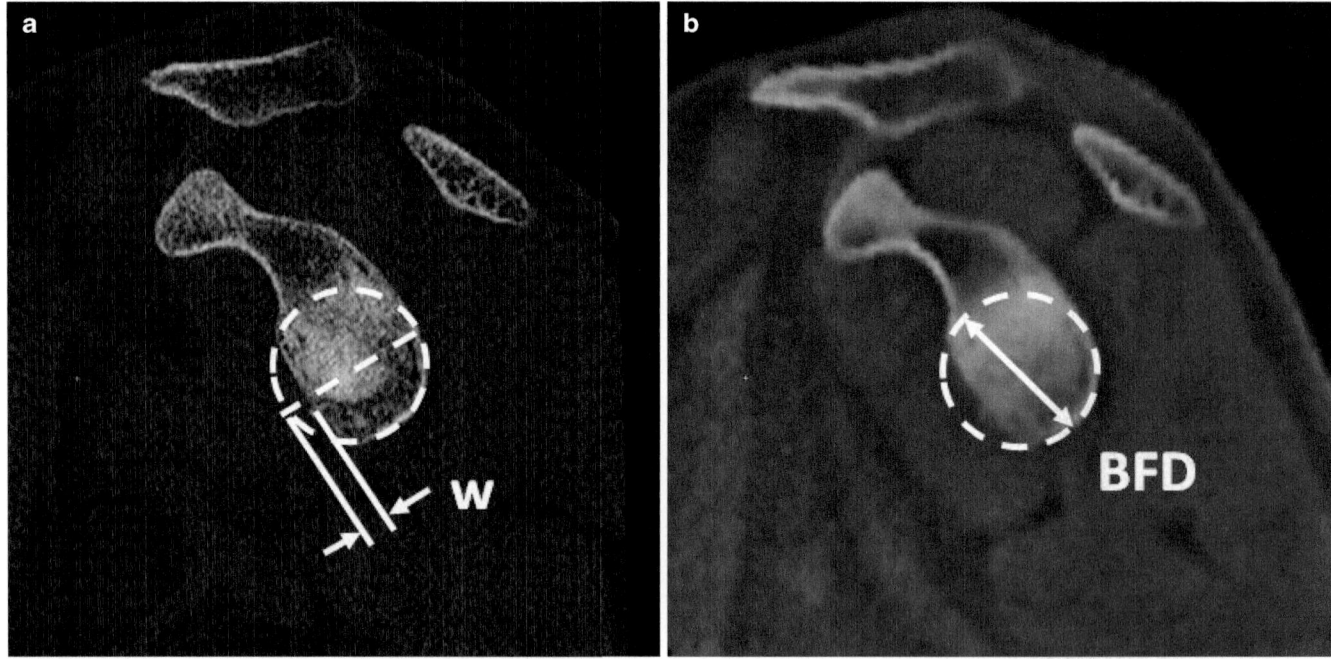

Fig. 44.3 En face MPR of glenoid showing Bankart lesion in (**a**) CT and (**b**) ZTE-MRI. *BFD* best-fit diameter; *w* defect width

width. Although the scope of measurements evaluated was limited to a single linear dimension (glenoid width), the study bore out the findings of earlier ZTE comparisons to CT in demonstrating strong agreement between measurements performed on images from the two modalities. A strength of this study was the additional assessment of ZTE across a range of resolutions (0.6–0.7, 0.8, and 1.00 mm³ voxels). Reported bias (from Bland–Altman analysis) was on the order of the voxel size (0.3–1.0 mm) for all readers between the two modalities, and intraclass correlation coefficients (ICC) demonstrated near-perfect agreement with CT at all evaluated ZTE resolutions

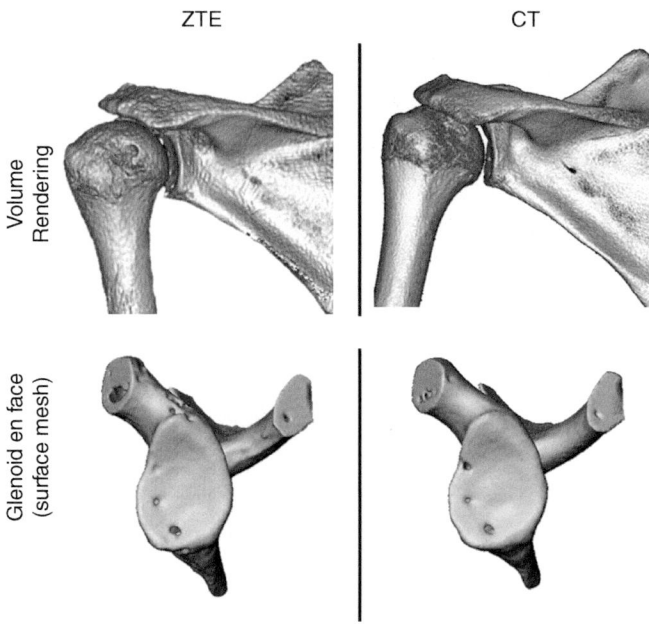

ZTE | CT

Volume Rendering

Glenoid en face (surface mesh)

Fig. 44.4 Volume renderings and surface meshes of bone surfaces from ZTE and CT

The Spine

Applications of ZTE imaging to the spine have also been pursued. Argentieri et al. [9] conducted a study comparing qualitative assessment of cervical neural foraminal stenosis (CNFS) between ZTE and CT imaging (Fig. 44.5) in a cohort of 34 patients. All six cervical motion segments were bilaterally evaluated using MPRs in the plane of each foramen, and substantial agreement between stenosis scores in the two modalities was demonstrated. A novel consideration of this study was the authors' accounting for differences in cervical spine posture between CT and MRI exams. Differences in the sagittal cervical curvature between exams were noted; however, the local cervical curvature of each motion segment was not associated with differences in the CNFS grade. Although ultimately not critical to the findings of the study, this aspect of the analysis emphasizes the potential value of concurrent imaging of bone and soft tissue imaging afforded by ZTE, which is absent with multimodal (MR and CT) imaging.

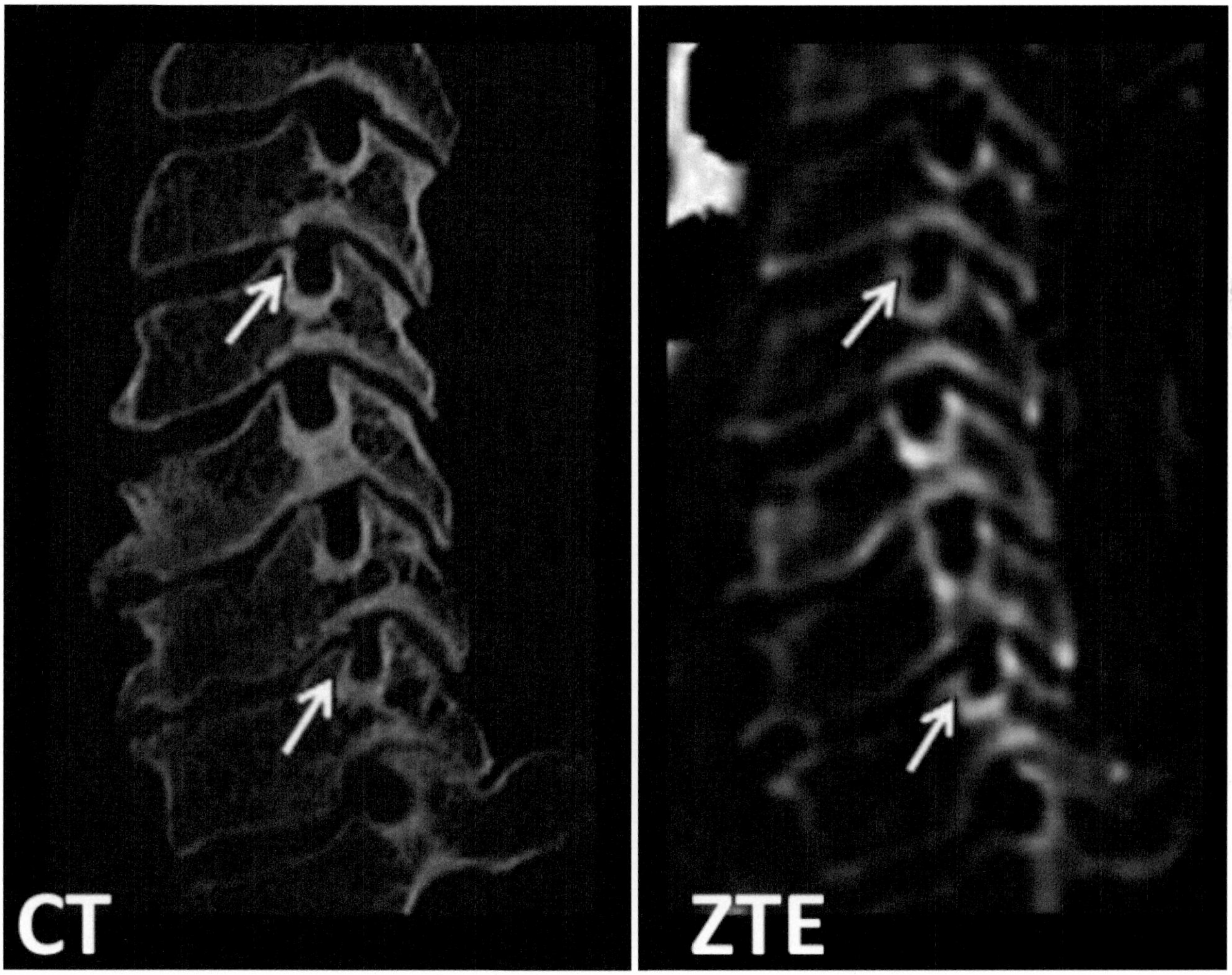

CT

ZTE

Fig. 44.5 Cervical neural foraminal stenosis comparison between CT (left) and ZTE-MRI (right)

Another spine study by Hou et al. [13] utilized spinal morphometry to assess agreement between CT and ZTE-MRI measuring axial orientation, foraminal diameter, pedicle width and height, and interarticular distance as well as osteoarthritis grades. Notably, this study also included a comparison of conventional MRI pulse sequences (proton density-weighted (PD-w), T_1-w, T_2-w, T_2-w fat-saturated) to CT and demonstrated stronger agreement ("substantial" to "near-perfect") between ZTE and CT than between conventional MRI and CT. While statistical differences were observed between conventional MRI and CT in the assessment of foraminal diameter and not between ZTE and CT, an equivalent resolution to ZTE was not utilized, so it cannot be ascertained whether the relative deficiency of conventional MRI was due to enhanced osseous contrast in ZTE or, more likely, the lower spatial resolution of the conventional sequences. Again, owing to radiosensitive tissues in the head, neck, and abdomen, applications of ZTE in the spine demonstrate opportunities for potential radiation dose mitigation.

The Hip/Pelvis

An additional area of interest for ZTE in orthopedics is imaging of the hips and pelvis. Many clinical concerns require radiological assessment of the hip and sacroiliac joints (SIJs). Of these, our site sought to evaluate the agreement between CT- and ZTE-based measurements of hip morphometry in assessment of developmental dysplasia of the hip (DDH) and femoroacetabular impingement (FAI) hip morphologies [8]. This subset of hip imaging patients is of particular interest, as the age of clinical presentation is younger, and these patients are often serially imaged (for follow-up and/or planning subsequent surgery). Furthermore, the anatomy of interest includes radiosensitive reproductive and intestinal tissues, which cannot be adequately shielded during CT imaging without obscuring the underlying osseous anatomy. In a sample of 38 hips from 23 patients, coronal and sagittal center-edge angles, femoral neck-shaft angle, acetabular version (at 1:00, 2:00, 3:00 positions), Tönnis angle, alpha angle, and modified beta-angle were measured on CT and ZTE images. Intraclass correlation coefficients demonstrated "good" (ICC = 0.60–0.74) to "excellent" (ICC = 0.75–1.00) agreement, and the magnitude of intermodal bias (Bland–Altman) was observed to be less than 3° for all but one measurement (modified beta-angle). Example images comparing ZTE and CT of the hip in axial views are shown in Fig. 44.6.

Another comparative study, by Wolharn et al. [14], of ZTE to CT in the lower torso focused on evaluation of the SIJ. Wolharn's study compared ZTE and CT assessment of 79 patients with a maximum of 12 months between imaging on the two modalities using ordinal grading (4-level "Likert" scale) for assessment of osteophytes, subchondral sclerosis, erosions, ankylosis, joint irregularities, joint widening, and vacuum sign in the SIJ. Good agreement was demonstrated in all assessed features, except vacuum sign, which reflects hypointense gas in the joint. Although this study did not utilize contrast inversion to produce "CT-like" contrast, the specific finding regarding vacuum sign/gas in the joint is notable as a minor limitation of utilizing ZTE in isolation from concurrent conventional MRI sequences.

The Knee

A qualitative study of ZTE for the assessment of bony abnormalities in the knee was also conducted [15]. In a cohort of 100 patients, this study evaluated osteophytosis, subchondral cysts, ossifications, and fractures. The study evaluated diagnostic confidence of readers in their evaluation of these osseous abnormalities in MRI exams, with and without ZTE. Raters scored their diagnostic confidence in osseous findings as higher with ZTE. Additionally, a spoiled gradient recalled echo (SPGR) sequence was also acquired for a subset of the patients ($N = 57$) and evaluated for its effect on diagnostic confidence. While both supplementary sequences were diagnostically useful, the addition of ZTE resulted in a greater improvement in reader confidence in osseous findings.

The Foot and Ankle

Our team also conducted a small study of the characterization of acute ankle fractures using ZTE [16]. A total of 14 acute ankle trauma cases were evaluated. Agreement in the diagnosis of fractures was assessed in the medial, lateral, and posterior malleolus, wherein raw agreements of 93%, 93%, and 100%, respectively, were observed across three readers. Additionally, fracture fragment size measurements were performed in a limited subset of these patients with concurrent CT. ICC values indicated excellent agreement between fragment measurements on the two modalities. Frequent concurrence of osseous and soft tissue injuries of the foot and ankle has led to our institution's rapid adoption of ZTE-MRI for foot and ankle trauma. ZTE is frequently requested as an addition to standard ankle MR examinations in the evaluation of malleolar fractures and associated ligament injuries. We have observed improved delineation of depressed tibial plafond fragments in posterior malleolar fractures (Fig. 44.7).

This summary of studies is not intended to be an exhaustive review of the extant literature on bone imaging with ZTE-MRI. Rather, these studies highlight the agreement of

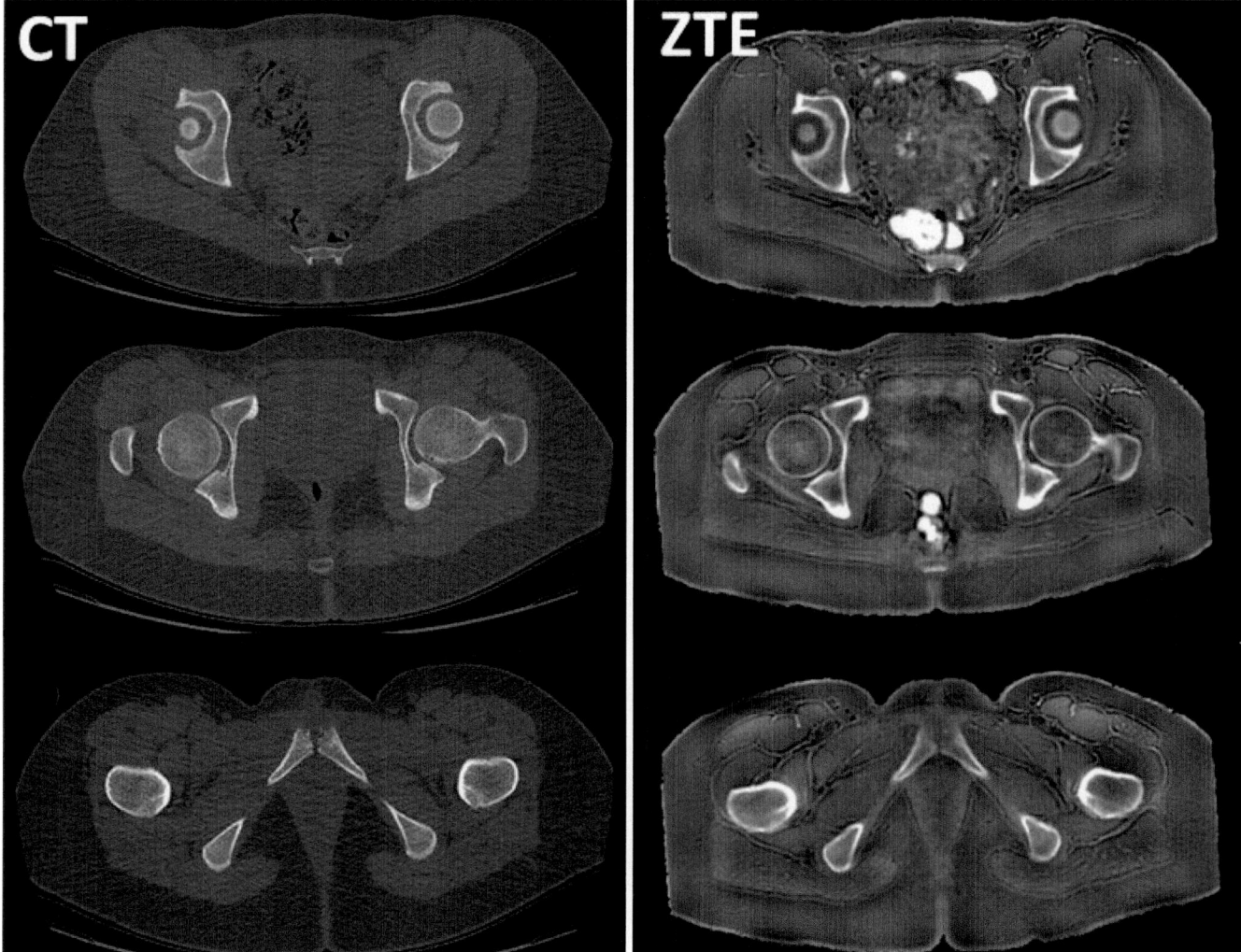

Fig. 44.6 Three axial views at descending locations through the pelvis in co-localized CT (left) and ZTE images (right)

ZTE with CT for diagnostic and morphometric tasks and instances where ZTE has been shown to provide added diagnostic value to MRI.

Limitations of ZTE-MRI for the Bone

Although the above examples demonstrate the application and suitability of ZTE for bone imaging in a broad array of anatomies, ZTE has several key limitations. As mentioned in the section "ZTE Image Acquisition and Post-processing," ZTE requires adequate and compatible hardware (scanner, coils) and software (pulse sequences, post-processing pipeline, etc.). In addition to the facility/site constraints on ZTE imaging, there are still limitations to what the pulse sequence can achieve, how it can be applied, and the contrast and resolution of the resulting images.

An abovementioned limitation of the contrast provided by ZTE is the potential mischaracterization of gases. In the section "The Hip/Pelvis," we summarized a study that showed poor agreement between ZTE and CT in assessing the presence of gas in the SIJ. Gases in joint spaces ("vacuum phenomena") manifest in acquired ZTE images as hypointense regions (or hyperintense on contrast-inverted images). Depending on its volume and diffuseness, the gas may be difficult to distinguish from adjacent bone. Although this limitation is inherent to the isolated assessment of a ZTE image series, the vacuum sign is distinguishable from adjacent bone when read with concurrent conventional MRI.

An additional limitation of ZTE is seen in the presence of other short-T_2/T_2^* tissues, such as fascia, which appears as hypointense on acquired images. The contrast between these tissues and adjacent muscle and fat are often accentuated by chemical shift artifacts. While these artifacts can be miti-

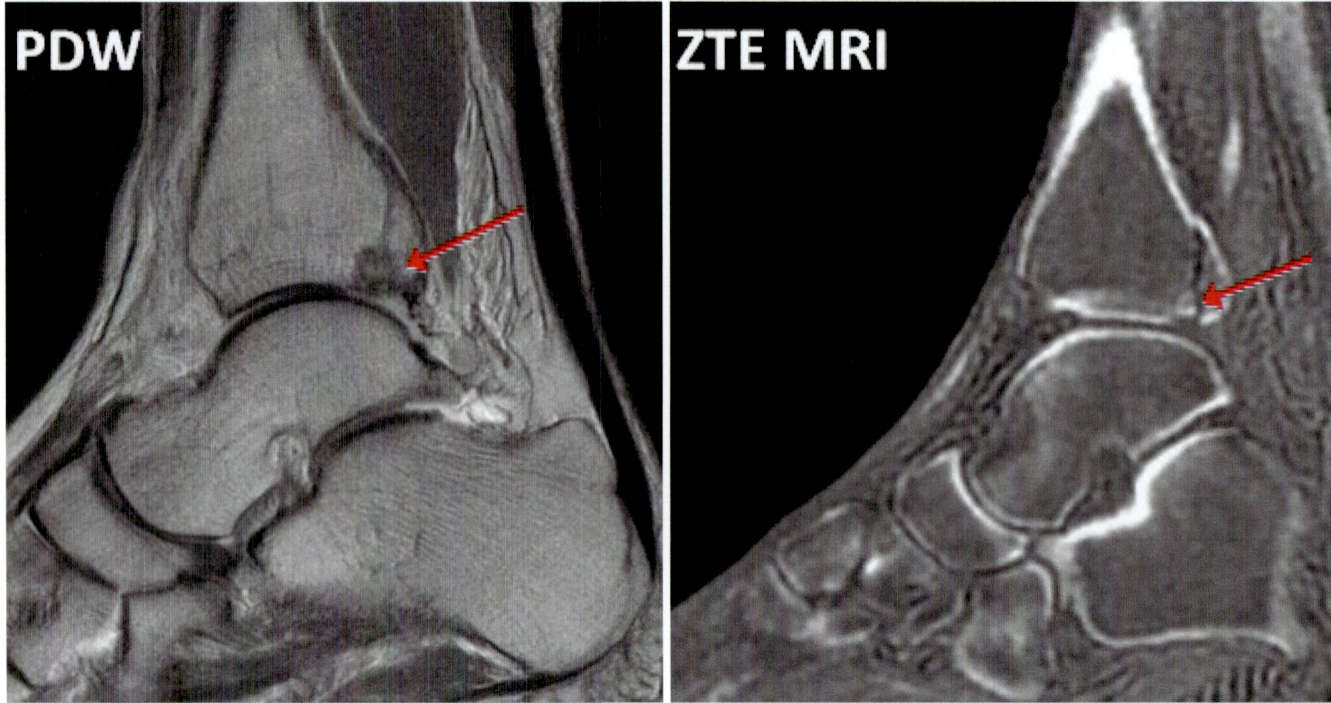

Fig. 44.7 PDW (left) and ZTE-MRI (right) of the same ankle showed clearer delineation of the tibial depressed plafond fragment and step-off from the tibia and distal fragment

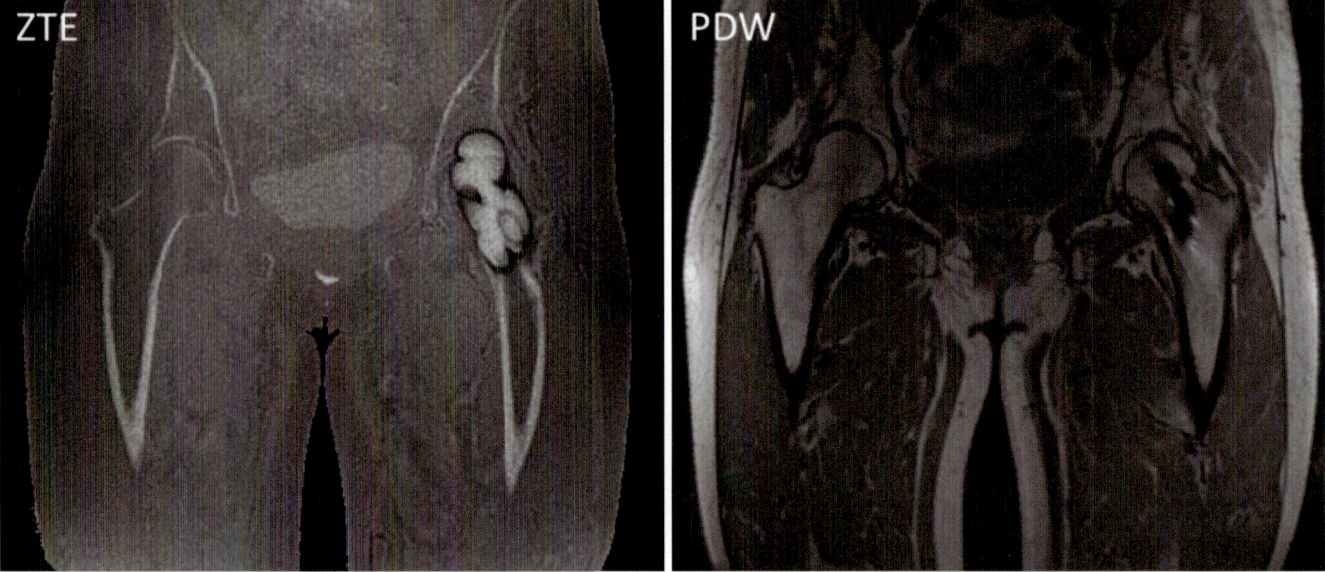

Fig. 44.8 The coronal view of the hips of a patient with unilateral (patient left) hardware. Colocalized slices in ZTE (left) and MAVRIC PDW MRI (right)

gated using greater receiver bandwidths, radiologists should be aware of them, particularly when they appear in proximity to anatomies of interest.

Imaging in the presence of metal remains a challenge for ZTE. Although metal artifact reduction strategies exist for some MRI pulse sequences (via slice encoding metal artifact correction (SEMAC) and multi-acquisition with variable resonance image combination (MAVRIC), there are currently no approaches implemented with ZTE acquisitions. An example showing the relative metal artifact in ZTE vs. colocalized proton density-weighted MAVRIC is shown in Fig. 44.8. The artifact is substantially larger and obscures and distorts the underlying osseous anatomy in ZTE, whereas the MAVRIC image shows the proximal femur with far less artifact, and the hip joint is visible.

Conclusions

ZTE-MRI is a robust pulse sequence that, when post-processed, yields images with CT-like contrast for bone. Numerous applications of ZTE imaging in orthopedic contexts have been explored, and studies have demonstrated good agreement with concurrent CT, suggesting that ZTE imaging not only provides better visualization of bone than conventional MRI but also affords sufficient osseous detail to replace CT in certain diagnostic and morphometric tasks. As demonstrated in several of the above studies, 3D visualization and modeling are possible with ZTE-MRI, opening a potential avenue for future work employing ZTE imaging in kinematic modeling of joint mechanics as well as an additional imaging modality for preoperative planning.

References

1. Weiger M, Brunner DO, Dietrich BE, Müller CF, Pruessmann KP. ZTE imaging in humans. Magn Reson Med. 2013;70(2):328–32.
2. Reichert IL, Robson MD, Gatehouse PD, He T, Chappell KE, Holmes J, Girgis S, Bydder GM. Magnetic resonance imaging of cortical bone with ultrashort TE pulse sequences. Magn Reson Imaging. 2005;23(5):611–8.
3. Aydıngöz Ü, Yıldız AE, Ergen FB. Zero echo time musculoskeletal MRI: technique, optimization, applications, and pitfalls. Radiographics. 2022;42(5):1398–414.
4. Engström M, McKinnon G, Cozzini C, Wiesinger F. In-phase zero TE musculoskeletal imaging. Magn Reson Med. 2020;83(1):195–202.
5. Lu A, Gorny KR, Ho M-L. Zero TE MRI for craniofacial bone imaging. Am J Neuroradiol. 2019;40(9):1562–6.
6. Tustison NJ, Cook PA, Gee JC. N4ITK: improved N3 bias correction. IEEE Trans Med Imaging. 2010;29(6):1310–20.
7. Breighner RE, Endo Y, Konin GP, Gulotta LV, Koff MF, Potter HG. Technical developments: zero echo time imaging of the shoulder: enhanced osseous detail by using MR imaging. Radiology. 2018;286(3):960–6.
8. Breighner RE, Bogner EA, Lee SC, Koff MF, Potter HG. Evaluation of osseous morphology of the hip using zero echo time magnetic resonance imaging. Am J Sports Med. 2019;47(14):3460–8.
9. Argentieri EC, Koff MF, Breighner RE, Endo Y, Shah PH, Sneag DB. Diagnostic accuracy of zero-echo time MRI for the evaluation of cervical neural foraminal stenosis. Spine (Phila Pa 1976). 2018;43(13):928–33.
10. Wiesinger F, Sacolick LI, Menini A, Kaushik SS, Ahn S, Veit-Haibach P, Delso G, Shanbhag DD. Zero TE MR bone imaging in the head. Magn Reson Med. 2016;75(1):107–14.
11. Cho SB, Baek HJ, Ryu KH, Choi BH, Moon JI, Kim TB, Kim SK, Park H, Hwang MJ. Clinical feasibility of zero TE skull MRI in patients with head trauma in comparison with CT: a single-center study. Am J Neuroradiol. 2019;40(1):109–15.
12. de Mello RAF, Ma Y-J, Ashir A, Jerban S, Hoenecke H, Carl M, Du J, Chang EY. Three-dimensional zero echo time magnetic resonance imaging versus 3-dimensional computed tomography for glenoid bone assessment. Arthroscopy. 2020;36(9):2391–400.
13. Hou B, Liu C, Li Y, Xiong Y, Wang J, Zhang P, Liu J, Liu WV, Li X. Evaluation of the degenerative lumbar osseous morphology using zero echo time magnetic resonance imaging (ZTE-MRI). Eur Spine J. 2022;31(3):792–800.
14. Wolharn L, Guggenberger R, Higashigaito K, Sartoretti T, Winklhofer S, Chung CB, Finkenstaedt T. Detailed bone assessment of the sacroiliac joint in a prospective imaging study: comparison between computed tomography, zero echo time, and black bone magnetic resonance imaging. Skelet Radiol. 2022;51(12):2307–15.
15. Bharadwaj UU, Coy A, Motamedi D, Sun D, Joseph GB, Krug R, Link TM. CT-like MRI: a qualitative assessment of ZTE sequences for knee osseous abnormalities. Skelet Radiol. 2022;51(8):1585–94.
16. Burge AJ, Breighner RE, Sahr M, Koff MF, Nwawka OK, Sneag DB, Konin K, Lin B, Helfet D, Potter HG. Utility of ZTE for the characterization of acute ankle fractures. Proc Intl Soc Mag Reson Med. 2018:1448.

MR-Based Attenuation Correction in PET–MRI

Tobias Schaeffter and Volkmar Schulz

Introduction

Medical imaging is the backbone of modern clinical diagnosis with more than five billion imaging investigations performed worldwide each year [1, 2]. Many radiological imaging modalities are based on high quality tomographic modalities such as computed tomography (CT), magnetic resonance imaging (MRI), ultrasound (US), and emission tomography, which provide complementary information of varying resolutions and sensitivities. In particular, MRI is a noninvasive technique without ionizing radiation, which provides both excellent soft tissue contrast visualization of morphology and a wide range of parameters for quantitative characterization of tissue properties and physiology. In distinction to this, emission tomography aims at imaging molecular processes using radioactively labeled molecules as the source of the imaging data. Such radiotracers are injected into the body and accumulate in regions of molecular and pathophysiological interest. In positron emission tomography (PET), the radioactive tracer decays to emit positrons that are annihilated by electron capture, resulting in the emission of a pair of nearly antiparallel 511-keV photons. These photons are measured in the detector ring of the PET system. Accurate information is important for solving the inverse problem of image reconstruction about how the photons in the body are attenuated on their way to the detectors since only a fraction of the emitted photons are detected. In conjunction with dedicated PET scans, CT scans are commonly used to help determine the attenuation values for the 511-keV photons and to obtain anatomical information.

Over the past decades, MR-compatible PET scanners have been developed [3–7] and have been used for clinical applications [8–11]. Like PET–CT scanners, PET–MRI scanners are capable of providing high-resolution anatomical information but with much improved soft tissue contrast and without ionizing radiation. In addition, MRI can provide additional functional information, such as perfusion or diffusion [9]. If the information from PET and MRI is accurately matched both spatially and temporally, then the MRI data can also be used to improve the accuracy of pharmacokinetic modeling, apply advanced motion compensation [12–15], and compensate for partial volume effects in PET data [16].

Unfortunately, the MR signal mainly depends on proton density and relaxation times rather than electron density and is thus not directly related to photon attenuation as it is in CT [17]. For example, bone and air have low intensity with conventional MR image measurements but very different attenuation coefficients with PET. Since the commercial introduction of PET–MRI, considerable effort has been made to develop reliable attenuation correction (AC) methods for PET–MRI. Another focus has been on the detection of tissues with ultrashort-T_2^*s such as cortical bone.

This chapter presents MR-based methods for deriving AC maps with the focus on ultrashort-T_2^* tissues. MR-specific challenges in determining attenuation corrections for ultrashort-T_2^* tissues are described. In addition, the relative impact on image quality and quantitative accuracy of AC compared to other correction techniques is presented. Finally, integration of AC into motion compensation and other areas for future work are discussed.

T. Schaeffter (✉)
Physikalisch-Technische Bundesanstalt (PTB),
Braunschweig and Berlin, Germany

Medical Engineering, Technical University of Berlin and Einstein Centre Digital Future, Berlin, Germany

Division of Imaging Sciences and Biomedical Engineering, King's College London, London, UK
e-mail: tobias.schaeffter@ptb.de

V. Schulz
Department of Physics of Molecular Imaging Systems, Institute for Experimental Molecular Imaging, RWTH Aachen University, Aachen, Germany

Institute of Physics IIIB, RWTH Aachen University, Aachen, Germany

Hyperion Hybrid Imaging Systems GmbH, Aachen, Germany

Fraunhofer Institute for Digital Medicine MEVIS, Aachen, Germany
e-mail: volkmar.schulz@pmi.rwth-aachen.de

Attenuation Correction in PET

PET measures the spatial distribution of injected radioactive tracers that emit positrons. After annihilation with electrons, 2 nearly antiparallel 511-keV γ-photons are emitted. These are then detected by a cylindrical ring of detectors around the patient. Hence, the annihilation is assumed to lie on the line connecting the two detected γ-photons, referred to as the line of response (LOR). Such coincidental events are stored in a sinogram, which shows the distribution of all LORs during a measurement. The name is due to the fact that a single voxel in the sinogram shows a sinusoidal curve. In recent decades, fast detectors have been developed that can measure the small (sub-nanosecond) time differences between the detection of the two γ-photons. This so-called time-of-flight (TOF) information can be used to determine the most likely location of the annihilation event along the LOR, resulting in a higher signal-to-noise ratio (SNR) in the reconstructed PET images.

Before the two photons reach the detector, they pass through the body and interact with the tissue, mainly by Compton scattering. In this process, photons interact with electrons and eject them from their atomic shells, resulting in a loss of energy and a change in photon direction. These two effects lead to a reduction in the number of photons observed along the LOR. In particular, the reduction increases exponentially as the length of the path increases. Photons that travel through more, or denser, tissue of the body to the detectors are more likely to be attenuated than those that travel through sparser, or less dense, tissues. Reconstruction of images from sinograms without AC, using the number of counts alone leads to inaccurate quantitation of tracer uptake. For instance, a higher number of counts could arise from lower attenuation in a tissue (e.g., lung) rather than because of a higher radiotracer uptake.

Therefore, it is essential to correct for attenuation effects. In former times, this was done using an external positron source that was rotated around the object and the attenuation of the transmitted photons was determined from such a transmission scan. However, nowadays, the majority of systems are hybrid PET–CT scanners, and CT provides not only images of the anatomy but also information on tissue attenuation values. The latter is possible because the signal intensity in CT is also due to photon attenuation. However, there is no unique relation between attenuation at the photon energies of CT (40–140 keV) and that of PET (511 keV). In particular, the attenuation of photons at the much lower CT energies has contributions from both Compton scattering and photoelectric absorption, which has a high dependence on the atomic number. As a result, photoelectric absorption in most soft tissues is a smaller effect than it is, for example, in

bone (due to its high calcium content), in metallic implants, and in contrast agents [18]. Therefore, it is possible for two distinct materials with the same value of attenuation coefficient at 511 keV to have different CT attenuation values, and errors in the AC derived from CT images will propagate to errors in PET images. A bilinear transform is often used to convert CT-derived attenuation coefficients to the equivalent values for PET [18, 19]. Often, there are also positional mismatches between the PET and CT images (i.e., emission and attenuation maps) due to patient motion. Furthermore, physiological motion introduces further artifacts and quantification errors in PET imaging when imaging the thoracic and abdominal regions.

MR Methods for Deriving Attenuation Correction Maps

Several approaches have been proposed to derive AC maps from MR images [20]. These can be broadly divided into registration-based and segmentation-based methods. In practice, combinations of both methods are usually used because there are device-related AC maps, such as a patient tables, covers, local receive coils, etc., and patient-related AC maps. There are other challenges related to AC maps for PET–MRI, such as attenuation correction of "invisible" MR coils and compensation for the limited field of view of MRI, which are not addressed in this chapter. In the following section, we focus on the estimation of AC maps in patients.

Registration-based methods for AC map creation use nonlinear image registration to transform an existing AC map to match the anatomy of a new patient. The key motivation behind this method is robust creation of an AC map. Registration-based methods were first proposed for standalone PET scanning to avoid the long acquisition times needed for transmission measurements [21]. For this, the transformation was determined by registering the acquired non-corrected PET image to a template of a previously acquired non-corrected PET image and then using the same transformation for warping the template attenuation coefficient map with the new anatomy. A similar approach has been used in a brain PET–MRI studies using MR images for registration and utilizing the higher spatial resolution and contrast of MRI [22, 23]. A more advanced method uses a larger number of available reference MR–CT datasets as an atlas [24]. In this approach, MR images of the atlas are co-registered to the actual MR image of the patient and the determined transformations are applied to the corresponding CT images of the atlas. A so-called pseudo-CT image is derived by taking a weighted average of all coregistered CT images, which is then used for determining AC maps.

Segmentation of Tissues

Although registration-based methods overcome the problem of the lack of dependence of the MR signal on photon attenuation, they may not be reliable in regions where there is a high degree of variability between patients. Therefore, segmentation-based methods based on images of the subject were proposed. These attempts to derive an AC map based on tissue classes for each voxel require image segmentation as an important post-processing step. In early work, MR images of the brain were segmented into air, brain tissue, skull, and scalp regions by fuzzy clustering means and AC values were assigned to different regions of the head [24]. Schulz et al. tested such a segmentation-based AC-based method in whole-body PET–MR applications for differentiating the three classes: air, lung, and soft tissue [17]. The methods used a free-breathing three-dimensional (3D) T_1-weighted spoiled gradient echo MR sequence with relatively large voxel sizes of $4 \times 4 \times 4$ mm^3. Identification of the lung tissue was performed using an adaptive lung surface model. The MR-based AC was compared to conventional AC derived from CT images. In most areas, the diagnostic value of the resulting PET images was rated as unaffected. However, an underestimation of activity was found in bone lesions showing the importance of bone in AC for accurate quantification of tracer activity. Similar findings have also been reported in another study in which the effect of replacing the AC measurement of bone with various constant values was investigated for PET activity quantification [25]. In addition to bone, the presence of adipose tissue in body PET–MR has been reported as a challenge, since the AC of fat differs from those of other soft tissues. Therefore, Martinez-Möller et al. have proposed the use of a so-called Dixon technique for MR-based AC [26] making use of the difference in Larmor frequency between protons in water and fat molecules. In their study, MR images were obtained with a two-point Dixon MR sequence. Subsequent thresholding for soft tissue and adipose tissue was applied. Segmentation artifacts arising from the lack of bone MR signal were corrected, and unclassified voxels were used for lung segmentation. The authors showed a maximum error of up to 13% by neglecting bone in the AC. Thus, MR methods for imaging cortical bone are highly desirable.

Segmentation of Tissues with Short T_2^*s

With conventional MRI, there is little or no contrast between air, parenchymal lung, and cortical bone due to the fast transverse relaxation (ultrashort T_2^*) of lung and cortical bone signals. One possible solution is to use ultrashort echo time (UTE) sequences that sample the free induction decay (FID) almost immediately after excitation so that the short-lived signals are sampled before they exponentially disappear into the noise background. UTE sequences were designed to visualize tissues with short- and ultrashort-T_2^* transverse relaxation times, such as tendons, ligaments, cortical bone, and lung tissue, as described in other chapters in this book. Most UTE sequences use the so-called dual-echo acquisitions: first, an FID image is acquired very quickly after radio frequency (RF) excitation with a nominal TE of 50–150 µs, and this is followed by a gradient echo acquisition after a few milliseconds (ms). Because tissues with short- and ultrashort-T_2^* are visible on the FID image but not on the subsequent gradient echo image, they can be distinguished from soft tissues with long T_2^*s (which are visible on both images) and air (not visible on either image). Such a dual-echo UTE sequence has been used by Catana et al. for bone–air segmentation in simultaneous PET–MRI of the human head [27]. An image intensity-based segmentation procedure was used to identify regions of air, soft tissue, and cortical bone in the acquired MR data and assign linear attenuation coefficients from the literature to these tissue types. The proposed method was tested on a brain PET insert inside an MR scanner using a UTE sequence with dual-echo times (TEs) of TE$_1$= 0.07 ms and TE$_2$= 2.4 ms. For comparison, CT scans were obtained to derive CT-based ACs as a reference. PET images were reconstructed both with UTE-MR- and CT-based attenuation corrections. However, the segmentation method used empirical thresholds for selecting tissue types, which might vary between scanners and with patient anatomy. This might be addressed via methods such as use of a Laplacian histogram, as proposed in Schulz et al. [17]. Keereman et al. proposed a quantitative UTE approach, which is less dependent on the MR system [28] (c.f. Figure 45.1). For this, dual-echo UTE images were used to roughly estimate the spatial distribution of R_2^* using logarithmic subtraction of the two acquired images $I_{TE1, 2}(x, y)$ at two TEs, TE$_1$ and TE$_2$:

$$R_2^* = \frac{\ln\left[I_{TE2}(x,y)\right] - \ln\left[I_{TE1}(x,y)\right]}{TE_2 - TE_1} \qquad (45.1)$$

In R_2^* maps, bone has a high R_2^* value, whereas soft tissues show low R_2^* values. In areas with no signal (e.g., air), R_2^* maps exhibit noise. R_2^* maps are used in a combined segmentation approach, where the thresholded FID image is used as a mask to preselect areas of soft tissue and bone. The mask is then used to remove noisy air regions on the R_2^* map, and two quantitative thresholds are applied to segment bone from soft tissue. The method was tested in R_2^* maps of the brain using TE$_1$= 0.14 ms and TE$_2$= 1.8 ms. AC maps derived from R_2^* maps and CT were applied to PET reconstruction and produced no large visual differences in the PET images.

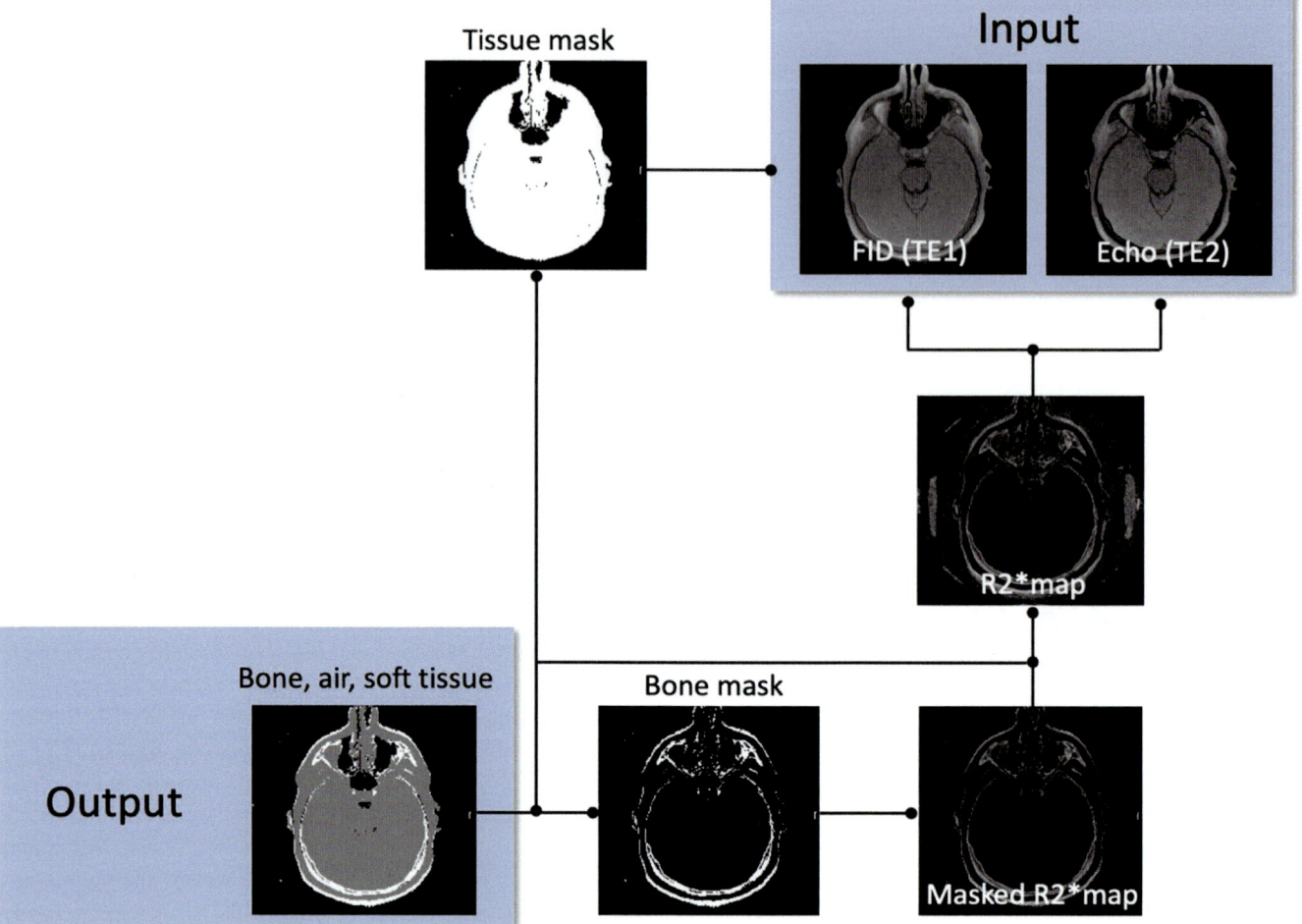

Fig. 45.1 Method for generating an AC map using a dual-echo UTE sequence. First, the FID image is thresholded to create a mask to segment air from other tissues (bone and soft tissue). Second, the FID and later echo images are used to estimate an R_2^* map. To exclude artifacts from air, the map is masked and then thresholded to separate bone from soft tissue. Finally, the two masks are combined to segment the different tissue classes and to produce an AC map. (Adapted with permission from Aitken [29])

A mean average relative difference of approximately 5% and a maximum difference of 20–40% were found.

Segmentation of Tissues with Short T_2^* from Water and Fat Soft Tissues

As discussed before, differentiation of adipose and water soft tissue is essential when highly accurate quantification of PET is desired because the ACs of adipose and water soft tissue differ by 10%. A combined MRI sequence for the discrimination of cortical bone, adipose tissue, air, and water soft tissue has been proposed by Berker et al. [30] and Han et al. [31]. This approach uses the acquisition of three signals, namely, one FID (I_{TE1}) and two echoes (I_{TE2} and I_{TE3}), and also uses appropriate longer TEs to encode for the chemical shift between fat and water (c.f. Figure 45.2a).

Berker et al. proposed an image processing pipeline that processes the magnitudes and phases of the three input images ($I_{TE1, 2, 3}$) to produce the desired attenuation map (c.f. Figure 45.3). The UTE(I_{TE1}) image and one echo image (I_{TE3}) were used to discriminate between cortical bone and air (I_{AIR}, I_{bone}), whereas the Dixon decomposition was applied to determine the water and fat fraction of each voxel from all three images. The segmented images were used to assign the classes to tissue-specific linear attenuation coefficients for 511-keV photons using literature values. In soft tissue voxels, the mean AC was calculated from the relative water–fat fraction r of the voxel using the linear mapping between the ACs of water soft tissue water μ_w and fat soft tissue fat μ_f:

$$\mu_r = \frac{1+r}{2}\mu_w + \frac{1-r}{2}\mu_f \qquad (45.2)$$

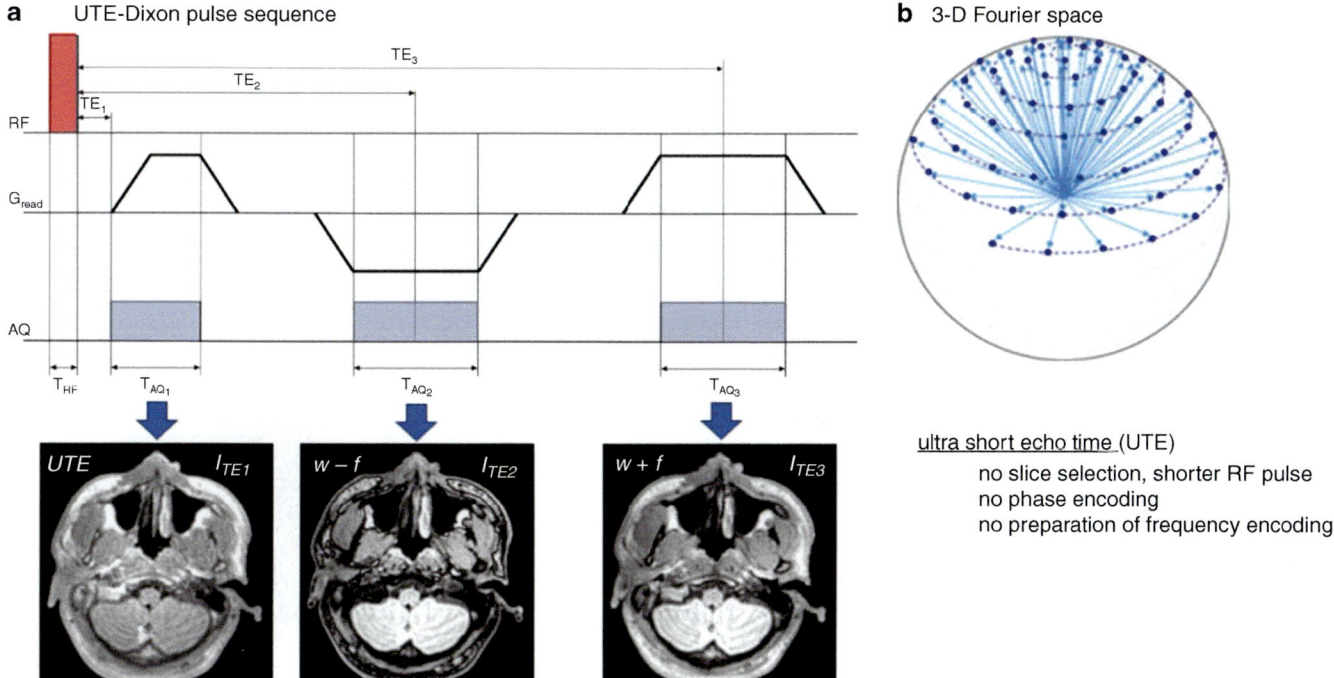

Fig. 45.2 (**a**) An MRI sequence timing diagram of a UTE-Dixon sequence (UTIL) from Berker et al. [30], showing RF excitation, read-out gradient (G_{read}), and data acquisition (AQ). The corresponding images are UTE: FID image, w-f: water and fat out of phase, and w + f: water and fat in phase. (**b**) The k-space acquisition scheme, showing the FID measurement based on the sampling from the k-space center to the surface of the sphere. (Adapted with permission from Berker et al. [30])

The method was tested in the head and neck region of patients by comparing AC maps and reconstructed PET images based on either CT- or MR-based AC maps. The average relative errors in PET activities were between −4.8% and +7.6% in eight volumes of interest in the brain using the four tissue classes for the AC. The proposed method showed better results than AC without water–fat discrimination (+11.4%) and in comparison excluding the UTE-based cortical bone discrimination (−14.1%).

UTE methods showed good performance in the head and neck for assigning regions with soft tissue, bone, and air. In principle, the transverse relaxation rate (R_2^*) measured with UTE allows a continuous determination of AC values [32]. This allows the estimation of bone mineral density and can thus address interpatient variations in bone AC due to differences in bone mineral density. However, UTE methods also detect other short-T_2^* tissues such as the tendons, which may be misclassified as bones. A modification of the 3D koosh ball acquisition toward two-dimensional (2D) stack-of-spirals allowed use of UTE with such trajectories [33]. An alternative method for bone detection was proposed, which uses

zero echo time (ZTE) MRI with proton density-weighted images [34–36]. The sequence employs RF excitation in the presence of the readout gradients. In comparison to UTE, this leads to two unique challenges. First, the excitation bandwidth of the RF pulse has to exceed the imaging bandwidth. Second, the switching time from RF transmit to receive mode causes some samples to be missed at the beginning of the readout and these need to be estimated in the reconstruction process. ZTE imaging can be combined with pre-pulses to influence image contrast. For instance, the water- and fat-suppressed proton projection MRI (WASPI) method allows generation of continuous-valued bone attenuation coefficients [36]. The limitations of the WASPI method are that the suppression pulses are sensitive to off-resonance effects at tissue–air interfaces, leading to unwanted suppression of bone signal and misclassification. Furthermore, two scans consisting of a ZTE and a two-point Dixon method have been proposed to classify bone, air, lung, and soft tissue [35]. This method uses ZTE for bone segmentation and Dixon MRI for classification of soft tissues. However, two scans have to be performed (Fig. 45.4).

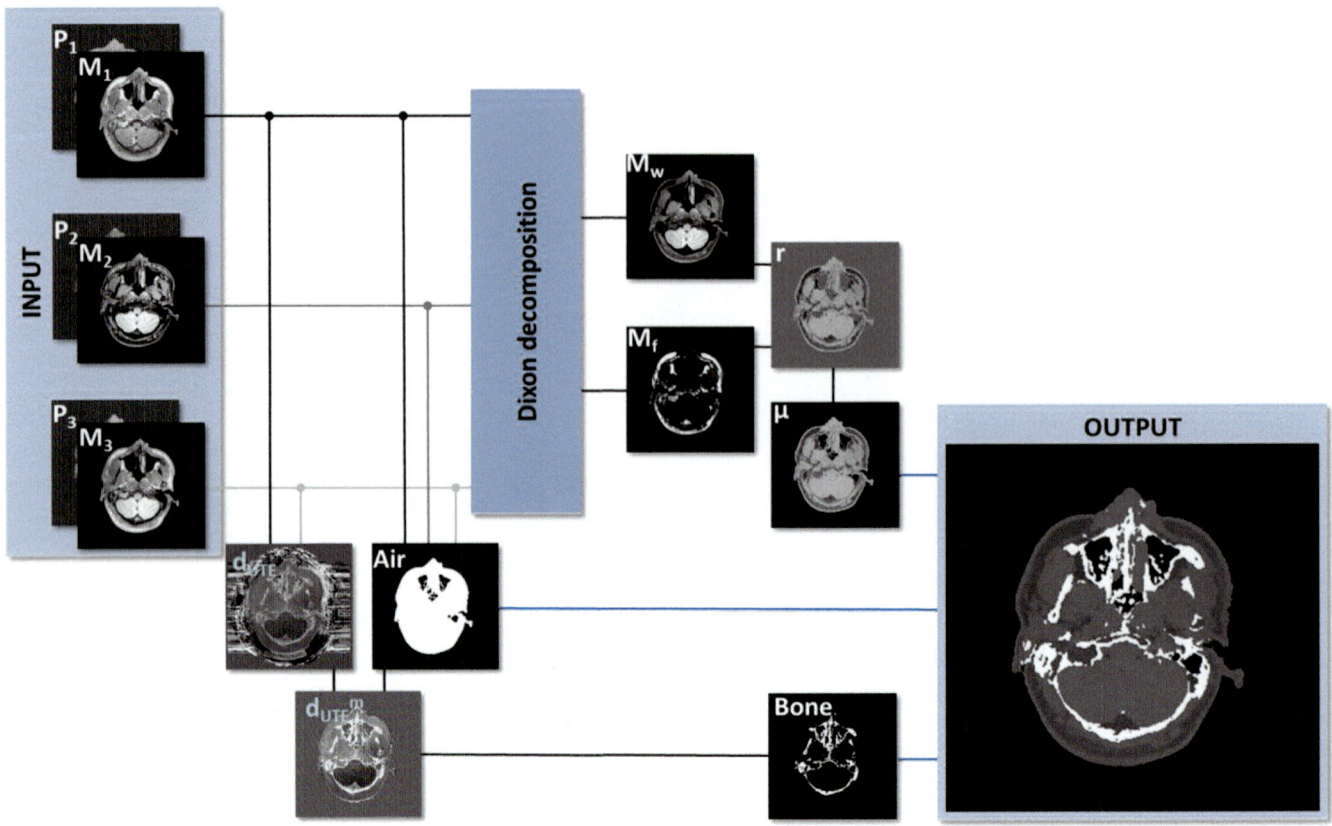

Fig. 45.3 A flowchart for image post-processing. The three input images were used to calculate the bone image, which is fused with the linear mapped attenuation image of water and fat. (Adapted with permission from Berker et al. [30])

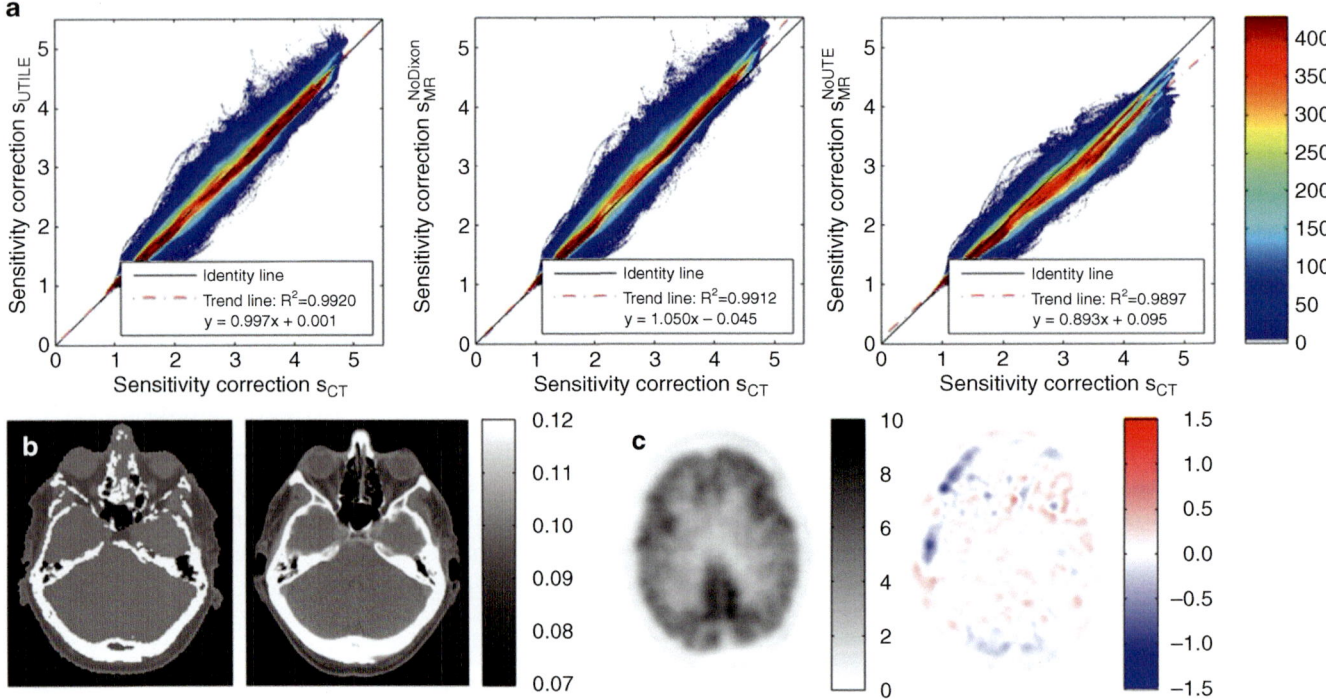

Fig. 45.4 (**a**) Joint histograms of sensitivity correction maps S_{UTILE} (left), embedded image (middle), and embedded image (right), all correlated with S_{CT} (aggregated over all patients). (**b**) Corresponding transverse slices of μUTILE (left) and micro-CT (μCT) (right) in inverse centimeters. (**c**) Corresponding transverse slices of PETUTILE (left) and difference image dUTILE (right) of a patient in SUV. (Reproduced with permission from Berker et al. [30])

System Imperfections

The robust derivation of AC maps from UTE sequences in regions of tissue interfaces remains challenging. Due to system imperfections, the required subtraction of the UTE and the gradient echo image can lead to artifacts when the images are separately scaled in intensity and differ in size. Consequently, boundaries between air and tissue often appear with high intensities in the subtraction images or related R_2^* maps, leading to misclassification in segmented AC maps. UTE acquisition parameters need to be carefully optimized so that the size of the imaged object is consistent across the UTE and the gradient echo acquisitions [37].

In UTE sequences, the rapidly decaying signal is measured while magnetic field gradients rapidly change. However, according to Faraday's law, ramping up gradients results in eddy currents in nearby conductors. These induced currents in turn generate magnetic fields that, according to Lenz's law, always oppose the original change in flux. This leads to deviations between the desired and the actual k-space trajectories and thus to degradation of the reconstructed images. Furthermore, system latencies lead to timing errors, which cause the k-space trajectories to be shifted, leading to further artifacts. For certain acquisition schemes, it is possible to estimate trajectory errors based on the data itself. For instance, a common approach for radial acquisitions is to correct the shifts of the k-space trajectories using a linear phase correction in the Fourier domain, i.e., in projection space.

Although the effects of eddy currents and delays can be partially corrected by gradient preemphasis and by shifting and scaling the k-space trajectories prior to reconstruction, some residual effects occur even with optimally configured systems. This is due in part to the fact that preemphasis waveforms are typically designed for conventional gradient echo imaging, where sampling occurs during the constant portion of the gradient waveform, rather than for ramp sampling as with UTE. The sampling strategy during ramping up is more susceptible to errors introduced by short-term eddy current behavior and is often not fully corrected by preemphasis. Furthermore, the effects of eddy currents can depend on the rate at which the gradient fields are ramped up ("slew rate"). The differences between UTE and conventional gradient echo imaging are particularly important when subtracting an FID image and a subsequent later echo image to estimate R_2^* maps, since differences between the two images lead to errors in the estimation. Thus, inconsistencies in the sampling need to be characterized and corrected.

One elegant way for characterization is the use of dynamic magnetic field monitoring using a field camera, which can measure eddy current effects on the sampling points in the k-space. For this, the effect of short- and long-term eddy currents on the actual k-space trajectory is measured in a separate calibration scan. This concept could be used with the so-called PET inserts, which usually have conductive surfaces, which form RF shields close to the object of interest. Gross-Weege et al. used the gradient impulse response function (GIRF) to measure and correct for these kinds of eddy currents [38]. In general, the deviation of trajectories results in image artifacts when using the nominal positions due to mis-sampling of the k-space center and incorrect distances between k-space points (c.f. Figure 45.5). The measured trajectories can then be used in MR reconstruction algorithms instead of using nominal trajectories. It has been shown in simulations and experiments that the approach improves the quality of AC maps. In particular, artifacts occurring at tissue interfaces lead to misclassification of bone, air, and, in particular, soft tissue as a bone in the nominal AC maps (c.f. Figure 45.6). The effect of erroneous AC maps was assessed in PET simulations showing errors in the uptake of $SUV_{max} = 7.17–12.19\%$ for simulated lesions in the range of $7.17–12.19\%$ using nominal trajectories, which were reduced to $SUV_{max} = -0.21$ to $+1.81\%$, if measured trajectories were used in the determination of AC maps.

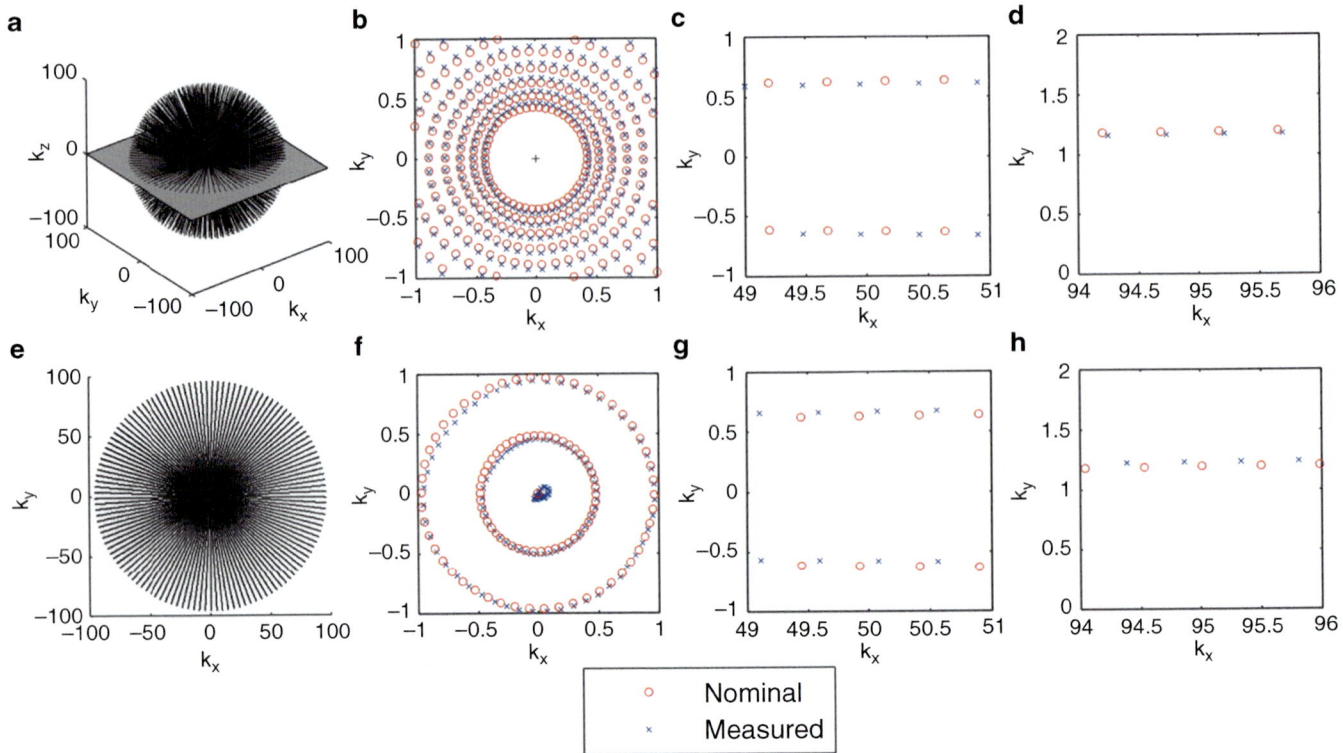

Fig. 45.5 Nominal (desired) and measured k-space trajectories for a 3D radial UTE scan. Several spokes from the 3D readout (**a**) are projected onto the k_x–k_y plane (**e**). The region of k-space center for FID (**b**) and echo (**f**). The radial trajectory results in a high sampling density in the k-space center. Only the second sampling is shown for simplicity. The zoomed region of k-space for FID (**c, d**) and echo (**g, h**) showing the deviation between the nominal and measured sampling point positions. (Reproduced with permission from Aitken et al. [37])

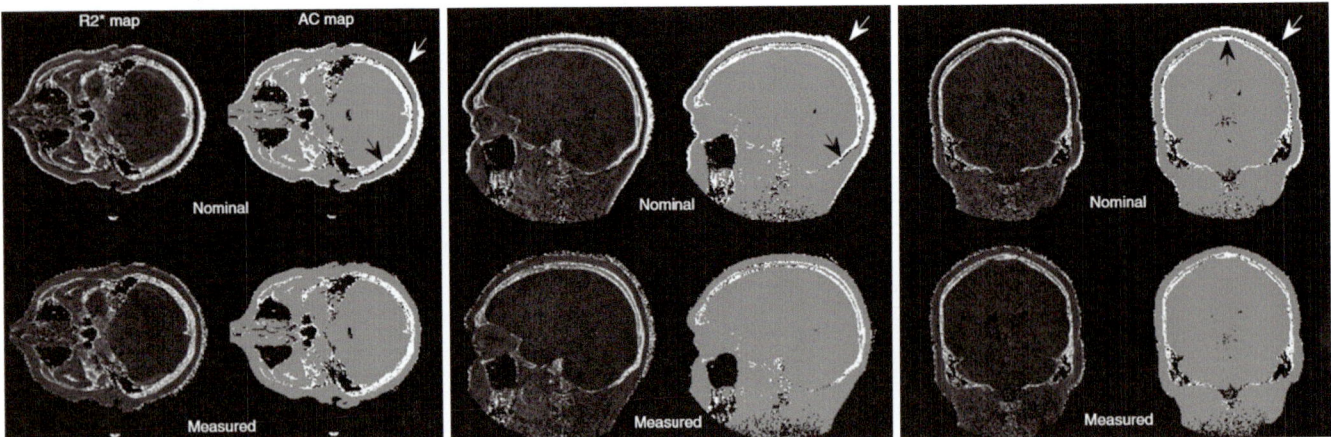

Fig. 45.6 Comparison of nominal k-space trajectories with measured trajectories derived from cranial UTE-MRI scans. The figures show the axial, sagittal, and coronal slices from 3D segmented AC maps (which were derived from R_2^* maps). Black arrows: hypointense artifacts at bone–soft tissue boundary, leading to misclassification of bone as air in nominal AC maps; white arrows: hyperintense artifacts at the boundary between air and soft tissue, leading to misclassification of soft tissue as bone in nominal AC maps. (Reproduced with permission from Aitken et al. [37])

Applications

Hybrid PET–MR imaging combines exquisite soft tissue information obtained by MRI with functional information provided by PET, including metabolic markers, perfusion, and target-specific binding tracers. While PET–MRI is clinically used in cardiology [39, 40] and oncology [41], the first PET–MRI human research images were of the brain [42]. Over the last decades, PET imaging has been used to study neurotransmitter activity and neuroinflammatory processes. Conversely, MRI has been the gold standard for the assessment of brain tumors, white matter (WM) disease, and stroke. As a result, hybrid PET–MR imaging has been of great interest for assessment of patients measuring many different tissue properties by MRI and PET. In particular, the combination of MR markers, such as structural information, connectivity, and perfusion, together with amyloid-specific PET tracers can assist the diagnosis and treatment of dementia in a single scan, thus simplifying workflow. Recently, a research dementia platform has been established at seven different sites in the United Kingdom to link PET–MRI scanners to support multicenter research and clinical trials in dementia [43]. Compared to other cerebral disorders (e.g., tumors, stroke), the diagnosis and treatment of dementia requires collaboration between different disciplines to identify characteristic patterns in the multiparametric findings, including integration of separate findings on MRI and PET images [44].

Oncology has been a major driver of hybrid PET–CT devices in the years since 2000, and PET–CT has largely replaced solitary PET scanners worldwide, which shows the widespread acceptance of hybrid imaging, especially in oncology. In pediatric neuro-oncology, PET–MRI provides excellent neuroimaging capabilities compared with CT as well as a lower radiation dose, which is relevant for follow-up studies in pediatric patients. In addition, MRI can provide additional information to assess lesions in the abdomen [45, 46] and breast [47]. Thus, simultaneous PET–MRI acquisitions are a powerful tool for the diagnostic assessment of tumors [48] and combine a variety of complementary functional and morphological imaging information. For instance, the assessment of cancer perfusion by dynamic contrast-enhanced MR (DCE-MR) imaging is one of the most widely used MR protocols [49]. It can provide parametric maps of contrast agent uptake using pharmacokinetic modeling. Such a quantitative imaging approach is of special interest in the detection and characterization of breast and hepatic malignancies. It can aid in treatment selection and the assessment of therapy. The introduction of hybrid scanners capable of performing simultaneous PET–MRI has improved anatomical localization and characterization of hepatic metastases as well as diagnostic accuracy in lesion detection [50]. The impact of accurate ACs has been demonstrated in patients with bone metastases using various radiotracers [51]. For this, a model-based segmentation approach has been used to determine five classes of tissues (including bone) from a whole-body Dixon scans [52].

In cardiology, combined PET–MRI has now been in routine clinical practice for almost 10 years [40]. Several cardiovascular applications have become established such as the detection of ischemia, viability, cardiomyopathy, inflammation of the myocardium, and atherosclerotic plaques. Simultaneous acquisition cardiac PET–MRI combines PET as a reference standard for myocardial perfusion with MRI as a reference standard for functional assessment. In addition, cardiac PET–MRI can characterize myocardial tissue by means of PET tracers and quantitative MRI methods like T_1, T_2 and extracellular volume fraction (ECF) measurements. Inflammatory processes are also an important target, which can be assessed through imaging of perfusion, edema, and molecular processes. In particular, vulnerable atherosclerotic plaque is an important cause of stroke and myocardial infarction requiring noninvasive imaging strategies for its early detection and characterization. The development of hybrid PET–MRI has opened new avenues for early diagnosis, improved risk stratification, and treatment evaluation of patients with atherosclerosis [53].

Limitations to the routine clinical use of PET–MR in the abdomen and the heart have been the need for robust MR-based AC to correct both PET and MRI. Lesion detectability and accurate uptake values are relevant in oncological applications, whereas improved spatial resolution is essential for some cardiovascular applications such as atherosclerotic plaque imaging. Respiratory and heart motion not only result in image artifacts with each modality (i.e., blurring and ghosting) but also lead to misalignments between the modalities and AC mismatches. The latter has a significant impact on quantification when different motion states in the AC and the emission data are used for the PET reconstruction. The impact of motion and errors in the AC map have been assessed in a PET simulation study using real MR data obtained from healthy volunteers demonstrating that both have a similar effect on standardized uptake values [54]. Furthermore, MR-based estimated motion fields (MFs) can be applied for nonrigid motion compensation of both imaging modalities. This can be done either in the image domain by warping PET and MR images to a common reference frame or by incorporating the motion information directly into an iterative image reconstruction algorithm [55]. The last few years have seen the development of novel MR acquisitions that provide both MR-based dynamic AC and displacement fields for motion-compensated PET–MRI reconstruction using the open-source Synergistic Reconstruction for Biomedical Imaging (SIRF) framework [56].

A 3D free-breathing AC-MRI acquisition scheme has been proposed for motion-corrected PET–MRI applications in the abdomen [57]. This technique provides dynamic respiratory and resolved MR-based AC maps and nonrigid respiratory motion fields (MFs), which can be utilized in motion-compensated reconstruction schemes for both MRI and PET. In order to evaluate the impact of registration accuracy on motion-compensated reconstruction algorithms, an open-source simulation framework for dynamic PET–MRI has been created [58]. MRI contrast and tracer kinetics can also be simulated together with motion fields as ground truth information. The motion-compensated reconstruction approach was tested in a clinical PET–MRI study in patients with hepatic metastases by obtaining DCE-MRI and PET data [59]. The nonrigid respiratory motion-cor-

rected framework made use of higher spatial resolution MR data for better motion correction. Quantitative evaluation of motion correction in PET images demonstrated average percentage increases in SUV_{mean} of 18% ± 6% and improved DCE-MRI parameter maps. The approach has also been tested in cardiac PET–MRI applications to enhance PET–MRI quality and improved the quantification of myocardial infarction [60]. Furthermore, it has been shown that motion-compensated PET–MRI reconstruction is highly beneficial in the detection of small atherosclerotic plaque lesions using [^{18}F]NaF as a plaque-specific PET tracer [61] (c.f. Figure 45.7), in which free-breathing 3D Dixon MR data were acquired and retrospectively binned into multiple respiratory and cardiac motion states to reconstruct respiratory and cardiac motion-resolved water–fat images. A nonrigid cardiorespiratory (cr) motion model and a motion-resolved AC map were also generated. The approach was tested in 10 patients, and the target-to-background ratios of identified plaques were improved by 7 ± 7%, con-

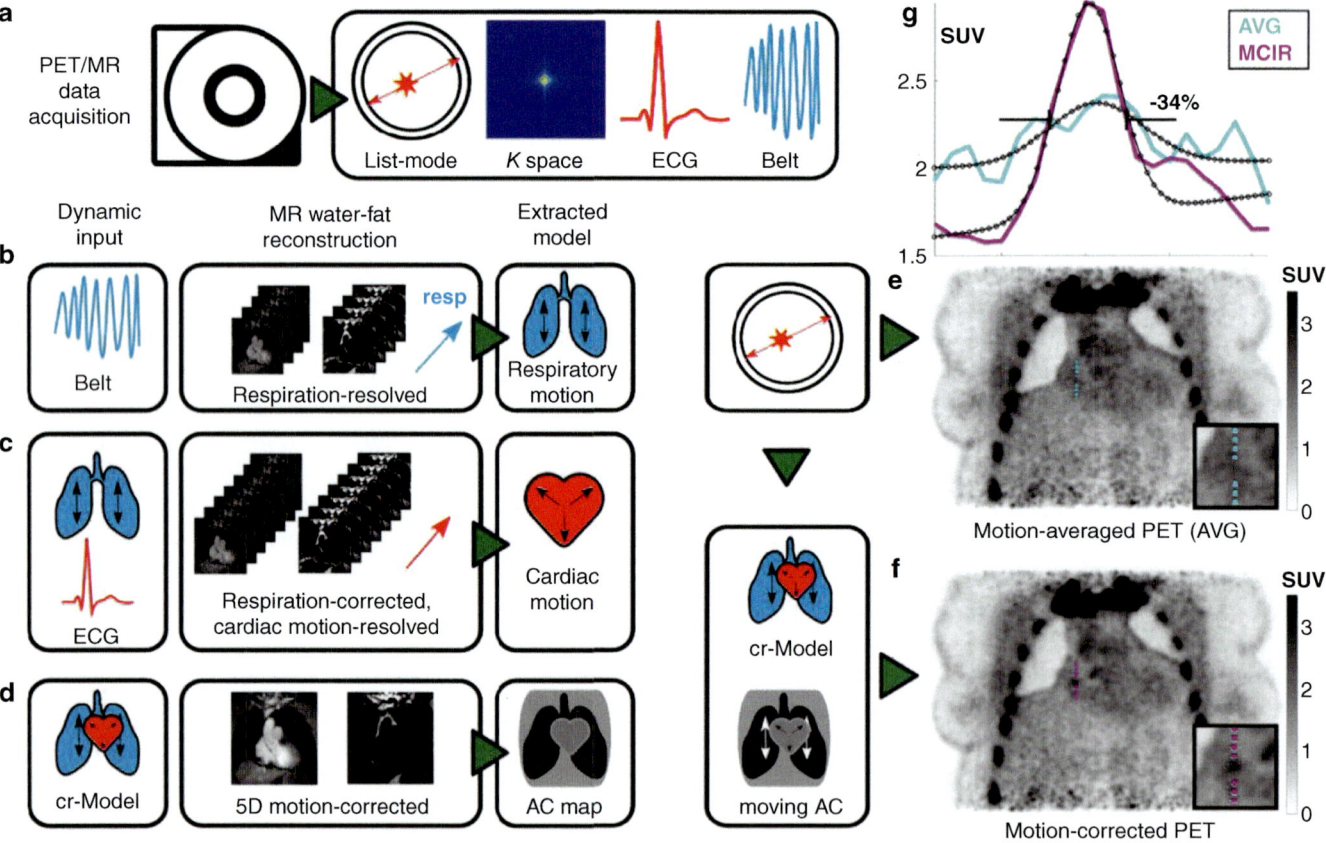

Fig. 45.7 Left: An overview of the reconstruction workflow. The acquired PET–MRI data (**a**) consist of list-mode and *k*-space data as well as the respiratory belt (**b**) and electrocardiogram (ECG) (**c**) as surrogate signals for the physiological motion model (**d**). A motion-averaged PET reconstruction shows a blurred lesion structure (**e**). Three MRI reconstructions (**b–d**) are performed from which motion information and an AC map are extracted. This information is incorporated into the PET reconstruction compensating both emission data

and attenuation map for motion, leading to cardiorespiratory(cr) motion-compensated PET images with improved sharpness of the lesion. Boxes indicate the enlarged areas of the lesion depicted in the lower right corner reconstruction with a SUV plot (**g**) showing improved contrast in motion-compensated image reconstruction (MCIR). (**f**) Motion-corrected PET (MCIR). (Adapted with permission from Mayer et al. [61])

trast-to-background ratios by 26 ± 38%, and the plaque diameter decreased by −22 ± 18%, providing sharper depiction of lesions.

Discussion

MR-based AC is an active field of research where different approaches have been proposed, and these have their advantages and disadvantages. A major aim is the discrimination of air, tissue, and cortical bone. Since the MRI signal of bone is extremely low on conventional MRI sequences, UTE-MRI-based AC methods have been proposed. Furthermore, in many applications, the separation of predominantly water-containing soft tissue and fat is necessary. Dixon-type MR sequences have been used to make use of the chemical shift between fat and water. However, the difference in the AC of bone and soft tissue is usually ignored, leading to errors. Therefore, the subsequent acquisition of Dixon and UTE sequences, or the combination of both, was proposed. Unfortunately, the acquisition times of many UTE sequences are extremely long for whole-body images. As a result, UTE-MR-based methods have mostly been applied to the head. There is a pressing need for faster acquisition strategies, such as compressed sensing and machine learning-based methods [62, 63], to accelerate the rather slow 3D radial acquisition schemes used with UTE sequences. Furthermore, appropriate calibration or measurement of k-space trajectories in UTE imaging is required for robust R_2^* maps and the related AC. Recently, the use of a simple measurement has been proposed to estimate the real readout gradient waveform and to use this knowledge in the reconstruction of high-resolution UTE images [38, 64]. Another possibility to avoid gradient imperfections is the use of ZTE imaging, which avoids the fast switching of gradients during the sampling. This technique has been used for MR-based AC in the brain [65] and pelvis [36]. For many applications in the abdomen, dynamic AC is highly important, i.e., adapting the AC map to the different motion states of the patient. Novel MRI techniques have been proposed to measure Dixon-based dynamic AC, and these have been used in several clinical applications. In principle, this can also be extended to UTE/ZTE-based techniques [66, 67], allowing reconstruction of high-resolution motion-compensated AC maps.

Conclusions

An overview of the current MR-based methods for deriving AC maps in simultaneous PET–MRI has been provided. The choice of the technique depends on the specific requirements of the application. MRI-based techniques for measuring bone with short T_2^*s are of great interest for the accurate quantification of PET tracer uptake in areas surrounded by bone. Such methods are prone to system imperfections, which need to be addressed to avoid inaccuracies in the AC. Furthermore, advanced MRI can provide AC and motion information from a single scan to address potential misalignment of AC and emission data. This information can also be used for motion-compensated reconstruction to improve PET–MR image quality and quantification, thus increasing the clinical potential of simultaneous PET–MRI.

References

1. Owens B. Scans: enhanced medical vision. Nature. 2013;502(7473):S82–3.
2. Roobottom C, Mitchell G, Morgan-Hughes G. Radiation-reduction strategies in cardiac computed tomographic angiography. Clin Radiol. 2010;65(11):859–67.
3. Shao Y, Cherry SR, Farahani K, Meadors K, Siegel S, Silverman RW, et al. Simultaneous PET and MR imaging. Phys Med Biol. 1997;42(10):1965.
4. Catana C, Wu Y, Judenhofer MS, Qi J, Pichler BJ, Cherry SR. Simultaneous acquisition of multislice PET and MR images: initial results with a MR-compatible PET scanner. J Nucl Med. 2006;47(12):1968–76.
5. Delso G, Fürst S, Jakoby B, Ladebeck R, Ganter C, Nekolla SG, et al. Performance measurements of the Siemens mMR integrated whole-body PET/MR scanner. J Nucl Med. 2011;52(12):1914–22.
6. Grant AM, Deller TW, Khalighi MM, Maramraju SH, Delso G, Levin CS. NEMA NU 2-2012 performance studies for the SiPM-based ToF-PET component of the GE SIGNA PET/MR system. Med Phys. 2016;43(5):2334–43.
7. Weissler B, Gebhardt P, Dueppenbecker PM, Wehner J, Schug D, Lerche CW, et al. A digital preclinical PET/MRI insert and initial results. IEEE Trans Med Imaging. 2015;34(11):2258–70.
8. Drzezga A, Souvatzoglou M, Eiber M, Beer AJ, Fürst S, Martinez-Möller A, et al. First clinical experience with integrated whole-body PET/MR: comparison to PET/CT in patients with oncologic diagnoses. J Nucl Med. 2012;53(6):845–55.
9. Ahn SJ, Park M-S, Kim KA, Park JY, Kim I, Kang WJ, et al. 18F-FDG PET metabolic parameters and MRI perfusion and diffusion parameters in hepatocellular carcinoma: a preliminary study. PLoS One. 2013;8(8):e71571.
10. Hectors SJ, Wagner M, Besa C, Huang W, Taouli B. Multiparametric FDG-PET/MRI of Hepatocellular Carcinoma: Initial Experience. Contrast Media Mol Imaging. 2018;2018:5638283. https://doi.org/10.1155/2018/5638283. PMID: 30402045; PMCID: PMC6192124.
11. Hirsch FW, Sattler B, Sorge I, Kurch L, Viehweger A, Ritter L, et al. PET/MR in children. Initial clinical experience in paediatric oncology using an integrated PET/MR scanner. Pediatr Radiol. 2013;43(7):860–75.
12. Munoz C, Kolbitsch C, Reader AJ, Marsden P, Schaefter T, Prieto C. MR-based cardiac and respiratory motion-compensation techniques for PET-MR imaging. PET clinics. 2016;11(2):179–91.
13. Tsoumpas C, Mackewn JE, Halsted P, King AP, Buerger C, Totman JJ, et al. Simultaneous PET–MR acquisition and MR-derived motion fields for correction of non-rigid motion in PET. Ann Nucl Med. 2010;24(10):745–50.
14. Guérin B, Cho S, Chun SY, Zhu X, Alpert NM, El Fakhri G, Reese T, Catana C. Nonrigid PET motion compensation in the lower

abdomen using simultaneous tagged-MRI and PET imaging. Med Phys. 2011;38(6):3025–38.

15. Fürst S, Grimm R, Hong I, Souvatzoglou M, Casey ME, Schwaiger M, et al. Motion correction strategies for integrated PET/MR. J Nucl Med. 2015;56(2):261–9.

16. Hutton BF, Thomas BA, Erlandsson K, Bousse A, Reilhac-Laborde A, Kazantsev D, Pedemonte S, Vunckx K, Arridge SR, Ourselin S. What approach to brain partial volume correction is best for PET/MRI? Nucl Instrum Methods Phys Res A. 2013;702:29–33.

17. Schulz V, Torres-Espallardo I, Renisch S, Hu Z, Ojha N, Börnert P, et al. Automatic, three-segment, MR-based attenuation correction for whole-body PET/MR data. Eur J Nucl Med Mol Imaging. 2011;38(1):138–52.

18. Kinahan PE, Townsend D, Beyer T, Sashin D. Attenuation correction for a combined 3D PET/CT scanner. Med Phys. 1998;25(10):2046–53.

19. Burger C, Goerres G, Schoenes S, Buck A, Lonn A, Von Schulthess G. PET attenuation coefficients from CT images: experimental evaluation of the transformation of CT into PET 511-keV attenuation coefficients. Eur J Nucl Med Mol Imaging. 2002;29(7):922–7.

20. Keereman V, Mollet P, Berker Y, Schulz V, Vandenberghe S. Challenges and current methods for attenuation correction in PET/MR. MAGMA. 2013;26(1):81–98.

21. Montandon M-L, Zaidi H. Atlas-guided non-uniform attenuation correction in cerebral 3D PET imaging. NeuroImage. 2005;25(1):278–86.

22. Malone IB, Ansorge RE, Williams GB, Nestor PJ, Carpenter TA, Fryer TD. Attenuation correction methods suitable for brain imaging with a PET/MRI scanner: a comparison of tissue atlas and template attenuation map approaches. J Nucl Med. 2011;52(7):1142–9.

23. Kops ER, Herzog H. Alternative methods for attenuation correction for PET images in MR-PET scanners. IEEE Nucl Sci Symp Conf Rec. 2007;6:4327–30.

24. Hofmann M, Steinke F, Scheel V, Charpiat G, Farquhar J, Aschoff P, et al. MRI-based attenuation correction for PET/MRI: a novel approach combining pattern recognition and atlas registration. J Nucl Med. 2008;49(11):1875–83.

25. Schleyer PJ, Schaeffter T, Marsden PK. The effect of inaccurate bone attenuation coefficient and segmentation on reconstructed PET images. Nucl Med Commun. 2010;31(8):708–16.

26. Martinez-Möller A, Souvatzoglou M, Delso G, Bundschuh RA, Chefd'hotel C, Ziegler SI, et al. Tissue classification as a potential approach for attenuation correction in whole-body PET/MRI: evaluation with PET/CT data. J Nucl Med. 2009;50(4):520–6.

27. Catana C, van der Kouwe A, Benner T, Michel CJ, Hamm M, Fenchel M, et al. Toward implementing an MRI-based PET attenuation-correction method for neurologic studies on the MR-PET brain prototype. J Nucl Med. 2010;51(9):1431–8.

28. Keereman V, Fierens Y, Broux T, De Deene Y, Lonneux M, Vandenberghe S. MRI-based attenuation correction for PET/MRI using ultrashort echo time sequences. J Nucl Med. 2010;51(5):812–8.

29. Aitken A. Advances in magnetic resonance imaging reconstruction methods incorporating prior knowledge. PhD thesis, King's College, London; 2014.

30. Berker Y, Franke J, Salomon A, Palmowski M, Donker HC, Temur Y, et al. MRI-based attenuation correction for hybrid PET/MRI systems: a 4-class tissue segmentation technique using a combined ultrashort-echo-time/Dixon MRI sequence. J Nucl Med. 2012;53(5):796–804.

31. Han PK, Horng DE, Gong K, Petibon Y, Kim K, Li Q, et al. MR-based PET attenuation correction using a combined ultrashort echo time/multi-echo dixon acquisition. Med Phys. 2020;47(7):3064–77.

32. Navalpakkam BK, Braun H, Kuwert T, Quick HH. Magnetic resonance–based attenuation correction for PET/MR hybrid imaging using continuous valued attenuation maps. Investig Radiol. 2013;48(5):323–32.

33. Qian Y, Boada FE. Acquisition-weighted stack of spirals for fast high-resolution three-dimensional ultra-short echo time MR imaging. Magn Reson Med. 2008;60(1):135–45.

34. Wiesinger F, Sacolick LI, Menini A, Kaushik SS, Ahn S, Veit-Haibach P, et al. Zero TE MR bone imaging in the head. Magn Reson Med. 2016;75(1):107–14.

35. Leynes AP, Yang J, Shanbhag DD, Kaushik SS, Seo Y, Hope TA, et al. Hybrid ZTE/Dixon MR-based attenuation correction for quantitative uptake estimation of pelvic lesions in PET/MRI. Med Phys. 2017;44(3):902–13.

36. Huang C, Ouyang J, Reese T, Wu Y, El Fakhri G, Ackerman J. Continuous MR bone density measurement using water-and fat-suppressed projection imaging (WASPI) for PET attenuation correction in PET-MR. Phys Med Biol. 2015;60(20):N369–81.

37. Aitken A, Giese D, Tsoumpas C, Schleyer P, Kozerke S, Prieto C, et al. Improved UTE-based attenuation correction for cranial PET-MR using dynamic magnetic field monitoring. Med Phys. 2014;41(1):012302.

38. Gross-Weege N, Nolte T, Schulz V. MR image corrections for PET-induced gradient distortions. Phys Med Biol. 2019;64(2):02NT03.

39. Rischpler C, Nekolla SG, Dregely I, Schwaiger M. Hybrid PET/MR imaging of the heart: potential, initial experiences, and future prospects. J Nucl Med. 2013;54(3):402–15.

40. Lau JM, Laforest R, Nensa F, Zheng J, Gropler RJ, Woodard PK. Cardiac applications of PET/MR imaging. Magn Reson Imaging Clin N Am. 2017;25(2):325–33.

41. Seifert R, Kersting D, Rischpler C, Opitz M, Kirchner J, Pabst KM, et al. Clinical use of PET/MR in oncology: an update. Semin Nucl Med. 2022;52(3):356–64.

42. Schlemmer H-PW, Pichler BJ, Schmand M, Burbar Z, Michel C, Ladebeck R, et al. Simultaneous MR/PET imaging of the human brain: feasibility study. Radiology. 2008;248(3):1028:1028.

43. Dimentias platform UK. https://www.dementiasplatform.uk.

44. Lorking N, Murray AD, O'Brien J. The use of PET/MRI in dementia: a literatur review. Int J Geriatr Psychiatry. 2021;36(10):1501–13.

45. Panda A, Goenka AH, Hope TA, Veit-Haibach P. PET/magnetic resonance imaging applications in abdomen and pelvis. Magn Reson Imaging Clin N Am. 2020;28(3):369–80.

46. Evangelista L, Zattoni F, Cassarino G, Artioli P, Cecchin D, Dal Moro F, et al. PET/MRI in prostate cancer: a systematic review and meta-analysis. Eur J Nucl Med Mol Imaging. 2021;48(3):859–73.

47. Fowler AM, Strigel RM. Clinical advances in PET–MRI for breast cancer. Lancet Oncol. 2022;23(1):e32–43.

48. Antoch G, Bockisch A. Combined PET/MRI: a new dimension in whole-body oncology imaging? Eur J Nucl Med Mol Imaging. 2009;36(1):S113–20.

49. Choyke PL, Dwyer AJ, Knopp MV. Functional tumor imaging with dynamic contrast-enhanced magnetic resonance imaging. J Magn Reson Imaging. 2003;17(5):509–20.

50. Beiderwellen K, Geraldo L, Ruhlmann V, Heusch P, Gomez B, Nensa F, et al. Accuracy of [18F] FDG PET/MRI for the detection of liver metastases. PLoS One. 2015;10(9):e0137285.

51. Grafe H, Lindemann ME, Ruhlmann V, Oehmigen M, Hirmas N, Umutlu L, et al. Evaluation of improved attenuation correction in whole-body PET/MR on patients with bone metastasis using various radiotracers. Eur J Nucl Med Mol Imaging. 2020;47(10):2269–79.

52. Paulus DH, Quick HH, Geppert C, Fenchel M, Zhan Y, Hermosillo G, et al. Whole-body PET/MR imaging: quantitative evaluation of a novel model-based MR attenuation correction method including bone. J Nucl Med. 2015;56(7):1061–6.

53. Aizaz M, Moonen RP, van der Pol JA, Prieto C, Botnar RM, Kooi ME. PET/MRI of atherosclerosis. Cardiovasc Diagn Ther. 2020;10(4):1120–39.

54. Buerger C, Tsoumpas C, Aitken A, King AP, Schleyer P, Schulz V, et al. Investigation of MR-based attenuation correction and motion compensation for hybrid PET/MR. IEEE Trans Nucl Sci. 2012;59(5):1967–76.

55. Polycarpou I, Tsoumpas C, Marsden PK. Analysis and comparison of two methods for motion correction in PET imaging. Med Phys. 2012;39(10):6474–83.

56. Brown R, Kolbitsch C, Delplancke C, Papoutsellis E, Mayer J, Ovtchinnikov E, et al. Motion estimation and correction for simultaneous PET/MR using SIRF and CIL. Philos Trans A Math Phys Eng Sci. 2021;379(2204):20200208.

57. Kolbitsch C, Neji R, Fenchel M, Mallia A, Marsden P, Schaeffter T. Respiratory-resolved MR-based attenuation correction for motion-compensated cardiac PET-MR. Phys Med Biol. 2018;63(13):135008.

58. Mayer J, Brown R, Thielemans K, Ovtchinnikov E, Pasca E, Atkinson D, et al. Flexible numerical simulation framework for dynamic PET-MR data. Phys Med Biol. 2020;65(14):145003.

59. Ippoliti M, Lukas M, Brenner W, Schatka I, Furth C, Schaeffter T, et al. Respiratory motion correction for enhanced quantification of hepatic lesions in simultaneous PET and DCE-MR imaging. Phys Med Biol. 2021;66(9):095012.

60. Kolbitsch C, Ahlman MA, Davies-Venn C, Evers R, Hansen M, Peressutti D, et al. Cardiac and respiratory motion correction for simultaneous cardiac PET/MR. J Nucl Med. 2017;58(5):846–52.

61. Mayer J, Wurster T-H, Schaeffter T, Landmesser U, Morguet A, Bigalke B, et al. Imaging coronary plaques using 3D motion-compensated [18F] NaF PET/MR. Eur J Nucl Med Mol Imaging. 2021;48(8):2455–65.

62. Chen Y, Ying C, Binkley MM, Juttukonda MR, Flores S, Laforest R, et al. Deep learning-based T_1-enhanced selection of linear attenuation coefficients (DL-TESLA) for PET/MR attenuation correction in dementia neuroimaging. Magn Reson Med. 2021;86(1):499–513.

63. Gong K, Han PK, Johnson KA, El Fakhri G, Ma C, Li Q. Attenuation correction using deep learning and integrated UTE/multi-echo Dixon sequence: evaluation in amyloid and tau PET imaging. Eur J Nucl Med Mol Imaging. 2021;48(5):1351–61.

64. Kronthaler S, Rahmer J, Börnert P, Makowski MR, Schwaiger BJ, Gersing AS, et al. Trajectory correction based on the gradient impulse response function improves high-resolution UTE imaging of the musculoskeletal system. Magn Reson Med. 2021;85(4):2001–15.

65. Sgard B, Khalifé M, Bouchut A, Fernandez B, Soret M, Giron A, et al. ZTE MR-based attenuation correction in brain FDG-PET/MR: performance in patients with cognitive impairment. Eur Radiol. 2020;30(3):1770–9.

66. Zhu X, Chan M, Lustig M, Johnson KM, Larson PE. Iterative motion-compensation reconstruction ultra-short TE (iMoCo UTE) for high-resolution free-breathing pulmonary MRI. Magn Reson Med. 2020;83(4):1208–21.

67. Ljungberg E, Wood TC, Solana AB, Williams SC, Barker GJ, Wiesinger F. Motion corrected silent ZTE neuroimaging. Magn Reson Med. 2022;88(1):195–210.

Zero Acoustic Noise with Zero TE MRI

David Grodzki and Florian Wiesinger

Introduction

Magnetic resonance imaging (MRI) is known to be notoriously noisy. It easily reaches acoustic noise levels of 95–110 dB(A) and more—corresponding to an airplane starting or a rock concert. High acoustic noise is one of the main reasons for patient discomfort and anxiety during an magnetic resonance (MR) examination, leading to increased motion and, occasionally, scan abortion [1–8].

Gradient activity is the major source of acoustic noise. During an MRI examination, gradient amplitudes are switched at a kilohertz frequency. The electrical currents required to generate the gradient fields apply strong Lorentz forces to the gradient coil, leading to vibrations and deformations of the coil. These mechanical forces coupled with the MRI system and the gradient coils effectively act as electromagnetic loudspeakers.

Since the invention of MRI, several approaches have been developed to reduce acoustic noise during MRI scans [9–16]. Initially, these techniques were hardware-based. The aim was to prevent and minimize the vibrations of the gradient coil and their transmission to the scanner. This included mechanical dampening and optimization of the system housing. In much more complex approaches, the gradient coil was placed in a vacuum chamber. Active noise cancellation methods have also been applied. All these approaches can decrease the overall acoustic noise generation of the MRI scanner, but they also increase system complexity and costs, making many of the approaches unattractive from a commercial point of view.

In 1995, Madio and Lowe, presented the ingenious rotating ultrafast imaging sequence (RUFIS), which reduces gradient switching to an absolute minimum (i.e., directional gradient updates using three-dimensional (3D) radial center-out imaging) [17–19], thereby opening the door to silent MR imaging. Following the invention of RUFIS, researchers were mainly interested in its other main characteristic, that of zero echo time (i.e., TE = 0) for imaging of short-lived signal structures ($T_2^* < 1$ ms), and, as a result, RUFIS became known as zero TE or ZTE. Nowadays, available ZTE implementations (i.e., water- and fat-suppressed proton projection MRI (WASPI) [20], pointwise encoding time reduction with radial acquisition (PETRA) [21], and hybrid filing (HYFI) [22]) are still largely based on the original RUFIS sequence with differences primarily related to the so-called "dead-time gap" filling. Due to its minimal gradient switching, ZTE implementations allow silent MR imaging with acoustic noise levels less than 5 dB(A) above ambient.

In order to be applicable in routine clinical imaging and to be accepted by radiologists, contrasts generated by ZTE need to match those used in conventional clinical MR imaging. In its native form, without any preparation pulses, ZTE produces spoiled gradient recalled echo (SPGR)-type contrast with proton density (PD) and T_1 weighting, dependent on the repetition time and flip angle settings. As described in the following sections, magnetization-prepared segmented ZTE can be used to generate routine clinical contrasts silently. To further expand the clinical coverage to include more comprehensive protocols, acoustic noise reduction (ANR) based on gradient attenuation and/or waveform smoothing have been implemented to provide quiet scanning with acoustic noise levels less than 25 dB(A) above ambient.

D. Grodzki (✉)
Siemens Healthineers, Erlangen, Germany

Department of Neuroradiology, Friedrich-Alexander-Universität Erlangen-Nuremberg, Erlangen, Germany
e-mail: David.Grodzki@siemens-healthineers.com

F. Wiesinger
GE Healthcare, Munich, Germany

Center for Neuroimaging, Institute of Psychiatry, Psychology & Neuroscience (IoPPN), King's College London, London, UK

© The Author(s), under exclusive license to Springer Nature Switzerland AG 2023
J. Du, G. M. Bydder (eds.), *MRI of Short- and Ultrashort-T₂ Tissues*, https://doi.org/10.1007/978-3-031-35197-6_46

Recap of ZTE: Quick and Quiet MRI with TE = 0

Within the large zoo of existing MR pulse sequences, RUFIS-type ZTE [17] can be considered the simplest, at least in terms of radiofrequency (RF) and gradient waveform complexity. As illustrated in the ZTE section of Fig. 46.1 (upper row), it consists of (1) extremely short, block-shaped RF hard pulses for signal excitation and constant amplitude readout gradients for image encoding. This leads to three-dimensional (3D), nonselective RF excitation followed by 3D center-out radial image encoding with a nominal echo time of TE = 0 (i.e., image encoding starting at the time of RF excitation). While the amplitude of the readout gradient remains constant (i.e., $|G_{read}| = (G_x^2 + G_y^2 + G_z^2)^{1/2}$), its direction changes between repetitions so that the endpoints of the 3D center-out radial spokes follow a smooth spiral trajectory along the surface of the spherical 3D-encoded k-space (with uniform angular sampling density). Accordingly, gradient switching is reduced to a minimum (because of the small directional gradient updates), hence enabling virtually silent MRI. Besides its main characteristics of TE = 0 and silent imaging, ZTE also offers highly efficient sampling (~95% of scan time is used for acquiring data) with exceptionally short repetition times (T_R) and robustness against eddy currents and patient motion.

Even though ZTE image encoding starts at the time of RF excitation, the MR system can only start sampling the free induction decay (FID) signal after the RF hardware changes from the transmit to the receive state. The finite time required for this transmit-receive switching results in a central, spherical k-space gap (often referred to as the dead-time gap). Nowadays, ZTE sequences are primarily distinguished by the way they (re-)acquire the center k-space gap, including WASPI [20] (which reacquires a limited number of spokes at a reduced gradient strength that fill in the missing gap), PETRA [21] (which samples the missing k-space using a Cartesian single-point scanning mode), and HYFI [22] (a combination of PETRA and WASPI). If the k-space gap is small, then parallel imaging can also be used to fill the missing k-space samples [23, 24].

Native ZTE: Illuminating the MR Invisible

The steady-state longitudinal magnetization ($M_{z,SPGR}$) of native ZTE is of the spoiled gradient recalled echo (SPGR) nature [6]:

$$M_{z,SPGR} = \frac{M_0 E_2^* (1 - E_1)}{1 - E_1 \cos(\alpha)} \cong \frac{M_0}{1 + \frac{T_1}{T_R}\frac{\alpha^2}{2}}, E_1 = e^{-\frac{T_R}{T_1}}, E_2^* = e^{-\frac{T_E}{T_2^*}} \cong 1 \tag{46.1}$$

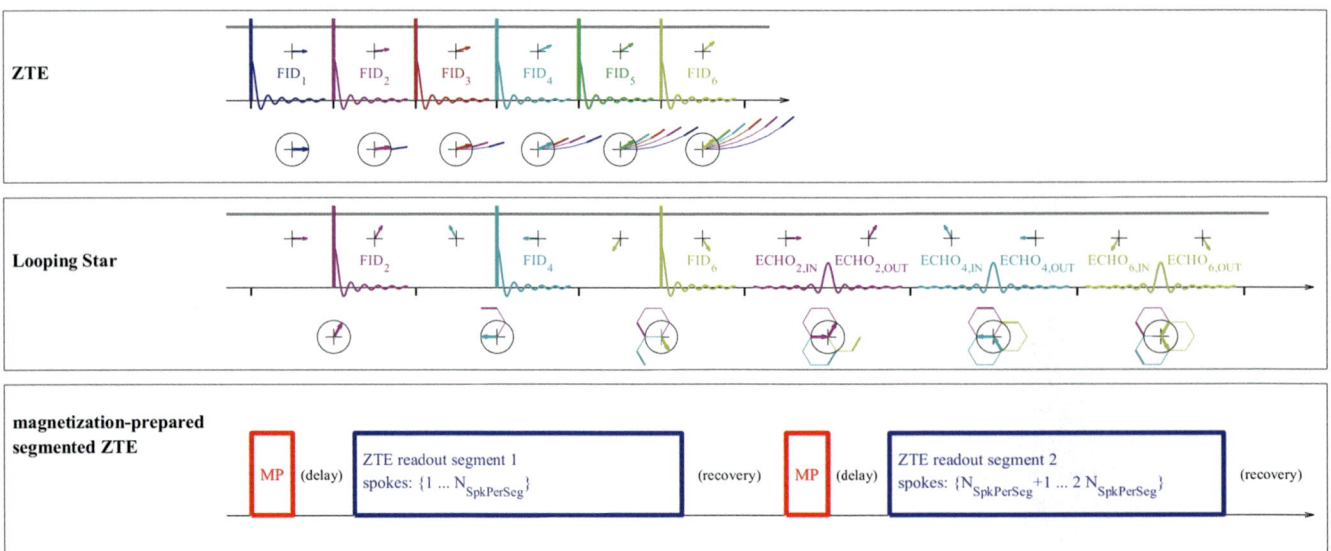

Fig. 46.1 A schematic illustration of native ZTE (top row), Looping Star (middle row), and magnetization-prepared segmented ZTE (bottom row)

with a signal-to-noise ratio (SNR)-optimal Ernst angle of $\alpha_{Ernst} = acos(E_1) \cong \sqrt{\dfrac{2T_R}{T_1}}$. The indicated approximation (i.e., $\alpha \ll 1$ rad and $T_R \ll T_1$) is appropriate for ZTE. For small flip angles (i.e., $\alpha^2 \ll \dfrac{2T_R}{T_1}$), T_1 saturation effects are negligible and ZTE permits direct measurement of the proton density (modulated by B_1 transmit-and-receive sensitivity profiles). The SPGR signal response can also be tuned for T_1 contrast and even quantitative T_1 parameter mapping using variable flip angle imaging [25]. While its short repetition times lead to comparatively low Ernst angles (e.g., $\alpha_{Ernst} = 2.5°$ for $T_R = 1$ ms and $T_1 = 1$ s), the maximum flip angle is constrained to only a few degrees because of its bandwidth (BW) dependence (i.e., $\alpha_{max} = \gamma B_{1,max}/BW$). This limitation can be stretched somewhat by correcting for slab-selective effects [26], using shaped (instead of hard) RF pulses [27, 28], and employing RF pulse encoding [29].

Because of its TE = 0 image encoding, ZTE allows depiction of short-lived structures (i.e., $T_2^* < 1$ ms) such as bone and lungs, which are otherwise difficult to depict using standard MR pulse sequences with TE ≥ 1 ms. As a result, native ZTE constitutes a radiation-free alternative for bone [30–38] and lung [39–44] imaging and provides valuable extra information in musculoskeletal and chest MR examinations.

ZTE Bone Imaging

The native ZTE section of Fig. 46.2 illustrates ZTE bone imaging of the head with cortical bone depicted in a similar way to computed tomography (CT) [30–38]. It is based on (1) minimal soft tissue contrast using proton density (PD)-weighted parameter settings (i.e., $\alpha = 1°$, bandwidth (BW) = ±100 kHz) and (2) contrast inversion (i.e., an inverse-linear or an inverse-logarithmic scale) [30, 32, 33, 37]. The latter provides CT-like contrast appearance with cortical bone appearing bright relative to the uniform low-signal, soft tissue background. Unlike CT, the air background appears bright as well. In order to minimize fat–water chemical shift artifacts associated with 3D radial image encoding (i.e., destructive signal interference at fat–water tissue interfaces), it is important to use a high imaging BW so that the readout duration is short relative to the fat–water out-phase TE (e.g., $TE_{OutPhase} = 1.15$ ms at 3 T) [37]. ZTE bone imaging has been demonstrated in musculoskeletal bone imaging applications [30–38] and for positron emission tomography (PET)/MR attenuation correction in PET/MR and MR-only radiation therapy planning [31, 33, 45–48]. The same imaging principles (i.e., PD-weighted, high-BW ZTE imaging) are also applicable to the depiction of vascular calcifications [49]. However, whether ZTE can provide calcification scoring similar to CT still remains to be seen.

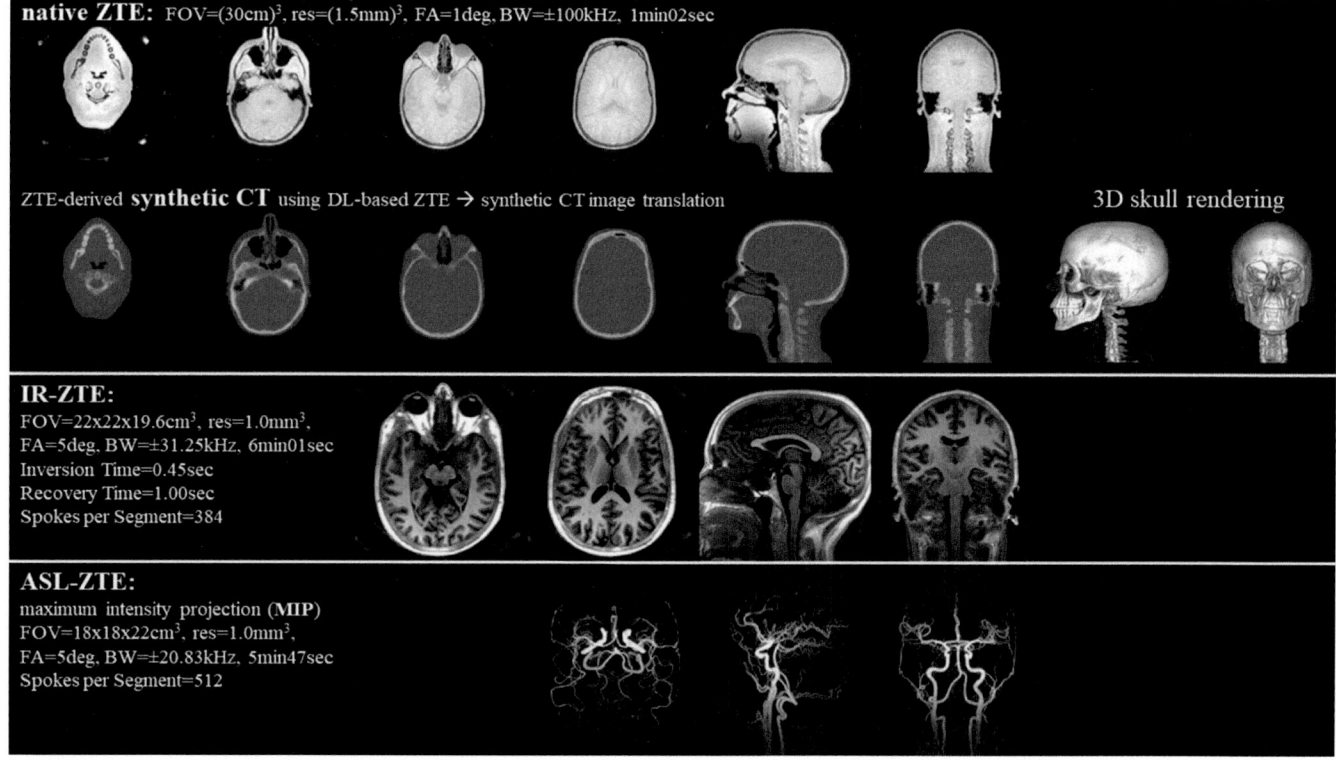

native ZTE: FOV=(30cm)^3, res=(1.5mm)^3, FA=1deg, BW=±100kHz, 1min02sec

ZTE-derived **synthetic CT** using DL-based ZTE → synthetic CT image translation   3D skull rendering

IR-ZTE:
FOV=22x22x19.6cm^3, res=1.0mm^3,
FA=5deg, BW=±31.25kHz, 6min01sec
Inversion Time=0.45sec
Recovery Time=1.00sec
Spokes per Segment=384

ASL-ZTE:
maximum intensity projection (**MIP**)
FOV=18x18x22cm^3, res=1.0mm^3,
FA=5deg, BW=±20.83kHz, 5min47sec
Spokes per Segment=512

Fig. 46.2 An illustration of native ZTE (top row), corresponding synthetic CT (second row), IR-prepared segmented ZTE (third row), and arterial spin labeling (ASL)-prepared segmented ZTE using maximum intensity projection (MIP, bottom row)

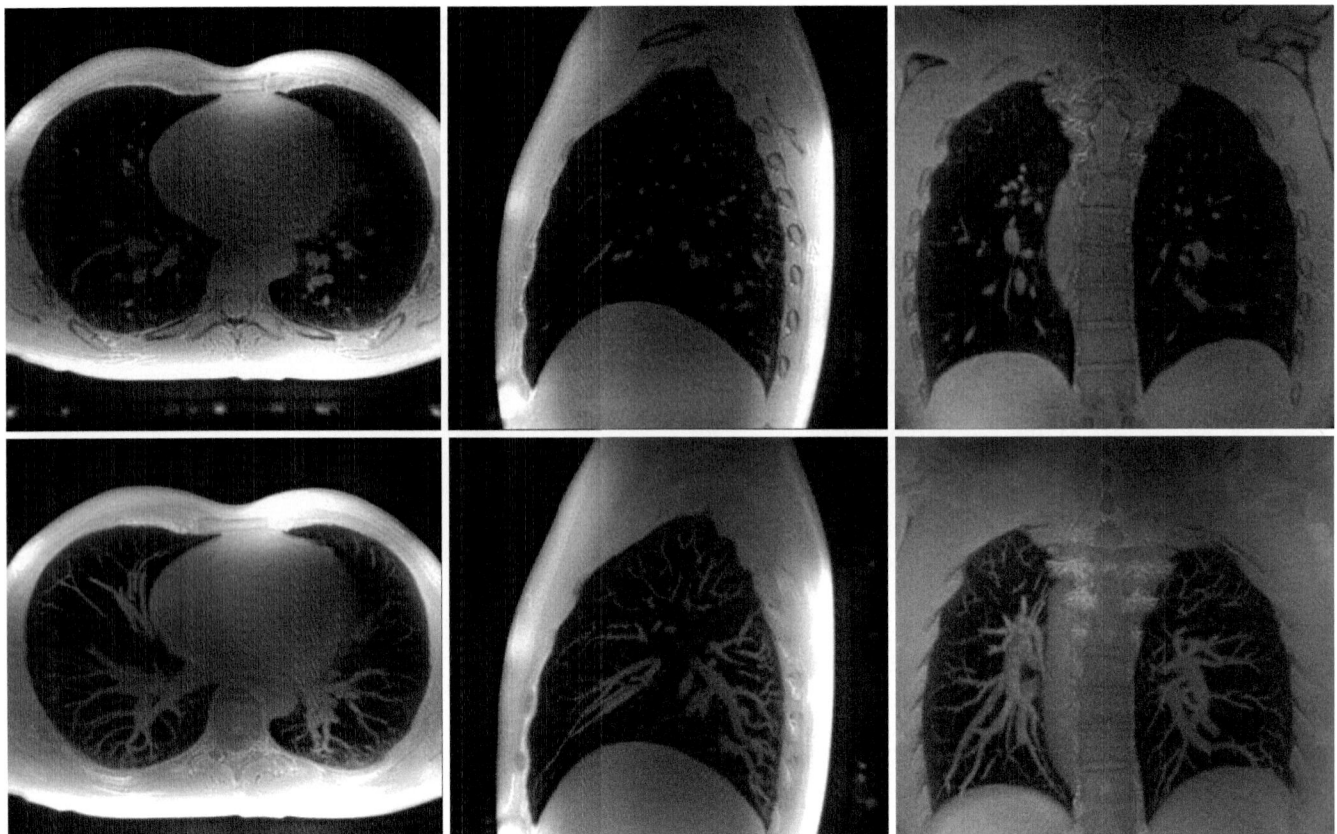

Fig. 46.3 Respiratory-triggered, submillimeter 3D ZTE lung imaging (i.e., resolution = (0.875 mm)^3, α = 1.2°, BW = ±62.5 kHz, 409,600 spokes, duration 8 min 53 s). The MIP (with 18-mm slab thickness) in the second row shows rich vascular information. (Reproduced with permission from Gibiino et al. [39])

ZTE Lung Imaging

Figure 46.3 illustrates respiratory-triggered, high-resolution, structural ZTE imaging of the lungs (i.e., with α = 1.2°, BW = ±62.5 kHz, and 409,600 spokes) [39]. The maximum intensity projection (MIP, bottom row) shows the rich vascular information contained in these images. The TE = 0 and 3D center-out radial sampling provide a robust imaging mechanism for depicting the heterogeneous anatomy of the lung (i.e., microscopic B_0 gradients at air–tissue interfaces leading to short-T_2^* signal lifetimes) and its periodic respiratory motion. Use of phyllotactic 3D spoke ordering [50, 51] (or other pseudo-randomized spoke orderings) allows continuous free-breathing acquisition with retrospective (self-) gating and/or respiratory motion correction. ZTE lung imaging has been demonstrated in numerous chest imaging studies, including depiction of small lung lesions in oncological imaging [40–43, 52].

Magnetization-Prepared ZTE: Beyond SPGR Contrast

Although interesting for certain applications, native ZTE alone is insufficient for MR radiological examinations, which require soft tissue contrast beyond that provided by SPGR T_1-weighting. An effective and flexible way of extending the contrast range and thereby the clinical applicability of silent ZTE imaging is to combine it with a magnetization preparation [53] similar to MP-RAGE (magnetization-prepared rapid gradient echo) [54]. As can be seen from the magnetization-prepared segmented ZTE section of Fig. 46.1 (bottom row), it consists of: (1) magnetization preparation (e.g., inversion recovery, arterial spin labeling (ASL), magnetization transfer (MT), T_2 preparation, diffusion preparation, fat saturation, etc.), which imprints the desired contrast weighting on the longitudinal magnetization; (2) an optional delay time; (3) segmented

ZTE imaging encoding (with each segment containing $N_{\mathrm{SpkPerSeg}}$ spokes), and (4) an optional T_1 recovery time. In order to maintain the overall silent imaging performance, all gradient aspects of the magnetization preparation module (and/or the surrounding spoiler gradients) must be silent as well. This can be achieved by limiting the gradient slew rate and/or gradient waveform smoothing (i.e., avoiding loud high-frequency gradient changes). It is important to note that because of its fast (i.e., $T_R \sim 1{-}2$ ms), efficient (i.e., sampling efficiency $\sim 95\%$), and silent performance, ZTE is ideally suited for magnetization-prepared 3D MRI.

The transient evolution of the longitudinal magnetization ($M_{z,n}$) during a ZTE readout segment follows a simple mathematical expression [6, 25]:

$$M_{z,n} = M_{z,\mathrm{PREP}} \left(E_1 \cos\alpha \right)^{n-1} + M_{z,\mathrm{SPGR}} \left[1 - \left(E_1 \cos\alpha \right)^{n-1} \right]$$

(46.2)

with $M_{z,\mathrm{PREP}}$ being the longitudinal magnetization just before the ZTE readout. Similarly, the average longitudinal magnetization ($<M_z>$, averaged over a segment containing $N = N_{\mathrm{SpkPerSeg}}$ spokes) equates to a weighted sum of $M_{z,\mathrm{PREP}}$ and $M_{z,\mathrm{SPGR}}$ according to

$$\langle M_z \rangle = \frac{\sum_{n=1}^{N} M_{z,n}}{N} = M_{z,\mathrm{PREP}} f + M_{z,\mathrm{SPGR}} \left(1 - f \right), \text{ with } f = \frac{1}{N} \frac{1 - \left(E_1 \cos\alpha \right)^N}{1 - E_1 \cos\alpha}$$

(46.3)

Inversion Recovery (IR)-Prepared ZTE

The IR-ZTE section of Fig. 46.2 (third row) illustrates silent 3D inversion recovery (IR)-prepared segmented ZTE imaging with image quality (i.e., contrast, resolution) and scan efficiency (i.e., SNR and scan time) similar to standard (i.e., loud) 3D MP-RAGE. Notably, the enhanced signal response from bone somewhat changes the image appearance between the brain and skin region, which can impact brain segmentation developed/trained for conventional 3D MP-RAGE. Similarly, T_1-prepared ZTE also captures short-lived myelin signals, which are invisible on standard MP-RAGE images with longer TEs [55]. To the best of our knowledge, there is no comprehensive study analyzing sequence parameters (inversion time, readout length, flip angles, delay times) for optimal contrast performance for silent T_1-prepared ZTE neuroimaging. Recently, Ljungberg et al. [51] have demonstrated self-navigated motion correction for IR-prepared ZTE using phyllotactic spoke ordering [50], thereby providing a comprehensive solution for two long standing problems of high-resolution T_1-weighted clinical neuroimaging (i.e., loud acoustic noise and patient motion). In recent years, silent T_1-prepared ZTE has been demonstrated in numerous studies mainly involving neuroimaging [56–58] but also including other body regions [59]. It is now commercially available on certain MR scanners.

Arterial Spin Labeling (ASL)-Prepared ZTE

The ASL-ZTE section of Fig. 46.2 (fourth row) illustrates silent MR angiography (MRA) using maximum intensity projection (MIP). Silent MRA is based on arterial spin labeling (ASL) magnetization preparation followed by a segmented ZTE readout. The TE = 0 characteristic provides accurate depiction of the vasculature and is robust against turbulent flow and stenosis. The latter is a unique advantage in favor of ZTE-MRA in addition to its intrinsic silent imaging. The advantage of TE = 0 for flow measurement was noted early on by Madio and Lowe [17, 18] and has been demonstrated more recently in numerous studies [60–67].

Other Preparations: T_2, Diffusion, Magnetization Transfer (MT), and Fat Saturation

Besides IR and ASL, other magnetization preparations have been explored to extend the contrast capabilities of silent ZTE imaging. These include T_2 [68], diffusion [69], and magnetization transfer (MT) preparations [70].

T_2 magnetization preparation consists of an RF pulse train, including (1) a tip-down pulse (i.e., exciting the magnetization), (2) one or more refocusing pulses (i.e., exposing the magnetization to T_2 relaxation), and (3) a tip-up pulse (i.e., turning the magnetization back into the longitudinal axis where its magnetization is stored for the segmented ZTE readout) [71]. For improved robustness to B_0 and B_1 inhomogeneity, adiabatic RF pulses are used for the refocusing and/or tip-up and tip-down pulses [72, 73].

T_2 preparation can be extended to diffusion preparation by adding diffusion gradients around the refocusing pules [74, 75]. To minimize acoustic noise, sinusoidal gradients are used during the diffusion preparation [69]. The diffusion preparation is known to be sensitive to motion and eddy currents, which are typically addressed via phase cycling, leading to an increase in scan time [75]. Compared to echo planar imaging (EPI) methods, diffusion-prepared ZTE provides undistorted and quiet 3D diffusion-weighted imaging.

MT (i.e., contrast dependent on interactions between bulk water protons and macromolecular protons) is typically encoded via magnetization preparation in the form of one (or multiple) off-resonant RF pulses [76, 77]. MT-prepared ZTE was first demonstrated by Holmes et al. [78] and extended to inhomogeneous MT (ihMT) by Wood et al. [70].

For musculoskeletal and body ZTE imaging, fat (or water) saturation provides another important magnetization preparation and additionally eliminates fat–water chemical shift artifacts, which are often problematic in 3D non-Cartesian images [37].

Quantitative Parameter Mapping

Magnetization-prepared ZTE can also be adapted for quantitative parameter mapping. For example, modified Look–Locker IR (MOLLI)-type [79, 80], silent ZTE-based T_1 mapping can be implemented using an IR preparation, followed by multiple ZTE readout segments (each segment containing $N_{\mathrm{SpkPerSeg}}$ spokes per segment). Quantitative PD and T_1 parameter maps can then be obtained by comparing the measured transient signals to the analytical IR-prepared SPGR signal equation (Eq. 46.3) using, e.g., least squares fitting or dictionary matching. For combined PD, T_1, and T_2 mapping (similar to magnetic resonance fingerprinting [81]), additional T_2 preparation can be incorporated in analogy to the so-called quantification using an interleaved Look–Locker acquisition sequence (QALAS) method [82, 83].

Figure 46.4 illustrates 3D silent quantitative PD, T_1, and T_2 parameter mapping in the brain [83]. Here, a transient T_1 and T_2 signal evolution is generated and encoded using (1) T_2 preparation followed by (2) a first ZTE segment, (3) IR preparation, and (4–6) three more ZTE segments. The PD map (including B_1 transmit and receive effects) can optionally be measured upfront using a separate low flip angle steady-state ZTE acquisition (i.e., $M_{z,SS} \cong M_0$ for $\alpha^2 \ll \dfrac{2 T_R}{T_1}$, cf. Eq. 46.1), which simplifies the problem to two-parameter (T_1 and T_2) least squares fitting. Additionally, the PD map can be used for ZTE bone imaging and/or as input for synthetic CT conversion.

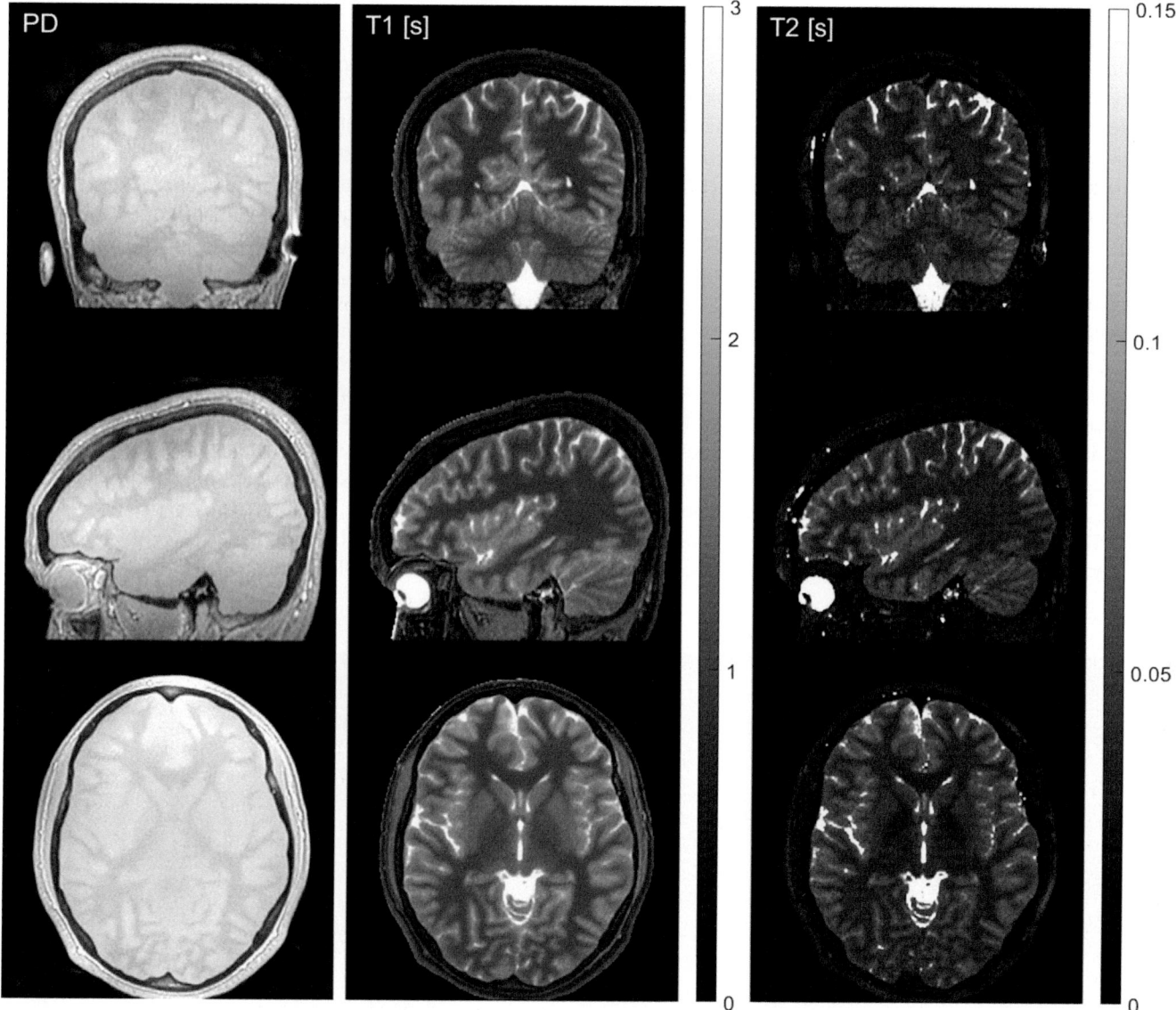

Fig. 46.4 3D silent parameter mapping (FOV = 192 × 192 × 160 mm³, res = (1.0 mm)³, BW = ±31.25 kHz, scan time = 8 min 44 s) showing PD (left column, including B_1 transmit and receiver effects), quantitative T_1 (middle column), and quantitative T_2 (right column)

Looping Star: Silent, Time-Multiplexed, Gradient Echo ZTE

Conventional multi-gradient-echo sequences for T_2^* and/or susceptibility-weighted imaging (SWI) and Dixon-type fat–water separation [84] rely on intensive gradient switching and are among the loudest and most unpleasant MR scans from a patient's perspective. Here, Looping Star [85, 86] offers a quiet, and hence much more pleasant, alternative.

Looping Star is best understood by considering gradient echo ZTE, where refocusing of a single FID signal is achieved using a sequence of self-refocusing spokes (e.g., six spokes following a hexagonal k-space trajectory) as illus-

trated in the Looping Star section of Fig. 46.1 (middle row). It is important to note that the original center-out FID signal is refocused into a full-diameter in-echo-out gradient echo. Looping Star can then be regarded as time-multiplexed, gradient-refocused ZTE, in which multiple MR signal coherences are excited (one after the other during the excitation phase) and refocused (one after the other during the refocusing phase). To avoid overlap of subsequent gradient echoes during the refocusing phase, only every other spoke is excited during the initial excitation phase. While the FID spokes are of center-out (i.e., half spoke) nature, the gradient echo spokes are full-diameter in-echo-out acquisitions. Like native ZTE, Looping Star is a highly efficient sequence with most of the sequence time spent encoding and acquiring FID and gradient echo data. Looping Star has been used for high spatial resolution structural imaging (T_2^* and SWI) and high spatiotemporal resolution functional blood oxygenation level-dependent (BOLD) functional MRI (fMRI) [85, 87, 88]. For a more detailed description of Looping Star, readers are referred to Chap. 10 (Looping Star: Time-Multiplexed, Gradient Echo, Zero TE MR Imaging).

Acoustic Noise Reduction via Gradient Attenuation

Native ZTE, magnetization-prepared ZTE, and Looping Star provide an arsenal of silent imaging methods with image quality and scan time comparable to conventional/loud sequences. These include high-resolution structural imaging (i.e., PD, T_1, T_2^*, SWI), functional BOLD fMRI, and quantitative (PD, T_1, T_2, T_2^*, QSM, apparent diffusion coefficient (ADC)) parameter mapping. In contrast, T_2-weighted imag-

ing and diffusion remain challenging because SPGR-type ZTE (even with magnetization preparation) cannot compete with fast/turbo spin echo (FSE/TSE) imaging. In order to "silence" these clinically important sequences and incorporate them into a comprehensive quiet neuroimaging exam, ANR based on gradient attenuation [89] and/or acoustic gradient waveform optimization [90, 91] can be used. Figures 46.5 and 46.6 show examples of quiet T_2-weighted FSE/TSE, diffusion-weighted, and susceptibility-weighted brain scans.

While the ZTE-based sequences (including Looping Star) are intrinsically silent with acoustic noise levels of less than 5 dB(A) above ambient noise, ANR is used to quietly scan clinical FSE/TSE and EPI sequences. Their acoustic noise can be reduced by 10–20 dB(A) or more. Together, ZTE and ANR enable comprehensive quiet neuroimaging examinations comprising all standard anatomical contrasts, quantitative parameter mapping, and functional BOLD fMRI [92]. Scan time and image quality (and thereby overall acceptance) can be improved using DL-based image reconstruction [93].

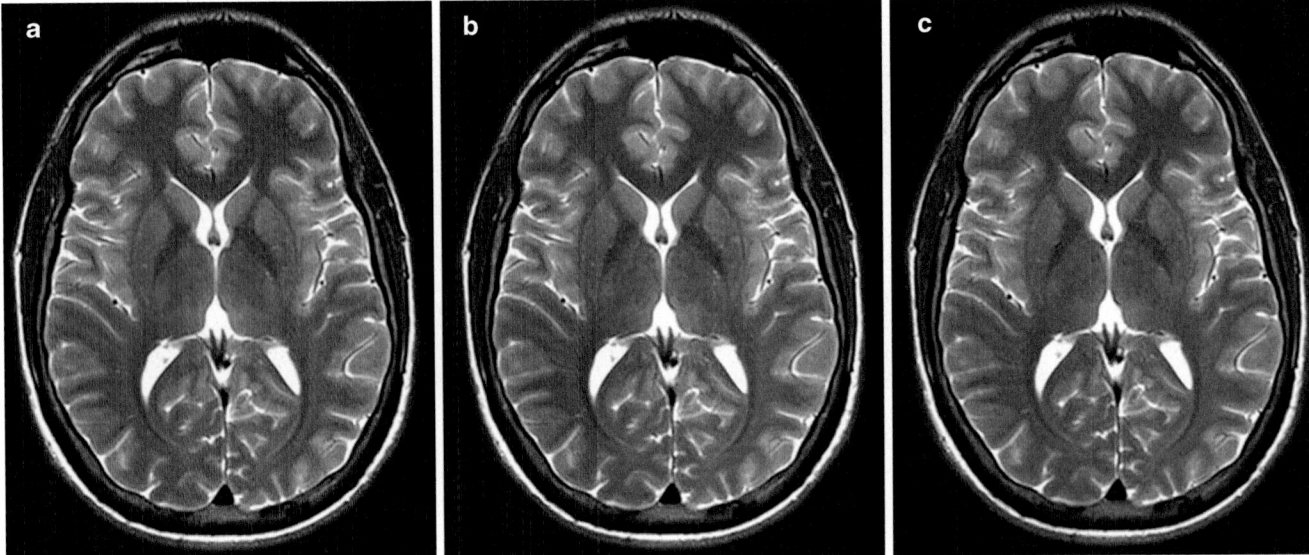

Fig. 46.5 An example 2D FSE/TSE protocol using the method described in Heismann et al. [90]. (**a**) Routine clinical implementation measured with an acoustic noise level of 88.8 dB(A), (**b**) the same pro-tocol using the described ANR at 82.5 dB(A), and (**c**) the same protocol with slightly increased readout BW (<10%) at a noise level of 74.4 dB(A). (Reproduced with permission from Heismann et al. [90])

Fig. 46.6 Single-shot EPI diffusion-weighted imaging (DWI) with $b = 1000$ s/mm^2 (**a**) with a corresponding ADC map (**b**) and quiet ANR sequence (**c**, **d**), showing a small acute infarction in the left putamen. Acoustic noise was reduced by 10.5 dB(A), which corresponds to a reduction of 70% in sound pressure. (Reproduced with permission from Ott et al. [91])

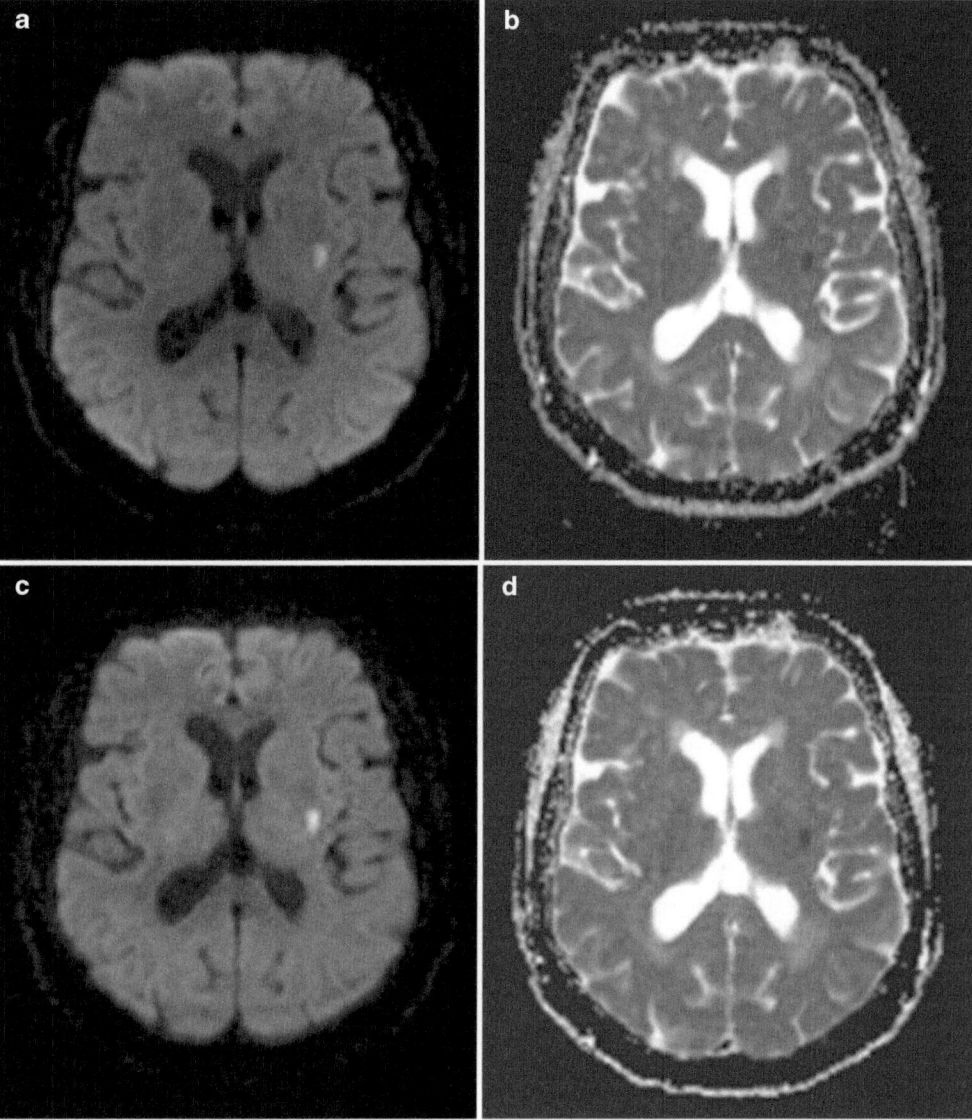

Outlook and Future Prospects

Several sequences introduced in this book such as ZTE, PETRA, and WASPI allow silent MRI within <5 dB(A) of ambient noise. Using dedicated preparation pulses with these sequences, routine clinical contrasts can be achieved and provide viable alternatives to loud standard sequences—with additional imaging advantages in some cases.

By combining ZTE with ANR techniques, it has been proven in several publications that comprehensive clinical protocols for brain, musculoskeletal, and other regions can be provided with acoustic noise reductions of 20 dB(A) or more. One obvious advantage is increased patient comfort. This increase in patient comfort can be especially beneficial for pediatric imaging, as described in Aida et al. [94] and Matsuo-Hagiyama et al. [95].

Generating ultralow acoustic noise MR images raised significant commercial and clinical interest in the early 2010s, as it is a topic that is easy to appreciate. This helped bring products such as SilenZ and Quiet Suite into clinical practice, and now they are broadly available for applications of ZTE as described in this book.

Even though reduction of acoustic noise was not the primary goal of ZTE scanning, it has opened new applications for ZTE sequences. Images may appear slightly different compared to conventional "loud" scans, but, in many investigations, they have proven their feasibility and reliability. From the authors' point of view, the obvious advantage in patient comfort due to noise reduction is reason enough to justify broad application of ZTE sequences in routine clinical imaging.

References

1. Brummett RE, Talbot JM, Charuhas P. Potential hearing loss resulting from MR imaging. Radiology. 1988;169(2):539–40.

2. Quirk ME, Letendre AJ, Ciottone RA, Lingley JF. Anxiety in patients undergoing MR imaging. Radiology. 1989;170(2):463–6.

3. Murphy KJ, Brunberg JA. Adult claustrophobia, anxiety and sedation in MRI. Magn Reson Imaging. 1997;15(1):51–4.

4. McJury M, Shellock FG. Auditory noise associated with MR procedures: a review. J Magn Reson Imaging. 2000;12(1):37–45.

5. Andoh J, Ferreira M, Leppert IR, Matsushita R, Pike B, Zatorre RJ. How restful is it with all that noise? Comparison of interleaved silent steady state (ISSS) and conventional imaging in resting-state fMRI. NeuroImage. 2017;147:726–35.

6. Ljungberg E, Damestani NL, Wood TC, et al. Silent zero TE MR neuroimaging: current state-of-the-art and future directions. Prog Nucl Magn Reson Spectrosc. 2021;123:73–93.

7. McJury MJ. Acoustic noise and magnetic resonance imaging: a narrative/descriptive review. J Magn Reson Imaging. 2022;55(2):337–46.

8. Grieder M, Koenig T. Effect of acoustic fMRI-scanner noise on the human resting state. Brain Topogr. 2022, Dec 19;36:32.

9. Hurwitz R, Lane SR, Bell RA, Brant-Zawadzki MN. Acoustic analysis of gradient-coil noise in MR imaging. Radiology. 1989;173(2):545–8.

10. Mansfield P, Chapman BL, Bowtell R, Glover P, Coxon R, Harvey PR. Active acoustic screening: reduction of noise in gradient coils by Lorentz force balancing. Magn Reson Med. 1995;33(2):276–81.

11. Cho ZH, Chung ST, Chung JY, et al. A new silent magnetic resonance imaging using a rotating DC gradient. Magn Reson Med. 1998;39(2):317–21.

12. Edelstein WA, Hedeen RA, Mallozzi RP, El-Hamamsy SA, Ackermann RA, Havens TJ. Making MRI quieter. Magn Reson Imaging. 2002;20(2):155–63.

13. Katsunuma A, Takamori H, Sakakura Y, Hamamura Y, Ogo Y, Katayama R. Quiet MRI with novel acoustic noise reduction. MAGMA. 2002;13(3):139–44.

14. Roozen NB, Koevoets AH, den Hamer AJ. Active vibration control of gradient coils to reduce acoustic noise of MRI systems. IEEE ASME Trans Mechatron. 2008;13(3):325–34.

15. Cooley CZ, Stockmann JP, Armstrong BD, et al. Two-dimensional imaging in a lightweight portable MRI scanner without gradient coils. Magn Reson Med. 2015;73(2):872–83.

16. Versteeg E, Klomp DWJ, Siero JCW. A silent gradient axis for soundless spatial encoding to enable fast and quiet brain imaging. Magn Reson Med. 2022;87(2):1062–73.

17. Madio DP, Lowe IJ. Ultra-fast imaging using low flip angles and fids. Magn Reson Med. 1995;34(4):525–9.

18. Madio DP, Gach HM, Lowe IJ. Ultra-fast velocity imaging in stenotically produced turbulent jets using RUFIS. Magn Reson Med. 1998;39(4):574–80.

19. Kuethe DO, Caprihan A, Lowe IJ, Madio DP, Gach HM. Transforming NMR data despite missing points. J Magn Reson. 1999;139(1):18–25.

20. Wu Y, Dai G, Ackerman JL, et al. Water- and fat-suppressed proton projection MRI (WASPI) of rat femur bone. Magn Reson Med. 2007;57(3):554–67.

21. Grodzki DM, Jakob PM, Heismann B. Ultrashort echo time imaging using pointwise encoding time reduction with radial acquisition (PETRA). Magn Reson Med. 2012;67(2):510–8.

22. Froidevaux R, Weiger M, Rösler MB, Brunner DO, Pruessmann KP. HYFI: hybrid filling of the dead-time gap for faster zero echo time imaging. NMR Biomed. 2021;34(6):e4493.

23. Pruessmann KP, Weiger M, Börnert P, Boesiger P. Advances in sensitivity encoding with arbitrary k-space trajectories: SENSE with arbitrary k-space trajectories. Magn Reson Med. 2001;46(4):638–51.

24. Wood T, Ljungberg E, Wiesinger F. Radial interstices enable speedy low-volume imaging. J Open Source Softw. 2021;6(66):3500.

25. Ljungberg E, Wood T, Solana AB, et al. Silent T_1 mapping using the variable flip angle method with B_1 correction. Magn Reson Med. 2020;84(2):813–24.

26. Grodzki DM, Jakob PM, Heismann B. Correcting slice selectivity in hard pulse sequences. J Magn Reson. 2012;214(1):61–7.

27. Li C, Magland JF, Seifert AC, Wehrli FW. Correction of excitation profile in zero echo time (ZTE) imaging using quadratic phase-modulated RF pulse excitation and iterative reconstruction. IEEE Trans Med Imaging. 2014;33(4):961–9.

28. Schieban K, Weiger M, Hennel F, Boss A, Pruessmann KP. ZTE imaging with enhanced flip angle using modulated excitation: ZTE imaging with modulated excitation. Magn Reson Med. 2015;74(3):684–93.

29. Froidevaux R, Weiger M, Pruessmann KP. Pulse encoding for ZTE imaging: RF excitation without dead-time penalty. Magn Reson Med. 2022;87(3):1360–74.

30. Wiesinger F, Sacolick L, Kaushik S, Ahn S, Delso G, Shanbhag D. Zero TE bone imaging. Proc Intl Soc Mag Reson Med. 2014:4261.

31. Delso G, Wiesinger F, Sacolick LI, et al. Clinical evaluation of zero-echo-time MR imaging for the segmentation of the skull. J Nucl Med. 2015;56(3):417–22.

32. Wiesinger F, Sacolick LI, Menini A, et al. Zero TEMR bone imaging in the head. Magn Reson Med. 2016;75(1):107–14.

33. Wiesinger F, Bylund M, Yang J, et al. Zero TE-based pseudo-CT image conversion in the head and its application in PET/MR attenuation correction and MR-guided radiation therapy planning. Magn Reson Med. 2018;80(4):1440–51.

34. Breighner RE, Endo Y, Konin GP, Gulotta LV, Koff MF, Potter HG. Technical developments: zero echo time imaging of the shoulder: enhanced osseous detail by using MR imaging. Radiology. 2018;286(3):960–6.

35. Cho SB, Baek HJ, Ryu KH, et al. Clinical feasibility of zero TE skull MRI in patients with head trauma in comparison with CT: a single-center study. AJNR Am J Neuroradiol. 2019;40(1):109–15.

36. Lu A, Gorny KR, Ho M-L. Zero TE MRI for craniofacial bone imaging. AJNR Am J Neuroradiol. 2019;40(9):1562–6.

37. Engström M, McKinnon G, Cozzini C, Wiesinger F. In-phase zero TE musculoskeletal imaging. Magn Reson Med. 2020;83(1):195–202.

38. Wiesinger F, Ho M-L. Zero-TE MRI: principles and applications in the head and neck. Br J Radiol. 2022;95(1136):20220059.

39. Gibiino F, Sacolick L, Menini A, Landini L, Wiesinger F. Free-breathing, zero-TE MR lung imaging. MAGMA. 2015;28(3):207–15.

40. Dournes G, Grodzki D, Macey J, et al. Quiet submillimeter MR imaging of the lung is feasible with a PETRA sequence at 1.5 T. Radiology. 2015;276(1):258–65.

41. Bae K, Jeon KN, Hwang MJ, et al. Comparison of lung imaging using three-dimensional ultrashort echo time and zero echo time sequences: preliminary study. Eur Radiol. 2019;29(5):2253–62.

42. Zeng F, Nogami M, Ueno YR, et al. Diagnostic performance of zero-TE lung MR imaging in FDG PET/MRI for pulmonary malignancies. Eur Radiol. 2020;30(9):4995–5003.

43. Boucneau T, Fernandez B, Besson FL, et al. AZTEK: adaptive zero TE k-space trajectories. Magn Reson Med. 2021;85(2):926–35.

44. Matsuo H, Nishio M, Nogami M, et al. Unsupervised-learning-based method for chest MRI–CT transformation using structure constrained unsupervised generative attention networks. Sci Rep. 2022;12(1):11090.

45. Yang J, Wiesinger F, Kaushik S, et al. Evaluation of sinus/edge-corrected zero-echo-time-based attenuation correction in brain PET/MRI. J Nucl Med. 2017;58(11):1873–9.

46. Leynes AP, Yang J, Wiesinger F, et al. Zero-echo-time and Dixon deep pseudo-CT (ZeDD CT): direct generation of pseudo-CT images for pelvic PET/MRI attenuation correction using deep convolutional neural networks with multiparametric MRI. J Nucl Med. 2018;59(5):852–8.

47. Blanc-Durand P, Khalife M, Sgard B, et al. Attenuation correction using 3D deep convolutional neural network for brain 18F-FDG PET/MR: comparison with atlas, ZTE and CT based attenuation correction. PLoS One. 2019;14(10):e0223141.

48. Kaushik S, Bylund M, Cozzini C, et al. Region of interest focused MRI to synthetic CT translation using regression and classification multi-task network. arXiv:2203.16288. 2022. https://doi.org/10.48550/arXiv.2203.16288.

49. Edelman RR, Flanagan O, Grodzki D, Giri S, Gupta N, Koktzoglou I. Projection MR imaging of peripheral arterial calcifications. Magn Reson Med. 2015;73(5):1939–45.

50. Piccini D, Littmann A, Nielles-Vallespin S, Zenge MO. Spiral phyllotaxis: the natural way to construct a 3D radial trajectory in MRI. Magn Reson Med. 2011;66(4):1049–56.

51. Ljungberg E, Wood TC, Solana AB, Williams SCR, Barker GJ, Wiesinger F. Motion corrected silent ZTE neuroimaging. Magn Reson Med. 2022;88(1):195–210.

52. Matsuo H, Nishio M, Nogami M, et al. Unsupervised-learning-based method for chest MRI-CT transformation using structure constrained unsupervised generative attention networks. Sci Rep. 2022;12(1):11090.

53. Haase A. Snapshot flash mri. Applications to T_1, T_2, and chemical-shift imaging. Magn Reson Med. 1990;13(1):77–89.

54. Mugler JP, Brookeman JR. Three-dimensional magnetization-prepared rapid gradient-echo imaging (3D MP RAGE). Magn Reson Med. 1990;15(1):152–7.

55. Jang H, Carl M, Ma Y, et al. Inversion recovery zero echo time (IR-ZTE) imaging for direct myelin detection in human brain: a feasibility study. Quant Imaging Med Surg. 2020;10(5):895–906.

56. Alibek S, Vogel M, Sun W, et al. Acoustic noise reduction in MRI using silent scan: an initial experience. Diagn Interv Radiol. 2014;20(4):360–3.

57. Ida M, Wakayama T, Nielsen ML, Abe T, Grodzki DM. Quiet T1-weighted imaging using PETRA: initial clinical evaluation in intracranial tumor patients. J Magn Reson Imaging. 2015;41(2):447–53.

58. Holdsworth SJ, Macpherson SJ, Yeom KW, Wintermark M, Zaharchuk G. Clinical evaluation of silent T_1-weighted MRI and silent MR angiography of the brain. AJR Am J Roentgenol. 2018;210(2):404–11.

59. Iwadate Y, Nozaki A, Nunokawa Y, Okuda S, Jinzaki M, Kabasawa H. Silent navigator-triggered silent MRI of the abdomen. Magn Reson Med. 2018;79(4):2170–5.

60. Irie R, Suzuki M, Yamamoto M, et al. Assessing blood flow in an intracranial stent: a feasibility study of MR angiography using a silent scan after stent-assisted coil embolization for anterior circulation aneurysms. AJNR Am J Neuroradiol. 2015;36(5):967–70.

61. Shang S, Ye J, Dou W, et al. Validation of zero TE-MRA in the characterization of cerebrovascular diseases: a feasibility study. AJNR Am J Neuroradiol. 2019;40(9):1484–90.

62. Koktzoglou I, Giri S, Piccini D, et al. Arterial spin labeled carotid MR angiography: a phantom study examining the impact of technical and hemodynamic factors. Magn Reson Med. 2016;75(1):295–301.

63. Fujiwara Y, Muranaka Y. Improvement in visualization of carotid artery uniformity using silent magnetic resonance angiography. Radiol Phys Technol. 2017;10(1):113–20.

64. Takano N, Suzuki M, Irie R, et al. Non-contrast-enhanced silent scan MR angiography of intracranial anterior circulation aneurysms treated with a low-profile visualized intraluminal support device. AJNR Am J Neuroradiol. 2017;38(8):1610–6.

65. Takano N, Suzuki M, Irie R, et al. Usefulness of non-contrast-enhanced MR angiography using a silent scan for follow-up after Y-configuration stent-assisted coil embolization for basilar tip aneurysms. AJNR Am J Neuroradiol. 2017;38(3):577–81.

66. Shang S, Ye J, Luo X, Qu J, Zhen Y, Wu J. Follow-up assessment of coiled intracranial aneurysms using zTE MRA as compared with TOF MRA: a preliminary image quality study. Eur Radiol. 2017;27(10):4271–80.

67. Heo YJ, Jeong HW, Baek JW, et al. Pointwise encoding time reduction with radial acquisition with subtraction-based MRA during the follow-up of stent-assisted coil embolization of anterior circulation aneurysms. AJNR Am J Neuroradiol. 2019;40(5):815–9.

68. Solana AB, Menini A, Sacolick LI, Hehn N, Wiesinger F. Quiet and distortion-free, whole brain BOLD fMRI using T_2-prepared RUFIS. Magn Reson Med. 2016;75(4):1402–12.

69. Yuan J, Hu Y, Menini A, et al. Near-silent distortionless DWI using magnetization-prepared RUFIS. Magn Reson Med. 2020;84(1):170–81.

70. Wood TC, Damestani NL, Lawrence AJ, et al. Silent myelin-weighted magnetic resonance imaging. Wellcome Open Res. 2020;5:74.

71. Brittain JH, Hu BS, Wright GA, Meyer CH, Macovski A, Nishimura DG. Coronary angiography with magnetization-prepared T_2 contrast. Magn Reson Med. 1995;33(5):689–96.

72. Garwood M, DelaBarre L. The return of the frequency sweep: designing adiabatic pulses for contemporary NMR. J Magn Reson. 2001;153(2):155–77.

73. Nezafat R, Ouwerkerk R, Derbyshire AJ, Stuber M, McVeigh ER. Spectrally selective B_1-insensitive T_2 magnetization preparation sequence. Magn Reson Med. 2009;61(6):1326–35.

74. Lee H, Price RR. Diffusion imaging with the MP-RAGE sequence. J Magn Reson Imaging. 1994;4(6):837–42.

75. Van AT, Cervantes B, Kooijman H, Karampinos DC. Analysis of phase error effects in multishot diffusion-prepared turbo spin echo imaging. Quant Imaging Med Surg. 2017;7(2):238–50.

76. Wolff SD, Balaban RS. Magnetization transfer contrast (MTC) and tissue water proton relaxation in vivo. Magn Reson Med. 1989;10(1):135–44.

77. Henkelman RM, Stanisz GJ, Graham SJ. Magnetization transfer in MRI: a review. NMR Biomed. 2001;14(2):57–64.

78. Holmes J, Samsonov A, Mossahebi P, Hernando D, Field A, Johnson K. Rapid, motion robust, and quiet quantitative magnetization transfer (qMT) imaging using a zero echo time (ZTE) acquisition. Proc Intl Soc Mag Reson Med. 2015:3358.

79. Messroghli DR, Radjenovic A, Kozerke S, Higgins DM, Sivananthan MU, Ridgway JP. Modified look-locker inversion recovery (MOLLI) for high-resolution T_1 mapping of the heart. Magn Reson Med. 2004;52(1):141–6.

80. Liu X, Gómez PA, Solana AB, Wiesinger F, Menzel MI, Menze BH. Silent 3D MR sequence for quantitative and multicontrast T_1 and proton density imaging. Phys Med Biol. 2020;65(18):185010.

81. Ma D, Gulani V, Seiberlich N, et al. Magnetic resonance fingerprinting. Nature. 2013;495(7440):187–92.

82. Kvernby S, Warntjes MJB, Haraldsson H, Carlhäll C-J, Engvall J, Ebbers T. Simultaneous three-dimensional myocardial T_1 and T_2 mapping in one breath hold with 3D-QALAS. J Cardiovasc Magn Reson. 2014;16(1):102.

83. Wiesinger F, McKinnon G, Kaushik S, et al. 3D silent parameter mapping: further refinements & quantitative assessment. Proc Intl Soc Mag Reson Med. 2021:1828.

84. Dixon WT. Simple proton spectroscopic imaging. Radiology. 1984;153(1):189–94.

85. Wiesinger F, Menini A, Solana AB. Looping Star. Magn Reson Med. 2019;81(1):57–68.

86. Wiesinger F, Solana AB. Looping star: revisiting echo in/out separation. Proc Intl Soc Mag Reson Med. 2020:3733.

87. Dionisio-Parra B, Wiesinger F, Sämann PG, Czisch M, Solana AB. Looping star fMRI in cognitive tasks and resting state. J Magn Reson Imaging. 2020;52(3):739–51.

88. Damestani NL, O'Daly O, Solana AB, et al. Revealing the mechanisms behind novel auditory stimuli discrimination: an evaluation of silent functional MRI using looping star. Hum Brain Mapp. 2021;42(9):2833–50.

89. Hennel F, Girard F, Loenneker T. "Silent" MRI with soft gradient pulses. Magn Reson Med. 1999;42(1):6–10.

90. Heismann B, Ott M, Grodzki D. Sequence-based acoustic noise reduction of clinical MRI scans. Magn Reson Med. 2015;73(3):1104–9.

91. Ott M, Blaimer M, Grodzki DM, et al. Acoustic-noise-optimized diffusion-weighted imaging. MAGMA. 2015;28(6):511–21.

92. Solana AB, Mandava S, Wang X, et al. AI-enhanced comprehensive quiet neuroimaging. Proc Intl Soc Mag Reson Med. 2023.

93. Lebel RM. Performance characterization of a novel deep learning-based MR image reconstruction pipeline. ArXiv:2008.06559. 2020. https://doi.org/10.48550/arXiv.2008.06559.

94. Aida N, Niwa T, Fujii Y, et al. Quiet T1-weighted pointwise encoding time reduction with radial acquisition for assessing myelination in the pediatric brain. AJNR Am J Neuroradiol. 2016;37(8):1528–34.

95. Matsuo-Hagiyama C, Watanabe Y, Tanaka H, et al. Comparison of silent and conventional MR imaging for the evaluation of myelination in children. Magn Reson Med Sci. 2017;16(3):209–16.

Current Status, Comparisons of Techniques, Challenges, and Future Directions for MRI of Short- and Ultrashort-T$_2$ Tissues

Jiang Du and Graeme M. Bydder

Introduction

The objectives of this book are to provide an accessible introduction to magnetic resonance imaging (MRI) of short- and ultrashort-T$_2$ tissues wherever possible written by active participants, outline important ideas in the field, and describe the current status of developments. This includes work conducted by individuals, groups, institutions, companies, and other organizations and covers many different activities. It reflects the fact that MRI of short- and ultrashort-T$_2$ tissues arose from a wide variety of sources, including conventional MRI, magnetic resonance spectroscopy (MRS), solid-state magnetic resonance (MR), contrast considerations, k-space mapping, and clinical needs.

Over the last 20 years, MRI of short- and ultrashort-T$_2$ tissues has moved from a few technical studies [1] to detailed understanding of the acquisition, contrast mechanisms, and quantification, with the next principal objective being increased clinical application. Commercial packages are now available on all the major manufacturers' systems, facilitating wider clinical use.

Formatting this book in relatively short chapters has made possible an overall progression of content from signal acquisition to clinical applications and has allowed inclusion of a broad range of views, but it has precluded in-depth reviews of

J. Du
Department of Radiology, University of California, San Diego, La Jolla, CA, USA

Department of Bioengineering, University of California, San Diego, La Jolla, CA, USA

VA San Diego Healthcare System, San Diego, CA, USA
e-mail: jiangdu@health.ucsd.edu

G. M. Bydder (✉)
Department of Radiology, University of California, San Diego, La Jolla, CA, USA

Mātai Medical Research Institute, Tairāwhiti Gisborne, New Zealand
e-mail: gbydder@health.ucsd.edu

particular subjects such as zero echo time (ZTE) and ultrashort echo time (UTE). To obtain more details about these topics, readers are referred to recent extensive reviews by Weiger et al. [2], Mastrogiacomo et al. [3], Afsahi et al. [4], and Ma et al. [5].

Notable work has been conducted within the scope of the title of this book, which has not been possible to include. Brief summaries of work in this category are included in the second section of this chapter.

Comparisons are made easier by presenting material in a uniform format within this book and by dividing this book into four sections. This is beneficial for assessing the pros and cons of UTE, ZTE, and variable echo time (vTE), for example. It also helps in understanding different contrast mechanisms and forms of quantitation and has allowed appreciation of both the advantages and disadvantages in different clinical applications as well as selection of techniques for particular purposes. Details of comparisons are included in the third section of this chapter. Challenges are dealt with in the penultimate fourth section, before future directions, which is divided into a general category considering progress in imaging in general and a specific category targeting MRI of short- and ultrashort-T$_2$ tissues.

Other Contributions to MRI of Short- and Ultrashort-T$_2$ Tissues

Although this book aims to provide a comprehensive assessment of data acquisition, contrast mechanisms, quantification, and applications, several major technical developments and clinical applications have not been included for a variety of reasons. Summaries of these contributions are included below.

First, a major data acquisition strategy, water- and fat-suppressed proton projection MRI (WASPI) [6], is not specifically included. Wu and Ackerman developed the WASPI technique and validated it in studies of bone and synthetic materials. They showed that the WASPI signal is highly correlated with organic matrix density in cortical and trabecular bone [7].

Second, Garwood and Idiyatullin pioneered the development of sweep imaging with Fourier transformation (SWIFT) [8], which has had widespread applications, including dental imaging [9], detection of iron oxide nanoparticles [10], and T_1 mapping of the osteochondral junction [11].

Third, Pauly and Nishimura pioneered the development of two-dimensional (2D) UTE imaging techniques and contrast mechanisms and later three-dimensional (3D) UTE imaging techniques [12–17].

Fourth, there are several other major contrast mechanisms. For example, the dual-band UTE technique as proposed by the Wehrli group for short-T_2 imaging in which a long dual-band saturation pulse is employed for more complete suppression of signals from long-T_2 species [18]. Short-T_2 signals may significantly decay during data acquisition, and an adaptive sampling strategy is extremely useful for minimizing spatial blurring, maximizing short-T_2 signal, and facilitating echo subtraction [19]. Off-resonance saturation contrast is another useful contrast mechanism that can be used with UTE [20], SWIFT, and other sequences to create contrast for the short-T_2 tissues or tissue components. The time-varying gradient-modulation SWIFT (GM-SWIFT) technique has also been implemented for short-T_2 imaging with much reduced peak and total radiofrequency (RF) power [21].

Fifth, there are several quantitative UTE-based techniques that are highly innovative but are not described in this book. For example, the Wehrli group proposed UTE mapping of bulk water in cortical bone [22] and, later, further developed a fast T_1-corrected volumetric bone water mapping algorithm [23]. The same group also developed innovative techniques to validate UTE and ZTE imaging of myelin in the white matter of the brain and spinal cord [24, 25].

Sixth, the Hargreaves group developed UTE-based double echo steady-state (DESS) imaging, including applications using diffusion weighting [26]. The UTE-type sequences can also be combined with the chemical exchange saturation transfer (CEST) technique to detect contrast agent uptake and probe pH changes [27, 28]. Furthermore, UTE sequences can be used to detect sodium in musculoskeletal [29], cardiac [30], and brain tissues [31] as well as phosphorus in the cortical and trabecular bone [32, 33].

Seventh, there are clinical applications not included. In the musculoskeletal system, the Chu group has conducted extensive research on UTE-T_2* mapping for evaluation of collagen structural integrity in articular cartilage and menisci and demonstrated elevated UTE-T_2* values in degeneration [34].

Eighth, the Gold group employed the dual-echo UTE subtraction technique to demonstrate cartilaginous endplate (CEP) morphology, where UTE-detected cartilaginous endplate abnormalities are significantly correlated with the Miyazaki grade [35]. The same group also performed UTE-based MRS on tendons and bone and helped pioneer the use of UTE sequences [36].

Ninth, in the respiratory system, Johnston et al. proposed an optimized 3D UTE sequence for pulmonary MRI, with relative signal difference between endobronchial air and adjacent lung tissue normalized to nearby vessels as a surrogate for lung tissue signal, which provides excellent depiction of interstitial fibrosis [37].

Tenth, in the gastrointestinal system, the Reeder group identified short- and ultrashort-T_2 components in the liver [38].

Eleventh, in the cardiovascular system, Robson et al. performed initial studies on variable echo time (TE) UTE chemical shift imaging (UTE-CSI) for mapping cardiac sodium distribution [39].

Twelfth, Kadbi et al. [40] and O'Brien et al. [41] employed UTE sequences to study blood flow in which a minimal TE was used to reduce artifacts associated with fast flow and turbulence.

Thirteenth, UTE is less sensitive to off-resonance artifacts from metallic implants and is therefore advantageous for imaging clipped aneurysms and coil embolization [42, 43].

Fourteenth, UTE allows direct imaging of vascular calcification, which may have T_2* values close to that of cortical bone and so may be invisible with conventional MRI [44–47].

Fifteenth, in the nervous system, long-T_2-saturated UTE imaging has been used to detect myelin loss in patients with multiple sclerosis [14]. UTE-magnetization transfer (UTE-MT) has been proposed for myelin imaging and quantification with UTE-based MT ratios (MTRs) showing a strong correlation ($R^2 = 0.71$) with the percentage coverage of myelin basic protein immunostaining [48]. Muller et al. also performed extensive studies of myelin with UTE at 7 T and characterized the tissue at this high field strength [49].

Sixteenth, UTE-type sequences have also been used in thermometry [50], stem cell tracking [51], and treatment monitoring.

Comparative Assessment of Techniques

Data Acquisition Techniques

All the major MR vendors have implemented UTE- and ZTE-type sequences on their equipment for research purposes and clinical applications. The first part of this book describes various data acquisition strategies for direct imaging of short- and ultrashort-T_2 tissues. Table 47.1 summarizes the techniques developed in recent years (not limited to those described in this book). These include single-point imaging (SPI) [52], single-point ramped imaging with T_1 enhancement (SPRITE) [53], 2D and 3D UTE [1, 5, 12, 16,

Table 47.1 Summary of short-T$_2$ imaging data acquisition strategies. These can be divided into five groups: the SPI group, which includes the basic SPI and SPRITE sequences; the UTE group, which includes 2D UTE sequences with radial or spiral trajectories as well as 3D UTE sequences with radial, TPI, or Cones trajectories; the ZTE group, which includes the 3D ZTE, WASPI, and Looping Star sequences; the hybrid group, which includes the PETRA, RHE, and HYFI sequences; and the SWIFT sequence. The technical performance in terms of sampling efficiency, short-T$_2$ spatial blurring, sensitivity to B_1 and B_0 inhomogeneities, sensitivity to eddy currents, and SNR efficiency as well as a summary of the significant advantages and disadvantages and related references for each technique are included. Technical performance (***high, **medium, *low)

Short-T$_2$ imaging data acquisition strategies		Technical performance (***high, **medium, *low)					Summary of significant advantages and disadvantages		Related references
		Sampling efficiency	Short-T$_2$ blurring	Sensitivity to B_1/B_0	Sensitivity to eddy currents	SNR efficiency	Advantages	Disadvantages	
SPI group	SPI	*	***	***	***	*	No short-T$_2$ spatial blurring, low sensitivity to B_1/B_0 and eddy currents	Extremely low sampling efficiency, extremely long scan time, extremely low SNR efficiency	[52]
	SPRITE	*	***	***	**	*	No blurring, low sensitivity to B_1/B_0 and eddy currents, solid and implant imaging	Low sampling efficiency, long scan time, low SNR efficiency	[53]
UTE group	2D radial	*	*	*	*	*	Relatively fast, flexible in choosing FAs and TEs	Short-T$_2$ blurring, highly sensitive to eddy currents as well as B_1/B_0 inhomogeneities	[1, 12, 65]
	2D spiral	*	*	*	*	*	Relatively fast, flexible in choosing FAs and TEs	Short-T$_2$ blurring, highly sensitive to eddy currents as well as B_1/B_0 inhomogeneities	[54]
	3D radial	**	**	*	**	**	Relatively fast, flexible in choosing FAs and TEs, good SNR efficiency	Short-T$_2$ blurring, highly sensitive to eddy currents as well as B_1/B_0 inhomogeneities	[19, 22, 66]
	3D TPI	***	*	*	**	***	Extremely efficient sampling, flexible in choosing FAs and TEs, high SNR efficiency	Short-T$_2$ blurring, highly sensitive to eddy currents as well as B_1/B_0 inhomogeneities	[55]
	3D Cones	***	*	*	**	***	Most efficient sampling, flexible in choosing FAs and TEs, high SNR efficiency	Short-T$_2$ blurring, highly sensitive to eddy currents as well as B_1/B_0 inhomogeneities	[16, 56]
vTE group	vTE	**	*	*	***	**	Relatively fast, flexible in choosing FAs, good SNR efficiency, robust to eddy currents	Short-T$_2$ blurring, difficult to vary TEs, inherently a longer, effective TE	[57]
	AWSOS	**	*	*	**	**	Efficient sampling, flexible in choosing FAs, high SNR efficiency	Short-T$_2$ blurring, longer, effective TE, sensitive to eddy currents, B_1/B_0 inhomogeneities	[58]

(continued)

Table 47.1 (continued)

Short-T$_2$ imaging data acquisition strategies		Technical performance (***high, **medium, *low)					Summary of significant advantages and disadvantages		Related references
		Sampling efficiency	Short-T$_2$ blurring	Sensitivity to B_1/B_0	Sensitivity to eddy currents	SNR efficiency	Advantages	Disadvantages	
ZTE group	ZTE	**	***	*	***	**	Reduced short-T$_2$ blurring, robust to eddy currents, silent, good SNR efficiency	Center of k-space resampling/compensation, low FAs, sensitive to B_1/B_0 inhomogeneities	[2, 61]
	WASPI	*	***	*	***	**	Reduced short-T$_2$ blurring, robust to eddy currents, silent, high contrast	Center of k-space resampling/compensation, low FAs, sensitive to B_1/B_0 inhomogeneities, long scan time	[6, 7]
	Looping Star	**	***	*	***	**	Reduced short-T$_2$ blurring, robust to eddy currents, silent, T$_2$*/phase information	Center of k-space resampling/compensation, low FAs, sensitive to B_1/B_0 inhomogeneities	[63]
Hybrid group	PETRA	**	***	*	***	**	Reduced short-T$_2$ blurring, insensitive to eddy currents, silent, good SNR efficiency	More complicated image reconstruction, sensitive to B_1/B_0 inhomogeneities	[59]
	RHE	**	***	*	***	**	Reduced short-T$_2$ blurring, insensitive to eddy currents, silent, good SNR efficiency	More complicated image reconstruction, sensitive to B_1/B_0 inhomogeneities	[60]
	HYFI	**	***	*	***	**	Reduced short-T$_2$ blurring, insensitive to eddy currents, silent, good SNR efficiency	More complicated image reconstruction, sensitive to B_1/B_0 inhomogeneities	[62]
SWIFT		*	***	**	***	**	Little short-T$_2$ blurring, robust to eddy currents and B_1/B_0 inhomogeneities	Little flexibility in FAs and TRs, more complicated image reconstruction	[8–10]

19, 22, 54–56], Cartesian variable TE (vTE) [57], WASPI [6], SWIFT [8], hybrid acquisition-weighted stack of spirals (AWSOS) [58], pointwise encoding time reduction with radial acquisition (PETRA) [59], ramped hybrid encoding (RHE) [60], ZTE [61], ZTE with hybrid filling (HYFI) [62], and Looping Star [63]. The technical performance in terms of data acquisition efficiency, short-T$_2$-related spatial blurring, sensitivity to eddy currents, sensitivity to B_1 and B_0 inhomogeneities, signal-to-noise ratio (SNR) efficiency, significant advantages and disadvantages, and related references for each data acquisition strategy are detailed in Table 47.1. Among the different data acquisition strategies, the SPI and SPRITE sequences are subjected to inherently low sampling efficiency [52, 53], which significantly limits their clinical applications. The 2D UTE sequence is highly sensitive to eddy currents due to its use of half-pulse excitations [1, 64]. 3D radial UTE acquisition is less sensitive to eddy currents than 2D UTE and works well for volumetric imaging of short- and ultrashort-T$_2$ species [5, 19]. The radial trajectory can be extended for twisted projection imaging (TPI) [55] or further twisted for more efficient 3D Cones imaging [16, 56]. The Cones trajectory is a generalization of the 3D radial trajectory in which spokes twist around one of the axes, resulting in longer readout times per repetition time (TR) and , therefore, a higher duty cycle and increased SNR efficiency [16]. 3D UTE sequences with twisted or Cones trajectories are more time-efficient but are also subjected to greater short-T$_2$ blurring. The vTE and AWSOS sequences are hybrid sequences largely based on the variable TE strategy in which shorter, effective TEs are used for low-frequency phase/slice encodings. A major limitation is short-T$_2$ spatial blurring associated with the longer, effective TEs for higher-frequency phase/slice encodings. ZTE, WASPI, and Looping Star are a group of sequences where k-space data are sampled after full ramp-up of the spatial encoding gradients, thus minimizing short-T$_2$ blurring. PETRA, RHE, and HYFI are a group of hybrid sequences combining SPI for the central k-space with ZTE sampling for outer k-space sampling. SWIFT is a different category of UTE imaging with a clear advantage in imaging ultrashort-T$_2$ species such as densely mineralized enamel and dentin [9]. Special reconstruction techniques are needed to generate 3D UTE images from radial or Cones sampling. UTE-type sequences repeatedly sample the center of the k-space, leading to reduced motion sensitivity compared with conventional Cartesian imaging.

Contrast Mechanisms and Their Clinical Applications

Table 47.2 summarizes morphological UTE- and ZTE-type imaging techniques detailed in the second part of this book.

The described contrast mechanisms include UTE- and ZTE-type data acquisitions combined with subtraction [1, 66], long-T$_2$ saturation [14], off-resonance saturation [20], adiabatic inversion recovery (IR)-based techniques [1, 5, 15, 65], adiabatic IR with echo subtraction [24, 67, 68], dual adiabatic IR [69, 70], adiabatic IR with fat saturation (FS) [71], short repetition time adiabatic inversion recovery (STAIR) [72–74], water–fat separation [75, 76], water excitation [77], UTE spectroscopic imaging (UTESI) [78], phase imaging [79], chemical shift artifacts [80], tissue property (TP) filters [81], and multiplied, added, subtracted, and/or divided IR (MASDIR) sequences [82]. Table 47.2 also lists technical performance in terms of B_1 and B_0 inhomogeneities, chemical shift artifacts, contrast-to-noise ratio (CNR) and SNR efficiencies, significant advantages and disadvantages, promising and challenging clinical applications, and related references for each contrast mechanism [5]. Among the different contrast mechanisms, dual-echo UTE with echo subtraction is the most time-efficient method [1], but it is sensitive to chemical shift, off-resonance, and susceptibility effects, leading to inefficient long-T$_2$ suppression [66]. A series of techniques have been developed based on various long-T$_2$ saturation contrast mechanisms, including T$_2$-selective RF excitation [13], dual-band UTE [14, 18], UTE with on-resonance or off-resonance saturation [20], and WASPI [6], but these are sensitive to B_1 and B_0 inhomogeneities that lead to incomplete long-T$_2$ signal suppression and therefore compromised short-T$_2$ contrast. UTESI- [78] and UTE-based water–fat separation techniques [75, 76, 83] have great potential for SNR-efficient imaging of short- and ultrashort-T$_2$ tissues by avoiding the short- and ultrashort-T$_2$ signal attenuation associated with chemical shift-based fat saturation pulses but lack long-T$_2$ water suppression. A variety of adiabatic IR-based techniques, including the basic IR sequence [15, 65, 84], dual IR [69, 70], IR with FS [71], and STAIR [72], appear more promising as they provide more uniform suppression of long-T$_2$ water and fat signals than other contrast mechanisms due in large part to the insensitivity of adiabatic inversion pulses to B_1 and B_0 inhomogeneities [85]. Overall, the IR-based techniques, especially STAIR-UTE, appear to be the most promising approach to high-contrast imaging of ultrashort-T$_2$* tissues such as those at the osteochondral junction, in the trabecular bone, and within myelin. Dual-echo UTE with echo subtraction works best for high-contrast imaging of short-T$_2$ tissues, which have relatively high ρ_ms (e.g., menisci, ligaments, and tendons); however, this technique is more difficult with ultrashort-T$_2$ tissues that have low ρ_ms (e.g., bone and myelin) where efficient long-T$_2$ suppression is of critical importance. The basic UTE and ZTE sequences appear to be the best option for high-resolution imaging of the lung [37, 86, 87], where motion compensation is the high priority.

Table 47.2 Summary of short- and ultrashort-T_2 imaging contrast mechanisms, including echo subtraction, long-T_2 saturation, off-resonance saturation, adiabatic IR, adiabatic IR with echo subtraction, dual adiabatic IR, adiabatic IR with fat saturation, short TR adiabatic IR, fat–water imaging, water excitation, and spectroscopic imaging, as well as technical performance in terms of B_1 inhomogeneity, B_0 inhomogeneity, fat-related chemical shift artifacts, CNR efficiency, SNR efficiency, a summary of the significant advantages and disadvantages, promising and challenging clinical applications, and related references for each technique. MSK musculoskeletal; OCJ osteochondral junction; CEP cartilaginous endplate. Technical performance (***high, **medium, *low)

| Short-T_2 imaging contrast mechanisms | Technical performance (***high, **medium, *low) | | | | | Summary of significant advantages and disadvantages | | Clinical applications | | Related references |
	B_1	B_0	Fat	CNR	SNR	Advantages	Disadvantages	Promising	Challenging	
Echo subtraction	**	*	*	*	***	High SNR, fast acquisition, easy to implement with UTE sequences	Low CNR, sensitive to B_0/susceptibility/off-resonance, strong fat signal, difficulty with ZTE/WASPI/SWIFT/PETRA sequences	Most MSK tissues, liver, lungs, iron overload, implants	Trabecular bone, myelin	[1, 19, 35, 54, 66]
Long-T_2 saturation	*	*	*	*	**	Medium SNR, variety of long-T_2 suppression pulses	Low CNR, sensitive to B_1/B_0/susceptibility/off-resonance, strong residual fat signal	Most MSK tissues	Trabecular bone, myelin	[13, 14, 18, 66]
Off-resonance saturation	**	**	***	**	*	High CNR, suitable for UTE, ZTE, SWIFT, PETRA	Low SNR, slow acquisition (need two acquisitions with and without saturation)	Most MSK tissues (CEP, OCJ, etc.)	Trabecular bone, myelin	[20]
Adiabatic inversion recovery	***	***	*	**	**	High CNR, robust to B_1/B_0 inhomogeneities, good for UTE, ZTE, SWIFT, PETRA	Low SNR, fat signal contamination, slow acquisition, difficulty in suppressing long-T_2 tissues with a broad range of T_1s	Most MSK tissues, iron overload	Trabecular bone, myelin	[5, 15, 24, 56, 65, 67]
Adiabatic inversion recovery + echo subtraction	***	**	**	***	*	High CNR, robust to B_1 inhomogeneity, magnitude, and complex subtraction	Low SNR, slow acquisition, difficulty in suppressing long-T_2 tissues with a broad range of T_1s	Most MSK tissues, iron overload, myelin	Trabecular bone	[24, 67, 68]
Dual adiabatic inversion recovery	***	**	**	***	*	High CNR, robust to B_1 inhomogeneity, suppression of long-T_2 water and fat	Sensitive to B_0 inhomogeneity, off-resonance, slow acquisition, difficulty in suppressing long-T_2 tissues with a broad range of T_1s	Most MSK tissues, especially the CEP, OCJ, etc.	Trabecular bone	[69, 70]
Adiabatic inversion recovery + fat saturation	***	**	**	***	*	High CNR, robust to B_1 inhomogeneity, suppression of long-T_2 water and fat	Sensitive to B_0 inhomogeneity, off-resonance, slow acquisition, difficulty in suppressing long-T_2 tissues with a broad range of T_1s	Most MSK tissues, especially the CEP, OCJ, etc.	Trabecular bone	[71]
Short TR adiabatic inversion recovery	***	***	***	***	*	High CNR, robust to B_1/B_0 inhomogeneities, suppression of water–fat regardless of T_1	Low SNR, slow acquisition, reduced performance when imaging tissues with slightly longer T_2*s and T_1s (e.g., meniscus, enthesis)	Cortical/trabecular bone, tendon, iron overload, myelin	Meniscus, enthesis	[72–74]
Fat–water imaging	**	**	**	*	***	High SNR, reasonable water–fat separation, fast acquisition	No long-T_2 suppression, low CNR for tissues with ultrashort T_2*, and low PD (e.g., bone, myelin)	Menisci, ligaments, enthesis, tendons	Trabecular bone, myelin	[75, 76]
Water excitation	*	*	**	**	***	High SNR, reasonable water–fat separation	No long-T_2 suppression, low CNR for tissues with ultrashort T_2*, and low PD (e.g., bone, myelin)	Menisci, ligaments, enthesis, tendons	Trabecular bone, myelin	[77]
Spectroscopic imaging	***	***	***	***	*	High CNR, excellent water–fat separation	No long-T_2 suppression, low CNR for tissues with ultrashort T_2*, and low PD (e.g., bone, myelin)	Menisci, ligaments, enthesis, tendons	Trabecular bone, myelin	[78]

Quantification Techniques and Their Clinical Applications

Quantitative techniques for MRI of short- and ultrashort-T$_2$ tissues include UTE-T$_1$ [88, 89], UTE-T$_2$* [90], UTE-T$_{1\rho}$ [91–93], UTE proton density (UTE-PD) [73, 94–96], UTE-MTR [48, 97, 98], UTE-MT modeling of macromolecular fraction (UTE-MMF) [99–101], UTE quantitative susceptibility mapping (UTE-QSM) [102–104], UTE perfusion [105–107], UTE diffusion [26, 108], and UTE-based deep learning methods [109, 110]. There are several other UTE-based imaging biomarkers, such as the porosity index (PI), which is defined as the ratio of signal intensities between a long TE and the shortest TE obtained by the UTE imaging [111], and the suppression ratio (SR), which is defined as the ratio between bone UTE signal without long-T$_2$ suppression and that with long-T$_2$ suppression [94]. Table 47.3 summarizes selected quantitative UTE-based imaging techniques described in the third part of this book. UTE-based quantitation involves short- and ultrashort-T$_2$ signal acquisition and suppression of unwanted long-T$_2$ signals. These quantitative UTE-type techniques have considerable potential for improv-ing diagnosis, as summarized in Table 47.3, which shows the targeted tissue component, the major confounding factor, i.e., the magic angle effect, changes with degeneration, and clinical applications for each biomarker [5]. UTE-based T$_2$* mapping allows quantitative evaluation of collagen degrada-tion in menisci, ligaments, and tendons [34]. UTE-based T$_{1\rho}$ mapping allows assessment of proteoglycan depletion in both short- and long-T$_2$ tissues [91, 93, 112]. UTE-MT imag-ing and signal modeling allow quantitative mapping of mac-romolecular fractions (MMFs) and changes in magnetization exchange in the menisci, ligaments, tendons, and bone [99–101, 113]. UTE-based quantitative susceptibility mapping (UTE-QSM) can directly quantify hemosiderin deposition in hemophilic joints and calcium in bone [102, 104, 114]. UTE-based perfusion permits robust separation of the red zone from the white zone in the meniscus, evaluation of bone physiology at the molecular level, and monitoring of bone fracture healing [105, 107]. UTE-based diffusion has the potential for assessment of early stage disease changes in highly ordered tissues such as the menisci, ligaments, and tendons [26, 108]. An important application of UTE diffu-sion techniques is the assessment of cartilaginous endplate

Table 47.3 Summary of quantitative short-T$_2$ imaging techniques, including UTE-based T$_1$, T$_2$*, T$_{1\rho}$, adiabatic T$_{1\rho}$, proton density (PD), magne-tization transfer ratio (MTR), macromolecular fraction (MMF), quantitative susceptibility (QSM), perfusion and diffusion, UTE-based porosity index (PI), and suppression ratio (SR), as well as the targeted tissue or component, the major confounding factor (usually the magic angle effect), changes with degeneration, clinical applications, and related references. UTE-AdiabT$_{1\rho}$, UTE adiabatic T$_{1\rho}$

Quantitative short-T$_2$ imaging technique	Target tissue component	Magic angle effect	Changes with degeneration	Clinical applications	Related references
UTE-T$_1$	Water	Minimal	Increase with degeneration/bone porosity	Osteoporosis, osteoarthritis, liver/joint iron, lung, etc.	[88, 89]
UTE-T$_2$*	Collagen	Strong	Increase or decrease with degeneration	Osteoarthritis, hemophilia, liver/joint iron, lung, etc.	[90]
UTE-T$_{1\rho}$	Proteoglycan	Strong	Increase with degeneration	Osteoarthritis, ankle/shoulder/spine degeneration, etc.	[91, 92]
UTE-AdiabT$_{1\rho}$	Proteoglycan	Minimal	Increase with degeneration	Osteoarthritis, ankle/shoulder/spine degeneration, etc.	[93]
UTE-PD	Water Myelin	Minimal	Increase with bone porosity Decrease in brain lesions	Bound/pore water mapping in osteoporosis Myelin in multiple sclerosis, Alzheimer's disease, etc.	[73, 94–96]
UTE-MTR	Collagen, myelin	Medium	Decrease with degeneration, bone porosity, demyelination	Osteoporosis, osteoarthritis, ankle/shoulder/spine degeneration, multiple sclerosis, Alzheimer's disease, etc.	[48, 97, 98]
UTE-MMF	Collagen, myelin	Minimal	Decrease with degeneration, demyelination	Osteoporosis, osteoarthritis, ankle/shoulder/spine degeneration, multiple sclerosis, Alzheimer's disease, etc.	[99–101]
UTE-QSM	Iron, calcium	Minimal	Increase with iron/calcium deposition	Osteoporosis, liver/joint iron, Parkinson's disease, etc.	[102–104]
UTE perfusion	Blood	Minimal	Increase with degeneration/fracture	Bone/tendons/ligaments fracture, meniscal tear, etc.	[105–107]
UTE diffusion	Collagen	Minimal	Increase with degeneration	Menisci/ligaments/tendons degeneration, etc.	[26, 108]
UTE-PI	Pore water	Minimal	Increase with bone porosity	Osteoporosis	[111, 117]
UTE-SR	Bound/pore water	Minimal	Decrease with bone porosity	Osteoporosis	[94, 118]

diffusivity, which is a crucial factor affecting spine disc degeneration [115], and may be used to evaluate intervertebral disc degeneration [116]. Direct quantitative UTE-T_2^* and diffusion imaging of the cartilaginous endplate may be extremely useful for diagnosing disc degeneration and associated back pain. PI is significantly correlated with microcomputed tomography (μCT)-based porosity, mechanical stiffness, age, and collagen estimation from near-infrared spectroscopy [117], whereas SR significantly correlates with bone porosity and age [118]. These UTE-based biomarkers are likely to have significant advantages over the current gold-standard dual-energy X-ray absorptiometry (DEXA) for measurement of bone mineral density (BMD). These quantitative imaging techniques can also be combined with other data acquisition strategies, such as ZTE, PETRA, RHE, vTE, AWSOS, etc., although the advantages and disadvantages of doing this remain to be investigated.

Clinical Applications

Promising and challenging clinical applications using contrast mechanisms and quantitation are summarized in Tables 47.2 and 47.3. In the musculoskeletal system, the most important tissues in order of their T_2s are cortical and trabecular bone, tendons, ligaments and menisci, fibrocartilage in the osteochondral junction, entheses and discs, and articular cartilage. Iron deposition in musculoskeletal tissues may place them under the short- and ultrashort-T_2 categories if they are not there already. Study of each of these tissues has pros and cons associated with it, but there is now a body of information on demonstrating morphological features and TPs in health and disease to assist informed decisions about clinical applications. Quantification of cortical bone is an obvious clinical application.

Myelin is the tissue most studied in the brain, and it is relatively easy to demonstrate its ultrashort-T_2 components with a T_2^* of ≈ 0.2 ms. This provides the basis for specific imaging of myelin and recognizing its diminution or loss in disease.

The lung has received attention from the beginning of clinical imaging of short- and ultrashort-T_2 components. Technical improvements in signal detection and motion artifact have made MRI more competitive with CT.

Iron imaging in the liver, particularly for high concentrations, is now validated and appears suitable for clinical applications.

There are areas such as the study of myofascial disease, fibrosis in many tissues, subclinical degeneration in tendons and ligaments as well as responses to treatment that also appear suitable for prime-time clinical research.

Challenges in MRI of Short- and Ultrashort-T_2 Tissues

Although extensive progress has been made in MRI of short- and ultrashort-T_2 tissues, including development of a variety of techniques for data acquisition, improving contrast, and quantitation, clinical applications are still limited. There are several major technical challenges to morphological and quantitative imaging of short- and ultrashort-T_2 tissues as described below:

First, imaging of short- and ultrashort-T_2 tissues is typically associated with spatial blurring and low SNR because of the fast signal decay during data sampling [19] and the relatively low ρ_ms of many short-T_2 species (e.g., bone, lung, myelin, etc.) [5]. A short sampling window is needed to minimize short-T_2 associated blurring, and this limits spatial resolution [19]. More advanced data acquisition and reconstruction strategies, stronger gradients and RF systems, and coils with improved SNR efficiency can all help in minimizing spatial blurring and improving the SNR of short- and ultrashort-T_2 tissue imaging.

Second, many UTE-type sequences are based on non-Cartesian sampling, which is more sensitive to eddy current effects than conventional Cartesian techniques [64]. Eddy currents can degrade the image quality and affect accuracy in quantitation, thereby limiting potential clinical applications. Eddy current compensation and k-space trajectory measurements are important in facilitating more reliable UTE imaging and quantification [119]. ZTE-type sequences are less sensitive to eddy currents because the k-space data are sampled after gradient ramp-up [2] and have many clinical applications such as bone imaging, which can outperform CT in detecting intraosseous lesions and cysts [120].

Third, quantitative imaging of short- and ultrashort-T_2 tissues is subjected to errors associated with long-T_2 fat signal contamination. Because long-T_2 tissues typically have higher proton densities, partial volume effects and other sources of long-T_2 signal contamination have a significant impact on the quantification accuracy in short- and ultrashort-T_2 imaging. This is especially the case for quantitative imaging of thin structures such as the osteochondral junction (0.1–0.2-mm thickness) [121] and the cartilaginous endplate (0.5–1-mm thickness) [122]. Myelin and trabecular bone are two extreme challenges for direct quantitative imaging. Myelin accounts for only a small fraction of the total UTE signal in the white matter of the brain and an even smaller fraction in the gray matter [123]. Trabecular bone imaging is complicated by its low ρ_m and the fact that it is surrounded by a large quantity of marrow fat and/or water. The combination of low ρ_m, ultrashort-T_2^*s, surrounding high signal from long-T_2 species, local susceptibility effects, and chemical shift effects make direct imaging of trabecular bone extremely challenging. Some simple contrast mechanisms, such as echo subtraction and long-T$_2$ saturation, are unlikely to provide selective imaging of myelin and trabecular bone. In fact, even adiabatic IR-based techniques, such as spectral presaturation with IR (SPIR) [124], may not be able to suppress signals from bone marrow fat efficiently. The residual fat signal can be higher than that from trabecular bone, as evidenced by the long-T$_2$* of 2.42 ± 0.56 ms at 3 T found with SPIR, which is much longer than the T$_2$* value of ~0.3 ms for trabecular bone measured with the STAIR-UTE technique at the same field strength [74]. There is a clear need for more robust long-T$_2$ suppression mechanisms, such as the STAIR approach, to accurately quantify short-T$_2$ and, especially, ultrashort-T$_2$ tissues such as trabecular bone and myelin.

Fourth, fat and related off-resonance artifacts can significantly reduce image contrast and are potential sources of error with quantitative UTE imaging of short- and ultrashort-T$_2$ tissues [66, 80, 125]. With T$_1$-weighted UTE imaging, fat appears as a high signal and can significantly reduce imaging contrast for tissue components of interest, such as cortical and trabecular bone, the osteochondral junction, and the cartilaginous endplate. Fat contamination and chemical shift artifacts can lead to significant errors in MR relaxation times (e.g., T$_1$, T$_2$, T$_2$*, T$_{1\rho}$) and other TPs (e.g., P$_m$, MTR, MMF, susceptibility, perfusion, diffusion). UTE sequences employ center-out radial or spiral mapping of the k-space, which may produce off-resonance-related spatial blurring due to the ring-shaped point spread function, an artifact that is notably different from those seen with a Cartesian sampling of the k-space [80]. Chemical shift-based artifacts in UTE imaging may mimic normal structures (e.g., the osteochondral junction) and/or diseases. On the other hand, conventional fat saturation pulses may significantly suppress signals from short- and ultrashort-T$_2$ tissues, which have broad spectral profiles and are subjected to direct saturation and MT effects [125]. Water excitation [77] and fat–water separation techniques [75, 76] may help preserve short-T$_2$ signals while improving contrast and quantification accuracy.

Fifth, the magic angle effect may affect both morphological and quantitative UTE imaging [126]. Most short- and ultrashort-T$_2$ tissues are collagen-rich, and, so, their UTE signal intensities can be highly fiber angle dependent [127]. Many biomarkers, including UTE-T$_2$* and UTE-T$_{1\rho}$, show strong angular dependence with values increased several fold due to the magic angle effect, which is far higher than changes due to degeneration [128, 129]. Largely, fiber angle independent biomarkers such as UTE-AdiabT$_{1\rho}$ [93, 112, 130] and UTE-MT modeling [99, 113, 131] may allow more reliable quantification of tissue degeneration. The magic angle effect of other biomarkers, such as UTE-QSM-derived

susceptibility [102–104] and UTE-DESS-derived apparent diffusion coefficient [26, 108], remains to be investigated.

Finally, the signal sources in direct UTE-type imaging of short- and ultrashort-T$_2$ tissues or tissue components need further investigation. There are some inconsistent results reported in the literature regarding morphological and quantitative imaging of ultrashort-T$_2$ tissues such as trabecular bone and myelin. For example, using SPIR-UTE for imaging of trabecular bone in the spine, Wurnig et al. measured T$_2$* values of ~2.42 ms, which is nearly 10 times longer than that reported for cortical bone, suggesting significant long-T$_2$ signal contamination [124]. Chao et al. reported that the WASPI signal was highly correlated ($r^2 = 0.97$ and $r^2 = 0.95$, respectively) to the true bone matrix mass density derived from gravimetric and amino acid analyses and hypothesized that the signal sources were collagen backbone protons, tightly bound water, and other immobile molecules [7]. Horch et al. investigated the proton nuclear magnetic resonance (NMR) signal resources in human cortical bone and identified five components, including collagen methylene (T$_2$ ~ 57 µs), collagen amides/hydroxides and mineral hydroxides water, collagen-bound water (T$_2$ ~ 416 µs), pore water, and lipid methylene (T$_2$ ~ 1–1000 ms) [132]. Siu et al. reported that UTE sequences could detect signals from collagen protons at 7 T [133]. Meanwhile, Ma et al. reported that 2D and 3D UTE sequences could not detect any signal from tendons and cortical bone after D$_2$O exchange and freeze-drying [134]. More recently, similar results have been found with a ZTE sequence, suggesting that collagen backbone protons have T$_2$s that are too short for direct imaging with UTE- or ZTE-type sequences using clinical whole-body scanners.

More debate exists regarding the signal source in direct imaging of myelin with UTE- and ZTE-type sequences. Direct MRI of myelin is technically challenging. Several groups have investigated the MR properties of nonaqueous myelin protons. Broad-line proton spectroscopic studies suggest that myelin is in a liquid–crystalline state [135]. Multicomponent analyses of spin echo or free induction decay (FID) of brain white matter samples have shown a broad range of extremely short-T$_2$ or short-T$_2$* values for nonaqueous myelin protons (e.g., ~50 µs [136], 7.5–101 µs [62], 50–1000 µs [137], 150–250 µs [123], etc.). NMR spectrometric studies demonstrate a wide distribution of T$_2$* values ranging from 8 µs to 26 ms in the spinal cord [24]. The T$_2$ spectrum of central and peripheral nerves and myelin phantoms has been used to characterize the biophysical origins of ultrashort-T$_2$ signals (50 µs < T$_2$ < 1 ms) in myelinated tissues [137]. HYFI imaging of D$_2$O-exchanged ex vivo porcine brain white matter samples suggests three signal components with T$_2$s of 7.5 µs (~85% of the total signal), 101 µs (~9%), and 50 ms (~6%), respectively [62]. Purified lyophilized bovine myelin extract powder, which is an organophilic extract of predominantly myelin-related brain lipids, shows zero signal with clinical gradient echo and spin echo sequences but a high signal with UTE sequences and demonstrates a short-T_2* of ~150 µs [138]. Similar short-T_2* values were demonstrated with STAIR-UTE imaging of the brain in vivo, showing that nonaqueous myelin protons are detectable with the STAIR-UTE sequence using clinical whole-body scanners [72]. More research is needed to investigate which group of nonaqueous myelin protons are detected by the STAIR-UTE sequence. Further research is also needed regarding the exact T_2* values for different groups of nonaqueous myelin protons in white matter in vivo.

MT modeling studies suggest that collagen backbone protons have extremely short T_2s of ~10 µs [99, 139, 140]. Our recent study has demonstrated that ZTE cannot detect collagen backbone protons in cortical bone and tendons, suggesting that ZTE is unable to directly image species with T_2s of ~10 µs. This result is inconsistent with the HYFI imaging of myelin with a T_2 of 7.5 µs. Furthermore, it is technically challenging to selectively image the super-short-T_2 (T_2 ~ 7.5 µs) myelin component by subtracting two HYFI datasets acquired with TEs of 15 and 460 µs, respectively [62], as the ultrashort-T_2 (e.g., T_2* ~0.2 ms) component detectable with STAIR-UTE [72] will likely show up in the subtraction image. More research is needed to clarify the exact signal sources in direct myelin imaging in vivo, especially using clinical whole-body scanners.

The Future of MRI of Short- and Ultrashort-T_2 Tissues

General Aspects of Imaging

The future of MRI of short- and ultrashort-T_2 tissues will be played out against a background of the future of medicine as a whole and that of imaging in particular [141].

In the imaging field, the general trends include improvement in system engineering that may take many different forms and is frequently incremental, but the overall results are continuing improvements in machine performance. These are often the overall sum of different advances but also arise from substantial specific achievements. The most important of these at the present time are artificial intelligence (AI) and quantification, including radiomics. These are being applied to all forms of imaging and at multiple levels. Substantial advantages have quite rapidly come to MRI from the use of AI in image reconstruction, and further progress is expected.

Quantification has taken a longer time and has concentrated on tissue properties such as T_1, T_2, and diffusion, but it is being incorporated into clinical practice on a broad front.

Radiomics is also being applied to recognize patterns that are not apparent on radiological inspection.

It is also important to be aware of advances in other forms of imaging of which the most notable at the present time are photon-counting computed tomography (CT), positron emission tomography (PET) labeled with prostate-specific membrane antigens (PSMAs) and fibroblast activation protein inhibitors (FAPIs) and theranostics. These techniques provide high contrast and highly specific images of prostate and breast tumors as well as fibrosis. [18]Fluorine-labeled PET also provides high contrast highly specific imaging of bone activity in disease. The techniques may provide performance beyond what is now possible with MRI. The advent of theranostics is also expanding imaging in a major way to include more therapeutic options, particularly in cancer.

General Aspects of MRI of Short- and Ultrashort-T_2 Tissues

Over the last 20 years, MRI of short- and ultrashort-T_2 tissues has moved from an experimental technique to one that is available on most clinical systems and appears likely to have an increasing role in clinical imaging. Future developments have been discussed in chapters throughout this book, but there are also specific examples below that may be important.

In terms of MR system design, a variety of niche options are now being pursued, but one particular system may be realizable without requiring radical system redesign. This is a head system that would also be suitable for peripheral musculoskeletal use as well as head and body studies in children. It would allow extremely high gradient performance due to the smaller bore size and permit machine performance greater than that of whole-body systems, e.g., at 3 T. It could be suitable for one-quarter to one-third of the patients normally scanned with whole-body systems but be cheaper and easier to install than those systems. Dedicated systems could be operated in conjunction with whole-body systems or for head-only studies in neurological clinics and peripheral musculoskeletal applications in orthopedic clinics.

In terms of new acquisitions, the double quantum-filtered and MT studies by Navon et al. may produce information not available otherwise [142].

On the contrast side, MASDIR sequences in the brain provide up to 15 times the T_1 contrast of conventional IR sequences, and this may have useful applications in many musculoskeletal tissues [82].

As far as quantitation is concerned, there may be renewed interest in T_1 because it is not subjected to magic angle effects, although specialized sequences are necessary to measure it accurately in short- and ultrashort-T_2 tissues.

In a number of situations, such as assessment of osteoporosis, the fundamental work of developing sequences and assessing their feasibility for clinical use has already been performed and what is required next is well organized clinical trials. This applies to other technical developments as well. As with oncology, and diseases of the nervous system, antibody-related therapeutics may become more important in the musculoskeletal system and require targeted forms of image acquisition, contrast, and quantitation to provide clinically useful data.

Specific Future Directions for MRI of Short- and Ultrashort-T$_2$ Tissues

The most significant obstacle in translating the various UTE-type sequences into clinical use is the limited signal and contrast with direct imaging of short- and ultrashort-T$_2$ tissues. The fast signal decay during data sampling may greatly reduce the achievable SNR and spatial resolution. An effective strategy is to develop stronger gradient and RF systems. For example, Weiger et al. employed a high-performance gradient insert that provided a maximum strength of 200 mT/m and a slew rate of 600 mT/m/ms, both of which are 4–5 times stronger than the typical gradient strength of ~40 mT/m and slew rate of ~150 mT/m/ms on clinical scanners [62]. The gradient inserts allowed ZTE imaging of myelin with higher spatial resolution, less blurring, and a higher SNR. A higher-power RF system also augments UTE imaging's capabilities as it is essential to minimize transverse relaxation during RF excitation for short-T$_2$ tissues. A shorter pulse with a higher power improves excitation efficiency and minimizes signal loss during RF excitation. The stronger gradient helps minimize the sampling window, thereby reducing short-T$_2$ signal loss during frequency encoding and eventually increasing the achievable SNR. Local parallel transmission is another approach to improve direct imaging of ultrashort-T$_2$ tissues or tissue components such as myelin and trabecular bone. The parallel transmission allows the use of shorter RF pulses with higher power but without SAR constraints [143], thereby significantly increasing the ultrashort-T$_2$ excitation efficiency. A major challenge in selective imaging of myelin and trabecular bone lies in the fact that complete suppression of long-T$_2$ signals from water and fat is extremely difficult. The STAIR contrast mechanism seems the most promising technique. However, STAIR-UTE works best with the shortest TR possible so that any long-T$_2$ signals, regardless of their T$_1$s, can be effectively suppressed [72, 74]. Stronger RF and gradient systems together with parallel transmission are expected to greatly reduce TR, therefore improving long-T$_2$ signal suppression in STAIR-UTE-type sequences and producing more accurate quantification (e.g., T$_2$* and P$_m$).

More contrast mechanisms and quantitation techniques have been developed for 2D and 3D UTE sequences. However, most contrast mechanisms can be easily combined with other data acquisition strategies. For example, STAIR contrast can be used with ZTE, PETRA, RHE, Looping Star, and other sequences for high contrast imaging of myelin and/or trabecular bone. On-resonance long-T$_2$ suppression or off-resonance short-T$_2$ saturation can be applied to WASPI, SWIFT, PETRA, SPI, RHE, and ZTE sequences, in which echo subtraction is not easily applicable for creating short-T$_2$ contrast. Various quantitative imaging techniques can also be implemented using ZTE, PETRA, and other data acquisition strategies. For example, UTE-QSM can be implemented with the Looping Star approach in which multi-echo ZTE data can be acquired for QSM processing [63].

UTE-type sequences allow direct imaging of both short- and long-T$_2$ tissues, which also means more comprehensive and time-consuming data analysis to investigate not just one specific tissue but all associated tissues and tissue components. Deep learning-based automatic segmentation and quantification [109, 110] may be especially helpful for this and facilitate translation of novel morphological and quantitative UTE-type techniques.

Direct imaging of short- and ultrashort-T$_2$ tissues can potentially improve the diagnosis of various diseases in the body's musculoskeletal, nervous, respiratory, gastrointestinal, and cardiovascular systems. UTE-type imaging with a high signal, spatial resolution, and contrast of otherwise "invisible" short- and ultrashort-T$_2$ tissues or tissue components will likely improve the classification and staging of diseases in a significant way. For example, human joints are composed of several different tissues (articular cartilage, synovium, menisci, ligaments, tendons, cortical and subchondral bone, bone marrow, etc.) that interact and allow joints to function over long periods of time. Degeneration of cartilage is generally considered the primary initiator of osteoarthritis (OA). However, recent understanding of OA has moved from a cartilage-centric focus to the concept of "whole-joint organ" disease [144]. When one tissue begins to deteriorate, it is likely to affect others and contribute to failure of the joint as a whole [145]. The WORMS (Whole-Organ MRI Score) scoring system is widely used to evaluate knee OA using clinical MR images [146], but many of the relevant joint tissues (e.g., menisci, ligaments, tendons, and bone) show little or no signal using this approach. UTE-type imaging of long-, short-, and ultrashort-T$_2$ tissues and tissue components in joints may significantly improve morphological assessment of joint degeneration.

Another example of the potential of UTE-type imaging to modify diagnosis and monitoring relates to the Pfirrmann grading system—a widely used method to evaluate intervertebral disk degeneration [147, 148]. The CEP plays a vital role in the transportation of oxygen and nutrients necessary to maintain disk health [116]; however, it is difficult to image this important structure with conventional MRI sequences. High contrast UTE-type imaging of the CEP is likely to improve the usefulness of the Pfirrmann grading system [115]. Thus, the power of combined morphological and quantitative UTE-type simultaneous imaging of long-, short-, and ultrashort-T_2 tissues facilitates a truly "whole-organ" approach for more comprehensive assessment of degeneration, thereby directly influencing the development and advancement of new grading systems not only for musculoskeletal diseases but also for other diseases of the body.

References

1. Robson MD, Gatehouse PD, Bydder M, Bydder GM. Magnetic resonance: an introduction to ultrashort TE (UTE) imaging. J Comput Assist Tomogr. 2003;27(6):825–46.
2. Weiger M, Pruessmann KP. Short-T(2) MRI: principles and recent advances. Prog Nucl Magn Reson Spectrosc. 2019;114-115:237–70.
3. Mastrogiacomo S, Dou W, Jansen JA, Walboomers XF. Magnetic resonance imaging of hard tissues and hard tissue engineered biosubstitutes. Mol Imaging Biol. 2019;21(6):1003–19.
4. Afsahi AM, Ma Y, Jang H, Jerban S, Chung CB, Chang EY, et al. Ultrashort echo time magnetic resonance imaging techniques: met and unmet needs in musculoskeletal imaging. J Magn Reson Imaging. 2022;55(6):1597–612.
5. Ma Y, Jang H, Jerban S, Chang EY, Chung CB, Bydder GM, et al. Making the invisible visible-ultrashort echo time magnetic resonance imaging: technical developments and applications. Appl Phys Rev. 2022;9(4):041303.
6. Wu Y, Chesler DA, Glimcher MJ, Garrido L, Wang J, Jiang HJ, et al. Multinuclear solid-state three-dimensional MRI of bone and synthetic calcium phosphates. Proc Natl Acad Sci U S A. 1999;96(4):1574–8.
7. Cao H, Ackerman JL, Hrovat MI, Graham L, Glimcher MJ, Wu Y. Quantitative bone matrix density measurement by water- and fat-suppressed proton projection MRI (WASPI) with polymer calibration phantoms. Magn Reson Med. 2008;60(6):1433–43.
8. Idiyatullin D, Corum C, Park JY, Garwood M. Fast and quiet MRI using a swept radiofrequency. J Magn Reson. 2006;181(2):342–9.
9. Idiyatullin D, Corum C, Moeller S, Prasad HS, Garwood M, Nixdorf DR. Dental magnetic resonance imaging: making the invisible visible. J Endod. 2011;37(6):745–52.
10. Zhou R, Idiyatullin D, Moeller S, Corum C, Zhang H, Qiao H, et al. SWIFT detection of SPIO-labeled stem cells grafted in the myocardium. Magn Reson Med. 2010;63(5):1154–61.
11. Nissi MJ, Lehto LJ, Corum CA, Idiyatullin D, Ellermann JM, Grohn OHJ, et al. Measurement of T(1) relaxation time of osteochondral specimens using VFA-SWIFT. Magn Reson Med. 2015;74(1):175–84.
12. Bergin CJ, Pauly JM, Macovski A. Lung parenchyma: projection reconstruction MR imaging. Radiology. 1991;179(3):777–81.
13. Sussman MS, Pauly JM, Wright GA. Design of practical T2-selective RF excitation (TELEX) pulses. Magn Reson Med. 1998;40(6):890–9.
14. Larson PE, Gurney PT, Nayak K, Gold GE, Pauly JM, Nishimura DG. Designing long-T_2 suppression pulses for ultrashort echo time imaging. Magn Reson Med. 2006;56(1):94–103.
15. Larson PE, Conolly SM, Pauly JM, Nishimura DG. Using adiabatic inversion pulses for long-T2 suppression in ultrashort echo time (UTE) imaging. Magn Reson Med. 2007;58(5):952–61.
16. Gurney PT, Hargreaves BA, Nishimura DG. Design and analysis of a practical 3D cones trajectory. Magn Reson Med. 2006;55(3):575–82.
17. Johnson EM, Vyas U, Ghanouni P, Pauly KB, Pauly JM. Improved cortical bone specificity in UTE MR imaging. Magn Reson Med. 2017;77(2):684–95.
18. Li C, Magland JF, Rad HS, Song HK, Wehrli FW. Comparison of optimized soft-tissue suppression schemes for ultrashort echo time MRI. Magn Reson Med. 2012;68(3):680–9.
19. Rahmer J, Bornert P, Groen J, Bos C. Three-dimensional radial ultrashort echo-time imaging with T_2 adapted sampling. Magn Reson Med. 2006;55(5):1075–82.
20. Du J, Takahashi AM, Bydder M, Chung CB, Bydder GM. Ultrashort TE imaging with off-resonance saturation contrast (UTE-OSC). Magn Reson Med. 2009;62(2):527–31.
21. Zhang J, Idiyatullin D, Corum CA, Kobayashi N, Garwood M. Gradient-modulated SWIFT. Magn Reson Med. 2016;75(2):537–46.
22. Techawiboonwong A, Song HK, Leonard MB, Wehrli FW. Cortical bone water: in vivo quantification with ultrashort echo-time MR imaging. Radiology. 2008;248(3):824–33.
23. Rad HS, Lam SC, Magland JF, Ong H, Li C, Song HK, et al. Quantifying cortical bone water in vivo by three-dimensional ultra-short echo-time MRI. NMR Biomed. 2011;24(7):855–64.
24. Wilhelm MJ, Ong HH, Wehrli SL, Li C, Tsai PH, Hackney DB, et al. Direct magnetic resonance detection of myelin and prospects for quantitative imaging of myelin density. Proc Natl Acad Sci U S A. 2012;109(24):9605–10.
25. Seifert AC, Li C, Wilhelm MJ, Wehrli SL, Wehrli FW. Towards quantification of myelin by solid-state MRI of the lipid matrix protons. NeuroImage. 2017;163:358–67.
26. Chaudhari AS, Sveinsson B, Moran CJ, McWalter EJ, Johnson EM, Zhang T, et al. Imaging and T(2) relaxometry of short-T(2) connective tissues in the knee using ultrashort echo-time double-echo steady-state (UTEDESS). Magn Reson Med. 2017;78(6):2136–48.
27. Soesbe TC, Togao O, Takahashi M, Sherry AD. SWIFT-CEST: a new MRI method to overcome T(2) shortening caused by PARACEST contrast agents. Magn Reson Med. 2012;68(3):816–21.
28. Ma YJ, High RA, Tang Q, Wan L, Jerban S, Du J, et al. AcidoCEST-UTE MRI for the assessment of extracellular pH of joint tissues at 3 T. Investig Radiol. 2019;54(9):565–71.
29. Zbyn S, Mlynarik V, Juras V, Szomolanyi P, Trattnig S. Sodium MR imaging of articular cartilage pathologies. Curr Radiol Rep. 2014;2(4):41.
30. Madelin G, Lee JS, Regatte RR, Jerschow A. Sodium MRI: methods and applications. Prog Nucl Magn Reson Spectrosc. 2014;79:14–47.
31. Riemer F, Solanky BS, Stehning C, Clemence M, Wheeler-Kingshott CA, Golay X. Sodium ((23)Na) ultra-short echo time imaging in the human brain using a 3D-cones trajectory. MAGMA. 2014;27(1):35–46.
32. Robson MD, Gatehouse PD, Bydder GM, Neubauer S. Human imaging of phosphorus in cortical and trabecular bone in vivo. Magn Reson Med. 2004;51(5):888–92.
33. Zhao X, Song HK, Seifert AC, Li C, Wehrli FW. Feasibility of assessing bone matrix and mineral properties in vivo by combined solid-state 1H and 31P MRI. PLoS One. 2017;12(3):e0173995.
34. Chu CR, Williams AA, West RV, Qian Y, Fu FH, Do BH, et al. Quantitative magnetic resonance imaging UTE-T_2* mapping of cartilage and meniscus healing after anatomic anterior cruciate ligament reconstruction. Am J Sports Med. 2014;42(8):1847–56.

35. Kim YJ, Cha JG, Shin YS, Chaudhari AS, Suh YJ, Hwan Yoon S, et al. 3D ultrashort TE MRI for evaluation of cartilaginous endplate of cervical disk in vivo: feasibility and correlation with disk degeneration in T2-weighted spin-echo sequence. AJR Am J Roentgenol. 2018;210(5):1131–40.

36. Gold GE, Pauly JM, Macovski A, Herfkens RJ. MR spectroscopic imaging of collagen: tendons and knee menisci. Magn Reson Med. 1995;34(5):647–54.

37. Johnson KM, Fain SB, Schiebler ML, Nagle S. Optimized 3D ultrashort echo time pulmonary MRI. Magn Reson Med. 2013;70(5):1241–50.

38. Zhu A, Hernando D, Johnson KM, Reeder SB. Characterizing a short T(2) * signal component in the liver using ultrashort TE chemical shift-encoded MRI at 1.5T and 3.0T. Magn Reson Med. 2019;82(6):2032–45.

39. Robson MD, Tyler DJ, Neubauer S. Ultrashort TE chemical shift imaging (UTE-CSI). Magn Reson Med. 2005;53(2):267–74.

40. Kadbi M, Negahdar M, Cha JW, Traughber M, Martin P, Stoddard MF, et al. 4D UTE flow: a phase-contrast MRI technique for assessment and visualization of stenotic flows. Magn Reson Med. 2015;73(3):939–50.

41. O'Brien KR, Myerson SG, Cowan BR, Young AA, Robson MD. Phase contrast ultrashort TE: a more reliable technique for measurement of high-velocity turbulent stenotic jets. Magn Reson Med. 2009;62(3):626–36.

42. Takano N, Suzuki M, Irie R, Yamamoto M, Teranishi K, Yatomi K, et al. Non-contrast-enhanced silent scan MR angiography of intracranial anterior circulation aneurysms treated with a low-profile visualized intraluminal support device. AJNR Am J Neuroradiol. 2017;38(8):1610–6.

43. Katsuki M, Narita N, Ozaki D, Sato Y, Iwata S, Tominaga T. Three tesla magnetic resonance angiography with ultrashort echo time describes the arteries near the cerebral aneurysm with clip and the peripheral cerebral arteries. Surg Neurol Int. 2020;11:224.

44. Chan CF, Keenan NG, Nielles-Vallespin S, Gatehouse P, Sheppard MN, Boyle JJ, et al. Ultra-short echo time cardiovascular magnetic resonance of atherosclerotic carotid plaque. J Cardiovasc Magn Reson. 2010;12(1):17.

45. Du J, Corbeil J, Znamirowski R, Angle N, Peterson M, Bydder GM, et al. Direct imaging and quantification of carotid plaque calcification. Magn Reson Med. 2011;65(4):1013–20.

46. Du J, Peterson M, Kansal N, Bydder GM, Kahn A. Mineralization in calcified plaque is like that of cortical bone—further evidence from ultrashort echo time (UTE) magnetic resonance imaging of carotid plaque calcification and cortical bone. Med Phys. 2013;40(10):102301.

47. Sharma S, Boujraf S, Bornstedt A, Hombach V, Ignatius A, Oberhuber A, et al. Quantification of calcifications in endarterectomy samples by means of high-resolution ultra-short echo time imaging. Investig Radiol. 2010;45(3):109–13.

48. Guglielmetti C, Boucneau T, Cao P, Van der Linden A, Larson PEZ, Chaumeil MM. Longitudinal evaluation of demyelinated lesions in a multiple sclerosis model using ultrashort echo time magnetization transfer (UTE-MT) imaging. NeuroImage. 2020;208:116415.

49. Muller M, Egger N, Sommer S, Wilferth T, Meixner CR, Laun FB, et al. Direct imaging of white matter ultrashort T(2)(*) components at 7 tesla. Magn Reson Imaging. 2022;86:107–17.

50. Rieke V, Butts PK. MR thermometry. J Magn Reson Imaging. 2008;27(2):376–90.

51. Kaggie JD, Markides H, Graves MJ, MacKay J, Houston G, El Haj A, et al. Ultra short echo time MRI of iron-labelled mesenchymal stem cells in an ovine osteochondral defect model. Sci Rep. 2020;10(1):8451.

52. Beyea SD, Balcom BJ, Prado PJ, Cross AR, Kennedy CB, Armstrong RL, et al. Relaxation time mapping of short T*$_2$ nuclei with single-point imaging (SPI) methods. J Magn Reson. 1998;135(1):156–64.

53. Balcom BJ, Macgregor RP, Beyea SD, Green DP, Armstrong RL, Bremner TW. Single-point ramped imaging with T$_1$ enhancement (SPRITE). J Magn Reson A. 1996;123(1):131–4.

54. Du J, Bydder M, Takahashi AM, Chung CB. Two-dimensional ultrashort echo time imaging using a spiral trajectory. Magn Reson Imaging. 2008;26(3):304–12.

55. Boada FE, Shen GX, Chang SY, Thulborn KR. Spectrally weighted twisted projection imaging: reducing T$_2$ signal attenuation effects in fast three-dimensional sodium imaging. Magn Reson Med. 1997;38(6):1022–8.

56. Carl M, Bydder GM, Du J. UTE imaging with simultaneous water and fat signal suppression using a time-efficient multi-spoke inversion recovery pulse sequence. Magn Reson Med. 2016;76(2):577–82.

57. Deligianni X, Bar P, Scheffler K, Trattnig S, Bieri O. High-resolution Fourier-encoded sub-millisecond echo time musculoskeletal imaging at 3 Tesla and 7 Tesla. Magn Reson Med. 2013;70(5):1434–9.

58. Qian Y, Williams AA, Chu CR, Boada FE. High-resolution ultrashort echo time (UTE) imaging on human knee with AWSOS sequence at 3.0 T. J Magn Reson Imaging. 2012;35(1):204–10.

59. Grodzki DM, Jakob PM, Heismann B. Ultrashort echo time imaging using pointwise encoding time reduction with radial acquisition (PETRA). Magn Reson Med. 2012;67(2):510–8.

60. Jang H, Wiens CN, McMillan AB. Ramped hybrid encoding for improved ultrashort echo time imaging. Magn Reson Med. 2016;76(3):814–25.

61. Weiger M, Pruessmann KP, Hennel F. MRI with zero echo time: hard versus sweep pulse excitation. Magn Reson Med. 2011;66(2):379–89.

62. Weiger M, Froidevaux R, Baadsvik EL, Brunner DO, Rosler MB, Pruessmann KP. Advances in MRI of the myelin bilayer. NeuroImage. 2020;217:116888.

63. Wiesinger F, Menini A, Solana AB. Looping Star. Magn Reson Med. 2019;81(1):57–68.

64. Lu A, Daniel BL, Pauly JM, Pauly KB. Improved slice selection for R$_2$* mapping during cryoablation with eddy current compensation. J Magn Reson Imaging. 2008;28(1):190–8.

65. Du J, Carl M, Bydder M, Takahashi A, Chung CB, Bydder GM. Qualitative and quantitative ultrashort echo time (UTE) imaging of cortical bone. J Magn Reson. 2010;207(2):304–11.

66. Du J, Bydder M, Takahashi AM, Carl M, Chung CB, Bydder GM. Short T$_2$ contrast with three-dimensional ultrashort echo time imaging. Magn Reson Imaging. 2011;29(4):470–82.

67. Waldman A, Rees JH, Brock CS, Robson MD, Gatehouse PD, Bydder GM. MRI of the brain with ultra-short echo-time pulse sequences. Neuroradiology. 2003;45(12):887–92.

68. Du J, Ma G, Li S, Carl M, Szeverenyi NM, VandenBerg S, et al. Ultrashort echo time (UTE) magnetic resonance imaging of the short T$_2$ components in white matter of the brain using a clinical 3T scanner. NeuroImage. 2014;87:32–41.

69. Du J, Takahashi AM, Bae WC, Chung CB, Bydder GM. Dual inversion recovery, ultrashort echo time (DIR UTE) imaging: creating high contrast for short-T(2) species. Magn Reson Med. 2010;63(2):447–55.

70. Du J, Carl M, Bae WC, Statum S, Chang EY, Bydder GM, et al. Dual inversion recovery ultrashort echo time (DIR-UTE) imaging and quantification of the zone of calcified cartilage (ZCC). Osteoarthr Cartil. 2013;21(1):77–85.

71. Ma YJ, Jerban S, Carl M, Wan L, Guo T, Jang H, et al. Imaging of the region of the osteochondral junction (OCJ) using a 3D adiabatic inversion recovery prepared ultrashort echo time cones (3D IR-UTE-cones) sequence at 3 T. NMR Biomed. 2019;32(5):e4080.

72. Ma YJ, Jang H, Wei Z, Cai Z, Xue Y, Lee RR, et al. Myelin imaging in human brain using a short repetition time adiabatic inversion recovery prepared ultrashort echo time (STAIR-UTE) MRI sequence in multiple sclerosis. Radiology. 2020;297(2):392–404.

73. Ma YJ, Jang H, Wei Z, Wu M, Chang EY, Corey-Bloom J, et al. Brain ultrashort T(2) component imaging using a short TR adiabatic inversion recovery prepared dual-echo ultrashort TE sequence with complex echo subtraction (STAIR-dUTE-ES). J Magn Reson. 2021;323:106898.

74. Ma YJ, Chen Y, Li L, Cai Z, Wei Z, Jerban S, et al. Trabecular bone imaging using a 3D adiabatic inversion recovery prepared ultrashort TE cones sequence at 3T. Magn Reson Med. 2020;83(5):1640–51.

75. Kronthaler S, Boehm C, Feuerriegel G, Bornert P, Katscher U, Weiss K, et al. Assessment of vertebral fractures and edema of the thoracolumbar spine based on water-fat and susceptibility-weighted images derived from a single ultra-short echo time scan. Magn Reson Med. 2022;87(4):1771–83.

76. Jang H, Carl M, Ma Y, Jerban S, Guo T, Zhao W, et al. Fat suppression for ultrashort echo time imaging using a single-point Dixon method. NMR Biomed. 2019;32(5):e4069.

77. Ma YJ, Jerban S, Jang H, Chang EY, Du J. Fat suppression for ultrashort echo time imaging using a novel soft-hard composite radiofrequency pulse. Magn Reson Med. 2019;82(6):2178–87.

78. Du J, Hamilton G, Takahashi A, Bydder M, Chung CB. Ultrashort echo time spectroscopic imaging (UTESI) of cortical bone. Magn Reson Med. 2007;58(5):1001–9.

79. Carl M, Chiang JT. Investigations of the origin of phase differences seen with ultrashort TE imaging of short T_2 meniscal tissue. Magn Reson Med. 2012;67(4):991–1003.

80. Bydder M, Carl M, Bydder GM, Du J. MRI chemical shift artifact produced by center-out radial sampling of k-space: a potential pitfall in clinical diagnosis. Quant Imaging Med Surg. 2021;11(8):3677–83.

81. Young IR, Szeverenyi NM, Du J, Bydder GM. Pulse sequences as tissue property filters (TP-filters): a way of understanding the signal, contrast and weighting of magnetic resonance images. Quant Imaging Med Surg. 2020;10(5):1080–120.

82. Ma YJ, Moazamian D, Cornfeld DM, Condron P, Holdsworth SJ, Bydder M, et al. Improving the understanding and performance of clinical MRI using tissue property filters and the central contrast theorem, MASDIR pulse sequences and synergistic contrast MRI. Quant Imaging Med Surg. 2022;12(9):4658–90.

83. Wang K, Yu H, Brittain JH, Reeder SB, Du J. K-space water-fat decomposition with T_2^* estimation and multifrequency fat spectrum modeling for ultrashort echo time imaging. J Magn Reson Imaging. 2010;31(4):1027–34.

84. Reichert IL, Robson MD, Gatehouse PD, He T, Chappell KE, Holmes J, et al. Magnetic resonance imaging of cortical bone with ultrashort TE pulse sequences. Magn Reson Imaging. 2005;23(5):611–8.

85. Garwood M, DelaBarre L. The return of the frequency sweep: designing adiabatic pulses for contemporary NMR. J Magn Reson. 2001;153(2):155–77.

86. Bae K, Jeon KN, Hwang MJ, Lee JS, Ha JY, Ryu KH, et al. Comparison of lung imaging using three-dimensional ultrashort echo time and zero echo time sequences: preliminary study. Eur Radiol. 2019;29(5):2253–62.

87. Burris NS, Johnson KM, Larson PE, Hope MD, Nagle SK, Behr SC, et al. Detection of small pulmonary nodules with ultrashort Echo time sequences in oncology patients by using a PET/MR system. Radiology. 2016;278(1):239–46.

88. Ma YJ, Lu X, Carl M, Zhu Y, Szeverenyi NM, Bydder GM, et al. Accurate T(1) mapping of short T(2) tissues using a three-dimensional ultrashort echo time cones actual flip angle imaging-variable repetition time (3D UTE-cones AFI-VTR) method. Magn Reson Med. 2018;80(2):598–608.

89. Ma YJ, Zhao W, Wan L, Guo T, Searleman A, Jang H, et al. Whole knee joint T(1) values measured in vivo at 3T by combined 3D ultrashort echo time cones actual flip angle and variable flip angle methods. Magn Reson Med. 2019;81(3):1634–44.

90. Williams A, Qian Y, Golla S, Chu CR. UTE-T_2 * mapping detects sub-clinical meniscus injury after anterior cruciate ligament tear. Osteoarthr Cartil. 2012;20(6):486–94.

91. Du J, Carl M, Diaz E, Takahashi A, Han E, Szeverenyi NM, et al. Ultrashort TE T1rho (UTE T1rho) imaging of the Achilles tendon and meniscus. Magn Reson Med. 2010;64(3):834–42.

92. Ma YJ, Carl M, Shao H, Tadros AS, Chang EY, Du J. Three-dimensional ultrashort echo time cones T(1rho) (3D UTE-cones-T(1rho)) imaging. NMR Biomed. 2017;30(6):e3709.

93. Ma YJ, Carl M, Searleman A, Lu X, Chang EY, Du J. 3D adiabatic T(1rho) prepared ultrashort echo time cones sequence for whole knee imaging. Magn Reson Med. 2018;80(4):1429–39.

94. Li C, Seifert AC, Rad HS, Bhagat YA, Rajapakse CS, Sun W, et al. Cortical bone water concentration: dependence of MR imaging measures on age and pore volume fraction. Radiology. 2014;272(3):796–806.

95. Manhard MK, Horch RA, Gochberg DF, Nyman JS, Does MD. In vivo quantitative MR imaging of bound and pore water in cortical bone. Radiology. 2015;277(3):221–9.

96. Jerban S, Ma Y, Li L, Jang H, Wan L, Guo T, et al. Volumetric mapping of bound and pore water as well as collagen protons in cortical bone using 3D ultrashort echo time cones MR imaging techniques. Bone. 2019;127:120–8.

97. Springer F, Martirosian P, Machann J, Schwenzer NF, Claussen CD, Schick F. Magnetization transfer contrast imaging in bovine and human cortical bone applying an ultrashort echo time sequence at 3 tesla. Magn Reson Med. 2009;61(5):1040–8.

98. Chang EY, Bae WC, Shao H, Biswas R, Li S, Chen J, et al. Ultrashort echo time magnetization transfer (UTE-MT) imaging of cortical bone. NMR Biomed. 2015;28(7):873–80.

99. Ma YJ, Chang EY, Carl M, Du J. Quantitative magnetization transfer ultrashort echo time imaging using a time-efficient 3D multispoke cones sequence. Magn Reson Med. 2018;79(2):692–700.

100. Xue YP, Ma YJ, Wu M, Jerban S, Wei Z, Chang EY, et al. Quantitative 3D ultrashort echo time magnetization transfer imaging for evaluation of knee cartilage degeneration in vivo. J Magn Reson Imaging. 2021;54(4):1294–302.

101. Zhang X, Ma YJ, Wei Z, Wu M, Ashir A, Jerban S, et al. Macromolecular fraction (MMF) from 3D ultrashort echo time cones magnetization transfer (3D UTE-cones-MT) imaging predicts meniscal degeneration and knee osteoarthritis. Osteoarthr Cartil. 2021;29(8):1173–80.

102. Dimov AV, Liu Z, Spincemaille P, Prince MR, Du J, Wang Y. Bone quantitative susceptibility mapping using a chemical species-specific R_2^* signal model with ultrashort and conventional echo data. Magn Reson Med. 2018;79(1):121–8.

103. Jang H, Lu X, Carl M, Searleman AC, Jerban S, Ma Y, et al. True phase quantitative susceptibility mapping using continuous single-point imaging: a feasibility study. Magn Reson Med. 2019;81(3):1907–14.

104. Jerban S, Lu X, Jang H, Ma Y, Namiranian B, Le N, et al. Significant correlations between human cortical bone mineral density and quantitative susceptibility mapping (QSM) obtained with 3D cones ultrashort echo time magnetic resonance imaging (UTE-MRI). Magn Reson Imaging. 2019;62:104–10.

105. Robson MD, Gatehouse PD, So PW, Bell JD, Bydder GM. Contrast enhancement of short T₂ tissues using ultrashort TE (UTE) pulse sequences. Clin Radiol. 2004;59(8):720–6.

106. Gatehouse PD, He T, Puri BK, Thomas RD, Resnick D, Bydder GM. Contrast-enhanced MRI of the menisci of the knee using ultrashort echo time (UTE) pulse sequences: imaging of the red and white zones. Br J Radiol. 2004;77(920):641–7.

107. Wan L, Wu M, Sheth V, Shao H, Jang H, Bydder G, et al. Evaluation of cortical bone perfusion using dynamic contrast enhanced ultrashort echo time imaging: a feasibility study. Quant Imaging Med Surg. 2019;9(8):1383–93.

108. Jang H, Ma Y, Carl M, Jerban S, Chang EY, Du J. Ultrashort echo time cones double echo steady state (UTE-cones-DESS) for rapid morphological imaging of short T(2) tissues. Magn Reson Med. 2021;86(2):881–92.

109. Xue YP, Jang H, Byra M, Cai ZY, Wu M, Chang EY, et al. Automated cartilage segmentation and quantification using 3D ultrashort echo time (UTE) cones MR imaging with deep convolutional neural networks. Eur Radiol. 2021;31(10):7653–63.

110. Byra M, Wu M, Zhang X, Jang H, Ma YJ, Chang EY, et al. Knee menisci segmentation and relaxometry of 3D ultrashort echo time cones MR imaging using attention U-net with transfer learning. Magn Reson Med. 2020;83(3):1109–22.

111. Rajapakse CS, Bashoor-Zadeh M, Li C, Sun W, Wright AC, Wehrli FW. Volumetric cortical bone porosity assessment with MR imaging: validation and clinical feasibility. Radiology. 2015;276(2):526–35.

112. Wu M, Ma YJ, Kasibhatla A, Chen M, Jang H, Jerban S, et al. Convincing evidence for magic angle less-sensitive quantitative T(1rho) imaging of articular cartilage using the 3D ultrashort echo time cones adiabatic T(1rho) (3D UTE cones-AdiabT(1rho)) sequence. Magn Reson Med. 2020;84(5):2551–60.

113. Ma YJ, Shao H, Du J, Chang EY. Ultrashort echo time magnetization transfer (UTE-MT) imaging and modeling: magic angle independent biomarkers of tissue properties. NMR Biomed. 2016;29(11):1546–52.

114. Jang H, von Drygalski A, Wong J, Zhou JY, Aguero P, Lu X, et al. Ultrashort echo time quantitative susceptibility mapping (UTE-QSM) for detection of hemosiderin deposition in hemophilic arthropathy: a feasibility study. Magn Reson Med. 2020;84(6):3246–55.

115. Fields AJ, Han M, Krug R, Lotz JC. Cartilaginous end plates: quantitative MR imaging with very short echo times-orientation dependence and correlation with biochemical composition. Radiology. 2015;274(2):482–9.

116. Fields AJ, Ballatori A, Liebenberg EC, Lotz JC. Contribution of the endplates to disc degeneration. Curr Mol Biol Rep. 2018;4(4):151–60.

117. Hong AL, Ispiryan M, Padalkar MV, Jones BC, Batzdorf AS, Shetye SS, et al. MRI-derived bone porosity index correlates to bone composition and mechanical stiffness. Bone Rep. 2019;11:100213.

118. Li C, Seifert AC, Rad HS, Bhagat YA, Rajapakse CS, Sun W, et al. Cortical bone water concentration: dependence of MR imaging measures on age and pore volume fraction. Radiology. 2016;280(2):796–806.

119. Duyn JH, Yang Y, Frank JA, van der Veen JW. Simple correction method for k-space trajectory deviations in MRI. J Magn Reson. 1998;132(1):150–3.

120. Breighner RE, Endo Y, Konin GP, Gulotta LV, Koff MF, Potter HG. Technical developments: zero echo time imaging of the shoulder: enhanced osseous detail by using MR imaging. Radiology. 2018;286(3):960–6.

121. Lane LB, Bullough PG. Age-related changes in the thickness of the calcified zone and the number of tidemarks in adult human articular cartilage. J Bone Joint Surg Br. 1980;62(3):372–5.

122. Berg-Johansen B, Han M, Fields AJ, Liebenberg EC, Lim BJ, Larson PE, et al. Cartilage endplate thickness variation measured by ultrashort echo-time MRI is associated with adjacent disc degeneration. Spine (Phila Pa 1976). 2018;43(10):E592–600.

123. Fan SJ, Ma Y, Zhu Y, Searleman A, Szeverenyi NM, Bydder GM, et al. Yet more evidence that myelin protons can be directly imaged with UTE sequences on a clinical 3T scanner: Bicomponent T₂* analysis of native and deuterated ovine brain specimens. Magn Reson Med. 2018;80(2):538–47.

124. Wurnig MC, Calcagni M, Kenkel D, Vich M, Weiger M, Andreisek G, et al. Characterization of trabecular bone density with ultra-short echo-time MRI at 1.5, 3.0 and 7.0 T—comparison with microcomputed tomography. NMR Biomed. 2014;27(10):1159–66.

125. Carl M, Nazaran A, Bydder GM, Du J. Effects of fat saturation on short T2 quantification. Magn Reson Imaging. 2017;43:6–9.

126. Bydder M, Rahal A, Fullerton GD, Bydder GM. The magic angle effect: a source of artifact, determinant of image contrast, and technique for imaging. J Magn Reson Imaging. 2007;25(2):290–300.

127. Fullerton GD, Cameron IL, Ord VA. Orientation of tendons in the magnetic field and its effect on T₂ relaxation times. Radiology. 1985;155(2):433–5.

128. Shao H, Pauli C, Li S, Ma Y, Tadros AS, Kavanaugh A, et al. Magic angle effect plays a major role in both T1rho and T2 relaxation in articular cartilage. Osteoarthr Cartil. 2017;25(12):2022–30.

129. Du J, Statum S, Znamirowski R, Bydder GM, Chung CB. Ultrashort TE T1rho magic angle imaging. Magn Reson Med. 2013;69(3):682–7.

130. Wu M, Ma Y, Wan L, Jerban S, Jang H, Chang EY, et al. Magic angle effect on adiabatic T(1rho) imaging of the Achilles tendon using 3D ultrashort echo time cones trajectory. NMR Biomed. 2020;33(8):e4322.

131. Zhu Y, Cheng X, Ma Y, Wong JH, Xie Y, Du J, et al. Rotator cuff tendon assessment using magic-angle insensitive 3D ultrashort echo time cones magnetization transfer (UTE-cones-MT) imaging and modeling with histological correlation. J Magn Reson Imaging. 2018;48(1):160–8.

132. Horch RA, Nyman JS, Gochberg DF, Dortch RD, Does MD. Characterization of 1H NMR signal in human cortical bone for magnetic resonance imaging. Magn Reson Med. 2010;64(3):680–7.

133. Siu AG, Ramadeen A, Hu X, Morikawa L, Zhang L, Lau JY, et al. Characterization of the ultrashort-TE (UTE) MR collagen signal. NMR Biomed. 2015;28(10):1236–44.

134. Ma YJ, Chang EY, Bydder GM, Du J. Can ultrashort-TE (UTE) MRI sequences on a 3-T clinical scanner detect signal directly from collagen protons: freeze-dry and D₂O exchange studies of cortical bone and Achilles tendon specimens. NMR Biomed. 2016;29(7):912–7.

135. Lecar H, Ehrenstein G, Stillman I. Detection of molecular motion in lyophilized myelin by nuclear magnetic resonance. Biophys J. 1971;11(2):140–5.

136. MacKay A, Laule C, Vavasour I, Bjarnason T, Kolind S, Madler B. Insights into brain microstructure from the T₂ distribution. Magn Reson Imaging. 2006;24(4):515–25.

137. Horch RA, Gore JC, Does MD. Origins of the ultrashort-T2 1H NMR signals in myelinated nerve: a direct measure of myelin content? Magn Reson Med. 2011;66(1):24–31.

138. Sheth V, Shao H, Chen J, Vandenberg S, Corey-Bloom J, Bydder GM, et al. Magnetic resonance imaging of myelin using ultrashort Echo time (UTE) pulse sequences: phantom, specimen,

volunteer and multiple sclerosis patient studies. NeuroImage. 2016;136:37–44.

139. Sled JG, Pike GB. Quantitative imaging of magnetization transfer exchange and relaxation properties in vivo using MRI. Magn Reson Med. 2001;46(5):923–31.

140. Henkelman RM, Huang X, Xiang QS, Stanisz GJ, Swanson SD, Bronskill MJ. Quantitative interpretation of magnetization transfer. Magn Reson Med. 1993;29(6):759–66.

141. Brink JA, Hricak H. Radiology 2040. Radiology. 2023;306(1):69–72.

142. Navon G, Shinar H, Eliav U, Seo Y. Multiquantum filters and order in tissues. NMR Biomed. 2001;14(2):112–32.

143. Zelinski AC, Angelone LM, Goyal VK, Bonmassar G, Adalsteinsson E, Wald LL. Specific absorption rate studies of the parallel transmission of inner-volume excitations at 7T. J Magn Reson Imaging. 2008;28(4):1005–18.

144. Hayashi D, Guermazi A, Hunter DJ. Osteoarthritis year 2010 in review: imaging. Osteoarthr Cartil. 2011;19(4):354–60.

145. Brandt KD, Radin EL, Dieppe PA, van de Putte L. Yet more evidence that osteoarthritis is not a cartilage disease. Ann Rheum Dis. 2006;65(10):1261–4.

146. Peterfy CG, Guermazi A, Zaim S, Tirman PF, Miaux Y, White D, et al. Whole-organ magnetic resonance imaging score (WORMS) of the knee in osteoarthritis. Osteoarthr Cartil. 2004;12(3):177–90.

147. Pfirrmann CW, Metzdorf A, Zanetti M, Hodler J, Boos N. Magnetic resonance classification of lumbar intervertebral disc degeneration. Spine (Phila Pa 1976). 2001;26(17):1873–8.

148. Griffith JF, Wang YX, Antonio GE, Choi KC, Yu A, Ahuja AT, et al. Modified Pfirrmann grading system for lumbar intervertebral disc degeneration. Spine (Phila Pa 1976). 2007;32(24):E708–12.

Index

Printed by Printforce, the Netherlands